A Manual of ACUPUNCTURE

Peter Deadman & Mazin Al-Khafaji

with Kevin Baker

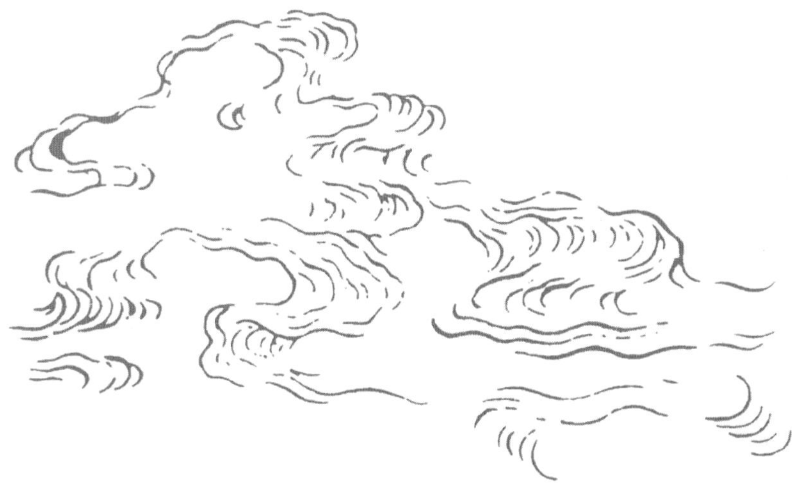

JOURNAL OF CHINESE MEDICINE PUBLICATIONS

Main text	Peter Deadman and Mazin Al-Khafaji
Point location text	Kevin Baker and Peter Deadman
Chinese translation	Mazin Al-Khafaji
Research into classical Chinese texts & commentaries	Mazin Al-Khafaji
Book design	John Chippindale, Peter Deadman and Simon Hedger
Brush calligraphy	A Hsiung Chen
Original illustrations	Marks Creative Consultants Barbara Loftus
Illustration commission and revision	Peter Deadman and Kevin Baker
Illustrations adapted by	Peter Deadman

Printed by Cushing Malloy, Inc., Ann Arbor, Michigan, USA

22 Cromwell Road
Hove
East Sussex
BN3 3EB
England

Fax : 01273-748588
e-mail : jcm@pavilion.co.uk
website : http://www.pavilion.co.uk/jcm/MOA.HOME.html

First published 1998 by Journal of Chinese Medicine Publications
Reprinted August 1998. Reprinted January 1999.

ISBN 0 9510546 7 8

Distributed in North America by Eastland Press,
1240 Activity Drive, #D Vista, California 92083, USA

The information given in this book is intended as a resource and guide to trained practitioners of acupuncture. It is not intended to substitute for such training and should not be considered to supplant the clinical judgement deriving from such training. Whilst every effort has been made to include cautions with regard to acupuncture treatment, the authors cannot accept responsibility for any treatment advice or information offered.

CONTENTS

CHAPTER CONTENTS

ACKNOWLEDGEMENTS

PETER DEADMAN

dedicates this book to his family, especially Jenny, Susie, Natasha and Noah and to his grandfather Professor Shmuel Eisenstadt, who died before he could complete his encyclopaedic dictionary of Hebrew Law.

MAZIN AL-KHAFAJI

dedicates this book to Pia Maria, Nadeem, Dina and Samir.

KEVIN BAKER

dedicates this book to his parents Mary and Tony.

With thanks to :

Tim Martin, who gave considerable assistance in the early stages of this book, Pia Maria Al-Khafaji, Fatima Bailey, Richard Blackwell, Shwu Ling Chern, Peter Eaton, Marian Fixler, Heiner Fruehauf, Oliver Hickey, Giovanni Maciocia, John O'Connor, Jacob Stevens, Rebecca Wilton, Allegra Wint.

INTRODUCTION

This book is deeply rooted in the classical tradition of Chinese acupuncture. The practice of acupuncture has grown spectacularly in the Western world over the last three or four decades. During the early period of this expansion there was scanty source material available. China was firmly closed to access by students of Chinese medicine, few textbooks were available in translation, and even fewer translators were skilled in the difficult task of rendering the terminology of Chinese medicine into other languages. As a result of these difficulties it was not easy to gain an understanding of the genuine and varied classical traditions of acupuncture, and there was inevitably a great deal of misunderstanding and much necessary invention to fill the gaps.

In addition to these factors, acupuncture is a forgiving and extremely flexible science. The insertion of a needle into the body in order to contact the qi will usually produce some changes, whichever the points selected. In current practice throughout the world, there is enormous variety in point selection. Indeed this 'fuzziness' is not confined to the Western world. Within modern and classical Chinese traditions there is also enormous variation in understanding and predicting the effects of needling different points, and a great variety of ways of treating different diseases.

Such variation in practice calls into question the idea that there are any universally agreed criteria for choosing points. This is a disturbing thought, especially in an age and a culture that calls for certainty, and is one that cannot be considered at length in these pages. It is our belief, however, that the nearest thing to an objective body of theoretical and clinical knowledge is found within the Chinese classical tradition. This is largely because it represents the slow accretion of observation, recording and testing over a largely unbroken period of over twenty centuries (surely one of the most remarkable recorded historical traditions in world medicine). Many of the texts used and referred to in this book, for example the *Systematic Classic of Acupuncture and Moxibustion* and the *Great Compendium of Acupuncture and Moxibustion* were largely a record of the clinical practice of their day. Each of these great encyclopaedic compilations carried forward the theory and practice of earlier works, yet added, modified and crafted them according to the practice of contemporary physicians. This is most clearly seen in the classical point prescriptions, many of which are recorded in this book. Some date back to the *Yellow Emperor's Inner Classic* and are found repeated through later compilations. Yet they often show modifications, for example the addition or subtraction of points and even the purpose for which they are used.

It is not our intention to present this traditional practice as cast in stone, as unchangeable, holy writ. The rapid development of acupuncture both within and outside China over the last few decades has itself led to great innovation in practice, and this is very much borne in mind in discussing the points. Furthermore, the enquiring and challenging nature of the modern Western mind can serve to dispel some of the rigid restraints of tradition, discarding what is not helpful and introducing new practice and perspective. It remains the case, however, that the historical tradition of Chinese acupuncture, this unique record of changing practice over two millennia, should serve as the foundation from which we work and develop.

Translation

As anyone who has attempted to translate from classical (and therefore often archaic) Chinese knows, the task is fraught with difficulty. There is much debate at present on how best to convey the meaning of many difficult terms and concepts found within traditional Chinese medicine. Like everyone else we have wrestled with these problems and have made the following decisions:

i. We have retained some Chinese (pinyin) terms which we feel are widely known, for example qi, yin, yang, jiao, Sanjiao, taiyang, yangming, shaoyang, taiyin, shaoyin, jueyin. We have kept these to a minimum, and the meaning of these terms is given in the glossary or within the text in case readers are not familiar with them. In some cases we have retained the Chinese term because there is not really any easy English alternative. Shan disorder, for example, is sometimes translated as hernia-like disorder in English texts. Hernia, however, only conveys one of three possible meanings of this term (see glossary).

ii. In translating the majority of terms, we have carefully consulted a variety of previous English translations and selected those renderings that seem to best convey the original meaning, yet are relatively easy to use in daily practice. Examples of these include atrophy disorder for 'wei zheng', painful obstruction for 'bi zheng' etc. We have also frequently stayed with terminology that is well known in order to make the text easier to read, for example we refer to the 'descending and dispersing' function of the Lung rather than recent alternatives such as 'depurative downbearing'.

iii. In many cases there does not seem to be any alternative but to adopt relatively new and unfamiliar terminology. This is especially the case with many of the indications of the points. Quite a few of these may be unfamiliar to most readers, for example sudden turmoil disorder, shan disorder, wind-taxation coughing, cold inversion, Lung atrophy etc. Although we recognise that this may present a steep learning curve for some readers, we feel that it is important to include these terms. Sudden turmoil disorder, for example, might be translated as cholera, but really refers to a wider variety of clinical situations where acute vomiting and diarrhoea present together, for example food poisoning. The simple fact is that disease description in classical Chinese texts is often different from a modern Western model, and yet may accurately convey clinical reality. In other words these terms are not just retained for reasons of historical accuracy. We hope that with continued use of this text and its glossary, many of these terms will in time become familiar.

iv. On occasions we have included purely Western medical terms. Hypertension, for example, has no equivalent in traditional Chinese medicine, and yet several acupuncture points have a demonstrable effect in reducing blood pressure. We have used the term erysipelas in place of the literal Chinese 'cinnabar toxin' as the meanings of the two terms are virtually identical.

v. As far as longer translated passages are concerned, the meaning of ancient texts written in classical Chinese is invariably open to some interpretation. We have consulted whichever commentaries are available and have generally chosen the most easily readable rendering.

The point actions

In general, it can be said that the ascribing of actions to acupuncture points is a modern (i.e. 20th century) practice, and one that draws from the Chinese herbal medicine tradition. Having said this, there is clear evidence of this practice in early texts. Among many examples, the *Systematic Classic of Acupuncture and Moxibustion* recommends Shangjuxu ST-37 for 'heat in the intestine' and the *Sagelike Prescriptions from the Taiping Era* recommends the same point for 'insufficiency of large intestine qi'. According to the *Essential Questions* Xiajuxu ST-39 'clears Stomach heat', whilst the *Great Compendium of Acupuncture and Moxibustion* recommends Sanyinjiao SP-6 for 'Spleen and Stomach deficiency'. Furthermore, in most cases ascribing actions to points is simply pragmatic. For example since Yinbai SP-1 is classically indicated for uterine bleeding, menorrhagia, blood in the urine, blood in the stool, vomiting blood, nosebleed and febrile disease with nosebleed, it is clear that it has the action of stopping bleeding. Lieque LU-7 is indicated for chills and fever and nasal congestion and discharge, and has clearly long been considered effective to release the exterior. Even a cursory examination of the classical indications of most points reveals such clear patterns of disharmony that can be summarised into point actions. Generalising the information in this way helps to clarify the welter of indications and simplify the learning process. It is not intended to replace a deeper study of the indications and influence of the points but rather to assist and complement it.

The point indications

The majority of the indications given in this text are taken from classical sources. Whilst not exhaustive, we have chosen to list them in greater number than most English texts. It is our observation that the more indications there are, the easier it is to form an impression of the nature and forte of each point. It is clear, also, that the recorded indications for the points represent an important record of clinical observation that is at least in part empirical rather than theoretical. In order to make the indications easier to absorb, we have chosen to group them according to type, and it should be stressed that these groupings are our own and are not found in classical texts.

The indications listed are not exclusively classical however. We have added modern indications when these clearly reflect current clinical practice. For example Zulinqi GB-41 is much used by contemporary doctors for one-sided headache, particularly in combination with Waiguan SJ-5 and especially for headaches associated with the menstrual cycle, despite the fact that all major classical references are to occipital pain, and pain of the vertex.

Finally we would like to stress that we have generally avoided adding indications to points when these are not listed in classical or modern Chinese texts. There has been a great deal of free interpretation in Western acupuncture, often based on supposition rather than either historical provenance or careful and lengthy clinical observation. One example of this process may be found with a point such as Shaofu HE-8. As the fire point of the Heart channel it is natural to assume that it clears Heart fire and thus that it would be indicated for disorders such as insomnia, mental agitation, sores in the mouth etc. and this is the impression given in a number of modern Western acupuncture books. In fact these indications are not found in classical Chinese texts and rarely in modern ones, and it is Laogong P-8 that has rather been used for these disorders. This is not to state categorically that Shaofu HE-8 does not have the ability to treat these disorders, only that it does not seem to have been used for this purpose. Our priority, therefore, has been to emphasise the historical records, not because we reject innovation and development, but rather because with a tradition as lengthy and unique as that of Chinese medicine, it is important first to establish what the tradition actually is, so as to innovate with care and respect.

The commentaries

The actions and indications of the points can be found in many acupuncture books. What has been lacking is a systematic attempt to clarify and explain how the point has been used through time and how we might better understand its range of actions and indications. In the commentaries on the major points we have endeavoured to draw together and elucidate a great range of information. This includes the major classical and modern indications, the classical combinations in which the point appears, commentaries on the points in a variety of texts, the point's location and its relationship to various channel pathways, the point's status (for example as a xi-cleft or jing-well point), the phase (according to five phase theory) to which it is ascribed etc. Having considered all these factors we have finally added our own interpretation and experience as practitioners of long standing. Interpretation necessarily requires making judgements, and we have tried to balance our own original contribution with respect for the available information.

There are many different traditional theories that can determine point selection. It could be, statistically-speaking, that the most commonly practised method throughout the world is the needling of acupuncture points simply because they are tender i.e. ahshi points. At a more complex level are five phase theory, five shu point theory, the theory of the back-shu and front-mu points, the combination of luo-connecting and yuan-source points and so on. Between these different theories, however, we often find major contradictions. Which of these theories will we try to apply, and how do we approach the contradictions? Some practitioners, favouring one particular theory, are happy to apply it in an absolute sense. Thus a close adherent of five phase theory might in all cases select a 'mother' point to tonify a particular channel and a 'child' point to reduce it. How can we determine whether the abstract application of a particular theory like this, as though it is always appropriate, can be supported? For example, Quchi L.I.-11 is the earth and hence 'mother' point of the Large Intestine channel, and should therefore have a reinforcing function. How do we then accommodate the fact that whilst indeed it is an important point to tonify qi and blood in the upper limb, it is otherwise used to drain excess heat, fire, wind and damp from the body as a whole, not to mention the fact that its recorded indications include very few intestinal disorders. Similarly, according to five phase theory, Jiexi ST-41 as the fire point of the earth Stomach channel should have a tonifying action, whereas all the recorded indications suggest it is used to reduce excess heat in both the Stomach channel and the Stomach fu.

As far as the five shu points are concerned, the *Classic of Difficulties* in the 68th Difficulty states that jing-river points should be needled for dyspnoea, cough, chills and fever. Should we take this to mean that all jing-river points have this effect, or that in these situations we should always needle the jing-river points? How do we combine this with the statement in the *Spiritual Pivot* that jing-river points should be needled in the late summer or for changes in the patient's voice? Or what of the *Spiritual Pivot* classification of the relative state of the qi and blood in the six channels? Yangming channel, for example, is abundant in qi and blood, and this theory is frequently called upon to explain the use of the Large Intestine and Stomach yangming channels in the treatment of atrophy disorder and painful obstruction. The *Spiritual Pivot* also states that taiyang and jueyin channels are abundant in blood, which helps to explain why points such as Weizhong BL-40 and Quze P-3 may be bled to clear heat from the body. What then of the contradictory clinical application of bleeding Shaoshang LU-11 in cases of sore throat, when the *Spiritual Pivot* states that taiyin channel is abundant in qi but not in blood?

Throughout the history of Chinese medicine, different theories have been developed, tested, contested, retained where useful and quietly dropped when not, and commonly kept in part when considered clinically or theoretically valuable. No matter that the theoretical body of acupuncture may contain contradictory theories. In certain situations one theory may be held to apply, in others not. In our commentaries on the points we have attempted to sift through these various theories and find those most relevant to understanding and explaining how a point has actually been used and tested in clinical practice, the final arbiter of such discussions.

The point combinations

The majority of the point combinations listed under each point in this book are taken from classical sources, and these are given in parentheses. We have taken the liberty of changing the order of the points listed so that the same combination will appear several times throughout the text, under different points listed in the combination. A small proportion of the combinations are modern, some taken from contemporary Chinese sources and some from our own clinical experience. In these cases no source is given.

Capitalisation

We have tried to keep capitalisation of words to a minimum. However we have kept the names of the zangfu (Lung, Stomach, Heart etc.) capitalised to distinguish them from the Western medicine names of the organs (lung, stomach, heart etc.)

Point locations

The locations given in this text are derived from a comprehensive review of the modern Chinese renderings of traditional sources, informed by the authors' clinical experience. We have made every effort to be as anatomically precise as possible and thus resolve the contradictions sometimes found in existing point location descriptions. Where there are in effect two alternative locations for a point this is clearly described in the text. The precision of anatomical description however does not relieve the practitioner of the responsibility for careful observation and palpation of the area to be needled so that relevant underlying structures such as blood vessels are protected and the fundamental importance of the role of palpation in point location is not neglected.

Location notes

These notes are derived from the authors' clinical experience taken together with the traditional sources. They are simply intended to facilitate the practitioner's ease of location of points in clinical practice.

Needling

The practitioner must remain aware that acupuncture is an invasive therapeutic procedure. The needling instructions given are intended to highlight the aspect of safety at least as much as that of therapeutic efficacy. To this end throughout the text specific cautions concerning the use of potentially harmful acupuncture points are clearly given.

Extra points

We have utilised the numbering system used in *Acupuncture: A Comprehensive Text*[1].

Errors

Every attempt has been made to reduce errors in this text. Such is the nature of human existence, however, that mistakes are unavoidable. In the interests of improving future editions, the authors would be grateful to have their mistakes pointed out.

Notes

1 *Acupuncture A Comprehensive Text*, Shanghai College of Traditional Medicine, translated and edited by John O'Connor and Dan Bensky, Eastland Press 1981.

THE CHANNELS AND COLLATERALS

"It is by virtue of the twelve channels that human life exists, that disease arises, that human beings can be treated and illness cured. The twelve channels are where beginners start and masters end. To beginners it seems easy; the masters know how difficult it is".

Spiritual Pivot Chapter 17.

"Qi cannot travel without a path, just as water flows or the sun and moon orbit without rest. So do the yin vessels nourish the zang and the yang vessels nourish the fu".

Spiritual Pivot Chapter 17.

INTRODUCTION

'Channels and collaterals' is a translation of the Chinese term 'jingluo'. 'Jing' has a geographical connotation and means a channel (e.g. a water channel) or longitude. In this book it is translated as 'channels', elsewhere as 'meridians'. Using the image of a tree, the 'jing' are like the trunk and main branches of the channel network. They generally run longitudinally through the body at a relatively deep level, and connect with the internal zangfu. Specifically they comprise the twelve primary channels, the eight extraordinary vessels and the twelve divergent channels. 'Luo' means 'to attach' or 'a net', and refers to the finer branches of the channel network which are more superficial and interconnect the trunk and main branches (jing), the connective tissues and cutaneous regions. In this book they are referred to in general as the collaterals, and more specifically as the luo-connecting channels. There are fifteen luo-connecting channels, the twelve that belong to the twelve primary channels, the luo-connecting channels of the Conception and Governing vessels, and the great luo-connecting channel of the Spleen. The general category of the collaterals also includes the myriad 'minute' collaterals that are distributed throughout the body. In addition to the jing and luo, there are twelve sinew channels and twelve cutaneous regions.

Whilst a typical chart of the acupuncture channels, therefore, illustrates only the superficial pathways of the twelve primary channels, we should remember that the channel network is considerably more complex than this, and there is no part of the body, no kind of tissue, no single cell, that is not supplied by the channels. Like a tree, the trunk and main branches define the main structure, whilst ever finer branches, twigs and leaves spread out to every part.

The study of the channels in traditional Chinese medicine can be said to be the equivalent of the study of anatomy in Western medicine. Chinese medicine paid scant attention to the physical structure of the interior of the body, and references to the shape and location of the internal zangfu in classical texts are few and very brief. Furthermore there was no study of the distribution of the nerves, or the origin and insertion of the muscles. Traditional Chinese medicine did, however, describe in minute detail the pathways of the wide variety of channels that serve to circulate the qi and blood to every part of the body. The channels penetrate the zangfu and the extraordinary fu in the deepest levels of the body and connect with the skin, muscles, flesh, tendons, and bones, the head, body and limbs, and the sense organs, linking all the tissues and structures of the body into an integrated whole.

HISTORY OF CHANNEL THEORY

Different theories have been advanced to explain the discovery of the channels. These theories may be summarised as being of two main kinds: i. points first, channels second, and ii. channels first, points second. According to the first theory, centuries of observation of the existence of tender spots on the body during the course of disease, and the alleviation of symptoms when they were stimulated by massage or heat, led to the gradual discovery of the acupuncture points. When sufficient points were known, they were linked into groups with common characteristics and effects, and aided by the observation of propagated sensation when they were stimulated, understanding of channel pathways followed. According to the second theory, propagated sensation during the course of massage and more especially the exploration of the internal landscape of the body through mediation and qigong practice, led to the discovery of the channel pathways, with the knowledge of specific points coming later. This second theory received strong confirmation from the significant discovery of a silk book during excavation of the Western Han tomb at Mawangdui[1], which describes the pathways of eleven channels but does not refer to any specific points.

THE FUNCTIONS OF THE CHANNELS

1 Transporting qi and blood throughout the body and rendering the body an integrated whole

It is by virtue of the complex interweaving network of the channels that the qi and blood is transported to every part of the body. All the organs, sense organs and tissues are nourished, energised and warmed by the qi and blood circulating through the channel network. Using the analogy of a plant, the zangfu may be perceived as the roots of the channels, the channels themselves as the stems, and the different body tissues, and especially the sense organs, as the flowers. Thus the Heart, for example, is said to 'flower' into the tongue. The zangfu, the channels passing through the limbs and body, and the tissues and sense organs which they nourish therefore constitute an integrated whole.

At the same time, by virtue of the interconnections between the channels, the zangfu themselves are linked with each other. For example, the primary channel of the Lung originates in the Stomach, and passes through the Large Intestine and diaphragm, whilst the primary channel of the Heart connects with the Small Intestine and Lung.

By virtue of their origin in the depths of the body and their emergence at the surface, the channels also link the interior with the exterior. Since they run bilaterally, or in the case of the Girdling vessel encircle the body, the primary, divergent, connecting and sinew channels as well as six of the extraordinary vessels, link the two sides of the body, and since they run vertically, the various channels link above with below. The theory of the channels, therefore, underlies one of the most significant discoveries of Chinese medicine; they form the physiological interconnections that render the body an integrated whole rather than a series of independent units.

2 Protecting the body

"When the pathogen comes to dwell as a guest, first it resides in the skin and body hair. If it remains and does not leave it will enter the minute connecting channels. If it remains and does not leave it will enter the luo-connecting channels. If it remains and does not leave it will enter the channels, reaching the five zang and spreading into the intestines and Stomach" *Essential Questions*[2].

The various kinds of channels occupy different depths within the body. As well as nourishing and energising these different layers of the body, the channels serve to prevent the penetration of pathogenic factors that may attack the body from the outside. Wind, cold, damp, heat, fire and dryness are important causes of disease according to Chinese medicine. When extreme, or when the body resistance is lowered, they can attack the body and easily penetrate to the deeper levels such as the zangfu and the bones and joints. The deeper the penetration towards the zangfu, the more serious the disease becomes. Part of the function of the channel network is to contain and repel these pathogenic factors, and prevent deeper penetration. Thus, for example, a person who sleeps in a draught may wake with a stiff and painful neck. The wind and cold will usually in this instance have injured only the more superficial portions of the channel network, i.e. the sinew channels, causing local stagnation of qi and blood. Treatment, whether by acupuncture, cupping or massage will relatively easily eliminate the pathogenic factor. If, however, a person is frequently exposed to wind, cold and damp, then over time the pathogenic factors will not be contained at the level of the superficial channels, but may penetrate deeper into the body, injuring the joints, sinews and bones. If even more prolonged, the pathogens may injure and weaken the zangfu, most commonly the Liver and Kidneys. Alternatively, an acute attack of wind and cold may induce the typical symptoms of chills, slight fever, headache, body aches, runny nose etc. Here, the pathogenic factors have injured and caused stagnation of the defensive and nutritive qi in the relatively superficial portion of the body. The treatment principle is to release the exterior. If, however, the pathogenic factors are not contained at the superficial level, but penetrate deeper, they may injure the zangfu, most commonly the Lung, Stomach, Spleen or intestines.

Most superficial

↑

Cutaneous regions
Minute collaterals
Sinew channels
Luo-connecting channels
Primary channels
Divergent channels
Extraordinary channels
Deep pathways of the primary and divergent channels

↓

Deepest

To summarise, the entire channel network serves as a series of barriers to prevent the deeper penetration of pathogenic factors from the exterior. When contained at the exterior, the disease is relatively less serious and easier to eliminate. When the body resistance is lowered, or the pathogenic factor is exceptionally strong or prolonged, and the channels cannot contain the pathogenic factors at the exterior, the disease is relatively more serious and harder to cure.

3 Responding to dysfunction in the body
When the harmony of the body is disrupted by any of the causes of disease, the channels can respond in a number of ways:

i. Disease of the channels themselves
The channels themselves can be diseased giving rise to local tenderness, pain, weakness, distention, numbness, tingling etc. Disease of the channels means impaired flow of qi and blood (i.e. stagnation) or insufficiency of qi and blood leading to malnourishment. For example:

- back sprain due to traumatic injury can give rise to pain, aching, tingling etc. in the channels in the lumbar region and leg.
- attack by pathogenic wind and cold into the muscle layers can give rise to stiffness, soreness and aching with points of local tenderness, whether acupuncture points or ahshi[3] points.
- prolonged exposure to wind-cold-damp may give rise to chronic pain and aching in the limbs and joints.
- previous injury or prolonged over-use of any part of the body may give rise either to stagnation or deficiency in the channels in a local area resulting in aching and pain.

ii. Disease of the zangfu reflecting onto the channels
When the zangfu are in disharmony internally, their related channels may also show signs of disorder, for example:

- stasis of Heart blood can give rise to pain which descends along the Heart channel in the arm, or ascends along the Heart channel to the throat.
- stagnation of Liver qi can lead to distention and pain in any portion of the Liver channel, or its interiorly-exteriorly related Gall Bladder channel, for example the genitals, lateral costal region, breasts, throat or head.
- Heat in the Stomach fu may give rise to symptoms such as excessive hunger and vomiting as well as transmitting to the Stomach channel in the head, giving rise to tooth abscess, bleeding gums, ulcers on the tongue etc.
- Liver fire can transmit via the Liver channel to the eyes and manifest as redness, soreness and pain.

iii. Disease transmitting via the channels
Disease can pass from one zangfu to another via the channels, or from one channel to another, for example:

- Heart fire can transmit from the Heart channel to its interiorly-exteriorly related hand Small Intestine channel, from the hand taiyang Small Intestine channel to the foot taiyang Bladder channel and thence to the Bladder fu.
- severe deficiency of Kidney yang and impaired transformation of body fluids can cause excessive water to overflow to the Lung and/or Heart, both linked to the Kidney via the internal pathway of its primary channel.

iv. Visibly showing disease
In some cases, the course of a diseased channel can be discoloured and therefore visible, whether purple showing stasis of blood, red indicating heat, or pale as a result of deficiency of qi and blood.

4 The channels serve to transmit qi to the diseased area
The channels serve to transmit acupuncture stimulation from the acupuncture point to the diseased area of the body, rendering acupuncture treatment effective. By stimulating an acupuncture point by some means, whether by needling, application of heat, pressure, massage or cupping, the qi and blood of the whole course of the channel may be regulated.

THE TWELVE PRIMARY CHANNELS

GENERAL DESCRIPTION

There are twelve primary channels running vertically, bilaterally, and symmetrically. Each channel corresponds to, and connects internally with, one of the twelve zangfu. The channels corresponding to the zang are yin, and the channels corresponding to the fu are yang. There are therefore six yin and six yang channels, three yin channels and three yang channels on the arm, and three yin channels and three yang channels on the leg.

To understand the pathways of the channels it is helpful to visualise a person standing with their arms by their sides, the palms facing the legs, rather than in the conventional anatomical position. The yang channels then traverse the outer surface of the arm or leg, travel to the head, and with the exception of the Stomach channel , the back. The yin channels traverse the inner surface of the limbs, and the abdomen and chest. More specifically:

- the three yin channels of the hand (Lung, Pericardium and Heart) begin on the chest and travel along the inner surface of the arm to the hand.
- the three yang channels of the hand (Large Intestine, Sanjiao and Small Intestine) begin on the hand and travel along the outer surface of the arm to the head.
- the three yang channels of the foot (Stomach, Gall Bladder and Bladder) begin on the face, in the region of the eye, and travel down the body and along the outer surface of the leg to the foot.
- the three yin channels of the foot (Spleen, Liver and Kidney) begin on the foot and travel along the inner surface of the leg to the chest or flank.

The course of each of the twelve channels comprises an internal and an external pathway. The external pathway is what is normally shown on an acupuncture chart and is relatively superficial. All the acupuncture points of a channel lie on its external pathway. The internal pathways are the deep course of the channel where it enters the body cavities. The superficial pathways of the twelve channels describe three complete circuits of the body

	Chest →	Hand →	Face →	Foot →	Chest
First circuit	Lung	Large Intestine	Stomach	Spleen	
Second circuit	Heart	Small Intestine	Bladder	Kidney	
Third circuit	Pericardium	Sanjiao	Gall Bladder	Liver	

NAMING OF THE TWELVE PRIMARY CHANNELS

The practice among English-speaking acupuncturists has been to use the same name for each zangfu and its related channel. Thus we talk of the Lung organ and the Lung channel. In practice this may blur the important distinction between the two, and serve to confuse when analysing the different clinical situations of disease of the channel alone, disease of the zangfu alone, or disease of both the zangfu and channel. In Chinese, each has a different name. Thus the Lung zang is known as 'fei' (Lung), whilst its related channel is known as shou taiyin fei jing (the hand taiyin Lung channel). This naming of each channel consists of three parts:

i. The zang or fu to which it belongs.
ii. The limb (upper or lower) through which it travels.
iii. Its yin or yang identity.

The twelve channels are paired with each other in two important ways:

Zangfu	Limb	Yin-yang identity	Zangfu	Limb	Yin-yang identity
Lung	hand	taiyin (supreme yin)	Small Intestine	hand	taiyang (supreme yang)
Spleen	foot	taiyin (supreme yin)	Bladder	foot	taiyang (supreme yang)
Large Intestine	hand	yangming (yang brightness)	Pericardium	hand	jueyin (absolute yin)
Stomach	foot	yangming (yang brightness)	Liver	foot	jueyin (absolute yin)
Heart	hand	shaoyin (lesser yin)	Sanjiao	hand	shaoyang (lesser yang)
Kidney	foot	shaoyin (lesser yin)	Gall Bladder	foot	shaoyang (lesser yang)

i. There is an 'exterior-interior' relationship between the yin and yang channels on the arm, and between the yin and yang channels on the leg, whereby each yang channel of the arm is paired with a yin channel of the arm, and each yang channel of the leg is paired with a yin channel of the leg. This 'interior-exterior' relationship expresses both an important physiological connection between the paired zang and fu, and an anatomical relationship between the channels. For example, when a person stands as described above, the Stomach channel of foot yangming occupies the anterior portion of the outer surface of the leg. It is 'interiorly-exteriorly' related to the Spleen channel of foot taiyin which occupies the anterior portion of the inner surface of the leg. At the same time, the Stomach function of 'rotting and ripening' food and drink is closely linked, physiologically, to the Spleen function of 'transporting and transforming' the products of digestion.

The interior-exterior relationships of the twelve primary channels are as follows:

Channel	Pathway	Channel	Pathway
Lung	anterior portion of the inside of the arm	Spleen	anterior portion of the inside of the leg
Large Intestine	anterior portion of the outside of the arm	Stomach	anterior portion of the outside of the leg
Pericardium	middle portion of the inside of the arm	Liver	middle portion of the inside of the leg
Sanjiao	middle portion of the outside of the arm	Gall Bladder	middle portion of the outside of the leg
Heart	posterior portion of the inside of the arm	Kidney	posterior portion of the inside of the leg
Small Intestine	posterior portion of the outside of the arm	Bladder	posterior portion of the outside of the leg

ii. The second pairing of the twelve primary channels results from a different perspective on their anatomical relationship, rather than the physiological functions of their related zangfu, although such a relationship often exists. In this pairing, a yang channel is paired with another yang channel, a yin channel with a yin channel. If a person stands normally, with their arms at their sides, the channel that occupies the anterior portion of the outer aspect of the arm is the Large Intestine channel of hand yangming. This is linked to the channel that occupies an anatomically similar position on the leg, i.e. the Stomach channel of foot yangming. The paired connection between these two channels is reflected in the fact that part of their name (yangming) is identical.

So important is this paired relationship, that they are often described as the 'six channels', each pair being referred to as a single channel. For example, yangming channel as a whole (meaning both Large Intestine and Stomach channels) is described as being 'abundant in qi and blood'. Similarly, the treatment principle for a patient presenting with pain in the lateral costal region as well as temporal headache may be to 'harmonise shaoyang channel'.

These two alternative ways of pairing the channels come together in the three main circuits of the flow of qi through the twelve primary channels. The flow of qi in each circuit begins in a yin channel on the chest and passes to the interiorly-exteriorly related yang channel at the hand. It then ascends along the yang channel to the face where it passes into the yang channel's paired yang channel according to six channel theory and descends to the foot where it passes to the interiorly-exteriorly related yin channel and ascends back to the chest before beginning a new circuit.

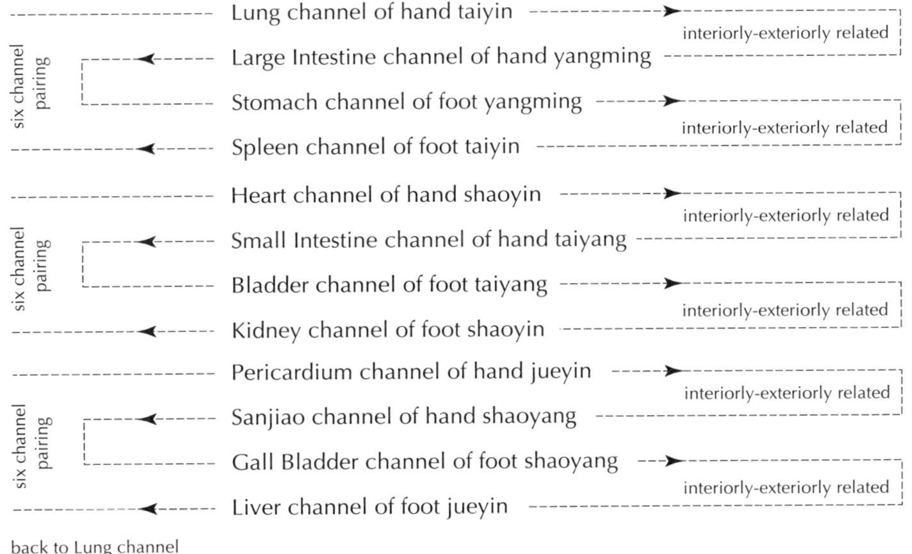

THE INTERIOR PATHWAYS OF THE PRIMARY CHANNELS

There is a tendency in studying the primary channels to focus on their superficial pathways, since this is where the acupuncture points lie. To understand the actions and indications of the points however, it is essential to know the deep pathways of the primary channels. For example:

- the Lung channel originates in the middle jiao, in the region of the Stomach, and most of the points of the Lung channel are able to treat disorders such as nausea and vomiting.
- the Stomach channel ascends to meet with the Governing vessel at points Shenting DU-24 and Renzhong DU-26. Since the Governing vessel enters the brain, this connection helps explain the important action of many Stomach channel points on disorders of the spirit.
- the affinity of Hegu L.I.-4 for treating pain both at the forehead and the side of the head reflects the fact that the internal pathway of the Large Intestine channel meets with the Gall Bladder channel at Yangbai GB-14, Xuanlu GB-5 and Xuanli GB-6.
- the internal pathway of the Pericardium channel descends through the middle jiao, enabling points such as Neiguan P-6 to treat nausea and vomiting.

THE TWELVE DIVERGENT CHANNELS

The twelve divergent channels branch out from the twelve primary channels and have no specific points of their own. It is important, however, to be familiar with the principal features of the divergent channels, since their pathways make internal linkages that may not be made by the primary channels, and therefore serve to explain the actions and indications of many points.

Most of the divergent channels belonging to the yang primary channels:

- separate from their yang primary channel on the limbs e.g. the Bladder channel at the popliteal fossa, the Stomach and Gall Bladder channels on the thigh, the Small Intestine channel at the shoulder, the Large Intestine channel on the hand.
- enter their related zang or fu as well as their internally-externally related zang or fu, for example the Bladder divergent channel travels to the Bladder fu and then to the Kidney zang; the Stomach divergent channel travels to the Stomach fu then to the Spleen zang etc.
- resurface at the supraclavicular fossa, neck or face and join their primary yang channel again.

The yin divergent channels belonging to the yin primary channels:

- separate from their yin primary channel on the limbs.
- sometimes enter their pertaining zang (Kidney, Heart, Lung).
- converge with their internally-externally related divergent channel.
- then join the primary yang channel itself.

FUNCTIONS AND CLINICAL SIGNIFICANCE OF THE DIVERGENT CHANNELS

1 The divergent channels strengthen the yin-yang relationship between internally-externally paired channels and zangfu

The interiorly-exteriorly related channels and zangfu are already linked by the primary and luo-connecting channels in the following ways:

- each primary channel precedes or follows its paired channel in the qi circuit, for example the Lung channel precedes the Large Intestine channel, the Spleen channel follows the Stomach channel.
- each primary channel internally links its own related zang or fu with the zang or fu corresponding to its paired channel, for example the Lung channel penetrates the Lung zang and the Large Intestine fu.
- the luo-connecting channels link the paired channels

Since the yang divergent channels further connect the paired zangfu and since the yin divergent channels intersect first with the yang divergent channels and then with the yang primary channels, the divergent channels are said to strengthen the bonds of paired yin and yang primary channels and the paired zangfu themselves.

2 The divergent channels distribute qi and blood to head and face

The six primary yang channels all circulate to the head and face, but of the yin primary channels only the Heart and Liver do so. By their link with the yang divergent and primary channels, the yin divergent channels provide a pathway for the yin channels to circulate qi and blood to the head and face. For example the Lung channel does not ascend higher than the throat region but Lung qi can circulate to the nose by virtue of the connection between the Lung divergent channel and the Large Intestine primary channel.

3 The divergent channels integrate areas of the body not supplied or interconnected by the primary channels
For example:

- great emphasis is placed on the important relationship between the Heart and the Kidneys (fire and water), yet although the primary channel of the Kidney connects with the Heart, the primary channel of the Heart does not connect with the Kidneys. The divergent channel of the Bladder (interiorly-exteriorly related to the Kidneys), however, travels from the Kidneys to the Heart, strengthening this bond.
- neither the Liver nor the Gall Bladder primary channels travel directly to the Heart, but the pathway of the Gall Bladder divergent channel to the Heart reinforces and helps explain the close physiological relationship between the Heart and the Liver and Gall Bladder.

4 The divergent channels help explain the clinical action of some commonly-used acupuncture points
For example:

- the Bladder divergent channel circulates through the rectal area, helping to explain the action of points such as Chengshan BL-57 and Feiyang BL-58 on the treatment of rectal diseases, especially haemorrhoids.
- the Stomach divergent channel enters the Heart, helping to explain the use of many Stomach channel points in the treatment of disorders of the spirit.
- the Bladder divergent channel links with the Heart helping to explain the effect of points of the Bladder channel in the treatment of disharmony of the Heart and spirit, for example Shenmai BL-62 for epilepsy, palpitations, insomnia and mania-depression disorder

The pathways of the divergent channels are illustrated in the main body of this text.

THE EIGHT EXTRAORDINARY VESSELS

The eight extraordinary vessels are the Conception (Ren), the Governing (Du), the Penetrating (Chong), the Girdling (Dai), the Yin Motility (Yin Qiao), the Yang Motility (Yang Qiao), the Yin Linking (Yin Wei) and the Yang Linking (Yang Wei). Of the eight, only the Conception and Governing vessels have points of their own and they are therefore sometimes included with the twelve primary channels in the term 'the fourteen channels'. The remaining six extraordinary vessels have no points of their own, but share points of the fourteen channels (known as the coalescent points). The eight extraordinary channels branch off from the trunks of the primary channels, and interlink the primary channels to each other. The pathways of the Conception and Governing vessels are discussed in detail in the main text of this book. The pathways of the remaining six extraordinary channels are given in the following pages.

FUNCTIONS OF THE EXTRAORDINARY VESSELS

1 The extraordinary vessels act as reservoirs
The *Classic of Difficulties*[4] compares the extraordinary channels to reservoirs which are able to absorb excessive qi and blood from the primary channels in the same way that reservoirs take excess water from canals and ditches at times of heavy rain.

2 The extraordinary vessels link the twelve primary channels

- the Governing vessel links all the yang channels at Dazhui DU-14, and is known as the 'sea of the yang channels', and helps regulate the qi of all the yang channels.
- the Conception vessel links all the yin channels, and is known as the 'sea of the yin channels' and helps regulate the qi of all the yin channels.
- the Penetrating vessel links the Stomach and Kidney channels as well as strengthening the link between the Conception and Governing vessels (like both of these vessels it originates in the pelvic cavity and ascends the front of the body as well as the spine). It is known as the 'sea of blood' or the 'sea of the twelve primary channels'.
- the Girdling vessel encircles the body at the waist, binding the vertical paths of the twelve primary channels in general and the Penetrating and Conception vessels and the Kidney, Liver and Spleen channels in particular.
- the Yin Motility vessel connects the Kidney and Bladder channels and is said to dominate quietness.
- the Yang Motility vessel connects the Bladder, Gall Bladder, Small Intestine, Large Intestine and Stomach channels and is said to dominate activity.
- the Yin Linking vessel connects the Kidney, Spleen and Liver channels and the Conception vessel and is said to dominate the interior of the whole body.
- the Yang Linking vessel connects the Bladder, Gall Bladder, Sanjiao, Small Intestine and Stomach channels and the Governing vessel, and is said to dominate the exterior of the whole body.

3 The extraordinary vessels protect the body

The Conception, Governing and Penetrating vessels circulate defensive qi over the chest, abdomen and back, helping to protect the body from exterior pathogenic factors. Since these three vessels originate in the pelvic cavity and are directly linked with the Kidneys, the storehouse of pre-heaven qi, this function demonstrates the relationship between constitutional vigour and defence against disease.

THE EXTRAORDINARY VESSELS HAVE THEIR OWN CONFLUENT POINTS

Each of the eight extraordinary channels has a confluent point on the limbs which is considered to have an effect on its extraordinary channel. These are listed and discussed in the Point Categories chapter.

THE PATHWAYS OF THE EIGHT EXTRAORDINARY VESSELS

For illustrations of the extraordinary channels discussed below, see the end of this chapter.

PENETRATING VESSEL

- originates inside the lower abdomen (in the uterus in women),
- emerges at the perineum (Huiyin REN-1),
- one branch ascends inside the spinal column,
- another branch emerges at Qichong ST-30, connects with the Kidney channel at Henggu KID-11 and ascends through the Kidney channel to Youmen KID-21, then disperses in the chest,
- from here, a third branch ascends alongside the throat, curves around the lips and terminates below the eye,
- a fourth branch emerges at Qichong ST-30, descends the medial aspect of the legs to the popliteal fossa, then descends the medial side of the lower leg, runs posterior to the medial malleolus and terminates on the sole of the foot
- a fifth branch separates from the leg branch at the heel, crosses the foot and terminates at the big toe.

Coalescent points: Huiyin REN-1, Yinjiao REN-7, Qichong ST-30, Henggu KID-11, Dahe KID-12, Qixue KID-13, Siman KID-14, Zhongzhu KID-15, Huangshu KID-16, Shangqu KID-17, Shiguan KID-18, Yindu KID-19, Futonggu KID-20, Youmen KID-21.

Pathological symptoms of the Penetrating vessel

Counterflow qi, abdominal urgency, dyspnoea, gynaecological disorders, atrophy disorder of the leg.

GIRDLING VESSEL

- originates in the region of Zhangmen LIV-13,
- circles round just below the hypochondriac region,
- runs obliquely downwards through Daimai GB-26, Wushu GB-27 and Weidai GB-28, encircling the waist like a belt.

Coalescent points: Daimai GB-26, Wushu GB-27 and Weidai GB-28.

Pathological symptoms of the Girdling vessel

Abdominal fullness, a sensation at the waist as though sitting in water, pain around the umbilicus, abdomen, waist and lumbar spine, red and white leucorrhoea, irregular menstruation, infertility, insufficient sperm, shan disorder.

YANG MOTILITY VESSEL

- originates at the lateral side of the heel at Shenmai BL-62,
- ascends along the lateral malleolus and the posterior border of the fibula,
- ascends the lateral side of the thigh to the hip (Juliao GB-29) and the postero-lateral costal region to the posterior axillary fold,
- zig-zags across the top of the shoulder,
- ascends across the neck to the corner of the mouth,
- ascends the cheek and alongside the nose to the inner canthus and communicates with the Yin Motility vessel and the Bladder channel at Jingming BL-1,
- continues upwards to the forehead then curves across the parietal region and descends to meet with Fengchi GB-20 and enters the brain "at the occiput between the two tendons".

Coalescent points: Shenmai BL-62, Pucan BL-61, Fuyang BL-59, Juliao GB-29, Naoshu SI-10, Jianyu L.I.-15, Jugu L.I.-16, Dicang ST-4, Juliao ST-3, Chengqi ST-1, Jingming BL-1 and Fengchi GB-20.

Pathological symptoms of the Yang Motility vessel

Daytime epilepsy, eye diseases, loss of consciousness, aversion to wind, hemiplegia, chronic painful obstruction, rigidity of the body, lumbar pain, contracted sinews, flaccidity of the muscles of the medial leg and tightness of the muscles of the lateral leg.

CHONG MAI SP4

THE PENETRATING VESSEL

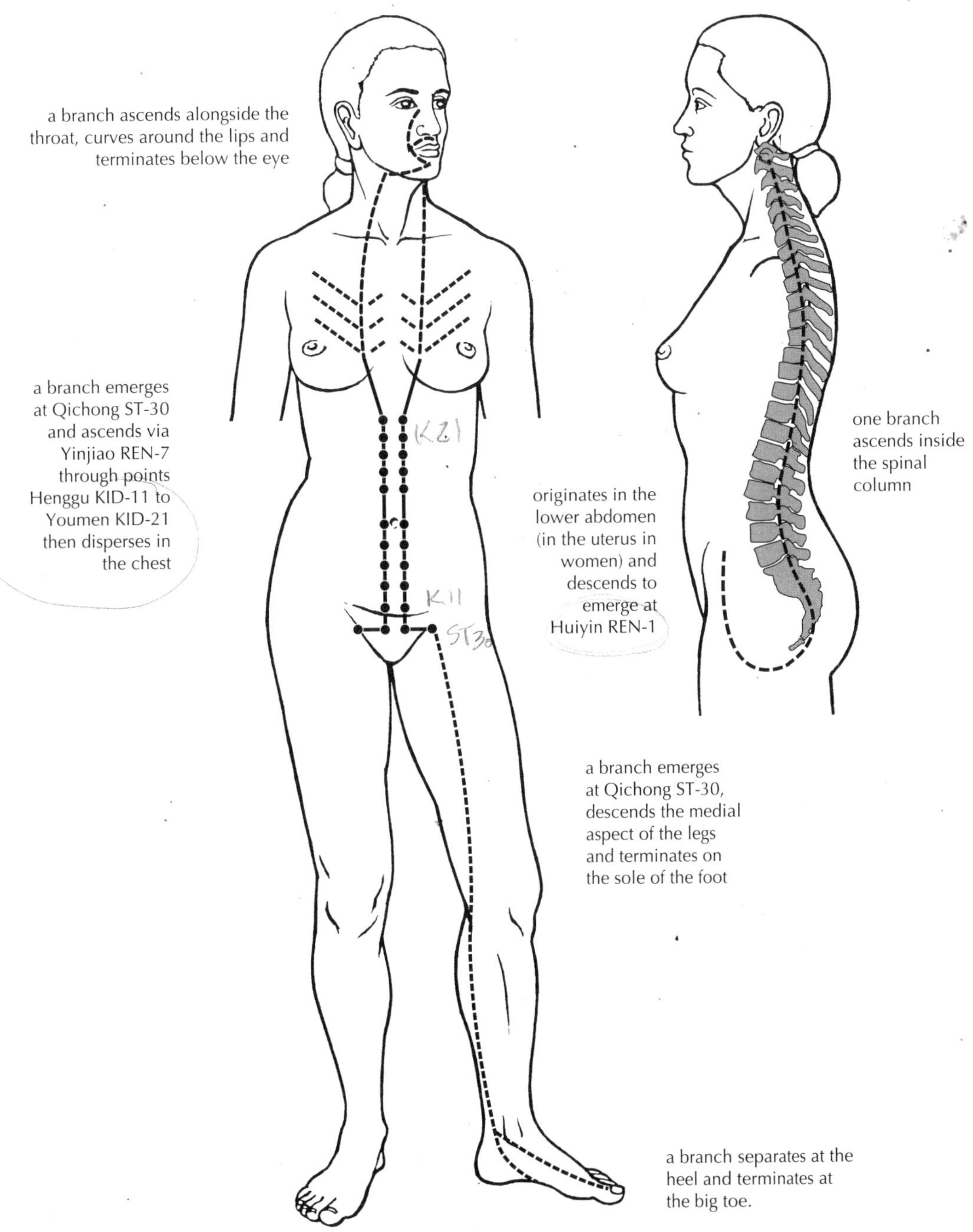
a branch ascends alongside the throat, curves around the lips and terminates below the eye
a branch emerges at Qichong ST-30 and ascends via Yinjiao REN-7 through points Henggu KID-11 to Youmen KID-21 then disperses in the chest
originates in the lower abdomen (in the uterus in women) and descends to emerge at Huiyin REN-1
one branch ascends inside the spinal column
a branch emerges at Qichong ST-30, descends the medial aspect of the legs and terminates on the sole of the foot
a branch separates at the heel and terminates at the big toe.

Coalescent points
Huiyin REN-1, Yinjiao REN-7, Qichong ST-30, Henggu KID-11, Dahe KID-12, Qixue KID-13, Siman KID-14, Zhongzhu KID-15, Huangshu KID-16, Shangqu KID-17, Shiguan KID-18, Yindu KID-19, Futonggu KID-20, Youmen KID-21.

Pathological symptoms of the Penetrating vessel
Counterflow qi, abdominal urgency, dyspnoea, gynaecological disorders, atrophy disorder of the leg.

THE GIRDLING VESSEL

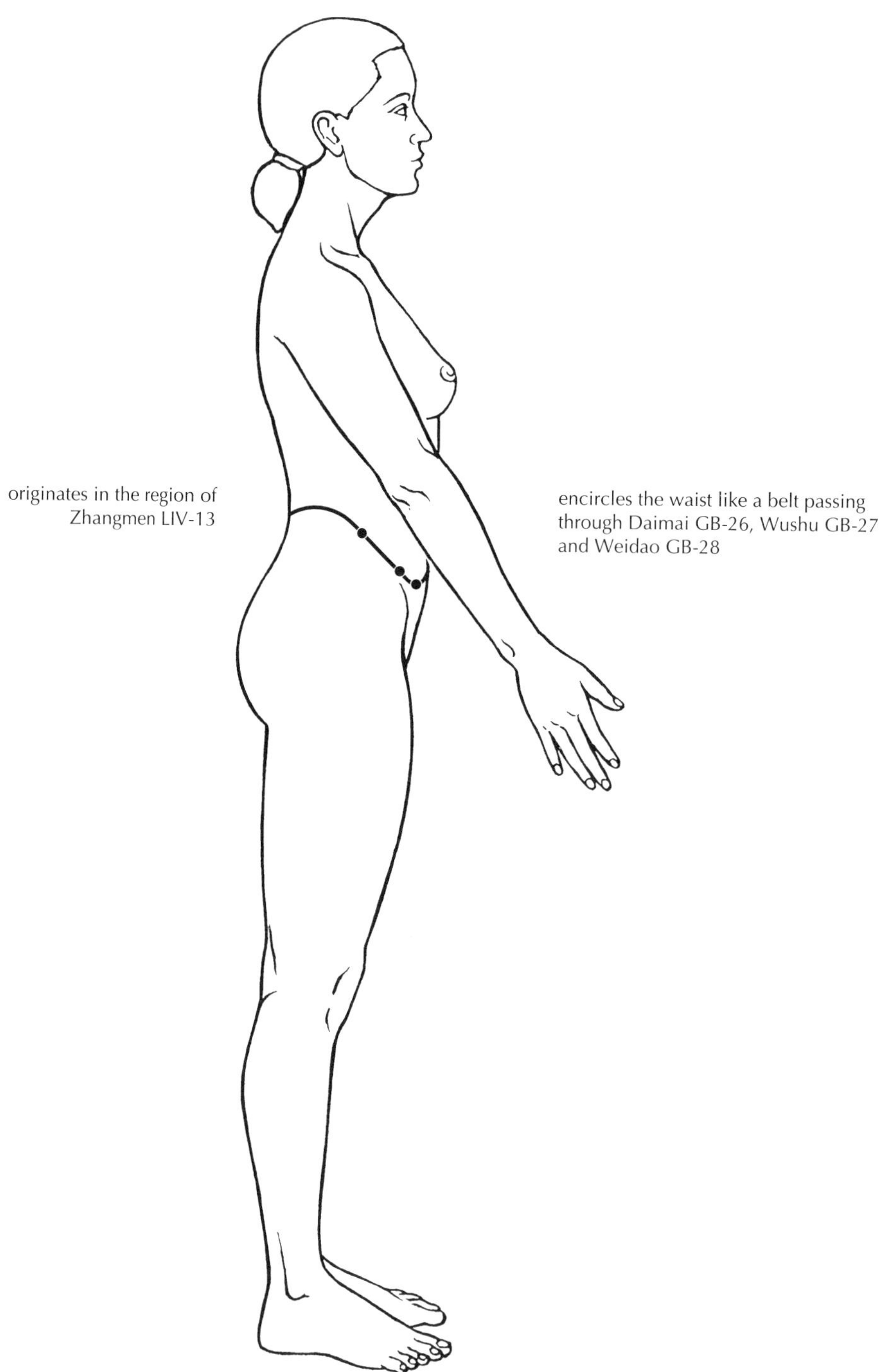

Coalescent points

Daimai GB-26, Wushu GB-27 and Weidao GB-28.

Pathological symptoms of the Girdling vessel

Abdominal fullness, a sensation at the waist as though sitting in water, pain around the umbilicus, abdomen, waist and lumbar spine, red and white leucorrhoea, irregular menstruation, infertility, insufficient sperm, shan disorder.

Qiao

THE YANG MOTILITY VESSEL

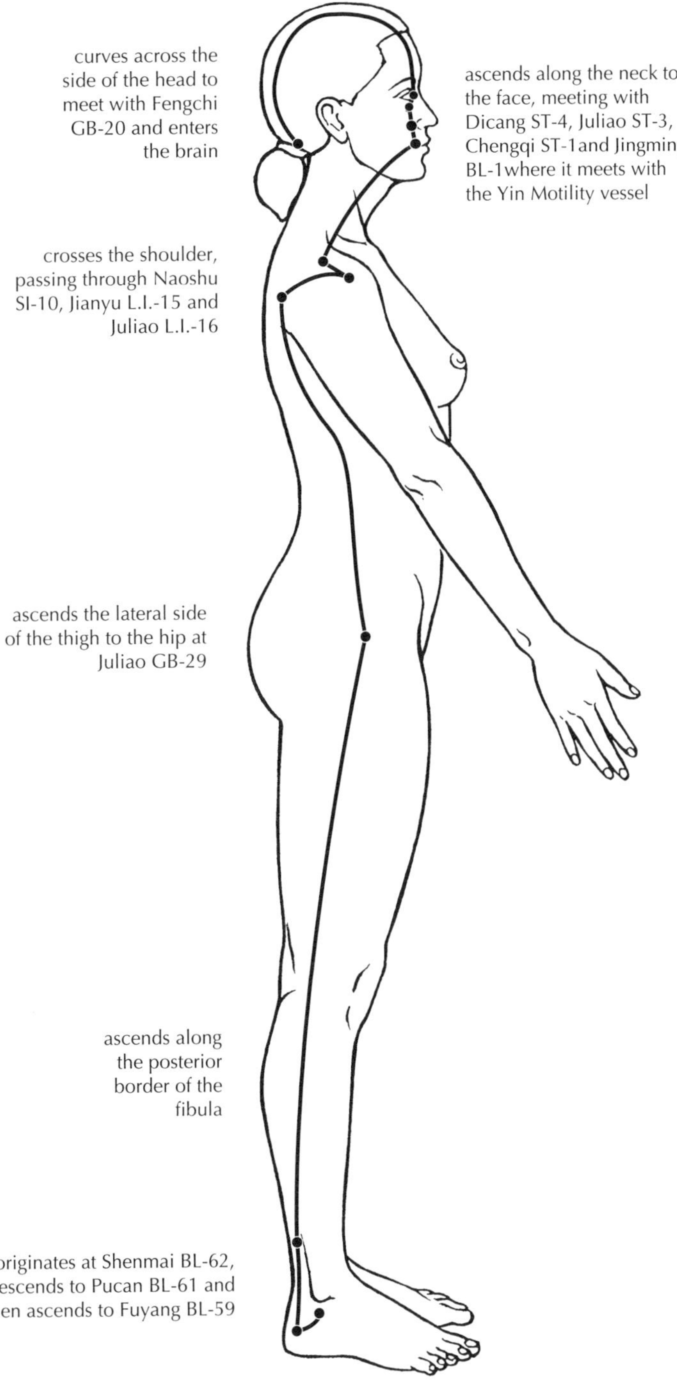
curves across the
side of the head to
meet with Fengchi
GB-20 and enters
the brain
ascends along the neck to
the face, meeting with
Dicang ST-4, Juliao ST-3,
Chengqi ST-1and Jingming
BL-1where it meets with
the Yin Motility vessel
crosses the shoulder,
passing through Naoshu
SI-10, Jianyu L.I.-15 and
Juliao L.I.-16
ascends the lateral side
of the thigh to the hip at
Juliao GB-29
ascends along
the posterior
border of the
fibula
originates at Shenmai BL-62,
descends to Pucan BL-61 and
then ascends to Fuyang BL-59

Coalescent points

Shenmai BL-62, Pucan BL-61, Fuyang BL-59, Juliao GB-29, Naoshu SI-10, Jianyu L.I.-15, Jugu L.I.-16, Dicang ST-4, Juliao ST-3, Chengqi ST-1, Jingming BL-1 and Fengchi GB-20.

Pathological symptoms of the Yang Motility vessel

Daytime epilepsy, eye diseases, loss of consciousness, aversion to wind, hemiplegia, chronic painful obstruction, rigidity of the body, lumbar pain, contracted sinews, flaccidity of the muscles of the medial leg and tightness of the muscles of the lateral leg.

YIN MOTILITY VESSEL

- originates below the medial malleolus at Zhaohai KID-6,
- ascends along the medial malleolus and the postero-medial surface of the lower leg and thigh to the external genitalia, then ascends the abdomen and chest to the supraclavicular fossa,
- ascends through the throat and emerges anterior to Renying ST-9,
- ascends beside the mouth and nose to the inner canthus where it meets with the Yang Motility vessel and Bladder channel at Jingming BL-1,
- then ascends with them to enter the brain.

Coalescent points: Zhaohai KID-6, Jiaoxin KID-8 and Jingming BL-1.

Pathological symptoms of the Yin Motility vessel
Night-time epilepsy, eye diseases, chills and fever, painful obstruction of the skin due to damp-heat, hypogastric pain, internal urgency, pain of the genitals, contracted sinews, shan disorder, uterine bleeding, leucorrhoea, flaccidity of the muscles of the lateral leg and tightness of the muscles of the medial leg.

YANG LINKING VESSEL

- originates near the heel at Jinmen BL-63 (at the junction of the leg yang channels),
- ascends along the lateral malleolus and the Gall Bladder channel of the leg to pass through the hip region,
- ascends along the postero-lateral costal region (posterior to the Yang Motility vessel) to the posterior axillary fold (Naoshu SI-10),
- crosses the top of the shoulder (Tianliao SJ-15 and Jianjing GB-21) and ascends along the neck and jaw, then passes anterior to the ear as far as the forehead (Benshen GB-13),
- crosses the parietal region through the points of the Gall Bladder channel as far as Fengchi GB-20, then connects with the Governing vessel at Fengfu DU-16 and Yamen DU-15.

Coalescent points: Jinmen BL-63, Yangjiao GB-35, Naoshu SI-10, Tianliao SJ-15, Jianjing GB-21, Touwei ST-8, Benshen GB-13, Yangbai GB-14, Toulinqi GB-15, Muchuang GB-16, Zhengying GB-17, Chengling GB-18, Naokong GB-19, Fengchi GB-20, Fengfu DU-16 and Yamen DU-15.

Pathological symptoms of the Yang Linking vessel
Visual dizziness, dyspnoea, acute and sudden pain and swelling of the lumbar region, chills and fever, dyspnoea with raised shoulders, fever and chills.

YIN LINKING VESSEL

- originates at the medial side of the leg at Zhubin KID-9 (at the junction of the leg yin channels),
- ascends along the medial aspect of the leg and thigh to the lower abdomen,
- ascends the ribs to Qimen LIV-14,
- ascends to the throat to meet the Conception vessel at Tiantu REN-22 and Lianquan REN-23.

Coalescent points: Zhubin KID-9, Chongmen SP-12, Fushe SP-13, Daheng SP-15, Fuai SP-16, Qimen LIV-14, Tiantu REN-22 and Lianquan REN-23.

Pathological symptoms of the Yin Linking vessel
Heart pain, pain of the chest, fullness and pain of the lateral costal region, lumbar pain.

THE YIN MOTILITY VESSEL

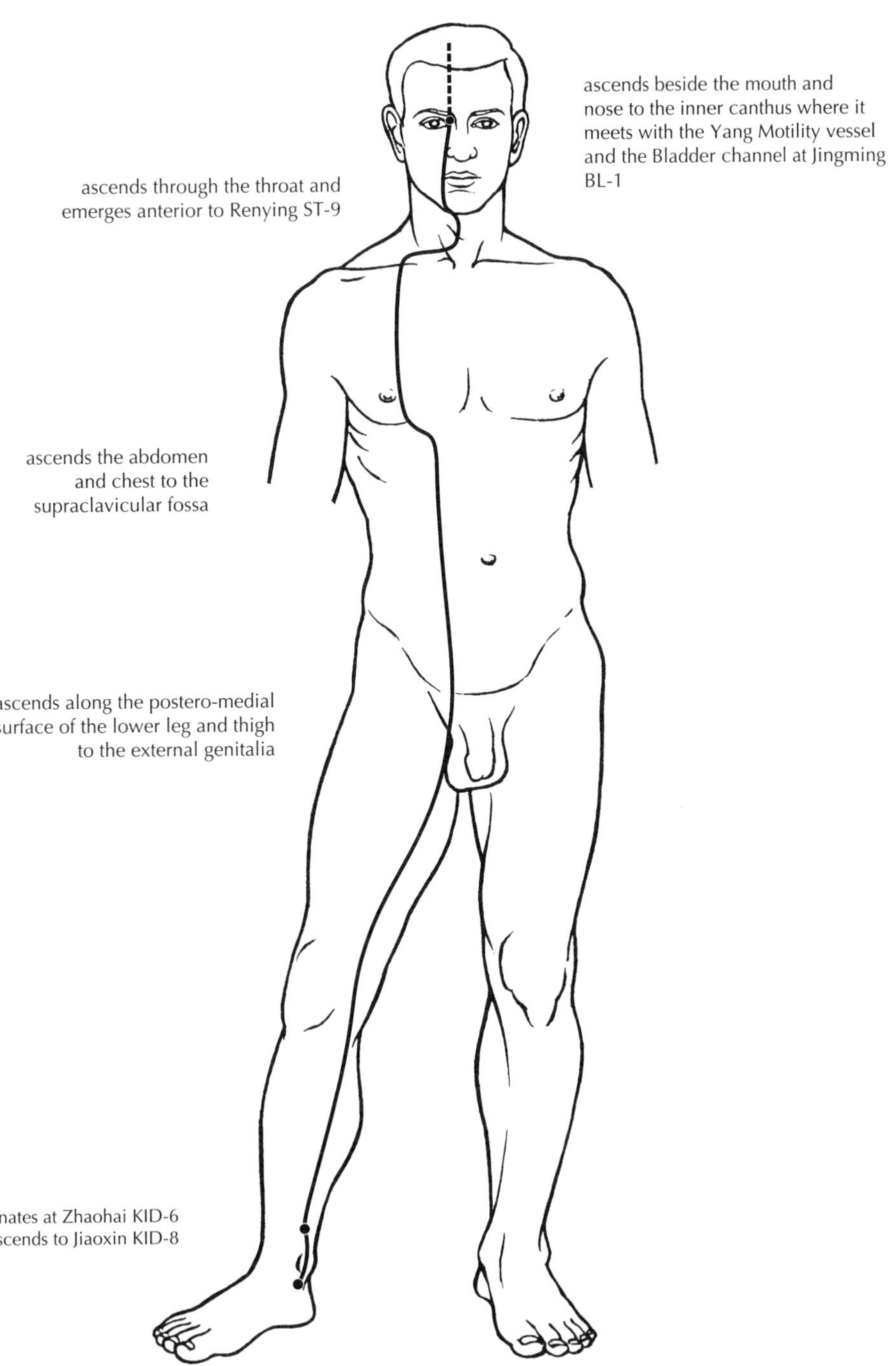

Coalescent points

Zhaohai KID-6, Jiaoxin KID-8 and Jingming BL-1.

Pathological symptoms of the Yin Motility vessel

Night-time epilepsy, eye diseases, chills and fever, painful obstruction of the skin due to damp-heat, hypogastric pain, internal urgency, pain of the genitals, contracted sinews, shan disorder, uterine bleeding, leucorrhoea, flaccidity of the muscles of the lateral leg and tightness of the muscles of the medial leg.

THE YANG LINKING VESSEL

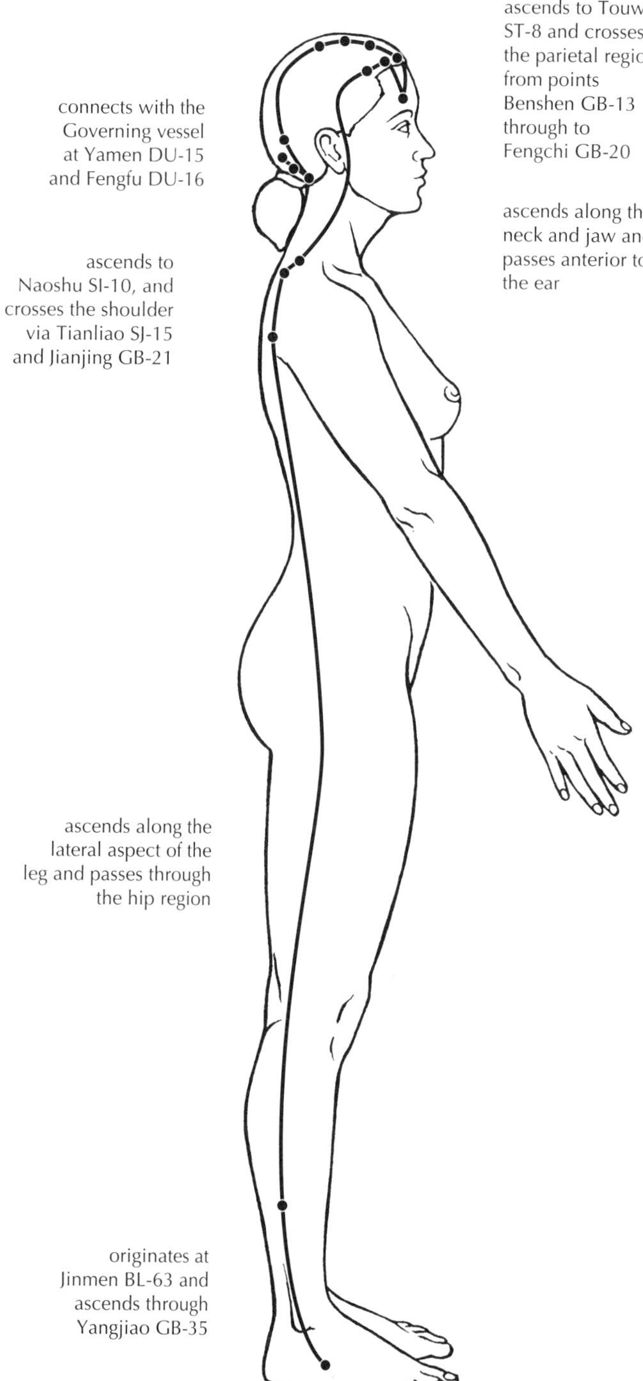

Coalescent points

Jinmen BL-63, Yangjiao GB-35, Naoshu SI-10, Tianliao SJ-15, Jianjing GB-21, Touwei ST-8, Benshen GB-13, Yangbai GB-14, Toulinqi GB-15, Muchuang GB-16, Zhengying GB-17, Chengling GB-18, Naokong GB-19, Fengchi GB-20, Fengfu DU-16 and Yamen DU-15.

Pathological symptoms of the Yang Linking vessel

Visual dizziness, dyspnoea, acute and sudden pain and swelling of the lumbar region, chills and fever, dyspnoea with raised shoulders.

THE YIN LINKING VESSEL

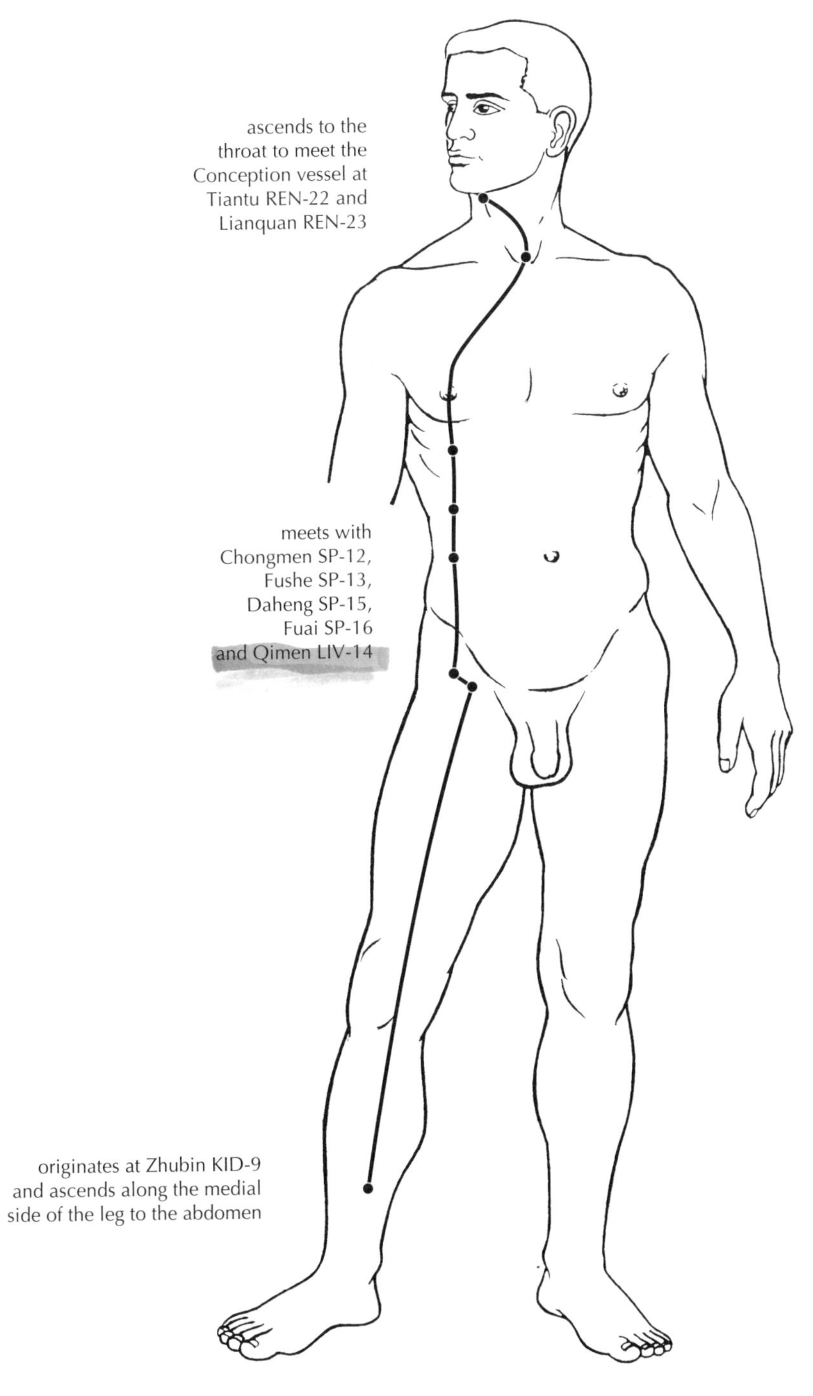

Coalescent points

Zhubin KID-9, Chongmen SP-12, Fushe SP-13, Daheng SP-15, Fuai SP-16, Qimen LIV-14, Tiantu REN-22 and Lianquan REN-23.

Pathological symptoms of the Yin Linking vessel

Heart pain, pain of the chest, fullness and pain of the lateral costal region, lumbar pain.

THE LUO-CONNECTING CHANNELS

There are fifteen principal luo-connecting channels which branch out from the primary channels and the extraordinary vessels and are distributed superficially over the body. The fifteen luo-connecting channels are made up of twelve from the twelve primary channels, one each for the Conception and Governing vessels, and the great luo-connecting channel of the Spleen.

PATHWAYS OF THE LUO-CONNECTING CHANNELS

The luo-connecting channels of the twelve primary channels spread from the luo-connecting point of their own channel to connect with their internally-externally paired channel. After joining with their paired channel they usually continue to follow their own pathways:

- Lung: from Lieque LU-7 the luo-connecting channel travels to the palm and thenar eminence.
- Large Intestine: from Pianli L.I.-6 the luo-connecting channel travels to the jaw, teeth and ear.
- Stomach: from Fenglong ST-40 the luo-connecting channel travels to the nape of the neck, head and throat.
- Spleen: from Gongsun SP-4 the luo-connecting channel travels to the abdomen, Stomach and intestines.
- Heart: from Tongli HE-5 the luo-connecting channel follows the Heart channel to the Heart, the base of the tongue and the eye.
- Small Intestine: from Zhizheng SI-7 the luo-connecting channel travels to the shoulder.
- Bladder: from Feiyang BL-58 the luo-connecting channel travels to the Kidney channel.
- Kidney: from Dazhong KID-4 the luo-connecting channel follows the Kidney channel to the perineum and lumbar vertebrae.
- Pericardium: from Neiguan P-6 the luo-connecting channel travels to the Pericardium and Heart.
- Sanjiao: from Waiguan SJ-5 the luo-connecting channel travels to meet the Pericardium channel at the chest.
- Gall-Bladder: from Guangming GB-37 the luo-connecting channel travels to the dorsum of the foot.
- Liver: from Ligou LIV-5 the luo-connecting channel travels to the genitals.

The pathways of the three remaining luo-connecting channels are as follows:

- Conception vessel: from Jiuwei REN-15 the luo-connecting channel spreads over the abdomen.
- Governing vessel: from Chengqiang DU-1 the luo-connecting channel travels up the sides of spine to the top of the head; at the shoulder blades it joins with the Bladder channel and threads through the spine.
- Spleen great luo-connecting channel: from SP-21 the luo-connecting channel spreads through the chest and lateral costal region.
- the *Essential Questions*[5] mentions a sixteenth luo-connecting channel known as the Stomach great luo-connecting channel which connects with the Lung and can be felt and sometimes seen 'throbbing ceaselessly' below the left breast.

FUNCTIONS OF THE LUO-CONNECTING CHANNELS

The luo-connecting channels strengthen the connection between internally-externally paired channels and zangfu. For a full discussion of the actions of the luo-connecting points, please refer to the chapter on Point Categories.

The pathways of the luo-connecting channels are illustrated in the main body of this text.

THE TWELVE SINEW CHANNELS

The twelve sinew channels:

- circulate on the periphery of the body.
- do not penetrate to the zangfu.
- are associated with and take their names from the twelve primary channels.
- all originate at the extremities (unlike the primary channels) and ascend to the head and trunk.
- broadly follow the course of their associated primary channels but are wider.
- are more superficial and follow the lines of major muscles and muscle groups, tendons, ligaments etc.

CLINICAL SIGNIFICANCE OF THE SINEW CHANNELS

The sinew channels can either reflect disturbances of the primary channels or can be injured themselves, mainly by traumatic injury or attack by exterior pathogens. There are no specific points which treat the sinew channels but they may be accessed by shallow needle insertions (especially at Ahshi points), and by relatively superficial techniques such as cupping, massage, plum blossom needling, dermal needling and guasha (skin scraping). The pathways of the sinew channels are illustrated in the main body of this text.

THE MINUTE COLLATERALS

Little is said about the minute collaterals in classical texts and it is possible that they derived their identity from observation of small blood vessels at the surface of the body. What is evident, however, is that for the qi and blood to reach every part of the body, the larger channels and collaterals need to branch into ever more minute channels, and it is this function that the minute collaterals serve.

THE TWELVE CUTANEOUS REGIONS

The twelve cutaneous regions are not channels as such, but skin regions overlying the broad network of superficial channels and linked to them. The cutaneous regions provide the theoretical foundation for the idea of invasion by exogenous pathogenic factors through the skin to the deeper layers of the jingluo system. Cutaneous regions also manifest disorders of the deep-lying channels, for example by abnormal skin sensations, skin lesions or discoloration:

- a blue-green (qing) colour indicates pain
- a red colour indicates heat
- a white colour indicates deficiency and cold

Finally, the cutaneous regions explain how treatment applied at the level of the skin (for example medicinal ointments, massage, cupping, plum blossom needling, skin scraping and dermal needling) is able to have a deep therapeutic effect. See overleaf for illustrations of the cutaneous regions.

NOTES

1 Silk scrolls describing the pathways of eleven channels and dating back to the 2nd century BCE were discovered during the excavation of tombs at Mawangdui, Hunan Province.

2 *Essential Questions* Chapter 63.

3 Ahshi points are points of tenderness that may or may not be standard acupuncture points of the fourteen channels.

4 *Classic of Difficulties* 27th Difficulty.

5 *Essential Questions* Chapter 18.

THE CUTANEOUS REGIONS

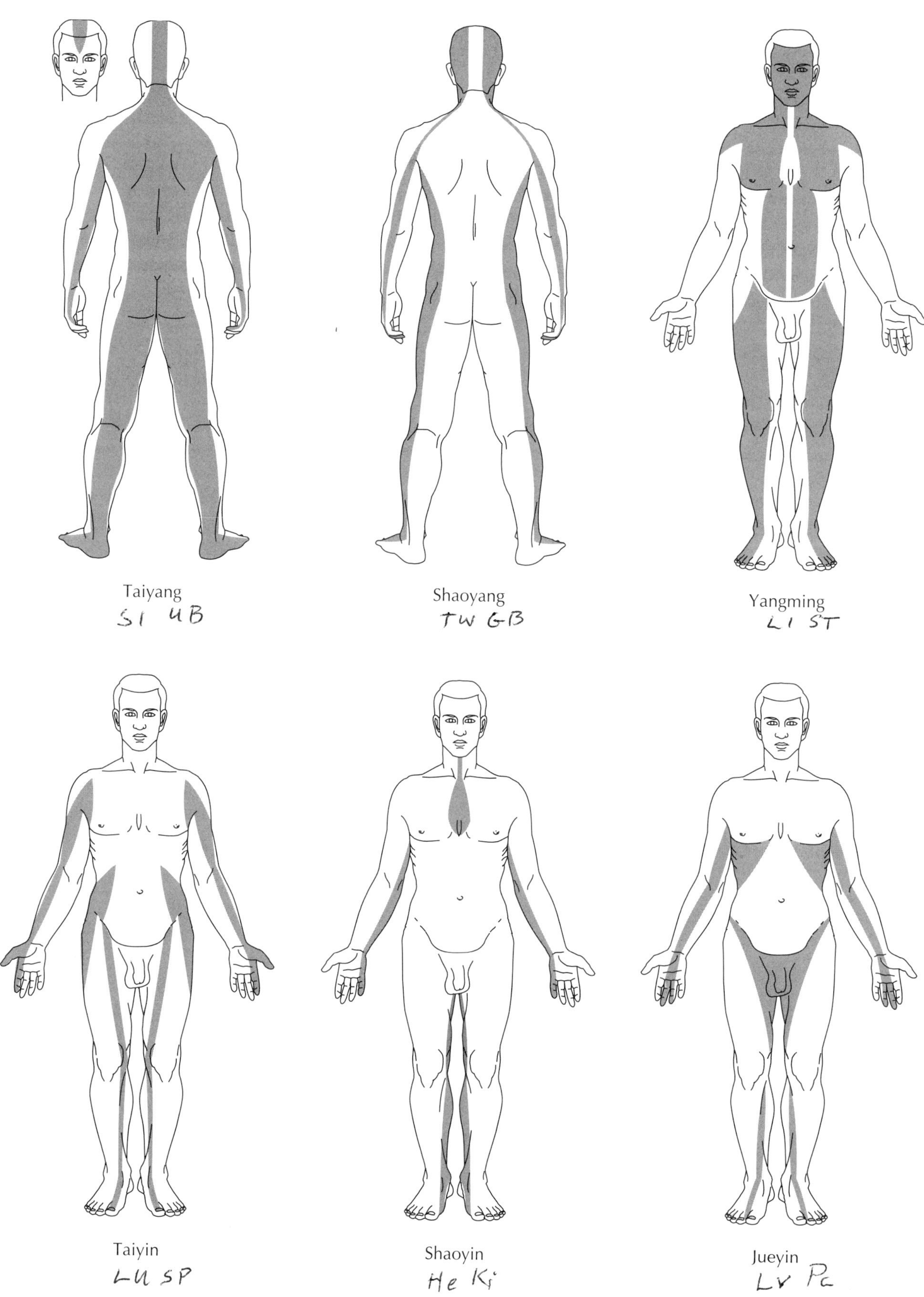

POINT CATEGORIES

THE FIVE SHU POINTS

The five shu-points (transporting points) are the jing-well, ying-spring, shu-stream, jing-river and he-sea points of the twelve primary channels and are one of the most important groups of acupuncture points. All are located at or distal to the elbow and knee joints. Since the qi flowing in these portions of the channels is passing through a particularly dynamic change in quality, the five shu-points play an important role in the formation of many acupuncture prescriptions. Historically, the naming of these points first dates back to the *Spiritual Pivot*[1]:

"The five zang have five shu [points] so in all there are twenty-five shu; the six fu have six shu [points], so in all there are thirty-six shu. There are twelve main channels and fifteen luo-connecting channels - a total of twenty-seven [channels of] qi running up and down [the body]. The point at which the qi emanates is known as the jing-well. The point at which the qi glides is known as the ying-spring. The point at which the qi pours through is known as the shu-stream. The point at which the qi flows is known as the jing-river and the point at which the qi enters inwards is known as the he-sea. Thus the flow of qi in the twenty-seven channels reaches each of the five shu-points".

It is interesting to note that at the time this passage was written, the Heart and Pericardium were not differentiated, which is why only five zang are mentioned. This is explained in the *Spiritual Pivot*[2] when the Yellow Emperor asks his adviser Qi Bo "Why does the hand shaoyin channel alone have no shu points"? Qi Bo replies:

"The shaoyin is the Heart vessel. The Heart is the great master of the five zang and six fu and is the abode of the essence-spirit. It stores so firmly that no pathogen can come to reside. If it does, then the Heart will be injured and the spirit will depart. If the spirit departs there is death. It is for this reason that the pathogens destined to attack the Heart will attack the Pericardium. The Pericardium is the channel that is controlled by the Heart. Therefore the Heart alone has no shu points".

The five shu-points points of the yin channels (and their corresponding phase)					
	Jing-Well (Wood)	**Ying-Spring (Fire)**	**Shu-Stream (Earth)**	**Jing-River (Metal)**	**He-Sea (Water)**
Lung	Shaoshang LU-11	Yuji LU-10	Taiyuan LU-9	Jingqu LU-8	Chize LU-5
Spleen	Yinbai SP-1	Dadu SP-2	Taibai SP-3	Shangqiu SP-5	Yinlingquan SP-9
Heart	Shaochong HE-9	Shaofu HE-8	Shenmen HE-7	Lingdao HE-4	Shaohai HE-3
Kidney	Yongquan KID-1	Rangu KID-2	Taixi KID-3	Fuliu KID-7	Yingu KID-10
Pericardium	Zhongchong P-9	Laogong P-8	Daling P-7	Jianshi P-5	Quze P-3
Liver	Dadun LIV-1	Xingjian LIV-2	Taichong LIV-3	Zhongfeng LIV-4	Ququan LIV-8

The five shu-points of the yang channels (and their corresponding phase)					
	Jing-Well (Metal)	**Ying-Spring (Water)**	**Shu-Stream (Wood)**	**Jing-River (Fire)**	**He-Sea (Earth)**
Large Intestine	Shangyang L.I.-1	Erjian L.I.-2	Sanjian L.I.-3	Yangxi L.I.-5	Quchi L.I.-11
Stomach	Lidui ST-45	Neiting ST-44	Xiangu ST-43	Jiexi ST-41	Zusanli ST-36
Small Intestine	Shaoze SI-1	Qiangu SI-2	Houxi SI-3	Yanggu SI-5	Xiaohai SI-8
Bladder	Zhiyin BL-67	Zutonggu BL-66	Shugu BL-65	Kunlun BL-60	Weizhong BL-40
Sanjiao	Guanchong SJ-1	Yemen SJ-2	Zhongzhu SJ-3	Zhigou SJ-6	Tianjing SJ-10
Gall Bladder	Zuqiaoyin GB-44	Xiaxi GB-43	Zulinqi GB-41	Yangfu GB-38	Yanglingquan GB-34

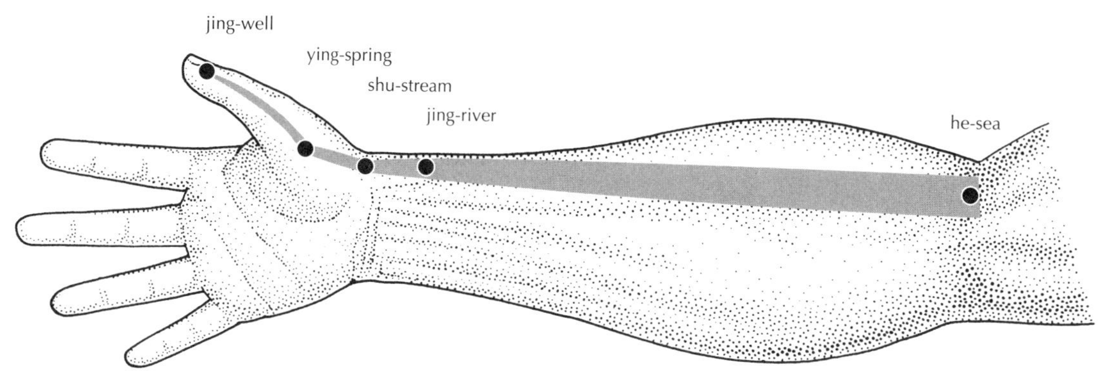

"The point at which the qi rises is known as the jing-well. The point at which the qi glides is known as the ying-spring. The point at which the qi pours through is known as the shu-stream. The point at which the qi flows is known as the jing-river. The point at which the qi enters inwards is known as the he-sea" (*Spiritual Pivot* Chapter 71).

Also, it is clear that the yuan-source points of the yang channels (belonging to the fu) were considered at this time to belong to the shu-point grouping, thus the yang channels were each considered to have six shu-points. On the yin channels (belonging to the zang), the yuan-source point is the same point as the shu-stream point, and thus each of the yin channels has only five shu-points.

The first passage from the *Spiritual Pivot* quoted above emphasises two further important aspects of the five shu-point classification:

- That portion of each of the twelve main channels that runs from the fingers or toes to the elbow joint or knee joint is compared to the flow of a river, emerging like a spring at the jing-well point and gradually growing in breadth and depth until it reaches the he-sea point at the elbow or knee.
- According to the five shu-point theory, the flow of qi along the channel is always from the extremities proximally to the elbow or knee. It will be seen from the tables above that the ascribing of five phase identities to the five shu-points also bears out this perception of the flow of qi from distal to proximal in all the twelve channels. In other words, although the yin channels begin with the wood point and the yang channels with the metal point, the progression through the five shu-points (always from distal to proximal) corresponds to the generating cycle of the five phases (i. wood, fire, earth, metal, water; ii. metal, water, wood, fire, earth).

By contrast, the theory of the circulation of the twelve channels (Lung to Large Intestine to Stomach to Spleen etc.) describes the three yin channels of the arm as flowing towards the hand from the chest, and the three yang channels of the leg as flowing towards the foot from the head. This perception of channel flow is given greater weight in the Western acupuncture tradition due to the method of numbering the acupuncture points, whereas in China the points are known by their names only.

These two different views of channel circulation suggest two different ways of understanding the movement of qi in the body. In both cases it is easier to imagine a person standing with their arms raised to the sky. In the centripetal flow embodied in the theory of the five shu-points, the macrocosmic qi is seen as entering the body via the extremities like a stream which widens into a river, flows into a broad and deep sea at the elbows and knees and unites and gathers deep within the body. In the second, the historically later concept of a self-contained energy circulation[3], the qi flows in continuous circuits around the body (from the chest to the hand, to the head, to the foot and back to the chest). This second view reflects the development of Chinese civilisation and agriculture, and especially the control and conservation of water through rivers, reservoirs, irrigation canals, ditches etc. upon which so much of acupuncture imagery is based. In this self-contained circulation, and most clearly seen by considering six channel theory, the yang channels descend from the hands to the feet in the same way that the yang heavenly qi radiates from above downwards, and the yin channels ascend from the feet to the hands, in the same way that the yin earthly qi rises upwards through the feet, like water through the roots of the tree. The yang channels move to and from the face which is circular like the symbol of heaven (yang), whilst the yin channels move to and from the chest which is square (a traditional symbol for earth).

Whilst these two different perceptions of channel flow are

another example of the readiness of Chinese medicine to embrace contradictory theories, we can say that the direction of flow in the five shu-point theory is not as important as the quality of energy described at each of the points. The jing-well points, for example, are situated on the tips of the fingers or toes (with the exception of Yongquan KID-1 which is located on the sole of the foot) where there is little flesh. The qi here is shallow and narrow, yet dynamic. The volatility of the qi at these points is emphasised by the fact that in the theory of the circulation of the twelve channels, it is at the extremities (jing-well points) that the qi changes direction and where yin and yang channels transform into each other. By contrast, the qi of the he-sea points, situated close to the large joints of the elbow and knee, runs deep and broad like an estuary flowing into the sea, preparing for its entry into the deepest levels of the body.

THE CLINICAL APPLICATION OF THE FIVE SHU-POINTS ACCORDING TO CLASSICAL THEORIES

During the long history of Chinese medicine, various attempts have been made to systematise the five shu-points in terms of their nature, their functions and their indications:

According to the *Classic of Difficulties*[4] the five shu-points are indicated in the following situations:

- jing-well points for fullness below the Heart.
- ying-spring points for heat in the body.
- shu-stream points for heaviness of the body and pain of the joints.
- jing-river points for cough and dyspnoea, chills and fever.
- he-sea points for counterflow qi and diarrhoea.

In his commentary on the above passage, Liao Run-hong of the Qing dynasty in *Compilation of Acupuncture and Moxibustion* related each of these indications to one of the zang (according to the five phase correspondences of the yin channels) as follows:

"Jing-well points are for fullness below the Heart, Liver pathogen; ying-spring points are for heat of the body, Heart pathogen; shu-stream points are for heaviness of the body, Spleen pathogen; jing-river points are for dyspnoea, cough, chills and fever, Lung pathogen; he-sea points are for counterflow qi and diarrhoea, Kidney pathogen".

The *Spiritual Pivot*[5] has two sets of indications for the five shu-points:

1 *According to the seasons*

- The five zang correspond to winter, in winter needle the jing-well points[6].
- The five colours correspond to spring, in spring needle the ying-spring points[7].
- The seasons correspond to summer, in summer needle the shu-stream points[8].
- The musical sounds correspond to late summer, in late summer needle the jing-river points[9].
- The flavours correspond to autumn, in autumn needle the he-sea points[10].

2 *According to symptomatology*

- When the disease is at the zang, needle the jing-well point.
- If manifesting as a change in the colour [complexion], needle the ying-spring point.
- When the disease attacks intermittently, needle the shu-stream point.
- When the disease manifests as changes in the patient's voice, needle the jing-river point.
- If there is disease of the Stomach and disorders resulting from irregular eating and drinking, needle the he-sea point.

The *Spiritual Pivot*[11] says;
"The divergent branches of the yang channels reach into the interior and connect with the fu ... the ying-spring and shu-stream points treat the channel, the he-sea points treat the fu".

The *Spiritual Pivot*[12] further distinguishes when to needle particular shu-points depending on the location and depth of the disease:

"There is yin within yin and yang within yang ... internally the five zang are yin whilst the six fu are yang; externally the sinews and bones are yin whilst the skin is yang. Thus it is said:

- When the disease is at the yin within yin (zang), needle the ying-spring and the shu-stream points of the yin channels.
- When the disease is at the yang within yang (skin), needle the he-sea points of the yang channels.
- When the disease is at the yin within yang (sinews and bones), needle the jing-river points of the yin channels.
- When the disease is at the yang within yin (fu), needle the luo-connecting points".

CLINICAL APPLICATION WITH REFERENCE TO CLASSICAL INDICATIONS

It is a commonplace that Chinese medicine allows (and indeed even embraces) contradiction much more readily than Western scientific thought. This is perhaps an inevitable feature of a system that has developed over such a long period of time, and in which no theory, if it offers something of clinical or philosophical value, need necessarily be abandoned in the light of a new and apparently contradictory one. Some of the classical theories on the use of the five shu-points are contradictory, some are scarcely borne out by clinical practice, and in some cases important clinical uses of these points are not referred to in the classical theories. In several instances, however, these theories have been clearly adopted into traditional and modern practice.

JING-WELL POINTS

"The point at which the qi emanates is known as the jing-well". The jing-well points ('jing' means 'well') are the first or last points of their respective channels. With the exception of Yongquan KID-1, all are located on the tips of the fingers or toes. According to the classical sources discussed above, the jing-well points are indicated for:

- fullness below the heart.
- diseases of the zang.

In the light of traditional and modern clinical application, the following observations may be made:

The jing-well points are used for clearing heat, restoring consciousness and rescuing collapse

This important use is not referred to in the classical theories given above. With the exception of Zuqiaoyin GB-44, Zhiyin BL-67 and Guanchong SJ-1 all the jing-well points are classically indicated for disorders such as coma, fainting and collapse, indeed all the twelve jing-well points in combination may be pricked and bled for collapse from windstroke or high fever. These actions reflect their particularly dynamic action on the qi.

The jing-well points treat the uppermost reaches of the channels

The jing-well points, situated at the extreme end of the channels, are in the main powerful points to clear heat and fullness from the uppermost reaches of their respective channel, particularly in acute disorders. For example:

- Shaoshang LU-11 for acute sore throat, throat painful obstruction and mumps.
- Shangyang L.I.-1 for throat painful obstruction, deafness, tinnitus and toothache.
- Lidui ST-45 for swelling of the face, toothache, lockjaw, throat painful obstruction, deviation of the mouth, nosebleed and yellow nasal discharge.
- Shaochong HE-9 for pain at the root of the tongue, swollen tongue, throat painful obstruction, heat in the mouth, pain and redness of the eyes.
- Shaoze SI-1 for headache, dizziness, red eyes, nosebleed, deafness, tinnitus, throat painful obstruction, curled tongue, stiff tongue, heat in the mouth, erosion of the mouth, mouth ulcers and drooling.
- Zhiyin BL-67 for vertex headache, occipital headache, nasal congestion, nosebleed, eye pain, pain of the inner canthus, deafness and tinnitus.
- Yongquan KID-1 for dizziness, vertex headache, throat painful obstruction, throat pain with inability to swallow, loss of voice, dry tongue and nosebleed.
- Zhongchong P-9 for pain at the root of the tongue, stiffness of the tongue and inability to speak.
- Guanchong SJ-1 for tinnitus, deafness, earache, stiff tongue, pain at the root of the tongue, dryness of the mouth, dry lips, bitter taste in the mouth, headache, redness of the eyes, throat painful obstruction and pain of the submandibular region.
- Zuqiaoyin GB-44 for headache, stabbing pain of the head, dizziness, sudden deafness, tinnitus, redness swelling and pain of the eyes, throat painful obstruction, stiffness of the tongue with inability to speak and curled tongue with dry mouth.
- Dadun LIV-1 for bitter taste in the mouth and ceaseless nosebleed.

These indications demonstrate clearly the principle that the most distal points on any channel are the strongest to clear excess and heat from the opposite end of the channel. It should be stressed that treating the channel in this context does not mean that these are important points for stiffness, pain and discomfort along the course of the channel as a whole, and thus the jing-well points are not generally indicated for painful obstruction, atrophy disorder or traumatic injury. A careful examination of the indications of the jing-well points, however, clearly contradicts the statement in the *Spiritual Pivot* that the jing-well points treat disorders of the zang.

The jing-well points treat fullness below the Heart

The term 'below the Heart' normally refers to the apex of the epigastrium. Examination of the indications of the jing-well points, however, show that many specifically treat stagnation and fullness throughout the chest region. This application does reflect Liao Run-hong's suggestion that they treat Liver pathogen, in other words Liver qi stagnation. For example:

- Shaoshang LU-11 for agitation [of the Heart] with cough and dyspnoea, fullness of the Heart with sweating and fullness below the Heart.
- Shangyang L.I.-1 for qi fullness of the chest radiating to the lateral costal region, dyspnoea and cough.
- Lidui ST-45 for fullness and distention of the chest and abdomen.
- Yinbai SP-1 for heat in the chest, fullness of the chest, dyspnoea and sighing.
- Shaochong HE-9 for Heart pain and pain of the chest and lateral costal region.
- Shaoze SI-1 for cold sensation below the Heart, agitation with Heart pain, oppression and pain of the chest and pain of the lateral costal region.
- Zhiyin BL-67 for pain of the lateral costal region and chest and agitation of the Heart.
- Yongquan KID-1 for Heart pain, cough and dyspnoea.
- Zhongchong P-9 for Heart pain, agitation of the Heart and oppression of the Heart with absence of sweating.
- Guanchong SJ-1 for congested heat of the upper jiao, oppression of the Heart with absence of sweating and Heart pain.
- Zuqiaoyin GB-44 for pain of the lateral costal region (with cough and inability to catch the breath).
- Dadun LIV-1 for sudden Heart pain.

The jing-well points treat disorders of the spirit

The jing-well points in the main share a common ability to regulate disorders of the spirit. For example, Shaoshang LU-11, Lidui ST-45, Yinbai SP-1, Shaochong HE-9, Shaoze SI-1, Yongquan KID-1 and Dadun LIV-1 are all indicated for various kinds of mania, and Lidui ST-45, Yinbai SP-1, Zuqiaoyin GB-44 and Dadun LIV-1 for various disorders of sleep such as insomnia, nightmares and somnolence.

YING-SPRING POINTS

"The point at which the qi glides is known as the ying-spring". The ying-spring points ('ying' means 'spring') are all located on the hands or feet and are the second or penultimate points of their respective channel. According to the classical sources discussed above, the ying-spring points are indicated for:

- heat in the body.
- changes in the colour (complexion).
- diseases of the yang channels.
- diseases of the zang (with the shu-stream point).

In the light of traditional and modern clinical application, the following observations may be made.

The ying-spring points clear heat

The ying-spring points without exception have an important effect on clearing heat from their respective zangfu or channel, especially, like the jing-well points, from the uppermost portion of the channel. Among the five shu-points they reflect the closest correspondence of classical shu-point theory, five phase theory and clinical practice. The ying-spring points of the yin channels belong to fire and those of the yang channels to water, and both may be reduced to clear heat and fire from the body. Among the most important of the ying-spring points with this effect are the following:

- Yuji LU-10 clears heat from the throat (the upper extremity of the Lung channel), clears dry heat from the Lung zang in cases of coughing (especially when accompanied by bleeding) and chest pain and clears heat transmitted from the Lung to the Stomach in the middle jiao and the Heart in the upper jiao.
- Erjian L.I.-2 and Neiting ST-44 treat heat disorders affecting the upper portion of the channel in the face and head, whilst Neiting ST-44 also clears heat and damp-heat from the intestines.
- Dadu SP-2 clears heat and damp-heat from the Spleen, Stomach and intestines giving rise to diarrhoea, constipation, vomiting and epigastric pain.
- Shaofu HE-8 treats Heart fire which transmits first to the Small Intestine and thence to the Bladder.
- Rangu KID-2 is the strongest point on the Kidney channel to clear deficiency heat from the Kidneys which either rises to the upper jiao and manifests as throat painful obstruction, coughing of blood and wasting and thirsting disorder, or blazes in the lower jiao giving rise to genital itching, uterine prolapse, infertility, irregular menstruation, difficult urination etc.
- Laogong P-8 is a powerful point to clear heat from the ying and blood levels and from the Pericardium during febrile diseases, to cool Heart fire in the upper jiao (for which purpose it is more strongly indicated than Shaofu HE-8), and to drain Stomach heat.
- Xiaxi GB-43 clears heat and stagnant heat (i.e. heat deriving from qi stagnation) from the head, ears, eyes, face, breast and lateral costal region, indeed the whole of the Gall Bladder channel.
- Xingjian LIV-2 is the principal acupuncture point to clear Liver fire affecting any part of the body, whether blazing upwards to the head and eyes, disturbing the Heart and spirit, transversely invading the Lungs or Stomach, entering the blood and causing reckless bleeding, or disturbing the lower jiao.

The ying-spring points treat changes in the complexion
As far as changes in the complexion are concerned, this theory may be explained by Liao Run-hong's statement "ying-spring points are for heat of the body, Heart pathogen", since it the Heart which manifests in the complexion. However the use of the ying-spring points in this way has little application in clinical practice.

The ying-spring points treat diseases of the yang channels and diseases of the zang (with the shu-stream point)
As far as acting on the yang channels is concerned, the ying-spring points of all the twelve channels (both yin and yang) have a strong action on clearing excess pathogenic factors, stagnation and heat from their respective channels, particularly, like the jing-well points, from the uppermost regions of the channel. In comparison with the jing-well points, however, they have a relatively greater action on disorders along the whole course of the channel (rather than just its upper end). Erjian L.I.-2, for example, in addition to its ability to treat disorders in the head and face, is also indicated for pain and stiffness of the shoulder and back, and cold and pain in the region of the point Jianyu L.I.-15. Similarly Qiangu SI-2, in addition to treating such disorders as mumps, swelling and pain of the neck and cheek, throat painful obstruction etc., also treats stiffness and pain of the neck and back and pain of the scapula, arm and wrist.

With reference to the combination of the ying-spring and shu-stream points referred to above, the following classical combinations indicate that this has been a commonly-used pairing:
- Pain of the Lung and Heart: Taiyuan LU-9 and Yuji LU-10 (*Systematic Classic*).
- Somnolence: Erjian L.I.-2 and Sanjian L.I.-3 (*Supplementing Life*).
- Deafness: Qiangu SI-2, Houxi SI-3 and Pianli L.I.-6 (*Supplementing Life*).
- Swelling of the inside of the throat: Rangu KID-2 and Taixi KID-3 (*Supplementing Life*).
- Ceaseless laughter: Daling P-7 and Laogong P-8 (*Supplementing Life*).
- Oppression of the Heart: Daling P-7 and Laogong P-8 (*Ode of the Jade Dragon*).
- Pain of the Liver and Heart: Xingjian LIV-2 and Taichong LIV-3 (*Thousand Ducat Formulas*).

SHU-STREAM POINTS

"The point at which the qi pours through is known as the shu-stream" ('shu' means 'to transport'). The shu-stream points of the three arm yin are all located at the flexure of the wrist. The shu-stream points of the other nine channels are all located proximal to the metacarpo-phalangeal or metatarso-phalangeal joints, with the exception of Taixi KID-3 which is located posterior to the medial malleolus. The shu-stream points of the six yin channels are also the yuan-source point of their respective channel. According to the classical sources discussed above, the shu-stream points are indicated for:

- disorders of the zang (with the ying-spring point).
- yang channel disorders (with the ying-spring point).
- heaviness of the body and pain of the joints.
- diseases which attack intermittently.

In the light of traditional and modern clinical use, the following observations may be made:

Disorders of the zang
The shu-stream points of the yin channels have to be viewed separately from the shu-stream points of the yang channels as their range of actions is quite different. The shu-stream points of the yin channels are the primary points for tonifying and harmonising their respective zang, and may therefore be considered as the single most important point of their respective channel:

- Taiyuan LU-9 is an essential point to tonify both Lung qi and yin.
- Taibai SP-3 strongly fortifies Spleen qi and yang.
- Shenmen HE-7 tonifies and nourishes the Heart in all kinds of deficiency, whether of qi, blood, yin or yang.
- Taixi KID-3 nourishes Kidney yin and tonifies Kidney qi and yang.
- Daling P-7 clears pathogenic factors from the Pericardium during the course of febrile diseases and strongly calms the spirit when disturbed by heat.
- Taichong LIV-3 is indicated for any pattern of the Liver zang whether deficient or excess.

This fully bears out the classical perspective that the shu-stream points treat disorders of the zang. This is partly determined, however, by the fact that on the yin channels they are the same point as the yuan-source point (where the original qi emerges on the channel) and according to the *Spiritual Pivot*[13] "When the five zang are diseased, select the yuan-source points".

The shu-stream points of the yang channels, by comparison, have relatively little action on zangfu disorders. However, Sanjian L.I.-3 is indicated for borborygmus and diarrhoea due to dampness, and Xiangu ST-43 for disorders of the Stomach and intestines.

Disorders of the yang channels
The shu-stream points of the yin channels, like all acupuncture points, have some action on regulating their respective channel but this action is overshadowed by their primary action on disorders of the zang. By contrast, the shu-stream points of the yang channels have important actions on their respective channels. Sanjian L.I.-3 clears wind and heat from the head, throat, teeth, eyes and mouth; Houxi SI-3 is a vital point for regulating disorders of the taiyang channel and the Governing vessel; Zhongzhu SJ-3 is important for disorders of shaoyang channel, especially affecting the ears; Zulinqi GB-41 has a particularly strong action on dispersing stagnation of Liver qi throughout the shaoyang channel.

Heaviness of the body and pain of the joints
According to the *Classic of Difficulties* shu-stream points are indicated for "heaviness of the body and pain of the joints". This is a clear reference to painful obstruction, especially when due to attack of dampness, reinforcing Liao Run-hong's observation that shu-stream points treat Spleen pathogen. Theoretically one would expect this observation to apply primarily to the yin channels whose shu-stream points pertain to earth, the phase associated with dampness. With the exception of Taibai SP-3 (pain of the knee and thigh, joint pains, lumbar pain, atrophy disorder), however, this is not borne out by the classical indications for the points. As far as the yang shu-stream points are concerned, there is relatively more evidence for this action. Sanjian L.I.-3 and Houxi SI-3 are both important points for disorders of the finger joints. Sanjian L.I.-3 is further indicated for shoulder and back pain from chronic painful obstruction leading to exhaustion of qi and blood, whilst Houxi SI-3 is an important distal point for all disorders of the neck as well as disorders of the shoulder, elbow, arm, lower back and knees. Xiangu ST-43 is frequently used in current practice for general aching due to wind, and for damp-heat painful obstruction.

Diseases manifesting intermittently
This is rather difficult to elucidate from examining the traditional indications. The classic intermittent disease, however, is malaria, and whilst this is a commonly found indication, no fewer than eight of the shu-stream points treat this disease (Sanjian L.I.-3, Xiangu ST-43, Shenmen HE-7, Houxi SI-3, Shugu BL-65, Taixi KID-3, Zhongzhu SJ-3 and Zulinqi GB-41).

JING-RIVER POINTS

"The point at which the qi flows is known as the jing-river". The jing-river points ('jing' means 'to pass through') are situated at or proximal to the wrist and ankle joints. According to the classical sources discussed above, the jing-river points are indicated for:

- cough and dyspnoea, chills and fever.
- diseases manifesting as changes in the patient's voice.
- diseases of sinews and bones (jing-river points of the yin channels).

In the light of traditional and modern clinical use, the following observations may be made:

Cough and dyspnoea, chills and fever
The proposition that the jing-river points are effective for treating cough and dyspnoea derives from the status of the jing-river points of the yin channels as metal points, (the Lung pertains to metal), hence Liao Run-hong's observation that they treat Lung pathogen. There is some evidence, however, that jing-river points of both the yin and yang channels have an action on either coughing and dyspnoea or chills and fever:

- Jingqu LU-8: cough, asthma, wheezing, dyspnoea, febrile disease with absence of sweating, febrile disease with breathlessness.
- Yangxi L.I.-5: cold cough, fever with absence of sweating.
- Jiexi ST-41: febrile disease with absence of sweating, malarial disorders.
- Shangqiu SP-5: chills and fever with vomiting, coughing and diarrhoea in children with no desire to eat, cough.
- Yanggu SI-5: febrile disease with absence of sweating, chills and fever.
- Kunlun BL-60: dyspnoea, cough, malaria, malaria with copious sweating.
- Fuliu KID-7: fever with absence of sweating.
- Jianshi P-5: aversion to wind and cold, febrile disease, malaria, obstruction of qi following windstroke leading to impaired breathing.
- Zhigou SJ-6: cough, cough with redness and heat of the face, febrile disease with absence of sweating.
- Yangfu GB-38: chills and fever, sweating with cold shivering, malaria.

Diseases manifesting in the patient's voice
This kind of indication is frequently found for the jing-river points:

- Yangxi L.I.-5: manic raving, propensity to laughter.
- Jiexi ST-41: Stomach heat with raving.
- Jianshi P-5: loss of voice, halting speech, manic raving as if seeing ghosts.

- Shangqiu SP-5: stiffness and pain of the root of the tongue, impaired speech, propensity to laughter, cold body with much sighing.
- Lingdao HE-4: sudden loss of voice.
- Fuliu KID-7: curled tongue with inability to speak, propensity to anger with incessant talking, propensity to laughter.
- Zhigou SJ-6: sudden loss of voice.
- Yangfu GB-38: sighing.
- Zhongfeng LIV-4: sighing.

Diseases of the sinews and bones
Several of the jing-river points have an important action on the sinews and bones, and this is not confined to the yin channels:
- Jiexi ST-41: sinew painful obstruction, damp painful obstruction, atrophy disorder of the leg.
- Shangqiu SP-5: pain and contraction of the sinews, bone painful obstruction, heavy body with painful joints.
- Lingdao HE-4: cold bones and marrow, clonic spasm.
- Yanggu SI-5: lockjaw, stiffness of the tongue in babies preventing suckling, clonic spasm.
- Kunlun BL-60: stiff neck, contraction of the shoulder and back, lumbar pain, sacral pain, pain of the coccyx, heel pain, ankle pain, lockjaw.
- Fuliu KID-7: cold and hot bones, atrophy disorder of the leg.
- Yangfu GB-38: wind painful obstruction with numbness, wandering pain of the joints, hemiplegia, contracted sinews, pain of the hundred joints (i.e. all the joints), lower limb painful obstruction, severe lumbar pain, lumbar pain like a small hammer in the middle of the back, pain of the lateral malleolus.
- Zhongfeng LIV-4: contracted sinews, lumbar pain.

HE-SEA POINTS

"The point at which the qi enters inwards is known as the he-sea". The he-sea points ('he' means 'to unite') of all the twelve channels are situated close to the elbow or knee joints. In addition to the twelve he-sea points, the Large Intestine, Small Intestine and Sanjiao (the three fu whose channel pathways lie on the upper limb) each have a lower he-sea point on the leg, namely Shangjuxu ST-37, Xiajuxu ST-39 and Weiyang BL-39. According to the classical sources discussed above, the he-sea points are indicated for:
- counterflow qi and diarrhoea.
- disease of the Stomach and disorders resulting from irregular eating and drinking.
- diseases of the fu.
- diseases of the skin (yang he-sea points only).

In the light of traditional and modern clinical use, the following observations may be made:

Counterflow qi and diarrhoea, disease of the Stomach & disorders resulting from irregular eating and drinking
The he-sea points of both the yin and yang channels as well as the lower he-sea points are among the most important acupuncture points for treating disorders of the Stomach and intestines. This reflects the principal that as the channels reach the elbow or knee, their points have a correspondingly greater effect on the centre of the body and thus the zangfu:
- Chize LU -5 is indicated for vomiting, diarrhoea and abdominal distention, reflecting the origin of the Lung channel in the middle jiao and its connection with the Large Intestine fu in the lower jiao.
- Quchi L.I.-11 is indicated for distention and pain of the abdomen, vomiting and diarrhoea and dysenteric disorder.
- Zusanli ST-36 is the foremost point on the body for harmonising the Stomach and fortifying the Spleen and is indicated for every kind of Stomach or Spleen disease, including nausea, vomiting and diarrhoea.
- Yinlingquan SP-9 is an important point for lack of appetite, diarrhoea, dysentery-like disorders and sudden turmoil disorder due to interior or exterior pathogenic dampness.
- Shaohai HE-3 is indicated for vomiting of foamy (watery) saliva.
- Weizhong BL-40 is indicated for sudden turmoil disorder with abdominal pain, vomiting and diarrhoea and dysenteric disorder.
- Fuliu KID-7 is indicated for diarrhoea, distention of the abdomen with borborygmus, dysenteric disorder and pus and blood in the stool.
- Quze P-3 is indicated for diarrhoea, dysentery-like disorders, and vomiting, especially when due to summer-heat.
- Tianjing SJ-10 is indicated for vomiting pus and blood, cough with fullness of the abdomen and no desire to eat or drink, and distention and pain of the lower abdomen.
- Yanglingquan GB-34 is especially indicated for vomiting due to shaoyang pattern or jaundice.
- Ququan LIV-8 is indicated for diarrhoea containing undigested food and diarrhoea containing blood and pus.
- Shangjuxu ST-37 is an essential point for regulating the intestines and clearing damp-heat and is much used for all intestinal diseases, whilst Xiajuxu ST-39, although less used, has a similar range of action.
- Weiyang BL-39 is indicated for distention and fullness of the lower abdomen and constipation.

Diseases of the fu

As we have seen above, many of the he-sea points have a strong action on the Stomach and intestines. As far as a wider action on the fu is concerned, this applies primarily to the he-sea points of the lower limb. Even the yang he-sea points of the Large and Small Intestines on the upper limb have relatively little action on the fu, and this reflects the general observation that the points of the three arm yang channels as a whole have scant action on their respective fu.

- On the lower limb, the yin he-sea points (Yinlingquan SP-9, Yingu KID-10, Ququan LIV-8) all strongly drain dampness and damp-heat from the fu or extraordinary fu in the lower jiao, specifically the Bladder, intestines and uterus.
- Yanglingquan GB-34 and Zusanli ST-36 are the most important points on their respective channels for treating disorders of their related fu (Gall Bladder and Stomach), equivalent in importance to the effect the shu-stream points of the yin channels have on their related zang.
- Shangjuxu ST-37 (lower he-sea point of the Large Intestine) is one of the most important distal points for treating disorders of the intestines.
- Weiyang BL-39 (the lower he-sea point of the Bladder) acts on the qi transforming action of the Bladder and is an important point in the treatment of retention of urine or difficult urination.

Diseases of the skin

Certain of the he-sea points are indicated for skin disorders, although this action is not limited to the yang he-sea points. However Quchi L.I.-11 and Weizhong BL-40 are probably the two most important acupuncture points for treating skin disorders:

- Quchi L.I.-11: erysipelas, urticaria, wind rash, dry skin, scaly skin, itching of the skin, shingles, pain and itching of the whole body as if bitten by insects, clove sores on the back.
- Weizhong BL-40: clove sores, erysipelas (cinnabar toxin), eczema, urticaria.
- Yingu KID-10: itching of the scrotum.
- Quze P-3: wind rash.
- Tianjing SJ-10: urticaria.
- Ququan LIV-8: itching of the genitals.

THE FIVE PHASE POINTS

The five phase properties of the five shu-points were established in the *Classic of Difficulties*[14]. On the yin channels, the jing-well point is ascribed to wood, the ying-spring point to fire and so on through the generating sequence (wood, fire, earth, metal and water) to the he-sea point which is ascribed to water. On the yang channels, the jing-well point is ascribed to metal, the ying-spring to water and so on through the generating sequence to the he-sea point which is ascribed to earth. Each phase is the 'child' of the one preceding it and the 'mother' of the one following it.

The *Classic of Difficulties*[15] says "In cases of deficiency reinforce the mother, in cases of excess reduce the child". This has been understood to describe the method of selecting points to tonify or reduce a channel or zangfu according to the generating sequence of the five phases. For example to tonify the Heart (fire) select the Heart channel point that belongs to the mother phase (wood) i.e. Shaochong HE-9; to reduce the Heart select the Heart channel point that belongs to the child phase (earth) i.e. Shenmen HE-7. The complete list of these mother and child points is as follows:

The mother-child points of the twelve channels

	Mother point	**Child point**
Lung	Taiyuan LU-9	Chize LU-5
Large Intestine	Quchi L.I.-11	Erjian L.I.-2
Stomach	Jiexi ST-41	Lidui ST-45
Spleen	Dadu SP-2	Shangqiu SP-5
Heart	Shaochong HE-9	Shenmen HE-7
Small Intestine	Houxi SI-3	Xiaohai SI-8
Bladder	Zhiyin BL-67	Shugu BL-65
Kidney	Fuliu KID-7	Yongquan KID-1
Pericardium	Zhongchong P-9	Daling P-7
Sanjiao	Zhongzhu SJ-3	Tianjing SJ-10
Gall Bladder	Xiaxi GB-43	Yangfu GB-38
Liver	Ququan LIV-8	Xingjian LIV-2

As might be expected from such a highly theoretical perspective, when we examine these mother and child points in the light of traditional point usage, some have indeed been used to tonify or reduce their related zangfu or channel, whilst in other cases there appears to have been no application of this kind:

- Taiyuan LU-9 (mother) is the principal point on the Lung channel to tonify any Lung deficiency, whilst Chize LU-5 (child) is important to reduce either excess or deficiency heat in the Lung.
- Quchi L.I.-11 (mother) is characterised primarily by its ability to clear a variety of excess pathogenic factors (heat, dampness etc.) from the body and its only

tonifying effect is on the flow of qi and blood in the upper limb, whilst Erjian L.I.-2 (child), as a distal point, is able to expel wind, clear heat and reduce swelling from the upper reaches of the channel.

- Both Jiexi ST-41 (mother) and Lidui ST-45 (child) act primarily to reduce excess pathogenic factors from the Stomach channel and zang, and the only tonifying effect of Jiexi ST-41, like that of Quchi L.I-11, is to benefit the flow of qi and blood in the limb.
- Dadu SP-2 (mother), like most of the shu-points of the Spleen channel, has some effect on tonifying the Spleen. Other points, however, such as Taibai SP-3 and Sanyinjiao SP-6 are considered superior for this purpose. Shangqiu SP-5 (child) is an important point to clear exterior or interior dampness deriving from Spleen deficiency.
- Shaochong HE-9 (mother) was, surprisingly in view of its status as a jing-well point, indicated in various classical texts for deficiency of the Heart. Shenmen HE-7 (child) is able to regulate all patterns of disharmony of the Heart zang, but as the shu-stream and yuan-source point is primarily used to tonify deficiency rather than drain excess.
- As emphasised throughout this text, the points of the three arm yang channels have little effect on their related fu, and Houxi SI-3 (mother) has no intestinal indications, whilst Xiaohai SI-8 (child) has only two. These points could in no sense, therefore, be said to tonify or reduce the Small Intestine fu. As far as the Small Intestine channel is concerned, both have a strong action on reducing heat, stagnation and pain from the channel and neither could be said to have any tonifying effect.
- As with the Small Intestine channel, neither Zhiyin BL-67 (mother) nor Shugu BL-65 (child) are significant points to treat their related fu, and both points primarily act to clear excess pathogenic factors from the channel.
- Fuliu KID-7 (mother) is an important point to strengthen the Kidney's function of dominating body fluids and regulating urination, whilst Yongquan KID-1 is able to help lower pathologically ascending heat, qi, yang and wind, especially when due to deficiency below.
- Zhongchong P-9 (mother) has no discernible action on tonifying the Pericardium or Heart zang or the Pericardium channel, whilst Daling P-7 (child) is an important point to clear heat from the Heart and Pericardium and to calm the spirit.
- Zhongzhu SJ-3 (mother) has no discernible action on tonifying any aspect of the Sanjiao function or channel, whilst Tianjing SJ-10 (child) has a strong action on resolving phlegm, descending rebellion of Lung and Stomach qi, and calming the spirit.
- Both Xiaxi GB-43 (mother) and Yangfu GB-38 (child), the water and fire points respectively of the Gall Bladder channel, are important to clear heat and uprising of yang from the Gall Bladder channel, and neither has any discernible tonifying effect.
- Although emphasised by some practitioners as a point to tonify the Liver yin and blood, Ququan LIV-8 (mother) is primarily used to clear damp-heat from the lower jiao and to resolve blood stasis in the uterus. Xingjian LIV-2 (child) is an important point to reduce excess in the form of fire, uprising yang and qi stagnation from the Liver zang and channel.

THE XI-CLEFT POINTS

The xi-cleft points of the twelve channels			
Lung	Kongzui LU-6	**Bladder**	Jinmen BL-63
Large Intestine	Wenliu L.I.-7	**Kidney**	Shuiquan KID-5
Stomach	Liangqiu ST-34	**Pericardium**	Ximen P-4
Spleen	Diji SP-8	**Sanjiao**	Huizong SJ-7
Heart	Yinxi HE-6	**Gall Bladder**	Waiqiu GB-36
Small Intestine	Yanglao SI-6	**Liver**	Zhongdu LIV-6

The xi-cleft points of the extraordinary channels			
Yang Motility	Fuyang BL-59	**Yang Linking**	Yangjiao GB-35
Yin Motility	Jiaoxin KID-8	**Yin Linking**	Zhubin KID-9

The xi-cleft points were first discussed in the *Systematic Classic of Acupuncture and Moxibustion*. The term 'xi' implies a cleft, crevice, hole or opening, and the xi-cleft points are where the qi and blood, which flow relatively superficially along the channels from the jing-well points, gather and plunge more deeply. The xi-cleft points in general are indicated in the treatment of acute conditions and pain, whilst the xi-cleft points of the yin channels have an additional action of treating disorders of blood. These theoretical concepts are clearly demonstrated by the clinical applications of these points:

- Kongzui LU-6 is an important point both for acute diseases of the Lung and for disorders of blood. It was traditionally indicated for attack by exterior pathogenic wind-heat or wind-dryness giving rise to febrile disease, acute cough and wheezing, swelling and pain of the throat and loss of voice and for coughing blood due to any aetiology. In modern clinical practice the principal use of this point is in the treatment of acute cough, wheezing or asthma of any pattern.

- Wenliu L.I.-7 is indicated in the treatment of acute disorders and pain affecting the Large Intestine channel, and can clear heat and detoxify poison in cases of clove sores, carbuncle and furuncle, throat painful obstruction, and heat and swelling of the face.
- Liangqiu ST-34 is unique among the xi-cleft points of the twelve channels in being located proximal to the knee or elbow. The Stomach channel passes through the breast and nipple, and Liangqiu ST-34 is traditionally indicated for acute disorders such as breast pain and breast abscess. In modern clinical practice it is also used for acute epigastric pain.
- Diji SP-8 has an important action on resolving blood stasis in the uterus and lower abdomen and is indicated in the treatment of dysmenorrhoea (especially when acute), irregular menstruation and abdominal masses in women due to this pathology.
- Yinxi HE-6 is indicated for severe and unbearable Heart pain due to blood stasis, and for bleeding disorders due to excessive heat agitating the blood. In current practice, however, Ximen P-4 (the xi-cleft point of the Pericardium channel) is more used for acute Heart pain. The relationship of Yinxi HE-6 to blood is also expressed via its effect on treating disorders of sweating (see commentary page xxx).
- Yanglao SI-6 is indicated for pain of the shoulder, scapula and arm that is so severe that it feels as if they are broken or dislocated. It is also used as a distal point for acute contraction and sprain of the lumbar region.
- Jinmen BL-63 is indicated for sudden onset of shan disorder, sudden turmoil disorder (acute vomiting and diarrhoea) with cramps, epilepsy and 'white tiger' joint pain (intense pain due to painful obstruction).
- Shuiquan KID-5 is indicated for a variety of menstrual disorders such as amenorrhoea, irregular menstruation, dysmenorrhoea and delayed menstruation, characterised either by deficiency of blood or stasis of blood.
- Ximen P-4 is the primary point for treating acute stasis of blood in the chest and Heart, giving rise to pain. It is also indicated for hot reckless bleeding in the upper jiao manifesting as nosebleed, and vomiting or coughing of blood.
- Huizong SJ-7 has no relevant indications and seems to have been little used in classical practice.
- Waiqiu GB-36 is indicated for painful skin associated with painful obstruction and atrophy disorder, as well as for rabies.
- Zhongdu LIV-6 is indicated for stasis of blood in the uterus, shan disorder and lower abdominal pain.
- Fuyang BL-59 is the xi-cleft point of the Yang Motility vessel but has few relevant indications.
- Jiaoxin KID-8 is the xi-cleft point of the Yin Motility vessel and is indicated for irregular menstruation, dysmenorrhoea, amenorrhoea and especially for uterine bleeding.
- Yangjiao GB-35 is the xi-cleft point of the Yang Linking vessel but has few relevant indications.
- Zhubin KID-9 is the xi-cleft point of the Yin Linking vessel and is traditionally indicated for acute and severe mental disorders such as madness, mania, mania depression disorder, raving, fury and cursing, vomiting of foamy (i.e. watery) saliva and tongue thrusting.

THE YUAN-SOURCE POINTS

Each of the twelve primary channels has a yuan-source point where it is said the original qi surfaces and lingers. The *Classic of Difficulties*[16] says:

"The dynamic qi below the navel, between the Kidneys [the basis] of human life, and the root of the twelve channels is known as the original [qi]. The Sanjiao is the envoy of the original qi, it dominates the movement of the three qi[17] and passes through the five zang and six fu. The term 'source' is an honorary name for the Sanjiao, therefore the places where it resides are known as the yuan-source [points]".

The yuan-source points of the twelve channels			
Lung	Taiyuan LU-9	**Bladder**	Jinggu BL-64
Large Intestine	Hegu L.I.-4	**Kidney**	Taixi KID-3
Stomach	Chongyang ST-42	**Pericardium**	Daling P-7
Spleen	Taibai SP-3	**Sanjiao**	Yangchi SJ-4
Heart	Shenmen HE-7	**Gall Bladder**	Qiuxu GB-40
Small Intestine	Wangu SI-4	**Liver**	Taichong LIV-3

The yuan-source points were first listed in Chapter 1 of the *Spiritual Pivot* as follows: Taiyuan LU-9 for the Lung, Daling P-7 for the Heart, Taibai SP-3 for the Spleen, Taichong LIV-3 for the Liver, Taixi KID-3 for the Kidney, Jiuwei REN-15 for the 'gao' (the area below the Heart) and Qihai REN-6 for the 'huang' (the area above the diaphragm). It is notable that in this passage, Daling P-7 is given as the yuan-source point of the Heart, and it was not until the *Systematic Classic of Acupuncture and Moxibustion* that the shu points (including the yuan-source point) of the Heart channel were first discussed. The yuan-source points of the six fu were given in Chapter 2 of the *Spiritual Pivot*.

On the yin channels only, the yuan-source points are the same as the shu-stream points. The *Spiritual Pivot* in Chapter 1 states "When the five zang are diseased, select the yuan-source points", whilst in Chapter 6 it recommends the use of the shu-stream points in the treatment of disorders of the zang. There is therefore considerable overlap in these two methods of classifying these points of the yin channels and we have seen in the discussion of the shu-stream points above that they are of fundamental importance in tonifying and regulating their respective zang, and are indeed the primary point on the yin channels for this purpose.

On the yang channels, however, the yuan-source points are discrete points lying between the shu-stream and jing-river points. They are usually the fourth point from the distal end of the channel, but in the case of the Gall Bladder channel, the fifth. In terms of their importance and indications they are quite different from the yuan-source points of the yin channels. They have a negligible tonifying effect and indeed have little ability to regulate their related fu, despite the fact that the *Classic of Difficulties*[18] says "When the ... six fu are diseased, select from the yuan-source points". Their principal actions are to dispel various kinds of excess pathogenic factors and to treat disorders along the pathway of their respective channels. Thus Hegu L.I.-4, for example, dispels exterior wind pathogen and regulates the whole course of the Large Intestine channel yet has negligible action on the Large Intestine fu, whilst Wangu SI-4 primarily treats contraction, stiffness and pain along the entire length of the Small Intestine channel, including the hand, elbow, arm, shoulder, neck and back.

Finally, the *Spiritual Pivot*[19] states:
"If the five zang are diseased, abnormal reactions will appear at the twelve yuan-source points; by knowing the correspondence of the yuan-source points to the relevant zang, the reaction can be seen, and thus one can identify which of the five zang are injured".

THE LUO CONNECTING POINTS

Each of the twelve primary channels has a luo-connecting channel which diverges from the primary channel at the luo-connecting point. In addition there are three further luo-connecting points: Jiuwei REN-15 (for the Conception vessel), Chengqiang DU-1 (for the Governing vessel) and Dabao SP-21 (the great luo-connecting point of the Spleen). The actions of the luo-connecting points may be summarised as: i. treating disorders of their interiorly-exteriorly related channel or zangfu, ii. treating disorders in regions reached by the luo-connecting channel, and iii. treating psycho-emotional disorders.

The luo-connecting points of the twelve channels			
Lung	Lieque LU-7	**Bladder**	Feiyang BL-58
Large Intestine	Pianli L.I.-6	**Kidney**	Dazhong KID-4
Stomach	Fenglong ST-40	**Pericardium**	Neiguan P-6
Spleen	Gongsun SP-4	**Sanjiao**	Waiguan SJ-5
Heart	Tongli HE-5	**Gall Bladder**	Guangming GB-37
Small Intestine	Zhizheng SI-7	**Liver**	Ligou LIV-5

Treating disorders of their interiorly-exteriorly related channel or zangfu

The *Guide to the Classic of Acupuncture* states "the luo-connecting points are located between two channels ... if they are punctured, symptoms of the exteriorly-interiorly related channels can be treated"[20]. In clinical practice, many of these points are used to treat disorders of both their corresponding zangfu and channel as well as their interiorly-exteriorly related zangfu or channel, for example:

- Lieque LU-7 is an important point in the treatment of headache, pain of the neck and nape, wind disorders which affect the head etc. despite the fact that the Lung channel does not ascend higher than the throat, and these indications are explained by the pathway of its interiorly-exteriorly related Large Intestine channel.
- Pianli L.I.-6 is used in the treatment of acute oedema which occurs when external wind disrupts the function of the Lung in regulating the water passages.
- Fenglong ST-40 is an essential point to assist the transformation of phlegm which accumulates when the Spleen's transportation and transformation function is impaired.
- Gongsun SP-4 is able to harmonise the function of the Stomach and intestines (which are governed by the

Spleen) and to treat both upper (Stomach) and lower (Spleen) abdominal pain.

- Zhizheng SI-7 has a pronounced effect on regulating and calming the Heart spirit and is indicated for a wide range of psycho-emotional disorders.
- Feiyang BL-58 is able to treat Kidney deficiency and cold in the lower part of the body (coldness and weakness of the legs, lumbar pain etc.) as well as uprising of yang along the Bladder channel to the head (headache, dizziness, heat etc.).
- Neiguan P-6 is universally known for its ability to treat nausea and vomiting. Both the Pericardium channel and its interiorly-exteriorly related Sanjiao channel descend through the upper, middle and lower jiao, reinforcing the ability of Neiguan P-6 to treat disorders of the middle jiao.
- Guangming GB-37 is much used in the treatment of eye disorders due to disharmony of the Liver.

Treating disorders in regions reached by the luo-connecting channel

- Lieque LU-7: the Lung luo-connecting channel spreads through the thenar eminence, and Lieque LU-7 is an important point in the treatment of thumb disorders.
- Pianli L.I.-6: the Large Intestine luo-connecting channel ascends to the ears, and Pianli L.I.-6 is especially applicable in the treatment of ear disorders such as tinnitus and deafness.
- Fenglong ST-40: the Stomach luo-connecting channel terminates at the throat and Fenglong ST-40 is indicated for swelling and pain of the throat, throat painful obstruction with sudden loss of voice, and plumstone throat.
- Gongsun SP-4: the Spleen luo-connecting channel enters the abdomen and connects with the intestines and Stomach, reinforcing the ability of Gongsun SP-4 to treat pain and disharmony in both these areas.
- Tongli HE-5: the Heart luo-connecting channel ascends to the root of the tongue and Tongli HE-5 is much used clinically to treat stiffness of the tongue and speech impairment, especially following windstroke.
- Dazhong KID-4: the Kidney luo-connecting channel ascends to a point below the Pericardium, and Dazhong KID-4 is indicated in the treatment of palpitations, restlessness and agitation of the Heart with fullness and vomiting.
- Ligou LIV-5: the Liver luo-connecting channel ascends to the genitals and Ligou LIV-5 is the primary point on the channel to treat a wide variety of disorders affecting this region.

Treating psycho-emotional disorders

Whilst it is true that classical texts include a variety of psycho-emotional indications for many of the acupuncture points, several of the luo-connecting points are particularly important in this respect, for example:

- Lieque LU-7: poor memory, propensity to laughter.
- Fenglong ST-40: mania-depression, mad laughter, great happiness, desires to ascend to high places and sing, discards clothing and runs around, seeing ghosts.
- Gongsun SP-4: mania-depression disorder, manic raving, insomnia and restlessness, Gall Bladder deficiency, much sighing.
- Tongli HE-5: frequent yawning and groaning with sadness, vexation and anger, sadness and fright, frequent agitation with burning sensation of the Heart, depressive disorder.
- Zhizheng SI-7: mania-depression, fear and fright, sadness and anxiety, restless zang disorder.
- Dazhong KID-4: palpitations, restlessness, dementia, mental retardation, somnolence, propensity to anger, fright, fear and unhappiness, desire to close the door and remain at home.
- Neiguan P-6: insomnia, the five types of epilepsy, mania, poor memory, apprehensiveness, fear and fright, sadness, loss of memory following windstroke.
- Ligou LIV-5: plumstone sensation in the throat, depression, fright palpitations, fear and fright, worried oppression.

In addition to the luo-connecting points of the twelve primary channels there are three further luo-connecting points:

- Jiuwei REN-15 is the luo-connecting point of the Conception vessel, from where the qi disperses and spreads down over the abdomen.
- Chengqiang DU-1 is the luo-connecting point of the Governing vessel, from where the qi ascends bilaterally along the sides of the spine to the nape of the neck and spreads over the occiput; at the scapular region it connects with the Bladder channel and threads through the spine.
- Dabao SP-21 is the great luo-connecting point of the Spleen, which emerges at three cun below the axilla spreading in the chest and lateral costal region.

THE METHOD OF COMBINING THE YUAN-SOURCE AND LUO-CONNECTING POINTS

The combination of the yuan-source and luo-connecting points in clinical practice is known as the 'host and guest combination'[21]. According to this theory, the yuan-source point of the first or primarily affected channel is combined with the luo-connecting point of its interiorly-exteriorly coupled channel. An examination of many classical point combinations shows that this method seems to have been little used (or at least recorded) through the centuries. It does, however, reflect some interesting combinations of points, some of which are frequently used in modern clinical practice:

- Hegu L.I.-4 and Lieque LU-7: this combination is frequently applied when exterior pathogenic wind invades the exterior of the body. Hegu L.I.-4 is able to expel the pathogen whilst Lieque LU-7 both assists in expelling the pathogen and restores the descending and disseminating functions of the Lung.
- Taiyuan LU-9 and Pianli L.I.-6: Pianli L.I.-6 is an important point to open and regulate the water passages and is indicated when pathogenic wind disrupts the function of the Lung resulting in acute oedema, especially of the upper part of the body, accompanied by absence of sweating and difficult urination. Since the root of this pattern is Lung deficiency, its combination with Taiyuan LU-9 is able to treat both the root and branch of this disorder.
- Taibai SP-3 and Fenglong ST-40: deficiency of the Spleen is the root cause of the formation of excessive phlegm. Taibai SP-3 is an important point to tonify the Spleen, whilst Fenglong ST-40 is the primary point on the body to resolve phlegm.
- Shenmen HE-7 and Zhizheng SI-7: Shenmen HE-7 is the principal point on the Heart channel to calm and regulate the spirit, and this is complemented by the strong action Zhizheng SI-7 has on treating psycho-emotional disorders.
- Taixi KID-3 and Feiyang BL-58: Taixi KID-3 is the main point on the Kidney channel to benefit Kidney yin below, whilst Feiyang BL-58 (Soaring Upwards) lowers excessive yang, which, not rooted and secured by deficient yin, rushes upwards to the head.
- Taichong LIV-3 and Guangming GB-37: the Liver 'opens into the eyes' and deficiency of Liver blood or yin, or blazing up of Liver fire or Liver yang may all give rise to eye disorders. Taichong LIV-3 is the primary point on the Liver channel to regulate these disharmonies of the Liver zang, whilst Guangming GB-37 (Bright Light) is an important point to benefit the eyes.

Some modern texts also refer to the combined use of the yuan-source and luo-connecting point of the same yin channel in the case of chronic diseases, for example Taiyuan LU-9 with Lieque LU-7 for chronic cough. This is based on the sayings "chronic disease often involves deficiency" and "at the outset disease is in the channels, later it will be in the luo-collaterals". For example, the yuan-source point (Taiyuan LU-9) is the main point on the Lung channel to tonify deficiency of the Lung, whilst Lieque LU-7, the luo-connecting point, is able to root out the disease from the luo-connecting channels.

THE BACK-SHU POINTS

The twelve back-shu points corresponding to the twelve zangfu lie along the Bladder channel on the back, 1.5 cun lateral to the midline. The term 'shu' means to transport and the name of each of the back-shu points is made up of the name of its corresponding zang or fu, followed by 'shu'. For example the back-shu point of the Heart (xin) is Xinshu BL-15, implying that the qi of the Heart is transported between the zang and this point.

The back-shu points of the twelve zangfu			
Lung	Feishu BL-13	**Bladder**	Pangguangshu BL-28
L. Intestine	Dachangshu BL-25	**Kidney**	Shenshu BL-23
Stomach	Weishu BL-21	**Pericardium**	Jueyinshu BL-14
Spleen	Pishu BL-20	**Sanjiao**	Sanjiaoshu BL-22
Heart	Xinshu BL-15	**Gall Bladder**	Danshu BL-19
S. Intestine	Xiaochangshu BL-27	**Liver**	Ganshu BL-18

The back-shu points lie at roughly the same anatomical level as their related zang or fu, thus Feishu BL-13, the back-shu point of the Lung, is the uppermost at the level of T3, then the Pericardium (Jueyinshu BL-14 at T4) and Heart (Xinshu BL-15 at T5) etc. The back-shu point of the Sanjiao (Sanjiaoshu BL-22) lies between the Stomach and the Kidney, i.e. between the middle and lower jiao. The back-shu points also lie more or less opposite their corresponding front-mu points, thus Feishu BL-13, the back-shu point of the Lung, lies both at the same level as the upper portion of the lung and at the level of its front-mu point, Zhongfu LU-1; Shenshu BL-23, the back-shu point of the Kidneys, lies at the same level as both Jingmen GB-25, its front-mu point, and the kidneys themselves.

In addition there are a number of other back-shu points which are independent of the zangfu, and therefore are not normally included in the listing of the back-shu points: Dushu BL-16 (Governing Shu), Geshu BL-17 (Diaphragm

Shu), Qihaishu BL-24 (Sea of Qi Shu), Guanyuanshu BL-26 (Gate of the Source Shu), Zhonglushu BL-29 (Mid-Spine Shu), Baihuanshu BL-30 (White Ring Shu) and Gaohuangshu BL-43 (Vital Region Shu).

The functions of the back-shu points

The first mention of the back-shu points is in the *Spiritual Pivot*[22]:

"The back-shu point for the centre of the thorax is below the tip of the big vertebra [C7], that for the Lungs is below the third vertebra, that for the Heart below the fifth vertebra, that for the diaphragm below the seventh vertebra, that for the Liver below the ninth vertebra, that for the Spleen below the eleventh vertebra, that for the Kidneys below the fourteenth vertebra, all of them are situated three cun from the spine. To locate the point accurately, press on the area, if the [original] pain is relieved, the point is correctly located".

This passage continues by saying that the back-shu points are contraindicated to needling and should only be treated by moxibustion. Later commentators, however, have interpreted this passage rather as warning against excessively deep needling.

The *Classic of Difficulties*[23] said:
"Yin diseases travel through the yang region and yang diseases travel through the yin region. The mu points are situated in the yin region, they may be used to treat yang diseases; the shu points are situated in the yang region, they may be used to treat yin diseases".

Taken together with the general concept "In diseases of yin, treat the yang"[24], these quotations suggest that the back-shu points should primarily be selected in cases of deficiency and cold (yin), and for diseases of the zang (yin) rather than the fu. It is certainly true that the classical indications for these points include many examples of deficiency and cold, for example:

- Feishu BL-13: cold Lung, Lung atrophy.
- Xinshu BL-15: Heart qi deficiency in children, frightened and cautious with Heart deficiency.
- Danshu BL-19: deficiency taxation.
- Pishu BL-20: Spleen qi cold.
- Weishu BL-21: Stomach cold and feeble.
- Shenshu BL-23: Kidney deficiency deafness, the five taxations and the seven injuries, taxation of the five zang, chronic cold of the water (Kidney) zang.

However it is equally true that there are numerous classical indications for excess disorders among the back-shu points, for example:

- Feishu BL-13: fullness of the chest, difficult breathing on lying down.
- Jueyinshu BL-14: oppression of the chest, pain of the chest and diaphragm due to accumulation of qi.
- Ganshu BL-18: pain and distention of the lateral costal region, hypogastric fullness and pain, fullness of the chest, much anger, mania-depression disorder, epilepsy.

In current clinical practice, and as far as we know for a long way back in the historical tradition, back-shu points have been selected equally for any pattern of their corresponding zangfu whether hot or cold, excess or deficient, and indeed have been considered vital points for these purposes. However it is probably true that most practitioners use the back-shu points of the zang more frequently than those of the fu, and this reflects the experience that whilst the back-shu points of the zang are of fundamental importance clinically, the front-mu points may be favoured for diseases of the fu.

Finally due to their location on the Bladder channel, the back-shu points, whilst treating the zangfu, clearly do not treat channel disorders (other than those of the Bladder channel). They are however indicated in some instances for disorders of the sense organs which pertain to the zangfu. Thus Ganshu BL-18 is much used for eye disorders, Shenshu BL-23 for ear disorders, and Xinshu BL-15 for "lack of strength in the root of the tongue".

THE FRONT-MU POINTS

There are twelve front-mu points, located on the chest or abdomen in close proximity to their respective zang or fu. All lie on the anterior of the body except Jingmen GB-25 which lies at the free end of the twelfth rib. Of the twelve points, only three lie on the channel corresponding to their related zang or fu (Zhongfu LU-1 front-mu point of

The front-mu points of the twelve zangfu

Lung	Zhongfu LU-1	**Bladder**	Zhongji REN-3
L. Intestine	Tianshu ST-25	**Kidney**	Jingmen GB-25
Stomach	Zhongwan REN-12	**Pericardium**	Shanzhong REN-17
Spleen	Zhangmen LIV-13	**Sanjiao**	Shimen REN-5
Heart	Juque REN-14	**Gall Bladder**	Riyue GB-24
S. Intestine	Guanyuan REN-4	**Liver**	Qimen LIV-14

the Lung, Qimen LIV-14 front-mu point of the Liver, and Riyue GB-24 front-mu point of the Gall Bladder). Of the remaining nine, six lie on the Conception vessel.

The term 'mu' means to gather or to collect, and the front-mu points are where the qi of the zangfu gathers and concentrates on the anterior surface of the body. There are few early classical references to these points.

The *Essential Questions* for example says:
"When a person is frequently indecisive, the Gall Bladder is deficient. The qi will flow upwards giving rise to a bitter taste in the mouth. To treat this use the front-mu and the back-shu of the Gall Bladder".

The *Classic of Difficulties*[25] says:
"The mu of the five zang are located at the yin [aspect], whilst the shu points are located at the yang [region]".

The *Classic of the Pulse* was the first text to list the front-mu points as a group, discussing ten points, and the *Systematic Classic of Acupuncture and Moxibustion* then added the front-mu points of the Sanjiao and Pericardium, completing this grouping as it is recognised today.

The *Classic of Difficulties*[26] says:
"Yin diseases travel through the yang region and yang diseases travel through the yin region. The mu points are situated in the yin region, they may be used to treat yang diseases; the shu points are situated in the yang region, they may be used to treat yin diseases."

We have seen that the back-shu points have a wide application in diseases of both the zang and the fu and the same is true for the front-mu points. Thus for example, Qimen LIV-14, the front-mu point of the Liver, is important for the treatment of Liver patterns, Juque REN-14 the front-mu point of the Heart for Heart patterns etc. Nor does it seem correct to say that the front-mu points are more used for yang diseases manifesting as acute, excess or hot patterns, for example points such as Zhangmen LIV-13, Zhongwan REN-12 or Tianshu ST-25 are equally applicable in excess or deficient, acute or chronic disorders. What is true, however, is that the front-mu points of the fu are located on the soft and unprotected regions of the abdomen, where needling can deeply reach them. These points (especially Tianshu ST-25, Zhongji REN-3, Guanyuan REN-4 and Zhongwan REN-12) are of particular importance in treating disorders of the intestines, Bladder and Stomach.

Few generalisations can therefore be made about the clinical application of these points, except for one obvious fact. With the exception of the three points mentioned above that do lie on their corresponding channel (Zhongfu LU-1, Qimen LIV-14 and Riyue GB-24), the front-mu points treat disorders of their respective zangfu but not their respective channel. In other words, whilst Juque REN-14, the front-mu point of the Heart, treats disorders of the Heart zang, it does not treat disorders of the Heart channel.

There are two other aspects of the back-shu and front-mu points that can be mentioned. The first is that they are likely to become tender in response to disharmony of their respective zang and fu, and thus can contribute towards making a diagnosis. The second is that they are commonly combined in treatment, for example Juque REN-14 and Xinshu BL-15 for the treatment of Heart patterns, and Pangguangshu BL-28 and Zhongji REN-3 for the Bladder.

THE HUI-MEETING POINTS

The hui-meeting points			
Zang	Zhangmen LIV-13	**Sinews**	Yanglingquan GB-34
Fu	Zhongwan REN-12	**Vessels**	Taiyuan LU-9
Qi	Shanzhong REN-17	**Bone**	Dazhu BL-11
Blood	Geshu BL-17	**Marrow**	Xuanzhong GB-39

The eight hui-meeting points were listed for the first time in the *Classic of Difficulties*[27].

- Zhangmen LIV-13 is both the hui-meeting point of the zang and the front-mu point of the Spleen. The *Standards of Patterns and Treatments* states "The essence of the five zang is all transported from the Spleen". Zhangmen LIV-13 is therefore an important point to tonify the Spleen itself as well as all the zang and the body as a whole.
- Zhongwan REN-12 is both the hui-meeting point of the fu and the front-mu point of the Stomach. As the origin of the post-natal qi, the Stomach (and Spleen) is considered to play a central role among the zangfu, transforming and distributing the essence of food and drink throughout the body. For this reason, the Stomach may be said to dominate the fu.
- Shanzhong REN-17 is the hui-meeting point of the qi and is also known as Shangqihai (Upper Sea of Qi). According to the *Spiritual Pivot*[28] Shanzhong REN-17 is the 'sea of qi' (linking with Dazhui DU-14, Yamen

DU-15 and Renying ST-9). Located in the centre of the chest, Shanzhong REN-17 has a strong effect on the gathering (zong) qi which in turn regulates both the Lung functions of dominating qi and controlling respiration and speech, and the Heart function of governing the blood and blood vessels.

- Geshu BL-17 is the hui-meeting point of blood and is the single most important acupuncture point for the treatment of any disorder arising from blood heat, blood stasis or blood deficiency.
- Yanglingquan GB-34 is the hui-meeting point of the sinews and has long been considered the main point to influence the sinews throughout the body, for example in cases of contraction of the sinews, stiffness of the neck and shoulders, stiffness and tightness of the muscles and joints, and most especially disorders of the leg such as knee pain, hemiplegia, atrophy disorder and painful obstruction.
- Taiyuan LU-9 is the hui-meeting point of the pulse and vessels. The *Classic of Difficulties*[29] states "The vessels gather at Taiyuan LU-9". Taiyuan LU-9 is an important point to harmonise the relationship between the gathering (zong) qi and the blood flowing in the vessels. When the gathering qi is deficient and fails to circulate the blood, it will pool and stagnate in the chest and Heart, giving rise to various manifestations of blood stasis. Taiyuan LU-9 is further indicated for disorders of the blood vessels in general such as vomiting, spitting or coughing blood and pulseless syndrome.
- Dazhu BL-11 is the hui-meeting point of bone and is indicated for various bone diseases and rigidity and pain of the neck, spine and lumbar region. In modern clinical practice it is used when painful obstruction penetrates deeply into the bones and joints causing deformity (known as bony painful obstruction).
- Xuanzhong GB-39 is the hui-meeting point of marrow, the origin of the bone marrow. It is able to benefit the sinews and bones and is indicated for a wide range of disorders characterised by weakness, flaccidity, contraction and pain of the limbs.

THE CONFLUENT POINTS OF THE EIGHT EXTRAORDINARY VESSELS

The confluent points of the extraordinary channels			
Conception	Lieque LU-7	**Yin Motility**	Zhaohai KID-6
Governing	Houxi SI-3	**Yang Motility**	Shenmai BL-62
Penetrating	Gongsun SP-4	**Yin Linking**	Neiguan P-6
Girdling	Zulinqi GB-41	**Yang Linking**	Waiguan SJ-5

There are two principal, and inter-related, ways that these points may be used: i. to activate their respective extraordinary channel, and ii. according to the *Ode of the Obstructed River*.

To activate their respective extraordinary channel

Lieque LU-7 (the Conception vessel)
The Conception vessel ascends along the anterior midline of the body and is closely related to the uterus and the genito-urinary organs. By opening and regulating the flow of qi in the Conception vessel, Lieque LU-7 is able to treat such symptoms as retention of the lochia and dead foetus, pain of the genitals and urinary disorders.

Zhaohai KID-6 (the Yin Motility vessel)
The regions traversed by the Yin Motility vessel include the medial aspect of the leg, the throat, the brain and the inner canthus. Zhaohai KID-6 is an important point for chronic throat disorders, and is indicated for a variety of eye disorders, day-time epilepsy, and tightness and contraction of the inner aspect of the leg, a traditional indication of disorder of the Yin Motility vessel.

Neiguan P-6 (the Yin Linking vessel)
According to the *Classic of Difficulties*[30] "When the Yin Linking vessel is diseased, Heart pain will result". Other traditional indications for this extraordinary channel include chest pain and fullness and pain of the lateral costal region. Neiguan P-6 is probably the single most important point for the treatment of pain of the Heart and chest, as well as pain of the lateral costal region, whatever the aetiology.

Gongsun SP-4 (the Penetrating vessel)
According to the *Classic of Difficulties*[31] "When the Penetrating vessel is diseased, counterflow qi and abdominal urgency will occur". The term abdominal urgency refers to a sensation of acute cramping abdominal pain, usually associated with dysenteric disorder, and Gongsun SP-4 is

an important point not only for this kind of abdominal pain but for distention and pain due to any aetiology in any area of the abdomen. As far as counterflow qi is concerned, Gongsun is indicated for rebellion of Stomach qi manifesting as vomiting and sudden turmoil disorder.

The Penetrating vessel ascends to the face, and Gongsun SP-4 is indicated for (and included in various classical combinations for) oedema, especially oedema of the face.

Despite the fact that the Penetrating vessel (Sea of Blood) originates in the uterus in females, it is notable that there are few gynaecological indications in either classical or modern texts for Gongsun SP-4.

Houxi SI-3 (the Governing vessel)

The Governing vessel ascends along the spinal column from the coccyx to the head, and Houxi SI-3 is an essential distal point in the treatment of occipital headache, and stiffness and pain of the neck, scapula and upper or lumbar spine.

The Governing vessel governs all the yang channels and hence the exterior portion of the body as a whole and Houxi SI-3 has a strong influence on dispelling febrile disease, especially malaria and attack by exterior pathogenic wind-cold or wind-heat which gives rise to chills and fever accompanied by severe neck pain or pain of the spine.

The Governing vessel enters the brain and Houxi SI-3 is an important point in the treatment of epilepsy.

Shenmai BL-62 (the Yang Motility vessel)

The Yang Motility vessel traverses the lateral side of the body and head, connects with the Gall Bladder channel at Fengchi GB-20 and enters the brain at Fengfu DU-16. Shenmai BL-62 is indicated for attack of exterior wind with stiff neck and headache, and for interior wind which rushes upwards to the head and brain giving rise to such symptoms as lockjaw, opisthotonos, upward staring eyes, deviation of the mouth and eyes, windstroke, hemiplegia and epilepsy. The Yang Motility vessel ascends to the inner canthus, and like the Yin Motility vessel is indicated for insomnia (excessive opening of the eyes).

Waiguan SJ-5 (the Yang Linking vessel)

The Yang Linking vessel links all the yang channels of the body, including the Governing vessel, and Waiguan SJ-5 is an important point to dispel pathogenic factors from the exterior (yang) portion of the body.

The forehead belongs to yangming channel, the temporal region to shaoyang channel and the occipital region to taiyang channel, whilst the Governing vessel ascends to the vertex. As a result of its influence on all these yang channels, Waiguan SJ-5 is indicated for temporal, frontal, occipital and vertex headaches.

Zulinqi GB-41 (the Girdling vessel)

The Girdling vessel encircles the waist and binds the Penetrating and Conception vessels and the Kidney, Liver and Spleen channels, whilst various pathways of the Gall Bladder channel traverse the chest region and breast. Zulinqi GB-41 is indicated for distention and pain of the breast, breast abscess, menstrual disorders and inhibited menstruation, and is particularly used in situations where Liver qi stagnation impairs the smoothness and regularity of the menstrual cycle.

According to the Ode of the Obstructed River

In the *Ode of the Obstructed River*, a passage on 'The Eight Therapeutic Methods' discusses the application of the eight confluent points of the extraordinary channels to affect specific symptoms and areas of the body:

- Lieque LU-7 for disorders of the head region, rebellion and blockage of phlegm and dry throat.
- Zhaohai KID-6 for throat wind (swelling and pain with difficulty in swallowing).
- Neiguan P-6 for disorders of the chest.
- Gongsun SP-4 for abdominal pain below the umbilicus.
- Houxi SI-3 for diseases of the Governing vessel and for mania-depression.
- Shenmai BL-62 to expel cold and heat and to treat one-sided and generalised head-wind and fright.
- Waiguan SJ-5 for injury by cold to the exterior accompanied by headache.
- Zulinqi GB-41 for disorders of the eyes.

THE TWELVE HEAVENLY STAR POINTS OF MA DAN-YANG

Ma Dan-yang, the great physician of the Jin dynasty, was the originator of the *Song of the Eleven Heavenly Star Points*, a list of what he considered to be the most important acupuncture points on the body. It first appeared in print in the *Classic of the Jade Dragon*. Xu Feng, who included this song in his work *Complete Collection of Acupuncture and Moxibustion* added a twelfth point (Taichong LIV-3) and this group of twelve points is nowadays known as the Twelve Heavenly Star Points of Ma Dan-yang.

The heavenly star points of Ma Dan-yang

Lieque LU-7	Neiting ST-44	Kunlun BL-60
Hegu L.I.-4	Tongli HE-5	Huantiao GB-30
Quchi L.I.-11	Weizhong BL-40	Yanglingquan GB-34
Zusanli ST-36	Chengshan BL-57	Taichong LIV-3

The points, with Ma Dan-yangs's (and in the case of Taichong LIV-3 Xu Feng's) indications are:

- Lieque LU-7: one-sided headache, wind painful obstruction and numbness of the whole body, obstruction of phlegm in the upper body, and lockjaw.
- Hegu L.I.-4: headache, swelling of the face, malaria with chills and fever, tooth decay, nosebleed and lockjaw with inability to speak.
- Quchi L.I.-11: aching elbow, hemiplegia with inability to close the hand, inability to draw a bow, flaccidity of the sinews so that a person cannot comb their hair, throat painful obstruction as if going to die, recurring fevers, skin disorders due to wind.
- Zusanli ST-36: cold Stomach, borborygmus and diarrhoea, swelling of the leg, soreness of the knee and calf, injury by cold, weakness, emaciation, parasitic infection of all types.
- Neiting ST-44: deathly chill in the hands and feet, dislike of voices, skin rashes, sore throat, continuous yawning, toothache, malaria with inability to eat.
- Tongli HE-5: inability to speak despite a desire to do so, vexation and anger, pounding of the Heart, when excess there is heaviness of the four limbs, the head, cheeks and face are red, when deficient there is inability to eat, sudden loss of voice and an expressionless face.
- Weizhong BL-40: lumbar pain with inability to straighten up, severe lumbar pain that radiates up the back with pain and stiffness of the sinews and bones, wind painful obstruction that frequently reoccurs, difficulty in stretching and bending the knee.
- Chengshan BL-57: lumbar pain, haemorrhoids, difficulty in defecation, leg qi, swelling of the knee, cramps and spasms and pain with cholera, tremors.
- Kunlun BL-60: cramping of the lumbar region and sacrum, sudden dyspnoea, fullness of the Heart, inability to walk or even take a step, as soon as he moves he groans.
- Huantiao GB-30: cold wind and damp painful obstruction, pain radiating from the hip to the calf, sighing with pain when turning over.
- Yanglingquan GB-34: swelling and numbness of the knee, cold painful obstruction, hemiplegia, inability to raise the leg
- Taichong LIV-3: fright epilepsy wind, distention of the throat and Heart, both legs unable to walk, the seven types of shan disorder, unilateral sagging and swelling of the testicle, cloudy vision, lumbar pain.

THE FOUR AND SIX COMMAND POINTS

This pre-Ming dynasty grouping of points first appeared in print in the *Glorious Anthology of Acupuncture and Moxibustion* by the Ming dynasty author Gao Wu. The four command points, which were clearly considered the four most useful and important of all the points, are:

- Zusanli ST-36 for disorders of the abdomen.
- Weizhong BL-40 for disorders of the lumbar region and back.
- Lieque LU-7 for disorders of the head and nape.
- Hegu L.I.-4 for disorders of the face and mouth.

These points can be used to treat any kind of disorder in these regions, whether deficient, excess, hot, cold, chronic or acute. Later generations added two more points to this grouping (thus known as the Six Command Points):

- Neiguan P-6 for disorders of the chest and lateral costal region
- Renzhong DU-26 for resuscitation.

POINTS OF THE FOUR SEAS

The *Spiritual Pivot*[32] describes four 'seas' in the human body. These are known as the sea of qi, the sea of blood, the sea of water and grain and the sea of marrow. This ancient classification gives symptoms of disorder of the four seas as follows:

The sea of qi

The points associated with the sea of qi are Renying ST-9, Shanzhong REN-17, Yamen DU-15 and Dazhui DU-14. The *Spiritual Pivot* says "When the sea of qi is in excess there is fullness in the chest, urgent breathing and a red complexion. When the sea of qi is insufficient, there is scanty energy insufficient for speech".

The sea of blood

The *Spiritual Pivot* says "The Penetrating vessel is the sea of the twelve channels. In the upper it is conveyed to Dazhu BL-11, and in the lower it emerges at both Shangjuxu ST-37 and Xiajuxu ST-39 ... When the sea of blood is in excess, there is a sensation as if the body were big; one feels disquiet, but does not know what disease there is; when the sea of blood is insufficient, one has the sensation of one's body being small; one feels reduced but does not know what could be the illness". Despite this passage it is worth noting that such indications are not found in subsequent discussions of these three points.

The sea of water and grain

Qichong ST-30 is given as the upper point of the 'sea of water and grain' and Zusanli ST-36 as its lower point. According to the *Spiritual Pivot* "when the sea of water and grain is in excess, there is abdominal fullness, and when it is deficient there is hunger with inability to eat".

The sea of marrow

The *Spiritual Pivot* says "Its point above is the top of the head; below it is Fengfu DU-16" and "When the sea of marrow is in excess then there is lightness of the body and much strength and a person's self exceeds the normal level; when the sea of marrow is insufficient there is a whirling sensation of the brain, dizziness, tinnitus, pain of the lower legs, impairment of vision, indolence and desire to sleep". The 'top of the head' is taken to be Baihui DU-20.

THE POINTS OF THE WINDOW OF HEAVEN

This is a group of ten points which have come to be known in Western acupuncture circles as 'Window of the Sky' points[33], or perhaps more suitably 'Window of Heaven' points. They are first referred to in the *Spiritual Pivot*[34] which says:

"Headache due to rebellion of yang, fullness of the chest with difficulty in breathing, choose Renying ST-9. Sudden loss of voice with fishbone [i.e. obstructed] qi in the throat, choose Futu L.I.-18 and bleed the root of the tongue. Sudden deafness with excess of qi, dimness of vision and hearing, select Tianyou SJ-16. Sudden twitching, epilepsy and dizziness, with inability of the legs to support the body, select Tianzhu BL-10. Sudden and severe thirst, internal rebellion, Liver and Lung struggle against each other, blood overflows from the mouth and nose, treat with Tianfu LU-3. These are the five regions of the window of heaven".

There is no further discussion of the significance of this grouping in this chapter, but Zhou Zhi-cong, in his commentary on this passage[35] stated:

"The points and the orifices of the head and face are like the great windows of a high pavilion by virtue of which qi moves. When there is inversion qi [i.e. chaotic and rebellious qi] below, then the channels in the upper region do not move and there is lack of clarity of vision and hearing, sudden loss of speech, convulsions and dizziness. The qi of speech of the three yang originates in the lower and emanates in the upper. Therefore, to summarise, it is said these are the five regions of the great window".

Inversion qi may be complicated by disharmony of yin and yang, disturbance in the flow of qi and blood, obstruction of turbid phlegm, obstruction and stagnation of food etc. It is said to arise suddenly at a time of change and transformation in the course of an illness, and can give rise to various new symptoms such as disturbance of the mental faculties as well as sudden fainting and inversion cold of the four limbs.

In Chapter 2, the *Spiritual Pivot* includes the five window of heaven points listed above in a list of ten points (with the addition of Tiantu REN-22, Tianchuang SI-16, Tianrong SI-17, Fengfu DU-16 and Tianchi P-1). This passage first discusses Tiantu REN-22, and then the six yang channel points as a sequence of vertical lines spreading from the Conception vessel and ending with Fengfu DU-16 on the Governing vessel, with Tianfu LU-3 and Tianchi P-1 as additional points.

The window of heaven points	
Tianfu LU-3	Tiantu REN-22
Renying ST-9	Tianchuang SI-16
Futu L.I.-18	Tianrong SI-17
Tianyou SJ-16	Fengfu DU-16
Tianzhu BL-10	Tianchi P-1

Later commentators (particularly Ma Shi, the great physician of the Ming dynasty and expert on the *Yellow Emperor's Inner Classic*[36]) pointed out that Tianrong SI-17 should in fact be Tianchong GB-9[37]. This is because the original passage, before listing Tianrong SI-17, says "the next slice is shaoyang", and of course Tianrong SI-17 belongs to taiyang channel not shaoyang. Replacing Tianrong SI-17 by Tianchong GB-9 would be more logical since each of the six yang channels would then be represented.

This passage from Chapter 2 of the *Spiritual Pivot* does not refer to this grouping as window of heaven points and offers no explanation or clinical or diagnostic application. The evidence for all ten points to be classified as window of heaven points is therefore very unclear, but there are a few interesting observations that can be made.

Firstly, most of the point names include the character 'tian' (Heaven, or Sky), in their name (although it should be stressed that there are other acupuncture points that also include this character, such as Tianquan P-2, Tianding L.I.-17, Tianzong SI-11 that are not included in this list). It is interesting, though, that an alternative name for Renying ST-9 is Tianwuhui (Heaven's Five Meetings).

Secondly, as indicated above, all but two of the ten points are located around the neck (the junction of the head and the body), whilst in terms of the human body, the heavenly region refers to the upper part or head.

Thirdly, there are some hints of a discernible pattern in their indications, the following appearing with some frequency:

- goitre or scrofula, or throat disorders.
- coughing, wheezing or chest oppression from rebellion of Lung qi.
- vomiting from rebellion of Stomach qi.
- headache and dizziness.
- heat, redness or swelling of the face or eyes.
- sudden onset of disorders.
- disorders of the sense organs.
- in some cases mental and emotional disorders.

When these observations are put together, we can suggest that the window of heaven points are indicated in the following situations:

Disharmony between the qi of the body and the head, with qi or blood rebelling upwards

If rebellious qi affects the Lung it gives rise to cough, wheezing or oppression of the chest. If it affects the Stomach there will be hiccup, nausea or vomiting. If it ascends to the head there may be headache and dizziness, heat, redness or swelling of the face, and disorders of the sense organs, especially the ears and eyes.

Thus, for example, Tianfu LU-3 is indicated for when Liver fire attacks the Lung causing an upsurge of reckless hot bleeding from the mouth and nose, and rebellion of Lung qi with wheezing and asthma. Renying ST-9 is indicated for wheezing, coughing and vomiting due to rebellion of Lung and Stomach qi as well as for red face, dizziness and headache. Tianzhu BL-10 is indicated for dizziness, headache, stiff neck, spasms and redness of the eyes in the upper body, and for deficiency below manifesting as inability of the legs to support the body. Fengfu DU-16 is indicated for stirring of interior wind which gives rise to headache, head wind, all types of wind disease, stiff neck, nosebleed, dizziness and 'the hundred diseases of the head'.

Window of heaven points Effect on cough or wheezing from rebellious Lung qi or vomiting from rebellious Stomach qi	
Tianfu LU-3	Wheezing, dyspnoea, cough, asthma, coughing blood
Futu L.I.-18	Cough, wheezing, asthma, coughing with much spittle
Renying ST-9	Fullness of the chest, shortness of breath, asthma, sudden turmoil disorder, vomiting
Tianrong SI-17	Chest fullness with difficulty in breathing, wheezing, cough, chest pain, vomiting foam
Tianchi P-1	Cough with copious phlegm, fullness of the chest, shortness of breath, uprising qi
Fengfu DU-16	Difficulty in breathing, heat in the chest, ceaseless vomiting
Tiantu REN-22	Obstruction in the chest, fullness of the chest, rebellious qi with cough, asthma, sudden dyspnoea, inability to breathe, abscess of the Lung with purulent bloody coughing, vomiting

Window of heaven points Effect on headache and dizziness and heat, redness or swelling of the face or eyes	
Tianfu LU-3	Dizziness
Renying ST-9	Headache, dizziness, red face
Tianchuang SI-16	Headache, swelling and pain of the cheek, heat sensation of the skin of the face
Tianrong SI-17	Swelling of the cheek
Tianzhu BL-10	Dizziness, redness of the eyes
Tianchi P-1	Headache
Tianyou SJ-16	Dizziness, headache, head wind, swollen face
Tiantu REN-22	Heat sensation of the skin of the face, red face
Fengfu DU-16	Headache, head wind, dizziness, the hundred diseases of the head

Scrofula and goitre

The majority of these points are indicated for scrofula (nodules which are mostly found on the sides of the neck) or goitre, as well as for swelling, pain and stagnation in the throat region. Whilst this may seem self-evident, as most are located in the neck region, it is worth noting that Tianfu LU-3 and Tianchi P-1, as well as Tianchong GB-9, which are located on the arm, chest and head respectively, also have these indications. Since stagnation of qi in the neck region is a major part of the pathogenesis of scrofula or goitre, once again these points demonstrate an ability to harmonise the flow of qi in this pivotal area between the head and body.

Window of heaven points Effect on goitre, scrofula or throat disorders	
Tianfu LU-3	Goitre, swelling of the throat
Futu L.I.-18	Goitre, scrofula, swelling and pain of the throat, rattling sound in the throat, difficulty in swallowing
Renying ST-9	Goitre, scrofula, swelling and pain of the throat, difficulty in swallowing
Tianchuang SI-16	Goitre, throat pain
Tianrong SI-17	Goitre, scrofula, throat painful obstruction, obstruction of the throat
Tianzhu BL-10	Swelling of the throat
Tianchi P-1	Scrofula of the neck
Tianyou SJ-16	Goitre, throat painful obstruction
Tiantu REN-22	Goitre, ulceration of the throat which prevents eating, swelling of the throat, cold sensation of the throat, dry throat, throat painful obstruction, rattling sound in the throat, accumulation of phlegm in the throat, plumstone qi
Fengfu DU-16	Swelling and pain of the throat

Sudden onset

Many of these points are indicated for sudden onset of disorders, reflecting their ability to treat the sudden chaos that arises during inversion qi disorders.

Window of heaven points Effect on sudden onset of disorders	
Futu L.I.-18	Sudden loss of voice
Renying ST-9	Sudden turmoil disorder
Tianchuang SI-16	Sudden loss of voice following windstroke, sudden loss of voice
Tianzhu BL-10	Epilepsy, sudden muscular contractions
Tianyou SJ-16	Sudden deafness
Tiantu REN-22	Sudden dyspnoea
Fengfu DU-16	Sudden inability to speak following windstroke

Psycho-emotional disorders

It is difficult to assess the importance of the mental and emotional disorders listed for some of these points. There is a tendency among some commentators, especially in the West, to ascribe important psycho-emotional effects to points which include the character tian (Heaven) in their name. However many points which are named in this way have few or no psycho-emotional disorders, whilst most of the powerful psycho-emotionally acting points do not include the name tian.

Window of heaven points Effect on emotional disorders	
Tianfu LU-3	Somnolence, sadness, weeping, disorientation and forgetfulness, absent-mindedness, insomnia, floating corpse ghost-talk, melancholy crying ghost talk
Tianchuang SI-16	Manic ghost talk, mania-depression
Tianzhu BL-10	Mania, incessant talking, seeing ghosts, epilepsy, childhood epilepsy
Tianyou SJ-16	Confused dreaming
Fengfu DU-16	Mania, incessant talking, mad walking and desire to commit suicide, sadness and fear with fright palpitations

Disorders of the sense organs

Finally, the ability of these points to regulate the flow of qi and blood to the head means that several of them are indicated for disorders of the sense organs.

Window of heaven points Effect on disorders of the sense organs	
Tianfu LU-3	Nosebleed, visual dizziness, short-sightedness
Renying ST-9	Visual dizziness
Tianchuang SI-16	Deafness, tinnitus, ear pain
Tianrong SI-17	Tinnitus and deafness
Tianzhu BL-10	Bursting eye pain, redness of the eyes, blurred vision, lacrimation, difficulty in speaking, nasal congestion, loss of sense of smell
Tianyou SJ-16	Impaired hearing, dimness of vision, pain of the eyes with inability to see, inability to open the eyes, lacrimation, rhinitis with nosebleed, loss of smell, stuffy nose
Fengfu DU-16	Flaccid tongue with inability to speak, visual dizziness, blurred vision, nosebleed
Tiantu REN-22	Inability to speak

THE THIRTEEN GHOST POINTS OF SUN SI-MIAO

The thirteen ghost points were listed in the *Thousand Ducat Formulas* by the great 7th century physician Sun Si-miao for the treatment of mania disorder and epilepsy. The thirteen ghost points are:

- Guigong (Ghost Palace) i.e. Renzhong DU-26.
- Guizhen (Ghost Pillow) i.e. Fengfu DU-16.
- Guitang (Ghost Hall) i.e. Shangxing DU-23.
- Guishi (Ghost Market) i.e. Chengqiang REN-24.
- Guixin (Ghost Faith) i.e. Shaoshang LU-11.

- Guitui (Ghost Leg) i.e. Quchi L.I.-11.
- Guichuang (Ghost's Bed) i.e. Jiache ST-6.
- Guilei (Ghost Fortress) i.e. Yinbai SP-1.
- Guixin (Ghost Heart) i.e. Daling P-7.
- Guicu (Ghost Cave) i.e. Laogong P-8.
- Guilu (Ghost Path) i.e. Shenmai BL-62.
- Guifeng (Ghost Seal) i.e. Haiquan (Extra) below the tongue.
- Guicang (Ghost Store) was also known as Yumentou (Extra) in women and Yinxiafeng (Extra) in men, both points more or less corresponding to Huiyin REN-1.

Historically however, there has been a certain amount of ambiguity concerning these points. Some authorities considered that Guixin was in fact Taiyuan LU-9 rather than Daling P-7, and that Guilu was either Jianshi P-5 or even Laogong P-8 rather than BL-62. Gao Wu's alternative list of these points in the *Glorious Anthology of Acupuncture and Moxibustion* included Shenting DU-24, Ruzhong ST-17, Yanglingquan GB-34 and Xingjian LIV-2 and omitted Shenmai BL-62, Shangxing DU-23, Quchi L.I.-11 and Yumentou/Yinxiafeng.

THE NINE NEEDLES FOR RETURNING THE YANG

The *Song of the Nine Needles for Returning the Yang*, a chapter in the *Glorious Anthology of Acupuncture and Moxibustion* lists nine points for the treatment of collapse of yang characterised by loss of consciousness, aversion to cold, cold counterflow of the limbs, purple lips etc. These are Hegu L.I.-4, Zusanli ST-36, Sanyinjiao SP-6, Yongquan KID-1, Taixi KID-3, Laogong P-8, Huantiao GB-30, Yamen DU-15 and Zhongwan REN-12.

MEETING POINTS OF MORE THAN ONE CHANNEL

In the course of the complex network of channel pathways, many of the channels intersect other channels at specific points. These points are thus able to influence more than one channel, and are frequently used for this purpose in clinical practice. For charts of the meeting points, please see the following pages.

NOTES

1 *Spiritual Pivot* Chapter 1.

2 *Spiritual Pivot* Chapter 71.

3 According to *The Practical Application of Meridian Style Acupuncture*, by John E. Pirog, Pacific View Press.

4 *Classic of Difficulties* 68th Difficulty.

5 *Spiritual Pivot* Chapter 44.

6 The *Classic of Difficulties* (74th Difficulty) says that in winter the he-sea points should be needled.

7 The *Classic of Difficulties* (74th Difficulty) says that in spring the jing-well points should be needled.

8 The *Classic of Difficulties* (74th Difficulty) says that in summer the ying-spring points should be needled.

9 The *Classic of Difficulties* (74th Difficulty) says that in late summer the shu-stream points should be needled.

10 The *Classic of Difficulties* (74th Difficulty) says that in autumn the jing-river points should be needled.

11 *Spiritual Pivot* Chapter 4.

12 *Spiritual Pivot* Chapter 6.

13 *Spiritual Pivot* Chapter 1.

14 *Classic of Difficulties* 64th Difficulty.

15 *Classic of Difficulties* 69th Difficulty.

16 *Classic of Difficulties* 66th Difficulty.

17 The three qi referred to here are considered by most authorities to refer to the nutritive qi, defensive qi and gathering qi.

18 *Classic of Difficulties* 66th Difficulty.

19 *Spiritual Pivot* Chapter 1.

20 Quoted in *Chinese Acupuncture and Moxibustion*, Foreign Languages Press, Beijing.

21 This appears to be a modern name and it is difficult to find any reference to this method of point combination in older sources.

22 *Spiritual Pivot* Chapter 51.

23 *Classic of Difficulties* 67th Difficulty.

24 *Essential Questions* Chapter 5.

25 *Classic of Difficulties* 67th Difficulty.

26 *Classic of Difficulties* 67th Difficulty.

27 *Classic of Difficulties* 45th Difficulty.

28 *Spiritual Pivot* Chapter 33.

29 *Classic of Difficulties* 45th Difficulty.

30 *Classic of Difficulties* 29th Difficulty.

31 *Classic of Difficulties* 29th Difficulty.

32 *Spiritual Pivot* Chapter 33.

33 They are listed, for example, in Felix Mann's *Treatment of Disease by Acupuncture* although no further information is given.

34 *Spiritual Pivot* Chapter 21.

35 *Yellow Emperor's Inner Classic*, Tianjing Scientific Publications, 1989, p195.

36 *Yellow Emperor's Inner Classic*, Tianjing Scientific Publications, 1989, p24.

37 In the *Spiritual Pivot* Tianrong was classified as a point of the Gall Bladder channel, whilst in the *Systematic Classic of Acupuncture and Moxibustion* it was listed as belonging to the Sanjiao channel. It was not until the 10th century classic *Necessities of a Frontier Official*, that Tianrong was finally ascribed to the Small Intestine channel.

MEETING POINTS OF THE CHANNELS

	Lung	Large Intestine	Stomach	Spleen	Heart	Small Intestine	Bladder	Kidney	Pericardium	Sanjiao	Gall Bladder	Liver	Conception v.	Governing v.	Yang Linking v.	Yin Linking v.	Yang Motility v.	Yin Motility v.	Penetrating v.	Girdling v.
LU-1	●			●																
L.I.-14		●				●	●													
L.I.-15		●															●			
L.I.-16		●															●			
L.I.-20		●	●																	
ST-1			●										●				●			
ST-3			●														●			
ST-4		●	●										●				●			
ST-7			●								●									
ST-8			●								●				●					
ST-9			●								●									
ST-12		●	●			●				●	●									
ST-30			●																●	
SP-6				●				●				●								
SP-12				●								●				●				
SP-13				●								●				●				
SP-15				●												●				
SP-16				●												●				
SI-10						●	●								●		●			
SI-12		●				●				●	●									
SI-18						●				●										
SI-19						●				●	●									
BL-1			●			●	●			●	●			●			●	●		
BL-11						●	●			●	●			●						
BL-12							●							●						
BL-31							●				●									
BL-32							●				●									
BL-33							●				●									
BL-34							●				●									
BL-41						●	●													

	Lung	Large Intestine	Stomach	Spleen	Heart	Small Intestine	Bladder	Kidney	Pericardium	Sanjiao	Gall Bladder	Liver	Conception v.	Governing v.	Yang Linking v.	Yin Linking v.	Yang Motility v.	Yin Motility v.	Penetrating v.	Girdling v.
BL-59							●										●			
BL-61							●										●			
BL-62							●										●			
BL-63							●								●					
KID-9								●										●		
KID-11								●											●	
KID-12								●											●	
KID-13								●											●	
KID-14								●											●	
KID-15								●											●	
KID-16								●											●	
KID-17								●											●	
KID-18								●											●	
KID-19								●											●	
KID-20								●											●	
KID-21								●											●	
P-1									●	●	●	●								
SJ-13										●					●					
SJ-15										●	●				●					
SJ-17										●	●									
SJ-20						●				●	●									
SJ-22						●				●	●									
GB-1						●				●	●									
GB-3			●							●	●									
GB-4			●							●	●									
GB-5		●	●							●	●									
GB-6		●	●							●	●									
GB-7							●				●									
GB-8							●				●									
GB-9							●				●									

	Lung	Large Intestine	Stomach	Spleen	Heart	Small Intestine	Bladder	Kidney	Pericardium	Sanjiao	Gall Bladder	Liver	Conception v.	Governing v.	Yang Linking v.	Yin Linking v.	Yang Motility v.	Yin Motility v.	Penetrating v.	Girdling v.
GB-10							●				●									
GB-11						●	●			●	●									
GB-12							●				●									
GB-13											●				●					
GB-14		●	●							●	●				●					
GB-15							●				●				●					
GB-16											●				●					
GB-17											●				●					
GB-18											●				●					
GB-19											●				●					
GB-20										●	●				●		●			
GB-21			●							●	●				●					
GB-23							●				●									
GB-24				●							●									
GB-26											●									●
GB-27											●									●
GB-28											●									●
GB-29											●						●			
GB-30							●				●									
GB-35											●				●					
LIV-13											●	●								
LIV-14				●								●				●				
DU-1								●			●		●	●						
DU-13							●							●						
DU-14		●	●			●	●			●	●			●						
DU-15														●	●					
DU-16														●	●					
DU-17							●							●						
DU-20							●			●	●	●		●						
DU-24			●				●							●						

	Lung	Large Intestine	Stomach	Spleen	Heart	Small Intestine	Bladder	Kidney	Pericardium	Sanjiao	Gall Bladder	Liver	Conception v.	Governing v.	Yang Linking v.	Yin Linking v.	Yang Motility v.	Yin Motility v.	Penetrating v.	Girdling v.
DU-26		●	●											●						
DU-28			●										●	●						
REN-1													●	●					●	
REN-2												●	●							
REN-3				●				●				●	●							
REN-4				●				●				●	●							
REN-7								●					●						●	
REN-10				●									●							
REN-12			●			●				●			●							
REN-13			●			●							●							
REN-17				●		●		●		●			●							
REN-22													●			●				
REN-23													●			●				
REN-24		●	●										●	●						

POINT SELECTION METHODS

SELECTING LOCAL POINTS

Local points are those which lie over, on, or in close proximity to the diseased area. This is perhaps the most obvious method of point selection, yet one which is of great importance in acupuncture treatment, and it should not be dismissed, as it sometimes is, as simplistic or symptomatic. Examination of the classical combinations found in this text in fact demonstrates that the use of local points has always been a fundamental principle of acupuncture.

Local points are much used in treating disorders of the zangfu, the extraordinary fu and the sense organs. Examples include:

- Tianshu ST-25 or Shenque REN-8 for diarrhoea.
- Zhongwan REN-12 for nausea.
- Shanzhong REN-17 for tightness of the chest.
- Guilai ST-29 for diseases of the uterus.
- Yingxiang L.I.-20 for diseases of the nose.
- Jingming BL-1 for diseases of the eyes.
- Tinggong SI-19 for diseases of the ears.

Equally commonly, local points - whether channel points, extraordinary points or ahshi[1] points - are needled in most cases of pain, and careful palpation of the affected area, as well as detailed questioning, should be used to determine the channels or points affected. The principal exception to the use of local points is in cases of acute pain or sprain when the practitioner might require the patient to mobilise the affected area during needling; in this case local needling is obviously impractical and the selection of distal points is favoured.

SELECTING ADJACENT POINTS

Adjacent points are points located near the affected area. Examples include:

- Xuehai SP-10, Liangqiu ST-34 or Yinlingquan SP-9 for diseases of the knee joint.
- Binao L.I.-14 for diseases of the shoulder.
- Jianjing GB-21 or Tianzong SI-11 for diseases of the breast.
- Yangbai GB-14 or Fengchi GB-20 for diseases of the eyes.
- Waiguan SJ-5 for diseases of the wrist joint.

SELECTING DISTAL POINTS

The use of distal points is the most frequently used method in acupuncture treatment. The *Ode to Elucidate Mysteries* refers to the 'four origins and three ends'. The four origins are the extremities of the limbs, whilst the three ends are the head, chest and abdomen. Points on the limbs (the four origins), especially in the area between the elbows and fingers and the knees and toes, therefore, are among the most important points on the body, and have a wide application in treating disorders of the head, chest, abdomen (the three ends) and additionally the back. Indeed there is no point distal to the elbow or knee that does not have an effect on these regions. So important are the distal points that it is said in relation to the theory of root (ben) and manifestation (biao) that the root is the lower and the manifestation is the upper, i.e. in the context of the channels, the extremities of the limbs are the root, and the head, shoulder, back and chest are the manifestation.

The primary principle of selecting distal points is to choose a point from the involved channel. Thus, for example, distal points from shaoyang channel (Sanjiao and Gall Bladder) will be selected for temporal headache, distal points from yangming channel (Large Intestine and Stomach) will be chosen for pain of the face and forehead, distal points from taiyang channel (Bladder and Small Intestine) will be selected for occipital headache and pain, and points from the jueyin Liver channel will be selected for vertex headache. The selection of distal points requires a good knowledge of the channels, not only the superficial and deep pathways of the primary channels, but also the pathways of the luo-connecting, divergent and muscle channels. For example, Taichong LIV-3 is selected as a distal point for vertex headache because the internal pathway of the Liver channel ascends to the vertex to meet Baihui DU-20. Several distal points of the Liver channel, which winds around the genitals, can be selected for genital disorders, but Ligou LIV-5, the luo-connecting point is favoured due to the pathway of the Liver luo-connecting channel which also ascends to the genitals. The point Chengshan BL-57 is much used for haemorrhoids due to the pathway of the Bladder divergent channel to the anus. Points of the Stomach channel are frequently used to treat disturbance of the spirit, since the Stomach divergent channel connects with the Heart, and the Stomach primary channel ascends to meet with the Du Mai at Shenting DU-24 and Renzhong DU-26 and hence affects the brain.

In the treatment of pain and disorders both of the zangfu and channels, it is common practice to combine the use of local, adjacent and distal points. Examples include:

- Shuaigu GB-8, Fengchi GB-20 and Xiaxi GB-43 for temporal headache.
- Rugen ST-18, Qimen LIV-14 and Zulinqi GB-41 for breast diseases.
- Zhongwan REN-12, Shanzhong REN-17 and Zusanli ST-36 for Stomach diseases.
- Jianyu L.I.-15, Binao L.I.-14 and Hegu L.I.-4 for disorders of the anterior shoulder.
- Naoshu SI-10, Bingfeng SI-12 and Houxi SI-3 for disorders of the posterior shoulder.

There are numerous examples of this method in the classical combinations given in this text.

SELECTING PROXIMAL POINTS

In disorders of the extremities, there are by definition no distal points, and in such cases some proximal points may be used, for example:

- Kongzui LU-6, Zhizheng SI-7, Yangxi L.I.-5, Jianyu L.I.-15 and Waiguan SJ-5 all treat disorders of the fingers and hand.
- Feiyang BL-58 treats disorders of the toes.
- Xiajuxu ST-39, Chengjin BL-56 and Chengshan BL-57 treat disorders of the heel, feet and soles.

SELECTING POINTS BELOW TO TREAT ABOVE

The principle of selecting points from the lower part of the body to treat diseases of the upper body shares a common approach with the method of selecting distal points, and is one of the key aspects of point selection. The six yang primary channels either begin or terminate on the face, the qi of the six yin primary channels reaches the head via their divergent channels, and the extraordinary channels, with the exception of the Girdling vessel, all ascend to the head.

The human body, having the characteristics of warmth, activity and transformation is yang by nature, and suffers from a tendency for its qi and yang to rise excessively. The principle of drawing down excess by selecting points in the lower body is therefore widely used. This is reflected in the *Yellow Emperor's Inner Classic*[2] which says "When the disease is above select [points] from below". Without exception, the points of the twelve primary channels distal to the elbows and knees treat disorders of the head, chest and upper back, since the upper jiao is 'above', whilst the distal points of the arm and leg channels are 'below'. Some distal points of the arm channels treat the middle jiao (for example Neiguan P-6) but these are exceptions, and it is rather the points that lie below these regions, those distal to the knee, that generally need to be selected to treat disorders of the middle and lower jiao (upper and lower abdomen, mid and lower back). This basic theory helps to explain one of the apparent contraindications of acupuncture practice, which is that few points of the Large and Small Intestine channels treat intestinal disorders. Since these fu lie in the lower jiao, the most effective points to treat them lie on the lower limbs, and the Large and Small Intestines are ascribed lower he-sea points (Shangjuxu ST-37 and Xiajuxu ST-39 respectively).

SELECTING POINTS ABOVE TO TREAT BELOW

The full quotation from the *Yellow Emperor's Inner Classic* given above continues "... if the disease is below, select points above". Whilst also an important principle of point selection, the use of points in the upper part of the body to treat disorders below is relatively less common than its opposite. Examples include:

- Dicang ST-4 for atrophy disorder with inability to walk and swelling of the leg.
- Renying ST-9 for vomiting and lumbar pain.
- Shuaigu GB-8 for incessant vomiting and cold in the Stomach.
- Fubai GB-10 for pain of the shoulder and arm, inability to raise the arm and flaccidity of the leg with inability to walk.
- Fengfu DU-16 for numbness of the legs
- Baihui DU-20 for oppression of the Heart, palpitations, rectal prolapse and prolapse of the uterus.
- Renzhong DU-26 for stiffness, sprain and pain of the spine.
- Huantiao GB-30 or Biguan ST-31 for disorders of the whole leg.
- Jianyu L.I.-15 for disorders of the whole arm.

SELECTING POINTS FROM THE FRONT TO TREAT THE BACK AND VICE-VERSA

"Yin diseases travel through the yang region and yang diseases travel through the yin region. The mu points are situated in the yin region, they may be used to treat yang disease; the shu points are situated in the yang region, they may be used to treat yin diseases". *Classic of Difficulties*[3].

"When the qi [gathers] in the chest, to prevent [disease use points on either side of the] breast and the shu point on the back [Feishu BL-13]; when the qi [gathers] in the abdomen, to prevent [disease use] the shu point on the back [Pishu BL-20] ... '. *Spiritual Pivot*[4]

Points on the back (principally the back-shu points) are commonly selected to treat disorders of the front of the body, for example Feishu BL-13, Jueyinshu BL-14, Xinshu

BL-15 and Geshu BL-17 all treat pain or oppression of the chest, points Ganshu BL-18, Danshu BL-19, Pishu BL-20 and Weishu BL-21 all treat abdominal disorders etc. Equally, points on the front of the body may be selected to treat disorders in the back, for example

- Zhongfu LU-1, Qihu ST-13, Burong ST-19 and Shiguan KID-18 treat pain of the mid or upper back
- Shuidao ST-28, Qichong ST-30, Qixue KID-13, Zhongzhu KID-15, Zhangmen LIV-13, Guanyuan REN-4, Yinjiao REN-7 and Shuifen REN-9 treat disorders of the lumbar spine.

For this reason, one method of point selection emphasises combining points of the front and back, often the front-mu and back-shu points, for example Juque REN-14 and Xinshu BL-15 for disorders of the Heart, Tianshu ST-25 and Dachangshu BL-25 for disorders of the Large Intestine fu etc.

SELECTING POINTS IN THE CENTRE TO TREAT THE EXTREMITIES

The selection of points in the centre to treat the extremities is relatively less common than its opposite. However, a number of points may be used in this way, for example:

- Rugen ST-18 for swelling and pain of the arm.
- Daju ST-27 for loss of use of the four limbs and hemiplegia.
- Daheng SP-15 for inability to raise and move the four limbs.
- Zhangmen LIV-13 for inability to raise the arm.
- Yaoyangguan DU-3 for inability to flex and extend the knee, pain of the outer aspect of the knee and inability to walk.
- Mingmen DU-4 for cold painful obstruction of the hands and feet.
- Zhongji REN-3 for exhaustion of the four limbs.
- Guanyuan REN-4 for tremor of the hands.

SELECTING POINTS FROM ONE CHANNEL TO TREAT ITS INTERIORLY-EXTERIORLY RELATED CHANNEL

Examples of this method, most commonly observed in relation to the luo-connecting points, include:

- selecting Hegu L.I.-4 to assist the Lung function of distributing defensive qi.
- selecting Pianli L.I.-6 to promote the Lung function of regulating the water passages when this is impaired by exterior wind.
- selecting Fenglong ST-40 to resolve phlegm due to disharmony of the Spleen.
- selecting Zhizheng SI-7 to regulate and calm the spirit when the Heart is in disharmony.

SELECTING POINTS FROM ONE PAIR OF THE SIX CHANNELS TO TREAT DISEASE OF THE OTHER

Examples include:

- selecting Zhigou SJ-6 from the hand shaoyang Sanjiao channel to treat hypochondriac pain due to disharmony of the foot shaoyang Gall Bladder channel.
- selecting Neiguan P-6 from the hand jueyin Pericardium channel to resolve stagnation of qi in the foot jueyin Liver channel in the chest and hypochondrium.

SELECTING POINTS ACCORDING TO CHANNEL CONNECTIONS

Examples include

- selecting Zhongfu LU-1 to regulate the function of the Stomach and treat nausea and vomiting, since the Lung primary channel originates in the middle jiao.
- selecting points of the Stomach or Bladder channels to regulate the spirit since both their divergent channels pass through the Heart.
- selecting Touwei ST-8 to treat headaches of the forehead, vertex or occiput because of its status as a meeting point of the Stomach channel with the Gall Bladder channel and the Yang Linking vessel (which itself links all the yang channels of the body including the Governing vessel and Bladder channel which together rule the vertex).
- selecting Sanyinjiao SP-6, the intersection of the Spleen, Liver and Kidney channels, to treat most diseases of the lower abdomen since all these channels pass through this area.
- selecting Dazhui DU-14, the meeting point of the Governing vessel with all the yang primary channels to release pathogenic factors from the (yang) exterior.

CROSS NEEDLING

Generally speaking, points are selected unilaterally from the affected side of the body, or else needled bilaterally, However, since the channels run bilaterally it is not uncommon to select points from one side of the body to treat disorders on the opposite side.

This principle of contralateral needling is discussed in the *Spiritual Pivot* which says "Contralateral insertion, that is, if the left is affected, the right is treated, and if the right affected, the left is needled"[5]. The *Treatise on Contralateral Insertion* in the *Essential Questions* says "When evils invade the channels, if the left side is in excess, the disease occurs on the right side, and vice versa ... for these conditions, contralateral insertion should be used"[6]. Among classical examples of this method, the *Great Compendium of Acupuncture and Moxibustion* recommended needling left Dicang ST-4 for diseases of the right side of the face, and vice-versa, and needling left Dadun LIV-1 for right-sided shan disorder and vice-versa, and the *Methods of Acupuncture and Moxibustion from the Golden Mirror of Medicine* by Wu Qian specified that moxa should be applied to right Tongtian BL-7 for disorders of the left nostril and vice-versa.

In modern clinical practice, chronic hemiplegia (of over three to six months duration) is often treated by first reducing points on the healthy side, then reinforcing points on the affected side. Contralateral needling is also commonly used either when the affected side is too painful to treat, or when, after needling, one wants the patient to mobilise the painful area. For example in cases of tennis elbow, the healthy side might be needled whilst the patient exercises the affected elbow.

Another form of cross-needling emphasised in acute painful disorders, especially sprain, selects points from the ankle to treat the opposite wrist (and vice-versa), from the knee to treat the opposite elbow (and vice-versa) and from the hip to treat the opposite shoulder (and vice-versa). In this case, the six channel relationships are called upon, for example right Qiuxu GB-40, a point of the foot shaoyang channel on the ankle joint would be selected to treat pain or sprain of the wrist joint in the area of left Yangchi SJ-4, a point of the hand shaoyang channel. Among classical applications of this method, Chize LU -5 at the elbow was traditionally indicated for crane's knee wind (swelling and pain of the knee, with atrophy above and below the joint).

Finally it should be noted that some channels cross the body. Examples are the Large Intestine primary channel which crosses to the opposite side of the face at Renzhong DU-26, and the Large Intestine sinew channel which crosses over the top of the head to connect with the mandible on the opposite side. For this reason some practitioners prefer to needle right Hegu L.I.-4 for disorders of the left side of the face and vice-versa.

SELECTION OF EMPIRICAL POINTS

The classical and modern use of acupuncture points can frequently be explained by reference to the channel pathways and the status of the point (for example jing-well, shu-stream, xi-cleft, hui-meeting point etc.). Frequently, however, the selection of distal points is determined by their historically established empirical effect. Examples of empirical point applications include:

- Naohui SJ-13, Tianfu LU-3 and Binao L.I.-14 are all used in the treatment of goitre and scrofula. Whilst all three channels do ascend to the neck or throat region, there is no simple explanation why these points on the upper arm, rather than the more powerful and distal shu-points should have this action.
- Tiaokou ST-38 is an important distal point in the treatment of shoulder pain, even though the Stomach channel does not pass through the shoulder region.
- Lingtai DU-10 is an empirical point in the treatment of carbuncles and furuncles and clove sores, although there is no obvious theoretical explanation why this should be so.
- Lieque LU-7 has traditionally been emphasised for the treatment of headache, even though the Lung channel does not ascend higher than the throat.
- Wangu SI-4 is traditionally indicated for jaundice, although there is no obvious theoretical explanation why this should be so.
- Waiqiu GB-36 was indicated for rabies in the *Illustrated Classic of Acupuncture Points on the Bronze Man* .

CHAIN AND LOCK POINT ASSOCIATION METHOD

The chain and lock point association method refers to the selection of points from the shoulder, elbow and hand or wrist to treat disorders of the upper limb and from the hip, knee and ankle to treat disorders of the lower limb. It is frequently used in the treatment of atrophy disorder and hemiplegia when points are primarily selected from yangming channels. Commonly, therefore, Jianyu L.I.-15, Quchi L.I.-11 and Hegu L.I.-4 are combined to treat the upper limbs, and Biguan ST-31, Zusanli ST-36 and Jiexi ST-41 for the lower limb. The method is not, however, confined to yangming channels, and a similar approach would combine Naoshu SI-10, Xiaohai SI-8 and Houxi SI-3 for pain of the posterior shoulder, or Chengfu BL-36, Weizhong BL-40 and Kunlun BL-60 for pain of the buttock and posterior leg.

ALTERNATING POINTS

When acupuncture is given frequently, for example in the treatment of hemiplegia following windstroke, or for any chronic and intractable disease, it is common practice to alternate points or point prescriptions to avoid over-stimulation of or damage to points. Thus, Jianyu L.I.-15, Quchi L.I.-11 and Hegu L.I.-4 may be substituted by Jianliao SJ-14, Shousanli L.I.-10 and Yangchi SJ-4 in the treatment of atrophy disorder of the arm, or Biguan ST-31, Zusanli ST-36 and Jiexi ST-41 may be substituted by Huantiao GB-30, Yanglingquan GB-34 and Qiuxu GB-40 for atrophy disorder of the leg. Similarly suitable points may be divided into two alternating prescriptions, one from the front and one from the back, for example in cases of epigastric pain due to attack on the Stomach by Liver qi,

Zhongwan REN-12, Zusanli ST-36, Qimen LIV-14 and Taichong LIV-3 may be alternated with Weishu BL-21, Ganshu BL-18, Yanglingquan GB-34 and Neiguan P-6.

POINT COMBINATIONS

Much space has been given in this text to point combinations from classical texts. Some of these combinations have a quite modern feel to them, in other words they might regularly be seen in use in clinical practice today. Others use what may seem to be obscure and unusual points from a current-day perspective.

It is well understood in Chinese herbal medicine that herbs in combination act synergistically, in other words that the sum effect of their combination is quite different from the sum of the actions and indications of the individual constituents. In the history of acupuncture, it is clear that a somewhat similar view was held. The majority of acupuncturists throughout the history of China were itinerant formula doctors[7] who memorised acupuncture prescriptions that were handed down in family lineages. These doctors often tended to specialise in the treatment of specific complaints, and the great acupuncture classics (for example the *Great Compendium of Acupuncture and Moxibustion*) were in part compilations of such acupuncture prescriptions, collected from the length and breadth of China. Many of these prescriptions appeared in early classical compilations and are found repeated in later classical sources. Some are still famous today, for example "Little sweating: reinforce Hegu L.I.-4, reduce Fuliu KID-7; much sweating: first reduce Hegu L.I.-4 then reinforce Fuliu KID-7"[8]. Many others have been forgotten. Some classical prescriptions seem well balanced, mixing local and distal points from the upper and lower body, for example "Head wind and dizziness: Fenglong ST-40, Hegu L.I.-4, Jiexi ST-41 and Fengchi GB-20"[9]. Others seem very unbalanced, for example "Vomiting with fullness of the chest: Shencang KID-25, Shufu KID-27, Lingxu KID-24 and Juque REN-14"[10].

Of course, whenever a practitioner selects a number of points to treat any patient, they by definition use a prescription of points, whether a classical one, a modern one as found in one of the current acupuncture texts on the treatment of disease, or one of their own choosing. Many factors go into the making of such a prescription. Some of these include:

- combining points from the upper and lower body.
- combining points from the left and right sides of the body.
- combining points from the front and back of the body.
- combining points to treat the root of the disorder and points to treat the manifestation.
- combining points from yin channels and points from yang channels.
- combining points from one channel with points from its interiorly-exteriorly coupled channel.
- combining points from one channel with points from its coupled channel according to six channel theory.

In clinical practice, when treating a long-standing disease, a patient may report that one point prescription, for example comprising points from the front of the body, seems to have a better effect than points from the back (or vice-versa). Sometimes a subtle change of point prescription will bring about a significant change or improvement. There are no hard and fast rules in the making of a point prescription.

It is the intention of this book to provide the practitioner with the maximum amount of information on the points in order to facilitate the best possible point prescription, and to give consideration and respect to the classical prescriptions which have stood the test of considerable periods of time.

NOTES

1 Ahshi points: points of local tenderness found on palpation which may, or may not, be regular acupuncture points. They are needled according to the concept that where there is pain, there is an acupuncture points.

2 *Spiritual Pivot* Chapter 9 and *Essential Questions* Chapter 70.

3 *Classic of Difficulties* 67th Difficulty.

4 *Spiritual Pivot* Chapter 52.

5 *Spiritual Pivot* Chapter 7.

6 *Essential Questions* Chapter 63.

7 According to Bob Flaws in Thoughts on Acupuncture, Internal Medicine and TCM in the West', *The Journal of Chinese Medicine*, Number 38, January 1992.

8 The *Great Compendium of Acupuncture & Moxibustion*.

9 The *Great Compendium of Acupuncture & Moxibustion*.

10 *Thousand Ducat Formulas*.

POINT LOCATION AND NEEDLING

CUN MEASUREMENTS

The human body has traditionally been measured according to proportional units known as cun. The cun measurement system is indispensable in accurate location of the acupuncture points. Since it is a proportional measurement system it is equally applicable to adults or children and to thin or obese subjects.

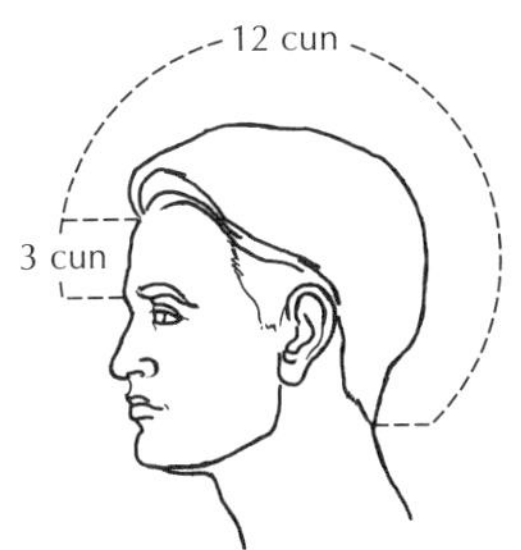

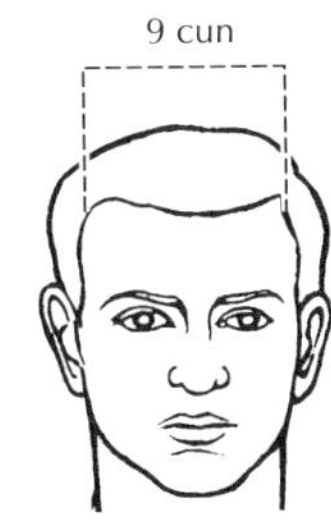

- The distance between the anterior and posterior hairlines is 12 cun.
- The distance between the glabella and the anterior hairline is 3 cun.
- The distance between the angles of the hairline is 9 cun.

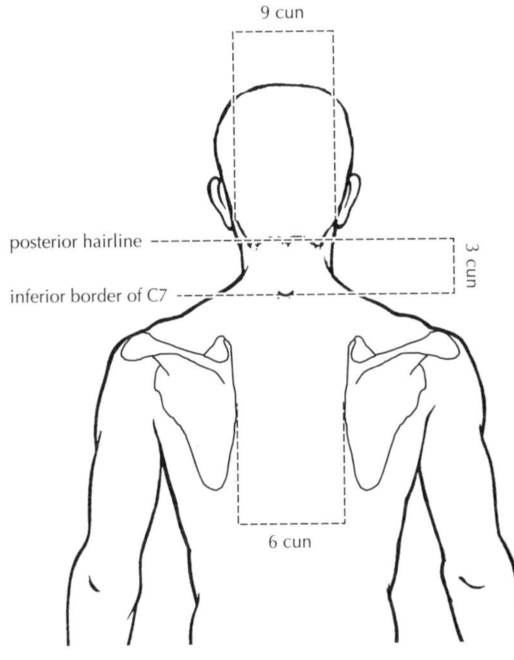

- The distance between the mastoid processes is 9 cun.
- The distance between the posterior hairline and the inferior border of the spinous process of C7 is 3 cun.
- The distance between the medial borders of the scapulae is 6 cun.

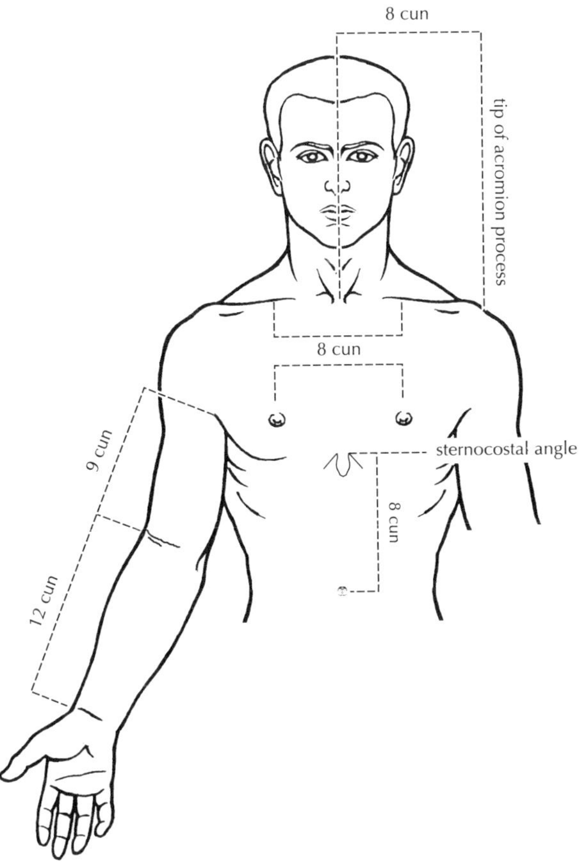

- The distance between the nipples is 8 cun.
- The distance between the midpoint of the clavicles is 8 cun.
- The distance between the tip of the acromion process and the midline of the body is 8 cun.
- The distance between the anterior axillary and cubital creases is 9 cun.
- The distance between the cubital crease and the wrist creases is 12 cun.
- The distance between the sternocostal angle and the umbilicus is 8 cun.

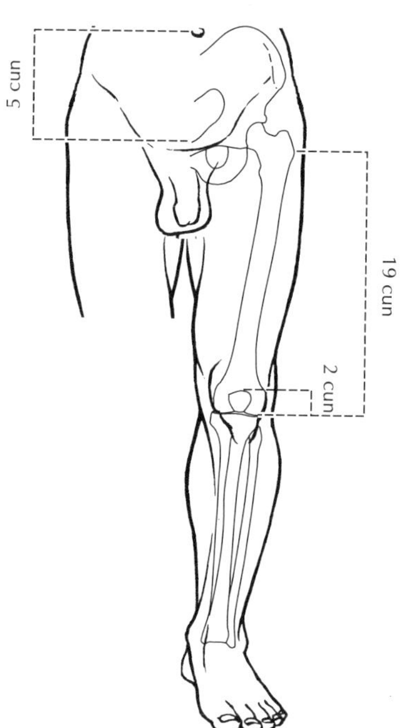

- The distance between the umbilicus and the pubic symphysis is 5 cun.
- The distance between the lateral prominence of the greater trochanter (approximately level with the inferior border of the pubic symphysis) and the popliteal crease is 19 cun.
- The height of the patella is 2 cun.

- The distance between the gluteal fold and the knee is 14 cun.
- The distance between the popliteal crease and the lateral malleolus is 16 cun.
- The distance between the popliteal crease and the medial malleolus is 15 cun.

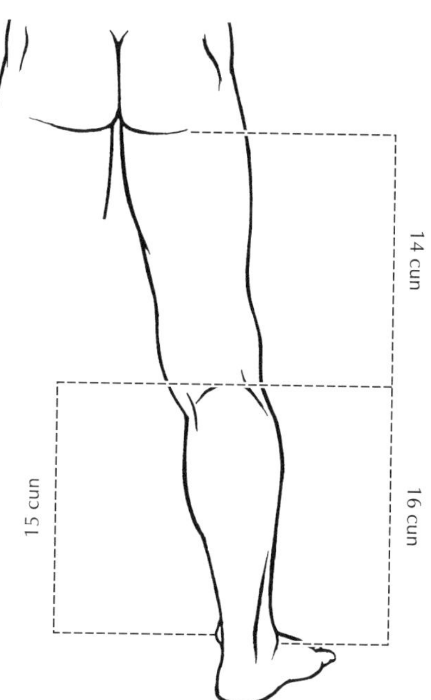

QUICK MEASUREMENTS

Generally speaking it is most accurate to locate points by using the above system of measurements. In practice, however, experienced practitioners often use hand measurements as follows. It is important to remember that it is the dimensions of the subject's hand, rather than the practitioner's, that should be used.

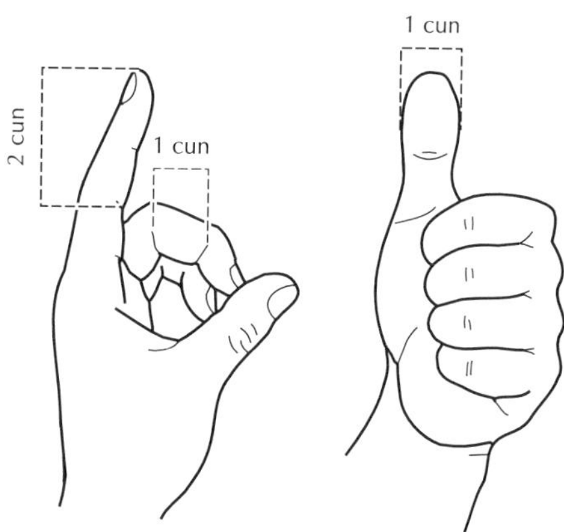

- The distance between the ends of the creases of the interphalangeal joints of the middle finger at their widest point is 1 cun.
- The distance between the proximal interphalangeal joint and the tip of the index finger is 2 cun.
- The width of the interphalangeal joint of the thumb is 1 cun.

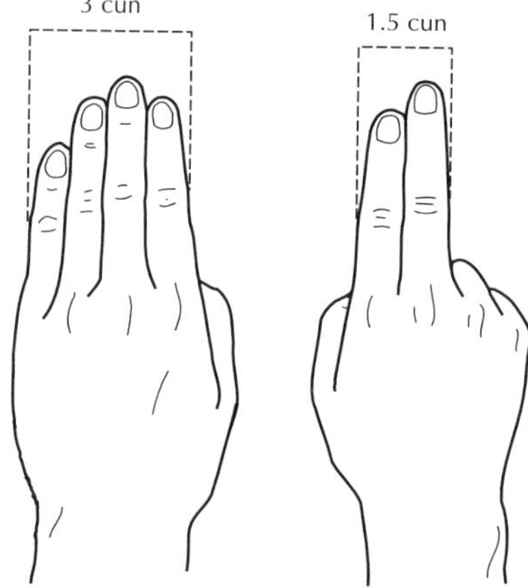

- The width of the four fingers held close together at the level of the dorsal skin crease of the proximal interphalangeal joint of the middle finger is 3 cun.
- The width of the index and middle fingers held close together at the level of the dorsal skin crease of the proximal interphalangeal joint of the middle finger is 1.5 cun.

NEEDLING

The needling directions used in this text are:

- Perpendicular: this denotes a 90 degree angle to the skin surface.
- Oblique: this denotes a 45 degree angle to the skin surface.
- Perpendicular-oblique: this denotes an angle of approximately 70 degrees to the skin surface.
- Transverse: this denotes an insertion parallel to the skin surface, through the subcutaneous tissue, after the dermal layer has been penetrated.
- Transverse-oblique: this denotes an angle of approximately 20 degrees to the skin surface.

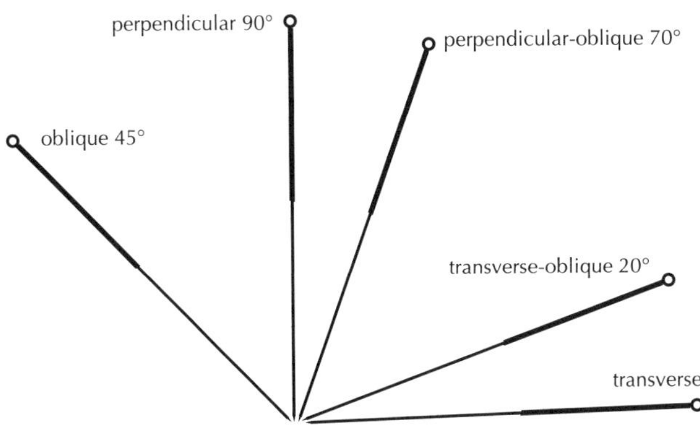

It is important to note that the needling directions are always relative to the skin surface rather than to absolute horizontal. For example when needling a point such as Zulinqi GB-41, the needle is inserted perpendicular to the skin surface, which may be at a 70 degree angle to the plane of the plantar surface of the foot.

DEPTH OF NEEDLING

The avoidance of injury is a fundamental principle of acupuncture in practice. Excessively deep needling or needling into major vessels or visceral organs can cause significant harm to the patient, and every care should be taken to prevent this happening. There is no substitute for clinical practice under expert supervision during the acupuncturist's training period. Increased safety and confidence will come with competent training. If in doubt, err on the side of caution. Every care has been taken in this text to recommend needling depths and points of caution in order to minimise risk. At the same time, where deeper needling is safe we have had no hesitation in recommending it, since it can make a significant difference to clinical outcome.

The following important cautions should be borne in mind:

Avoidance of pneumothorax

Perpendicular or deep oblique needling should not be used anywhere over the thoracic cavity, whether on the chest, back or supraclavicular area. This is in order to avoid the risk of pneumothorax. Pneumothorax should be considered a possibility if any of the following symptoms occur: chest pain, chest tightness, cough or shortness of breath. A substantial pneumothorax will also result in tachycardia, hypotension, excessive sweating or impaired consciousness. Pneumothorax constitutes a medical emergency and expert assistance should be summoned in any case where this is suspected. It is important to note that the clinical effects of pneumothorax can be delayed, and the same procedures should be adopted if a patient reports any of the above symptoms within a few hours of needling.

Needling the abdomen

Whilst in Chinese practice it is not considered problematic to needle into the peritoneal cavity, the approach followed in this text is to avoid penetration into the peritoneal cavity, and needle depths for points on the abdomen have been recommended with this in mind. However, the practitioner must use their discretion when needling thin or emaciated patients or children.

Needling close to major organs

Where acupuncture points lie over or close to major organs, this is specified in the text, and greater caution should be applied when needling such points. The relevant organs are the pleura, lungs, heart, liver, spleen, kidneys and bladder. The following illustrations show the location of these organs.

The pleura exists in two layers: i. the parietal pleura covers the inside of the thoracic cavity, including the upper surface of the diaphragm and the lateral surfaces of the mediastinum (containing the heart and great vessels), and ii. the visceral pleura covers each lung separately. The pleural cavity is the potential space that exists between these two layers. Penetration of this space either with or without penetration of underlying lung tissue may induce a pneumothorax. The pleural cavity extends from the supraclavicular fossa superiorly, down to the eighth rib in the mid-clavicular line, to the tenth rib in the mid-axillary line, and to the twelfth rib at the lateral border of the erector spinae muscles. Anteriorly the two pleural reflections (right and left) extend more or less to the midline behind the sternum. Posteriorly the two pleural

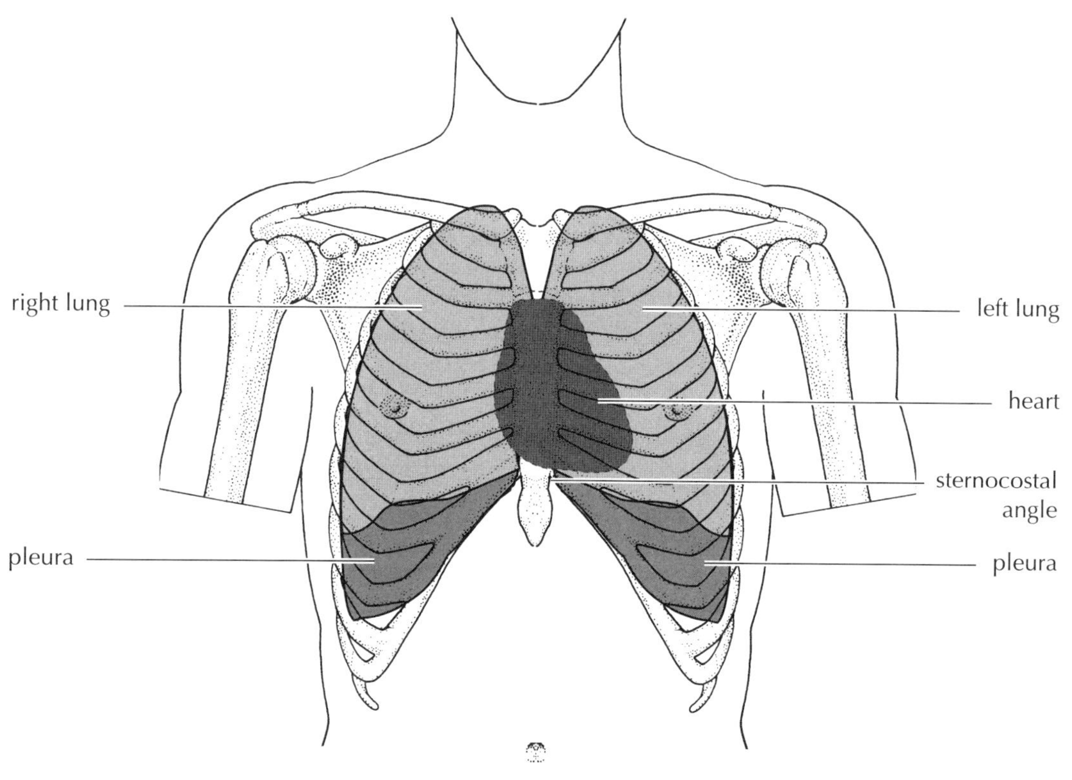
right lung
left lung
heart
sternocostal angle
pleura
pleura

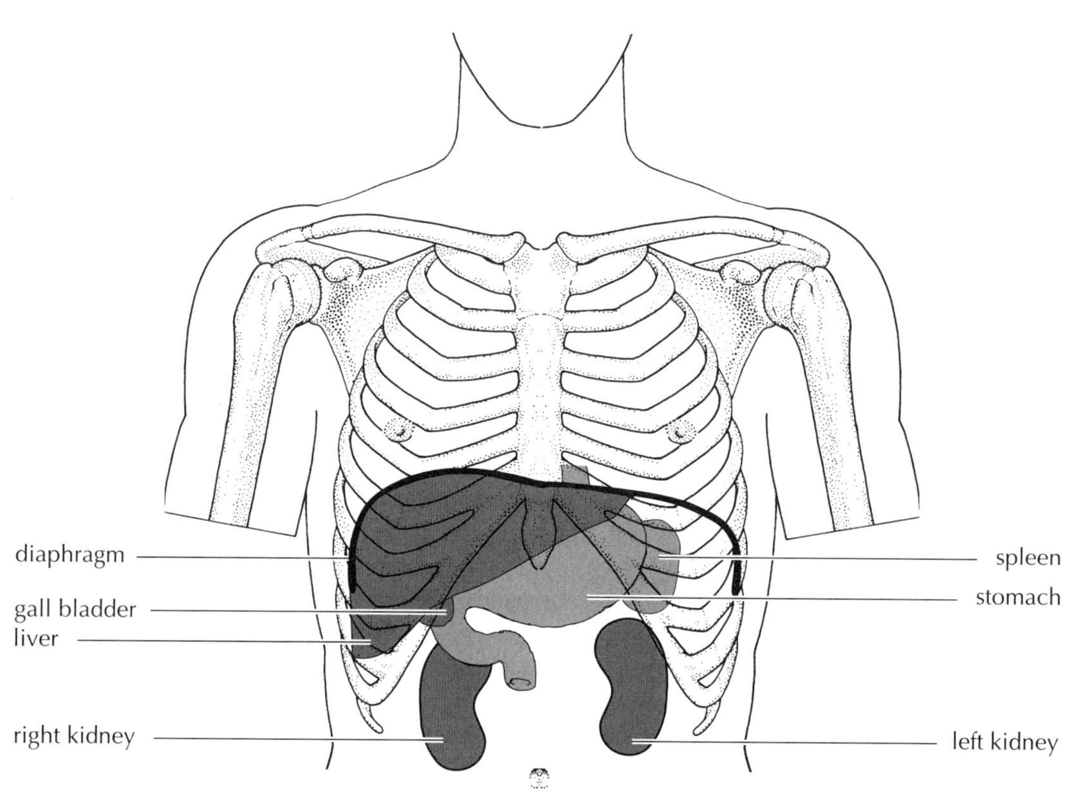
diaphragm
spleen
gall bladder
stomach
liver
right kidney
left kidney

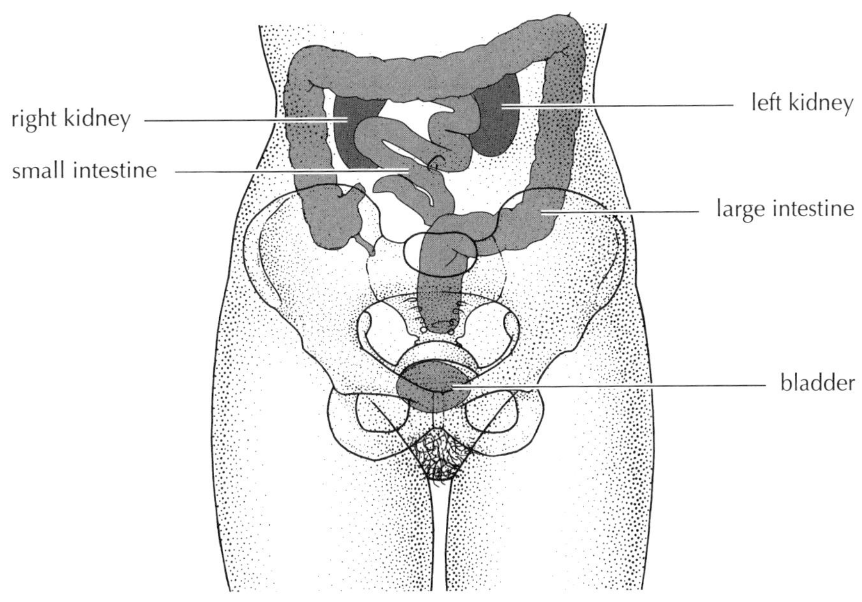
right kidney
small intestine
left kidney
large intestine
bladder

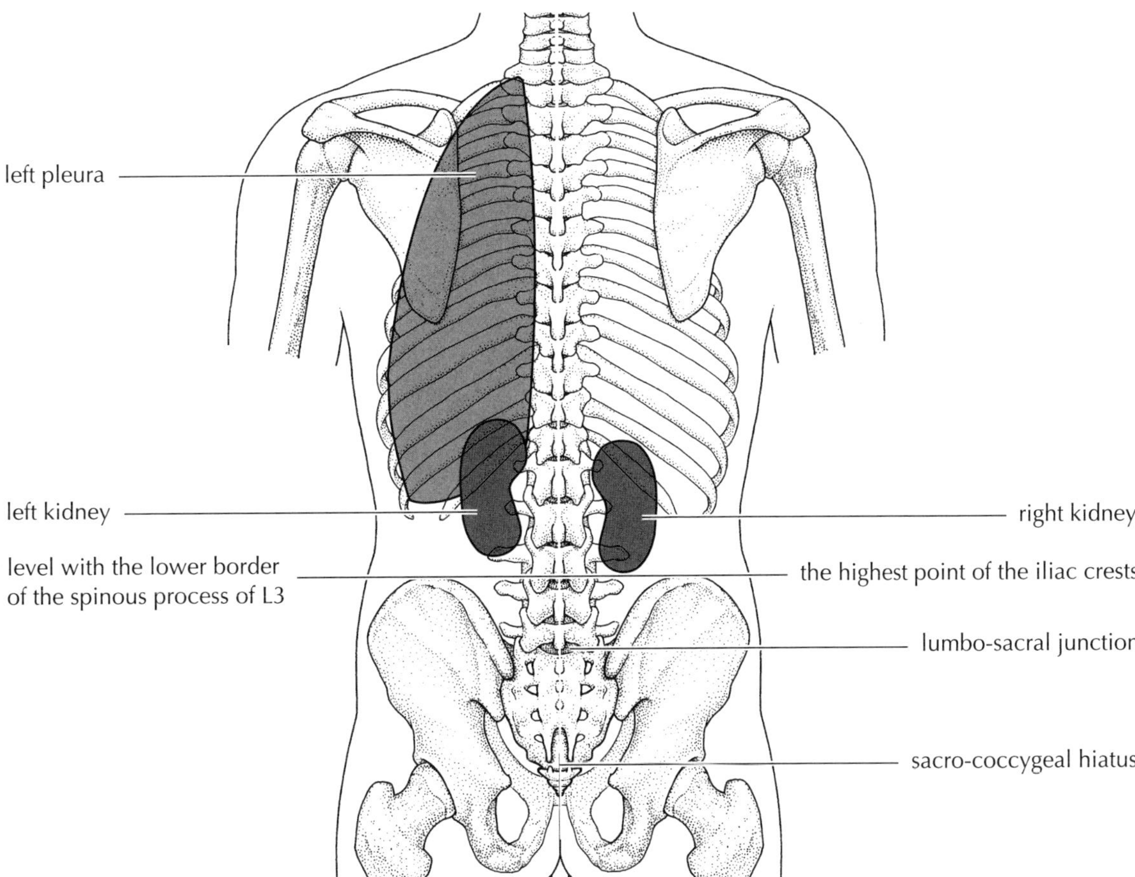
left pleura
left kidney
right kidney
level with the lower border
of the spinous process of L3
the highest point of the iliac crests
lumbo-sacral junction
sacro-coccygeal hiatus

reflections run vertically alongside the thoracic vertebral bodies from T1 extending down to T12. Essentially, any points lying over the thoracic cage if needled injudiciously have the potential to induce pneumothorax. For advice on which specific points may cause a pneumothorax please consult the cautionary advice given in the needling instruction.

The lung organ itself extends from the supraclavicular fossa to fill the pleural cavities as far as the diaphragm. The level of the lower border of the lung varies according to the stage of respiration. In the resting position, this level lies two rib spaces above the pleural reflection anteriorly, medially and laterally.

The cardiac outline extends from the second to the sixth intercostal spaces, and from the right parasternal area across almost to the left mamillary line. The inferior surface of the heart rests on the diaphragm and particularly if the heart is enlarged, it is possible with deep needling to damage the heart muscle using acupuncture points in the epigastric area (e.g. Juque REN-14, Jiuwei REN-15, Youmen KID-21, Burong ST-19).

The liver is situated under the diaphragm, in the right subcostal area, and extends across the midline in the epigastric area. If enlarged, it emerges below the costal margin on the right side, and also extends more widely into the epigastric area.

The spleen lies beneath the ninth, tenth and eleventh ribs on the left side of the abdominal cavity, deep to the postero-lateral aspect of the ribcage. If the spleen enlarges, it extends anteriorly and inferiorly, and the tip emerges beneath the left costal margin at the front, and in extreme cases it may extend as far as the right iliac fossa.

The kidneys lie on the posterior abdominal wall, deep to the paravertebral muscles, between the twelfth thoracic and the third lumbar vertebrae. For this reason, Bladder channel points above Qihaishu BL-24 should be needled obliquely towards the spine rather than perpendicularly.

The bladder lies behind the pubic symphysis, and if full it will extend upwards into the hypogastric area, possibly as far as Guanyuan REN-4. It is advisable to ask the patient to empty their bladder prior to needling in this area.

Needling close to major blood vessels
Where acupuncture points lie over or close to major blood vessels, this is specified in the text. In general, the risk of penetration of blood vessels can be minimised by paying attention to the sensation induced by needle insertion. Whilst the desired sensation of the arrival of qi (deqi) is characterised chiefly by heaviness, numbness or aching, penetration of blood vessels is likely to result in sharp and painful sensations (more so for arteries than veins). If this happens, it is advisable to withdraw the needle, re-check the location of the point, and re-insert the needle in a different direction with caution. If on withdrawal of a needle significant bleeding is evident (either under the skin or through the skin) then pressure should be applied with a cotton wool ball. In the case of venous bleeding (generally slower and darker haemorrhage), pressure should be applied for one minute. In the case of arterial bleeding (generally more rapid and brighter-red haemorrhage), pressure should be applied for a minimum of three minutes.

Needling close to major nerves
Where acupuncture points lie over or close to major nerves, this is specified in the text, and greater caution should be applied when needling such points. The risk of damage to nerves can be minimised by paying attention to the sensation induced by needle insertion. Whilst an electric sensation is considered an acceptable form of arrival of qi sensation (deqi), it does indicate direct stimulation of a nerve, and further manipulation should be avoided. It is not generally necessary to withdraw the needle should this occur.

SURFACE ANATOMY

How to locate and count the ribs

- The ribs are best counted downwards from the second rib, the costal cartilage of which is level with the palpable sternal angle.
- To locate the free end of the eleventh rib, place the entire hand on the upper abdomen and with gentle finger pressure palpate downwards along the costal margin, until the end of the rib is located just above the level of the umbilicus. Maintaining contact with the whole hand will help reduce hypersensitivity. To locate the free end of the twelfth rib, continue to palpate along the inferior margin of the ribcage until the free end is palpated in the lateral lumbar region.

How to locate C7
Run your finger down the neck along the midline. The first palpable vertebral spinous process is that of C6; if the subject extends their neck, this process becomes impalpable. The next vertebra down is C7 which is much more readily palpable, and remains palpable on extension of

the neck. Ask the subject to prop themselves up on their elbows and rotate their neck from side to side. This vertebra will be felt to rotate slightly. T1, which is the most prominent vertebra at the base of the neck, will not be felt to move on rotation of the neck. The vertebrae from T1 to approximately T9 are counted downwards from C7.

How to locate L3 and L5

Place the hands at the sides of the pelvis and feel the highest point of the iliac crests; the line connecting these two points is level with the lower border of the spinous process of L3. To locate the lumbo-sacral junction (inferior to L5) count two intervertebral spaces down from the lower border of L3. Alternatively run your finger up the back of the sacrum into the first palpable intervertebral space. The lumbo-sacral junction is generally felt as a pronounced depression.

To facilitate location of points of the lumbo-sacral region, it is helpful to place a pillow under the subject's lower abdomen. This will serve to open up the intervertebral spaces and is more comfortable for the subject.

Note that in some subjects, the first sacral vertebra becomes 'lumbarised', i.e. it separates from the rest of the sacrum and is hence palpable as an additional lumbar vertebra. In other cases, the fifth lumbar vertebra becomes 'sacralised', i.e. it fuses with the rest of the sacrum.

The vertebrae from L4 to T10 are generally counted upwards from L5.

How to locate the sacral foramina

The sacral foramina are not always easy to locate. There are, however, some helpful guidelines

First locate the lumbo-sacral junction and the sacro-coccygeal hiatus at the midline. Divide this line into five equal spaces using the four fingertips of one hand. Each fingertip should then lie on one of the four sacral spinous processes which are sometimes palpable. The foramina lie lateral to the processes, at the same level, and at approximately half the distance (i.e. 0.75 cun) between the midline and the Bladder back-shu point line. Note that the line of the sacral foramina runs slightly towards the midline as it descends. Note also that the foramina may be palpable in some subjects, and that pressure applied to them may induce a deqi sensation (slight tingling etc.).

The second sacral foramen lies at approximately the midpoint of a line drawn between the posterior superior iliac spine and the sacro-coccygeal hiatus.

The inner Bladder back-shu point line

All the back-shu points are defined as lying 1.5 cun lateral to the midline. In practice, however, they are located on the line which runs along the highest points of the paraspinal muscles. Their actual distance from the spine therefore varies somewhat, being shorter in the upper thoracic, lower lumbar and sacral regions, and longer in the mid-thoracic region.

How to locate the sternocostal angle

Many of the points of the upper abdomen are located using the sternocostal angle (xiphi-sternal junction) as a reference point. In order to locate the sternocostal angle, run the forefinger upwards along the lower margin of the ribcage into the depression immediately below the solid bony part of the sternum. It is here that the cartilaginous xiphoid process meets the bony sternum. The xiphoid process can vary in size substantially and may either be visible and palpable, or invisible and impalpable. In older individuals, the xiphoid may calcify and hence it is important not to confuse the lower level of the sternum with the lower level of the xiphoid process.

Palmaris longus

This tendon is absent in one or both arms in approximately 20% of subjects. In the absence of the palmaris longus tendon, locate points of the Pericardium channel on the ulnar side of the tendon of flexor carpi radialis.

手太陰肺經

THE LUNG CHANNEL OF HAND TAIYIN

THE LUNG CHANNEL OF HAND TAIYIN

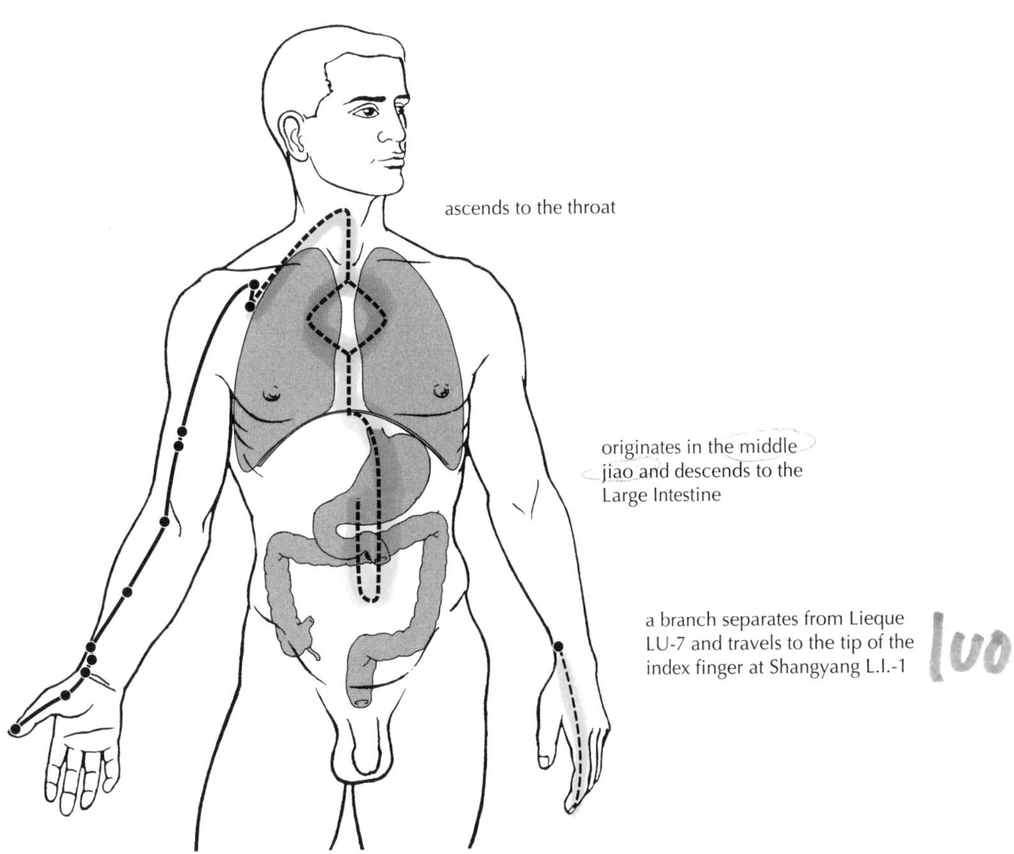

The Lung primary channel

THE LUNG PRIMARY CHANNEL

- originates in the middle jiao, in the region of the Stomach,
- descends to connect with the Large Intestine,
- returns upwards to pass the cardiac orifice of the Stomach and traverses the diaphragm,
- penetrates the Lung,
- ascends to the throat region,
- passes obliquely downwards towards Zhongfu LU-1 where the channel emerges,
- ascends one rib space to Yunmen LU-2 in the centre of the hollow of the delto-pectoral triangle,
- descends along the antero-lateral aspect of the upper arm, lateral to the Heart and Pericardium channels, to the cubital fossa of the elbow at Chize LU-5,
- passes along the antero-lateral aspect of the forearm towards the styloid process of the radius,
- follows the lateral border of the radial artery to the wrist at Taiyuan LU-9,
- traverses the thenar eminence to terminate at the radial side of the thumbnail at Shaoshang LU-11.
- a branch separates from the main channel at Lieque LU-7, at the styloid process, and travels directly to the radial side of the tip of the index finger, where it links with the Large Intestine channel at Shangyang L.I.-1.

The Lung primary channel connects with the following zangfu: Stomach, Large Intestine, Lung.

The Lung primary channel meets with other channels at the following points: None.

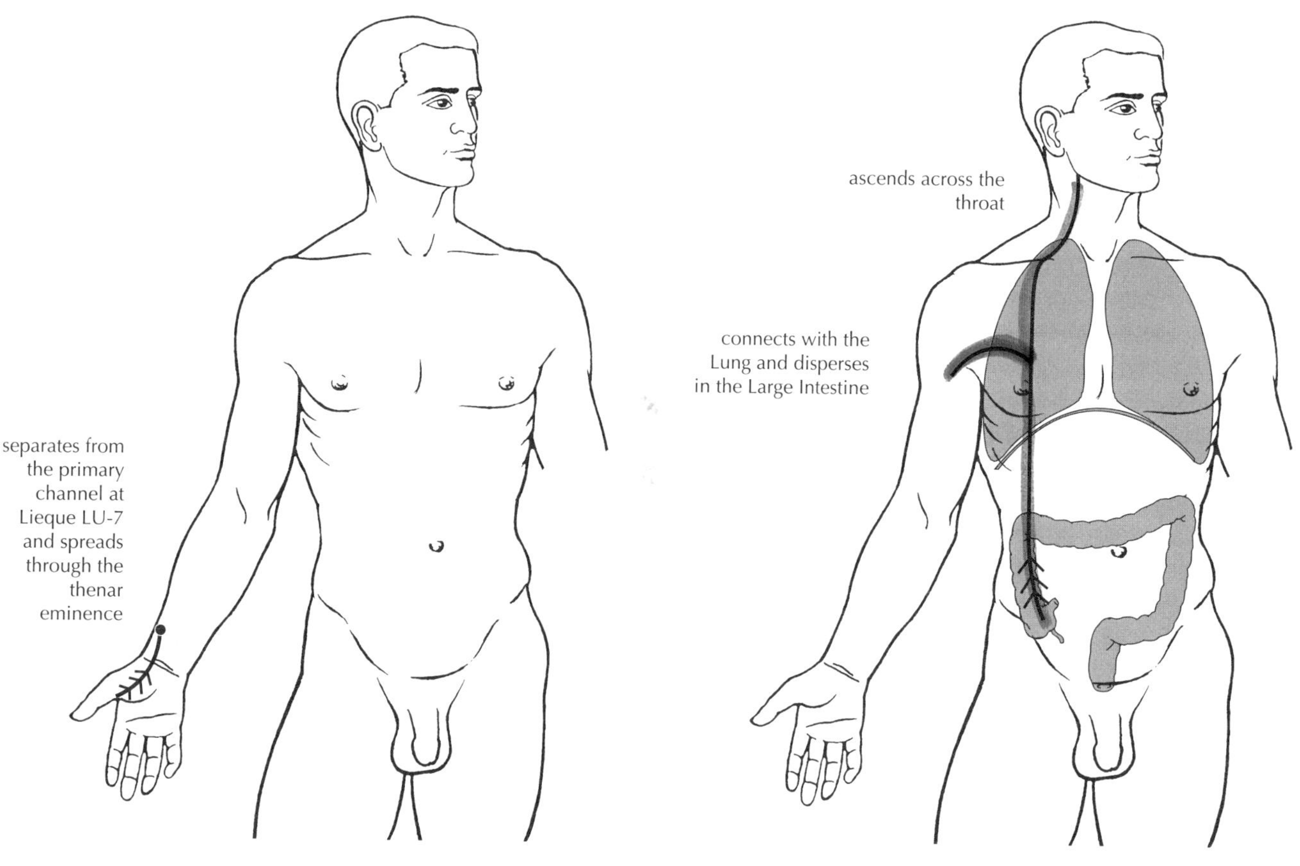

The Lung luo-connecting channel

The Lung divergent channel

THE LUNG LUO-CONNECTING CHANNEL

- separates from the Lung primary channel at Lieque LU-7,
- follows the Lung channel into the palm and spreads through the thenar eminence,
- connects with the Lung channel's interiorly-exteriorly related Large Intestine channel.

THE LUNG DIVERGENT CHANNEL

- diverges from the Lung primary channel at the axilla and passes anterior to the Heart channel in the chest,
- connects with the Lung and disperses in the Large Intestine,
- a branch ascends from the Lung, emerges at the supraclavicular fossa, ascends across the throat and converges with the Large Intestine channel.

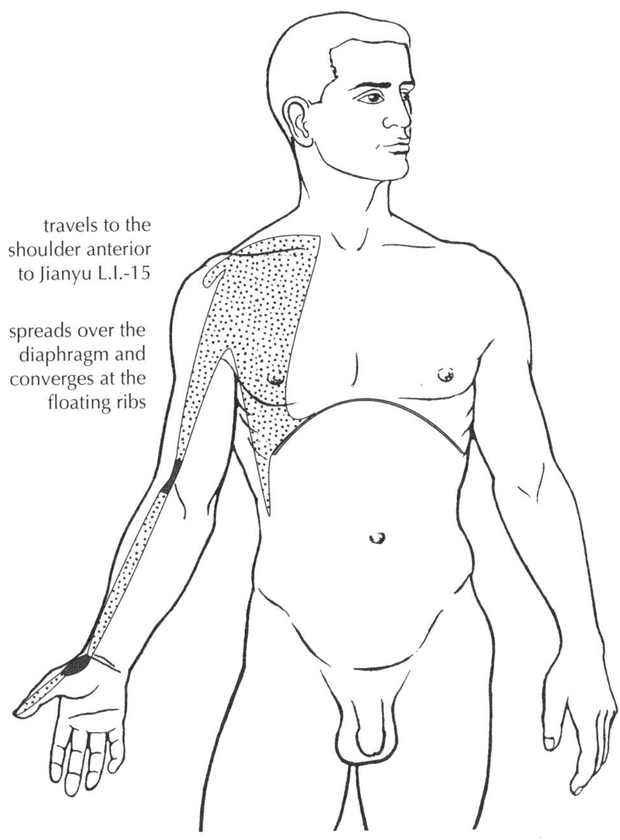

The Lung sinew channel

THE LUNG SINEW CHANNEL

- originates on the thumb at Shaoshang LU-11 and ascends to bind at the thenar eminence,
- follows the radial pulse and ascends the flexor aspect of the forearm to bind at the centre of the elbow,
- continues along the antero-lateral aspect of the upper arm to enter the chest below the axilla,
- emerges in the region of Quepen ST-12 and travels laterally to the shoulder, anterior to L.I.-15,
- returns to the supraclavicular (Quepen ST-12) region and descends into the chest,
- spreads over the diaphragm and converges in the region of the floating ribs.

Pathological symptoms of the Lung sinew channel

Cramping and pain along the course of the channel. When severe there is accumulation of lumps below the right lateral costal region, tension along the lateral costal region and spitting of blood.

DISCUSSION

The Lung channel of hand taiyin is interiorly-exteriorly coupled with the Large Intestine channel, and paired with the Spleen channel according to six channel theory. The Lung-Large Intestine relationship is further strengthened by the fact that:

- the interior pathway of the Lung primary channel descends to the Large Intestine fu.
- a branch of the Lung primary channel separates from Lieque LU-7 to connect with Shangyang L.I.-1.
- the Lung luo-connecting channel connects with the Large Intestine channel.
- the Lung divergent channel descends to the Large Intestine fu and connects with the Large Intestine channel in the neck.

In addition, it is helpful to note that:

- the Lung primary channel originates in the middle jiao in the region of the Stomach.
- the Lung primary and divergent channels ascend to the throat.
- the Lung channel does not connect directly with the nose, but does so indirectly via the Large Intestine channel.

The Lung has five principal functions:

- governing qi and controlling respiration.
- controlling disseminating and descending.
- regulating the water passages.
- controlling the skin and body hair.
- opening into the nose.

It is by virtue of these functions, as well as the channel pathways discussed above, that many of the actions and indications of the points of the Lung channel can be explained. These can be summarised as:

- treating rebellion of Lung qi manifesting as respiratory disorders such as coughing, dyspnoea, wheezing, asthma and shortness of breath.
- restoring the Lung's disseminating function when this is impaired by exterior pathogenic factors which lodge in the superficial portion of the body.
- treating nasal disorders, including nosebleed and nasal obstruction.
- treating disorders of the throat such as dryness, soreness, congestion, swelling and pain.
- treating oedema and obstructed urination when this is caused by impairment of the Lung's function of regulating the water passages and controlling disseminating and descending.
- treating vomiting due to rebellion of Stomach qi.

ZHONGFU LU-1

中府

Middle Palace

Front-Mu point of the Lung
Meeting point of the Lung and Spleen channels

LOCATION

On the lateral aspect of the chest, in the first intercostal space, 6 cun lateral to the midline, 1 cun inferior to Yunmen LU-2.

LOCATION NOTE

i. Ask the patient to extend their hand forwards whilst you apply resistance to their hand, in order to emphasise the delto-pectoral triangle. First locate Yunmen LU-2 in the centre of the triangle, then locate Zhongfu LU-1 in the intercostal space approximately one cun inferior and slightly lateral to it; ii. To locate the first intercostal space, first locate the costal cartilage of the second rib which is level with the sternal angle, then locate the first intercostal space above it.

NEEDLING

Transverse-oblique insertion 0.5 to 1 cun medially along the intercostal space.

Caution: deep perpendicular or oblique insertion carries a substantial risk of causing a pneumothorax.

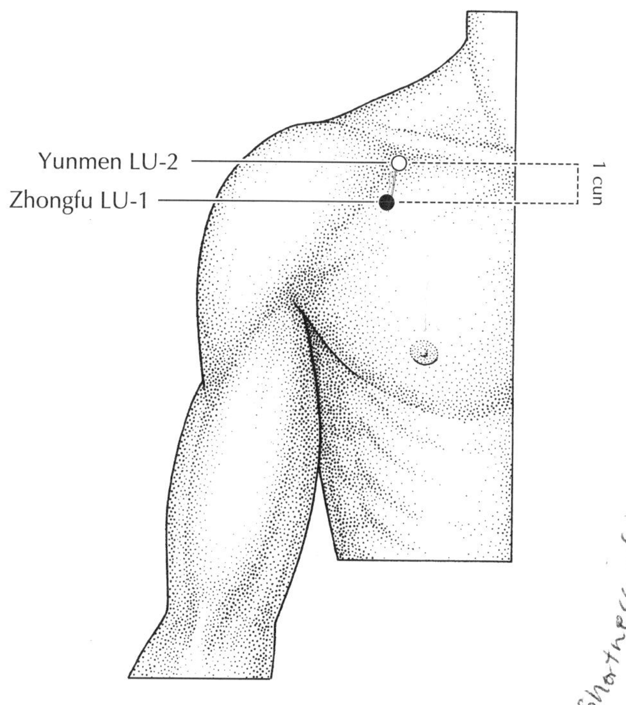

ACTIONS

Disseminates and descends Lung qi and alleviates cough and wheezing
Transforms phlegm, clears heat and regulates the water passages
Descends Stomach qi

INDICATIONS

- Cough, coughing turbid phlegm, coughing blood and pus, dyspnoea, wheezing, asthma, fullness of the chest, chest pain, breathing with raised shoulders, oppression of the chest and difficulty in breathing, diminished qi with inability to lie down.
- Heat in the chest, aversion to cold, chills and fever, sweating.
- Throat painful obstruction, nasal congestion, swelling of the face.
- Difficult ingestion, vomiting, Gall Bladder heat vomiting, retching, abdominal distention.
- Skin pain, running piglet qi with lumbar pain, goitre, pain of the upper back and shoulder.

COMMENTARY

Zhongfu LU-1 is the front-mu point of the Lung. The term 'mu' means to gather or to collect, and the front-mu points are where the qi of the zangfu gathers and concentrates on the anterior surface of the body. Zhongfu LU-1, like all the front-mu points, therefore acts primarily on the Lung zang rather than the Lung channel.

According to the *Spiritual Pivot*[1] "The Lung is the canopy of the five zang and the six fu". As the uppermost zang, the Lung receives via respiration the clear qi of heaven (qing qi) in the same way that the canopy of a forest receives the light and air essential for life. Through inhalation, the Lung descends the qi to the Kidneys, and through exhalation, the Lung disseminates qi to the surface of the body and expels waste qi. The Lung is therefore said to dominate respiration and to both descend and disseminate the qi.

These functions may be impaired either when the Lung qi is deficient, or when excess pathogenic factors (whether internally or externally generated) obstruct the Lung. The forte of Zhongfu LU-1 is to clear excess of all kinds from the Lung, whether due to exterior pathogenic factors (e.g. wind-cold or wind-heat) which penetrate to the Lung zang, or to internally generated disharmony (e.g. turbid phlegm or phlegm-heat, qi stagnation etc.). In all such cases there will be dyspnoea, coughing or wheezing and an oppressive full sensation of the chest, thus the *Spiritual Pivot*[2] says "The Lung stores the qi ... when excess there is dyspnoea and fullness of the chest with an upturned face". These symptoms will often be exacerbated on lying down, which places more strain on the Lung descending function as well as allowing phlegm to accumulate, thus the *Essential Questions*[3] says "The Lung is the canopy of the zang. When Lung qi is abundant, the mai [pulse] is large; when the mai is large, [the patient] is unable to lie flat".

According to the *Spiritual Pivot*[4] "Lung qi opens into the nose; when the Lung is in harmony, the nose will distinguish the fragrant from the foul". Zhongfu LU-1, although primarily used to regulate the Lung zang, is indicated when excess type Lung patterns are accompanied by such Lung channel disorders as nasal obstruction and throat painful obstruction.

According to a saying of Chinese medicine "The Lung is the upper source of water". The Lung can be compared to a lid, for example the lid of a teapot. When the lid is too tight, the tea cannot pour, and when the Lung in the upper body is in excess, the fluids remain above and are not excreted below. Zhongfu LU-1 is indicated for acute swelling of the face which occurs when exterior pathogenic wind obstructs the Lung's function of regulating the water passages and descending body fluids.

The Lung and the Stomach both dominate descending, and disharmony of one may affect the other. If Lung qi accumulates above, it may adversely influence the descending function of the Stomach, giving rise to difficult ingestion, vomiting, retching, and abdominal distention. Conversely, obstruction in the Stomach may impair the Lung descending function leading to cough, dyspnoea and wheezing. In *Essential Questions*[5] Qi Bo, the Yellow Emperor's minister, explains that cough may originate in any of the zangfu and says "When cold food and drink enters the Stomach, it may rise upwards by way of the Lung channel to the Lung, leading to cold in the Lung". The name of this point 'Middle Palace' refers to the origin of the Lung channel, which arises in the middle jiao (in the region of the Stomach) and descends to the Large Intestine before ascending to emerge at Zhongfu LU-1. Zhongfu LU-1, therefore, is especially indicated in this dual disharmony of the Lung and Stomach. Interestingly, Zhongfu LU-1 is also indicated for Gall Bladder heat vomiting, perhaps reflecting the five phase theory that metal (the Lung) is able to control wood (Gall Bladder).

According to the *Essential Questions*[6] "The Lung dominates the skin ... of the entire body". The *Spiritual Pivot*[7] states "when the pathogen is in the Lung there will be painful skin, chills and fever, rebellious qi, dyspnoea and sweating." Zhongfu LU-1 is one of the few acupuncture points indicated for the painful skin which can commonly accompany extrerior diseases. Finally, the *Essential Questions*[8] includes Zhongfu LU-1 among the eight points to clear heat from the chest (bilateral Quepen ST-12, Dazhu BL-11, Zhongfu LU-1 and Fengmen BL-12).

COMBINATIONS

- Fullness of the chest with oesophageal constriction: Zhongfu LU-1 and Yishe BL-49 (*One Hundred Patterns*).
- Chest pain: Zhongfu LU-1, Yunmen LU-2, Feishu BL-13, Qimen LIV-14, Yinbai SP-1, Hunmen BL-47 and Daling P-7 (*Thousand Ducat Formulas*).
- Swelling of the face and abdomen: Zhongfu LU-1, Jianshi P-5 and Hegu L.I.-4 (*Thousand Ducat Formulas*).
- Enuresis: Zhongfu LU-1, Guanmen ST-22 and Shenmen HE-7 (*Thousand Ducat Formulas*).
- Abdominal fullness, shortness of breath with a rattling sound: moxa Zhongfu LU-1, Shanzhong REN-17 and Shenque REN-8 (*Thousand Ducat Formulas*).
- Difficult ingestion: Zhongfu LU-1, Kunlun BL-60, Chengman ST-20, Yuji LU-10 and Zhourong SP-20 (*Supplementing Life*).
- Oesophageal constriction, with difficult ingestion and vomiting: Zhongfu LU-1 and Zhongting REN-16 (*Thousand Ducat Formulas*).

YUNMEN LU-2

Cloud Gate

雲門

LOCATION

On the antero-lateral aspect of the chest, below the lateral extremity of the clavicle, 6 cun lateral to the midline, in the centre of the hollow of the delto-pectoral triangle.

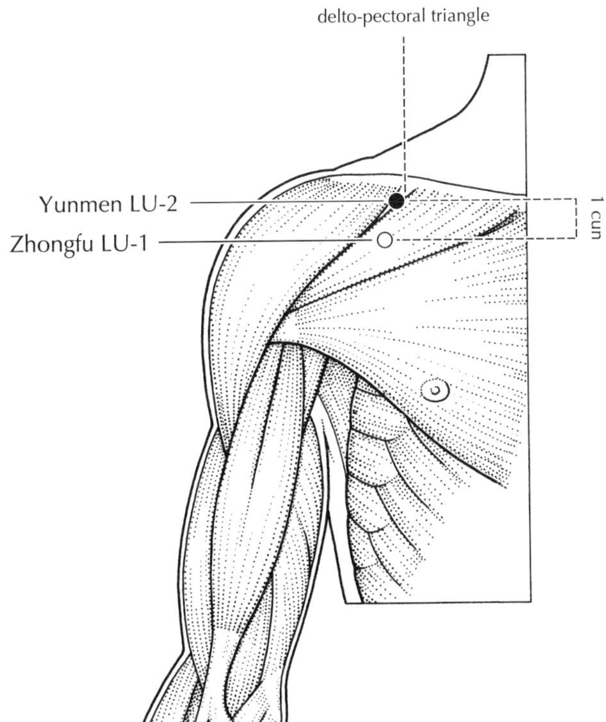

LOCATION NOTE

Ask the patient to extend their hand forwards whilst you apply resistance to their hand, in order to emphasise the delto-pectoral triangle, and locate Yunmen LU-2 at its centre.

NEEDLING

Transverse-oblique insertion 0.5 to 1 cun.
Caution: deep perpendicular or oblique insertion carries a substantial risk of causing a pneumothorax.

ACTIONS

Clears Lung heat and disseminates and descends Lung qi
Dispels agitation and fullness

INDICATIONS

- Cough, wheezing, asthma, dyspnoea with inability to lie down, shortness of breath, oppressive and agitated sensation in the chest, heat in the chest, oppression and pain in the chest, upsurging of qi to the Heart, sudden pain of the Heart and abdomen.
- Pain of the lateral costal region and back, pain of the back and shoulders, pain of the shoulder with inability to raise the arm, pain of the supraclavicular fossa.
- Interrupted pulse which cannot be felt at the cun position, throat painful obstruction, goitre, injury by cold giving rise to persistent heat in the limbs.

COMMENTARY

According to the *Essential Questions*[9] Yunmen LU-2 is one of the eight points for draining heat from the extremities (although in fact only seven are listed, since Yaoshu DU-2 is on the midline) namely Yunmen LU-2, Jianyu L.I.-15, Weizhong BL-40 and Yaoshu DU-2. This is reflected in the indication for this point found in the *Great Compendium of Acupuncture and Moxibustion* "injury by cold giving rise to persistent heat in the limbs".

COMBINATIONS

- Chest pain: Yunmen LU-2, Zhongfu LU-1, Yinbai SP-1, Qimen LIV-14, Feishu BL-13, Hunmen BL-47 and Daling P-7 (*Thousand Ducat Formulas*).
- Pain of the shoulder with inability to raise the arm: Yunmen LU-2 and Bingfeng SI-12 (*Supplementing Life*).
- Dyspnoea with rebellious qi, breathing with raised shoulders, inability to taste food: Yunmen LU-2, Qihu ST-13, Tianfu LU-3 and Shenmen HE-7 (*Thousand Ducat Formulas*).
- Throat painful obstruction: Yunmen LU-2, Zhongfu LU-1, Jianyu L.I.-15, Weizhong BL-40, Fuliu KID-7 and Fubai GB-10 (*Supplementing Life*).

TIANFU LU-3

Palace of Heaven

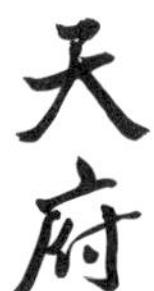

Point of the Window of Heaven

LOCATION

On the antero-lateral aspect of the upper arm, 3 cun inferior to the axillary fold and 6 cun superior to Chize LU-5, in the depression between the lateral border of the biceps brachii muscle and the shaft of the humerus.

LOCATION NOTE

Divide the distance between the axillary fold and the cubital crease of the elbow into equal thirds. Tianfu LU-3 is at the junction of the upper and middle third.

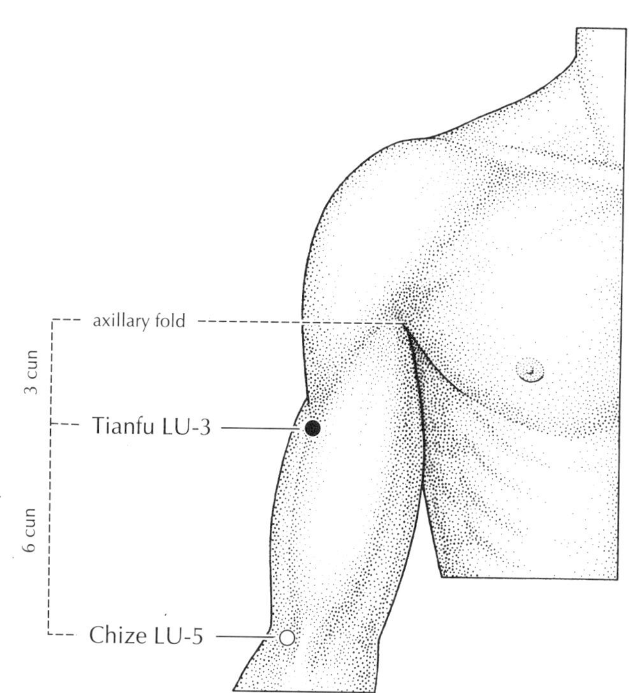

NEEDLING

Perpendicular insertion 0.5 to 1 cun. **Note**: according to several classical texts, this point is contraindicated to moxibustion. The *Systematic Classic of Acupuncture and Moxibustion* says that if moxa is used it will cause counterflow and disordered qi.

ACTIONS

Clears Lung heat and descends Lung qi
Cools blood and stops bleeding
Calms the corporeal soul (po)

INDICATIONS

- Wheezing, dyspnoea, cough, asthma, nosebleed, spitting blood, coughing blood, much spittle.
- Somnolence, insomnia, sadness, weeping, disorientation and forgetfulness, floating corpse ghost-talk, melancholy crying ghost talk.
- Goitre, swelling of the throat, pain of the inner (antero-lateral) aspect of the upper arm, dizziness, swelling and distention of the body, malaria, purple-white wind blotches (pityriasis versicolor), visual dizziness, short-sightedness.

COMMENTARY

According to the *Discourse Into the Origins and Development of Medicine* "The Lung is the delicate zang, neither heat nor cold is appropriate ... too hot and the fire will melt the metal and the blood will stir". As early as the *Spiritual Pivot*[10] Tianfu LU-3 was indicated for "Sudden and severe thirst, internal rebellion, Liver and Lung struggle against each other, blood overflows from the mouth and nose". This quotation is a clear reference to the pattern of Liver fire attacking the Lung. A branch of the Liver channel crosses the diaphragm and scatters in the Lung, and if Liver fire rushes upwards and scorches the Lung it may injure both the blood vessels (causing reckless pouring of blood from the mouth and nose), and the fluids (giving rise to thirst). At the same time there will usually be cough, which is characterised in this pattern by bouts of spasmodic coughing with a red face, or dyspnoea or asthma which is typically induced or worsened by frustration or anger.

The above passage in the *Spiritual Pivot* lists Tianfu LU-3 among five 'Window of Heaven' points (for a fuller discussion see page 48). Tianfu LU-3 shares with these points the common actions of i. treating goitre due to stagnation of qi and phlegm in the neck region, ii. descending the qi of the Lung, and iii. benefiting the sensory orifices, in this case the eyes (visual dizziness and short-sightedness). It is also interesting to note that its ability to treat goitre as well as eye diseases is shared by three points of the upper arm, Tianfu LU-3, Binao L.I.-14 and Naohui SJ-13. There is no apparent explanation why these points, rather than more distal ones, should have such an action, and this is predominantly a reflection of empirical observation.

According to Chinese medicine the Lung stores the corporeal soul (po), one of the five aspects of the spirit (when this term is used in its widest sense). Tianfu LU-3 'Palace of Heaven' is indicated for a range of psycho-emotional disorders characterised by sadness, weeping, disorientation and forgetfulness as well as for somnolence and insomnia.

Tianfu LU-3 is also indicated for 'floating corpse ghost talk'. This term probably refers to the delirious speech seen in the terminal stages of pulmonary tuberculosis. Sun Si-miao in his *Thousand Ducat Formulas* specifically refers to 'melancholy crying ghost talk' in relation to this point, and it was this great physician himself who classified pulmonary tuberculosis (known at that time as feishi - flying corpse) as a disease of the Lung rather than one involving demonic possession. An alternative explanation is that the term does in fact refer to raving or nonsensical speech attributed to demonic possession. A contemporary book on Chinese folk beliefs[11] explains "In cases where the ghost's (i.e. evil spirit's) influence was the result of a gradual process, the victim would initially be sad, sensitive, and withdrawn. As the ghost's powers over the victim's mind became stronger, he would begin to behave as if he were in a dream, talk about ghostly matters, or act as if he were conversing with ghosts".

COMBINATIONS

- Rebellious qi with dyspnoea and inability to catch the breath: Tianfu LU-3, Shufu KID-27 and Shencang KID-25 (*Supplementing Life*).
- Dyspnoea with rebellious qi, breathing with raised shoulders, inability to taste food: Tianfu LU-3, Qihu ST-13, Yunmen LU-2 and Shenmen HE-7 (*Thousand Ducat Formulas*).
- Nosebleed: Tianfu LU-3 and Hegu L.I.-4 (*One Hundred Symptoms*).
- Goitre, tumour of the neck and swollen throat: Tianfu LU-3 and Naohui SJ-13 (*Thousand Ducat Formulas*).
- Goitre, tumour of the neck and swollen throat: Tianfu LU-3, Qishe ST-11 and Naohui SJ-13 (*Supplementing Life*).
- Painful obstruction with difficulty bending and extending the elbow joint, pain and heaviness of the arm with acute pain of the axilla: Tianfu LU-3, Naohui SJ-13 and Qishe ST-11 (*Thousand Ducat Formulas*).
- Purple-white wind blotches (pityriasis versicolor): Tianfu LU-3 and Xiabai LU-4 (*Investigation Into Points Along the Channels*).

XIABAI LU-4
Clasping the White

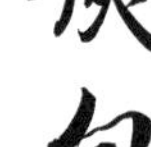

LOCATION
On the antero-lateral aspect of the upper arm, 4 cun inferior to the axillary fold and 5 cun superior to Chize LU-5, in the depression between the lateral border of the biceps brachii muscle and the shaft of the humerus.

LOCATION NOTE
Divide the distance between the axillary fold and the cubital crease of the elbow into equal thirds and locate Xiabai LU-4 one cun inferior to the junction of the upper and middle third (Tianfu LU-3).

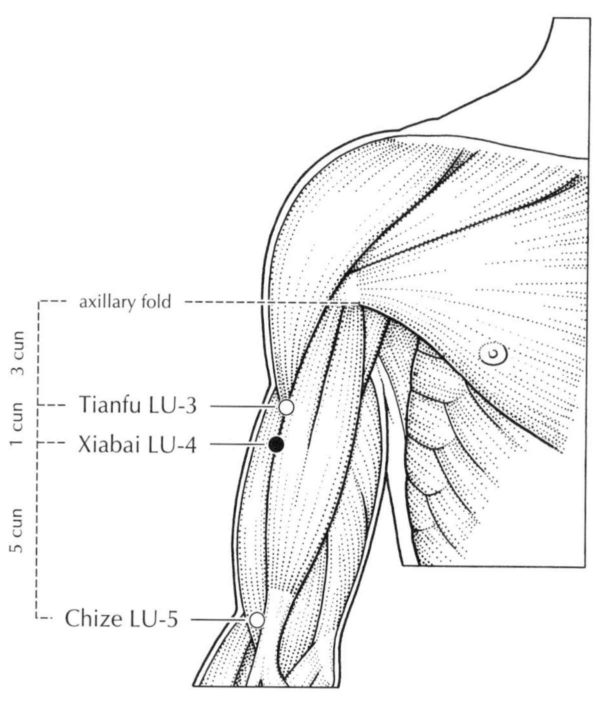

NEEDLING
Perpendicular insertion 0.5 to 1 cun.

ACTIONS
Descends Lung qi
Regulates qi and blood in the chest

INDICATIONS
- Cough, dyspnoea, asthma, shortness of breath.
- Heart pain, palpitations, agitation and fullness, retching.
- Pain in the medial aspect of the arm, purple-white wind blotches (pityriasis versicolor).

COMBINATIONS
- Pain of the Heart with shortness of breath: Xiabai LU-4, Qimen LIV-14, Changqiang DU-1, Tiantu REN-22 and Zhongchong P-9 (*Thousand Ducat Formulas*).
- Purple-white wind blotches (pityriasis versicolor): Xiabai LU-4 and Tianfu LU-3 (*Investigation Into Points Along the Channels*).

CHIZE LU-5
Cubit Marsh

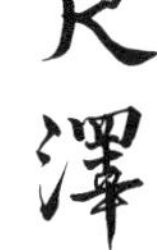

He-Sea and Water point of the Lung channel

LOCATION
On the cubital crease of the elbow, in the depression at the radial side of the tendon of biceps brachii.

LOCATION NOTE
i. Locate slightly lateral to the tendon rather than immediately next to it; ii. Locate and needle with the elbow slightly flexed, avoiding the cubital vein.

NEEDLING
Perpendicular insertion 0.5 to 1 cun.

ACTIONS
Clears heat from the Lung and descends rebellious qi
Regulates the water passages
Activates the channel
Relaxes the sinews and alleviates pain

INDICATIONS
- Cough, coughing phlegm, asthma, wheezing, dyspnoea, shortness of breath, agitation and fullness of the chest.
- Tidal fever, taxation fever, shivering, malaria, dry mouth and tongue, throat painful obstruction, tendency to sneeze.
- Spitting blood, coughing blood, nosebleed, vomiting blood.
- Vomiting, diarrhoea, abdominal distention.
- Swelling of the four limbs, enuresis, frequent urination.
- Pain of the lateral costal region, Heart pain, agitation of the Heart, sobbing with grief, acute and chronic childhood fright wind, epilepsy, clonic spasm.
- Coldness of the shoulder, pain of the upper arm and shoulder, inability to raise the arm to the head, wandering painful obstruction of the elbow and upper arm, restricted movement of the elbow, elbow pain, difficulty in opening and extending the hand, the five types of lumbar pain, crane's knee swelling and pain.

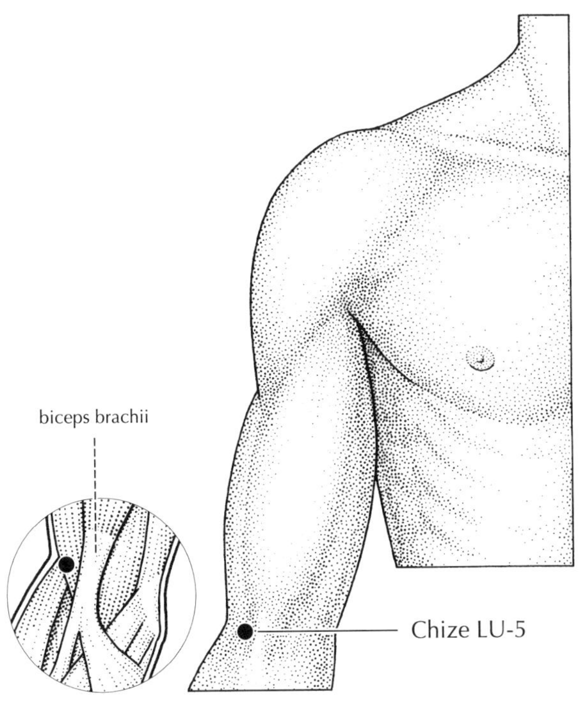

COMMENTARY

Chize LU-5 is the water and he-sea point of the Lung channel. Its principal action is to clear all forms of heat (whether excess or deficient) from the Lung, and to descend Lung qi.

Excess heat in the Lung may be due to interior or exterior factors. Interior factors include smoking, overconsumption of rich, greasy, spicy food and alcohol, transformation of long-standing retention of phlegm-damp into phlegm-heat, and invasion by Liver fire. Exterior factors include pathogenic wind-cold or wind-heat which penetrate the Lung zang and transform into heat. Deficiency heat in the Lung may be due either to depletion and exhaustion of Lung and Kidney yin, or to damage to Lung yin by long-standing or repeated attacks of excess heat. The presence of any form of heat in the Lung will disturb its function of descending qi and lead to such symptoms of rebellion of Lung qi as coughing, shortness of breath, wheezing and asthma. In the case of excess heat there may be coughing of phlegm and agitation and fullness of the chest, whilst in cases of deficiency heat there may be tidal fever or taxation fever and dry mouth and tongue.

Whilst equally applicable to cases of both excess and deficiency heat, the appropriate combination of Chize LU-5 with other points will determine the different approach required in the treatment of these two conditions. In the case of excess heat, characterised by fullness in the chest and expectoration of yellow, green or brown phlegm, it may be combined with points to transform phlegm and clear heat such as Fenglong ST-40 and Zhongfu LU-1. In the case of deficiency heat, characterised by dry mouth and tongue and tidal fever or taxation fever, it may be combined with points to nourish yin and moisten the Lung such as Taiyuan LU-9, Gaohuangshu BL-43 and Taixi KID-3.

According to the *Classic of Difficulties*[12] he-sea points are indicated for "counterflow qi and diarrhoea", whilst the *Spiritual Pivot* says "in disorders of the Stomach and in disorders resulting from irregular eating and drinking, select the he-sea point"[13]. The Lung and Stomach both dominate descending whilst the Lung channel arises in the middle jiao, in the region of the Stomach. In addition to descending rebellious Lung qi, Chize LU-5 also treats vomiting due to rebellious Stomach qi, as well as diarrhoea and abdominal distention.

The *Discourse Into the Origins and Development of Medicine* says "The Lung is the delicate zang, neither heat nor cold is appropriate ... too hot and the fire will melt the metal and the blood will stir". Heat in the Lung, whether of deficient or excess type, may injure the blood vessels and give rise to reckless bleeding, characterised by coughing or spitting of blood or nosebleed. As well as being indicated for heat-induced bleeding from the Lung, due to its secondary action of descending Stomach qi Chize LU-5 may also be used for vomiting blood. The *Song of Points for Miscellaneous Diseases* states uncompromisingly "In cases of vomiting blood the action of Chize LU-5 is without comparison"[14].

The close relationship of the Lung to body fluids is emphasised in two sayings of Chinese medicine "The Lung is the upper source of water" and "The Lung dominates the movement of water". If exterior pathogenic wind obstructs the Lung's function of regulating the water passages and descending body fluid, there may be urinary retention as well as swelling of the four limbs. If the Lung is deficient, there may be enuresis or frequent urination. Chize LU -5 is indicated in both these patterns.

The Lung and Heart dominate the upper jiao and share an intimate relationship. The *Warp and Woof of Warm Febrile Disease* says "The Lung and Heart are mutually connected; when there is Lung heat it most easily enters the Heart". When Lung heat transmits to the Heart there will be agitation, whilst if heat condenses the blood and gives rise to blood stasis, there will be Heart pain. In both these situations Chize LU-5 is indicated.

Occupying a central position along the Lung channel, Chize LU-5 has an important effect on the whole upper limb, and is indicated for disorders of the channel in the shoulder, upper arm, elbow and hand characterised by pain and restricted motion. Migratory pain due to attack of pathogenic wind-damp is known as wandering painful obstruction or wind painful obstruction, and as well as being indicated for wandering painful obstruction of the upper arm and elbow, Chize LU-5 appears in classical combinations for wind painful obstruction of the whole body. Many classical sources particularly mention the ability of Chize LU-5 to relax contraction of the sinews, for example the *Song of the Jade Dragon* says "In contraction of the sinews with difficulty in opening and extending the hand, the use of Chize LU-5 should always be emphasised". Its use in the treatment of pain and contraction of the elbow is self-evident, and it is especially useful in the treatment of tennis elbow in preference to Quchi L.I.-11, as a needle inserted at Chize LU-5 can be more easily directed towards the area of acute focalised tenderness. Chize LU-5 is also indicated for swelling and pain of the knee (crane's knee wind) reflecting the commonly used 'cross-connection' method of needling the equivalently positioned joint in the upper limb to treat disorders of the lower limb and vice-versa (see page 59).

Interestingly, Chize LU-5 also treats 'the five types of lumbar pain'. In a sense this point, located in the flexure of the elbow joint, can be viewed as the equivalent on the upper limb of Weizhong BL-40 which is located in the flexure of the knee joint and is much used for lumbar pain.

COMBINATIONS

- Shortness of breath, pain of the lateral costal region and agitation of the Heart: Chize LU-5 and Shaoze SI-1 (*Thousand Ducat Formulas*).
- Shortness of breath: Chize LU-5 and Daling P-7 (*Great Compendium*).
- Any type of spitting blood: reinforce Chize LU-5 and reduce Yuji LU-10 (*Systematic Classic*).
- Wind painful obstruction: Chize LU-5 and Yangfu GB-38 (*Great Compendium*).
- Wind painful obstruction: Chize LU-5, Tianjing SJ-10, Shaohai HE-3, Weizhong BL-40 and Yangfu GB-38 (*Great Compendium*).
- Contraction of the arm with tightness of the sinews of both hands resulting in inability to open the hands: Chize LU-5, Quchi L.I.-11, Yangchi SJ-4, Hegu L.I.-4 and Zhongzhu SJ-3 (*Great Compendium*).
- Contraction and cold of the shoulder and back, with pain of the inner aspect of the scapula: Chize LU-5, Geshu BL-17, Yixi BL-45 and Jinmen BL-63 (*Thousand Ducat Formulas*).
- Contraction of the elbow with pain: Chize LU-5 joined to Quchi L.I.-11 (*Ode of the Jade Dragon*).
- Pain of the lumbar and lateral costal regions due to sprain: Chize LU-5, Renzhong DU-26 and Weizhong BL-40; afterwards needle Kunlun BL-60, Shugu BL-65, Zhigou SJ-6 and Yanglingquan GB-34 (*Great Compendium*).

KONGZUI LU-6

Maximum Opening

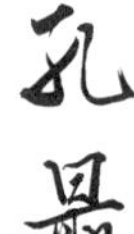

Xi-Cleft point of the Lung channel

LOCATION

On the flexor aspect of the forearm, 7 cun proximal to Taiyuan LU-9, on the line connecting Taiyuan LU-9 with Chize LU-5.

LOCATION NOTE

Divide the distance between Taiyuan LU-9 and Chize LU-5 into half. Kongzui LU-6 is in a palpable depression 1 cun proximal to this midpoint.

NEEDLING

Perpendicular or oblique insertion 0.5 to 1.5 cun.

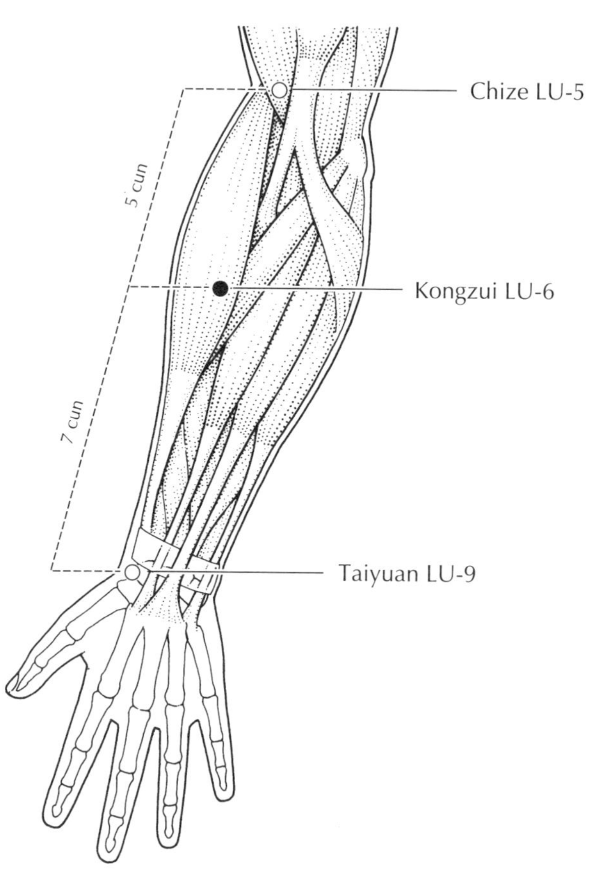

ACTIONS

Disseminates and descends Lung qi
Clears heat and moistens the Lung
Clears heat and stops bleeding
Moderates acute conditions

INDICATIONS

- Cough, wheezing, asthma, chest pain, swelling and pain of the throat, loss of voice, febrile disease with absence of sweating.
- Coughing blood, spitting blood, vomiting blood, hiccup.
- Severe pain of the elbow and upper arm, inability to raise the arm above the head, difficulty in flexing and extending the fingers, epigastric pain, haemorrhoids, headache, clonic spasm.

COMMENTARY

Kongzui LU-6 is the xi-cleft point of the Lung channel. The xi-cleft points are where the qi and blood, which flow relatively superficially along the channels from the jing-well points, gather and plunge more deeply. The xi-cleft points in general are indicated in the treatment of acute conditions and pain, whilst the xi-cleft points of the yin channels have an additional action of treating disorders of blood. Kongzui LU-6 is an important point both for acute diseases of the Lung, and for disorders of blood.

Kongzui LU-6 is particularly indicated for attack by exterior pathogenic wind-heat or wind-dryness which i. lodge in the superficial layer and obstruct the normal functioning of the pores, giving rise to febrile disease with absence of sweating, or ii. penetrate the Lung zang and channel giving rise to acute cough and wheezing, swelling and pain of the throat and loss of voice. In modern clinical practice, however, the principal use of this point is in the treatment of acute cough, wheezing or asthma of any aetiology.

As the Lung channel xi-cleft point, Kongzui LU-6 is also particularly indicated for all kinds of bleeding from the Lung whether due to wind-dryness, wind-heat, phlegm-heat, Liver-Lung disharmony or yin deficiency.

Finally, Kongzui LU-6 is indicated for obstruction of qi along the Lung channel with such symptoms as severe pain of the elbow and upper arm, difficulty in flexing and extending the fingers, and inability to raise the arm above the head.

COMBINATIONS

- Febrile disease with absence of sweating: Kongzui LU-6 and Shangliao BL-31 (*Systematic Classic*).
- Loss of voice: Kongzui LU-6 and Yamen DU-15 (*Supplementing Life*).
- Spitting blood: Kongzui LU-6, Quze P-3 and Feishu BL-13 (*Classic of Supplementing Life*).
- Headache: Kongzui LU-6, Houxi SI-3, Tianzhu BL-10, Taodao DU-13 and Dazhu BL-11 (*Thousand Ducat Formulas*).
- Acute asthma: Kongzui LU-6 and Dingchuan (M-BW-1).

LIEQUE LU-7

Broken Sequence

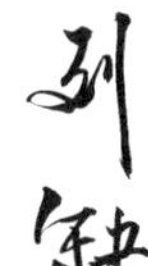

Luo-Connecting point of the Lung channel
Confluent point of the Conception vessel
Gao Wu Command point
Ma Dan-yang Heavenly Star point

LOCATION

On the radial aspect of the forearm, approximately 1.5 cun proximal to Yangxi L.I.-5, in the cleft between the tendons of brachioradialis and abductor pollicis longus.

LOCATION NOTE

If the forefinger is placed at Yangxi L.I.-5, in the anatomical snuffbox, and moved directly proximally over the full extent of the styloid process of the radius, the finger falls into the cleft between the two tendons.

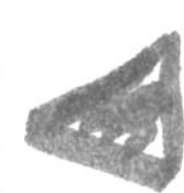

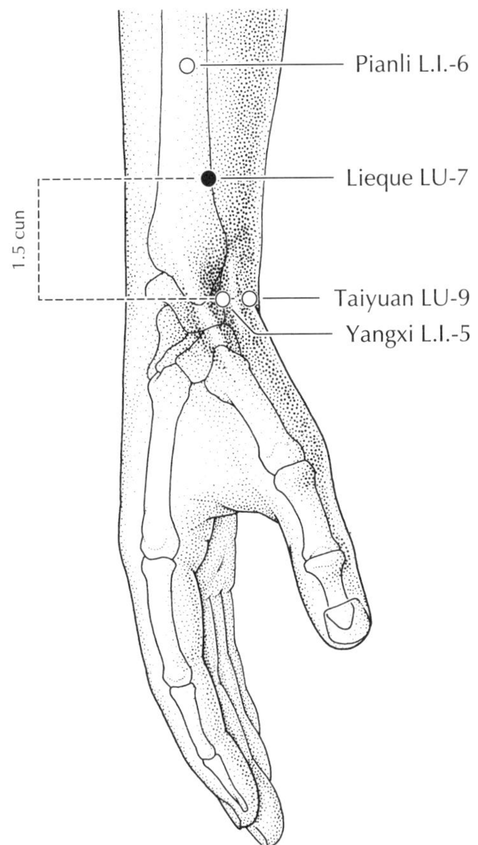

NEEDLING

With the fingers of one hand pinch up the skin over the point, and with the other hand needle transversely in a proximal or distal direction, 0.5 to 1 cun, avoiding the cephalic vein.

ACTIONS

Releases the exterior and expels wind
Promotes the descending function of the Lung
Pacifies wind and phlegm
Benefits the head and nape
Opens and regulates the Conception vessel
Regulates the water passages
Activates the channel and alleviates pain

INDICATIONS

- Chills and fever, nasal congestion and discharge, nasal polyps, flaring of the nostrils, throat painful obstruction, cough, coughing up phlegm, wheezing, dyspnoea, asthma, diminished qi and shortness of breath, heat of the chest and back, shivering and cold of the chest and back, sweating, sudden swelling of the four limbs, thirst, inversion counterflow of the four limbs.
- Headache and stiffness of the neck and nape, one-sided headache, lockjaw, hemiplegia, deviation of the mouth and eye, toothache, epilepsy, childhood fright-epilepsy, acute childhood fright wind, loss of consciousness, vomiting of foamy (watery) saliva, wind painful obstruction, hypertension.
- Retention of lochia, retention of the dead foetus, post-partum inability to speak, blood in the urine, hot and painful urination, difficult urination, pain of the penis, pain of the genitals, seminal emission.
- Poor memory, palpitations, propensity to laughter, frequent yawning and stretching, tension of the chest and back, fullness of the lateral costal region, breast abscess.
- Weakness or pain of the wrist and hand, pain of the thumb, shoulder pain, heat in the palm, malaria.

COMMENTARY

The name of this point 'Broken Sequence' is an ancient term for lightning. This name may be understood in three ways: i. the electric sensation that may be generated when needling this point, ii. the ability of Lieque LU-7 to clear heaviness and oppression of the chest in the way that a lightning storm clears the sky, and iii. the sudden fork in the Lung channel at this point. It is notable that several of the luo-connecting points (for example Fenglong ST-40, Feiyang BL-58, Dazhong KID-4) are located at sites where the channel suddenly changes direction, and in the case of Lieque LU-7 this fork takes it almost as far as the pathway of the Large Intestine channel, emphasising the close affinity of this point to the Lung's paired yang channel.

Lieque LU-7 was included by Ma Dan-yang, the great physician of the Jin dynasty, among the 'eleven heavenly star points'[15] his grouping of the most vital acupuncture points, and was indicated by him for one-sided headache, wind painful obstruction and numbness of the whole body, obstruction of phlegm in the upper body, and lockjaw. The *Glorious Anthology of Acupuncture and Moxibustion* by the Ming dynasty author Gao Wu includes Lieque LU-7 among the 'four command points' (for disorders of the head and nape). In the *Ode Of The Obstructed River* the use of Lieque LU-7 is referred to as one of 'the eight therapeutic methods'. In this description of the application of the eight confluent points of the extraordinary vessels to affect specific symptoms and areas of the body, Lieque LU-7 is indicated for disorders of the head region, rebellion and blockage of phlegm and dry throat.

The clear emphasis on the ability of Lieque LU-7 to treat the head and neck region in each of these three point groupings is surprising since the Lung channel does not ascend higher than the throat. The effect of Lieque LU-7 on the head region as a whole can, however, be explained by the following factors: i. the action of Lieque LU-7 on expelling and pacifying wind whose nature is to attack the upper portion of the body, and ii. the close connection between Lieque LU-7, the luo-connecting point of the Lung channel, and its interiorly-exteriorly related Large Intestine channel which does ascend to the head.

Lieque LU-7 is an important point in the treatment of wind disorders, whether of exterior or interior origin. According to both the *Spiritual Pivot*[16] and the *Essential Questions*[17] "Taiyin is the opening, jueyin is the closing and shaoyin is the pivot". The Lung (taiyin), which communicates directly with the exterior via respiration, and indirectly through its close relationship with the skin of the whole body, is the most open and vulnerable of the zang to attack by exterior pathogens. When exterior pathogenic wind, in combination with heat, cold or dryness, attacks the superficial portion of the body, it has three principal effects: i. it may obstruct the defensive qi and impair the disseminating function of the Lung, giving rise to the classic signs of an exterior pattern such as chills and fever, headache, aches and pains in the neck, shoulders and back etc., ii. it may impair the descending function of the Lung, resulting in coughing, wheezing and asthma, and iii. it may interfere with the Lung's function of regulating the water passages and descending fluids to the Bladder, resulting in acute swelling of the limbs. Lieque LU-7 is not only the luo-connecting point of the Lung channel, communicating with the yang Large Intestine channel, but is also the point where a branch of the Lung primary channel diverges to link with Shangyang L.I.-1 on the index finger. Due to this close connection with the Lung channel's yang (exterior) paired channel, Lieque LU-7 is the most exterior-acting of the Lung channel points and is the principal point on the channel to release the exterior, promote the function of the Lungs in dispersing and descending, and regulate the water passages.

"Wind is characterised by upward and outward dispersion". This saying of Chinese medicine means that wind tends to attack both the upper and exterior portions of the body. As well as releasing wind from the exterior, Lieque LU-7 is able to clear both exterior and interior wind from the head and upper body in the treatment of disorders such as facial paralysis, lockjaw, epilepsy, toothache and headache. Its ability to treat the head, and in particular the yangming facial area, again reflects its close connection with the Large Intestine channel, a concept emphasised in the *Guide to the Classic of Acupuncture* which states "the luo-connecting points are located between two channels ... if they are punctured, symptoms of the interiorly-exteriorly related channels can be treated"[18]. The wind-expelling action of Lieque LU-7 is also reflected in its classical use in the treatment of wind painful obstruction and numbness of the whole body.

The ability of Lieque LU-7 to pacify interior wind is complemented by its action of descending phlegm. Wind-phlegm (the combination of interior wind and phlegm) is a common pattern underlying disorders such as epilepsy, lockjaw, facial paralysis and hemiplegia for which this point is indicated. In Lung disorders, failure of the Lung to disseminate and descend body fluids results in accumulation of phlegm in the chest and Lieque LU-7 is also indicated for coughing phlegm and vomiting of foamy (watery) saliva.

From the earliest times Lieque LU-7 has been an important point in the treatment of headaches, for example the *Ode of Spiritual Brightness* states "in treating headache, whether one-sided or not, reduce Lieque LU-7". Whilst this action can in part be explained by the ability of Lieque LU-7 to expel and pacify wind, as well as by its connection with the Large Intestine channel, this is predominantly an example of the fruits of long empirical observation.

Lieque LU-7 is the confluent point of the Conception vessel, which ascends along the anterior midline of the body and is closely related to the uterus and the genito-urinary organs. By opening and regulating the flow of qi in the Conception vessel, Lieque LU-7 is able to treat such symptoms as retention of the lochia and dead foetus, pain of the genitals and urinary disorders. Its effect on a wide range of urinary disorders such as blood in the urine, and hot, painful and difficult urination, further reflects the important function of the Lung in regulating the water passages, especially descending fluids to the Bladder.

Lieque LU-7 shares with the other luo-connecting points of the yin channels (Gongsun SP-4, Tongli HE-5, Dazhong KID-4, Ligou LIV-5 and Neiguan P-6) the special ability to treat psycho-emotional disorders, and is indicated for propensity to laughter, frequent yawning and stretching and especially for poor memory.

As far as disorders of the Lung channel are concerned, Lieque LU-7 treats heat in the palms and shoulder pain, but is particularly important for pain of the thumb joint and index finger. For this purpose it is needled towards the hand and manipulated to transmit sensation to the diseased area, whilst for all other purposes, Lieque LU-7 is generally needled proximally towards the elbow.

Finally the *Great Compendium of Acupuncture and Moxibustion* gives specific indications for excess and deficiency of the luo-connecting points. In the case of Lieque LU-7, these are heat of the chest and back, sweating, sudden swelling of the four limbs (excess); shivering and cold of the chest and back, diminished qi and shortness of breath (deficiency).

COMBINATIONS

- Acute dyspnoea: Lieque LU-7 and Zusanli ST-36 (*Song of Points*).
- Oedema: Lieque LU-7, Yanggu SI-5, Hegu L.I.-4, Jianshi P-5, Yanglingquan GB-34, Yingu KID-10, Zusanli ST-36, Ququan LIV-8, Jiexi ST-41, Xiangu ST-43, Fuliu KID-7, Gongsun SP-4, Lidui ST-45, Chongyang ST-42, Yinlingquan SP-9, Weishu BL-21, Shuifen REN-9 and Shenque REN-8 (*Great Compendium*).
- One-sided wind (hemiplegia): Lieque LU-7 and Chongyang ST-42 (*Great Compendium*).
- One-sided or generalised headache: Lieque LU-7 and Taiyuan LU-9 (*Ode of Xi-hong*).
- Deviation of the mouth: Lieque LU-7 and Dicang ST-4 (*Supplementing Life*).
- Deviation of the mouth and face: Lieque LU-7 and Wangu GB-12 (*Supplementing Life*).
- Childhood fright-epilepsy: Lieque LU-7 and the luo-connecting point of the yangming (*Systematic Classic*).
- Pain of the genitals: Lieque LU-7, Yinlingquan SP-9 and Shaofu HE-8 (*Formulas for the Living*).
- Heat in the palms: Lieque LU-7, Jingqu LU-8 and Taiyuan LU-9 (*Great Compendium*).
- Malaria with chills and fever: Lieque LU-7, Houxi SI-3, Qiangu SI-2 and Shaoze SI-1 (*Thousand Ducat Formulas*).
- Poor memory: Lieque LU-7, Gaohuangshu BL-43, Shendao DU-11 and Youmen KID-21 (*Supplementing Life*).
- Poor memory: Lieque LU-7, Xinshu BL-15, Shenmen HE-7, Zhongwan REN-12, Zusanli ST-36, Shaohai HE-3 and moxa Baihui DU-20 (*Outline of Medicine*).
- Frequent laughter: Lieque LU-7, Daling P-7, Renzhong DU-26 and Yangxi L.I.-5 (*Great Compendium*).
- Stabbing qi pain of the two breasts: Taiyuan LU-9 and Lieque LU-7 (*Song of Points*).

JINGQU LU-8

Channel Gutter

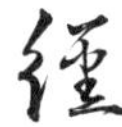
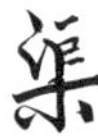

Jing-River and Metal point of the Lung channel

LOCATION

Above the wrist, 1 cun proximal to Taiyuan LU-9, on the line connecting Taiyuan LU-9 with Kongzui LU-6, in the depression at the base of the styloid process of the radius and on the radial side of the radial artery.

LOCATION NOTE

If the forefinger is placed on Taiyuan LU-9 and moved proximally over the palpable styloid process of the radius, it will naturally fall into the depression where Jingqu LU-8 is located.

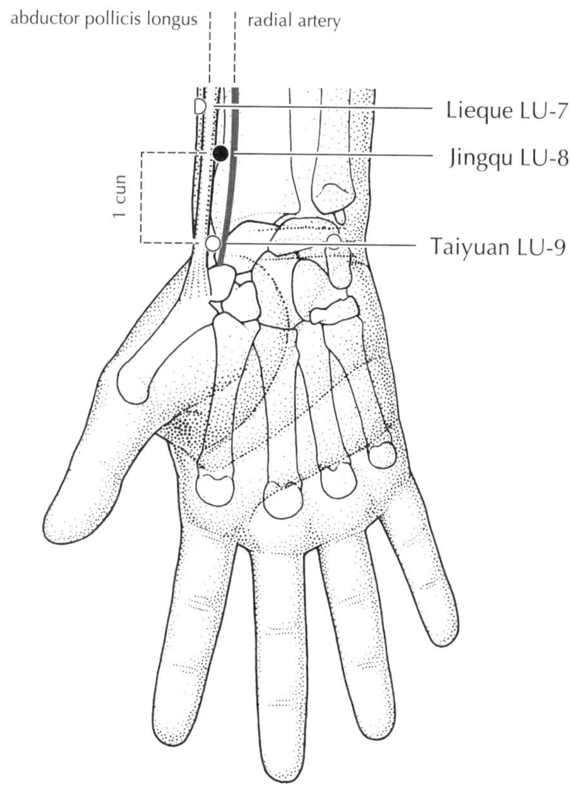

NEEDLING

Oblique proximal or perpendicular insertion 0.3 to 0.5 cun, avoiding the radial artery.

ACTIONS

Descends Lung qi and alleviates cough and wheezing

INDICATIONS

- Cough, asthma, wheezing, dyspnoea, distention and pain of the chest and upper back, sore throat, throat painful obstruction, febrile disease with absence of sweating, febrile disease with breathlessness, heat in the palms.
- Heart pain with vomiting, wrist pain, malaria, much yawning, pain in the soles of the feet.

COMMENTARY

According to the *Classic of Difficulties*[19] jing-river points are indicated for "cough and dyspnoea, chills and fever". Jingqu LU-8, the jing-river point of the Lung channel, is primarily indicated for excess type cough, dyspnoea and wheezing with fullness and pain of the chest and upper back, and for febrile disease with absence of sweating.

An unusual indication for Jingqu LU-8 found in the *Classic of Supplementing Life with Acupuncture and Moxibustion* is pain in the region of Yongquan KID-1. Pain in the sole is usually due either to deficiency of the Kidneys or to phlegm and dampness pouring downwards.

It should be emphasised, however, that in modern clinical practice Jingqu LU-8 is infrequently used.

COMBINATIONS

- Tension of the chest and back with a swollen sensation of the chest: Jingqu LU-8 and Qiuxu GB-40 (*Thousand Ducat Formulas*).
- Febrile disease with absence of sweating: Jingqu LU-8 and Dadu SP-2 (*One Hundred Symptoms*).

TAIYUAN LU-9

Supreme Abyss

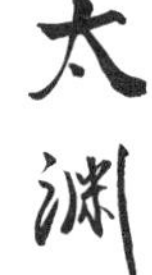

Shu-Stream, Yuan-Source and Earth point of the Lung channel
Hui-Meeting point of the Vessels

LOCATION

At the wrist joint, in the depression between the radial artery and the tendon of abductor pollicis longus, level with Shenmen HE-7 (the proximal border of the pisiform bone).

LOCATION NOTE

The location of this point is normally given in relation to the crease of the wrist. Since wrist creases are a superficial and variable anatomical feature, it is better to locate this point in relation to the nearby pisiform bone: first locate Shenmen HE-7 at the lower border of the pisiform bone, then find Taiyuan LU-9 at the same level.

NEEDLING

Perpendicular insertion 0.3 to 0.5 cun, avoiding the radial artery.

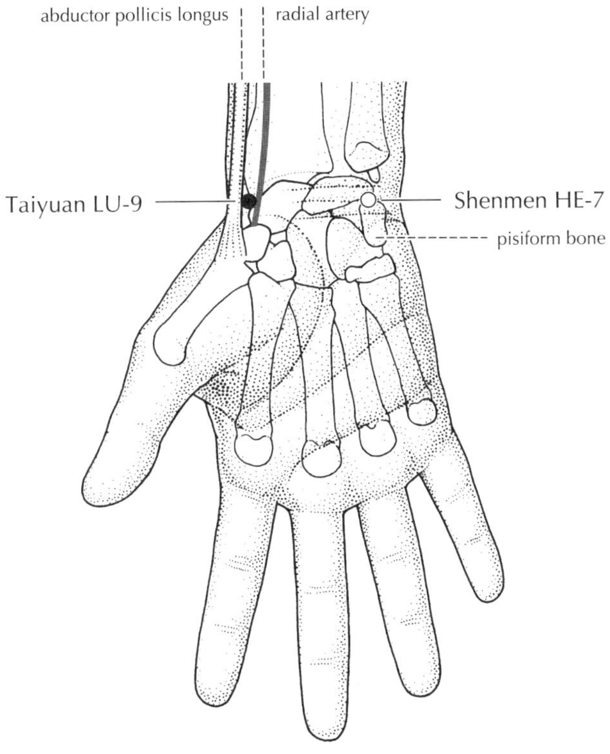

ACTIONS

Tonifies the Lung and transforms phlegm
Promotes the descending function of the Lung
Regulates and harmonises the one hundred vessels
Activates the channel and alleviates pain

INDICATIONS

- Cough, cough with watery phlegm, asthma, wheezing, dyspnoea, shortness of breath, much yawning, heat in the palms, dry throat, oppression and agitation of the chest with difficult breathing and inability to lie down.
- Spitting blood, coughing blood, vomiting blood, agitation with Heart pain accompanied by choppy pulse, manic raving, pulseless syndrome.
- Rebellion of Stomach qi, belching, superficial visual obstruction, redness and pain of the eyes, cold shivering, cold inversion, toothache, head wind, swelling of the face.
- Weakness or pain of the wrist, pain of the shoulder and back, pain of the supraclavicular fossa, pain in the inner aspect of the arm, breast pain.

COMMENTARY

Taiyuan LU-9 is the shu-stream, yuan-source and earth point of the Lung channel. The *Spiritual Pivot* in Chapter Six, recommends the use of the shu-stream points in the treatment of disorders of the zang, whilst in Chapter 1 it says "When the five zang are diseased, select [from] the twelve yuan-source [points]". Furthermore, the *Classic of Difficulties*[20] states "in cases of deficiency reinforce the mother" (according to five phase theory Taiyuan LU-9 is the earth, and thus mother, point of the metal zang). Taiyuan LU-9 therefore is the single most important point on the Lung channel to tonify the Lung qi or yin, the two principal patterns of Lung deficiency.

Taiyuan LU-9 is indicated for Lung deficiency characterised by chronic weak coughing or wheezing. In the case of Lung qi deficiency there may also be shortness of breath and much yawning, whilst in the case of Lung yin deficiency there may be heat in the palms and spitting of blood. Taiyuan LU-9 will also assist in the transformation of phlegm which arises due to deficiency. If Lung qi is too weak to move the fluids in the Lung there may be copious watery phlegm, whilst if Lung yin is deficient, and the consequent heat condenses the fluids, there may be scanty dry phlegm with dryness of the throat. As well as tonifying deficiency, Taiyuan LU-9 is able to promote the descending function of the Lung and is indicated for fullness and oppression of the chest with inability to lie down.

According to the *Classic of Difficulties*[21] "the vessels gather at Taiyuan LU-9", whilst the *Classic of Categories* states "The flow of the channels [must] follow the qi, the qi is dominated by the Lung, therefore it is the meeting of the hundred vessels". These statements refer to the important relationship between the qi and the blood, expressed in the saying "The qi is the commander of blood", and the further statement in the *Classic of Categories* that "The vessels are the pathways of the blood qi; the circulation of the vessels is dependent on qi". In other words, the blood moves through the blood vessels by virtue of the movement of qi, and in the chest and Heart region especially, the circulation of the blood is dependent on the gathering qi [formed from the combination of air inhaled by the Lung and the grain qi of food and drink]. Taiyuan LU-9, the hui-meeting point of the vessels, is therefore an important point to harmonise the relationship between the gathering qi and the blood. When the gathering qi is deficient and fails to circulate the blood, it will pool and stagnate in the chest and Heart, giving rise to oppression and fullness, agitation, Heart pain with a choppy pulse, and in severe cases manic raving. Taiyuan LU-9 is further indicated for disorders of the blood vessels in general such as vomiting, spitting or coughing blood and pulseless syndrome.

The Lung channel has its origin in the middle jiao, and in common with many points of the channel Taiyuan LU-9 is able to harmonise the Stomach, being indicated for rebellion of Stomach qi with belching, as well as for Stomach channel heat symptoms such as toothache, superficial visual obstruction, redness and pain of the eyes and breast pain.

Finally, Taiyuan LU-9 is indicated for pain affecting various portions of the Lung channel including the supraclavicular fossa, the shoulder and back, the inner aspect of the arm and the wrist. It should be noted that the Chinese reference to the 'inner' aspect of the arm in respect of the Lung channel assumes a standing posture with the palms hanging facing the sides. In terms of the Western anatomical position used throughout this book, the Lung channel occupies the antero-lateral position on the arm.

COMBINATIONS

- Lung distention: Taiyuan LU-9 and Feishu BL-13 (*Systematic Classic*).
- Pain of the Lung and Heart: Taiyuan LU-9 and Yuji LU-10 (*Systematic Classic*).
- Dry throat: Taiyuan LU-9 and Yuji LU-10 (*Great Compendium*).
- Manic raving: Taiyuan LU-9, Yangxi L.I.-5, Xialian L.I.-8 and Kunlun BL-60 (*Great Compendium*).
- Agitation and oppression with inability to sleep: Taiyuan LU-9, Gongsun SP-4, Yinbai SP-1, Feishu BL-13, Yinlingquan SP-9 and Sanyinjiao SP-6 (*Great Compendium*).
- Belching: Taiyuan LU-9 and Shenmen HE-7 (*Great Compendium*).
- Stabbing qi pain of the two breasts: Taiyuan LU-9 and Lieque LU-7 (*Song of Points*).

YUJI LU-10

Fish Border

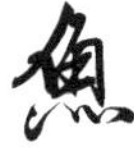
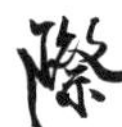

Ying-Spring and Fire point of the Lung channel

LOCATION

On the thenar eminence of the hand, in a depression between the midpoint of the shaft of the first metacarpal bone and the thenar muscles.

LOCATION NOTE

Locate and needle close to the border of the metacarpal bone.

NEEDLING

Perpendicular insertion 0.5 to 1 cun.

ACTIONS

Benefits the throat
Clears Lung heat
Descends rebellious qi
Harmonises the Stomach and Heart

INDICATIONS

- Throat painful obstruction, sore throat, dry throat, loss of voice.
- Cough with absence of sweating, cough leading to hypogastric or sacral pain, cough accompanied by hiccup, shortness of breath with Heart painful obstruction, diminished qi with Heart painful obstruction, chest painful obstruction with inability to catch the breath.
- Deficiency heat, heat in the body, aversion to cold, attack of wind and cold after intake of alcohol leading to chills and fever.
- Coughing blood, vomiting blood, blood in the urine.
- Agitation of the Heart, sadness and fear, anger and mania, sadness and anger with counterflow qi, Heart painful obstruction with fear and fright.
- Yellow tongue coating, breast abscess, toothache, lacrimation, visual dizziness, genital damp itching, impotence with abdominal distention, headache, malaria, tetany.
- Abdominal pain with inability to eat or drink, sudden turmoil disorder, oesophageal constriction due to middle jiao deficiency, vomiting, childhood nutritional impairment.
- Heat and pain of the palm and thumb, contraction of the elbow with distention and fullness of the arm.

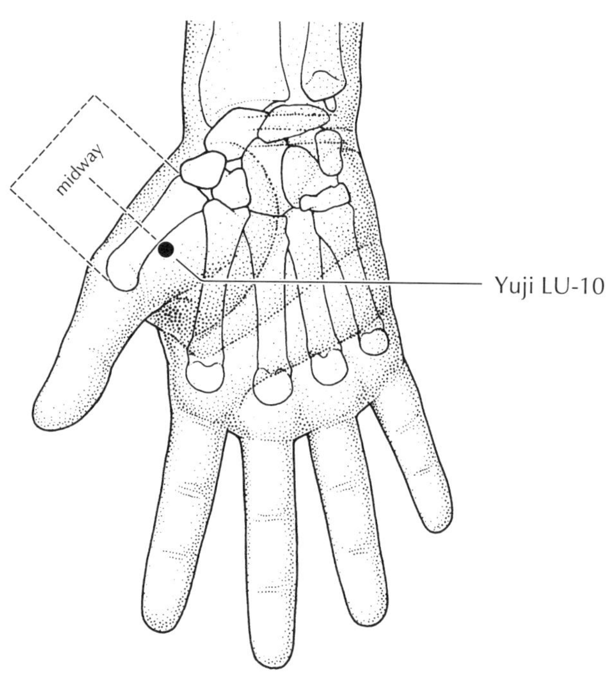

COMMENTARY

Yuji LU-10 is the ying-spring and fire point of the Lung channel. According to the *Classic of Difficulties*[22] ying-spring points are indicated for "heat in the body", and Yuji LU-10 is effective to clear heat from both the Lung channel and the Lung zang.

It is a general characteristic of the more distal points of the channels that they treat disorders of the upper end of the channel. The internal pathway of the Lung channel rises to the throat, and Yuji LU-10 is a major point for a wide range of throat disorders characterised by heat and dryness, whether due to deficiency or excess, and is indicated for pain, swelling, congestion and dryness of the throat and loss of voice.

Excess heat in the Lung zang may be subdivided into predominance of heat or predominance of phlegm. Yuji LU-10 is indicated in the former, whilst points such as Zhongfu LU-1 and Chize LU-5 are preferable for the latter. If heat lodged in the Lung obstructs the descent of Lung qi, it will lead to coughing. If the fluids of the Lung are vaporised by heat, there will be sweating, whilst if Lung heat has scorched and consumed the fluids there will be coughing with absence of sweating. The extent of the sweating, therefore, indicates the severity of the heat. By virtue of its action on clearing heat, Yuji LU-10 is equally effective in clearing Lung heat deriving from deficiency of yin.

Yuji LU-10 is indicated for bleeding disorders affecting all three jiao. Lung heat may injure the vessels of the Lung causing coughing of blood, transmit to the origin of the Lung channel in the Stomach causing vomiting of blood, or transmit to the Heart and thence the Small Intestine and Bladder giving rise to blood in the urine (which may be accompanied by genital damp itching or impotence).

Yuji LU-10 is able to harmonise the relationship of the Lung and Heart on the one hand, and the Lung and Stomach on the other. According to the *Warp and Woof of Warm Febrile Disease* "The Lung and Heart are mutually connected, thus when there is Lung heat it most easily enters the Heart". If Lung heat agitates in the upper jiao therefore, it may transmit to the Heart causing agitation and mental disturbance such as anger and mania. Alternatively, if the gathering qi is deficient, then the qi of both the Lung and Heart will be deficient and unable to circulate the blood through the Heart with consequent stasis of Heart blood. Yuji LU-10 is indicated for diminished qi, shortness of breath and Heart painful obstruction.

The Lung channel originates in the middle jiao in the region of the Stomach. Yuji LU-10 is able to: i. clear heat which transmits to the Stomach channel giving rise to toothache, lacrimation or breast abscess, ii. counter dual rebellion of Lung and Stomach qi manifesting as cough with hiccup, and iii. treat various disorders of the Stomach fu including abdominal pain with inability to eat or drink, vomiting, childhood nutritional impairment and oesophageal constriction due to middle jiao deficiency.

Finally, Yuji LU-10 is an important local point in the treatment of pain and heat of the thumb joint.

COMBINATIONS

- Throat pain: Yuji LU-10 and Yemen SJ-2 (*One Hundred Symptoms*).
- Dry throat: Yuji LU-10 and Taiyuan LU-9 (*Great Compendium*).
- Stiffness of the tongue: Yuji LU-10, Shaoshang LU-11, Yamen DU-15, Erjian L.I.-2, Zhongchong P-9, Yingu KID-10 and Rangu KID-2 (*Great Compendium*).
- Headache: Yuji LU-10, Hegu L.I.-4, Tianchi P-1, Tongziliao GB-1, Sibai ST-2, Tianchong GB-9, Sanjiaoshu BL-22 and Fengchi GB-20 (*Systematic Classic*).
- Any type of spitting blood: reduce Yuji LU-10 and reinforce Chize LU-5 (*Systematic Classic*).
- Vomiting blood: Yuji LU-10, Quze P-3 and Shenmen HE-7 (*Great Compendium*).
- Pain of the Lung and Heart: Yuji LU-10 and Taiyuan LU-9 (*Systematic Classic*).
- Heart painful obstruction, sadness and fear: Yuji LU-10, Shenmen HE-7 and Dadun LIV-1 (*Great Compendium*).
- Manic raving, fear and fright: Yuji LU-10, Zhizheng SI-7, Hegu L.I.-4, Shaohai HE-3, Quchi L.I.-11 and Wangu SI-4 (*Thousand Ducat Formulas*).
- Pain of the penis: Yuji LU-10, Taixi KID-3, Zhongji REN-3 and Sanyinjiao SP-6 (*Great Compendium*).
- Enuresis: Yuji LU-10, Shenmen HE-7, Taichong LIV-3, Dadun LIV-1 and Guanyuan REN-4 (*Great Compendium*).
- Breast abscess: Yuji LU-10, Xiajuxu ST-39, Zusanli ST-36, Xiaxi GB-43, Weizhong BL-40, Zulinqi GB-41 and Shaoze SI-1 (*Great Compendium*).
- Difficult ingestion: Yuji LU-10, Zhongfu LU-1, Kunlun BL-60, Chengman ST-20 and Zhourong SP-20 (*Supplementing Life*).
- Difficult ingestion: Yuji LU-10, Neiguan P-6 and Zusanli ST-36 (*Great Compendium*).
- Contraction of the elbow: Yuji LU-10, Chize LU-5, Jianyu L.I.-15, Xiaohai SI-8, Jianshi P-5, Daling P-7 and Houxi SI-3 (*Great Compendium*).

SHAOSHANG LU-11

少商

Lesser Shang

Jing-Well and Wood point of the Lung channel
Sun Si-miao Ghost point

LOCATION

On the extensor aspect of the thumb, at the junction of lines drawn along the radial border of the nail and the base of the nail, approximately 0.1 cun from the corner of the nail.

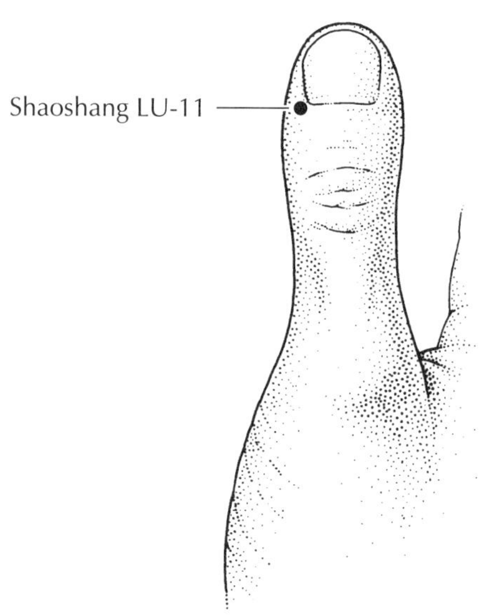

NEEDLING

Perpendicular or oblique insertion directed proximally 0.1 to 0.2 cun, or prick to bleed.

ACTIONS

Revives consciousness
Clears heat and benefits the throat

INDICATIONS

- Loss of consciousness from windstroke, loss of consciousness, cold inversion, hot inversion.
- Sore throat, throat painful obstruction, childhood throat moth, mumps, lotus flower tongue, nosebleed, dry lips with desire to drink, febrile disease with cold shivering.
- Agitation (of the Heart) with cough and dyspnoea, fullness of the Heart with sweating, fullness below the Heart, mania, childhood fright wind, malaria, vomiting.
- Pain and contraction of the wrist, pain of the thumb, heat of the palms, painful obstruction of the upper arm, pain of the front of the ear.

COMMENTARY

Shaoshang LU-11[23] is the jing-well point of the Lung channel, and in common with many of the jing-well points is an important point to revive collapse, being indicated for loss of consciousness (from windstroke) and cold or hot inversion.

The internal pathway of the Lung channel ascends, at its highest point, to the throat. As the terminal point of the Lung channel, Shaoshang LU-11 has a particularly strong action on the opposite end of the channel and may be needled or pricked to bleed in all acute disorders of the throat and surrounding tissues due to excess heat and fire poison. As well as simple sore throat due to attack by exterior wind-heat, Shaoshang LU-11 is indicated for mumps and 'childhood throat moth', a traditional disease category more or less corresponding to tonsillitis. To induce bleeding more easily from Shaoshang LU-11, the thumb and index fingers of one hand are used to grasp and engorge the patient's thumb, whilst using the other hand to prick the point. According to Master Zhu Dan-xi[24] of the Jin-Yuan dynasty "recuperation instantly follows bleeding". Both Shaoshang LU-11 and Yuji LU-10 have an important effect on the throat. In comparison with Yuji LU-10, which is indicated for both excess and deficiency heat, Shaoshang LU-11 is generally used for more extreme conditions due only to excess.

The *Classic of Difficulties*[25] states that jing-well points treat "fullness below the Heart". The region 'below the Heart' specifically refers to the apex of the epigastrium, but many of the jing-well points in fact treat stagnation and fullness throughout the chest region. Shaoshang LU-11 is indicated for fullness of the Heart and of the region below the Heart, accompanied by sweating. Its ability to treat stasis and heat in the Heart is further reflected by its indications for mania and agitation of the Heart. For this reason it was included under its alternative name of Gui-xin (Ghost Faith) among Sun Si-miao's 'thirteen ghost points' for the treatment of mania disorder and epilepsy.

COMBINATIONS

- Swollen and painful throat: Shaoshang LU-11, Tiantu REN-22 and Hegu L.I.-4 (*Great Compendium*).
- Coughing and dyspnoea: Shaoshang LU-11 and Daling P-7 (*Thousand Ducat Formulas*).
- Stiffness of the tongue: Shaoshang LU-11, Yuji LU-10, Yamen DU-15, Erjian L.I.-2, Zhongchong P-9, Yingu KID-10 and Rangu KID-2 (*Great Compendium*).
- Rattling sound in the throat: Shaoshang LU-11, Taichong LIV-3 and Jingqu LU-8 (*Thousand Ducat Formulas*).
- Blood deficiency thirst: Shaoshang LU-11 and Quze P-3 (*One Hundred Symptoms*).

- Vomiting: Shaoshang LU-11 and Laogong P-8 (*Thousand Ducat Formulas*).
- Dementia: Shaoshang LU-11, Shenmen HE-7, Yongquan KID-1 and Xinshu BL-15 (*Great Compendium*).

NOTES

1 *Spiritual Pivot* Chapter 1.
2 *Spiritual Pivot* Chapter 8.
3 *Essential Questions* Chapter 46.
4 *Spiritual Pivot* Chapter 17.
5 *Essential Questions* Chapter 38.
6 *Essential Questions* Chapter 44.
7 *Spiritual Pivot* Chapter 20.
8 *Essential Questions* Chapter 61.
9 *Essential Questions* Chapter 61.
10 *Spiritual Pivot* Chapter 21.
11 *Nourishment of Life*, Health in Chinese Society, Linda C. Koo, The Commercial Press, Hong Kong p. 123.
12 *Classic of Difficulties* 68th Difficulty.
13 *Spiritual Pivot* Chapter 44.
14 It should, however, be pointed out that the terms coughing blood and vomiting blood were used interchangeably in the *Essentials from the Golden Cabinet*, and some later writers also did not differentiate clearly between them, therefore failing to distinguish the origin of the bleeding.
15 Ma Dan-yang was the originator of the *Song of the Eleven Heavenly Star Points*. They first appeared in print in the 12th century CE *Classic of the Jade Dragon*. Xu Feng included this text in his work *Complete Collection of Acupuncture and Moxibustion* and added a twelfth point, Taichong LIV-3.
16 *Spiritual Pivot* Chapter 5.
17 *Essential Questions* Chapter 6.
18 Quoted in *Chinese Acupuncture and Moxibustion*, Foreign Languages Press, Beijing.
19 *Classic of Difficulties* 68th Difficulty.
20 *Classic of Difficulties* 69th Difficulty.
21 *Classic of Difficulties* 45th Difficulty.
22 *Classic of Difficulties* 68th Difficulty.
23 'Shang' is the note associated with the metal phase in an ancient musical annotation system.
24 *The Heart & Essence of Dan-xi's Methods of Treatment*, A Translation of Zhu Dan-xi's Dan Xi Zhi Fa Xin Yao, Blue Poppy Press, p. 304.
25 *Classic of Difficulties* 68th Difficulty.

手陽明大腸經

THE LARGE INTESTINE CHANNEL OF HAND YANGMING

THE LARGE INTESTINE CHANNEL OF HAND YANGMING

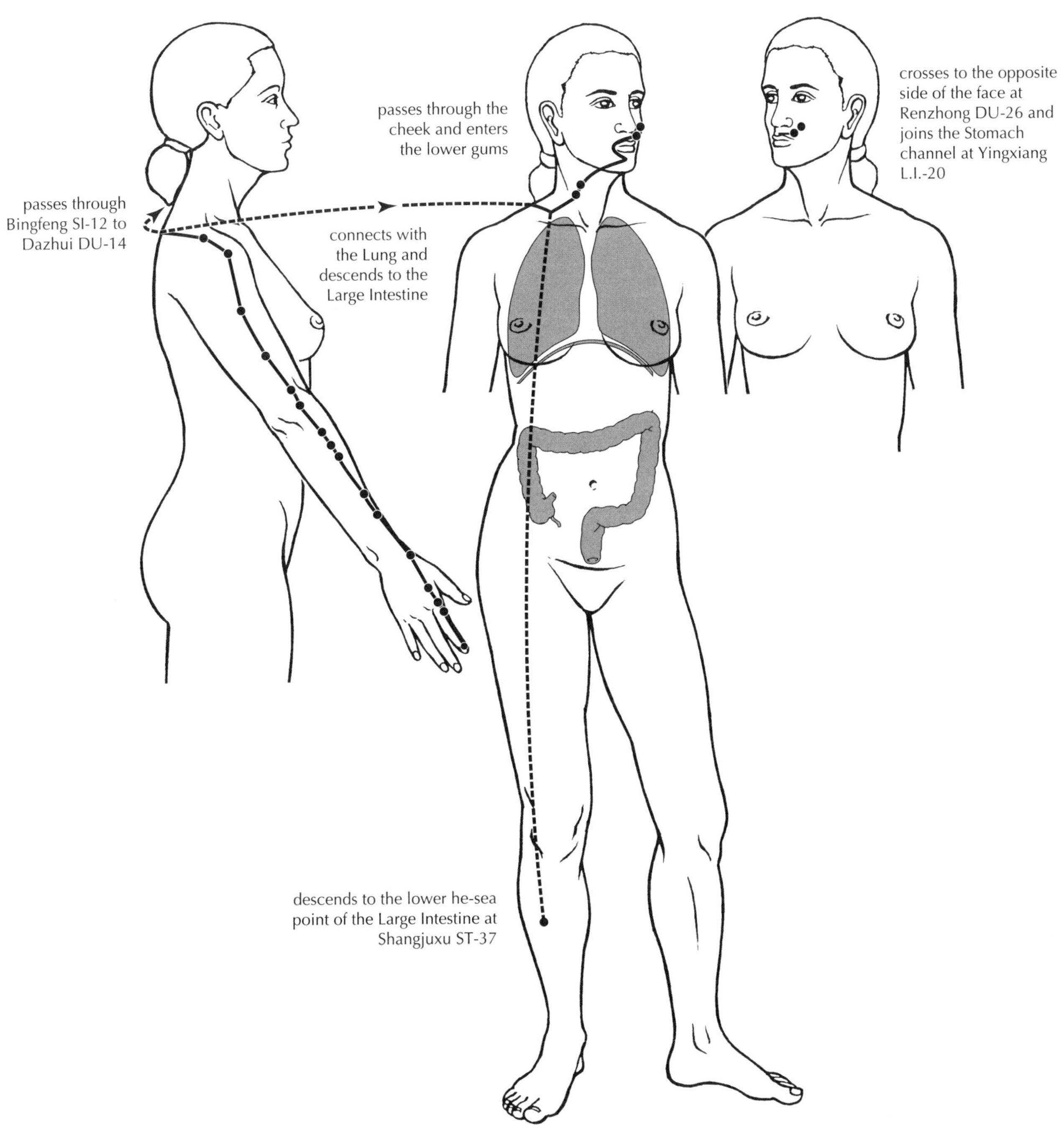
passes through the
cheek and enters
the lower gums
crosses to the opposite
side of the face at
Renzhong DU-26 and
joins the Stomach
channel at Yingxiang
L.I.-20
passes through
Bingfeng SI-12 to
Dazhui DU-14
connects with
the Lung and
descends to the
Large Intestine
descends to the lower he-sea
point of the Large Intestine at
Shangjuxu ST-37

The Large Intestine primary channel

THE LARGE INTESTINE PRIMARY CHANNEL

- begins at the radial side of the tip of the index finger,
- runs proximally along the radial side of the index finger and passes through the interspace between the first and second metacarpal bones at Hegu L.I.-4,
- reaches the depression between the tendons of extensor pollicis longus and brevis (anatomical snuff-box) where Yangxi L.I.-5 is situated,
- continues along the lateral aspect of the forearm to the lateral aspect of the elbow at Quchi L.I.-11,
- rises along the lateral aspect of the upper arm to the shoulder joint at Jianyu L.I.-15,
- crosses behind the shoulder to the depression between the scapular spine and the lateral extremity of the clavicle (Jugu L.I.-16),
- travels in a medial direction, passing through Bingfeng SI-12 (in the centre of the suprascapular fossa) to Dazhui DU-14 (just below the spinous process of the vertebra of C7) where it meets with the other five yang channels of the hand and foot,
- from Dazhui DU-14 it enters the supraclavicular fossa in the region of Quepen ST-12 and connects with the Lung before descending through the diaphragm to join with the Large Intestine,
- another branch ascends from the supraclavicular fossa along the lateral aspect of the neck, passes through the cheek, and enters the lower gums.
- from the gums the channel passes through Dicang ST-4, curves around the upper lip and crosses to the opposite side of the body at Renzhong DU-26, at the philtrum,
- from Renzhong DU-26, the left channel travels to the right and the right channel travels to the left to terminate either side of the nose at Yingxiang L.I.-20,
- at Yingxiang L.I.-20 the Large Intestine channel joins with the Stomach channel.
- According to the *Spiritual Pivot*[1] a branch of the Large Intestine primary channel descends to Shangjuxu ST-37.

The Large Intestine primary channel connects with the following zangfu: Large Intestine, Lung.

The Large Intestine primary channel meets with other channels at the following points: Dicang ST-4, Quepen ST-12, Bingfeng SI-12, Dazhui DU-14, Renzhong DU-26, Chengjiang REN-24. Note that although Xuanlu GB-5, Xuanli GB-6 and Yangbai GB-14 are classically listed as meeting points with the Large Intestine channel, illustrations of the channel do not normally show these connections.

Note: i. According to descriptions of the Lung primary channel pathway, a branch of the channel runs from Lieque LU-7 to Shangyang L.I.-1. This latter point however is not classified as a meeting point of the Large Intestine and Lung channels. ii. Chengjiang REN-24 is classified as a meeting point of the Conception vessel with the Large Intestine channel. This connection is not conventionally mentioned however, in descriptions of the pathway of the Large Intestine primary channel.

THE LARGE INTESTINE LUO-CONNECTING CHANNEL

- begins at Pianli L.I.-6,
- joins with its interiorly-exteriorly associated Lung channel three cun above the wrist,
- ascends the arm through Jianyu L.I.-15 to the jaw and cheek, where it divides, one branch connecting with the teeth, the other entering the ear to join the 'zong mai' (where the channels of the Large Intestine, Stomach, Small Intestine, Gall Bladder and Sanjiao gather and collect at the ear).

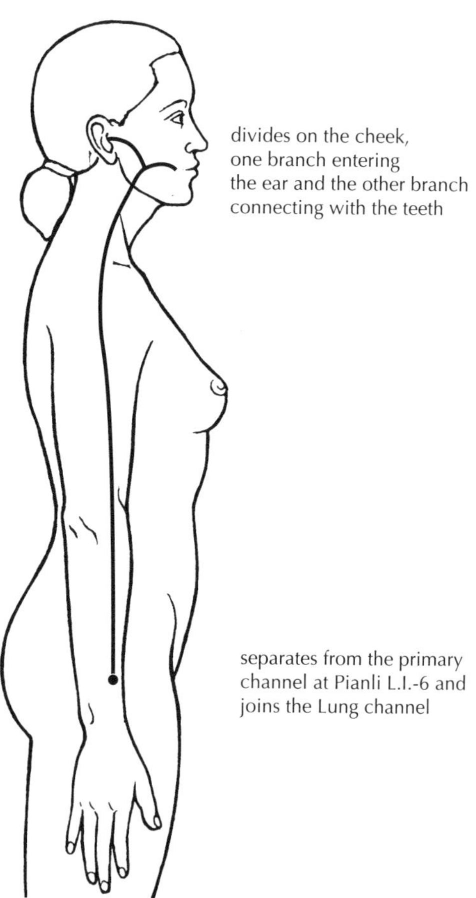
divides on the cheek, one branch entering the ear and the other branch connecting with the teeth
separates from the primary channel at Pianli L.I.-6 and joins the Lung channel

The Large Intestine luo-connecting channel

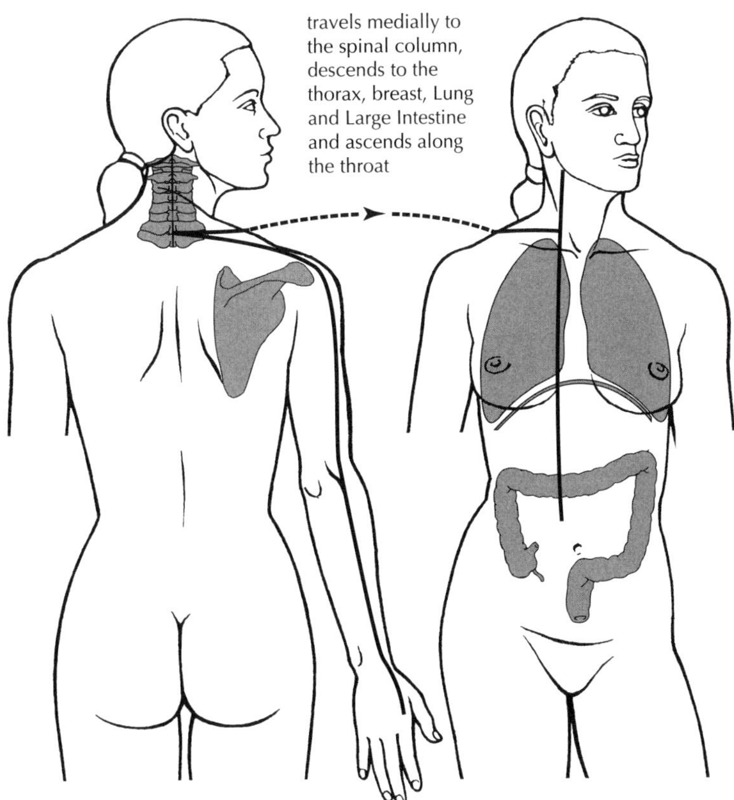

The Large Intestine Divergent channel

THE LARGE INTESTINE DIVERGENT CHANNEL

- separates from the Large Intestine primary channel on the hand,
- ascends the arm to the shoulder at Jianyu L.I.-15,
- travels medially to the spinal column,
- crosses to the supraclavicular fossa and descends to the thorax, breast, Lung and Large Intestine,
- a branch ascends from the supraclavicular fossa along the throat and unites with the Large Intestine primary channel.

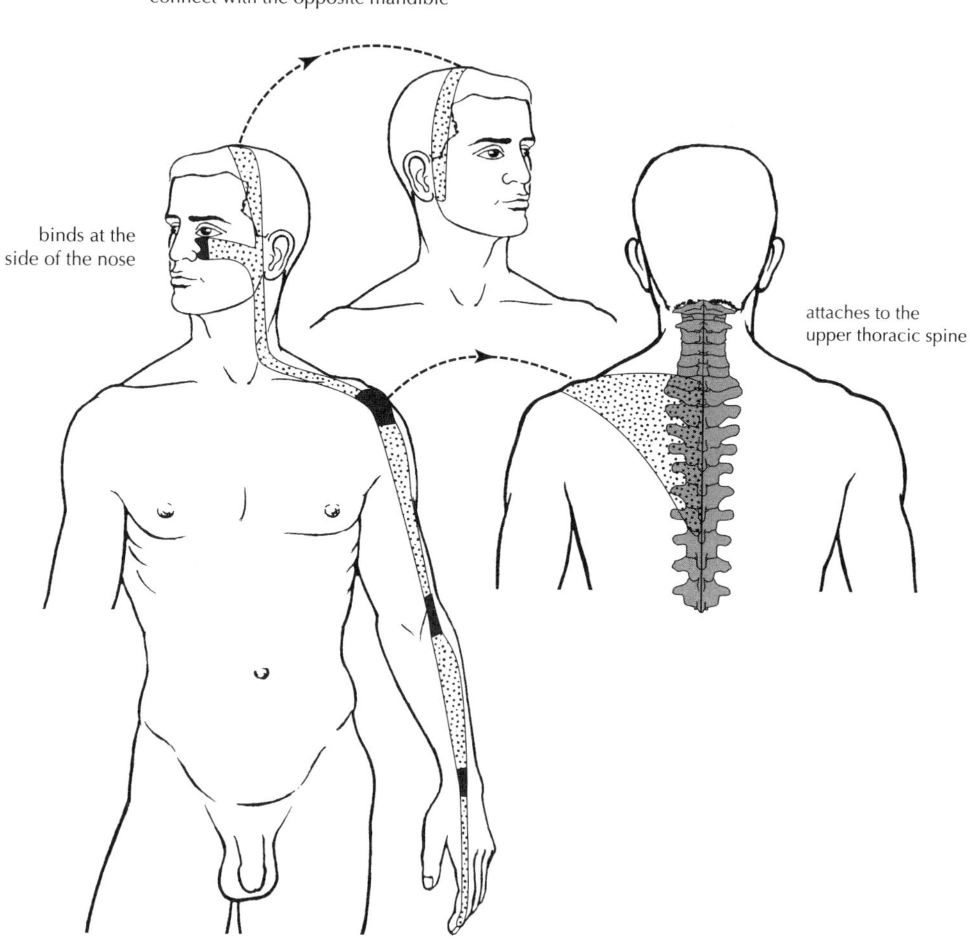

The Large Intestine sinew channel

THE LARGE INTESTINE SINEW CHANNEL

- begins at the tip of the index finger at Shangyang L.I.-1 and binds at the dorsum of the wrist,
- ascends the forearm and binds at the lateral aspect of the elbow,
- ascends the upper arm to bind at the shoulder,
- a branch winds around the scapula and attaches to the upper thoracic spine,
- from the shoulder the main channel ascends to the neck from where a branch ascends across the cheeks to bind at the side of the nose, whilst,
- the main channel ascends anterior to the Small Intestine sinew channel, crosses the temple to the corner of the forehead, and crosses over the top of the head to connect with the mandible on the opposite side.

Pathological symptoms of the Large Intestine sinew channel
Cramping and pain along the course of the channel, inability to raise the shoulder, inability to turn the neck to the left or to the right.

DISCUSSION

The Large Intestine channel of hand yangming is interiorly-exteriorly coupled with the Lung channel of hand taiyin, and paired with the Stomach channel of foot yangming according to six channel theory. The Large Intestine-Lung relationship is further strengthened by the fact that:

- both the interior pathway of the Large Intestine channel as well as the Large Intestine divergent channel enter the Lung zang.
- the Large Intestine luo-connecting channel from Pianli L.I.-6 joins with the Lung channel.

In addition it is clinically valuable to note that:

- the Large Intestine primary channel enters the gums of the lower teeth.
- the Large Intestine primary channel crosses to the contralateral side of the face at Renzhong DU-26.
- the Large Intestine sinew channel ascends to the corner of the forehead and crosses over the top of the head to connect with the opposite mandible.
- the Large Intestine luo-connecting channel enters the ear as well as the teeth.
- the Large Intestine divergent channel descends to the breast.
- the Large Intestine sinew channel attaches to the upper thoracic spine and the divergent channel travels medially to the spinal column.

The function of the Large Intestine fu is to receive waste material sent down from the Small Intestine, absorb its fluid content and form the remainder into faeces to be excreted. Despite this, although several points of the Large Intestine channel have an action on the intestines and lower abdomen (particularly in the treatment of borborygmus and diarrhoea), in clinical practice they are considerably less used than points of the Spleen and Stomach channels. Also there is no Large Intestine channel point indicated for difficult defecation or constipation. This paucity of Large Intestine indications is not surprising in view of the fact that whilst the channel traverses the upper body, the fu lies in the lower abdomen.

According to the *Spiritual Pivot*[2] "Yangming channel is abundant in qi and blood". Points of both the arm and leg portions of yangming channel are therefore much used clinically to regulate qi and blood in the limbs and treat atrophy disorder and painful obstruction, hemiplegia and pain of all kinds.

In the Chinese tradition 'the sage faces South' and thus the light and warmth of the sun fall on the front of the body. The yangming channels, on the anterior of the limbs, receive the full intensity of the sun, as does the abdominal and chest portion of the foot yangming Stomach channel, the only yang channel to run along the anterior of the body. For this reason, yangming or 'yang brightness' is considered to be particularly replete with yang qi. Points of the Large Intestine channel, therefore, are among the most important points to clear excess of yang in the form of heat and fever, notably Hegu L.I.-4 and Quchi L.I.-11.

Apart from the above, the primary actions and indications of the points of the Large Intestine channel can be summarised as:

- treating all disorders of the yangming channel in the head; this area includes the face and cheeks, forehead, eyes, nose, lips, gums and teeth.
- treating disorders of the ear (Large Intestine luo-connecting channel).
- expelling wind, cold and heat from the exterior portion of the body.
- clearing wind-heat, interior heat and fire poison from the areas traversed by the channel, especially in the head.
- clearing yangming fire which disturbs the Heart and spirit.
- assisting the Lung in its function of opening the water passages.

SHANGYANG L.I.-1

Shang Yang

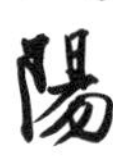

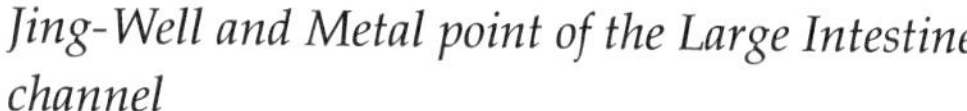

Jing-Well and Metal point of the Large Intestine channel

LOCATION

On the dorsal aspect of the index finger, at the junction of lines drawn along the radial border of the nail and the base of the nail, approximately 0.1 cun from the corner of the nail.

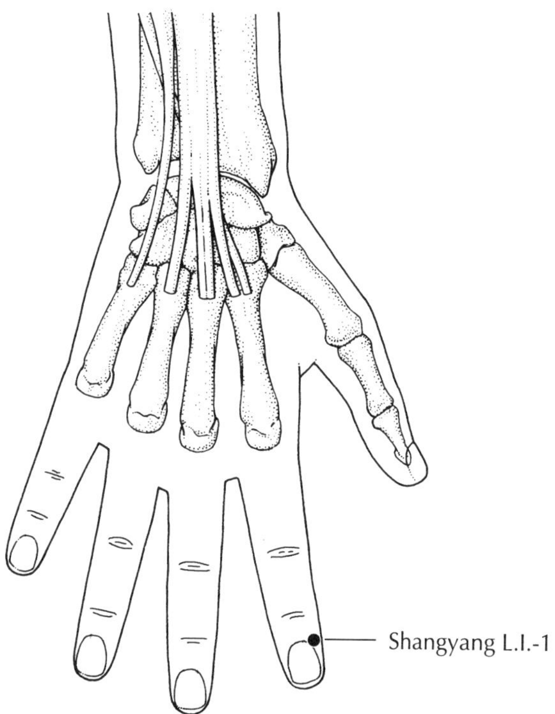

NEEDLING

Perpendicular or oblique insertion directed proximally 0.1 to 0.2 cun, or prick to bleed.

ACTIONS

Clears heat, reduces swelling and alleviates pain
Revives consciousness

INDICATIONS

- Throat painful obstruction, toothache of the lower jaw, pain of the lower cheek, swelling of the submandibular region, dry mouth, deafness, tinnitus.
- Loss of consciousness from windstroke, loss of consciousness, qi fullness of the chest radiating to the lateral costal region, dyspnoea and cough, febrile disease with absence of sweating, hot malaria.
- Pain of the shoulder and back that radiates to the supraclavicular fossa, numbness and heat of the fingers.

COMMENTARY

The term 'shang' in the name of this point is the note associated with the metal phase in an ancient musical notation system, whilst 'yang' denotes the yang channel and serves to differentiate this point from Shaoshang LU-11 'Lesser Shang'. Shangyang L.I.-1 is the metal point of the Large Intestine metal channel.

As the most distal point of the Large Intestine channel, Shangyang L.I.-1 has an urgent effect on resolving heat, swelling and pain at the opposite end of the channel, most frequently due to attack of wind-heat or accumulation of fire poison. According to the *Ode to Elucidate Mysteries* "the root of the hand yangming is Shangyang L.I.-1 and it knots at Futu L.I.-18 and Pianli L.I.-6". This statement emphasises the special affinity of this point for the ear (which is reached by the Large Intestine luo-connecting channel from Pianli L.I.-6), reflected in its indications for tinnitus and deafness. In addition, the Large Intestine primary channel traverses the lower part of the cheek and enters the lower jaw, whilst the Large Intestine divergent channel ascends along the throat. Shangyang L.I.-1 is therefore used for disorders of these regions characterised by severe and sudden swelling, heat and pain, for example toothache of the lower jaw, throat painful obstruction and swelling of the submandibular region. The ability of Shangyang L.I.-1 to dynamically clear heat has a wider application in the treatment of febrile diseases, and especially malaria.

In common with the other jing-well points, Shangyang L.I.-1 is used to revive from collapse and is indicated for loss of consciousness (from windstroke).

A branch of the Lung channel terminates at Shangyang L.I.-1 and as the metal point of the yang metal channel, it is indicated for fullness characterised by qi stagnation in the Lung, which may i. radiate to the lateral costal region, and ii. give rise to dyspnoea and coughing. In respect of this ability to clear fullness from the chest region, Shangyang L.I.-1 is typical of the jing-well points.

Finally the Large Intestine muscle and divergent channels both connect with the spine, and Shangyang L.I.-1 is indicated for pain of the shoulder and back which radiates to the supraclavicular fossa.

COMBINATIONS

- Febrile disease with absence of sweating: Shangyang L.I-1, Hegu L.I-4, Yangxi L.I.-5, Xiaxi GB-43, Lidui ST-45, Laogong P-8 and Wangu SI-4 (*Great Compendium*).
- Cold malaria: Shangyang L.I-1 and Taixi KID-3 (*One Hundred Symptoms*).
- Malaria with generalised fever: Shangyang L.I.-1, Sanjian L.I.-3 Zhongzhu SJ-3, Yindu KID-19 and Shaohai HE-3 (*Supplementing Life*).

- Chronic malaria: Shangyang L.I.-1, Zhongzhu SJ-3 and Qiuxu GB-40 (*Great Compendium*).
- Tinnitus: Shangyang L.I.-1, Pianli L.I.-6, Yangxi L.I.-5, Luoque BL-8, Wangu SI-4 and Qiangu SI-2 (*Supplementing Life*).
- Deafness: Shangyang L.I.-1, Zhongzhu SJ-3, Waiguan SJ-5, Erheliao SJ-22, Tinghui GB-2, Tinggong SI-19, Hegu L.I.-4 and Zhongchong P-9 (*Precious Mirror*).
- Dry mouth and tongue with difficult ingestion: Shangyang L.I.-1, Danshu BL-19 and Xiaochangshu BL-27 (*Thousand Ducat Formulas*).
- Swelling of the supraclavicular fossa [Quepen ST-12]: Shangyang L.I.-1, Taixi KID-3 and Zulinqi GB-41 (*Great Compendium*).

ERJIAN L.I.-2

二間

Second Space

Ying-Spring and Water point of the Large Intestine channel

LOCATION

On the radial border of the index finger, in a depression just distal to the metacarpo-phalangeal joint.

LOCATION NOTE

This point will be easier to find if the index finger is relaxed in a slightly flexed position.

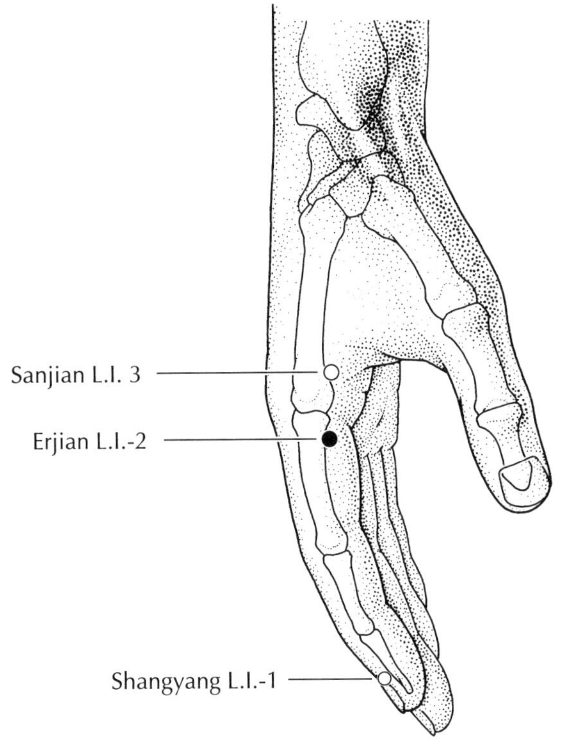

NEEDLING

i. Oblique proximal or distal insertion 0.2 to 0.3 cun; ii. Perpendicular-oblique insertion towards the palm, 0.5 cun.

ACTIONS

Expels wind, clears heat and reduces swelling
Alleviates pain

INDICATIONS

- Toothache, pain and swelling of the lower cheek, acute weeping eczema of the face, deviation of the mouth and eye, nosebleed, rhinitis, throat painful obstruction, dry mouth, cloudy vision, eye diseases, yellow eyes.
- Febrile disease, cold shivering, acute food stagnation.
- Injury by cold with water binding the chest and lateral costal region, propensity to fright, somnolence.
- Pain and stiffness of the shoulder and back, cold and pain at the point Jianyu L.I.-15.

COMMENTARY

According to the *Classic of Difficulties*[3] ying-spring points are indicated for "heat in the body". Erjian L.I.-2, the ying-spring point of the Large Intestine channel, clears heat and expels wind from the upper reaches of the channel in the teeth, nose, face, throat and eyes.

It is useful to view the Large Intestine channel in relationship both to the Lung channel, with which it is interiorly-exteriorly coupled, and to the Stomach channel with which it is paired according to six channel theory (yangming). The Large Intestine channel may be seen as the exterior reflection of the Lung, and its distal points such as Erjian L.I.-2 are used to expel wind-heat from the exterior portion of the Lung, especially the throat and nose, being indicated for sore throat, rhinitis and nosebleed accompanied by fever and shivering. As far as the Stomach is concerned, accumulated heat in the Stomach and Large Intestine may be transmitted along the hand yangming channel and give rise to inflammation of the throat, dry mouth and toothache. Various classical sources have emphasised the use of Erjian L.I.-2 for toothache, rather than the more commonly-used Hegu L.I.-4, which may be seen as a reflection of the dynamic and urgent quality of the more distal point. Although the Large Intestine channel does not reach the eye, its coupled yangming Stomach channel originates at the eye and this explains the ability of Erjian L.I.-2 to treat eye diseases.

The indications for Erjian L.I.-2 include propensity to fright and somnolence. It also appears in combination for toothache with lumbar pain, and, with several points of the Kidney channel, for somnolence. These indications hint at Kidney disharmony, and it may be that as the water point of the Large Intestine metal channel, Erjian L.I.-2 was considered effective in the treatment of deficiency patterns of the Kidneys.

Finally the Large Intestine muscle and divergent channels both connect with the spine, and Erjian L.I.-2 is indicated for pain and stiffness of the shoulder and back.

COMBINATIONS

- Toothache and lumbar pain accompanied by throat painful obstruction: Erjian L.I.-2 and Yangxi L.I.-5 (*Ode of Xi-hong*).
- Toothache of the lower jaw: Erjian L.I.-2, Shangyang L.I.-1, Yanggu SI-5, Yemen SJ-2 and Sidu SJ-9 (*Thousand Ducat Formulas*).
- Toothache: Erjian L.I.-2 and Quanliao SI-18 (*Systematic Classic*).
- Rhinitis with nose bleed: Erjian L.I.-2, Yingxiang L.I.-20 and Fengfu DU-16 (*Great Compendium*).
- Pain of the eye: Erjian L.I.-2, Yangxi L.I.-5, Daling P-7, Sanjian L.I.-3, Qiangu SI-2 and Shangxing DU-23 (*Great Compendium*).
- Somnolence: Erjian L.I.-2, Shouwuli L.I.-13, Taixi KID-3, Dazhong KID-4 and Zhaohai KID-6 (*Supplementing Life*).
- Somnolence: Erjian L.I.-2, Sanjian L.I.-3, Taixi KID-3, Zhaohai KID-6, Baihui DU-20, Tianjing GB-21, Lidui ST-45 and Ganshu BL-18 (*Great Compendium*).
- Excessive fright: Erjian L.I.-2, Yinxi HE-6, Jianshi P-5 and Lidui ST-45 (*Supplementing Life*).

SANJIAN L.I.-3

Third Space

三
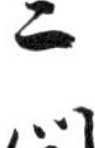

Shu-Stream and Wood point of the Large Intestine channel

LOCATION

On the radial side of the index finger, in the substantial depression proximal to the head of the second metacarpal bone.

LOCATION NOTE

This point is easier to locate when the hand is made into a loose fist.

NEEDLING

Perpendicular insertion 0.5 to 2 cun, directed towards Houxi SI-3. **Note:** needle with the hand in a loose fist position, with the metacarpal bones lying in the same plane. This is especially important when needling deeply towards the opposite side of the hand.

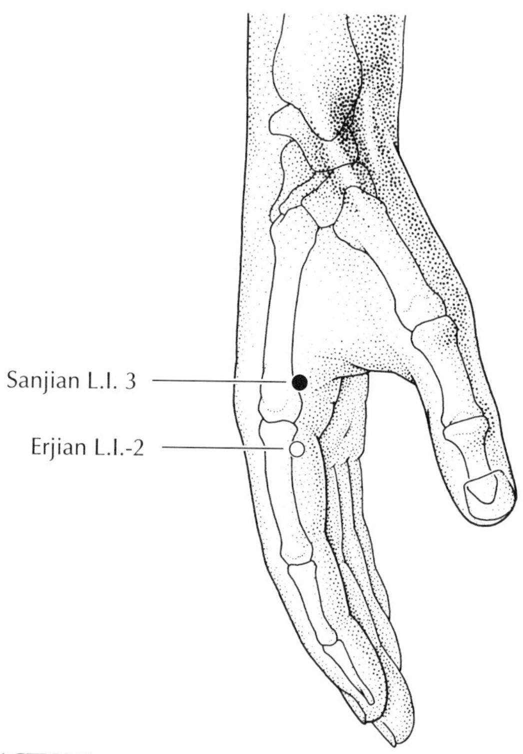

ACTIONS

Expels wind and heat
Clears heat and benefits the throat and teeth
Dispels fullness and treats diarrhoea

INDICATIONS

- Throat painful obstruction, obstruction of the throat, toothache of the lower jaw, pain from decaying teeth, tongue thrusting, acute eye pain, dry scorched lips and mouth, nosebleed, rhinitis, tinnitus, chills and fever.
- Cold or damp (dong) diarrhoea, borborygmus, somnolence, injury by cold with water binding the chest and lateral costal region, fright, fullness of the chest, malaria.
- Acute stiff neck, redness and swelling of the dorsum of the hand, difficulty in flexing and extending the fingers.

COMMENTARY

In common with many of the distal points of the Large Intestine channel, Sanjian L.I.-3 expels wind-heat and yangming channel heat from the upper reaches of the channel, being indicated for symptoms such as pain and swelling of the throat, dry scorched lips and mouth, chills and fever and nosebleed. As far as toothache and pain from tooth decay is concerned, Zhu Dan-xi of the Jin-Yuan dynasty recommended applying moxibustion to Sanjian L.I.-3 for toothache of the lower jaw (and to Shousanli L.I.-10 for toothache of the upper jaw[4]), whilst in modern clinical practice, some Chinese practitioners favour Sanjian L.I.-3 over Hegu L.I.-4 for the treatment of severe or recalcitrant toothache.

It is a characteristic of the three yang channels of the hand (Large and Small Intestines and Sanjiao) that relatively few of their points are indicated for disorders of their corresponding fu, for example points of the Small Intestine channel are notable for the absence of indications of intestinal disorders. By contrast, the lower he-sea points which are ascribed to these three channels on the lower limb (Shangjuxu ST-37 for the Large Intestine, Xiajuxu ST-39 for the Small Intestine and Weiyang BL-39 for the Sanjiao) are much used clinically for disorders of the fu. In the case of the Large Intestine channel however, several points including Sanjian L.I.-3 are classically indicated for borborygmus and diarrhoea. Nevertheless, points of the Large Intestine channel are little used for this purpose in clinical practice, and they appear in relatively few classical combinations for the treatment of intestinal disorders.

According to the *Classic of Difficulties*[5] the shu-stream points are indicated for "heaviness of the body and pain of the joints". Sanjian L.I.-3 is an important local point for treating disorders of the fingers (especially the index and middle fingers) and dorsum of the hand. It is often combined with Houxi SI-3 in the treatment of stiffness, swelling and pain of the five fingers, and like Houxi SI-3, whose location it mirrors, is also indicated (although less used clinically) for acute stiff neck.

Finally, like Erjian L.I.-2, Sanjian L.I.-3 is indicated for such symptoms as somnolence and fright.

COMBINATIONS

- Pain from tooth decay: Sanjian L.I.-3, Daying ST-5 and Zhengying GB-17 (*Preserving Life*).
- Erosion, heat and dryness of the mouth: Sanjian L.I.-3, Laogong P-8, Shaoze SI-1 and Taichong LIV-3 (*Thousand Ducat Formulas*).
- Obstruction of the throat: Sanjian L.I.-3 and Jianshi P-5 (*Great Compendium*).
- Somnolence: Sanjian L.I.-3 and Erjian L.I.-2 (*Supplementing Life*).
- Somnolence with no desire to move the four limbs: Sanjian L.I.-3, Sanyangluo SJ-8, Tianjing SJ-10, Zuwuli LIV-10 and Lidui ST-45 (*Thousand Ducat Formulas*).
- Borborygmus and diarrhoea: Sanjian L.I.-3, Shenque REN-8 and Shuifen REN-9 (*Great Compendium*).
- Pain of the shoulder and back, wind-taxation [chronic painful obstruction leading to exhaustion of qi and blood]: Sanjian L.I.-3 and Shenshu BL-23 (*Ode of Xi-hong*).

HEGU L.I.-4

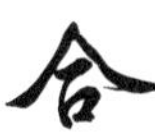

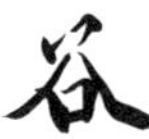

Joining Valley

Yuan-Source point of the Large Intestine channel
Gao Wu Command point
Ma Dan-yang Heavenly Star point

LOCATION

On the dorsum of the hand, between the first and second metacarpal bones, at the midpoint of the second metacarpal bone and close to its radial border.

LOCATION NOTE

Ask the patient to squeeze the thumb against the base of the index finger, and locate Hegu L.I.-4 at the highest point of the bulge of the muscle and approximately level with the end of the crease.

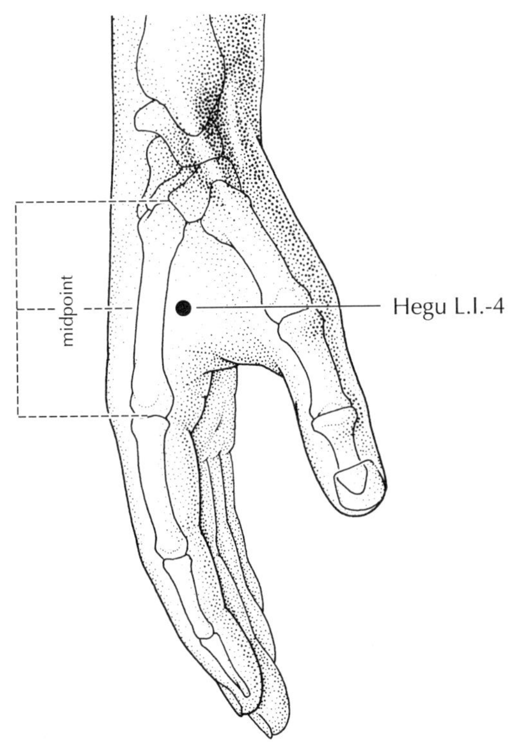

NEEDLING

i. Perpendicular insertion 0.5 to 1 cun; ii. Oblique insertion directed proximally 1 to 1.5 cun.
Caution: contraindicated in pregnancy.

ACTIONS

Regulates the defensive qi and adjusts sweating
Expels wind and releases the exterior
Regulates the face, eyes, nose, mouth and ears
Activates the channel and alleviates pain
Induces labour
Restores the yang

INDICATIONS

- Exterior wind-cold pattern, chills and fever, injury by cold with great thirst, copious sweating, absence of sweating, febrile disease with absence of sweating, floating pulse.
- Headache, one-sided headache, headache of the whole head, hypertension.
- Redness, swelling and pain of the eyes, dimness of vision, superficial visual obstruction.
- Nosebleed, nasal congestion and discharge, rhinitis, sneezing.
- Toothache or pain of tooth decay in the lower jaw, mouth ulcers, lotus flower tongue, cracked tongue, rigid tongue, lips do not close, tightness of the lips.
- Throat painful obstruction, childhood throat moth, mumps, loss of voice.
- Swelling of the face, deviation of the face and mouth, lockjaw, deafness, tinnitus.
- Amenorrhoea, prolonged labour, delayed labour, retention of dead foetus.
- Dysenteric disorder, childhood nutritional impairment, childhood fright wind, wind rash, malaria, mania.
- Painful obstruction and atrophy disorder of the four limbs, hemiplegia, pain of the sinews and bones, pain of the arm, contraction of the fingers, pain of the lumbar spine.

COMMENTARY

Hegu L.I.-4 was included by Ma Dan-yang, the great physician of the Jin dynasty, among the 'eleven heavenly star points'[6], his grouping of the most vital acupuncture points, and was indicated by him for headache, swelling of the face, malaria with chills and fever, tooth decay, nosebleed and lockjaw with inability to speak. The Ming dynasty author Gao Wu in his work *Glorious Anthology of Acupuncture and Moxibustion* also recognised the supreme importance of this point and included it among his 'four command points' (for the face and mouth). Some hundreds of years later it is still probably the best known and most commonly used of the acupuncture points.

Hegu L.I.-4 is a primary point to expel wind-cold or wind-heat and to release the exterior. It may be useful in this respect to view the yang Large Intestine channel as the exterior reflection of the yin Lung channel with which it is coupled. The Lung dominates the exterior by virtue of its function of controlling the skin and body hair and spreading the defensive qi. Attack by exterior pathogenic wind-cold or wind-heat which disrupts the exterior portion of the Lung system therefore, may be treated via points of the Large Intestine channel, most notably by Hegu L.I.-4. Thus the *Great Compendium of Acupuncture and Moxibustion* recommends this point for "injury by cold, headache, rigid spine, and absence of sweating". This is the classic presentation of wind-cold binding the exterior portion of the body. The basic principle in Chinese medicine for the treatment of this condition is to release the exterior by inducing sweating, thereby expelling the pathogen along with the sweat and facilitating the circulation of defensive qi. In fact, Hegu L.I.-4 may also be used for injury by any exterior pathogenic factor which is accompanied by sweating (in this case pathological sweating which does not serve to expel the pathogenic factor). This dual action of Hegu L.I.-4 on both inducing and stopping sweating is reflected by the advice given in the *Great Compendium of Acupuncture and Moxibustion* to reinforce Hegu L.I.-4 and reduce Fuliu KID-7 if there is no sweating, and to reduce Hegu L.I.-4 and reinforce Fuliu KID-7 in cases with copious sweating. The explanation of this apparently contradictory function is that Hegu L.I.-4 is able to regulate defensive qi and hence adjust the pores, whatever the pattern, indeed some authorities go so far as to attribute to Hegu L.I.-4 the ability to tonify the defensive qi.

The passage from the *Great Compendium of Acupuncture and Moxibustion* quoted above includes the symptom of 'great thirst', which is clearly not typical of exterior patterns (where the fever and thirst are still relatively mild). This does, however, reflect the common use of Hegu L.I.-4, especially in combination with Quchi L.I.-11, to reduce high fever of whatever aetiology.

Hegu L.I.-4 is the single most important point to treat disorders of the face and sense organs. This has been emphasised in numerous classics, for example the *Classic of the Jade Dragon* states "Hegu L.I.-4 treats all diseases of the head, face, ears, eyes, nose, cheeks, mouth and teeth". This point is essential in the treatment of any disorder affecting these areas - whether acute or chronic, hot or cold, deficient or excess - but is least used clinically for disorders of the ears. As far as headaches are concerned, Hegu L.I.-4 is considered appropriate in the treatment of headache in any location due to attack by exterior pathogens, and most particularly any frontal (yangming channel) headache. In clinical practice, however, it is used even more widely, for example the *Classic of the Jade Dragon* recommended Hegu L.I.-4 for one-sided or generalised headache, whilst the *Ode of the Jade Dragon* more specifically recommended Hegu L.I.-4 for head wind without phlegm, and Fengchi GB-20 for head wind with phlegm. The affinity of Hegu L.I.-4 for both the forehead and the side of the head reflects the fact that the internal pathway of the Large Intestine channel meets with the Gall Bladder channel at Yangbai GB-14, Xuanlu GB-5 and Xuanli GB-6.

Hegu L.I.-4 is considered to have a particular ability to ease pain, especially in the areas discussed above, and is a commonly used point in acupuncture analgesia. According to Chinese medicine, pain of excess type arises when impaired circulation of qi and blood leads to stagnation. This is expressed in the saying "without movement there is pain, with movement there is no pain". The special ability of Hegu L.I.-4 to treat pain is explained by the statement in the *Spiritual Pivot*[7] "Yangming channel is abundant in qi and blood". This emphasises the particular ability of points on the Large Intestine and Stomach (yangming) channels to promote circulation of qi and blood, and thus dispel obstruction and stop pain, for example in painful disorders such as painful obstruction. However the abundance of qi and blood in the arm and foot yangming channels means that their points are not only important to dispel stagnation, but also to tonify qi and blood in the channels and thus bring nourishment to the limbs in case of atrophy disorder and hemiplegia. In practice, Hegu L.I.-4 is commonly combined with Jianyu L.I.-15 and Quchi L.I.-11 in the 'chain and lock' point association method for pain, paralysis or atrophy of the upper limb.

Bilateral Hegu L.I.-4 and Taichong LIV-3 are known as the Four Gates. This combination first appeared in the *Ode to Elucidate Mysteries* which said "for cold and heat with painful obstruction, open the Four Gates". The text goes on to imply that the yuan-source points of the six yang channels emerge at the four gates. Since a fundamental principle for treating painful obstruction is to select points from yang channels, this helps to explain why these two points are considered so effective in treating painful obstruction. Subsequently, the use of the Four Gates has been extended to treat a variety of disorders involving pain and spasm. This is an elegant combination. Hegu L.I.-4 on the upper extremity lies in the wide valley between the first and second metacarpals, whilst Taichong LIV-3 on the lower extremity lies in the wide valley between the first and second metatarsals. Hegu L.I.-4, the yuan-source point, belongs to yangming channel which is 'abundant in qi and blood' whilst Taichong LIV-3, the shu-stream and yuan-source point of the Liver channel, has the function of spreading the qi. Together they are able to activate the qi and blood and ensure their free and smooth passage throughout the body.

Hegu L.I.-4 has a strong action on promoting labour. The *Ode to Elucidate Mysteries* tells how the Song dynasty Crown Prince, in a dispute with the doctor Xu Wen-bai over whether a pregnant woman was carrying a girl or twins, ordered her belly to be cut open to find out. Xu Wen-bai begged to use his needles instead, and on reducing Zusanli ST-36 and reinforcing Hegu L.I.-4 two babies emerged. Due to its strong action of inducing labour, and even promoting the expulsion of a dead foetus, Hegu L.I.-4 is contraindicated in pregnancy.

Finally Hegu L.I.-4 is cited in the *Song of the Nine Needles for Returning the Yang*, for the treatment of collapse of yang characterised by loss of consciousness, aversion to cold, cold counterflow of the limbs, purple lips etc.

COMBINATIONS

- Little sweating: reinforce Hegu L.I.-4, reduce Fuliu KID-7. Copious sweating: first reduce Hegu L.I.-4 then reinforce Fuliu KID-7 (*Great Compendium*).
- Injury by cold with absence of sweating: Hegu L.I.-4 (reinforce), Neiting ST-44 (reduce), Fuliu KID-7 (reduce) and Bailao (M-HN-30) (*Great Compendium*).
- Injury by cold with sweating: Hegu L.I.-4 (reduce), Neiting ST-44 (reduce), Fuliu KID-7 (reinforce) and Bailao (M-HN-30) (*Great Compendium*).
- Injury by cold with great heat that does not recede: reduce Hegu L.I.-4, Quchi L.I.-11, Xuanzhong GB-39, Zusanli ST-36, Dazhui DU-14 and Yongquan KID-1 (*Great Compendium*).
- Diseases of the head, face, ears, eyes, mouth and nose: Hegu L.I.-4 and Quchi L.I.-11 (*Miscellaneous Diseases*).
- Headache: Hegu L.I.-4, Tianchi P-1, Tongziliao GB-1, Yuji LU-10, Sibai ST-2, Tianchong GB-9, Sanjiaoshu BL-22 and Fengchi GB-20 (*Systematic Classic*).
- One-sided or generalised headache: Hegu L.I.-4, Sizhukong SJ-23 and Fengchi GB-20 (*Great Compendium*).
- One-sided or generalised head wind: Hegu L.I.-4, Baihui DU-20, Qianding DU-21, Shenting DU-24, Shangxing DU-23, Sizhukong SJ-23, Fengchi GB-20, Zanzhu BL-2 and Touwei ST-8 (*Great Compendium*).
- Head wind and dizziness: Hegu L.I.-4, Fenglong ST-40, Jiexi ST-41 and Fengchi GB-20 (*Great Compendium*).
- Head wind with splitting sensation, pain between the eyebrow and the eye: Hegu L.I.-4, Yangbai GB-14 and Jiexi ST-41 (*Classic of the Jade Dragon*).
- Pain of the head and nape: Hegu L.I.-4, Houding DU-19 and Baihui DU-20 (*Great Compendium*).
- Dimness of vision: Hegu LI-4, Yanglao SI-6 and Quchai BL-4 (*Supplementing Life*).
- Internal eye obstruction: Hegu L.I.-4, Tongziliao GB-1, Zulinqi GB-41 and Jingming BL-1 (*Great Compendium*).
- "When Jingming BL-1 is ineffective in treating diseases of the eye, combine it with Hegu L.I.-4 and Guangming GB-37" (*Ode of Xi-hong*).
- Superficial visual obstruction: Hegu L.I.-4, Jingming BL-1 and Sibai ST-2 (*Great Compendium*).
- Loss of voice: Hegu L.I.-4, Yongquan KID-1 and Yangjiao GB-35 (*Systematic Classic*).
- Swollen painful throat: Hegu L.I.-4, Shaoshang LU-11 and Tiantu REN-22 (*Great Compendium*).

- Nasal polyps and nasal congestion and discharge: Hegu L.I.-4 and Taichong LIV-3 (*Song of Points*).
- Red eyes and nosebleed: Hegu L.I.-4, Toulinqi GB-15 and Taichong LIV-3 (*Song of Points*).
- Bleeding from the nose: Hegu L.I.-4 and Tianfu LU-3 (*One Hundred Symptoms*).
- Rhinitis with clear nasal discharge: Hegu L.I.-4, Fengmen BL-12, Shenting DU-24, Zanzhu BL-2, Yingxiang L.I.-20, Zhiyin BL-67 and Futonggu KID-20 (*Thousand Ducat Formulas*).
- Deafness: Hegu L.I.-4, Zulinqi GB-41 and Jinmen BL-63 (*Song of Points*).
- Purulent ear sores with discharge: Hegu L.I.-4, Yifeng SJ-17 and Ermen SJ-21 (*Great Compendium*).
- Swelling, pain and redness of the ear: Hegu L.I.-4, Tinghui GB-2 and Jiache ST-6 (*Great Compendium*).
- Itching and swelling of the face: Hegu L.I.-4 and Yingxiang L.I.-20 (*Ode of Xi-hong*).
- Swelling of the face and abdomen: Hegu L.I.-4, Zhongfu LU-1 and Jianshi P-5 (*Thousand Ducat Formulas*).
- Deviation of the mouth and eye: Hegu L.I.-4, Jiache ST-6, Dicang ST-4, Renzhong DU-26, Chengjiang REN-24 and Tinghui GB-2 (*Illustrated Supplement*).
- Sudden mania: Hegu L.I.-4, Jianshi P-5 and Houxi SI-3 (*Great Compendium*).
- Manic raving with fear and fright: Hegu L.I.-4, Yuji LU-10, Zhizheng SI-7, Shaohai HE-3, Quchi L.I.-11 and Wangu SI-4 (*Thousand Ducat Formulas*).
- Lockjaw following windstroke: reduce Hegu L.I.-4, Jiache ST-6, Renzhong DU-26, Baihui DU-20 and Chengjiang REN-24 (*Great Compendium*).
- Loss of consciousness from windstroke: Hegu L.I.-4, Renzhong DU-26 and Zhongchong P-9. If this is ineffective, needle Yamen DU-15 and Dadun LIV-1 (*Great Compendium*).
- Difficult delivery: reinforce Hegu L.I.-4, reduce Sanyinjiao SP-6 and Taichong LIV-3 (*Great Compendium*).
- Absence of lactation: Hegu L.I.-4, Shaoze SI-1 and Shanzhong REN-17 (*Great Compendium*).
- Prolapse of the rectum: Hegu L.I.-4, Dachangshu BL-25, Baihui DU-20, Changqiang DU-1, Jianjing GB-21 and Qichong ST-30 (*Compilation*).
- Dysenteric disorder: Hegu L.I.-4 and Zusanli ST-36; if severe add Zhonglushu BL-29 (*Song of Points*).
- "For cold and heat with painful obstruction, open the Four Gates" [Hegu L.I.-4 and Taichong LIV-3] (*Ode to Elucidate Mysteries*).
- Unendurable pain of the arm that radiates to the shoulder and spine: Hegu L.I.-4 and Taichong LIV-3 (*Ode of Xi-hong*).
- Acute dysmenorrhoea: Hegi L.I.-4 and Diji SP-8.

YANGXI L.I.-5
Yang Stream

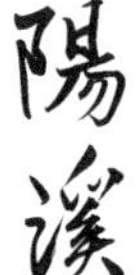

Jing-River and Fire point of the Large Intestine channel

LOCATION
On the radial side of the wrist, in the centre of the hollow formed by the tendons of extensor pollicis longus and brevis (anatomical snuffbox).

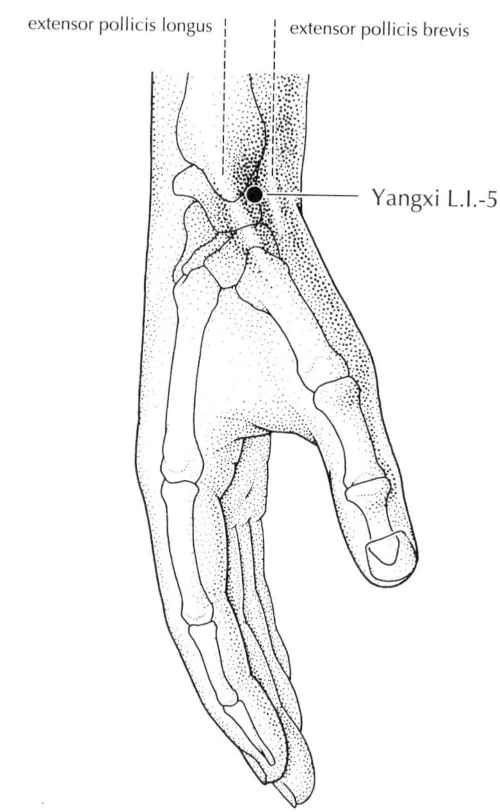

LOCATION NOTE
i. Ask the subject to extend the thumb to emphasise the hollow of the anatomical snuffbox; ii. Look carefully to locate the cephalic vein which runs through the anatomical snuffbox in order to avoid needling through the vein.

NEEDLING
Perpendicular insertion 0.5 to 1 cun.

ACTIONS
Clears heat and alleviates pain
Clears yangming fire
Calms the spirit
Benefits the wrist joint

INDICATIONS

- Rhinitis, nosebleed, tinnitus, deafness, ear pain, redness, swelling and pain of the eyes, superficial visual obstruction, lacrimation, toothache, pain from tooth decay, headache, chronic headache, frontal headache, throat painful obstruction, pain of the root of the tongue.
- Mania-depression, febrile disease with agitation of the Heart, manic raving, propensity to laughter, seeing ghosts, fright.
- Cold cough, vomiting of foam, urticaria, malaria, fever with absence of sweating.
- Weakness and pain of the wrist, contraction of the five fingers, heat in the palms, difficulty in raising the elbow.

COMMENTARY

Yangxi L.I.-5 is the jing-river and fire point of the Large Intestine channel, and in common with the fire points of all the twelve channels, has a strong action on clearing heat. Thus whilst its area of action (nose, ears, eyes, teeth, head and throat etc.) is similar to that of Hegu L.I.-4, its action is primarily to clear heat and fire in these areas. When heat obstructs the nose there will be bleeding or rhinitis; when heat ascends to the ears there will be tinnitus, deafness and pain; when heat obscures the eyes there will be redness, swelling and pain of the eyes, superficial visual obstruction and lacrimation; when yangming channel heat inflames the teeth and gums there will be toothache, and when heat accumulates in the throat there will be swelling and congestion.

The Large Intestine and Stomach belong to yangming. Exuberant fire in yangming may easily transmit to the Heart and disrupt the spirit, whether in the form of the irritability and delirium that may occur during the course of a yangming stage fever, or in the form of the long-term Stomach fire or phlegm-fire seen in many serious emotional disorders. This important relationship is explained by the fact that although they are not linked by the primary channels, the Stomach divergent channel connects with the Heart, whilst the Stomach primary channel meets with the Governing vessel (and thus the brain) at Shenting DU-24 and Renzhong DU-26. Yangxi L.I.-5, the fire point of the hand yangming channel, is therefore indicated for febrile disease with agitation of the Heart, mania-depression, 'seeing ghosts', fright, manic raving and propensity to laughter. The last two indications may further reflect its status as a jing-river point which, according to the *Spiritual Pivot*[8] should be needled when there are "diseases manifesting in the patient's voice".

Finally, Yangxi L.I.-5 is an important point in the treatment of wrist disorders, and like Wangu SI-4, its corresponding point on the ulnar side of the wrist, is indicated for contraction of all the five fingers. In learning the names of the points of the yang channels at the wrist, it is helpful to remember the similarity between their names: Yangxi L.I.-5 (Yang Stream), Yanggu SI-5 (Yang Valley) and Yangchi SJ-4 (Yang Pool).

COMBINATIONS

- Pain of the eye: Yangxi L.I.-5, Erjian L.I.-2, Daling P-7, Sanjian L.I.-3, Qiangu SI-2 and Shangxing DU-23 (*Great Compendium*).
- Tinnitus and deafness: Yangxi L.I.-5, Xiaguan ST-7, Guanchong SJ-1, Yemen SJ-2 and Yanggu SI-5 (*Systematic Classic*).
- Tinnitus: Yangxi L.I.-5, Shangyang L.I.-1, Pianli L.I.-6, Luoque BL-8, Wangu SI-4 and Qiangu SI-2 (*Supplementing Life*).
- Ear pain, deafness and tinnitus: Yangxi L.I.-5, Tianchuang SI-16, Guanchong SJ-1, Yemen SJ-2 and Zhongzhu SJ-3 (*Thousand Ducat Formulas*).
- Urticaria from extreme heat: Yangxi L.I.-5 and Jianyu L.I.-15 (*One Hundred Symptoms*).
- Toothache and lumbar pain accompanied by throat painful obstruction: Yangxi L.I.-5 and Erjian L.I.-2 (*Ode of Xi-hong*).
- Vomiting phlegm and watery saliva, dizziness that does not cease: Yangxi L.I.-5, Gongsun SP-4, Fenglong ST-40 and Shanzhong REN-17 (*Complete Collection*).
- Frequent laughter: Yangxi L.I.-5, Lieque LU-7, Daling P-7 and Renzhong DU-26 (*Great Compendium*).
- Manic raving, seeing ghosts: Yangxi L.I.-5, Pucan BL-61 and Wenliu L.I.-7 (*Supplementing Life*).
- Manic raving: Yangxi L.I.-5, Taiyuan LU-9, Xialian L.I.-8 and Kunlun BL-60 (*Great Compendium*).
- Fright palpitations: Yangxi L.I.-5 and Danshu BL-19 (*Divine Moxibustion*).

PIANLI L.I.-6

Veering Passage

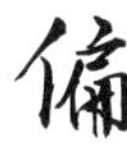

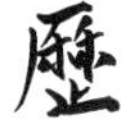

Luo-Connecting point of the Large Intestine channel

LOCATION

3 cun proximal to Yangxi L.I.-5 on the line connecting Yangxi L.I.-5 with Quchi L.I.-11.

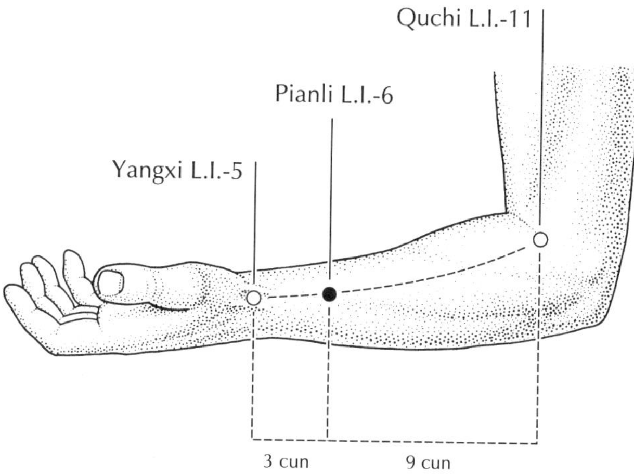

LOCATION NOTE

i. Locate with the elbow flexed and with the radial side of the arm upwards; ii. Divide the distance between Yangxi L.I.-5 and Quchi L.I.-11 into half, and then halve the distance between this midpoint and Yangxi L.I.-5.

NEEDLING

Transverse-oblique insertion, 0.5 to 1 cun.

ACTIONS

Expels wind and clears heat
Opens and regulates the water passages

INDICATIONS

- Tinnitus, deafness, toothache, tooth decay, cold teeth, redness and pain of the eyes, dimness of vision, blurred vision, rhinitis, nosebleed, dry throat, throat painful obstruction, deviation of the mouth, swelling of the cheek.
- Difficult urination, oedema, ascites, obstruction of the diaphragm, borborygmus with oedema, attack by wind with absence of sweating.
- Malaria, manic raving.
- Pain of the wrist, elbow and upper arm.

COMMENTARY

Pianli L.I.-6 is the luo-connecting point of the Large Intestine channel from where the luo-connecting channel diverges, hence the name 'Veering Passage'. From this point the luo-connecting channel ascends to the jaw and ears, whilst the Large Intestine primary channel traverses the lower jaw, nose and face, before joining with the Stomach channel which connects to the eye. Like many distal points of the Large Intestine channel, Pianli L.I.-6 is effective in clearing wind and heat from all these areas (e.g. toothache, redness and pain of the eyes, nosebleed, rhinitis etc.) and is especially applicable for ear disorders such as tinnitus and deafness due to attack of exterior pathogenic wind and heat.

The luo-connecting channel from Pianli L.I.-6 joins with its interiorly-exteriorly coupled Lung channel. The *Guide to the Classics of Acupuncture* states "the luo-connecting points are located between two channels ... if they are punctured, symptoms of the interiorly-exteriorly related channels can be treated[9]". The yang Large Intestine channel may be seen as the outer reflection of its coupled yin Lung channel, and its points are frequently used to release the exterior portion of the Lung system. When external wind disrupts the function of the Lung in regulating the water passages, there may be acute oedema, especially of the upper part of the body, accompanied by absence of sweating and difficult urination. Pianli L.I.-6 is the primary point on the Large Intestine channel to open and regulate the water passages and thus treat such symptoms as difficult urination, oedema, ascites and borborygmus with oedema.

Finally the *Great Compendium of Acupuncture and Moxibustion* gives specific indications for excess and deficiency of the luo-connecting points. In the case of Pianli L.I.-6, these are tooth decay and deafness (excess); cold teeth and obstruction of the diaphragm (deficiency).

COMBINATIONS

- Tinnitus: Pianli L.I.-6, Yangxi L.I.-5, Shangyang L.I.-1, Luoque BL-8, Wangu SI-4 and Qiangu SI-2 (*Supplementing Life*).
- Deafness: Pianli L.I.-6, Qiangu SI-2 and Houxi SI-3 (*Supplementing Life*).
- Deafness due to Kidney deficiency: Pianli L.I.-6, Shenshu BL-23 and Tinghui GB-2 (*Illustrated Supplement*).
- Rhinitis with nose bleed: Pianli L.I-6, Hegu L.I-4, Sanjian L.I-3, Kunlun BL-60 and Zutonggu BL-66 (*Supplementing Life*).
- Dry throat: Pianli L.I.-6, Jiquan HE-1, Taiyuan LU-9, Taichong LIV-3 and Tiantu REN-22 (*Supplementing Life*).
- Soreness and pain of the elbow and forearm with difficulty in extending and flexing: Pianli L.I.-6 and Shousanli L.I.-10 (*Supplementing Life*).

WENLIU L.I.-7

Warm Flow

温溜

Xi-Cleft point of the Large Intestine channel

LOCATION

5 cun proximal to Yangxi L.I.-5 on the line connecting Yangxi L.I.-5 with Quchi L.I.-11.

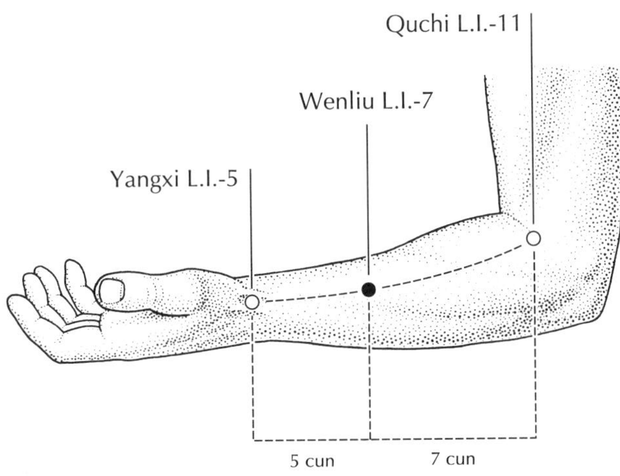

LOCATION NOTE

i. Locate with the elbow flexed and with the radial side of the arm upwards; ii. Divide the distance between Yangxi L.I.-5 and Quchi L.I.-11 into two equal parts, then locate Wenliu L.I.-7 one cun distal to this midpoint.

NEEDLING

Transverse-oblique insertion, 0.5 to 1 cun.

ACTIONS

Clears heat and detoxifies poison
Moderates acute conditions
Regulates and harmonises the intestines and Stomach
Clears yangming fire and calms the spirit

INDICATIONS

- Headache, deviation of the face and mouth, redness, swelling and pain of the face, clove sores, carbuncle and furuncle, pain of the teeth and mouth, tongue thrusting, throat painful obstruction with loss of voice.
- Borborygmus with abdominal pain, abdominal distention, vomiting of watery saliva and foam, sudden swelling of the four limbs.
- Frequent laughter, raving, seeing ghosts.
- Pain and difficulty in raising the shoulder and arm.

COMMENTARY

Wenliu L.I.-7 is the xi-cleft point of the Large Intestine channel. The xi-cleft points are where the qi and blood, which flow relatively superficially along the channels from the jing-well points, gather and plunge more deeply. The xi-cleft points in general are indicated in the treatment of acute conditions and pain, and this is reflected in the ability of Wenliu L.I.-7 to clear heat and detoxify poison in cases of clove sores, carbuncles and furuncles, throat painful obstruction, and heat and swelling of the face. Clove sores are small hard deep-rooted clove-shaped purulent lesions. They are primarily due to unregulated diet or external wind and fire poison which invade the superficial portion of the body. The condition tends to develop very rapidly with severe localised pain, redness and swelling, often accompanied by fever.

One notable feature of the hand yang channels (Large Intestine, Sanjiao and Small Intestine) is that relatively few of their points treat disorders of their corresponding fu. As far as the Large Intestine channel is concerned, Wenliu L.I.-7 and its following points Xialian L.I.-8 and Shanglian L.I.-9, however, are indicated for disorders of the intestines and Stomach (in the case of Wenliu L.I.-7 for borborygmus accompanied by abdominal pain, abdominal distention, and vomiting of foam or watery saliva). This follows the general principle of all the yang channels, most clearly seen on the leg yang, that as the points approach the elbow or knee they begin to have a greater action on their corresponding fu. It should be noted, however, that in clinical practice points of the Large Intestine channel are rarely used for disorders of the intestines, and this is borne out by the absence of Wenliu L.I.-7 in combinations for this purpose in any of the major classics.

The action of Wenliu L.I.-7 on clearing yangming fire and calming the spirit, and thus treating frequent laughter, raving and 'seeing ghosts', is similar to that of Yangxi L.I-5.

COMBINATIONS

- Throat painful obstruction with loss of voice: Wenliu L.I.-7 and Quchi L.I.-11 (*Systematic Classic*).
- Stiff tongue, tongue thrusting: Wenliu L.I.-7, Huaroumen ST-24 and Shaohai HE-3 (*Supplementing Life*).
- Manic raving, seeing ghosts: Wenliu L.I.-7, Yangxi L.I.-5 and Pucan BL-61 (*Supplementing Life*).
- Stiffness of the nape of the neck due to injury by cold: Wenliu L.I.-7 and Qimen LIV-14 (*One Hundred Symptoms*).

XIALIAN L.I.-8

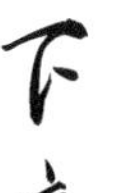

Lower Angle

LOCATION
On the radial side of the forearm, 4 cun distal to Quchi L.I.-11, on the line connecting Quchi L.I.-11 with Yangxi L.I.-5.

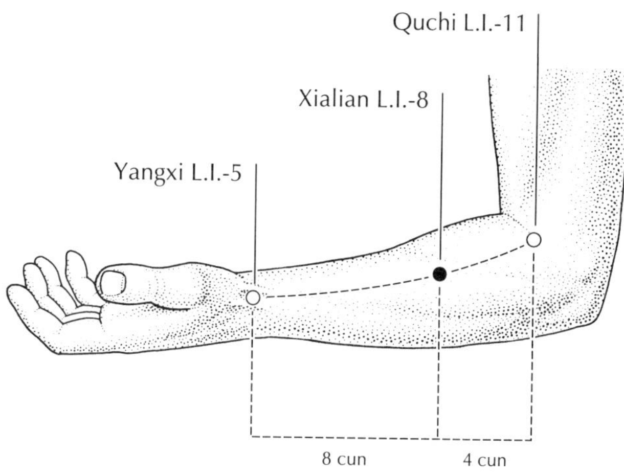

LOCATION NOTE
i. Locate with the elbow flexed and with the radial side of the arm upwards; ii. Divide the distance between Yangxi L.I.-5 and Quchi L.I.-11 into three equal parts. Xialian L.I.-8 is located at the junction of the proximal and middle thirds.

NEEDLING
Perpendicular or oblique insertion 0.5 to 1.5 cun.

ACTIONS
Harmonises the Small Intestine
Expels wind and clears heat
Clears yangming fire and calms the spirit

INDICATIONS
- Abdominal pain, lower abdominal distention, fullness and pain of the abdomen and lateral costal region, periumbilical pain, insufficiency of Small Intestine qi, diarrhoea containing undigested food, blood in the stool, dark urine.
- Headache, head wind, dizziness, pain of the eye, dry lips with drooling, breast abscess, dyspnoea.
- Manic raving, mad walking.
- Hemiplegia, wind-damp painful obstruction, cold painful obstruction, pain of the elbow and arm.

COMMENTARY
Xialian L.I.-8 (Lower Angle) and Shanglian L.I.-9 (Upper Angle) are a reflection on the upper limb of the points Xiajuxu ST-39 (Lower Great Hollow) and Shangjuxu ST-37 (Upper Great Hollow), the he-sea points of the Small and Large Intestines respectively, on the lower limb. Xialian L.I.-8 is therefore indicated for disorders of the intestines, particularly the Small Intestine, manifesting as fullness, distention and pain of the abdomen, periumbilical pain, insufficiency of Small Intestine qi, blood in the stool and diarrhoea containing undigested food. In clinical practice, however, the points on the lower limb are much more frequently used to treat intestinal disorders.

The Large Intestine divergent channel descends to the breast, and Xialian L.I.-8 is indicated for breast abscess, the only point on the Large Intestine channel with this indication.

The action of Xialian L.I.-8 on clearing yangming fire and calming the spirit, and thus treating manic raving and mad walking, is similar to that of Yangxi L.I.-5.

COMBINATIONS
- Hot Stomach with no pleasure in eating: Xialian L.I.-8 and Xuanzhong GB-39 (*Supplementing Life*).
- Diarrhoea due to injury by food: Xialian L.I.-8 and Shanglian L.I.-9 (*Great Compendium*).
- Manic raving: Xialian L.I.-8, Taiyuan LU-9, Yangxi L.I.-5 and Kunlun BL-60 (*Great Compendium*).
- Wind damp painful obstruction: Xialian L.I.-8 and Weizhong BL-40 (*Supplementing Life*).
- Pain and cold of the arm: Xialian L.I.-8, Quchi L.I.-11 and Jianjing GB-21 (*Great Compendium*).
- Difficult and dark urination: Xialian L.I.-8 and Shanglian L.I.-9 (*Thousand Ducat Formulas*).

SHANGLIAN L.I.-9

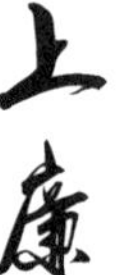

Upper Angle

LOCATION
On the radial side of the forearm, 3 cun distal to Quchi L.I.-11, on the line connecting Quchi L.I.-11 with Yangxi L.I.-5.

LOCATION NOTE
i. Locate with the elbow flexed and with the radial side of the arm upwards; ii. Divide the distance between Yangxi L.I.-5 and Quchi L.I.-11 into half, and then halve the distance between this midpoint and Quchi L.I.-11.

NEEDLING
Perpendicular or oblique insertion 0.5 to 1.5 cun.

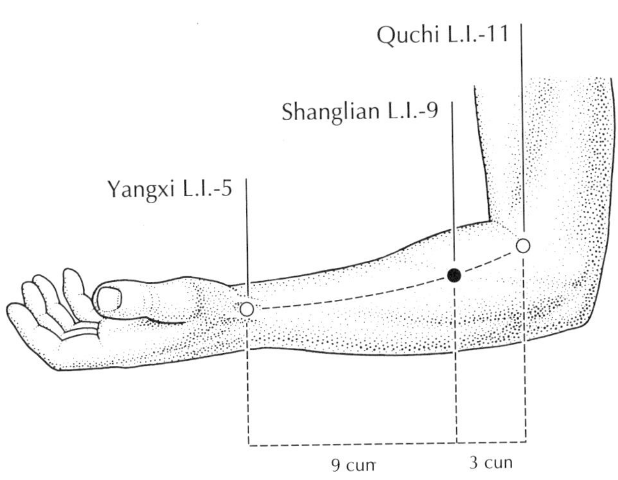

ACTIONS

Harmonises the Large Intestine
Activates the channel and alleviates pain

INDICATIONS

- Borborygmus, Large Intestine qi stagnation, abdominal pain, difficult and dark urination.
- Chest pain, dyspnoea, brain wind, headache.
- Pain or numbness of the shoulder, elbow and arm, numbness of the limbs, hemiplegia from windstroke, cold sensation of the bone marrow.

COMMENTARY

See discussion of Xialian L.I.-8 above.

COMBINATIONS

- Fullness of the abdomen and lateral costal region: Shanglian L.I.-9, Yanglingquan GB-34 and Zulinqi GB-41 (*Great Compendium*).
- Dyspnoea with inability to walk: Shanglian L.I.-9, Qimen LIV-14 and Zhongwan REN-12 (*Great Compendium*).

SHOUSANLI L.I.-10

Arm Three Miles

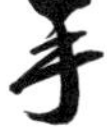

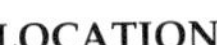

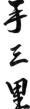

LOCATION

On the radial side of the forearm, 2 cun distal to Quchi L.I.-11, on the line connecting Quchi L.I.-11 with Yangxi L.I.-5.

LOCATION NOTE

i. Locate with the elbow flexed and with the radial side of the arm upwards; ii. First locate Shanglian L.I.-9, then locate Shousanli L.I.-10 one cun proximal to it; iii. This point is usually significantly tender to palpation.

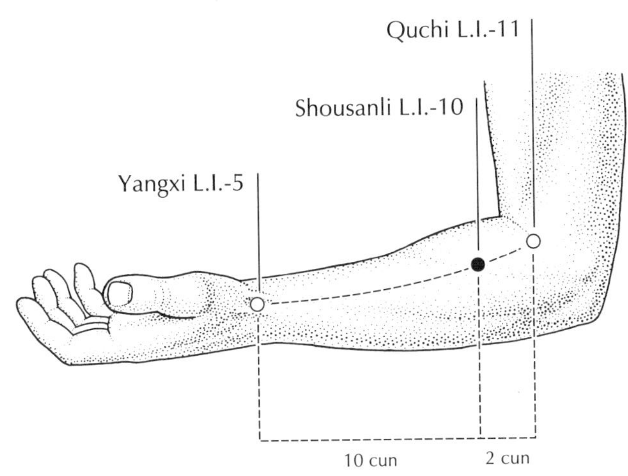

NEEDLING

Perpendicular or oblique insertion 0.5 to 1.5 cun.

ACTIONS

Regulates qi and blood, activates the channel and alleviates pain
Harmonises the intestines and Stomach

INDICATIONS

- Pain and immobility of the arm and shoulder, windstroke, paralysis of the arm, numbness of the arm, atrophy disorder, hemiplegia, contraction and inflexibility of the elbow, lumbar pain with inability to lie down.
- Abdominal pain, vomiting and diarrhoea, periodic sensation of cold in the intestines, sudden turmoil disorder.
- Toothache with swelling of the cheek, deviation of the mouth, loss of voice, scrofula.

COMMENTARY

Shousanli L.I.-10 (Arm Three Miles), just distal to the elbow joint, mirrors the location of Zusanli ST-36 (Leg Three Miles) on the leg and shares its name. Although both points have the action of harmonising the Stomach and intestines, this is a secondary and relatively minor action of Shousanli L.I.-10.

Yangming channels are "abundant in qi and blood"[10], and in the same way that Zusanli ST-36 is a primary point to treat disorders of the lower limb, the main clinical application of Shousanli L.I.-10 is to invigorate and regulate the circulation of qi and blood in the upper limb as a whole. It is much used in the treatment of both atrophy disorder and painful obstruction, as well as pain, immobility and numbness of the arm, in which case it is often combined with such points as Jianyu L.I.-15 and Hegu L.I.-4 in the 'chain and lock' point combination method.

Shousanli L.I.-10 is often alternated with Quchi L.I.-11 in the treatment of chronic and long-standing disorders of the channels such as hemiplegia and atrophy disorder, to avoid over-needling the same few points. Shousanli L.I.-10 is also often clinically combined with Quchi L.I.-11 as an adjacent point for diseases of the elbow, particularly tennis elbow.

As far as the treatment of toothache is concerned, Zhu Dan-xi of the Jin-Yuan dynasty recommended applying moxibustion to Shousanli L.I.-10 for toothache of the upper jaw (and to Sanjian L.I.-3 for toothache of the lower jaw)[11].

COMBINATIONS

- Stubborn numbness of both forearms: Shousanli L.I.-10 and Shaohai HE-3 (*One Hundred Symptoms*).
- Pain of the forearm: Shousanli LI-10, Quchi LI-11 and Houxi SI-3 (*Supplementing Life*).
- Soreness and pain of the elbow and forearm with difficulty in extending and flexing: Shousanli L.I.-10 and Pianli L.I.-6 (*Supplementing Life*).
- Contraction and inability to extend the arm and elbow: Shousanli L.I.-10 and Zuqiaoyin GB-44 (*Supplementing Life*).
- Head wind, visual dizziness and stiffness of the nape of the neck: Shousanli L.I.-10, Shenmai BL-62 and Jinmen BL-63 (*Miscellaneous Diseases*).
- Scrofula: Shousanli L.I.-10, Shaohai HE-3, Tianchi P-1, Zhangmen LIV-13, Zulinqi GB-41, Zhigou SJ-6, Yangfu GB-38 and Jianjing GB-21 (*Great Compendium*).

QUCHI L.I.-11

Pool at the Crook

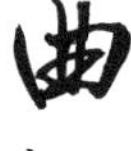

He-Sea and Earth point of the Large Intestine channel
Sun Si-miao Ghost point
Ma Dan-yang Heavenly Star point

LOCATION

At the elbow, midway between Chize LU-5 and the lateral epicondyle of the humerus, at the lateral end of the transverse cubital crease.

LOCATION NOTE

This point should be located with the elbow flexed.

NEEDLING

Perpendicular insertion 1 to 1.5 cun, or joined by through-needling to Shaohai HE-3.

ACTIONS

Clears heat
Cools the blood, eliminates wind, drains damp and alleviates itching
Regulates qi and blood
Activates the channel and alleviates pain

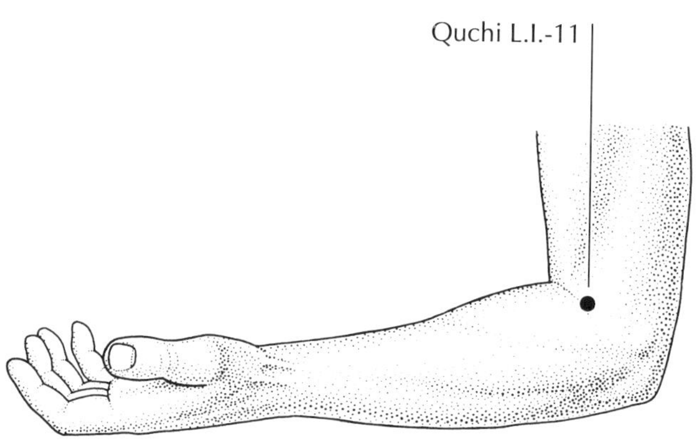

INDICATIONS

- High fever that does not recede, injury by cold with residual fever that does not recede, thirst with sweating on drinking and dry and hot skin when does not drink, malaria.
- Throat painful obstruction, loss of voice, toothache, redness and pain of the eyes, lacrimation, pain in the front of the ear.
- Agitation and oppression of the chest, manic disorders, poor memory, tongue thrusting, dizziness, hypertension, goitre, scrofula.
- Erysipelas (cinnabar toxin), urticaria, wind rash, dry skin, scaly skin, itching of the skin, shingles, pain and itching of the whole body as if bitten by insects, clove sores on the back.
- Distention and pain of the abdomen, vomiting and diarrhoea, dysenteric disorder, amenorrhoea.
- Numbness of the upper arm, painful obstruction, wind painful obstruction, hemiplegia, clonic spasm, contraction, immobility and pain of the elbow and shoulder, emaciation and weakness of the elbow, redness and swelling of the arm, atrophy disorder of the lower limbs, pain and swelling of the ankle.

COMMENTARY

Quchi L.I.-11 was included by Ma Dan-yang, the great physician of the Jin dynasty, among the 'eleven heavenly star points'[6], his grouping of the most vital acupuncture points. It is a powerful and essential point in the treatment of fevers and heat in the body, skin diseases, hypertension and disorders of the arm.

Yangming or 'yang brightness' channel is considered to be particularly replete with yang qi, and points of the Large Intestine channel are among the most important points to clear excess of yang in the form of heat. Quchi L.I.-11 is the principal point on the channel, and indeed one of the foremost points on the body, to clear heat and fire. It is used in all cases of fever due to excess heat when pathogenic factors have penetrated to the yangming or qi levels, and chills are no longer present. In this respect it may be compared to Hegu L.I.-4 which is mainly used when the pathogenic factors are still on the exterior in the form of wind-cold or wind-heat, when the fever is moderate, and when chills are still present. In clinical practice both points are commonly used together to control many different kinds of fever. Like Hegu L.I.-4 and other points of the Large Intestine channel, Quchi L.I.-11 is also used to clear heat from the yangming channel in the head, whether it affects the throat, eyes or teeth, and it is indicated for swelling and pain of the throat, redness and pain of the eyes, lacrimation and toothache. Like Yangxi L.I.-5, it is able to clear yangming fire which transmits to the Heart and spirit, and it is indicated for agitation and oppression of the chest, mania disorder and tongue thrusting. For this reason, under its alternative name of Guitui (Ghost Leg) Quchi L.I.-11 was included by Sun Si-miao among his 'thirteen ghost points' for the treatment of mania disorder and epilepsy.

According to the *Spiritual Pivot*[12] "When the disease is at the yang within yang [skin], needle the he-sea points of the yang channels". Whilst this is not applicable in all cases, it is notable that Quchi L.I.-11 and Weizhong BL-40, the he-sea points of the Large Intestine and Bladder channels respectively, are two of the most important points in the treatment of skin diseases. Quchi L.I.-11 is classically indicated for a variety of skin disorders such as erysipelas (cinnabar toxin), urticaria, wind rash, shingles, clove sores and dry, scaly, and itchy skin. This reflects the ability of Quchi L.I.-11 to expel wind, resolve damp, and clear heat, fire and fire-poison, the main components of excess-type skin disorders. In modern clinical practice, however, acupuncture is used as a primary therapy in relatively few dermatological diseases (pride of place being given to herbal medicine), and is considered to be of value principally in the treatment of urticaria, herpes zoster and itching of the skin.

According to the *Classic of Difficulties*[13] he-sea points are effective in the treatment of "counterflow qi and diarrhoea" whilst the *Spiritual Pivot* says "in disorders of the Stomach and in disorders resulting from irregular eating and drinking, select the he-sea point"[14]. Although not having such a wide application in the treatment of these disorders as Shangjuxu ST-37, the lower he-sea point of the Large Intestine, Quchi L.I.-11 is indicated for vomiting and diarrhoea, as well as abdominal pain, and is an essential point in the treatment of dysenteric disorder, especially when accompanied by fever. In modern clinical practice it is much used for bacillary dysentery.

In recent times, Quchi L.I.-11 has been widely used in the treatment of hypertension, often in combination with Zusanli ST-36. Hypertension as a category did not exist in traditional medicine, its clinical manifestations being included in the categories of headache, dizziness etc., and the effect of reducing these points to lower excessively high blood pressure is a modern interpretation of the statement in the *Spiritual Pivot*[15] "Yangming channels are abundant in qi and blood".

Quchi L.I.-11 is a major point in the treatment of disorders of the whole upper limb. According to Ma Dan-yang "Quchi L.I.-11 is excellent for treating pain of the elbow, hemiplegia with inability to close the hand, inability to draw a bow, and flaccidity of the sinews so that a person cannot comb their hair". Quchi L.I.-11 can both resolve obstruction in the channel resulting in pain and painful obstruction, and by regulating qi and blood can strengthen and nourish in all cases of weakness of the arm such as atrophy disorder. It is a vital point in the treatment of hemiplegia following windstroke, and for clonic spasm of the upper limb of any aetiology, and for this purpose is i. commonly combined with Jianyu L.I.-15 and Hegu L.I.-4 in the 'chain and lock' point association method, and ii. joined by through-needling to Shaohai HE-3. This latter technique reflects the importance of Shaohai HE-3 as a point to treat disorders of the arm, as well as the clinical observation that while points from the yang channels are emphasised in the treatment of atrophy disorder and hemiplegia, better results are obtained when some points from yin channels are also included in the point prescription.

Finally it is worth noting that despite its status as the 'mother' point of the Large Intestine channel, the only tonifying application of Quchi L.I.-11 is in nourishing the upper limb in this way, all its other actions being to reduce excess pathogenic factors of various kinds.

COMBINATIONS

- Fever: Quchi L.I.-11 and Shaochong HE-9 (*One Hundred Symptoms*).
- Injury by cold with great heat which does not recede: reduce Quchi L.I.-11, Xuanzhong GB-39, Zusanli ST-36, Dazhui DU-14, Yongquan KID-1 and Hegu L.I.-4 (*Great Compendium*).
- Malaria with much heat and little cold: Quchi L.I.-11, Dazhui DU-14, Houxi SI-3 and Jianshi P-5 (*Great Compendium*).

- Malaria with much cold and little heat: Quchi L.I.-11 Dazhui DU-14 and Houxi SI-3 (*Great Compendium*).
- Diseases of the head, face, ears, eyes, mouth and nose: Quchi L.I.-11 and Hegu L.I.-4 (*Miscellaneous Diseases*).
- Toothache with aversion to cold: Quchi L.I.-11, Daying ST-5, Quanliao SI-18 and Tinghui GB-2 (*Thousand Ducat Formulas*).
- Manic raving, fear and fright: Quchi L.I.-11, Yuji LU-10, Zhizheng SI-7, Hegu L.I.-4, Shaohai HE-3 and Wangu SI-4 (*Thousand Ducat Formulas*).
- Hemiplegia: Quchi L.I.-11 and Yanglingquan GB-34 (*One Hundred Symptoms*).
- One-sided wind (hemiplegia): Quchi L.I.-11, Yanglingquan GB-34 and Huantiao GB-30 (*Supplementing Life*).
- Windstroke with one-sided withering and incessant pain: Quchi L.I.-11, Jianyu L.I.-15, Xuanzhong GB-39, Taixi KID-3, Zusanli ST-36 and Kunlun BL-60 (*Great Compendium*).
- Atrophy disorder and numbness of the arm: Quchi LI-11, Waiguan SJ-5 and Tianjing SJ-10 (*Thousand Ducat Formulas*).
- Pain of the elbow, at times cold: Quchi L.I.-11, Guanchong SJ-1, Shousanli L.I.-10, Zhongzhu SJ-3, Yanggu SI-5 and Chize LU-5 (*Thousand Ducat Formulas*).
- Pain and cold of the arm: Quchi L.I.-11, Xialian L.I.-8 and Jianjing GB-21 (*Great Compendium*).
- Pain and heaviness of the shoulder with inability to raise the arm: Quchi L.I.-11 and Tianliao SJ-15 (*Supplementing Life*).
- Inability to bend the elbow and fingers: Quchi L.I.-11, Shousanli L.I.-10, Waiguan SJ-5 and Zhongzhu SJ-3 (*Great Compendium*).
- Contraction of the arm with tightness of the sinews of both hands resulting in inability to open the hands: Quchi L.I.-11, Chize LU-5, Yangchi SJ-4, Hegu L.I.-4 and Zhongzhu SJ-3 (*Great Compendium*).
- Contraction of the elbow with pain: Chize LU-5 joined to Quchi L.I.-11 (*Ode of the Jade Dragon*).
- Pain of the forearm: Quchi L.I.-11 and Jianjing GB-21 (*Ode to Elucidate Mysteries*).
- Pain of the forearm: Quchi LI-11, Shousanli LI-10 and Houxi SI-3 (*Supplementing Life*).
- Hypertension: Quchi L.I.-11, Renying ST-9 and Zusanli ST-36.
- Hypertension: Quchi L.I.-11, Renying ST-9, Baihui DU-20 and Taichong LIV-3.
- Bacillary dysentery: Quchi L.I.-11, Shangjuxu ST-37 and Tianshu ST-25.

ZHOULIAO L.I.-12

Elbow Crevice

肘髎

LOCATION

When the elbow is flexed, this point is located in the depression 1 cun proximal to and 1 cun lateral to Quchi L.I.-11.

LOCATION NOTE

When the elbow is flexed, this point may be found directly above the lateral epicondyle of the humerus, just anterior to the lateral supracondylar ridge.

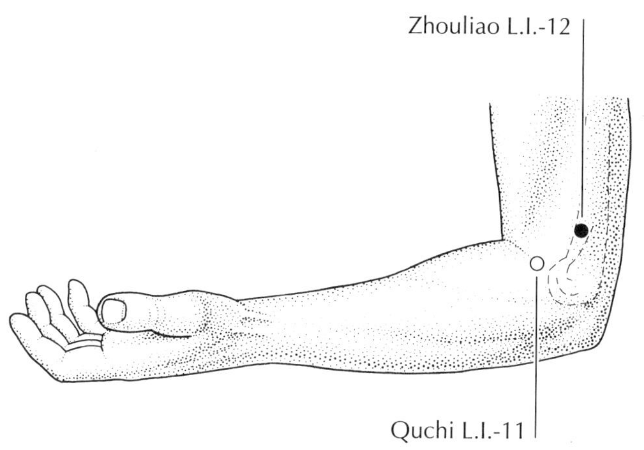

NEEDLING

Perpendicular insertion 0.5 to 1 cun.

ACTIONS

Activates the channel and alleviates pain
Benefits the elbow joint

INDICATIONS

- Wind-taxation with somnolence, contraction, numbness and immobility of the upper arm, pain and stiffness of the elbow.

COMMENTARY

Zhouliao L.I.-12 is primarily used as a local point for disorders of the elbow (for example in the treatment of tennis elbow when pain radiates upwards towards the shoulder).

COMBINATIONS

- Swelling and redness of the arm with elbow pain: Zhouliao L.I.-12, Jianyu L.I.-15 and Wangu SI-4 (*Great Compendium*).
- Pain and inability to raise the arm: Zhouliao L.I.-12 and Binao L.I.-14 (*Preserving Life*).

SHOUWULI L.I.-13

Arm Five Miles

手五里

LOCATION

On the lateral side of the upper arm, 3 cun proximal to Quchi L.I.-11, on the line connecting Quchi L.I.-11 with Jianyu L.I.-15.

LOCATION NOTE

i. Locate approximately one handbreadth superior to Quchi L.I.-11, in the depression between the lateral border of biceps brachii and the humerus; ii. Locate at one third of the distance between Quchi L.I.-11 and the axillary fold.

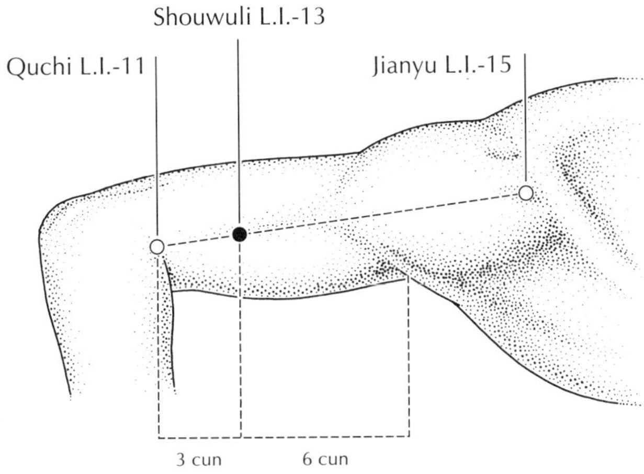

NEEDLING

Perpendicular insertion 1 to 1.5 cun.

ACTIONS

Activates the channel and alleviates pain
Alleviates coughing
Regulates qi, drains damp and transforms phlegm

INDICATIONS

- Pain, numbness or contraction of the elbow and upper arm, inability to raise the arm, shoulder pain, wind-taxation with fear and fright.
- Cough, difficulty in breathing, vomiting blood.
- Scrofula, desire to sleep, diminished qi, inability to move the four limbs, yellow body with intermittent low-grade fever, malaria, blurred vision, fullness and distention below the Heart, fear and fright.

COMBINATIONS

- Scrofula: Shouwuli L.I.-13 and Binao L.I.-14 (*One Hundred Symptoms*).
- Scrofula: moxa Shouwuli L.I.-13 and Renying ST-9 thirty times (*Thousand Ducat Formulas*).

BINAO L.I.-14

Upper Arm

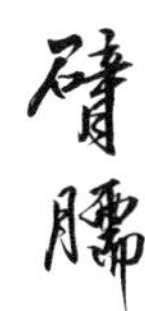

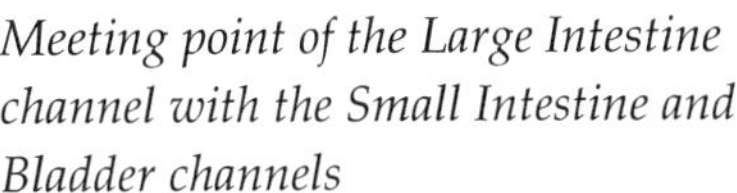
Meeting point of the Large Intestine channel with the Small Intestine and Bladder channels

LOCATION

On the lateral side of the upper arm, in the visible and tender depression formed between the distal insertion of the deltoid muscle and the brachialis muscle, approximately three fifths of the distance along the line drawn between Quchi L.I.-11 and Jianyu L.I.-15.

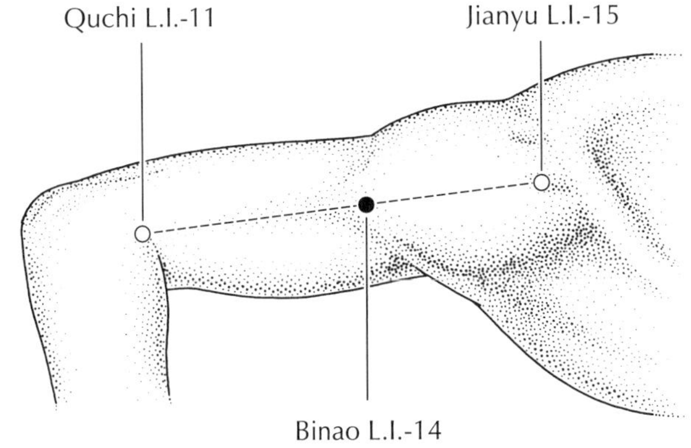

LOCATION NOTE

This point is easier to locate if the muscles of the upper arm are tensed.

NEEDLING

Oblique insertion 1 to 1.5 cun.

ACTIONS

Activates the channel and alleviates pain
Regulates qi and dissipates phlegm nodules
Benefits the eyes

INDICATIONS

- Pain, numbness and painful obstruction of the upper arm and shoulder, wasting and weakness of the upper arm, inability to raise the arm, contraction and stiffness of the neck.
- Scrofula, goitre, chest pain.
- Redness swelling and pain of the eyes.

COMMENTARY

Although not a major point, Binao L.I.-14 is frequently employed for channel disorders in the upper arm, especially when pain radiates either downwards from the shoulder towards the elbow, or upwards from the elbow towards the shoulder.

Like several points of the Large Intestine and Sanjiao channels located between the elbow and the shoulder, Binao L.I.-14 is also indicated for scrofula and goitre. Scrofula and goitre, although different in aetiology, always involve phlegm, combined either with stagnant qi or with heat. In the case of Binao L.I.-14, its ability to treat these disorders derives mainly from the course of the Large Intestine channel through the lateral side of the neck, rather than a special ability to transform phlegm, and the action of 'regulating qi and transforming phlegm' in this context therefore only applies to scrofula and goitre. The explanation of why several points of the upper arm have this special action whilst the more distal shu-points do not, is unclear (see also Tianfu LU-3, Jianyu L.I.-15, Shouwuli L.I.-13, Tianjing SJ-10 and Naohui SJ-13).

Finally, Binao L.I.-14 also shares with several points of the upper arm the ability to treat disorders of the eyes, in this case redness, swelling and heat.

COMBINATIONS

- Pain and inability to raise the arm: Binao L.I.-14 and Zhouliao L.I.-12 (*Preserving Life*).
- Wasting and weakness of the arm with inability to raise the arm to the head: Binao L.I.-14 and Jianyu L.I.-15 (*Preserving Life*).
- Scrofula: Binao L.I.-14 and Shouwuli L.I.-13 (*One Hundred Symptoms*).

JIANYU L.I.-15

Shoulder Bone

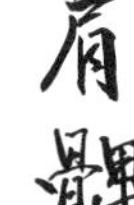

Meeting point of the Large Intestine channel with the Yang Motility vessel

LOCATION

In the depression which lies anterior and inferior to the acromion, at the origin of the deltoid muscle. (**Note:** Jianliao SJ-14 is located in the depression which lies posterior and inferior to the acromion).

LOCATION NOTE

If the arm is abducted, the two hollows will be more easily palpable and are often visible.

NEEDLING

i. With the arm abducted, perpendicular insertion directed towards the centre of the axilla, 1 to 1.5 cun; ii. Transverse-oblique insertion directed distally towards the elbow, 1.5 to 2 cun.

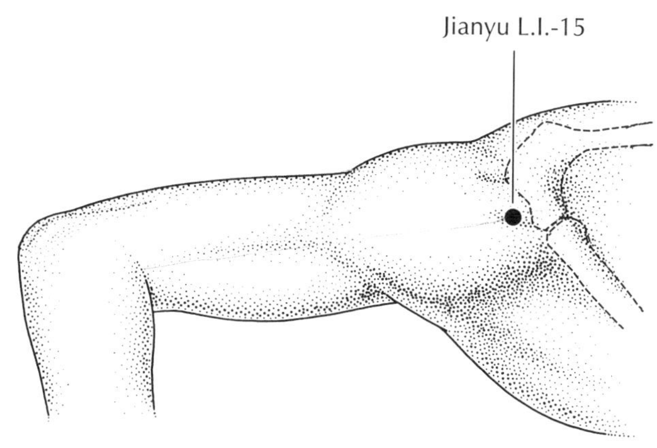

ACTIONS

Dispels wind-damp, alleviates pain and benefits the shoulder joint

Eliminates wind and regulates qi and blood

Regulates qi and dissipates phlegm nodules

INDICATIONS

- Shoulder pain, weakness of the shoulder, wind-damp of the shoulder, heat sensation in the shoulder, redness and swelling in the shoulder, inability to raise the arm to the head, contraction and numbness of the arm, hemiplegia, wind paralysis, windstroke, wind atrophy disorder, wind disease, heat in the four limbs, inability to turn the head, painful obstruction of the fingers.
- Wind-heat urticaria, injury by cold with heat that does not dissipate.
- Scrofula, goitre, seminal emission due to taxation, hypertension.

COMMENTARY

Jianyu L.I.-15, a meeting point of the Large Intestine channel with the Yang Motility vessel, is also reached by the Lung and Bladder sinew channels, the Large Intestine divergent channel and the Small Intestine luo-connecting channel. Jianyu L.I.-15 is considered the pre-eminent point for treating the shoulder, and clinically the majority of shoulder disorders affect this region.

Stiffness, pain, immobility or weakness of the shoulder or frozen shoulder may derive from: i. injury by exterior pathogenic wind, cold, damp or heat, i.e. painful obstruction, ii. stagnation of qi and blood from traumatic injury, misuse or overuse, or iii. deficiency of qi and blood from overuse, old age or prolonged obstruction of the channel. In all these cases Jianyu L.I.-15 may be used, and in clinical practice is commonly combined with Jianliao SJ-14. As far as needling is concerned, there are two principal methods. For pain and immobility of the shoulder joint, the arm should be abducted as far as is comfortable and supported on a rolled pillow, whilst the needle is directed into the shoulder joint towards the centre of the axilla. For pain extending down the arm, however, Jianyu L.I.-15 is usually needled with a transverse-oblique insertion towards the elbow joint.

The shoulder joint is the pivot of the arm. As Jianyu L.I.-15 is the foremost point affecting the shoulder, lies on yangming channel which is "abundant in qi and blood", and is a meeting point with the Lung sinew and Small Intestine luo-connecting channels, it is a vital point to promote circulation of qi and blood in the upper limb as a whole, and is indicated for all kinds of atrophy disorder and painful obstruction and hemiplegia. For this purpose it is commonly combined in the 'chain and lock' method with points Quchi L.I.-11 and Hegu L.I.-4.

Jianyu L.I.-15 is also indicated in the treatment of urticaria due to attack of exterior wind-heat. This highlights the action of Jianyu L.I.-15 in eliminating wind, which is emphasised in a variety of classical references to wind paralysis, windstroke, wind atrophy disorder and more generally simply 'wind disease'. Like Binao L.I.-14, Jianyu L.I.-15 is also indicated for scrofula and goitre.

Finally, according to the *Essential Questions*[16] Jianyu L.I.-15 is one of the 'eight points for draining heat from the extremities' (although in fact only seven are listed) namely bilateral Yunmen LU-2, bilateral Jianyu L.I.-15, bilateral Weizhong BL-40 and Yaoshu DU-2.

COMBINATIONS

- Wasting and weakness of the arm with inability to raise the arm to the head: Jianyu L.I.-15 and Binao L.I.-14 (*Preserving Life*).
- Redness and swelling of the upper arm with pain of the joint: Jianyu L.I.-15, Zhouliao L.I.-12 and Wangu SI-4 (*Great Compendium*).
- Heat sensation of the shoulder with inability to turn the head: Jianyu L.I.-15, Jianzhen SI-9 and Guanchong SJ-1 (*Thousand Ducat Formulas*).
- Contraction of the elbow: Jianyu L.I.-15, Chize LU-5, Xiaohai SI-8, Jianshi P-5, Daling P-7, Houxi SI-3 and Yuji LU-10 (*Great Compendium*).
- Windstroke with one-sided withering and incessant pain: Jianyu L.I.-15, Xuanzhong GB-39, Taixi KID-3, Quchi L.I.-11, Zusanli ST-36 and Kunlun BL-60 (*Great Compendium*).
- Urticaria from extreme heat: Jianyu L.I.-15 and Yangxi L.I.-5 (*One Hundred Symptoms*).

JUGU L.I.-16

Great Bone

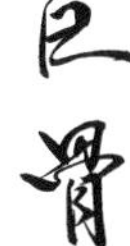

Meeting point of the Large Intestine channel with the Yang Motility vessel

LOCATION

On the upper aspect of the shoulder, in the depression medial to the acromion process and between the lateral extremity of the clavicle and the scapular spine.

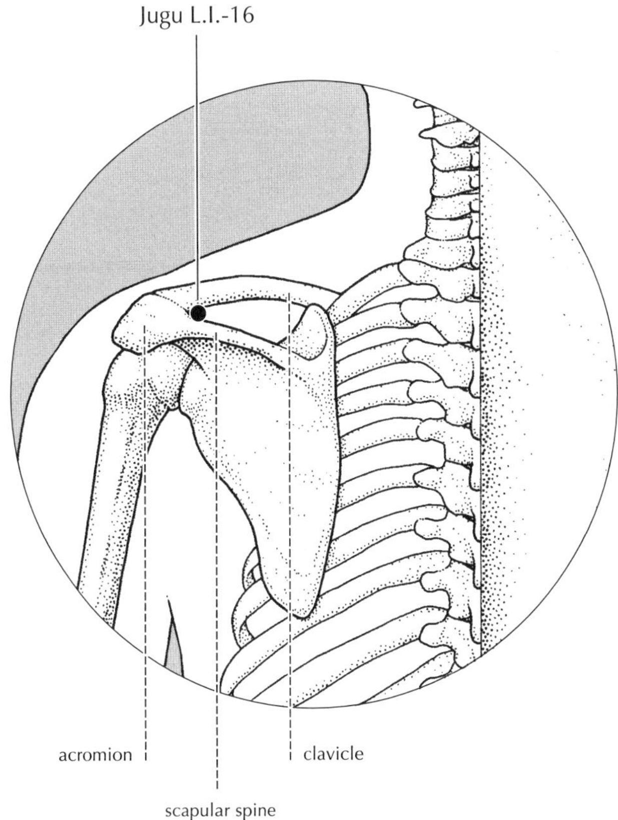

NEEDLING

Perpendicular or oblique insertion 0.5 to 1 cun.

Caution: deep medial insertion carries a risk of causing a pneumothorax, particularly in thin patients.

ACTIONS

Activates the channel, alleviates pain and benefits the shoulder joint

Regulates qi and blood and dissipates phlegm nodules

INDICATIONS

- Pain of the shoulder and back, blood stasis in the shoulder, difficulty in moving or raising the arm, pain of the upper arm.
- Fright epilepsy, vomiting of copious quantities of blood, blood stasis in the chest, scrofula, goitre.

COMMENTARY

Jugu L.I.-16 is frequently used as an adjacent point in the treatment of shoulder disorders, and in such cases should always be palpated for tenderness. The use of Jugu L.I.-16 is particularly emphasised when the shoulder disorder is chronic and recalcitrant, reflected by the indication for blood stasis in the shoulder. This is explained by the saying "Chronic disease is frequently [due to] stasis". Its action on treating disorders of blood also extends to blood stasis in the chest and vomiting blood.

Like Shouwuli L.I.-13, Binao L.I.-14 and Jianyu L.I.-15, Jugu L.I.-16 is indicated for scrofula.

COMBINATIONS

- Inability to raise the arm: Jugu L.I.-16 and Qiangu SI-2 (*Supplementing Life*).
- Pain of the shoulder and back: Jugu L.I.-16, Tianyou SJ-16, Quepen ST-12, Shendao DU-11, Dazhu BL-11, Tiantu REN-22 and Shuidao ST-28 (*Thousand Ducat Formulas*).

TIANDING L.I.-17

Heaven's Tripod

天鼎

LOCATION

On the lateral side of the neck, 1 cun inferior to Futu L.I.-18, on the posterior border of the sternocleidomastoid muscle.

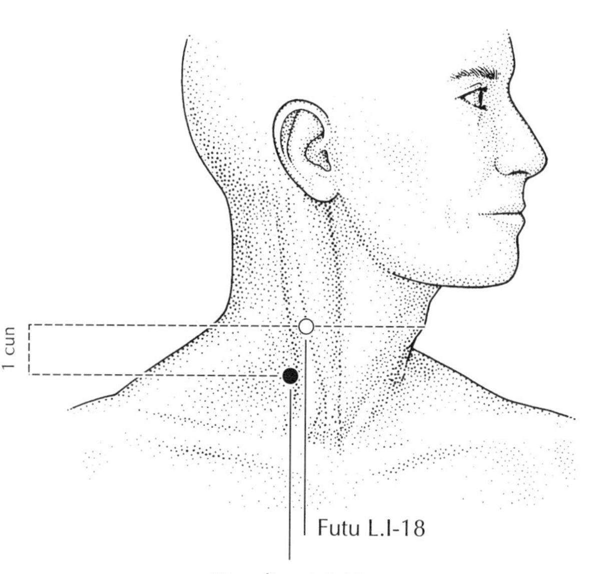

NEEDLING

i. Perpendicular insertion 0.3 to 0.5 cun; ii. Oblique insertion 0.5 to 0.8 cun.

Caution: deeper needling may puncture the carotid artery or jugular vein.

ACTIONS

Benefits the throat and voice

INDICATIONS

- Sudden loss of voice, throat painful obstruction, rattling sound in the throat, goitre, scrofula, difficulty in breathing, difficult ingestion.

COMBINATIONS

- Halting speech and loss of voice: Tianding L.I.-17 and Jianshi P-5 (*One Hundred Symptoms*).

FUTU L.I.-18

Support the Prominence

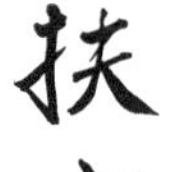
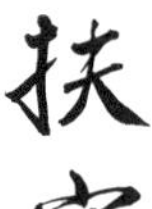

Point of the Window of Heaven

LOCATION

On the lateral side of the neck, level with the tip of the laryngeal prominence, between the sternal and clavicular heads of the sternocleidomastoid muscle.

LOCATION NOTE

i. Palpation of the sternal and clavicular heads is made easier if the patient turns their head away from the side to be needled, whilst you apply resistance at the chin; ii. In females the laryngeal prominence is not as pronounced as in males. If it is indistinct, palpate the depression formed by the lower border of the hyoid bone and the upper border of the thyroid cartilage at the midline. The laryngeal prominence lies just below this; iii. This point may be located approximately 3 cun (one handbreadth) lateral to the laryngeal prominence.

NEEDLING

i. Perpendicular insertion 0.3 to 0.5 cun; ii. Oblique insertion 0.5 to 0.8 cun.

Caution: deeper needling may puncture the carotid artery or jugular vein.

ACTIONS

Benefits the throat and voice

Alleviates cough and wheezing

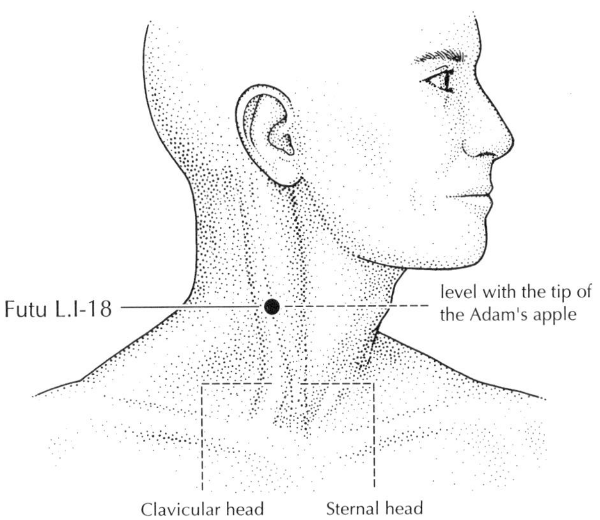

INDICATIONS
- Swelling and pain of the throat, sudden loss of voice, rattling sound in the throat, goitre, scrofula, difficulty in swallowing.
- Cough, coughing with much spittle, wheezing, asthma, hypotension.

COMMENTARY
In Chapter 21 of the *Spiritual Pivot* Futu L.I.-18 is included in a list of five points known as 'Window of Heaven' (literally 'five regions of the Window of Heaven') points. This passage states "Sudden loss of voice with obstructed qi in the throat, choose Futu L.I.-18 and bleed the root of the tongue". Futu L.I.-18 shares certain important characteristics of this grouping in that it treats goitre and scrofula due to stagnation of qi and phlegm in the pivotal neck region, and sudden loss of voice, coughing and wheezing due to inversion qi. For a fuller discussion of the points of the 'Window of Heaven' see page 48.

In clinical practice, Futu L.I.-18 is frequently used as an alternative to (or in combination with) Renying ST-9, in the treatment of difficulty in swallowing (especially following windstroke) and chronic disorders of the vocal cords.

COMBINATIONS
- Sudden loss of voice: Futu L.I.-18, Tianchuang SI-16, Zhigou SJ-6, Qubin GB-7 and Lingdao HE-4 (*Thousand Ducat Formulas*).
- Bleeding from the root of the tongue: Futu L.I.-18, Dazhong KID-4 and Touqiaoyin GB-11 (*Thousand Ducat Formulas*).
- Cough with rebellious qi, dyspnoea, vomiting of foam and clenched teeth: Futu L.I.-18, Tianrong SI-17, Lianquan REN-23, Pohu BL-42, Qishe ST-11 and Yixi BL-45 (*Thousand Ducat Formulas*).

KOUHELIAO L.I.-19
Mouth Grain Crevice

禾髎

LOCATION
Below the lateral margin of the nostril, 0.5 cun lateral to Renzhong DU-26.

LOCATION NOTE
Renzhong DU-26 is located above the upper lip on the midline, at the junction of the upper third and lower two thirds of the philtrum.

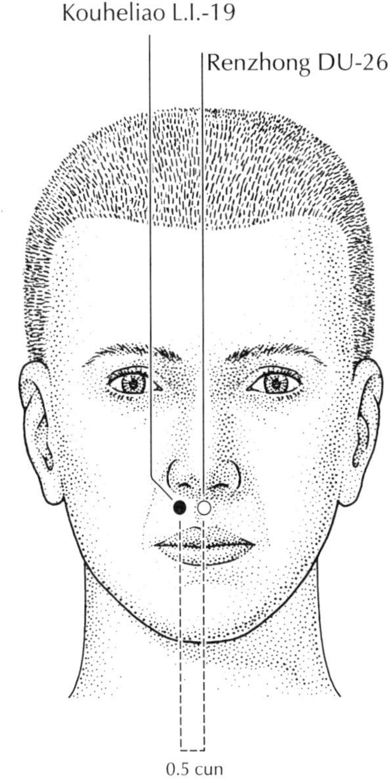

NEEDLING
Oblique insertion 0.3 to 0.5 cun. **Note**: according to some classical and modern texts, this point is contraindicated to moxibustion.

ACTIONS
Eliminates wind and opens the nasal passages

INDICATIONS
- Nasal congestion and discharge, loss of sense of smell, nasal sores, nasal polyps, rhinitis with nosebleed.
- Lockjaw, deviation of the mouth, loss of consciousness.

COMBINATIONS
- Nosebleed: Kouheliao L.I.-19 and Shangxing DU-23 (*Miscellaneous Diseases*).
- Incessant nosebleed: Kouheliao L.I.-19, Duiduan DU-27 and Laogong P-8 (*Supplementing Life*).
- Nasal congestion with inability to distinguish the fragrant from the foul: Kouheliao L.I.-19, Yingxiang L.I.-20, Shangxing DU-23 and Wuchu BL-5 (*Great Compendium*).

YINGXIANG L.I.-20
Welcome Fragrance

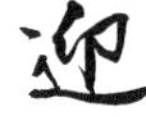
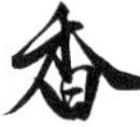

Meeting point of the Large Intestine and Stomach channels

LOCATION
In the naso-labial groove, at the level of the midpoint of the lateral border of the ala nasi.

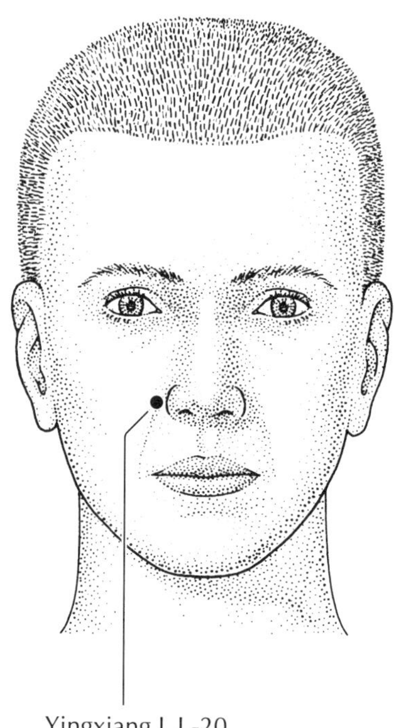
Yingxiang L.I.-20

NEEDLING
Transverse insertion medio-superiorly 0.3 to 0.5 cun or join to Bitong (M-HN-14) at the highest point of the naso-labial groove. **Note**: according to some classical and modern texts, this point is contraindicated to moxibustion.

ACTIONS
Opens the nasal passages
Expels wind and clears heat

INDICATIONS
- Nasal congestion, nasal congestion and discharge, rhinitis, profuse nasal discharge, loss of sense of smell, nasal polyps, nasal sores, sneezing, nosebleed.
- Deviation of the mouth, swelling and itching of the face, pain and swelling of the lip, heat and redness of the eyes, dyspnoea, round worms in the bile duct.

COMMENTARY
As its name 'Welcome Fragrance' implies, Yingxiang L.I.-20 is the foremost local point for treating all disorders of the nose. As such it is the primary local point for treating the Chinese disease categories of 'bi yuan', 'bi qiu', nasal polyps and sores. Bi yuan (literally 'nose pool' but translated in this text as nasal congestion and discharge) more or less corresponds to sinusitis and encompasses symptoms such as thin or thick nasal discharge and blocked and stuffy nose, commonly accompanied by pain and loss of sense of smell and taste. Bi qiu (translated in this text as rhinitis) also includes allergic rhinitis and encompasses such symptoms as sneezing, nasal discharge and itching.

Yangming channel governs the facial area, and Yingxiang L.I.-20, a meeting point of the Large Intestine and Stomach channels, is able to expel wind and heat from the face as a whole. It is particularly indicated for swelling and itching of the face, as well as for pain and swelling of the lip, heat and redness of the eyes and deviation of the mouth.

In recent years this point, needled to join with Sibai ST-2, has been much used to control the pain of biliary ascariasis. This disorder, which is endemic in China, is passed by eating contaminated raw vegetables fertilised by human 'night soil'. If the worms, which grow in the gall bladder, pass into the biliary duct, there is severe pain which is similar to that of cholelithiasis. The first step in treatment is to needle from Yingxiang L.I.-20 through to Sibai ST-2 with strong manipulation. This is usually effective to control the pain within one or two minutes. Additional points on the body are used to consolidate the effect, whilst herbal medicine is used subsequently to eliminate the worms.

COMBINATIONS
- Nasal congestion with inability to distinguish the fragrant from the foul: Yingxiang L.I.-20, Shangxing DU-23, Wuchu BL-5 and Kouheliao L.I.-19 (*Great Compendium*).
- Rhinitis with clear nasal discharge: Yingxiang L.I.-20, Hegu L.I.-4, Fengmen BL-12, Shenting DU-24, Zanzhu BL-2, Zhiyin BL-67 and Futonggu KID-20 (*Thousand Ducat Formulas*).

- Rhinitis with nose bleed: Yingxiang L.I.-20, Erjian L.I.-2 and Fengfu DU-16 (*Great Compendium*).
- Itching and swelling of the face: Yingxiang L.I.-20 and Hegu L.I.-4 (*Ode of Xi-hong*).

NOTES

1 *Spiritual Pivot* Chapter 4.

2 *Spiritual Pivot* Chapter 9.

3 *Classic of Difficulties* 68th Difficulty.

4 *The Heart & Essence of Dan-xi's Methods of Treatment*, A Translation of Zhu Dan-xi's Dan Xi Zhi Fa Xin Yao, Blue Poppy Press, p. 310.

5 *Classic of Difficulties* 68th Difficulty.

6 Ma Dan-yang was the originator of the *Song of the Eleven Heavenly Star Points*. They first appeared in print in the 12th century CE *Classic of the Jade Dragon*. Xu Feng included this text in his work *Complete Collection of Acupuncture and Moxibustion* and added a twelfth point, Taichong LIV-3.

7 *Spiritual Pivot* Chapter 9.

8 *Spiritual Pivot* Chapter 44.

9 Quoted in *Chinese Acupuncture and Moxibustion*, Foreign Languages Press, Beijing.

10 *Spiritual Pivot* Chapter 9.

11 *The Heart & Essence of Dan-xi's Methods of Treatment*, A Translation of Zhu Dan-xi's Dan Xi Zhi Fa Xin Yao, Blue Poppy Press, p. 310.

12 *Spiritual Pivot* Chapter 6.

13 *Classic of Difficulties* 68th Difficulty.

14 *Spiritual Pivot* Chapter 44.

15 *Spiritual Pivot* Chapter 9.

16 *Essential Questions* Chapter 61.

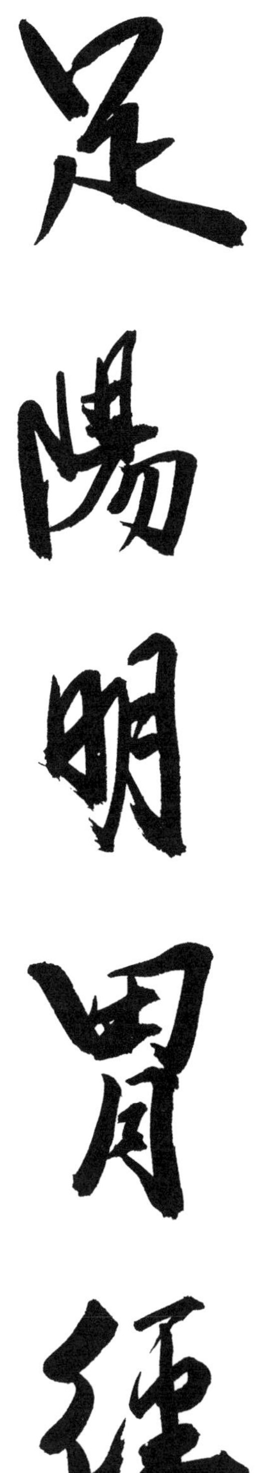

THE STOMACH CHANNEL OF FOOT YANGMING

THE STOMACH CHANNEL OF FOOT YANGMING

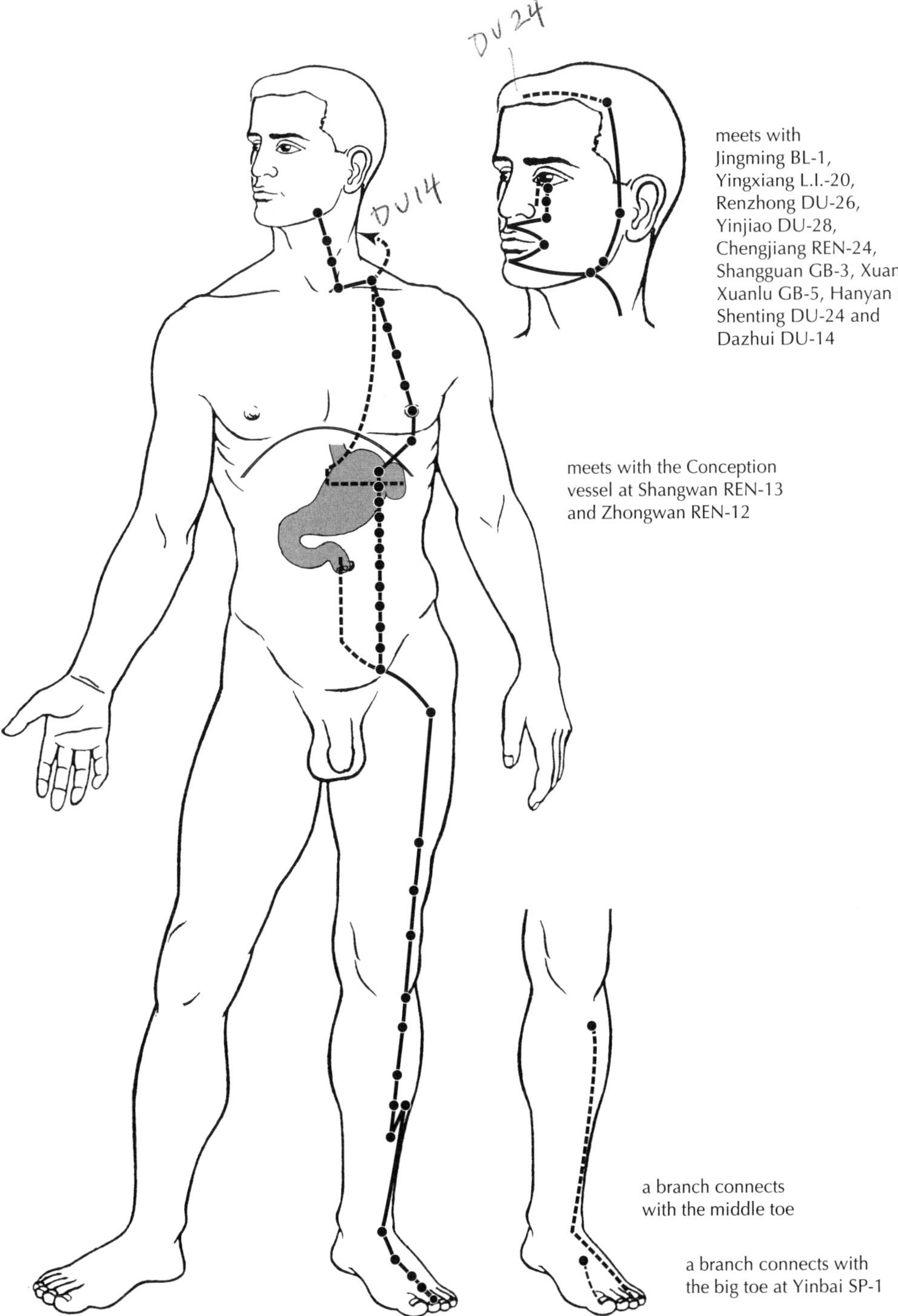
meets with
Jingming BL-1,
Yingxiang L.I.-20,
Renzhong DU-26,
Yinjiao DU-28,
Chengjiang REN-24,
Shangguan GB-3, Xuanli GB-6,
Xuanlu GB-5, Hanyan GB-4,
Shenting DU-24 and
Dazhui DU-14
meets with the Conception
vessel at Shangwan REN-13
and Zhongwan REN-12
a branch connects
with the middle toe
a branch connects with
the big toe at Yinbai SP-1

THE STOMACH PRIMARY CHANNEL

- begins at the lateral side of the nose at Yingxiang L.I.-20,
- ascends to the medial canthus where it meets the Bladder channel at Jingming BL-l,
- descends laterally along the infra-orbital ridge to Chengqi ST-l,
- descends to enter the upper gum and curves to meet with Yinjiao DU-28 and Renzhong DU-26,
- circles around the lips and meets the Conception vessel at Chengjiang REN-24 in the mento-labial groove of the chin,
- runs laterally across the cheeks to Daying ST-5 and to Jiache ST-6 at the angle of the mandible,

- ascends anterior to the ear passing via Xiaguan ST-7 to Shangguan GB-3,
- ascends within the hairline of the temporal region to Touwei ST-8, passing via Xuanli GB-6, Xuanlu GB-5 and Hanyan GB-4,
- follows the hairline to meet the Governing channel at Shenting DU-24.

A branch

- separates at Daying ST-5 and descends along the anterior border of the sternocleidomastoid muscle in the throat region to enter the supraclavicular fossa at Quepen ST-12,
- travels posteriorly to the upper back where it meets the Governing channel at Dazhui DU-14,
- descends through the diaphragm, linking with Shangwan REN-13 and Zhongwan REN-12 to enter the Stomach and connect with the Spleen.

A further branch

- descends from Quepen ST-12 along the mamillary line, 4 cun lateral to the midline as far as Rugen ST-18, then passes 2 cun lateral to the midline and descends alongside the umbilicus to Qichong ST-30 in the inguinal region.

A further branch

- originates from the pyloric orifice of the Stomach, descends within the abdomen and meets with the previous portion of the channel at Qichong ST-30.

From the inguinal region at Qichong ST-30 the channel

- travels laterally to Biguan ST-31 on the antero-lateral aspect of the thigh,
- descends along the lateral margin of the femur to the patella and alongside the lateral margin of the tibia to the dorsum of the foot, terminating at the lateral side of the tip of the second toe at Lidui ST-45.

A further branch

- separates from the main channel at Zusanli ST-36, three cun below the knee, and terminates at the lateral aspect of the middle toe.

A further branch

- separates on the dorsum of the foot at Chongyang ST-42 and terminates at the medial side of the tip of the big toe at Yinbai SP-l where it links with the Spleen channel.

The Stomach primary channel connects with the following zangfu: Stomach and Spleen.

The Stomach primary channel meets with other channels at the following points: Yingxiang L.I.-20, Jingming BL-1, Shangguan GB-3, Hanyan GB-4, Xuanlu GB-5, Xuanli GB-6, Dazhui DU-14, Shenting DU-24, Renzhong DU-26, Yinjiao DU-28, Zhongwan REN-12, Shangwan REN-13, Chengjiang REN-24. Note that Yangbai GB-14 and Jianjing GB-21 are also known as meeting points of the Gall Bladder and Stomach channels, but illustrations of the Stomach channel do not normally show these connections. By contrast, although a branch of the Stomach channel connects Chongyang ST-42 with Yinbai SP-1, the latter point is not described as a meeting point of the Spleen and Stomach channels.

THE STOMACH LUO-CONNECTING CHANNEL

- originates on the lateral side of the lower leg at Fenglong ST-40,
- travels to the medial aspect of the lower leg to join with the Spleen channel,
- ascends the leg and trunk to the nape of the neck and head where it converges with the qi of the other yang channels,
- then travels internally to terminate at the throat.

THE STOMACH DIVERGENT CHANNEL

- branches from the primary channel in the middle of the thigh,
- ascends and enters the abdomen,
- travels to the Stomach and disperses in the Spleen,
- ascends to penetrate the Heart,
- ascends along the oesophagus and emerges at the mouth,
- continues along the nose to connect with the eye and then unites with the primary Stomach channel.

THE STOMACH SINEW CHANNEL

- begins at the middle three toes and binds on the dorsum of the foot,
- ascends along the lateral aspect of the tibia and binds at the lateral aspect of the knee, connecting with the Gall Bladder sinew channel,
- ascends to bind at the hip joint,
- passes through the lower ribs into the spine.

A branch

- runs along the tibia and binds at the knee,
- ascends the thigh and binds in the pelvic region above the genitals,
- ascends the abdomen and chest and binds at Quepen ST-12,
- ascends the neck to the jaw, mouth and side of the nose and binds below the nose,
- joins with the Bladder sinew channel to form a muscular net around the eye, known as the 'lower net' (the Bladder sinew channel forms the 'upper net').

A sub-branch

- separates at the jaw and binds in front of the ear.

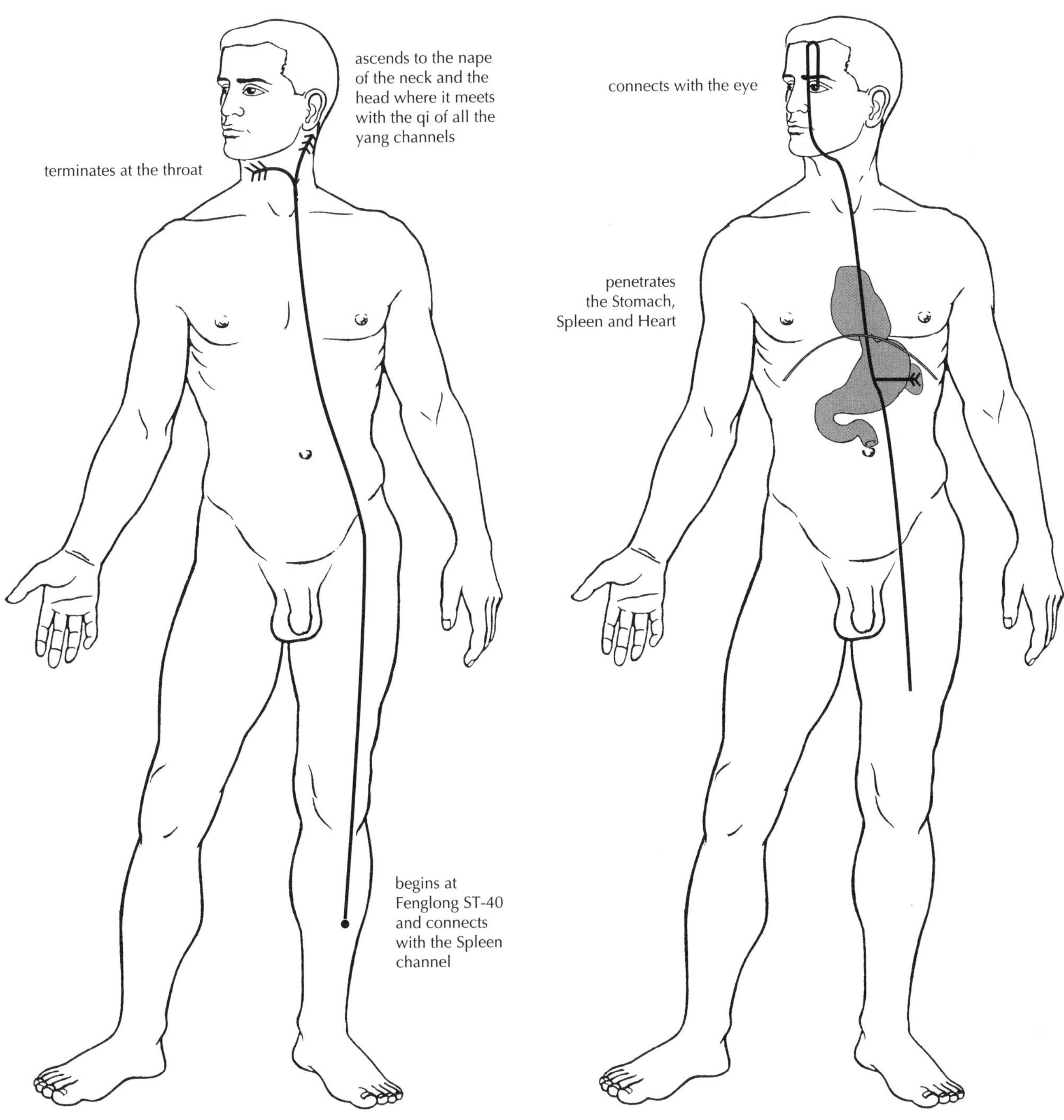
ascends to the nape of the neck and the head where it meets with the qi of all the yang channels
terminates at the throat
begins at Fenglong ST-40 and connects with the Spleen channel
connects with the eye
penetrates the Stomach, Spleen and Heart

The Stomach luo-connecting channel

The Stomach divergent channel

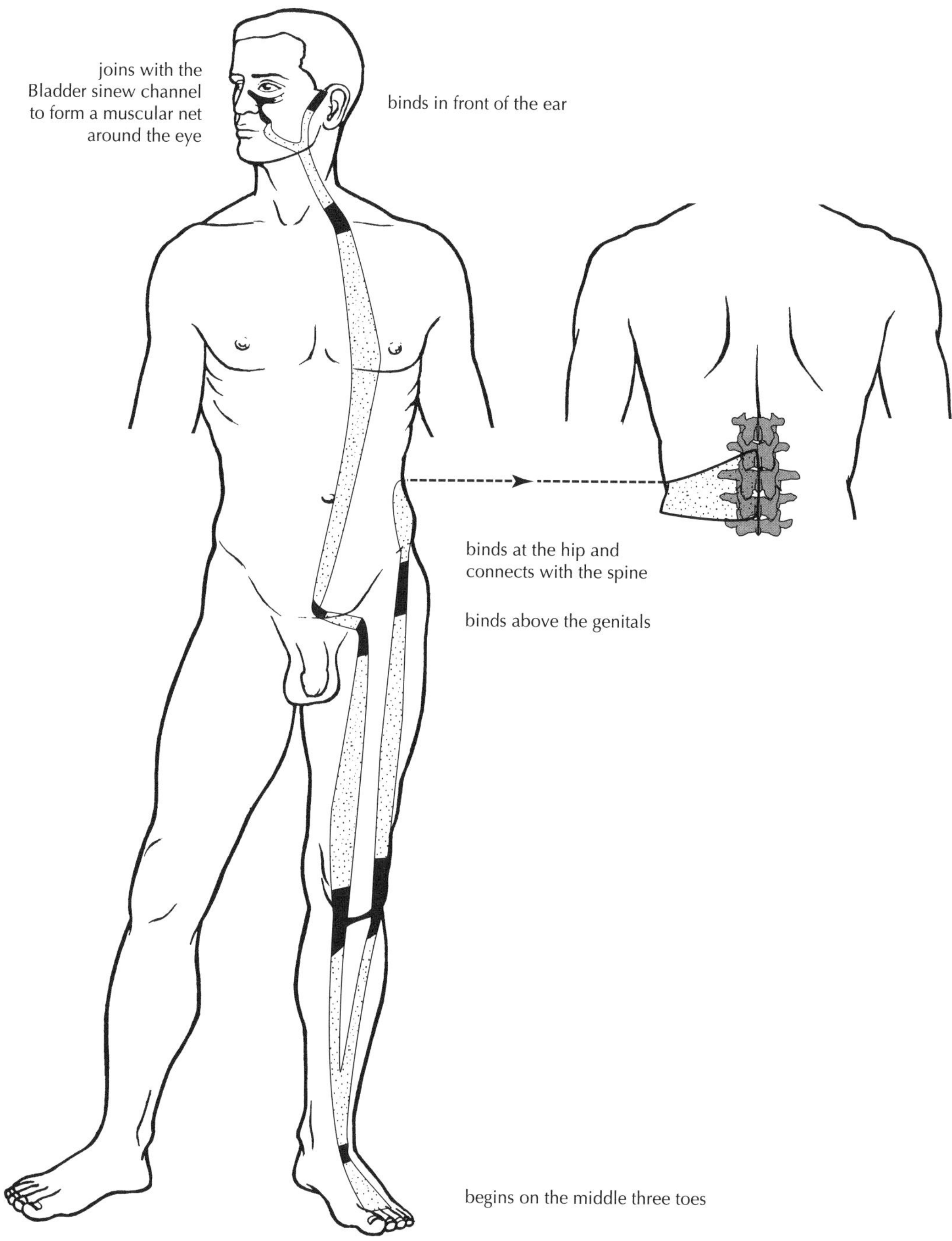
joins with the
Bladder sinew channel
to form a muscular net
around the eye
binds in front of the ear
binds at the hip and
connects with the spine
binds above the genitals
begins on the middle three toes

The Stomach sinew channel

Pathological symptoms of the Stomach sinew channel
Strained middle toe, cramping of the lower leg, spasmodic twitching and hardness of the muscles of the foot, spasm of the thigh, swelling of the anterior inguinal region, shan disorder, abdominal sinew spasm that extends to the Quepen [supraclavicular fossa] region and cheek, sudden deviation of the mouth, [if cold] inability to close the eye, [if hot] laxity of the sinews and the eye cannot be opened. If the cheek sinew has cold, it will be tense and pull the cheek, and the mouth will be deviated; if there is heat then the sinews become flaccid and this will result in deviation of the mouth.

DISCUSSION

The Stomach channel of foot yangming is interiorly-exteriorly coupled with the Spleen channel of foot taiyin, and paired with the Large Intestine channel of hand yangming according to six channel theory. The Stomach-Spleen relationship is further strengthened by the fact that:

- the Stomach primary channel enters the Spleen.
- the Stomach divergent channel disperses in the Spleen.
- the Stomach luo-connecting channel from Fenglong ST-40 joins with the Spleen channel.

In addition it is clinically valuable to note that:

- the Stomach primary channel enters the upper gum, then joins with the Governing vessel at Renzhong DU-26, circles the lips and joins with the Conception vessel at Chengjiang REN-24, thus connecting with both the upper and lower teeth.
- the Stomach channel ascends in front of the ear and meets with the Gall Bladder channel (which enters the ear) at Xiaguan ST-7.
- the Stomach luo-connecting channel terminates at the throat whilst the Stomach primary channel descends through the throat region.
- the Stomach divergent channel penetrates the Heart, whilst the Stomach primary channel ascends to meet the Governing vessel at both Shenting DU-24 and Renzhong DU-26.
- the Stomach primary channel descends through the breast and nipple.
- the Stomach primary channel descends to cross the chest, epigastrium and upper and lower abdomen.
- a branch of the primary channel terminates at the lateral side of the middle toe, the only channel to go to this toe.

The functions of the Stomach fu are to control the 'rotting and ripening' of food, to control descending and to act as the first stage in the digestion of fluids. Disharmony of the Stomach therefore manifests as i. disorders of appetite and digestion, ii. distention and pain in the epigastrium due to failure of the Stomach qi to descend, or iii. belching, nausea or vomiting due to rebellious ascent of Stomach qi. Many points of the Stomach channel, both local abdominal points and the more distal points, are used to treat such disorders.

According to the *Spiritual Pivot*[1] "Yangming channel is abundant in qi and blood". Points of foot yangming channel are therefore much used clinically to regulate qi and blood in the lower limb and to treat atrophy disorder and painful obstruction, hemiplegia and pain of all kinds.

In the Chinese tradition the 'sage faces South', and thus the light and warmth of the sun fall on the front of the body. The yangming channels on the anterior of the limbs receives the full intensity of the sun, as does the abdominal and chest portion of the foot yangming Stomach channel, the only yang channel to run along the anterior of the body. For this reason, yangming or 'yang brightness' is considered to be particularly full of yang qi. Points of the Stomach channel, therefore, are among the most important points to clear excess of yang in the form of febrile heat, or heat which rises to disturb the Heart and spirit.

Apart from the above, the primary actions and indications of the points of the Stomach channel can be summarised as:

- treating all disorders of the yangming channel in the head including the eyes, face and cheeks, forehead, nose, lips, gums and teeth.
- treating disorders of the ear.
- treating disorders of the throat.
- regulating the function of the intestines.
- treating disorders of the upper, middle and lower jiao, especially the Lung, Heart, chest, epigastrium, Stomach, Spleen, uterus and Bladder.
- tonifying qi, blood, yin and yang.
- treating both acute and chronic disorders of the breast.
- treating disturbance of the spirit, especially mania-depression.

CHENGQI ST-1

Container of Tears

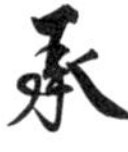
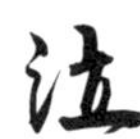

Meeting point of the Stomach channel with the Yang Motility and Conception vessels

LOCATION

With the eyes looking directly forwards, this point is located directly below the pupil between the eyeball and the infraorbital ridge.

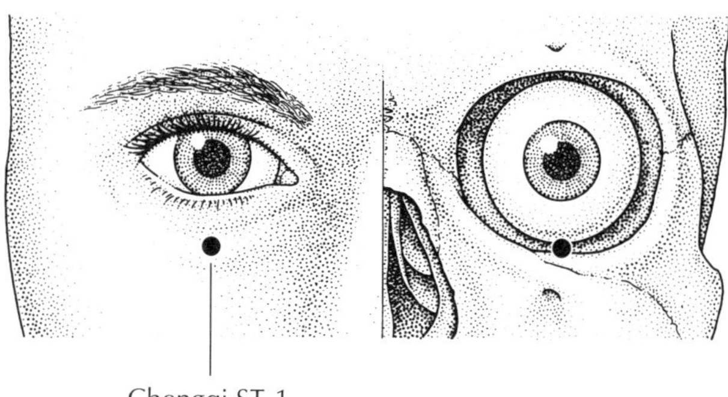

Chengqi ST-1

NEEDLING

Ask the patient to close their eyes and look upwards. Use a finger to push the eyeball upwards and insert the needle, first slightly inferiorly, then perpendicularly, between the eyeball and the inferior wall of the orbit, 0.5 to 1 cun. **Note**: according to several classical texts, this point is contraindicated to moxibustion.

Caution: i. the needle should be inserted slowly without lifting, thrusting or rotating; ii. immediately on withdrawal of the needle, press firmly with a cotton wool ball for about a minute to prevent haematoma; iii. this needling method should not be attempted by those who have not had appropriate clinical supervision.

ACTIONS

Benefits the eyes and stops lacrimation

Eliminates wind and clears heat

INDICATIONS

- Redness, swelling and pain of the eyes, lacrimation on exposure to wind, cold lacrimation, hot lacrimation, superficial visual obstruction, dimness of vision, short sightedness, visual dizziness, night blindness, itching of the eyes, upward staring eyes, twitching of the eyelids.
- Deviation of the mouth and eye, inability to speak, deafness and tinnitus.

COMMENTARY

Chengqi ST-1 is one of the two principal local points of the primary channels for the treatment of eye diseases (the other being Jingming BL-1), and is the meeting of a network of channels. The Stomach primary channel meets the Bladder channel at Jingming BL-1 before descending along the infraorbital ridge to Chengqi ST-1, the Stomach divergent channel connects with the eye, and the Stomach sinew channel joins with the Bladder sinew channel to form a muscular net around the eye.

The aetiology and pathology of eye disorders is complex and varied but may be simplified into i. attack by exterior pathogenic wind-heat or wind-cold, ii. interior disharmony (primarily flaring of Liver fire, uprising of Liver yang or deficiency of Liver yin and blood), or iii. a combination of both interior disharmony and exterior pathogens. Not only is Chengqi ST-1 able to dispel pathogenic factors such as wind, cold and heat from the eye, but by strongly invigorating and stimulating the qi and blood of the local area it is equally applicable for disorders due to any kind of interior disharmony, and is therefore indicated for the fullest range of eye diseases. This includes the traditional categories of redness, swelling and pain, lacrimation, superficial visual obstruction, dimness of vision, short sightedness, night blindness, itching of the eyes, upward staring eyes, visual dizziness and twitching of the eyelids. In terms of modern disease categories, Chengqi ST-1 is indicated for acute and chronic conjunctivitis, myopia, glaucoma, astigmatism, colour blindness, neuritis of the optic nerve, keratitis, and blepharospasm.

As the name 'Container of Tears' suggests, Chengqi ST-1 is especially important in the treatment of excessive lacrimation, which is classically subdivided into cold or hot types, in both cases complicated by exterior wind. The cold type may be due to deficiency and cold of the Liver channel or exhaustion of the Liver and Kidneys, whilst the hot type may be due to Liver channel wind-heat or Liver yin deficiency with heat.

COMBINATIONS

- Deviation of the mouth with inability to speak: Chengqi ST-1, Sibai ST-2, Juliao ST-3, Kouheliao L.I.-19, Shangguan GB-3, Daying ST-5, Quanliao SI-18, Qiangjian DU-18, Fengchi GB-20, Yingxiang L.I.-20 and Renzhong DU-26 (*Supplementing Life*).
- Short-sightedness: Chengqi ST-1, Jingming BL-1, Fengchi GB-20, Guangming GB-37, Taichong LIV-3 and Hegu L.I.-4.
- Redness, swelling and pain of the eye: Chengqi ST-1, Zanzhu BL-2, Fengchi GB-20, Taiyang (M-HN-9), Hegu L.I.-4 and Xingjian LIV-2.

SIBAI ST-2

Four Whites

四白

LOCATION

With the eyes looking directly forwards, this point is located 1 cun directly below the pupil, in the depression at the infraorbital foramen.

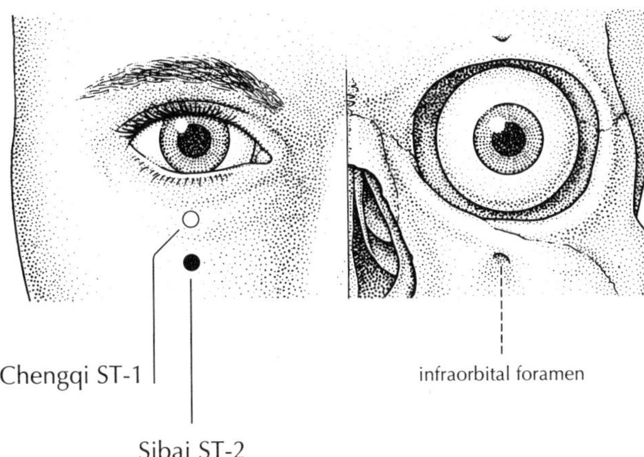

LOCATION NOTE

The infraorbital foramen can be felt by palpating downwards from the edge of the orbital bone, about 0.3 cun below the edge.

NEEDLING

i. Perpendicular insertion 0.2 to 0.4 cun; ii. Transverse insertion to join with such points as Quanliao SI-18, Yingxiang L.I.-20 etc; iii. Oblique insertion supero-laterally, along the infraorbital foramen, 0.3 to 0.5 cun. **Note**: according to several classical texts, this point is contraindicated to moxibustion.

Caution: i. deep insertion along the foramen may injure the eyeball; ii. manipulation by lifting and thrusting is contraindicated due to the risk of damaging the infraorbital nerve which emerges from the foramen.

ACTIONS

Eliminates wind, clears heat and benefits the eyes

INDICATIONS

- Redness and pain of the eyes, superficial visual obstruction, dimness of vision, visual dizziness, itching eyes, excessive lacrimation, deviation of the mouth and eye, twitching of the eyelids, headache.
- Round worms in the bile duct.

COMMENTARY

Although not a major point, Sibai ST-2 may be used in the following three clinical situations: i. as a substitute for Chengqi ST-1 in the treatment of eye diseases for those who have not mastered the more difficult technique of needling the latter point, ii. as a local point - often joined to adjacent points - for facial pain and paralysis, and iii. in the treatment of round worms in the bile duct (see Yingxiang L.I.-20).

COMBINATIONS

- Superficial visual obstruction: Sibai ST-2, Jingming BL-1 and Hegu L.I.-4 (*Great Compendium*).
- Headache and visual dizziness: Sibai ST-2, Yongquan KID-1 and Dazhu BL-11 (*Supplementing Life*).

JULIAO ST-3

Great Crevice

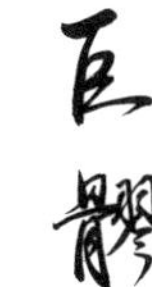

Meeting point of the Stomach channel with the Yang Motility vessel

LOCATION

With the eyes looking directly forwards, this point is located directly below the pupil, level with the lower border of the ala nasi, on the lateral side of the naso-labial groove.

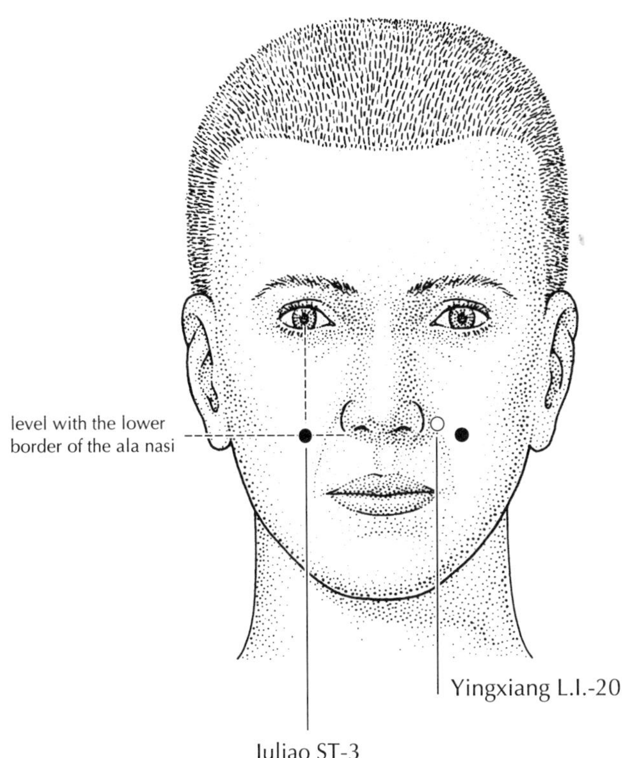

NEEDLING
i. Perpendicular insertion 0.3 to 0.4 cun; ii. Transverse insertion to join with such points as Dicang ST-4, Quanliao SI-18 etc.

ACTIONS
Eliminates wind, dissipates swelling and alleviates pain

INDICATIONS
- Pain and swelling of the external nose and cheek, nosebleed, toothache, swelling and pain of the lips and cheek, deviation of the mouth, aversion to wind and cold in the face and eyes, superficial visual obstruction, excessive lacrimation, clonic spasm.
- Leg qi, swelling of the knee.

COMBINATIONS
- Pain and swelling of the cheek: Juliao ST-3 and Tianchuang SI-16 (*Supplementing Life*).

DICANG ST-4
Earth Granary

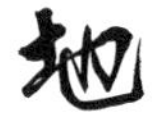
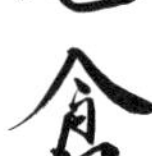

Meeting point of the Stomach and Large Intestine channels with the Yang Motility and Conception vessels

LOCATION
0.4 cun lateral to the corner of the mouth.

LOCATION NOTE
This point lies in the continuation of the naso-labial groove; ask the patient to smile if the groove is not visible.

NEEDLING
Transverse insertion to join with such points as Jiache ST-6, Yingxiang L.I.-20, Chengqiang REN-24 etc.

ACTIONS
Eliminates wind from the face
Activates the channel and alleviates pain

INDICATIONS
- Deviation of the mouth, pain of the cheek, trigeminal neuralgia, drooling, food and drink leak out of the mouth, numbness of the lips and face, toothache, contraction of the facial muscles, loss of speech.
- Ceaseless movement of the eyeball, inability to close the eye, twitching of the eyelids, itching of the eye, blurring of distant objects, night blindness.
- Atrophy disorder with inability to walk, swelling of the leg, inability to eat.

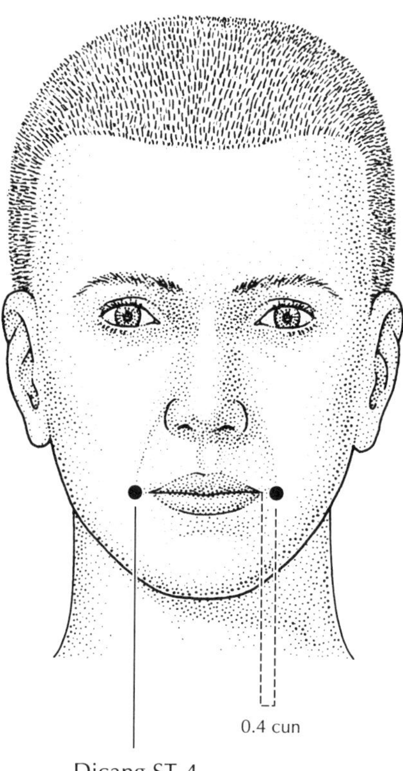

COMMENTARY
The 12th century classic *Secret Writings of Bian Que* states "use Dicang ST-4 in all cases where treacherous wind enters the ear, mouth and eye and leads to deviation". Dicang ST-4 is an important local point to eliminate wind from the face and is frequently used in the treatment of facial paralysis, whether due to exterior pathogenic wind or the sequelae of windstroke, particularly when the mouth is affected with symptoms such as drooling and deviation. Dicang ST-4 is also important in the treatment of facial pain such as trigeminal neuralgia. Pain of the face is usually differentiated into: i. invasion of the channels of the face by wind and cold, ii. flaring up of Stomach and Liver fire, and iii. heat due to yin deficiency. Due to its location, Dicang ST-4 may be needled whatever the pattern.

For both these applications, Dicang ST-4 is commonly joined to points such as Jiache ST-6, Quanliao SI-18, Yingxiang L.I.-20 and Chengjiang REN-24 by transverse needling. The *Great Compendium of Acupuncture and Moxibustion* recommends needling left Dicang ST-4 for diseases of the right side of the face, and vice-versa. This principle of contralateral needling is discussed in the *Spiritual Pivot*[2] which states "Contralateral insertion, that is, if the left is affected, the right is treated, and if the right affected, the left is needled", and the *Essential Questions*[3] which says "When evils invade the channels, if the left side is in excess, the disease occurs on the right side, and vice versa ... for these conditions, contralateral insertion should be used". Although common practice emphasises needling the diseased side, these statements underline the important principle of treating the healthy side, where the qi is plentiful, in chronic cases and those involving great deficiency.

It is interesting to note the use of Dicang ST-4 for leg disorders, reflecting the principle stated in the *Yellow Emperor's Inner Classic*[4] "When the disease is below select [points] from above". Whilst the use of points on the lower body to treat diseases of the upper body is extremely common, the reverse is relatively rare. Other examples are Baihui DU-20 for anal disorders, Renzhong DU-26 and Renying ST-9 for lumbar pain, and Shuaigu GB-8 for vomiting.

COMBINATIONS

- Deviation of the mouth: Dicang ST-4 and Jiache ST-6 (*Ode of the Jade Dragon*).
- Deviation of the mouth: Dicang ST-4 and Lieque LU-7 (*Supplementing Life*).
- Deviation of the mouth and eye: Dicang ST-4, Jiache ST-6, Renzhong DU-26, Chengjiang REN-24, Tinghui GB-2 and Hegu L.I.-4 (*Illustrated Supplement*).
- Legs withered and lame: Dicang ST-4 and Taiyuan LU-9 (*Thousand Ducat Formulas*).

DAYING ST-5

Great Welcome

大迎

LOCATION

Directly anterior to the angle of the jaw, in a depression at the anterior border of the masseter muscle.

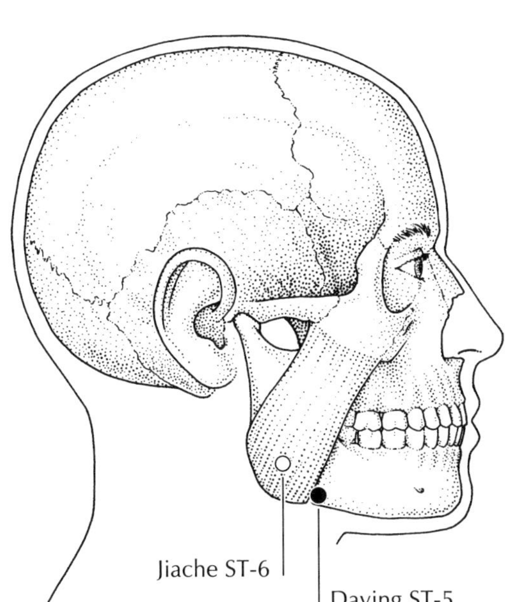

LOCATION NOTE

Ask the patient to clench the jaw before locating.

NEEDLING

i. Oblique insertion 0.3 to 0.5 cun; or ii. Transverse insertion to join with such points as Dicang ST-4, Jiache ST-6 etc.

Caution: vigorous manipulation is contraindicated to avoid the risk of damaging the facial artery and vein.

ACTIONS

Eliminates wind and reduces swelling

INDICATIONS

- Wind tetany with lockjaw, deviation of the mouth, twitching of the lips, toothache of the lower jaw, frequent yawning, stiffness of the tongue with inability to speak, inability to close the eyes accompanied by pain of the eyes.
- Swelling of the face and lower cheek, wind obstructing the face leading to swelling, mumps, scrofula, neck pain with chills and fever, aversion to cold.

COMBINATIONS

- Toothache with aversion to cold: Daying ST-5, Quanliao SI-18, Tinghui GB-2 and Quchi L.I.-11 (*Thousand Ducat Formulas*).
- Pain from tooth decay: Daying ST-5, Sanjian L.I.-3 and Zhengying GB-17 (*Supplementing Life*).
- Toothache and tooth decay: Daying ST-5, Xiaguan ST-7, Yifeng SJ-17 and Wangu SI-4 (*Supplementing Life*).
- Deviation of the mouth with inability to speak: Daying ST-5, Chengqi ST-1, Sibai ST-2, Juliao ST-3, Kouheliao L.I.-19, Shangguan GB-3, Quanliao SI-18, Qiangjian DU-18, Fengchi GB-20, Yingxiang L.I.-20 and Renzhong DU-26 (*Supplementing Life*).

JIACHE ST-6

Jaw Bone

頰車

Sun Si-miao Ghost point

LOCATION

Approximately 1 fingerbreadth anterior and superior to the angle of the jaw at the prominence of the masseter muscle.

LOCATION NOTE

Ask the patient to clench the jaw before locating.

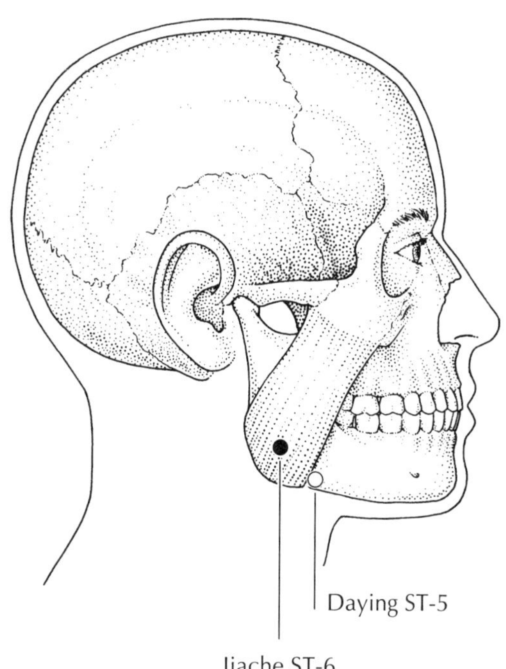

NEEDLING

i. Perpendicular insertion 0.5 cun; ii. Transverse insertion to join with such points as Dicang ST-4, Daying ST-5, Xiaguan ST-7 etc.; iii. Transverse insertion towards the upper or lower jaw for toothache.

ACTIONS

Eliminates wind and benefits the jaw and teeth
Activates the channel and alleviates pain

INDICATIONS

- Deviation of the mouth and eye, swelling of the cheek, toothache, gum disorders, lockjaw, tension and pain of the jaw, inability to chew, inability to open the mouth following windstroke.
- Stiffness and pain of the neck, mumps, loss of voice.

COMMENTARY

Jiache ST-6 (Jaw Bone) is an important point in the treatment of a wide range of local disorders affecting the jaw, including inability to chew, inability to open the mouth after windstroke, lockjaw, and tension, pain or paralysis of the jaw. Its range of action extends upwards along the Stomach channel into the face for deviation of the mouth and eye and swelling of the cheek, and downwards along the channel for mumps, and stiffness and pain of the neck. The predominant pathogenic factor in all these different disorders is wind, whether of external or internal origin. Jiache ST-6 is also a major point in the treatment of disorders of the gum and teeth of the lower jaw.

Jiache ST-6 is one of the 'thirteen ghost points', listed under its alternative name Guichuang (Ghost's Bed) in the *Supplement to the Thousand Ducat Formulas* by Sun Simiao. This grouping of points was used to treat mania and epilepsy, and it is unclear why Jiache ST-6 was ascribed this action, especially in the light of the fact that there are no indications of this kind listed for the point. One possible explanation is the fear that epileptics might bite off their tongue while gnashing their teeth during a fit, in which case Jiache ST-6 would be included in a prescription for epilepsy in order to relax the jaw.

COMBINATIONS

- Pain and deviation of the mouth, aversion to wind and cold, inability to chew: Jiache ST-6 and Quanliao SI-18 (*Thousand Ducat Formulas*).
- Deviation of the mouth and eye: Jiache ST-6, Dicang ST-4, Renzhong DU-26, Chengjiang REN-24, Tinghui GB-2 and Hegu L.I.-4 (*Illustrated Supplement*).
- Lockjaw following windstroke: reduce Jiache ST-6, Renzhong DU-26, Baihui DU-20, Chengjiang REN-24 and Hegu L.I.-4 (*Great Compendium*).
- Lockjaw: Jiache ST-6, Shangguan GB-3 and Ahshi points (*Compilation*).
- Inability to chew: Jiache ST-6 and Jiaosun SJ-20 (*Thousand Ducat Formulas*).
- Swelling, pain and redness of the ear: Jiache ST-6, Tinghui GB-2 and Hegu L.I.-4 (*Great Compendium*).

XIAGUAN ST-7

Below the Joint

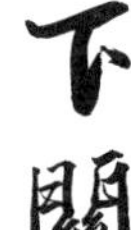

Meeting point of the Stomach and Gall Bladder channels

LOCATION

At the lower border of the zygomatic arch, in the depression anterior to the condyloid process of the mandible.

LOCATION NOTE

Although this point is needled with the mouth closed, it is helpful to ask the patient to open the mouth to better locate the condyloid process. If the finger rests on the condyloid process when the mouth is open, it will fall into Xiaguan ST-7 when the mouth is closed.

NEEDLING

i. Perpendicular insertion slightly inferiorly 0.5 to 1 cun; ii. Transverse insertion to join with such points as Tinggong SI-19, Jiache ST-6, Quanliao SI-18 etc. for diseases of the ear, teeth, face and jaw.

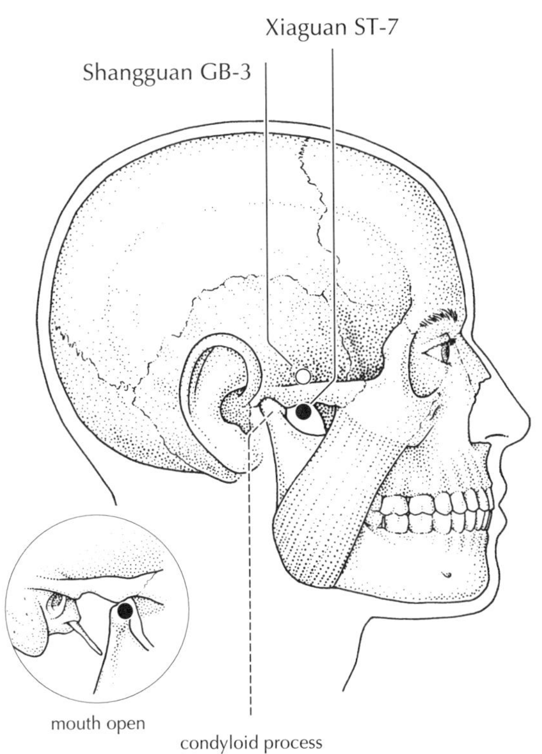

ACTIONS

Benefits the ears, jaw and teeth
Activates the channel and alleviates pain

INDICATIONS

- Deafness, tinnitus, ear pain, itching and purulent discharge from the ear.
- Lockjaw, dislocation of the jaw.
- Toothache, pain of the teeth of the lower jaw, swelling and pain of the gums (of the lower jaw), pain of the cheek and face, swelling of the cheek, yawning, deviation of the mouth and eye, visual dizziness.

COMMENTARY

Xiaguan ST-7 is an important and commonly used point for the treatment of local disorders affecting the ear (deafness, tinnitus, pain and discharge), cheek (pain and swelling), teeth (toothache, swelling and pain of the gum) and upper jaw (lockjaw and dislocation). Its ability to treat ear disorders is explained both by its location, and by the fact that the Gall Bladder channel, which enters the ear, meets with the Stomach channel at this point.

In the treatment of facial pain and trigeminal neuralgia Xiaguan ST-7 is sometimes needled 0.5 cun anterior to its textbook location.

COMBINATIONS

- Tinnitus and deafness: Xiaguan ST-7, Yangxi L.I.-5, Guanchong SJ-1, Yemen SJ-2 and Yanggu SI-5 (*Systematic Classic*).
- Deafness: Xiaguan ST-7, Huizong SJ-7 and Yifeng SJ-17 (*Systematic Classic*).
- Toothache and tooth decay: Xiaguan ST-7, Daying ST-5, Yifeng SJ-17 and Wangu SI-4 (*Supplementing Life*).
- Hemiplegia with deviation of the mouth and eye: Xiaguan ST-7 and Shangguan GB-3 (*Supplementing Life*)
- Yawning and pain of the lower teeth: Xiaguan ST-7, Daying ST-5 and Yifeng SJ-17 (*Thousand Ducat Prescriptions*).
- Facial paralysis: Xiaguan ST-7, Yifeng SJ-17, Dicang ST-4, Jiache ST-6, Sibai ST-2 and Hegu L.I.-4.

TOUWEI ST-8

Head's Binding

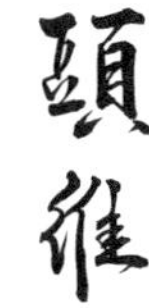

Meeting point of the Stomach and Gall Bladder channels with the Yang Linking vessel

LOCATION

At the corner of the forehead, 4.5 cun lateral to Shenting DU-24 and 0.5 cun within the anterior hairline.

LOCATION NOTE

There are three methods to locate this point: i. Find the meeting point of a horizontal line drawn 0.5 cun within the anterior hairline, and a vertical line drawn 0.5 cun posterior to the hairline of the temple; ii. Locate Toulinqi GB-15 which lies directly above the pupil when the patient is looking directly forwards, and Shenting DU-24 which lies on the midline, 0.5 cun posterior to the anterior hairline. Touwei ST-8 lies on the continuation of a line drawn between these two points and twice its distance; iii. 0.5 cun superior to the upper line of origin of the temporalis muscle, 0.5 cun posterior to a vertical line drawn directly above Taiyang (M-HN-9).

NEEDLING

Transverse insertion 0.5 to 1 cun. **Note**: according to several classical texts, this point is contraindicated to moxibustion.

ACTIONS

Eliminates wind and alleviates pain
Benefits the eyes

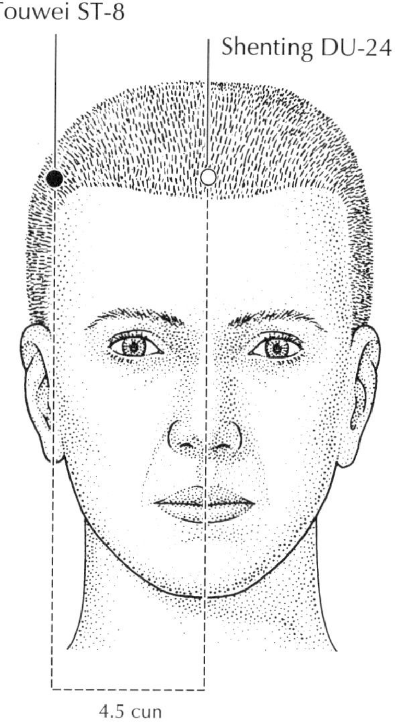

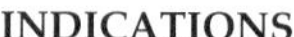
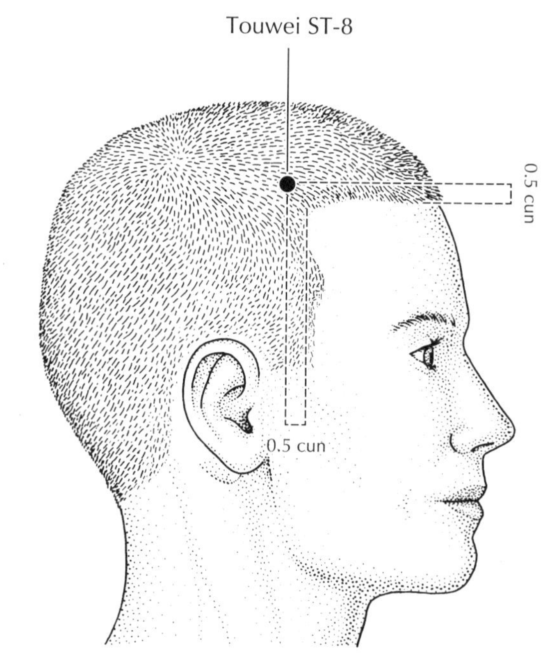

INDICATIONS

- Headache, splitting headache with chills and fever, dizziness, vomiting.
- Dimness of vision, bursting eye pain, lacrimation on exposure to wind, twitching of the eyelids.
- Dyspnoea with agitation and oppression, hemiplegia.

COMMENTARY

Touwei ST-8 is an important point to treat headaches. Located at the corner of the forehead, it is a meeting point of the Stomach channel with the Gall Bladder channel and the Yang Linking vessel. This meeting of three channels which have such influence on the head is reflected in the name of this point 'Head's Binding'. The Stomach channel belongs to yangming which rules the forehead, the Gall Bladder channel belongs to shaoyang which rules the temporal region, whilst the Yang Linking vessel links all the yang channels of the body including the Governing vessel and the Bladder channel which rule the vertex. Whilst the forte of Touwei ST-8 is the treatment of frontal headaches, with different needle direction it may also be used for temporal and vertex headaches.

Touwei ST-8 is particularly indicated in headaches and eye disorders due to wind, whether exterior pathogenic wind invading the channels of the head, or internally generated wind. As far as exterior headaches are concerned, although it is suitable for both wind-cold and wind-heat, many classics stress its use in the treatment of splitting headaches with bursting eye pain, symptoms more usually associated with wind-heat. Heat is a yang pathogen and its nature is to flare upwards and expand, obstructing the collaterals and leading to a distending and splitting sensation of the head. In the treatment of headache accompanied by pain or twitching of the eyes, Touwei ST-8 is frequently combined in classical prescriptions with Zanzhu BL-2. Touwei ST-8 is also indicated for severe headache accompanied by vomiting, and is especially suitable for migraine headache with nausea or vomiting and dimness of vision or bursting pain of the eyes. The ability of Touwei ST-8 to clear internally generated wind from the head is reflected not only in its use for this kind of headache, but also for dizziness and hemiplegia.

COMBINATIONS

- Headache with eye pain: Touwei ST-8 and Zanzhu BL-2 (*Ode of the Jade Dragon*).
- Head wind with splitting pain, bursting pain of the eyes and lacrimation: Touwei ST-8 and Zanzhu BL-2 (*Golden Mirror*).
- Pain between the eyebrows: Touwei ST-8 and Zanzhu BL-2 (*Song of the Jade Dragon*)
- Twitching of the eyelids: Touwei ST-8 and Zanzhu BL-2 (*Great Compendium*).
- Splitting headache with bursting eye pain: Touwei ST-8 and Daling P-7 (*Thousand Ducat Formulas*).
- One-sided or generalised head wind: Touwei ST-8, Baihui DU-20, Qianding DU-21, Shangxing DU-23, Shenting DU-24, Sizhukong SJ-23, Fengchi GB-20, Hegu L.I.-4 and Zanzhu BL-2 (*Great Compendium*).
- Lacrimation on exposure to wind: Touwei ST-8, Jingming BL-1, Fengchi GB-20 and Toulinqi GB-15 (*Great Compendium*).

RENYING ST-9

Man's Welcome

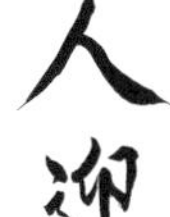

Meeting point of the Stomach and Gall Bladder channels
Point of the Window of Heaven
Point of the Sea of Qi

LOCATION

Level with the tip of and 1.5 cun lateral to the laryngeal prominence, in the depression between the anterior border of the sternocleidomastoid muscle and the lateral border of the thyroid cartilage. **Note:** the carotid artery lies just deep to, and can be readily palpated at, the anterior border of the sternocleidomastoid muscle. This point therefore lies between the carotid artery and the lateral border of the thyroid cartilage.

LOCATION NOTE

i. Ask the patient to lie flat and remove any pillow. Palpate the laryngeal prominence, and then, laterally, the lateral border of the thyroid cartilage. A little more laterally than this, the carotid artery may be felt. Use the index finger of one hand to define and enlarge the space between the lateral border of the thyroid cartilage and the artery and needle into this space with the other hand; ii. In females the laryngeal prominence is not as pronounced as in males. If it is indistinct, palpate the depression formed by the lower border of the hyoid bone and the upper border of the thyroid cartilage at the midline. The laryngeal prominence lies just below this.

NEEDLING

Perpendicular insertion 0.5 to 1 cun. **Note:** according to most classical texts, this point is contraindicated to moxibustion. **Caution:** care should be taken to avoid puncturing the carotid artery which must be palpated and then held laterally during needling, by using the index finger and thumb of one hand, above and below the point. This needling method should not be attempted by those who have not had appropriate clinical supervision.

ACTIONS

Regulates qi and blood and lowers rebellion
Benefits the throat and neck
Alleviates pain

INDICATIONS

- Headache, dizziness, visual dizziness, red face, fullness of the chest, shortness of breath, asthma, sudden turmoil disorder, vomiting, pulseless syndrome, hypertension, hypotension.
- Swelling and pain of the throat, scrofula, goitre, difficulty in swallowing.
- Lumbar pain.

COMMENTARY

Renying ST-9 is also known by its alternative name Tianwuhui (Heaven's Five Meetings). It is one of five points known as 'window of heaven' (literally 'five regions of the window of heaven') points in the *Spiritual Pivot*[5] which states "headache due to rebellion of yang,

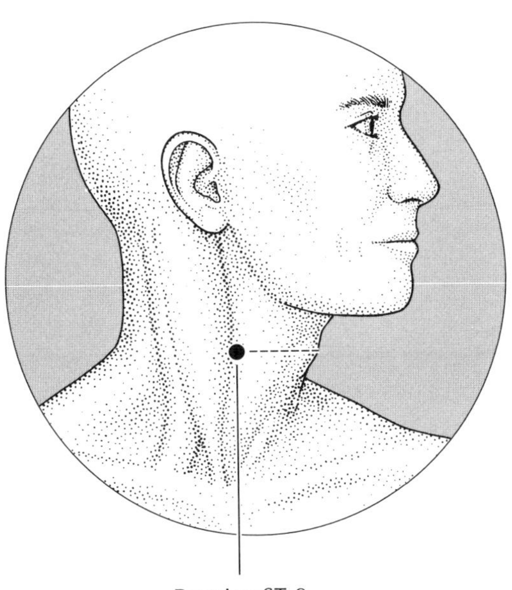

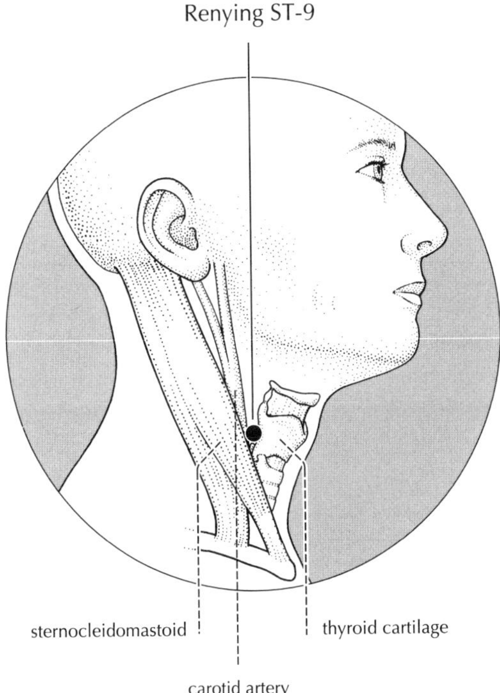

fullness of the chest with difficulty in breathing, choose Renying ST-9". Located in the pivotal neck region, Renying ST-9 dramatically illustrates the characteristic ability of this group of points to re-establish harmony in the flow of qi between the body and the head. The rebellion of qi, which arises when the qi in the lower regions is disordered and chaotic, may manifest in various ways. In the head it gives rise to headache, dizziness and redness of the face; in the neck region it stagnates giving rise to scrofula and goitre; in the middle and upper jiao it injures the normal descent of Stomach and Lung qi and gives rise to vomiting, sudden turmoil disorder, wheezing, asthma and fullness of the chest.

According to Zhou Zhi-cong's commentary on the above passage from the *Spiritual Pivot*, the condition known as inversion qi (disordered, chaotic and rebellious qi) underlies the clinical manifestations of all the points of the window of heaven. One of the manifestations of inversion qi is sudden acute pain, and this echoes the important modern use of Renying ST-9 for acute lumbar sprain, as well as sprain and severe pain in any region of the body. The ability of Renying ST-9 to reorder rebellion and upsurge of qi also explains its strong action in reducing hypertension.

According to the chapter 'Discourse On the Seas' of the *Spiritual Pivot*[6] Renying ST-9 (along with Shanzhong REN-17, Yamen DU-15 and Dazhui DU-14) is a point of the 'sea of qi'. This passage gives the following indications for insufficiency and excess of the sea of qi "When the sea of qi is in excess there is fullness in the chest, urgent breathing and a red complexion. When the sea of qi is insufficient, there is scanty energy insufficient for speech". The dual and overlapping properties of Renying ST-9 as a point of the sea of qi and a point of the window of heaven underline its importance in harmonising and redistributing disordered qi in the body.

As long ago as the *Yellow Emperor's Inner Classic*, observation and palpation of the pulse at Renying ST-9 was considered an important diagnostic method. The *Essential Questions*[7] in discussing obstructed urination describes a pattern of "heat in the body like charcoal, the neck and chest are obstructed as if separated, a restless and abundant pulse at Renying ST-9 and dyspnoea with counterflow qi". Elsewhere in the *Essential Questions* great diagnostic significance is ascribed to the relative strengths of the pulses at the wrist and at Renying ST-9, whilst Zhang Zhong-jing refers to three methods of pulse diagnosis (Renying ST-9 in the upper, the wrist pulse in the middle and Chongyang ST-42 in the lower). Because of the complications inherent in these methods, they were abandoned relatively early in the history of Chinese medicine in favour of focusing on the wrist pulse.

COMBINATIONS

- Sudden turmoil disorder, headache, chest pain and dyspnoeic rales: Renying ST-9, Neiguan P-6, Guanchong SJ-1, Sanyinjiao SP-6 and Zusanli ST-36 (*Compilation*).
- Scrofula: moxa Renying ST-9 and Shouwuli L.I.-13 thirty times (*Thousand Ducat Formulas*).
- Tinnitus with lumbar pain: first needle Renying ST-9, then needle Ermen SJ-21 and Zusanli ST-36 (*Secrets of the Celestial Star*).
- Hypertension: Renying ST-9, Quchi L.I.-11 and Zusanli ST-36.
- Hypertension: Renying ST-9, Baihui DU-20, Quchi L.I.-11 and Taichong LIV-3.
- Acute lumbar sprain or any acute pain: Renying ST-9 bilaterally or on the affected side.

SHUITU ST-10

Water Prominence

水突

LOCATION

On the neck, at the anterior border of the sternocleidomastoid muscle, midway between Renying ST-9 and Qishe ST-11.

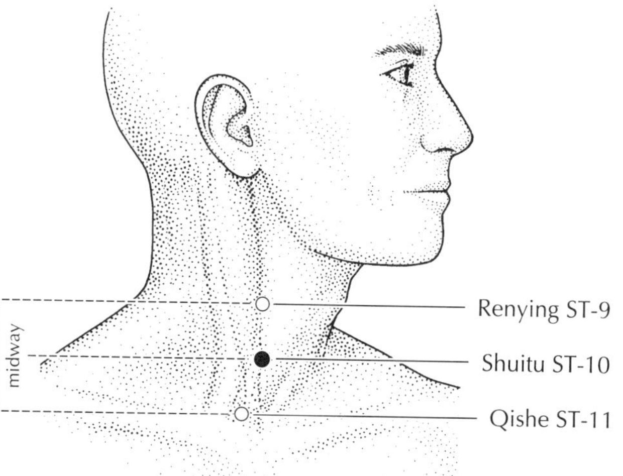

LOCATION NOTE

To identify the anterior border of the muscle, ask the patient to turn their head away from the side to be needled, whilst you apply resistance at the chin.

NEEDLING

Perpendicular-oblique insertion directed medially to avoid the carotid artery, 0.5 to 1 cun.
Caution: see Renying ST-9.

ACTIONS
Benefits the throat and neck
Descends Lung qi

INDICATIONS
- Swelling and pain of the throat, goitre, scrofula.
- Cough, whooping cough, shortness of breath, dyspnoea, swelling and pain of the shoulder.

COMBINATIONS
- Swelling of the throat: Shuitu ST-10 and Qishe ST-11 (*Supplementing Life*).

QISHE ST-11
Abode of Qi

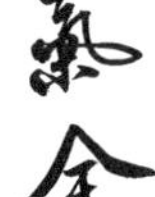

LOCATION
At the root of the neck, superior to the medial end of the clavicle, directly below Renying ST-9 in the depression between the sternal and clavicular heads of the sternocleidomastoid muscle.

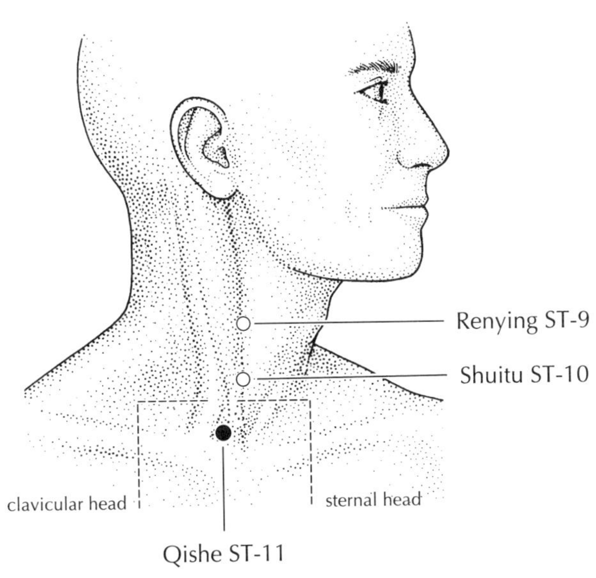

LOCATION NOTE
Palpation of the sternal and clavicular heads is made easier if the patient turns their head away from the side to be needled, whilst you apply resistance at the chin.

NEEDLING
Perpendicular insertion 0.3 to 0.5 cun.
Caution: deep insertion may puncture the lung.

ACTIONS
Benefits the throat and neck and descends qi

INDICATIONS
- Swelling and pain of the throat, scrofula, goitre, stiffness of the neck with inability to turn the head.
- Dyspnoea, difficult ingestion, hiccup.

COMBINATIONS
- Goitre, tumours of the neck and swollen throat: Qishe ST-11, Tianfu LU-3 and Naohui SJ-13 (*Supplementing Life*).
- Rebellious qi coughing: Qishe ST-11 and Pohu BL-42 (*Systematic Classic*).
- Cough with rebellious qi, dyspnoea, vomiting of foam and clenched teeth: Qishe ST-11, Pohu BL-42, Futu L.I.-18, Tianrong SI-17, Lianquan REN-23 and Yixi BL-45 (*Thousand Ducat Formulas*).

QUEPEN ST-12
Empty Basin

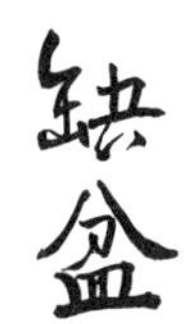

Meeting point of the Stomach, Large Intestine, Small Intestine, Sanjiao and Gall Bladder channels

LOCATION
In the supraclavicular area, posterior to the superior border of the clavicle and at its midpoint, 4 cun lateral to the midline, on the mamillary line.

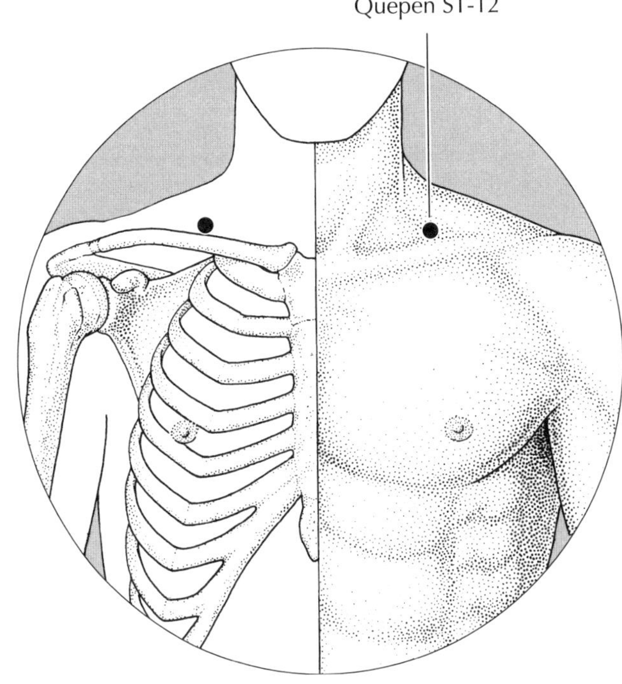

LOCATION NOTE
This point should be located and needled behind the clavicle, paying strict attention to the caution below.

NEEDLING
Perpendicular insertion 0.3 to 0.5 cun along the posterior border of the clavicle. **Note**: according to the *Systematic Classic of Acupuncture and Moxibustion* and the *Illustrated Supplement to the Classic of Categories* this point is contraindicated in pregnancy.
Caution: deep or posterior insertion may injure the subclavian vessels or puncture the lung.

ACTIONS
Descends Lung qi and clears heat from the chest
Activates the channel and alleviates pain

INDICATIONS
- Cough, coughing blood, dyspnoea, fullness of the chest, heat and fullness in the chest, chills and fever with sweating, absence of sweating, oedema, scrofula, throat painful obstruction.
- Pain of the supraclavicular fossa, pain of the shoulder that radiates to the neck, numbness and painful obstruction of the upper limb, inability to raise the arm, lumbar pain with inability to turn.

COMMENTARY
Quepen ST-12, is a meeting point of the Stomach channel with all the primary yang channels except the Bladder, and its principal function is to descend rebellion of qi. This is reflected both by its ability to treat rebellion of Lung qi manifesting as cough, dyspnoea and fullness of the chest, as well as by the traditional observation that it is contraindicated in pregnancy. The *Essential Questions*[8] includes Quepen ST-12 among the eight points (bilateral Quepen ST-12, Dazhu BL-11, Zhongfu LU-1 and Fengmen BL-12) to clear heat from the chest.

Quepen ST-12 is also indicated for pain of the supraclavicular fossa, pain of the shoulder that radiates to the neck, and numbness and pain of the upper limb.

COMBINATIONS
- Cough: Quepen ST-12, Shanzhong REN-17 and Juque REN-14 (*Thousand Ducat Formulas*).
- Coughing and spitting blood: Quepen ST-12, Xinshu BL-15, Ganshu BL-18, Juque REN-14 and Jiuwei REN-15 (*Supplementing Life*).
- Heat in the chest: Quepen ST-12 and Qimen LIV-14 (*Thousand Ducat Formulas*).
- Pain of the shoulder and back: Quepen ST-12, Tianyou SJ-16, Shendao DU-11, Dazhu BL-11, Tiantu REN-22, Shuidao ST-28 and Jugu L.I.-16 (*Thousand Ducat Formulas*).

QIHU ST-13
Qi Door

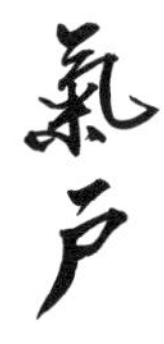

LOCATION
At the top of the chest, directly below Quepen ST-12, on the inferior border of the clavicle, 4 cun lateral to the midline, on the mamillary line.

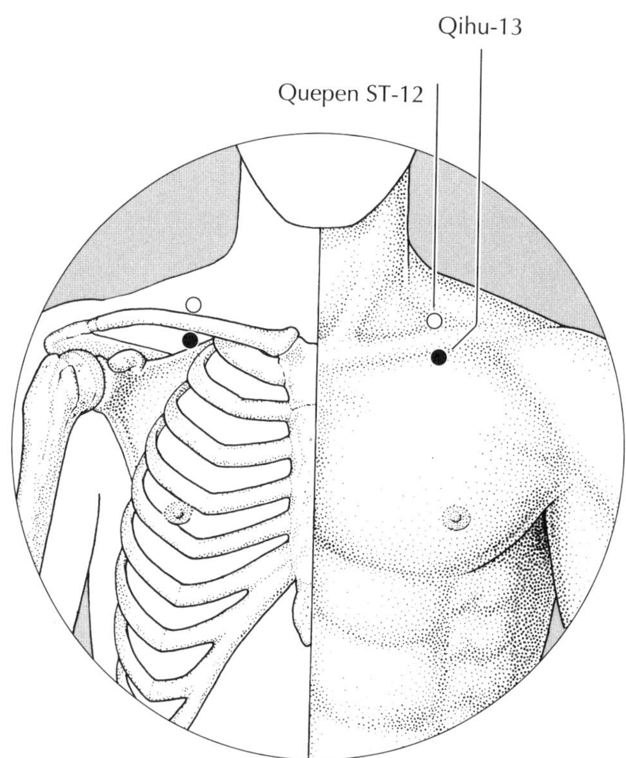

NEEDLING
Transverse-oblique insertion laterally or medially, 0.5 to 0.8 cun, or transverse insertion inferiorly along the channel. **Caution:** deep or perpendicular insertion carries a substantial risk of puncturing the lung or injuring the subclavian vessels.

ACTIONS
Descends rebellious qi and unbinds the chest

INDICATIONS
- Fullness and distention of the chest and lateral costal region, pain of the chest and upper back, cough, dyspnoea, asthma, wheezing, vomiting blood, hiccup, inability to taste food, stiffness of the neck with inability to turn the head.

COMBINATIONS
- Chronic pain of the lateral costal region: Qihu ST-13 and Huagai REN-20 (*One Hundred Symptoms*).

- Dyspnoea with rebellious qi, breathing with raised shoulders, inability to taste food: Qihu ST-13, Yunmen LU-2, Tianfu LU-3 and Shenmen HE-7 (*Thousand Ducat Formulas*).

KUFANG ST-14

庫房

Storehouse

LOCATION

On the chest, in the first intercostal space, 4 cun lateral to the midline (Huagai REN-20), on the mamillary line.

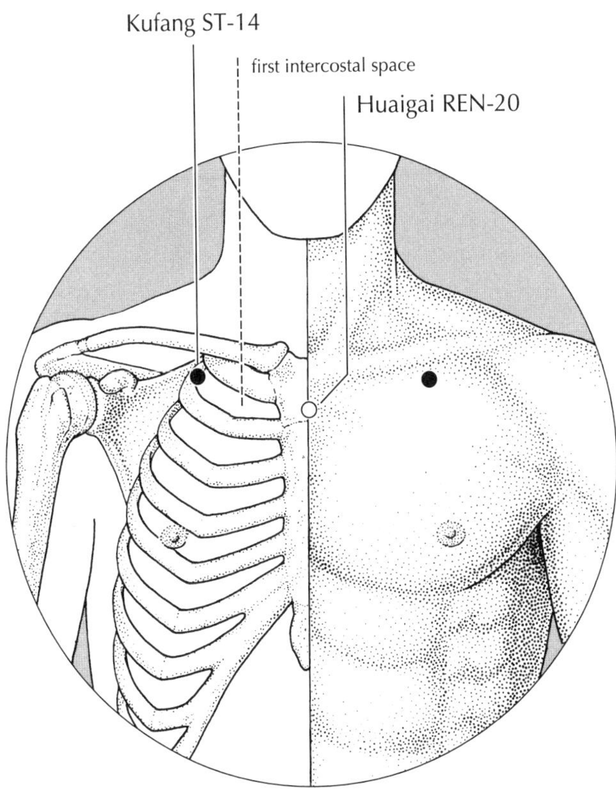

LOCATION NOTE

i. First locate the costal cartilage of the second rib which is level with the sternal angle, then locate the first intercostal space above it; ii. Note that in males the nipple lies in the fourth intercostal space; iii. Note that the intercostal space curves upwards laterally, so that Kufang ST-14 will lie superior to the level of Huagai REN-20.

NEEDLING

Transverse-oblique insertion laterally or medially along the intercostal space 0.5 to 0.8 cun, or transverse insertion superiorly or inferiorly along the channel.

Caution: deep or perpendicular insertion carries a substantial risk of puncturing the lung.

ACTIONS

Descends rebellious qi and unbinds the chest

INDICATIONS

- Distention and fullness of the chest and lateral costal region, cough, coughing of pus and blood, dyspnoea.

COMBINATIONS

- Cough: Kufang ST-14, Wuyi ST-15 and Gaohuangshu BL-43 (*Supplementing Life*).

WUYI ST-15

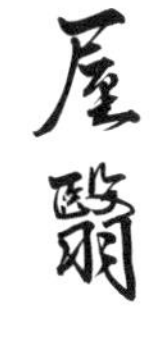

Room Screen

LOCATION

On the chest, in the second intercostal space, 4 cun lateral to the midline (Zigong REN-19), on the mamillary line.

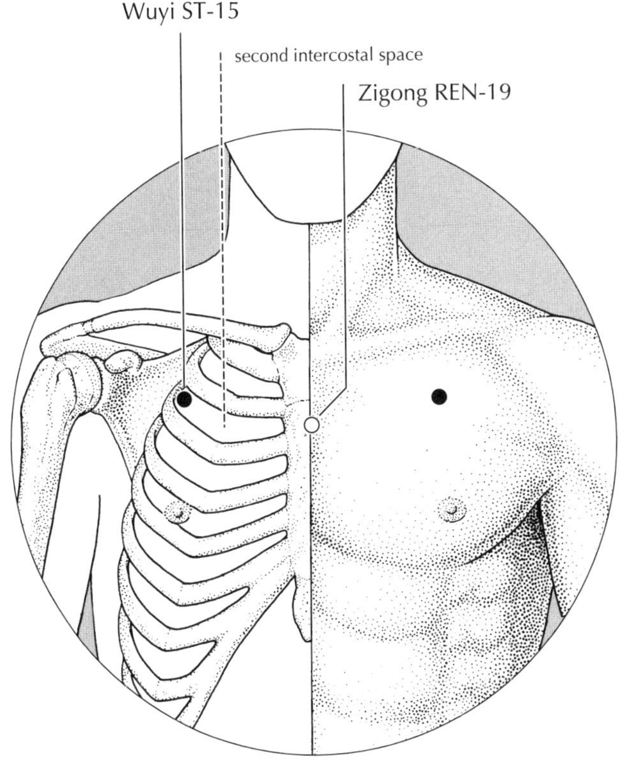

LOCATION NOTE

i. First locate the costal cartilage of the second rib which is level with the sternal angle, then locate the second intercostal space below it; ii. Note that in males the nipple lies in the fourth intercostal space; iii Note that the intercostal space curves upwards laterally, so that Wuyi ST-15 will lie superior to the level of Zigong REN-19.

NEEDLING
Transverse-oblique insertion laterally or medially along the intercostal space 0.5 to 0.8 cun, or transverse insertion superiorly or inferiorly along the channel.
Caution: deep or perpendicular insertion carries a substantial risk of puncturing the lung.

ACTIONS
Descends rebellious qi and unbinds the chest
Benefits the breasts
Alleviates pain and itching of the skin

INDICATIONS
- Cough, wheezing, dyspnoea, shortness of breath, coughing of pus and blood, distention and pain of the chest and lateral costal region.
- Breast pain, breast abscess.
- Pain of the skin making wearing of clothes unbearable, generalised itching, heaviness of the body, swollen body, pain and weakness of the limbs.

COMBINATIONS
- Itching with much pain: Wuyi ST-15 and Zhiyin BL-67 (*One Hundred Symptoms*).

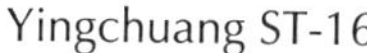

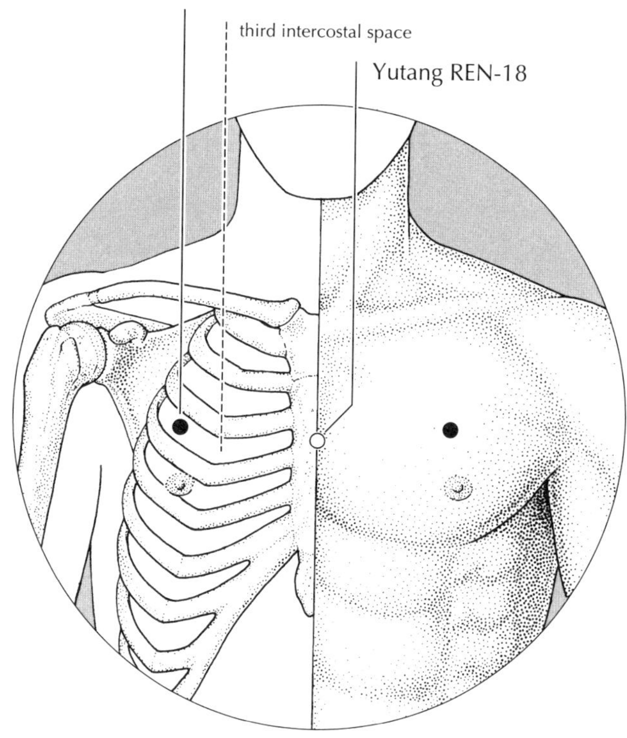

YINGCHUANG ST-16
Breast Window

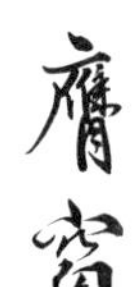

LOCATION
On the chest, in the third intercostal space, 4 cun lateral to the midline (Yutang REN-18), on the mamillary line.

LOCATION NOTE
i. First locate the second intercostal space (see Wuyi ST-15 above), then find the third intercostal space below it; ii. Note that in males the nipple lies in the fourth intercostal space.

NEEDLING
Transverse-oblique insertion laterally or medially along the intercostal space 0.5 to 0.8 cun, or transverse insertion superiorly or inferiorly along the channel.
Caution: deep or perpendicular insertion carries a substantial risk of puncturing the lung.

ACTIONS
Alleviates cough and wheezing
Benefits the breasts

INDICATIONS
- Cough, fullness of the chest with shortness of breath, restless sleep, fever and chills, swelling of the lips, borborygmus and watery diarrhoea.
- Breast abscess.

COMBINATIONS
- Swelling of the lips: Yingchuang ST-16 and Taichong LIV-3 (*Supplementing Life*).
- Breast abscess, chills and fever with shortness of breath, restless sleep: Yingchuang ST-16 and Shenfeng KID-23 (*Supplementing Life*).

RUZHONG ST-17
Middle of the Breast

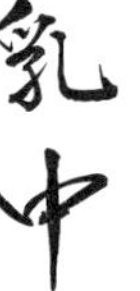

LOCATION
At the centre of the nipple, in the fourth intercostal space, 4 cun lateral to the midline.

NEEDLING
This point is contraindicated to both needling and moxibustion, and is used simply as a reference point.

RUGEN ST-18

Root of the Breast

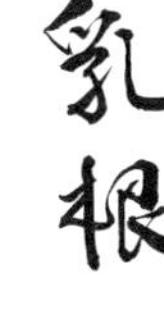

LOCATION

Directly below the nipple, in the fifth intercostal space.

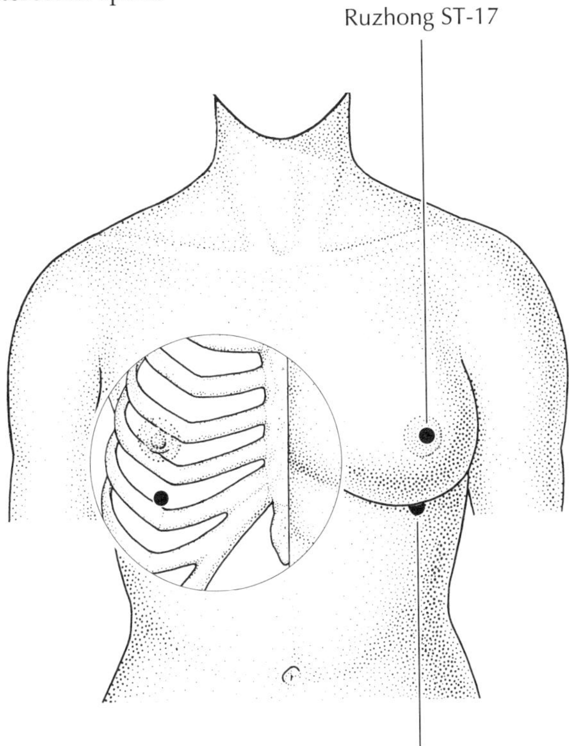

LOCATION NOTE

i. First locate the second intercostal space (see Wuyi ST-15 above), then find the fifth intercostal space, three spaces below it; ii. In males the nipple lies in the fourth intercostal space; iii. On a woman, this point lies at the root of the breast, inferior to the breast tissue itself; in females the nipple is unlikely to lie 4 cun lateral to the midline and should not be used as a reference point.

NEEDLING

Transverse-oblique insertion laterally or medially along the intercostal space 0.5 to 1 cun, or transverse insertion superiorly or inferiorly along the channel.

Caution: deep or perpendicular insertion carries a substantial risk of puncturing the lung.

ACTIONS

Benefits the breasts and reduces swelling

Unbinds the chest and alleviates cough and wheezing

INDICATIONS

- Breast abscess, breast pain, scanty lactation, difficult labour.
- Cough, dyspnoea, oppression and pain below the chest, oppression of the diaphragm, oesophageal constriction with difficult ingestion, sudden turmoil disorder with cramps, inversion counterflow of the four limbs, swelling and pain of the arm.

COMMENTARY

Rugen ST-18 is the principle local point for treating disorders of the breast. According to Zhu Dan-xi of the Jin-Yuan dynasty "The breasts are where the yangming passes, and the nipples are ascribed to the jueyin"[9]. Disharmony of the Stomach yangming or Liver jueyin channels is therefore involved in all breast disorders. Since Rugen ST-18 regulates the qi and blood of the breast area as a whole, it may be used for any excess type breast disorder characterised by pain, distention, swelling or abscess, whether due to Stomach fire or oppression and stagnation of Liver qi (the two main excess interior pathological factors in breast disease).

Nursing mothers are particularly prone to breast disorders. Zhu Dan-xi went on to say "If the breast-feeding mother has thick flavoured [food] or bears indignation or grudges, qi will therefore stop circulating and the portals will become blocked. [Because] milk is no longer able to come out, the blood of the yangming becomes hot and transforms into pus"[10]. As well as breast abscess due to these internal factors, Rugen ST-18 is also indicated when exposure of the breast to exterior pathogenic factors, improper suckling, or even, according to Zhu Dan-xi, the burning hot breath of the new-born baby blowing onto the breast, lead to heat, stagnation and swelling. As far as scanty lactation is concerned, this is most commonly due to stagnation of Liver qi resulting in failure of free flow, or to insufficiency of qi and blood, mainly due to deficiency of the Stomach and Spleen. Rugen ST-18 is indicated whatever the pattern.

According to the *Great Compendium of Acupuncture and Moxibustion* Rugen ST-18 is recommended for "pain of the chest, diaphragm qi". This refers to oppression of the chest with shortness of breath due to stagnation of Liver qi. Rugen ST-18 may also be used more widely for cough or asthma.

Finally, according to the *Ode of Xi-hong*, Rugen ST-18 may be used to promote and hasten labour, although it is not traditionally contraindicated in pregnancy.

COMBINATIONS

- Coughing and wheezing with phlegm: Rugen ST-18 and Shufu KID-27 (*Ode of the Jade Dragon*).
- Breast abscess: Rugen ST-18, Yingchuang ST-16, Xiajuxu ST-39, Taichong LIV-3 and Fuliu KID-7 (*Compilation*).

BURONG ST-19
Not Contained

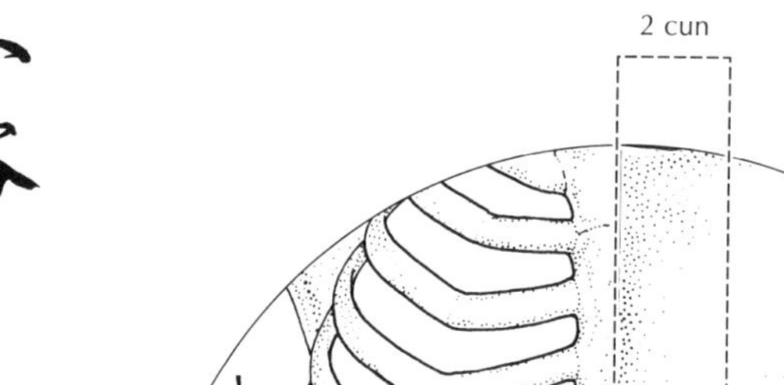

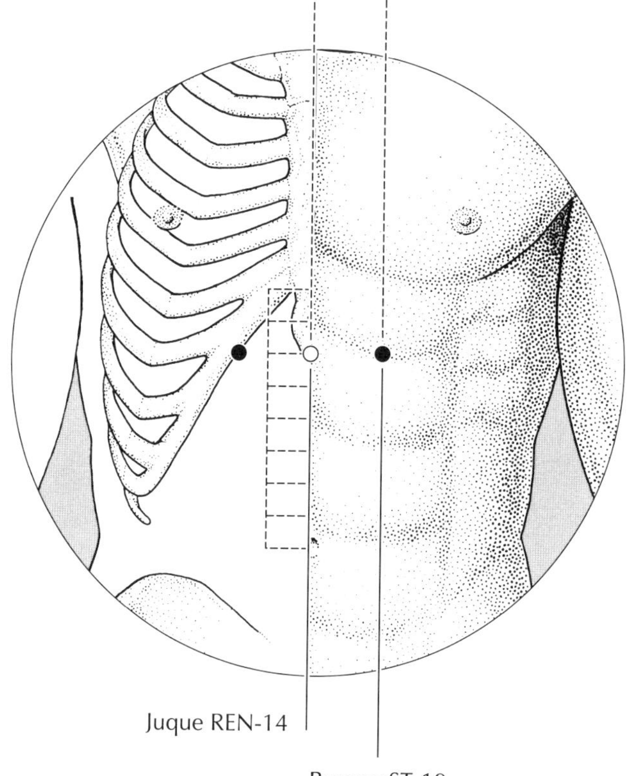

LOCATION
On the abdomen, 2 cun lateral to the midline and 6 cun superior to the umbilicus, level with Juque REN-14.

LOCATION NOTE
i. The 2 cun line is located halfway between the midline and the palpable lateral border of the rectus abdominis muscle; ii. In some patients with a narrow subcostal angle, this point may fall on the costal margin. The options then are to a. locate more medially, b. needle transversely on the costal margin, c. select a different point.

NEEDLING
Perpendicular insertion 0.5 to 0.8 cun.
Caution: deep insertion may injure the heart on the left or the liver on the right if either of these organs is enlarged.

ACTIONS
Harmonises the middle jiao and lowers rebellion
Descends qi and alleviates cough and wheezing

INDICATIONS
- Abdominal distention, epigastric pain, vomiting, vomiting blood, poor appetite, abdominal deficiency borborygmus.
- Cough, dyspnoea, difficult breathing with raised shoulders, pain of the chest, back, shoulder and intercostal region, pain of the Heart, dry mouth.

COMMENTARY
Because of its location, Burong ST-19 is sometimes selected for the treatment of hypochondriac pain, nausea and vomiting due to cholecystitis or cholelithiasis. Its name 'Not Contained' or 'Uncontainable' refers to the inability of the Stomach to retain its contents.

COMBINATIONS
- Vomiting: Burong ST-19, Shangwan REN-13 and Daling P-7 (*Supplementing Life*).
- Stabbing pain of the Heart: Burong ST-19 and Qimen LIV-14 (*Thousand Ducat Formulas*).
- Fullness of the chest and lateral costal region: Burong ST-19 and Zhangmen LIV-13 (*One Hundred Symptoms*).
- Acute pain of cholelithiasis: Burong ST-19 (right), Dannangxue (M-LE-23), Yanglingquan GB-34 (left), Qimen LIV-14 (right), Zhongwan REN-12, Hegu L.I.-4 and Taichong LIV-3.

CHENGMAN ST-20
Supporting Fullness

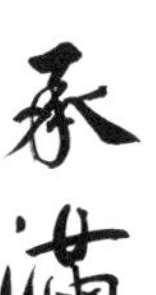

LOCATION
On the abdomen, 2 cun lateral to the midline and 5 cun superior to the umbilicus, level with Shangwan REN-13.

LOCATION NOTE
i. The 2 cun line is located halfway between the midline and the palpable lateral border of the rectus abdominis muscle; ii. In some patients with a narrow subcostal angle, this point may fall on the costal margin. The options then are to a. locate more medially, b. needle transversely on the costal margin, c. select a different point.

NEEDLING
Perpendicular insertion 0.5 to 1 cun.
Caution: i. in thin subjects, deep needling may penetrate the peritoneal cavity; ii. deep needling at right Chengman ST-20 may penetrate an enlarged liver.

ACTIONS
Harmonises the middle jiao
Descends rebellion of the Lung and Stomach

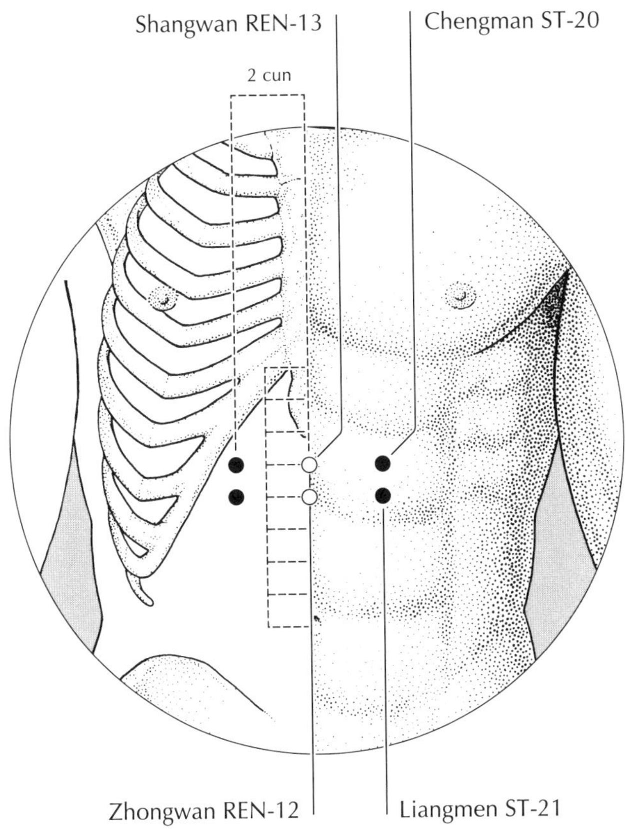

INDICATIONS

- Epigastric pain, vomiting, vomiting blood, spitting blood, hiccup, difficult ingestion, poor appetite, abdominal distention, borborygmus, diarrhoea, hardness and pain of the lateral costal region.
- Shortness of breath, wheezing, difficult breathing with raised shoulders.

COMBINATIONS

- Difficult ingestion: Chengman ST-20, Zhongfu LU-1, Kunlun BL-60, Yuji LU-10 and Zhourong SP-20 (*Supplementing Life*).
- Hardness and pain of the lateral costal region: Chengman ST-20 and Zhongwan REN-12 (*Thousand Ducat Formulas*).

LIANGMEN ST-21

Beam Gate

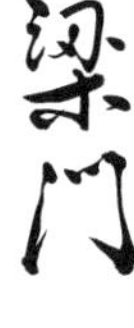

LOCATION

On the abdomen, 2 cun lateral to the midline and 4 cun superior to the umbilicus, level with Zhongwan REN-12.

LOCATION NOTE

i. The 2 cun line is located halfway between the midline and the palpable lateral border of the rectus abdominis muscle; ii. In some patients with a narrow subcostal angle, this point may fall on the costal margin. The options then are to a. locate more medially, b. needle transversely on the costal margin, c. select a different point.

NEEDLING

Perpendicular insertion 1 to 1.5 cun.

Caution: i. in thin subjects, deep needling may penetrate the peritoneal cavity; ii. deep needling at right Liangmen ST-21 may penetrate an enlarged liver.

ACTIONS

Regulates qi and alleviates pain
Harmonises the middle jiao and transforms stagnation
Raises the qi and stops diarrhoea

INDICATIONS

- Epigastric pain, qi accumulation in the lateral costal region, qi accumulation below the chest, abdominal distention.
- Vomiting, poor appetite, borborygmus, slippery diarrhoea, undigested food (in the stool).

COMMENTARY

Liangmen ST-21 is an important point for treating distention and pain due to stagnation of qi, especially in the lateral abdomen and the lateral costal region. It is used in preference to, or in combination with, Zhongwan REN-12 when there is severe epigastric and abdominal pain, particularly in these lateral regions.

More widely, Liangmen ST-21 is able to regulate the Stomach and Spleen and transform food accumulation, being indicated for vomiting, poor appetite, borborygmus, undigested food in the stool and diarrhoea, especially slippery diarrhoea. This term refers to diarrhoea which, because of its persistent and chronic nature, leads to downward collapse of qi. The collapse of qi in turn leads to a worsening of the diarrhoea which becomes ceaseless both at night and during the day, and is accompanied by symptoms such as shortness of breath, loss of appetite, emaciation etc.

The term 'liang' in the name of Liangmen ST-21 refers to one of the 'five accumulations' discussed in the *Classic of Difficulties*. This form of accumulation is said to pertain to the Heart and is characterised by a palpable mass in the region below the Heart (epigastrium), and the use of Liangmen ST-21 is emphasised in various classics for epigastric pain and qi accumulation below both the chest and lateral costal region.

GUANMEN ST-22

Pass Gate

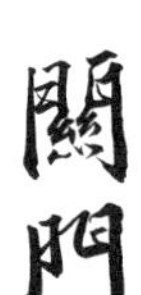

LOCATION

On the abdomen, 2 cun lateral to the midline and 3 cun superior to the umbilicus, level with Jianli REN-11.

LOCATION NOTE

The 2 cun line is located halfway between the midline and the palpable lateral border of the rectus abdominis muscle.

NEEDLING

Perpendicular insertion 1 to 1.5 cun.
Caution: in thin subjects, deep needling may penetrate the peritoneal cavity.

ACTIONS

Regulates qi and alleviates pain
Regulates the intestines and benefits urination

INDICATIONS

- Abdominal qi accumulation, sensation of qi moving in the abdomen, abdominal pain, abdominal distention and fullness, acute periumbilical pain.
- Constipation, borborygmus, diarrhoea, dysenteric disorder, poor appetite, oedema, enuresis, phlegm malaria with cold shivering.

COMMENTARY

Guanmen ST-22 is included in two elegant combinations for the treatment of enuresis. Both also include Shenmen HE-7, reflecting the principle that the involuntary discharge of urine, especially during sleep, indicates a disorder of the spirit as much as a disorder of the urinary system.

COMBINATIONS

- Enuresis: Guanmen ST-22, Shenmen HE-7 and Weizhong BL-40 (*Systematic Classic*).
- Enuresis: Guanmen ST-22, Zhongfu LU-1 and Shenmen HE-7 (*Thousand Ducat Formulas*).

TAIYI ST-23

Supreme Unity

太乙

LOCATION

On the abdomen, 2 cun lateral to the midline and 2 cun superior to the umbilicus, level with Xiawan REN-10.

LOCATION NOTE

The 2 cun line is located halfway between the midline and the palpable lateral border of the rectus abdominis muscle.

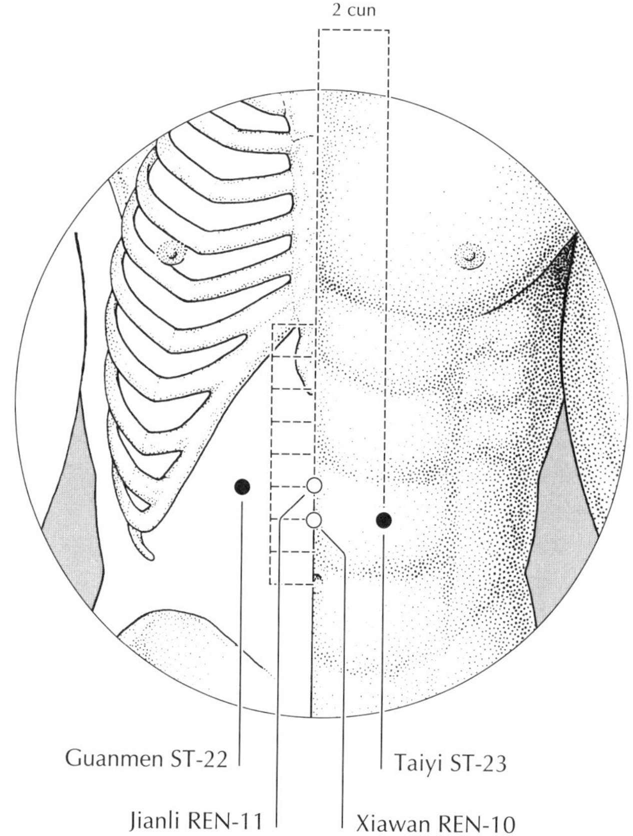

NEEDLING

Perpendicular insertion 1 to 1.5 cun.
Caution: in thin subjects, deep needling may penetrate the peritoneal cavity.

ACTIONS

Transforms phlegm and calms the spirit
Harmonises the middle jiao

INDICATIONS

- Mania-depression, agitation, tongue thrusting, mad walking.
- Epigastric pain, abdominal pain, poor appetite, diarrhoea, shan disorder.

COMMENTARY

The action of this point on calming the spirit and treating psycho-emotional disorders (recorded in various classics) is attributable to three factors: i. its ability, like several points of the Stomach channel (most notably Fenglong ST-40) to assist the Spleen in transforming phlegm, ii. the internal connection between the Stomach divergent channel and the Heart zang, and iii. the meeting of the Stomach channel with the Governing vessel (and thus the brain) at points Shenting DU-24 and Renzhong DU-26, both of which strongly influence the brain and spirit.

Although there are many causes for the formation of phlegm, disharmony of the Stomach and Spleen is the most common. Once formed, phlegm or phlegm-heat may rise to veil the portals of the Heart and disturb the spirit, leading to such symptoms as mania-depression, agitation, and mad walking. The Heart channel ascends to the root of the tongue. When phlegm blocks the Heart there may be tongue thrusting, where the tongue is repeatedly thrust out of the mouth like a snake's tongue. This symptom is most commonly seen in the pattern of phlegm-heat accumulated in the Spleen and Heart, although it is also differentiated into Spleen and Kidney deficiency heat and may be seen in epilepsy. It is frequently accompanied by a red distended tongue, ulceration of the tongue, and thirst with desire for cold fluids.

The name 'Taiyi' (Supreme Unity) refers to the state of undifferentiated oneness that according to Daoist theory existed before the arising of yin and yang duality and the separation of heaven and earth. One explanation of the naming of this point is that Taiyi ST-23 lies close to that region of the abdomen that brings about separation of the pure and impure contents of the digestion, but where this process has not yet taken place.

The dual action of Taiyi ST-23 on psycho-emotional and abdominal disorders (such as pain and diarrhoea) renders it especially suitable for conditions where both present together. This combination of symptoms is commonly encountered in patients who present with anxiety focused both on the chest and abdomen, accompanied by palpitations, tightness of the chest, abdominal pain and diarrhoea.

COMBINATIONS

- Mania-depression with tongue thrusting: Taiyi ST-23 and Huaroumen ST-24 (*Systematic Classic*).
- Madness and mania disorder with tongue thrusting: Taiyi ST-23, Feiyang BL-58 and Huaroumen ST-24 (*Thousand Ducat Formulas*).
- Tongue thrusting: Taiyi ST-23 and Zhubin KID-9 (*Supplementing Life*).

HUAROUMEN ST-24

Slippery Flesh Gate

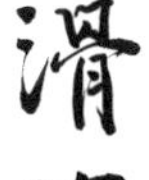
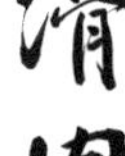
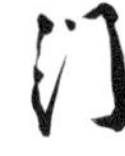

LOCATION

On the abdomen, 2 cun lateral to the midline and 1 cun superior to the umbilicus, level with Shuifen REN-9.

LOCATION NOTE

The 2 cun line is located halfway between the midline and the palpable lateral border of the rectus abdominis muscle.

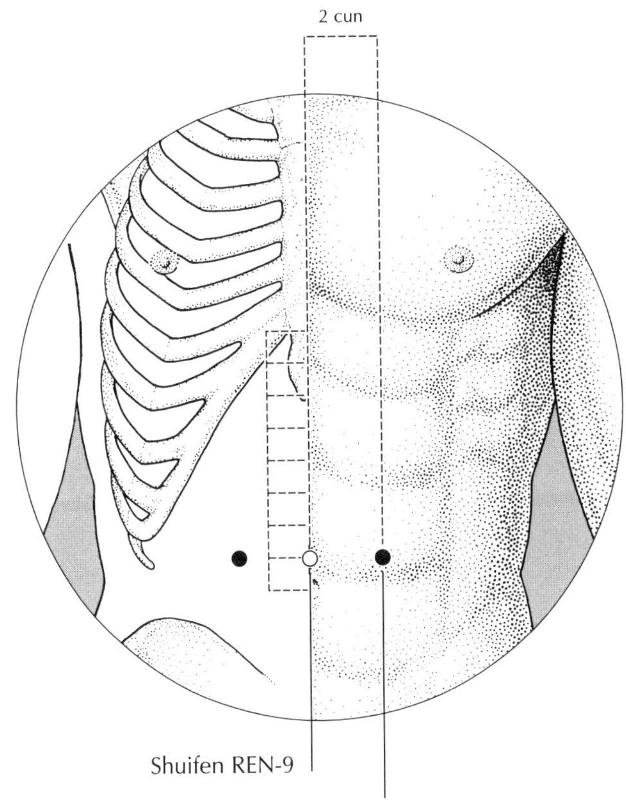

NEEDLING

Perpendicular insertion 1 to 1.5 cun.
Caution: in thin subjects, deep needling may penetrate the peritoneal cavity.

ACTIONS

Transforms phlegm and calms the spirit
Harmonises the Stomach and alleviates vomiting

INDICATIONS

- Mania-depression, tongue thrusting, stiff tongue, lotus flower tongue.
- Vomiting, vomiting of blood, epigastric pain.

COMMENTARY

See Taiyi ST-23 above.

COMBINATIONS

- Stiff tongue, tongue thrusting: Huaroumen ST-24, Shaohai HE-3 and Wenliu L.I.-7 (*Supplementing Life*).

TIANSHU ST-25

Heaven's Pivot

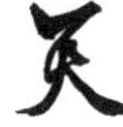

Front-Mu point of the Large Intestine

LOCATION

On the abdomen, 2 cun lateral to the umbilicus.

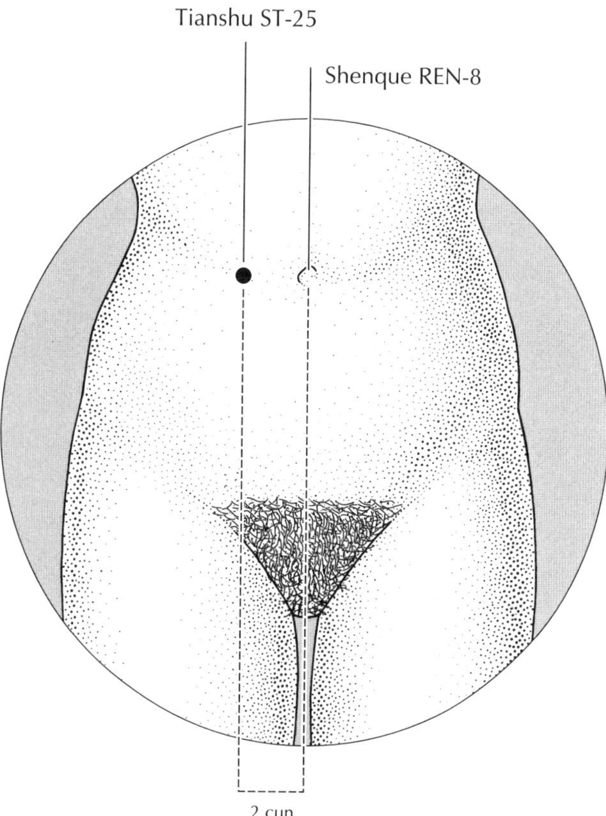

LOCATION NOTE

The 2 cun line on the abdomen is located halfway between the midline and the palpable lateral border of the rectus abdominis muscle.

NEEDLING

i. Perpendicular insertion 1 to 1.5 cun; ii. oblique inferior insertion towards the uterus for diseases of the uterus. **Caution:** in thin subjects, deep needling may penetrate the peritoneal cavity.

ACTIONS

Regulates the intestines
Regulates the Spleen and Stomach
Resolves dampness and damp-heat
Regulates qi and blood and eliminates stagnation

INDICATIONS

- Diarrhoea, Spleen-diarrhoea, persistent diarrhoea with undigested food (in the stool), dysenteric disorder, borborygmus, lower yuan (origin) deficient and cold, constipation.
- Oedema, drum distention, swelling of the face, turbid painful urinary dysfunction.
- Vomiting, retching, difficult ingestion, poor appetite, sudden turmoil disorder.
- Abdominal pain, abdominal distention with laboured breathing, intestinal abscess, generalised swelling with severe cutting periumbilical pain, umbilical shan disorder with localised pain that periodically surges up to the Heart, shan disorder, running piglet qi.
- Abdominal (zheng jia) masses in women, pain of the uterus, dysmenorrhoea, irregular menstruation, infertility, red and white leucorrhoea.
- Cold shivering from malaria, severe heat with manic raving.

COMMENTARY

The close relationship between the Stomach and intestines is emphasised in the *Spiritual Pivot*[11] which states "the Small and Large Intestines both pertain to the Stomach". Furthermore, the Stomach is interiorly-exteriorly coupled with the Spleen which dominates transportation and transformation and plays an important role in regulating the intestines. Tianshu ST-25 is the front-mu point of the Large Intestine, located on the Stomach channel, and is thus the point where the qi of the Large Intestine gathers and concentrates on the anterior surface of the body.

Tianshu ST-25, located on either side of the umbilicus, was said by the *Ode to Elucidate Mysteries* to dominate the middle region[12], and its name 'Heaven's Pivot' or 'Celestial Pivot' refers to its central position between the upper and lower abdomen, the Stomach and the intestines. The *Essential Questions* states "[The area] above the celestial pivot is ruled by celestial qi; [the area] below the celestial pivot is ruled by the earthly qi. The place where these qi intersect is the origin of man's qi and the ten thousand things"[13].

The two principal actions of Tianshu ST-25 are i. treating intestinal disorders, and ii. regulating qi and eliminating stasis in the lower abdomen. Tianshu ST-25 is the single most important point for the treatment of the widest variety of intestinal disorders. Due to its ability to regulate the Spleen and transform dampness, its forte is in the treatment of diarrhoea; indeed the *Ode of the Jade Dragon* states "The pattern of Spleen diarrhoea, look no further, needle bilateral Tianshu ST-25". Diarrhoea and dysenteric disorder may be acute and due to accumulation of cold-damp, damp-heat or fire-poison, or may be chronic and due to deficiency of the Spleen and Kidneys or disharmony of the Liver and Spleen. Whatever the aetiology, Tianshu ST-25 should form a pivotal role in the prescription, in combination with other suitable points selected according to differentiation. In modern practice Tianshu ST-25 is much used in the treatment of bacillary dysentery and acute simple appendicitis in combination with such points as Shangjuxu ST-37 and Quchi L.I.-11. Although an important local point in the treatment of constipation, many authorities consider the more lateral Daheng SP-15 to be more effective.

The damp draining action of Tianshu ST-25 is further evidenced by its indications for oedema, swelling of the face, drum distention and turbid painful urinary dysfunction.

Because of its central position between the upper and lower abdomen, the effect of Tianshu ST-25 extends upwards to the Stomach. It is indicated for vomiting, retching and sudden turmoil disorder in which vomiting is accompanied by diarrhoea. Various classics also emphasise the ability of Tianshu ST-25 to tonify deficiency, the *Investigation Into Points Along the Channels* recommending it for 'lower yuan (origin) deficient and cold' and the *Ode to Elucidate Mysteries* for 'deficiency damage'.

Tianshu ST-25 also has an important action on regulating qi and eliminating stagnation in the lower abdomen. It is indicated for a wide range of problems including distention and pain of the abdomen, intestinal abscess, shan disorder, severe cutting periumbilical pain etc., as well as the treatment of menstrual disorders and abdominal or uterine masses due to stasis of either qi or blood.

COMBINATIONS

- Ceaseless diarrhoea: Tianshu ST-25, Zhongwan REN-12 and Zhongji REN-3 (*Great Compendium*).
- Undigested food (in the stool), no pleasure in eating, periumbilical pain: Tianshu ST-25, Neiting ST-44 and Lidui ST-45 (*Supplementing Life*).
- Red (bloody) dysenteric disorder: Tianshu ST-25, Neiting ST-44, Yinbai SP-1, Qihai REN-6, Zhaohai KID-6 and Neiguan P-6 (*Great Compendium*).
- Vomiting and sudden turmoil disorder: Tianshu ST-25 and Zhigou SJ-6 (*Supplementing Life*).
- Irregular menstruation: Tianshu ST-25 and Shuiquan KID-5 (*One Hundred Symptoms*).
- Umbilical shan disorder: Tianshu ST-25, Shenque REN-8 and Shimen REN-5 (*Supplementing Life*).
- Hypogastric shan disorder: Tianshu ST-25, Shimen REN-5, Qihai REN-6 and Shenque REN-8 (*Thousand Ducat Formulas*).
- Facial swelling: Tianshu ST-25, Fenglong ST-40, Chongyang ST-42, Xiangu ST-43 and Lidui ST-45 (*Thousand Ducat Formulas*).

WAILING ST-26

Outer Mound

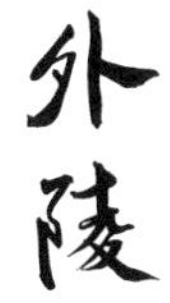

LOCATION

On the lower abdomen, 2 cun lateral to the midline and 1 cun inferior to the umbilicus, level with Yinjiao REN-7.

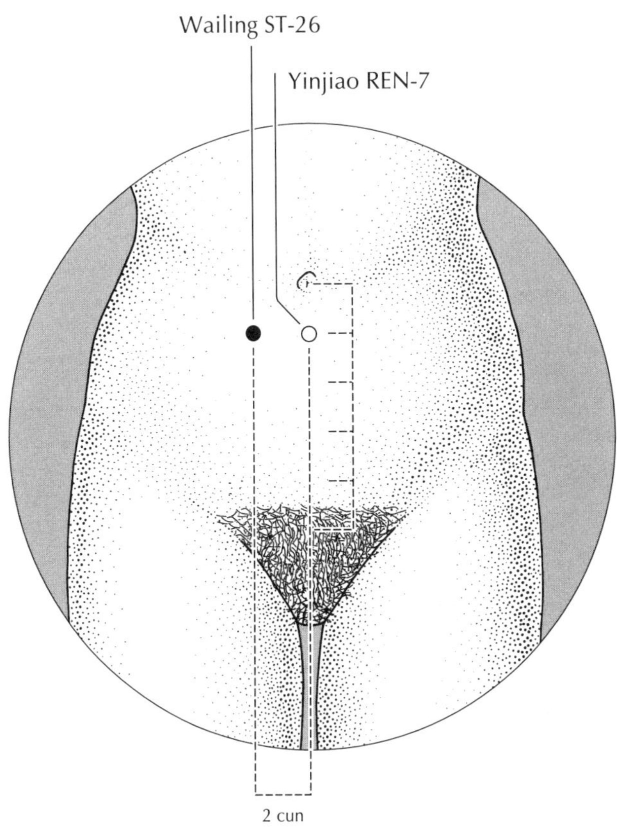

LOCATION NOTE

The 2 cun line is located halfway between the midline and the palpable lateral border of the rectus abdominis muscle.

NEEDLING

Perpendicular insertion 1 to 1.5 cun. **Caution:** in thin subjects, deep needling may penetrate the peritoneal cavity.

ACTIONS

Regulates qi and alleviates pain

INDICATIONS

- Severe abdominal pain, abdominal distention, shan disorder.
- Dysmenorrhoea, amenorrhoea.

COMBINATIONS

- Severe abdominal pain: Wailing ST-26 and Tianshu ST-25 (*Supplementing Life*).

DAJU ST-27

大巨

The Great

LOCATION

On the lower abdomen, 2 cun lateral to the midline and 2 cun inferior to the umbilicus, level with Shimen REN-5.

LOCATION NOTE

The 2 cun line is located halfway between the midline and the palpable lateral border of the rectus abdominis muscle.

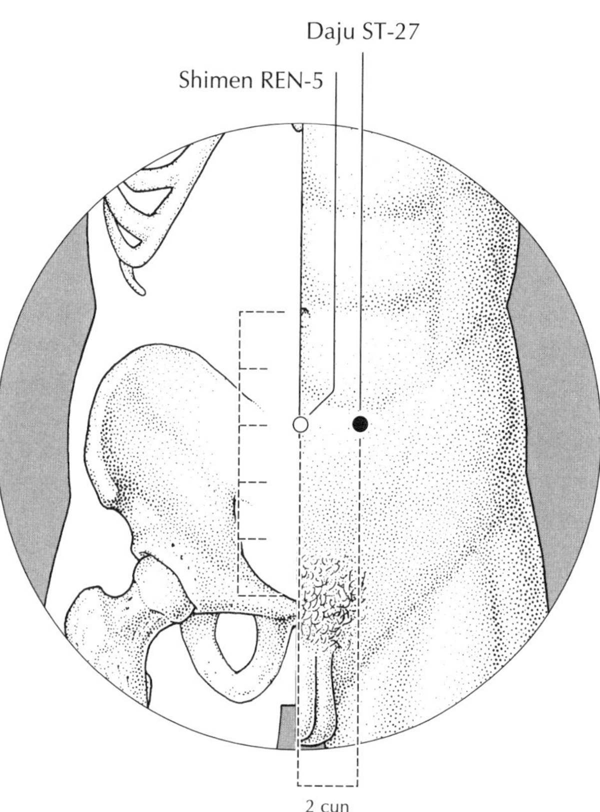

NEEDLING

Perpendicular insertion 1 to 1.5 cun.
Caution: in thin subjects, deep needling may penetrate the peritoneal cavity.

ACTIONS

Benefits the Kidneys and firms essence
Regulates qi and promotes urination

INDICATIONS

- Premature ejaculation, seminal emission, irregular menstruation, difficult urination, retention of urine.
- Fright palpitations and insomnia, propensity to fright, agitation with thirst, loss of use of the four limbs, hemiplegia.
- Lower abdominal distention and fullness, shan disorder.

COMBINATIONS

- Cold-damp shan disorder: Daju ST-27, Diji SP-8 and Zhongdu LIV-6 (*Systematic Classic*).
- Palpitations and insomnia: Daju ST-27, Qihai REN-6 and Sanyinjiao SP-6 (*Supplementing Life*).

SHUIDAO ST-28

水道

Water Passage

LOCATION

On the lower abdomen, 2 cun lateral to the midline and 3 cun inferior to the umbilicus, level with Guanyuan REN-4.

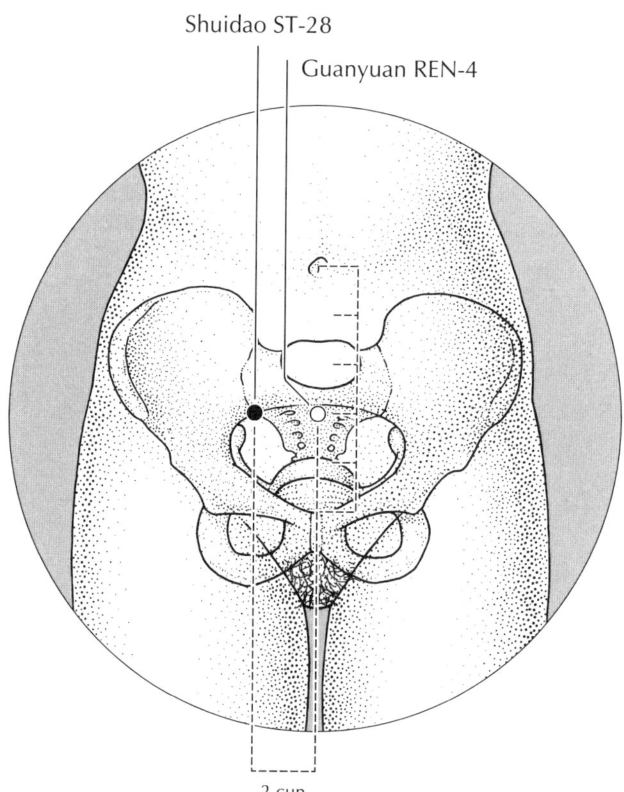

LOCATION NOTE

The 2 cun line is located halfway between the midline and the palpable lateral border of the rectus abdominis muscle.

NEEDLING

Perpendicular insertion 1 to 1.5 cun. **Caution:** deep insertion may penetrate the peritoneal cavity in thin patients or may penetrate a full bladder; the patient should therefore be asked to empty the bladder before needling.

ACTIONS

Regulates the lower jiao and dispels stagnation
Benefits the Bladder and the uterus

INDICATIONS

- Retention of urine and faeces, oedema, cold in the Bladder, distention and fullness of the lower abdomen, shan disorder.
- Hypogastric pain in women extending to the genitals, dysmenorrhoea, infertility, cold in the uterus that radiates down the thigh to the knee, uterine (jia) masses, retention of dead foetus, retention of the placenta, lumbar pain accompanying menstruation, heat binding the three jiao.
- Pain of the lumbar vertebrae, pain of the shoulder and back.

COMMENTARY

Although this point is most commonly known as *Shuidao* (Water Passage), the great 7th century physician Sun Simiao referred to left Shuidao as *Baomen* (Gate of the Uterus) and right Shuidao as *Zihu* (Child's Door)[14], emphasising its action on gynaecological disorders. These two ways of naming this point reflect its dual actions of clearing stasis from the Bladder and promoting urination on the one hand, and clearing stasis of qi and blood from the uterus on the other. As far as the former action is concerned, Shuidao ST-28 is indicated when excess pathogenic factors obstruct the qi transformation function of the Bladder leading to retention of urine. As for the latter action, Shuidao ST-28 is particularly indicated for cold congealing the uterus (see Guilai ST-29 for a fuller discussion) and giving rise to obstruction of blood, manifesting with a variety of symptoms of blood stasis such as dysmenorrhoea, infertility, menstrual pain radiating to the lumbar region or down the thighs, and retention of the placenta or retention of dead foetus. It is also specifically indicated for uterine (jia) masses, implying masses of indefinite form and changing location, primarily due to qi stagnation. The unifying factor between these two spheres of action is obstruction, emphasising that this point is almost exclusively used for excess patterns.

Shuidao ST-28 is also indicated for pain of the lumbar region and pain of the shoulder and back and appears in at least two classical combinations for this purpose. This is an example of the method of selecting points from the front of the body to treat the back, and also reflects the fact that the Stomach sinew channel passes through the lower ribs and connects with the spine.

COMBINATIONS

- Stiffness of the spine: Shuidao ST-28 and Jinsuo DU-8 (*One Hundred Symptoms*).
- Pain of the shoulder and back: Shuidao ST-28, Tianyou SJ-16, Quepen ST-12, Shendao DU-11, Dazhu BL-11, Tiantu REN-22 and Jugu L.I.-16 (*Thousand Ducat Formulas*).

GUILAI ST-29

Return

歸來

LOCATION

On the lower abdomen, 2 cun lateral to the midline and 4 cun inferior to the umbilicus, level with Zhongji REN-3.

LOCATION NOTE

The 2 cun line is located halfway between the midline and the palpable lateral border of the rectus abdominis muscle.

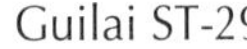

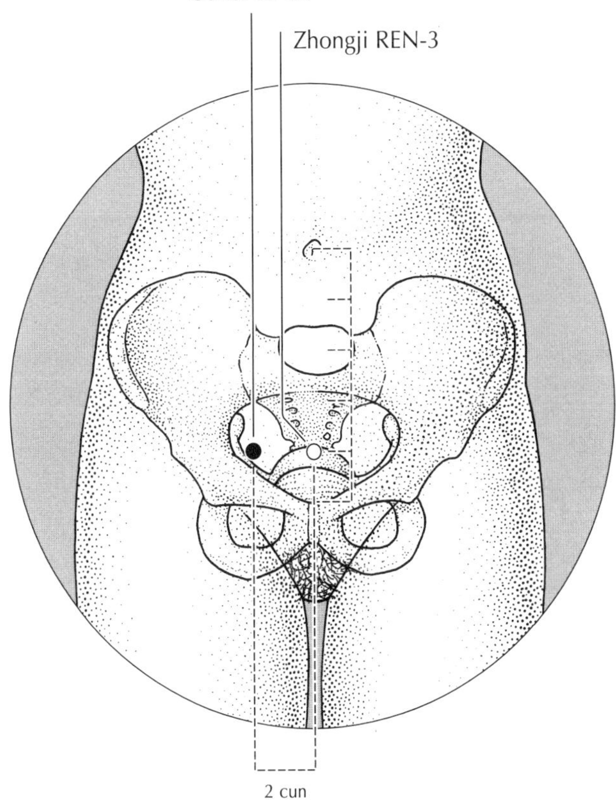

NEEDLING

Perpendicular insertion 1 to 1.5 cun. **Caution:** deep insertion may penetrate the peritoneal cavity in thin patients or may penetrate a full bladder; the patient should therefore be asked to empty the bladder before needling.

ACTIONS

Warms the lower jiao

Regulates menstruation and benefits the genital region

INDICATIONS

- Amenorrhoea, irregular menstruation, uterine (ji) masses, uterine prolapse, swelling, pain and cold of the vagina, infertility, leucorrhoea.

- Retraction of the testicles, pain of the penis, impotence, seminal emission, nocturnal urination, the seven kinds of shan disorder, running piglet qi, hypogastric pain.

COMMENTARY

The name of this point 'Guilai' (Return) is normally understood to refer to its ability to restore the condition of the uterus and genitals to normal.

According to the *Essential Questions*[15] "qi and blood desire warmth and dislike cold; when [there is] cold they coagulate; when [there is] warmth they disperse and flow". The *Spiritual Pivot*[16] states "The blood [vessels], nutritive and defensive [qi] of man circulate without stopping, in the same way that the stars do in the upper region and the rivers in the lower region. When a cold pathogen comes to reside in the channels as a guest, the blood will coagulate; when the blood coagulates the channels do not move".

The over-riding action of Guilai ST-29 is to warm the lower jiao, most particularly the uterus in women and the genital region in both men and women. Cold may be excess or deficient in nature. As far as excess cold is concerned, the uterus (along with the Stomach, Spleen and intestines) belongs to that group of the zangfu or extra fu that can suffer from direct penetration by exterior pathogenic cold (i.e. without initial symptoms and signs of an exterior pattern such as chills and fever, body aches etc.). Injury of the uterus by cold may be due to inadequate clothing or sitting on cold ground, or over-consumption of cold foods and drinks, especially during menstruation or after childbirth. Pathogenic cold causes stagnation of qi and coagulation of blood in the uterus and disrupts the function of the Conception and Penetrating vessels, giving rise to disorders such as amenorrhoea, irregular menstruation, uterine masses etc. Guilai ST-29 is one of the primary points to warm the uterus and drive out pathogenic cold.

As far as deficiency cold is concerned, Guilai ST-29 is also an important point for treating disorders due to decline of Kidney yang which generates cold, giving rise to irregular menstruation, amenorrhoea, infertility etc. The ability of Guilai ST-29 to treat such disorders derives from its action of warming and benefiting the uterus rather than by directly tonifying Kidney yang. Guilai ST-29 is also indicated for running piglet qi which may arise when Kidney yang deficiency leads to accumulation of cold in the lower jiao (see Qichong ST-30).

Amenorrhoea may be due to either excess or deficient patterns (stagnation of qi and stasis of blood, pathogenic cold, phlegm stagnation, blood deficiency, Kidney deficiency or heat pathogen which consumes yin blood). Due to its action of 'returning' the menstruation, Guilai ST-29 is commonly used in the treatment of amenorrhoea due to any of these patterns.

The genital region in both men and women is equally susceptible to attack by pathogenic cold, giving rise to a variety of symptoms characterised by pain and retraction of the testicles, penis or vagina. As well as being able to warm and scatter excess cold in this region, Guilai ST-29 can firm and warm the lower jiao and is used in the treatment of disorders such as impotence, seminal emission, leucorrhoea and nocturnal urination due to decline of ming men fire.

Although the clinical manifestations will be somewhat different in each of the above situations, most will be characterised by aversion to cold and preference for and amelioration with heat. Since Guilai ST-29 is mainly indicated for cold patterns it is particularly suited to treatment by combined needling and moxibustion.

COMBINATIONS

- Sagging and swollen testicle without pain: Guilai ST-29, Dadun LIV-1 and Sanyinjiao SP-6 (*Great Compendium*).
- Retracted testicle: Guilai ST-29 and Wushu GB-27 (*Supplementing Life*).

QICHONG ST-30

Rushing Qi

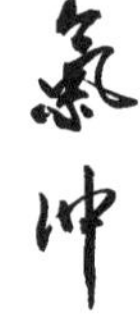

Meeting point of the Stomach channel with the Penetrating vessel
Point of the Sea of Water and Grain

LOCATION

On the lower abdomen, 2 cun lateral to the midline, level with the superior border of the pubic symphysis (Qugu REN-2).

LOCATION NOTE

The 2 cun line may be located halfway between the midline and the palpable lateral border of the rectus abdominis muscle.

NEEDLING

Perpendicular insertion 1 to 1.5 cun.
Caution: in thin patients, i. deep insertion in a superior direction may penetrate the peritoneal cavity or a full bladder (the patient should therefore be asked to empty the bladder before needling); ii. deep insertion in an inferior direction in the male may penetrate the spermatic cord.

ACTIONS

Regulates qi in the lower jiao
Regulates the Penetrating vessel
Subdues running piglet qi

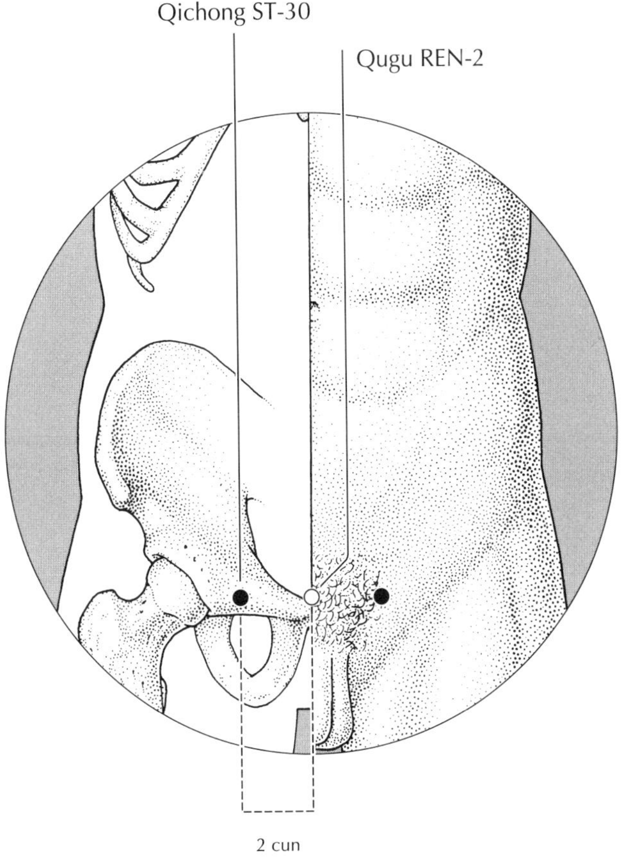

INDICATIONS

- Hypogastric pain, sudden fullness and distention of the abdomen, fullness of the abdomen with inability to lie down, twisting pain of the abdomen, heat in the abdomen, heat in the body with abdominal pain, hardness below the umbilicus, retention of urine and faeces, heat in the Large Intestine, prolapse of the rectum, injury by cold leading to heat in the Stomach, hot painful urinary dysfunction, stone oedema.
- Irregular menstruation, sudden amenorrhoea, abnormal uterine bleeding, infertility, disorders related to childbirth, retention of the placenta, difficult lactation.
- Swelling and pain of the external vagina, swelling and pain of the penis, pain of the testicles, retraction and pain of both testicles, shan disorder, impotence, pain of the lumbar region with difficulty in turning, fullness of the lateral costal region.
- Running piglet qi, qi rushing upwards to attack the Heart, foetus (foetal qi) rushes up to attack the Heart.

COMMENTARY

The name of this point Qichong may be translated as 'Rushing Qi' or 'Pouring Qi'. The character 'chong' is the same as in the Penetrating vessel (chong mai). This name reflects both the ability of Qichong ST-30 to regulate the circulation of qi in the lower abdomen and its status as the point where the Penetrating vessel emerges on the abdomen. Qichong ST-30 has a broad action in treating many disorders affecting this area. By regulating qi, Qichong ST-30 may be used to disperse stagnation, pain, cold and heat in the genital region, intestines, Bladder and the abdomen as a whole, and is indicated for such disorders as pain, fullness and distention of the lower abdomen, abdominal heat, twisting pain of the abdomen, heat in the Large Intestine, retention of urine and faeces, hot painful urinary dysfunction, stone oedema etc.

The Penetrating vessel emerges at the perineum and meets the Stomach yangming channel at Qichong ST-30. The Penetrating vessel influences the lower abdomen as a whole, including the genital organs, and especially helps regulate the function of the uterus and menstruation. Qichong ST-30 is therefore indicated for such genital disorders as swelling and pain of the penis and vagina, pain and retraction of the testicles, impotence etc., and such gynaecological and obstetrical disorders as irregular menstruation, sudden amenorrhoea, abnormal uterine bleeding, infertility, retention of the placenta and difficult lactation.

According to the *Classic of Difficulties*, when the Penetrating vessel is diseased, there will be upsurging qi and acute abdominal disturbance. Qichong ST-30, located on the lower abdomen and the point where the Penetrating vessel emerges, is the single most important point in the treatment of running piglet qi. According to the *Essentials from the Golden Cabinet* "Running piglet disorder arises from the lower abdomen; it rushes up to the throat with such ferocity that the patient feels he is close to death. It attacks and then remits. It is brought about by fear and fright". Running piglet qi primarily arises when stagnant Liver qi transforms to heat, or when Kidney yang deficiency leads to accumulation of cold in the lower jiao. In both cases, qi is violently discharged and rushes upwards along the Penetrating vessel causing great agitation and anxiety. Qichong ST-30 is also indicated for foetal qi rushing up to the Heart. This condition, described by Zhu Dan-xi, manifests as distention, fullness and pain of the abdomen and Heart in a pregnant woman.

In the chapter 'Discourse On the Seas' in the *Spiritual Pivot*[17] Qichong ST-30 is given as the upper point of the 'sea of water and grain' (Zusanli ST-36 is the lower point). According to this passage, when the sea of water and grain is in excess, there is abdominal fullness, and when it is deficient there is hunger with inability to eat. Finally, the *Essential Questions*[18] includes Qichong ST-30 among the eight points to clear heat from the Stomach (bilateral Qichong ST-30, Zusanli ST-36, Shangjuxu ST-37 and Xiajuxu ST-39).

COMBINATIONS

- Insomnia: Qichong ST-30 and Zhangmen LIV-13 (*Supplementing Life*).
- Prolapse of the rectum: Qichong ST-30, Dachangshu BL-25, Baihui DU-20, Changqiang DU-1, Jianjing GB-21 and Hegu L.I.-4 (*Compilation*).
- Stone oedema of the upper abdomen: moxa Qichong ST-30, Rangu KID-2, Siman KID-14 and Zhangmen LIV-13 (*Thousand Ducat Formulas*).

BIGUAN ST-31

Thigh Gate

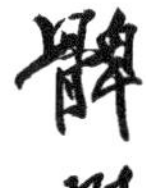

LOCATION

On the upper thigh, in a depression just lateral to the sartorius muscle, at the junction of a vertical line drawn downward from the anterior superior iliac spine, and a horizontal line drawn level with the lower border of the pubic symphysis.

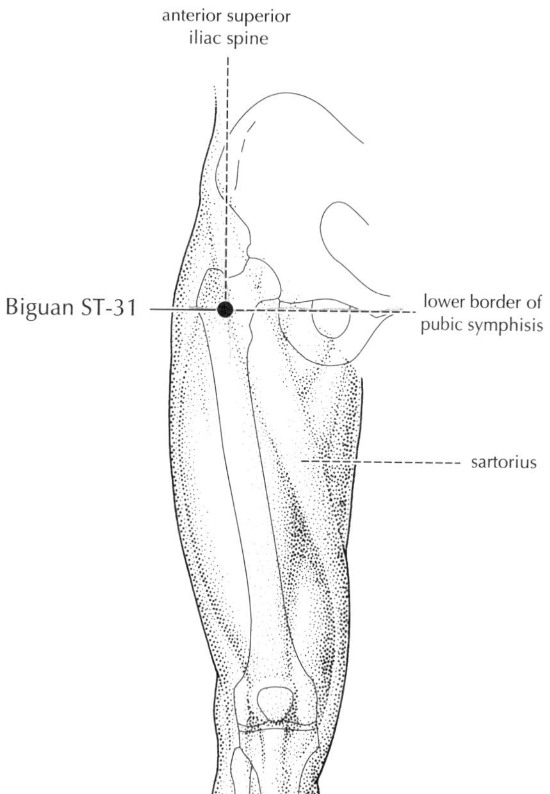

LOCATION NOTE

The horizontal level may also be taken as approximately the most prominent point of the greater trochanter.

NEEDLING

Perpendicular or oblique insertion 1 to 2 cun.

ACTIONS

Activates the channel and alleviates pain
Dispels wind-damp

INDICATIONS

- Atrophy disorder and painful obstruction of the lower limb, hemiplegia, numbness of the legs, cold damp leg qi, pain of the hip joint, pain of the thigh, sciatica, contraction of the thigh muscles, cold painful obstruction of the knees, inability to extend and bend the knee, lumbar pain, jaundice.

COMMENTARY

Biguan ST-31 (Thigh Gate) is located close to the pivotal hip region, the 'gate' of the lower limb. According to the *Spiritual Pivot*[19] "Yangming channel is abundant in qi and blood", and points of both arm and foot yangming channel are much used clinically to promote the circulation of qi and blood in the extremities, rendering them ideal for treating numbness, paralysis, stiffness and pain in the four limbs.

Biguan ST-31 is an important point to regulate the circulation of qi and blood in the leg as a whole, and in the Stomach channel in particular. In this respect it may be viewed as the equivalent point on the lower limb of Jianyu L.I.-15 on the upper limb. Its main applications are in the treatment of atrophy disorder, hemiplegia and painful obstruction of the whole leg, or in the treatment of pain from the hip radiating down the Stomach channel. In such cases it is frequently combined in the 'chain and lock' method with Zusanli ST-36 and Jiexi ST-41. A number of classics also specifically recommend Biguan ST-31 for cold painful obstruction of the knees and for lumbar pain.

COMBINATIONS

- Numbness of the knee: Biguan ST-31, Dubi ST-35, and Yanglingquan GB-34 (*Supplementing Life*).
- Weakness and paralysis of the legs: Biguan ST-31, Zusanli ST-36, Yanglingquan GB-34, Xuanzhong GB-39 and Jiexi ST-41.

FUTU ST-32
Crouching Rabbit

伏兔

LOCATION

On the thigh, on a line drawn between the lateral border of the patella and the anterior superior iliac spine, in a depression 6 cun proximal to the superior border of the patella.

LOCATION NOTE

Divide the distance between the prominence of the greater trochanter and the upper border of the patella into thirds; this point is located just superior to the junction of the lower and middle thirds.

prominence of greater trochanter
11 cun
Futu ST-32
6 cun
superior border of the patella

NEEDLING

Perpendicular or oblique insertion 1 to 2 cun.

ACTIONS

Activates the channel and alleviates pain
Dispels wind-damp

INDICATIONS

- Painful obstruction and atrophy disorder of the lower limb, leg qi, pain, numbness and contraction of the muscles of the thigh, coldness and pain of the knee, weakness of the knee, lumbar pain, contraction of the arm.
- Shan disorder, abdominal distention with diminished qi, diseases of the eight regions in women, mania, ghost talk, urticaria, heavy head.

COMMENTARY

Although principally used for channel disorders of the lower limb, the *Sagelike Prescriptions from the Taiping Era* recommends Futu ST-32 for diseases of the eight regions in women. These are i. the external genitals, ii. the breast, iii. disorders of pregnancy, iv. post-partum disorders, v. uterine bleeding, vi. leucorrhoea, vii. menstruation and viii. abdominal masses.

COMBINATIONS

- Wind leg qi: first moxa Fengshi GB-31 then moxa Futu ST-32 (*Thousand Ducat Formulas*).

YINSHI ST-33
Yin Market

陰市

LOCATION

On the thigh, on a line drawn between the lateral border of the patella and the anterior superior iliac spine, in a depression 3 cun proximal to the superior border of the patella.

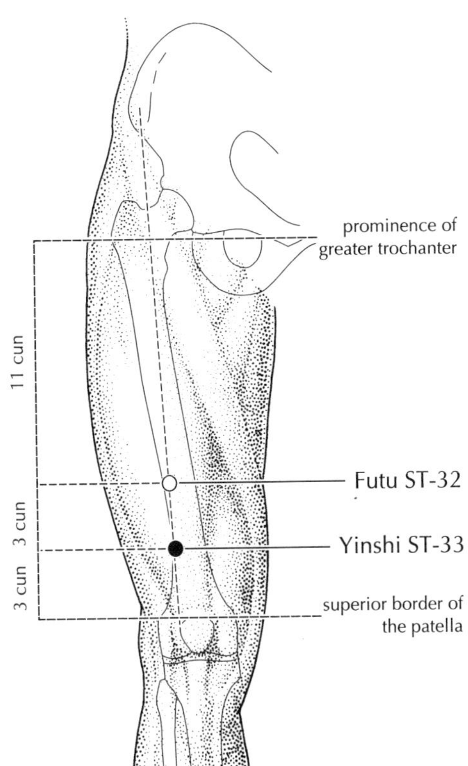

LOCATION NOTE

i. Locate Yinshi ST-33 one handbreadth proximal to the upper border of the patella; ii. Locate Yinshi ST-33 midway between Futu ST-32 and the upper border of the patella.

NEEDLING

Perpendicular or oblique insertion 1 to 1.5 cun.

ACTIONS

Activates the channel and alleviates pain
Dispels wind-damp

INDICATIONS

- Sensation like cold water in the lumbar region and legs, difficulty in stretching and bending the leg, atrophy disorder and painful obstruction of the leg, leg qi, weakness of the leg and knee, pain of the thigh and knee.
- Wasting and thirsting disorder, cold shan disorder, distention and pain of the abdomen, oedema with enlarged abdomen.

COMBINATIONS

- Lack of strength in the legs: Yinshi ST-33 and Fengshi GB-31 (*Ode of the Jade Dragon*).
- Pain of the legs and lumbar region: Yinshi ST-33, Huantiao GB-30, Fengshi GB-31, Weizhong BL-40, Kunlun BL-60, Chengshan BL-57 and Shenmai BL-62 (*Great Compendium*).
- Redness, swelling and pain of the knees: Yinshi ST-33, Xiguan LIV-7, Weizhong BL-40 and Zusanli ST-36 (*Great Compendium*).
- Disorders of the knee and the region above the knee: moxa Yinshi ST-33 and Huantiao GB-30 (*Great Compendium*).
- Cold abdominal shan disorder: Yinshi ST-33, Ganshu BL-18 and Taixi KID-3 (*Great Compendium*).

LIANGQIU ST-34

Ridge Mound

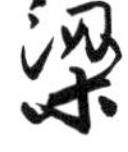

Xi-Cleft point of the Stomach channel

LOCATION

On the thigh, on a line drawn between the lateral border of the patella and the anterior superior iliac spine, in a depression 2 cun proximal to the superior border of the patella.

LOCATION NOTE

Since the height of the patella is measured as 2 cun, this point may be located one patella's length above its superior border.

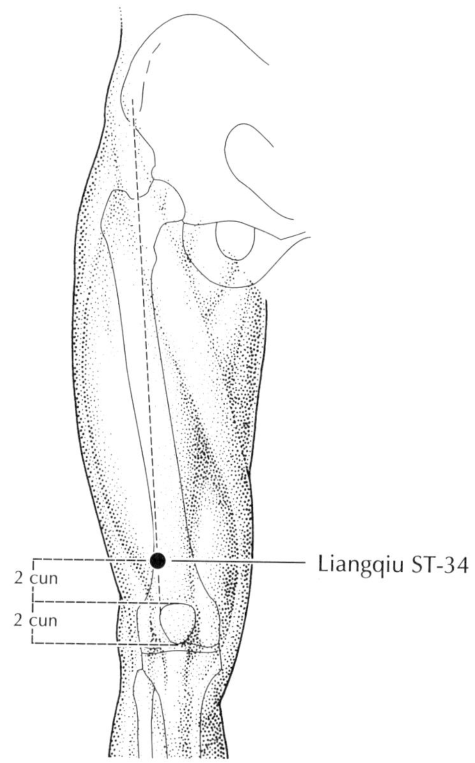

NEEDLING

Perpendicular or oblique insertion 1 to 1.5 cun.

ACTIONS

Activates the channel and alleviates pain
Harmonises the Stomach and alleviates pain
Moderates acute conditions

INDICATIONS

- Swelling and pain of the knee, difficulty in flexing and extending the knee, pain of the knee and leg, crane's knee wind, difficulty in walking, painful obstruction of the shin, cold painful obstruction with numbness, cold of the legs and feet, lumbar pain.
- Epigastric pain, acid regurgitation, breast abscess, pain and swelling of the breast, 'big fright'.

COMMENTARY

Liangqiu ST-34 is the xi-cleft point of the Stomach channel and is the only one of the xi-cleft points of the twelve primary channels which is located proximal to the knee or elbow. It is an important adjacent point in the treatment of knee disorders (often combined with such points as Xiyan (MN-LE-16), Xuehai SP-10, Yinlingquan SP-9 and Yanglingquan GB-34) and for painful obstruction, cold and pain of the leg.

The xi-cleft points are where the qi and blood, which flow relatively superficially along the channels from the jing-well points, gather and plunge more deeply. The xi-cleft points in general are indicated in the treatment of acute conditions and pain. The yangming Stomach channel traverses the breast and passes through the nipple, and Liangqiu ST-34 is classically indicated for such acute disorders of the breast as swelling, pain and abscess. In clinical practice it is also used for acute epigastric pain, although this seems to be a modern rather than traditional usage.

COMBINATIONS
- Breast abscess: Liangqiu ST-34 and Diwuhui GB-42 (*Supplementing Life*).
- Contracted sinews with difficulty in flexing and extending the knee, and inability to walk: Liangqiu ST-34, Ququan LIV-8 and Xiyangguan GB-33 (*Thousand Ducat Formulas*).
- Acute epigastric pain: Liangqiu ST-34 and Liangmen ST-21.
- Stiffness, soreness and pain of the knee: Liangqiu ST-34, Xuehai SP-10, Xiyan (MN-LE-16), Yanglingquan GB-34 and Yinlingquan SP-9.

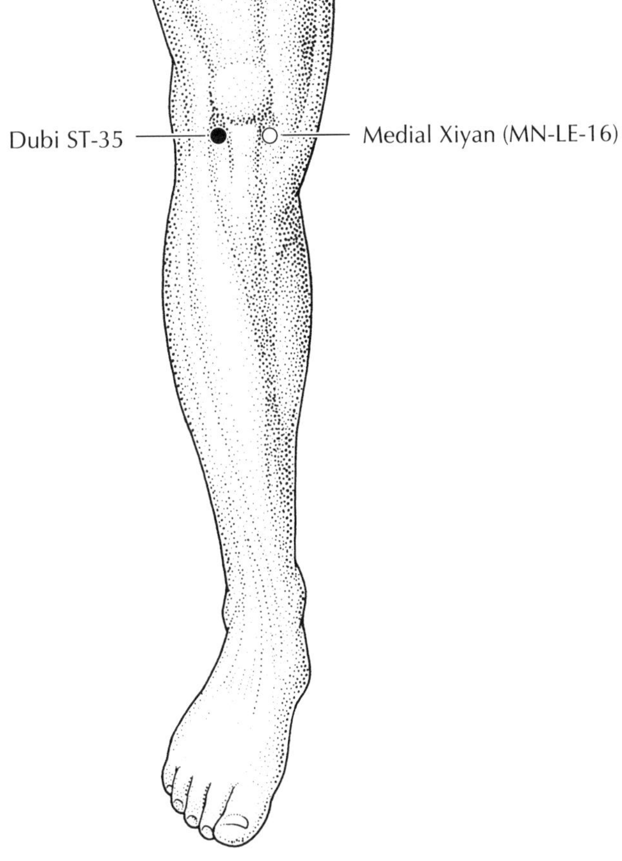

DUBI ST-35

Calf's Nose

犢鼻

LOCATION
On the knee, in the hollow formed when the knee is flexed, immediately below the patella and lateral to the patellar ligament.

LOCATION NOTE
This point is also known as lateral Xiyan, forming a pair with medial Xiyan (MN-LE-16) [see Extra points] which lies immediately below the patella and medial to the patellar ligament.

NEEDLING
With the knee flexed and supported by a rolled pillow, i. Perpendicular insertion, directed towards Weizhong BL-40, 1 to 2 cun; ii. Oblique insertion in a medial and superior direction, behind the patella 1 to 2 cun, iii. Behind the patellar ligament to join with medial Xiyan (MN-LE-16).

ACTIONS
Dispels wind-damp and reduces swelling
Activates the channel and alleviates pain

INDICATIONS
- Swelling and pain of the knee joint, difficulty in flexing and extending the knee, weakness of the knee joint, numbness of the knee, numbness of the lower limb, atrophy disorder of the lower limb, leg qi.

COMMENTARY
Dubi ST-35, located in the lateral visible hollow below the patella, is an essential point in the treatment of all knee disorders, whether due to deficiency or excess, heat or cold. In clinical practice it is frequently combined with the extra point medial Xiyan (located in the medial visible hollow below the patella), and is therefore most often known as lateral Xiyan.

COMBINATIONS
- Disorders of the knee and below the knee: moxa Dubi ST-35, Xiguan LIV-7, Zusanli ST-36 and Yanglingquan GB-34 (*Supplementing Life*).
- Numbness of the knee: Dubi ST-35, Biguan ST-31 and Yanglingquan GB-34 (*Supplementing Life*).

ZUSANLI ST-36

Leg Three Miles

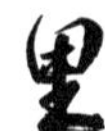

He-Sea and Earth point of the Stomach channel
Gao Wu Command point
Ma Dan-yang Heavenly Star point
Point of the Sea of Water and Grain

LOCATION

Below the knee, 3 cun inferior to Dubi ST-35, one finger-breadth lateral to the anterior crest of the tibia.

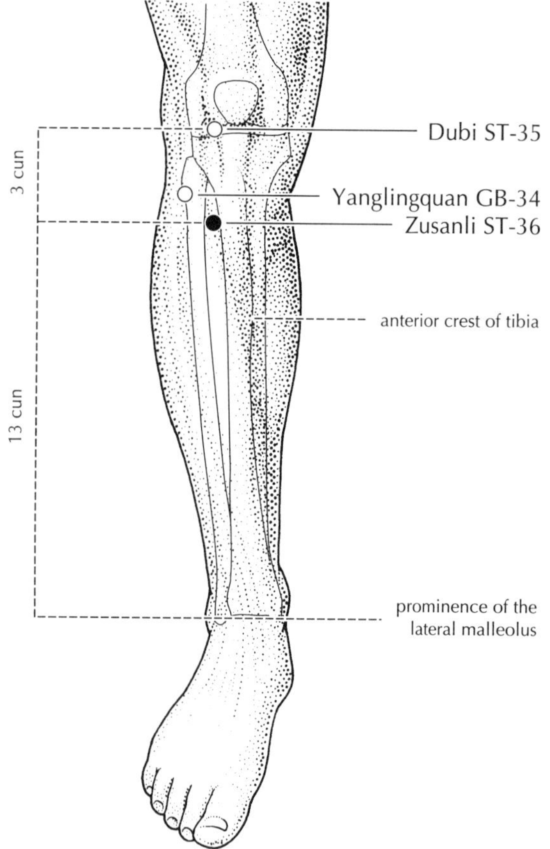

LOCATION NOTE

i. First locate Yanglingquan GB-34. Zusanli ST-36 lies one cun inferior to Yanglingquan GB-34 and one finger-breadth lateral to the anterior crest of the tibia; ii. Locate one handbreadth below Dubi ST-35.

NEEDLING

Perpendicular insertion 1 to 1.5 cun.

ACTIONS

Harmonises the Stomach
Fortifies the Spleen and resolves dampness
Supports the correct qi and fosters the original qi
Tonifies qi and nourishes blood and yin
Clears fire and calms the spirit
Activates the channel and alleviates pain
Revives the yang and restores consciousness

INDICATIONS

- Epigastric pain, nausea, vomiting, bitter vomiting, vomiting pus and blood, hiccup, belching, distention and pain of the abdomen, fullness and distention of the Heart and abdomen, heat in the middle jiao with propensity to hunger, hunger without desire to eat, poor appetite, difficult ingestion.
- Borborygmus, flatulence, diarrhoea and dysenteric disorder, undigested food (in the stool), cold in the middle jiao with borborygmus, cold in the intestines, chronic diarrhoea, sudden turmoil disorder, leg qi, oedema, heaviness of the four limbs, lower abdominal pain and swelling with inability to urinate, jaundice.
- The five taxations and the seven injuries, insufficiency of original qi, insufficiency of yin qi, insufficiency of zang qi, insufficiency of Stomach qi, deficient dyspnoea, shortness of breath and cough, dyspnoea with inability to stand for long.
- Dizziness, post-partum blood dizziness, dimness of vision, tinnitus, palpitations, hypertension.
- Mania-depression, manic singing, raving, abusive talk, anger and fright, tendency to sadness, outrageous laughter, agitation with heat in the body.
- Throat painful obstruction with inability to speak, chills and fever, febrile disease with absence of sweating, febrile disease with heavy head and pain of the forehead, headache, cold nose, pain of the brain, pain of the lateral costal region, blood stasis in the interior, blood stasis in the chest, sudden Heart pain, fullness of the chest and lateral costal region, qi rushing up to the chest.
- Lockjaw, clonic spasm, loss of consciousness.
- Breast abscess, swelling of the breast, pain of the knee and shin, pain of the thigh and shin, windstroke, hemiplegia, muscle pain, chronic painful obstruction, lumbar pain with inability to turn, shan disorder.

COMMENTARY

Zusanli ST-36 (Leg Three Miles) is the he-sea and earth point of the Stomach earth channel. It was included by Ma Dan-yang, the great physician of the Jin dynasty, among the 'eleven heavenly star points'[20], his grouping of the most vital acupuncture points, and was indicated by him for cold in the Stomach, borborygmus and diarrhoea, swelling of the leg, pain of the knee, emaciation due to injury by cold and all parasitic diseases. The *Glorious Anthology of Acupuncture and Moxibustion* by the Ming dynasty author Gao Wu includes Zusanli ST-36 among the 'four command points' (for disorders of the abdomen). Qin Cheng-zu of the Song dynasty declared that by using the point Zusanli ST-36 "all diseases can be treated".

The term 'li' in the name Zusanli may variously be interpreted as meaning a measure of distance (a Chinese mile) or as a homonym for 'to rectify'. The former interpretation reflects the idea that stimulating Zusanli ST-36 would enable a person to walk a further three li, even when exhausted, as well as that the point is located three cun below the knee. The latter interpretation reflects the concept that Zusanli ST-36 is able to rectify either the three vital zangfu (Stomach, Spleen and Kidneys) or the three jiao (upper, middle and lower).

The *Classic of Difficulties*[21]recommended the use of the he-sea points for "counterflow qi and diarrhoea", whilst the *Spiritual Pivot*[22] not only recommended their use for diseases of the internal fu, but also stated "in disorders of the Stomach and in disorders resulting from irregular eating and drinking, select the he-sea point". Zusanli ST-36 may be used in the treatment of any disorder of the Stomach fu, whether due to cold or heat, deficiency or excess, stagnation and retention of food, fluid or blood etc. Under normal conditions the Stomach has the function of receiving food and drink, "rotting and ripening" them, and descending the products of digestion. When these functions are impaired, which can be due to any of the above patterns, two principal disharmonies may appear: i. Stomach qi may fail to descend, leading to stagnation of qi and food and giving rise to epigastric or abdominal fullness, distention and pain, poor appetite etc. or ii. Stomach qi may rebel upwards giving rise to nausea, vomiting, belching, hiccup and difficult ingestion. In the case of Stomach heat there may be excessive hunger, whilst in the case of Stomach yin deficiency there may be hunger without desire to eat. In any one of these possible disorders of the Stomach, Zusanli ST-36 is indicated.

Zusanli ST-36, the earth point of the Stomach channel, also has a profound effect on regulating its coupled earth zang, the Spleen, and is able to strengthen the Spleen's function of transforming and transporting both food essence and fluid. As such it is an important point for the treatment of diarrhoea or dysenteric disorder, borborygmus, oedema, inability to urinate and heaviness of the limbs. Its important action on all disorders of the intestines, which are dominated by the Spleen, is reflected in the *Spiritual Pivot*[23] which advises the use of Zusanli ST-36 "when the intestines do not function correctly; if it is full reduce it, if it is empty reinforce it". It should be emphasised that the ability of Zusanli ST-36 to transform damp derives from its primary action of tonifying the Spleen. This differentiates Zusanli ST-36 from a point such as Yinlingquan SP-9 where the action of transforming damp is primary.

The Stomach and Spleen in the middle jiao are the root of the post-heaven qi and the prime source for the production of qi and blood and the continual supplementation of the pre-heaven essence. This vital role is emphasised in countless statements found in the ancient classics such as "The Stomach is the root of the zangfu"[24], "The five zang and six fu all receive qi from the Stomach"[25], "The Stomach is the sea of qi and blood"[26], as well as traditional sayings such as "Stomach qi is the root of man". Another saying "With Stomach qi there is life, without Stomach qi there is death" emphasises the vital importance of assessing the state of the Stomach qi (manifested by the patient's appetite and digestion) in prognosis. It is said that even in serious disease, strong Stomach qi is an encouraging prognostic sign, whilst in a less serious disease, exhaustion of Stomach qi is a poor prognostic sign. This principle is reinforced in the *Essential Questions*[27] which says "Water and grain are the root of human life; without water and grain a person will die, as one will die when Stomach qi is absent from the pulse". In the chapter 'Discourse On the Seas' in the *Spiritual Pivot*[28], Zusanli ST-36 is given as the lower point of the 'sea of water and grain' (Qichong ST-30 is the upper point). According to this passage, when the sea of water and grain is in excess, there is abdominal fullness, and when it is deficient there is hunger with inability to eat.

Zusanli ST-36 is the single most important point in the body to stimulate the action of the Stomach and Spleen in generating qi and blood. The post-heaven qi derives from the interaction of the grain qi (extracted from food and drink by the Spleen and Stomach) and the clear qi of air (transformed by the Lung), with the assistance of the original qi. Zusanli ST-36 alone is an important point to tonify the qi of the whole body, or in combination with Taiyuan LU-9 (the earth point of the Lung metal channel) to tonify the Lung qi according to the principle of 'cultivating the earth to generate metal'. It is indicated for insufficiency of original qi, deficient dyspnoea, dyspnoea with inability to stand for long, coughing and shortness of breath. By virtue of its action of tonifying qi, Zusanli ST-36 is also able to nourish the blood and is indicated for palpitations, dimness of vision, dizziness and post-partum blood dizziness.

Zusanli ST-36 is also renowned for its ability to support the correct qi. This is expressed in the recommendation by

Sun Si-miao to apply regular moxibustion to Zusanli ST-36 to preserve and maintain health, and in the ancient proverb (quoted for example by the 13th century doctor Wang Zhi-zhong) "if you wish to be safe never allow Sanli (ST-36) to become dry", referring to the prophylactic use of moxibustion. This saying implies that a constant suppurating sore should be maintained at Zusanli ST-36 through the repeated use of burning moxibustion. The *Great Compendium of Acupuncture and Moxibustion* also emphasises the profound tonifying effect of this point by stating "frequently moxa Zusanli ST-36 and Qihai REN-6 in young people whose qi is feeble" whilst Ma Dan-yang advocates regular needling and moxibustion at Zusanli ST-36 for those who have passed the age of thirty. It is sometimes suggested that Zusanli ST-36 should not be needled in case of attack by exterior pathogens, since its effect of reinforcing the correct qi may also reinforce the pathogen. In this respect, however, it is interesting to note that Zusanli ST-36 is classically indicated for chills and fever, febrile disease with absence of sweating, and febrile disease with heavy head and pain of the forehead.

The great Han dynasty physician Hua Tuo is said to have valued the use of Zusanli ST-36 to treat the five taxations and the seven injuries. The five taxations as discussed in the *Spiritual Pivot*[29] are i. excessive use of the eyes which injures the blood, ii. excessive lying down which injures the qi, iii. excessive sitting which injures the flesh, iv. excessive standing which injures the bones, and v. excessive walking which injures the sinews. In later texts, the concept of the five taxations was also used to refer to taxation of each of the five zang[30]. Although also referring to a range of male genital disorders (see glossary), the seven injuries in this context are i. overeating which injures the Spleen, ii. great anger which injures the Liver, iii. heavy lifting or prolonged sitting on damp ground which injure the Kidneys, iv. pathogenic cold which injures the Lung, v. worry and anxiety which injure the Heart, vi. wind, rain, cold and summer-heat which injure the body, and vii. excessive fear which injures the emotions.

Zusanli ST-36 is also indicated classically for insufficiency of both original qi and yin. Original qi originates in the Kidneys but is dependent on the post-heaven qi of the Stomach and Spleen. The *Treatise on the Spleen and Stomach* by Li Dong-yuan says "Sufficiency of original qi is dependent on the qi of the Spleen and Stomach being free of injury; only then can the original qi be supplemented and nourished". As far as deficiency of yin is concerned, according to *Secrets of a Frontier Official* "When a person passes the age of thirty, if moxa is not applied to Zusanli ST-36 then the qi will rise and rush to the eyes". This statement emphasises that Zusanli ST-36 is also able to supplement the inevitable decline of Kidney yin that occurs with advancing age, and thus prevent pathologically ascending yang from rushing to the head and eyes.

The Stomach divergent channel connects with the Heart, whilst the Stomach primary channel meets with the Governing vessel (and thus the brain) at Shenting DU-24 and Renzhong DU-26. If yangming fire blazes out of control it may be transmitted along these channels to the Heart and brain and agitate the spirit. Heart fire may be complicated by phlegm, which usually derives from prolonged dampness or from condensation of body fluids by fire. Zusanli ST-36 is able to clear yangming fire and, due to its influence on the Spleen, to resolve dampness and transform phlegm. This renders it effective in treating a wide variety of mental disturbances, especially those characterised by manic behaviour, for example mania-depression, manic singing, raving, abusive talk, anger and fright and outrageous laughter. One alternative name for Zusanli ST-36 given in the *Illustrated Supplement to the Classic of Categories* is Guixie (Ghost Evil), underlining its ability to treat mental disorders. In addition, since blood is the material basis for the Heart to house the spirit, the blood enhancing property of Zusanli ST-36 also renders it effective to treat emotional disorders arising from Heart blood deficiency. More widely, due to the pathway of the Stomach channel in the upper body, Zusanli ST-36, like Fenglong ST-40, is indicated for pain of the Heart and chest, especially when due to blood stasis.

Zusanli ST-36 is an important point to treat disorders of the Stomach channel, including swelling, pain and abscess of the breast as well as pain of the thigh and shin. The fact that yangming channel is abundant in qi and blood, allied with the inherent nourishing quality of this point, renders Zusanli ST-36 a vital point in the treatment of disorders of the lower limb as a whole, especially atrophy disorder and hemiplegia. This is emphasised in the *Essential Questions* which states "When there is illness in the Spleen it fails to transport body fluids for the Stomach. The four limbs do not receive the nourishment of water and grain and therefore become weak. There is no free flow through the vessel-pathways and there is no qi to engender the sinews, bones and muscles which therefore cannot function"[31]. Zusanli ST-36 is no less important in the treatment of painful obstruction due to cold and dampness, especially when chronic in nature. The *Spiritual Pivot*[32] says "for damp painful obstruction that is not expelled, for chronic cold that does not cease, choose Zusanli ST-36". In the treatment of atrophy disorder and painful obstruction, Zusanli ST-36 is frequently combined in the chain and lock method with other points of the Stomach yangming channel such as Biguan ST-31 and Jiexi ST-41.

Zusanli ST-36 is cited in the *Song of the Nine Needles for Returning the Yang* for the treatment of collapse of yang characterised by loss of consciousness, aversion to cold, cold counterflow of the limbs, purple lips etc. The *Essential Questions*[33] includes Zusanli ST-36 among the eight points to clear heat from the Stomach (bilateral Qichong ST-30, Zusanli ST-36, Shangjuxu ST-37 and Xiajuxu ST-39).

In conclusion, such is the range of actions and indications of this singular point, that it barely seems an exaggeration to state, as did Qin Cheng-zu nearly a thousand years ago, that by the use of Zusanli ST-36 "all diseases can be treated".

COMBINATIONS

- Internal injury by accumulation of food in the Stomach: Zusanli ST-36 and Xuanji REN-21 (*Miscellaneous Diseases*).
- Accumulation in the Stomach: Zusanli ST-36 and Xuanji REN-21 (*Ode of Xi-hong*).
- Obstruction of food in the Stomach: Zusanli ST-36 and Xuanji REN-21 (*Heavenly Star Points*).
- Stagnation of food in the mid-abdomen, stabbing pain that does not cease: Zusanli ST-36, Gongsun SP-4, Jiexi ST-41 and Zhongwan REN-12 (*Complete Collection*).
- Difficult ingestion: Zusanli ST-36, Yuji LU-10 and Neiguan P-6 (*Great Compendium*).
- Abdominal fullness: Zusanli ST-36 and Yixi BL-45 (*Supplementing Life*).
- Abdominal pain: Zusanli ST-36, Neiguan P-6 and Zhongwan REN-12 (*Great Compendium*).
- Sudden turmoil disorder: Zusanli ST-36 and Yingu KID-10 (*One Hundred Symptoms*).
- Sudden turmoil disorder, headache, chest pain and dyspnoeic rales: Zusanli ST-36, Renying ST-9, Neiguan P-6, Guanchong SJ-1 and Sanyinjiao SP-6 (*Compilation*).
- Undigested food (in the stool), vomiting immediately after ingestion: first needle Xiawan REN-10, then reduce Zusanli ST-36 (*Thousand Ducat Formulas*).
- Undigested food (in the stool): Zusanli ST-36, Dachangshu BL-25, Sanyinjiao SP-6, Xiawan REN-10, Sanjiaoshu BL-22, Xuanshu DU-5 and Liangmen ST-21 (*Supplementing Life*).
- All types of diarrhoea and abdominal disorders: Zusanli ST-36 and Neiting ST-44 (*Miscellaneous Diseases*).
- Dysenteric disorder: Zusanli ST-36 and Hegu L.I.-4; if severe add Zhonglushu BL-29 (*Song of Points*).
- Blood in the stool: Zusanli ST-36, Zhongwan REN-12 and Qihai REN-6 (*Glorious Anthology*).
- Deficiency constipation: reduce Zusanli ST-36 and reinforce Zhigou SJ-6 (*Song of Points*).
- Difficult urination or retention of urine: Zusanli ST-36 and Shaofu HE-8 (*Thousand Ducat Formulas*).
- Jaundice with weakness of the four limbs: Zusanli ST-36 and Zhongwan REN-12 (*Classic of the Jade Dragon*).
- Acute dyspnoea: Zusanli ST-36 and Lieque LU-7 (*Song of Points*).
- Liver blood deficiency with cloudy vision: reduce Zusanli ST-36 and reinforce Ganshu BL-18 (*Song of the Jade Dragon*).
- Post-partum dizziness: Zusanli ST-36, Zhigou SJ-6 and Sanyinjiao SP-6 (*Great Compendium*).
- To hasten delivery: Zusanli ST-36 and Zhiyin BL-67 (*Miscellaneous Diseases*).
- Haemorrhage: moxa Zusanli ST-36 and needle Yinbai SP-1 (*Glorious Anthology*).
- Breast abscess: Zusanli ST-36, Yuji LU-10, Xiajuxu ST-39, Xiaxi GB-43, Weizhong BL-40, Zulinqi GB-41 and Shaoze SI-1 (*Great Compendium*).
- Feebleness of the legs: Zusanli ST-36, Weizhong BL-40 and Chengshan BL-57 (*Great Compendium*).
- Atrophy disorder: moxa Zusanli ST-36 and Feishu BL-13, needle Zhongdu GB-32 and Huantiao GB-30, (*Glorious Anthology*).
- Cold damp leg qi: Zusanli ST-36 and Sanyinjiao SP-6 (*Song of the Jade Dragon*).
- Leg qi: Zusanli ST-36, Xuanzhong GB-39 and Sanyinjiao SP-6 (*Ode of the Jade Dragon*).
- Pain and soreness of leg qi: first needle Jianjing GB-21, then needle Zusanli ST-36 and Yanglingquan GB-34 (*Celestial Star*).
- Redness, swelling and pain of the knees: Zusanli ST-36, Yinshi ST-33, Xiguan LIV-7 and Weizhong BL-40 (*Great Compendium*).
- Inability to walk: Zusanli ST-36, Taichong LIV-3 and Zhongfeng LIV-4 (*Ode of the Jade Dragon*).
- Disorders of the knee and below the knee: moxa Zusanli ST-36, Dubi ST-35, Xiguan LIV-7 and Yanglingquan GB-34 (*Supplementing Life*).
- Windstroke with one-sided withering and incessant pain: Zusanli ST-36, Jianyu L.I.-15, Xuanzhong GB-39, Taixi KID-3, Quchi L.I.-11 and Kunlun BL-60 (*Great Compendium*).
- Mania: Zusanli ST-36, Jianshi P-5, Baihui DU-20, Fuliu KID-7 and Yingu KID-10 (*Illustrated Supplement*).
- Injury by cold with great heat that does not recede: reduce Zusanli ST-36, Hegu L.I.-4, Quchi L.I.-11, Xuanzhong GB-39, Dazhui DU-14 and Yongquan KID-1 (*Great Compendium*).

SHANGJUXU ST-37

Upper Great Void

上巨虛

Lower He-Sea point of the Large Intestine
Point of the Sea of Blood

LOCATION

On the lower leg, 3 cun inferior to Zusanli ST-36, one finger-breadth lateral to the anterior crest of the tibia.

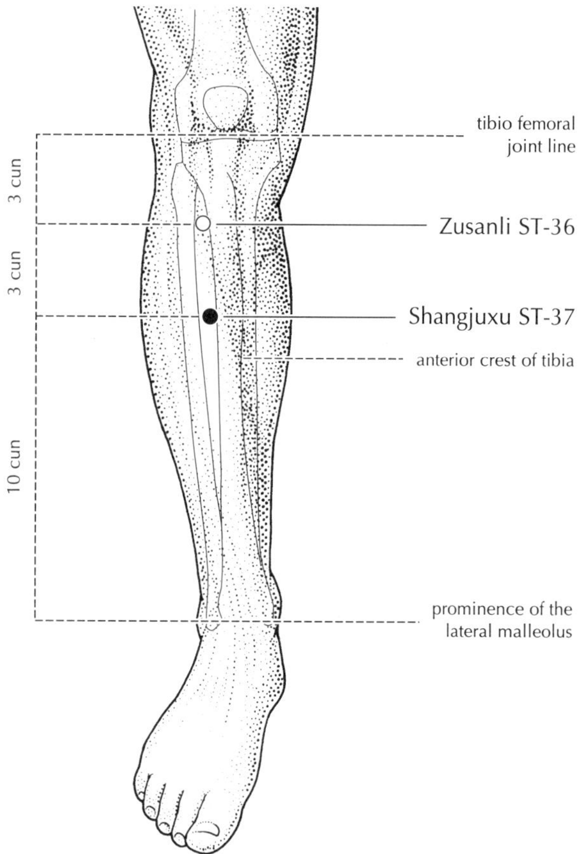

LOCATION NOTE

Locate one handbreadth below Zusanli ST-36.

NEEDLING

Perpendicular or oblique insertion 1 to 1.5 cun.

ACTIONS

Regulates the intestines and transforms stagnation
Clears damp heat and alleviates diarrhoea and dysenteric disorder
Regulates the Spleen and Stomach
Activates the channel and alleviates pain

INDICATIONS

- Borborygmus, diarrhoea, diarrhoea containing undigested food, diarrhoea due to attack of cold in winter, dysenteric disorder, heat in the Large Intestine, cold of the Large Intestine, deficiency of Large Intestine qi, intestinal abscess, cutting pain of the intestines, constipation, abdominal pain, abdominal distention, periumbilical pain with inability to stand for long, dark urine.
- Heat in the Stomach, deficiency and weakness of the Spleen and Stomach, insufficiency of zang qi, consumption, shortness of breath, dyspnoea with difficulty in walking, qi rushes up to the chest, fullness of the chest and lateral costal region, swelling of the face.
- Mania, aversion to the sound of people talking.
- Hemiplegia, leg qi, numbness and painful obstruction of the lower limb, coldness and pain of the bone marrow, weakness of the leg, contraction and pain of the front of the shin, swelling of the knee.

COMMENTARY

The *Yellow Emperor's Inner Classic* stated "The Large and Small intestines fall under the influence of the Stomach"[34] and classified Shangjuxu ST-37 as the lower he-sea point of the Large Intestine. The three yang channels of the arm (Large Intestine, Small Intestine and Sanjiao) are unique in that whilst the channels traverse the upper jiao, their respective fu belong to the lower jiao. Thus although the *Spiritual Pivot* states that the "He-sea points treat disorders of the internal fu", the he-sea points of these three channels (Quchi L.I.-11, Xiaohai SI-8, and Tianjing SJ-10 respectively) have relatively little action on their related fu. The Large and Small Intestines and the Sanjiao, however, each have a lower he-sea point (Shangjuxu ST-37, Xiajuxu ST-39 and Weiyang BL-39) which predominantly treat disorders of their respective fu.

Shangjuxu ST-37 is an important point in the treatment of a wide range of intestinal disorders. It is especially effective in the treatment of diarrhoea and dysenteric disorder, whether due to deficiency, cold, dampness, or damp-heat, and in recent times has been much used in the treatment of bacillary dysentery. Shangjuxu ST-37 is also used in the treatment of stagnation and obstruction of the intestines, giving rise to distention and pain of the abdomen, constipation and intestinal abscess. This comprehensive ability of Shangjuxu ST-37 to regulate the intestines was referred to in the earliest classics. For example, the *Systematic Classic of Acupuncture and Moxibustion* recommends Shangjuxu ST-37 for "heat in the Large Intestine, diarrhoea containing undigested food and borborygmus", whilst the tenth century classic *Sagelike Prescrip-*

tions from the Taiping Era recommends it for insufficiency of Large Intestine qi.

Some classics ascribe qi tonifying actions to this point, for example "deficiency and weakness of Spleen and Stomach, insufficiency of zang qi, shortness of breath etc." These may be explained by the beneficial effect that firming the intestines in cases of loose stool and diarrhoea will have on the transportation and transformation function of the Spleen. It is also worth noting that acupuncture points immediately distal or proximal to very powerful points, often share some of their functions and indications. It is as though the influence of Zusanli ST-36 is so great that it can resonate onto Shangjuxu ST-37.

According to the *Spiritual Pivot*[35] Shangjuxu ST-37 is a point of the 'sea of blood'. This passage says "The Penetrating vessel is the sea of the twelve channels (i.e. the sea of blood). In the upper it is conveyed to Dazhu BL-11, and in the lower it emerges at both Shangjuxu ST-37 and Xiajuxu ST-39 ... When the sea of blood is in excess, there is a sensation as if the body were big; one feels disquiet, but does not know what disease there is; when the sea of blood is insufficient, one has the sensation of one's body being small; one feels reduced but does not know what could be the illness". Despite this passage it is worth noting that such indications are not found in later texts.

In common with many points of the Stomach channel, Shangjuxu ST-37 is especially effective in treating disorders of the lower limb as a whole. This action is explained by the saying "Yangming channels are abundant in qi and blood". The ability of Shangjuxu ST-37 to promote the flow of smooth qi and blood throughout the leg renders it effective in the treatment of hemiplegia, leg qi, weakness of the leg, swelling of the knee and all kinds of atrophy disorder and painful obstruction, whether due to excess or deficiency patterns.

Finally, the *Essential Questions*[36] includes Shangjuxu ST-37 among the eight points to clear heat from the Stomach (bilateral Qichong ST-30, Zusanli ST-36, Shangjuxu ST-37 and Xiajuxu ST-39).

COMBINATIONS

- Yellow and difficult urination: Shangjuxu ST-37 and Xiajuxu ST-39 (*Systematic Classic*).
- Bacillary dysentery: Shangjuxu ST-37, Tianshu ST-25 and Quchi L.I.-11.

TIAOKOU ST-38

Lines Opening

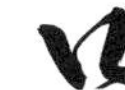

LOCATION

On the lower leg, midway between the tibiofemoral joint line (level with the popliteal crease) and the prominence of the lateral malleolus, one fingerbreadth lateral to the anterior crest of the tibia.

NEEDLING

Perpendicular or oblique insertion 1 to 1.5 cun.

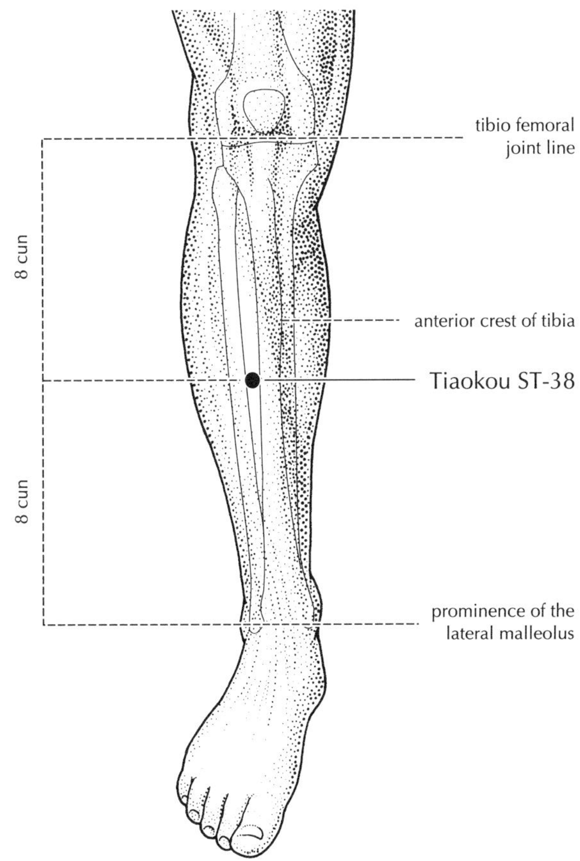

ACTIONS

Expels wind-damp and alleviates pain
Benefits the shoulder

INDICATIONS

- Atrophy disorder and painful obstruction of the lower limb, damp painful obstruction, numbness, coldness, swelling and pain of the shin, inability to stand for long, swelling of the thigh and knee, heat in the soles of the feet.
- Pain and stiffness of the shoulder, abdominal pain.

COMMENTARY

Tiaokou ST-38 is either used as a local point in the treatment of a variety of disorders of the leg, or more commonly as an important empirical point in the treatment of shoulder disorders. For this latter use, Tiaokou ST-38 is normally needled on the affected side, with the patient sitting. After qi is obtained, the patient is asked to move the shoulder around the area of pain whilst the needle is manipulated at Tiaokou ST-38. In most cases, pain will be relieved and mobility increased immediately. This procedure is normally followed by needling of appropriate local and distal points. Although the ability of this point to treat shoulder disorders with great effectiveness may be partially explained by the close link between the Stomach and Large Intestine channels, this is first and foremost an example of the empirical use of acupuncture points.

COMBINATIONS

- Heat in the sole of the foot with inability to stand for long: Tiaokou ST-38, Zusanli ST-36, Chengshan BL-57 and Chengjin BL-56 (*Thousand Ducat Formulas*).
- Flaccidity of the legs with difficulty in walking: first needle Xuanzhong GB-39 then needle Tiaokou ST-38 and Chongyang ST-42 (*Secrets of the Heavenly Star*).
- Shoulder pain: Tiaokou ST-38 and local points.

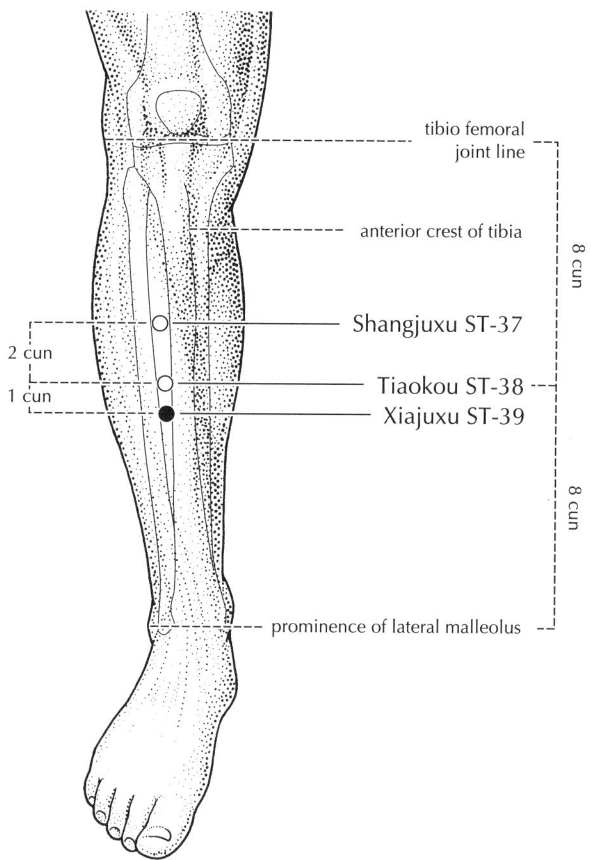

XIAJUXU ST-39

Lower Great Void

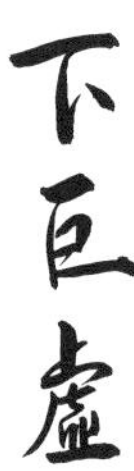

Lower He-Sea point of the Small Intestine
Point of the Sea of Blood

LOCATION

On the lower leg, 3 cun inferior to Shangjuxu ST-37, one finger-breadth lateral to the anterior crest of the tibia.

LOCATION NOTE

Divide the distance between the tibiofemoral joint line (level with the popliteal crease) and the prominence of the lateral malleolus into two equal parts. The midpoint is Tiaokou ST-38; Xiajuxu ST-39 is located 1 cun below Tiaokou ST-38.

NEEDLING

Perpendicular or oblique insertion 1 to 1.5 cun.

ACTIONS

Moves Small Intestine qi and transforms stagnation
Regulates and harmonises the intestines and clears damp-heat
Activates the channel and alleviates pain

INDICATIONS

- Lower abdominal pain, lumbar pain that radiates to the testicles.
- Diarrhoea, diarrhoea containing undigested food, dysenteric disorder, pus and blood in the stool, insufficiency of Small Intestine qi, dark urine.
- Breast abscess, manic raving, sudden fright, drooling, dry lips, throat painful obstruction, absence of sweating, no pleasure in eating, pallor.
- Painful obstruction and atrophy disorder of the lower limb, hemiplegia of the leg, atrophy disorder of the foot, pain of the heel, extreme sensation of cold and heat in the shoulder, heat sensation in the area between the ring and little fingers, burning sensation in front of the ears.

COMMENTARY

The *Yellow Emperor's Inner Classic* stated "The Large and Small intestines fall under the influence of the Stomach"[37] and classified Xiajuxu ST-39 as the lower he-sea point of the Small Intestine. The three yang channels of the arm (Large Intestine, Small Intestine and Sanjiao) are unique in that whilst the channels traverse the upper jiao, their respective fu belong to the lower jiao. Thus although the

Spiritual Pivot states that the "He-sea points treat disorders of the internal fu", the he-sea points of these three channels (Quchi L.I.-11, Xiaohai SI-8, and Tianjing SJ-10 respectively) have relatively little action on their related fu. The Large and Small Intestines and the Sanjiao, however, each have a lower he-sea point (Shangjuxu ST-37, Xiajuxu ST-39 and Weiyang BL-39) which predominantly treat disorders of their respective fu.

Xiajuxu ST-39 may be used in two principal patterns of the Small Intestine, namely Small Intestine qi pain and Small Intestine deficient and cold. The former is characterised by severe pain of the lower abdomen which radiates to the waist and lumbar region and down to the testicles. The latter is characterised by (dull) lower abdominal pain (which is improved with warmth and pressure) and chronic diarrhoea or dysenteric disorder etc. Xiajuxu ST-39 is further able to treat diarrhoea and dysenteric disorder due to damp heat which give rise to pus and blood in the stool.

The *Essential Questions*[38] includes Xiajuxu ST-39 among the eight points to clear heat from the Stomach, emphasising that as well as being the he-sea point of the Small Intestine, this point lies on the Stomach channel and is indicated for heat in the channel giving rise to disorders such as breast abscess, dry lips and throat painful obstruction. Unusually, Xiajuxu ST-39 is also clearly ascribed some ability to regulate the Small Intestine channel, reflected in such indications as extreme sensation of cold and heat in the shoulder, heat sensation in the area between the ring and little fingers, and burning sensation in front of the ears.

For a discussion of Xiajuxu ST-39 as a point of the 'sea of blood' refer to the commentary on Shangjuxu ST-37.

Finally, Xiajuxu ST-39 belongs to yangming channel which is abundant in qi and blood, and is similar to points such as Zusanli ST-36 and Shangjuxu ST-37 in its ability to treat disorders of the lower limb. It is indicated for painful obstruction and atrophy disorder of the lower limb and foot, hemiplegia and heel pain.

COMBINATIONS

- Diarrhoea and dysenteric disorder with pus and blood: Xiajuxu ST-39, Youmen KID-21 and Taibai SP-3 (*Supplementing Life*).
- Manic raving: Xiajuxu ST-39 and Qiuxu GB-40 (*Thousand Ducat Formulas*).
- Fullness of the chest and lateral costal region radiating to the abdomen: Xiajuxu ST-39, Qiuxu GB-40, Xiaxi GB-43 and Shenshu BL-23 (*Great Compendium*).
- Breast abscess: Xiajuxu ST-39, Zusanli ST-36, Xiaxi GB-43, Yuji LU-10, Weizhong BL-40, Zulinqi GB-41 and Shaoze SI-1 (*Great Compendium*).

FENGLONG ST-40

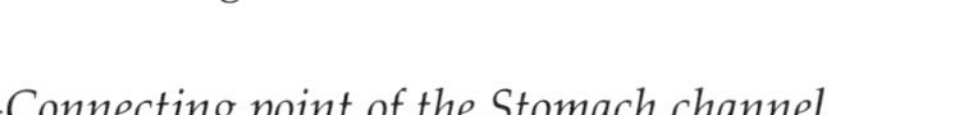

Abundant Bulge

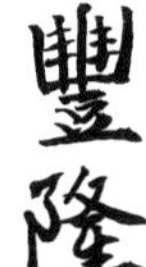

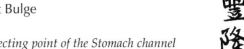

Luo-Connecting point of the Stomach channel

LOCATION

On the lower leg, midway between the tibiofemoral joint line (level with the popliteal crease) and the lateral malleolus, two finger-breadths lateral to the anterior crest of the tibia (i.e. one finger-breadth lateral to Tiaokou ST-38).

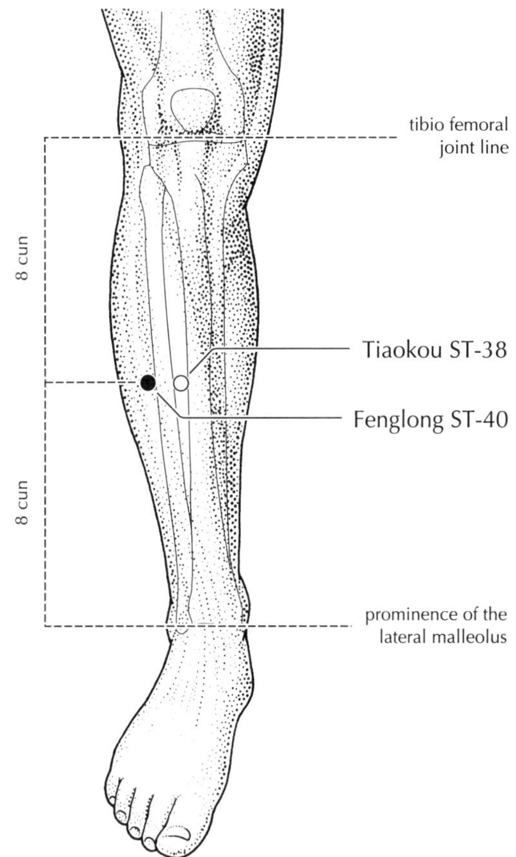

NEEDLING

Perpendicular or oblique insertion 1 to 1.5 cun.

ACTIONS

Transforms phlegm and dampness
Benefits the chest
Clears phlegm from the Lung and alleviates cough and wheezing
Clears phlegm from the Heart and calms the spirit
Activates the channel and alleviates pain

INDICATIONS

- Copious phlegm, fullness, oppression and pain of the chest, stabbing pain of the chest, cutting pain of the abdomen, swelling of the face, dizziness, headache, wind-phlegm headache, plumstone qi (globus hystericus), swelling and pain of the throat, throat painful obstruction with sudden loss of voice.
- Damp body, slackness and heaviness of the body.
- Cough and shortness of breath, cough with copious phlegm, wheezing, dyspnoea, asthma.
- Mania-depression, mad laughter, great happiness, desires to ascend to high places and sing, discards clothing and runs around, restlessness, seeing ghosts, indolence, epilepsy, hypertension.
- Constipation, difficulty in passing urine and stools.
- Atrophy disorder and painful obstruction of the lower limb, pain of the knee and leg, difficulty in flexing and extending the knee, lack of control of the legs, withering of the lower legs.

COMMENTARY

Fenglong ST-40 is the single most important acupuncture point to transform phlegm in the body, whatever its origin. Phlegm may be formed when i. stagnation of Liver qi impairs the circulation of fluids which then congeal into phlegm, ii. excess or deficiency heat condense body fluids (phlegm is known as the 'substantial part of fire', and fire the 'non-substantial part of phlegm') or iii. any or all of the three zang responsible for fluid transformation and transportation are deficient (the Lung in the upper jiao, the Spleen in the middle jiao and the Kidneys in the lower jiao). Of all these, disharmony of the transportation and transformation function of the Spleen is clinically the most important, thus the *Essential Questions*[39] says "The Spleen is the origin of phlegm" and "When water, grain and body fluids do not flow, they will accumulate and form phlegm-fluid (tanyin)". When the Spleen transportation and transformation function is impaired, therefore, body fluids collect and over time transform to phlegm, which may then transmit to other zangfu and regions of the body. Furthermore, it is a general treatment principle that the Spleen should be regulated in the treatment of phlegm of any aetiology, to assist in its transformation. Fenglong ST-40 is the point from which the Stomach luo-connecting channel connects with its associated Spleen channel. The *Guide to the Classics of Acupuncture* states "the luo-connecting points are located between two channels ... if they are punctured, symptoms of the interiorly-exteriorly related channels can be treated"[40]. Traditionally, Fenglong ST-40 has been used to treat any accumulation of phlegm, especially affecting the Lung, Heart, throat and head.

According to a saying of Chinese medicine, "The Spleen is the origin of phlegm and the Lung is the container of phlegm". When phlegm obstructs the descent of Lung qi, or when Lung qi deficiency is unable to descend the fluids, there may be coughing, wheezing and asthma characterised by copious expectoration of phlegm. When cold predominates, the phlegm will be clear or white, whilst when heat predominates, the phlegm will be yellow, green or brown. Whether cold or hot, Fenglong ST-40 is an essential point to transform phlegm in the Lung.

Both the primary and sinew channels of the Stomach pass through the chest, and Fenglong ST-40 has long been considered a pre-eminent point in the treatment of chest pain. If phlegm obstructs the free movement of qi and blood in the chest there may be fullness, oppression and stabbing pain. Such is its affinity for the chest, however, that Fenglong ST-40 may be used in the treatment of any kind of chest pain including sprain and injury of the chest muscles.

The pattern of phlegm or phlegm-fire misting or deranging the Heart and spirit principally occurs when severe emotional depression leads to stagnation of qi. Stagnant qi can no longer distribute body fluids, which coagulate to form phlegm. Phlegm then obstructs the portals of the Heart, disrupting the spirit. Pronounced or prolonged stagnation of qi and phlegm may transform into fire resulting in phlegm-fire, which may be further complicated by over-consumption of greasy and spicy food and alcohol. When the fire aspect of phlegm-fire is intense, the patient suffers from 'kuang', or mania disorder, with such symptoms as mad laughter and wild and intense behaviour. When the phlegm aspect predominates, with relatively less fire, the patient suffers from 'dian', characterised by mental confusion, lethargy and stupor. The ability of Fenglong ST-40 to transform phlegm, combined with the fact that the Stomach divergent channel connects with the Heart, and the Stomach primary channel with the Governing vessel (and thus the brain) at Shenting DU-24 and Renzhong DU-26, renders it particularly suitable in treating these disorders.

The Stomach luo-connecting channel from Fenglong ST-40 joins with all the yang channels in the head region. If phlegm-damp obstructs the upper jiao and the head, it may impair the ascent of clear yang to the head and sensory orifices, giving rise to dizziness and headache characterised by a heavy and clouded sensation. If interior wind rushes upwards, carrying phlegm with it, this is known as wind-phlegm and may give rise to such symptoms as epilepsy and severe dizziness. The Stomach luo-connecting channel terminates at the throat, and if stagnant qi impairs the ability of the Lung and Stomach to descend the fluids, phlegm is formed and combines with stagnant qi to obstruct the throat, giving rise to plumstone qi (globus hystericus) a sensation of throat blockage which worsens or ameliorates according to fluctuations in the emotional state and which is normally associated with stagnation of qi and phlegm.

A great variety of disorders affecting any region of the body may be caused by phlegm. This is expressed in the Chinese medicine sayings "There is no place that phlegm cannot reach", "The hundred diseases all pertain to phlegm", "Strange diseases often involve phlegm", and "Chronic disease often involves phlegm". Whatever the manifestations, if phlegm is a component of the pathology, Fenglong ST-40 is indicated.

Like many points of the foot yangming Stomach channel which is abundant in qi and blood, Fenglong ST-40 is indicated for channel disorders such as atrophy disorder and painful obstruction of the lower leg. Due to its ability to transform phlegm, Fenglong ST-40 is especially indicated in the treatment of hemiplegia due to wind-phlegm in the channels.

Finally the *Great Compendium of Acupuncture and Moxibustion* gives specific indications for excess and deficiency of the luo-connecting points. In the case of Fenglong ST-40, these are mania-depression (excess); lack of control of the legs and withering of the lower legs (deficiency).

COMBINATIONS

- All phlegm disease, head wind, dyspnoea and cough, all types of phlegm-fluid (tanyin): Fenglong ST-40 and Zhongwan REN-12 (*Outline of Medicine*).
- Cough with phlegm: Fenglong ST-40 and Feishu BL-13 (*Ode of the Jade Dragon*).
- Vomiting phlegm and watery saliva, dizziness that does not cease: Fenglong ST-40, Yangxi L.I.-5, Gongsun SP-4 and Shanzhong REN-17 (*Complete Collection*).
- Stabbing pain of the chest: Fenglong ST-40 and Qiuxu GB-40 (*Thousand Ducat Formulas*).
- Headache that is difficult to endure: Fenglong ST-40 and Qiangjian DU-18 (*One Hundred Symptoms*).
- Head wind and dizziness: Fenglong ST-40, Hegu L.I.-4, Jiexi ST-41 and Fengchi GB-20 (*Great Compendium*).
- Facial swelling: Fenglong ST-40, Tianshu ST-25, Lidui ST-45, Xiangu ST-43 and Chongyang ST-42 (*Thousand Ducat Formulas*).
- Mania disorder with rash behaviour, desires to ascend to high places and sing, discards clothing and runs around: Fenglong ST-40 and Chongyang ST-42 (*Thousand Ducat Formulas*).
- Loss of voice: Fenglong ST-40, Tiantu REN-22, Rangu KID-2, Yingu KID-10, Fuliu KID-7 and Lingdao HE-4 (*Illustrated Supplement*).

JIEXI ST-41

Stream Divide

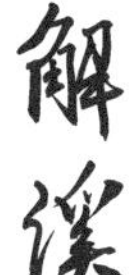

Jing-River and Fire point of the Stomach channel

LOCATION

On the ankle, level with the prominence of the lateral malleolus, in a depression between the tendons of extensor hallucis longus and extensor digitorum longus.

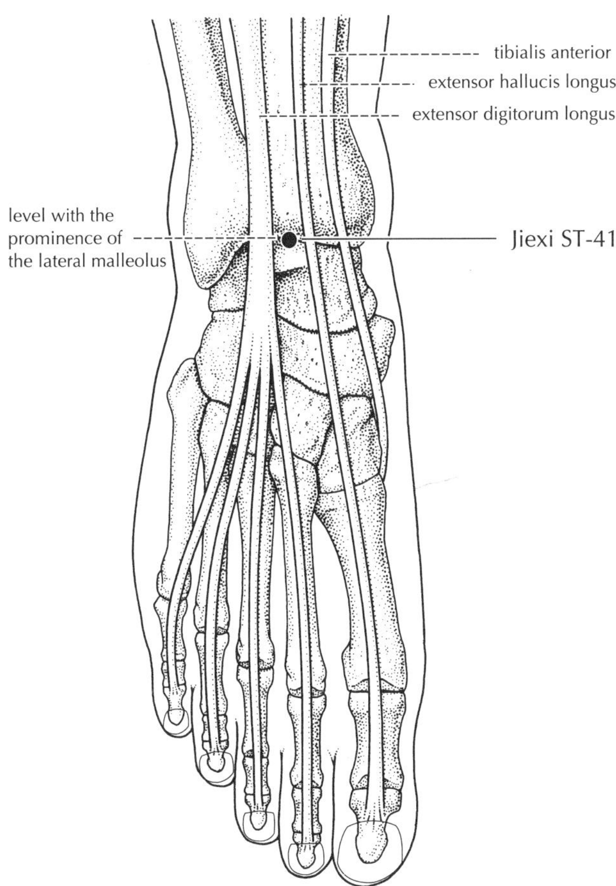

LOCATION NOTE

Ask the patient to extend the big toe against resistance in order to define the tendon of extensor hallucis longus, and locate Jiexi ST-41 lateral to this tendon and level with the prominence of the lateral malleolus. If in doubt, ask the patient to extend the remaining toes against resistance to define the tendon of extensor digitorum longus; Jiexi ST-41 is located between the two tendons.

NEEDLING

i. Perpendicular insertion 0.5 cun; ii. Oblique insertion beneath the tendons to join with Shangqiu SP-5 medially or Qiuxu GB-40 laterally.

Caution: the anterior tibial vessels and nerve lie deep to this point.

ACTIONS
Clears heat from the Stomach channel and fu
Calms the spirit
Activates the channel and alleviates pain

INDICATIONS
- Swelling of the face and head, frontal headache, pain of the eyebrow, head wind, redness of the face and eyes, visual dizziness, dizziness, pain in the mouth, biting of the tongue.
- Abdominal distention, abdominal distention after eating, belching with abdominal distention and fullness, hunger with inability to eat, constipation.
- Febrile disease with absence of sweating, malarial disorders, sudden turmoil disorder with cramps.
- Epilepsy, clonic spasm, mania, agitation, sadness and weeping, fright palpitations, Stomach heat with raving, seeing ghosts, hypertension.
- Swelling and pain of the ankle joint, drop-foot, atrophy disorder of the leg, heaviness of the knee and thigh, sciatica, sinew painful obstruction, damp painful obstruction, injury of the big toe.

COMMENTARY
It is an important principal of the five shu points that the more distal they are (i.e. close to the fingers or toes), the stronger their effect on treating their corresponding channel as a whole, and the opposite end of the channel in particular, whilst the more proximal they are (close to the knee and elbow), the more pronounced their action on the internal fu and the trunk and body portion of the channel. In terms of the Stomach channel Jiexi ST-41, the jing-river and fire point, lying as it does between the two extremes, has an equally important effect on clearing heat from both the channel and the fu.

The effectof Jiexi ST-41 on clearing heat from the Stomach channel, especially the upper part, is reflected in its ability to treat pain, swelling and inflammation in the yangming portion of the head, manifesting as frontal headache, redness of the face and eyes, mouth pain etc. Although swelling of the face is usually differentiated as either Spleen yang deficiency, or Lung qi deficiency complicated with invasion of exterior wind, Jiexi ST-41 is indicated here by virtue of its action of clearing the yangming channel which governs the face.

When heat accumulates in the Stomach fu it may: i. impair the descending function of the Stomach giving rise to abdominal distention and belching, ii. cause excessive hunger due to hyperactivity of yang, or iii. dessicate the fluids in the Stomach and intestines leading to hunger with inability to eat and constipation. Jiexi ST-41 is indicated in all three patterns.

Stomach fire may ascend along the Stomach divergent channel to the Heart, and along the Stomach primary channel which connects with the Governing vessel (and thus the brain) at Shenting DU-24 and Renzhong DU-26. The resulting disturbance of the spirit and Heart may give rise to various emotional disorders, especially of the manic kind, and palpitations associated with emotional changes such as fright. Jiexi ST-41 has a dual ability to clear heat from the Stomach and to calm and sedate the spirit.

Finally, Jiexi ST-41 is an important and much-used point in disorders of the lower leg. It is frequently combined with Biguan ST-31 and Zusanli ST-36 in the 'chain and lock' method for the treatment of atrophy disorder and hemiplegia. It may also be used as a distal point for disorders of the knee joint, and is important in the treatment of local disorders of the foot and ankle. For this purpose it may be directed laterally towards Qiuxu GB-40 for disorders of the middle and lateral portions of the ankle, and towards Shangqiu SP-5 for disorders of the middle and medial portions of the ankle. Needling to join with Shangqiu SP-5 is also applied for dual disharmony of the Stomach and Spleen.

COMBINATIONS
- Head wind with a splitting sensation, pain between the eyebrow and the eye: Jiexi ST-41, Hegu L.I.-4 and Yangbai GB-14 (*Classic of the Jade Dragon*).
- Head wind, redness of the face and eyes: Jiexi ST-41 and Tongli HE-5 (*Great Compendium*).
- Head wind and dizziness: Jiexi ST-41, Hegu L.I.-4, Fenglong ST-40 and Fengchi GB-20 (*Great Compendium*).
- Stagnation of food in the mid-abdomen, stabbing pain that does not cease: Jiexi ST-41, Zusanli ST-36, Gongsun SP-4 and Zhongwan REN-12 (*Complete Collection*).
- Sudden turmoil disorder: Jiexi ST-41, Juque REN-14, Guanchong SJ-1, Zhigou SJ-6 and Gongsun SP-4 (*Systematic Classic*).
- Sudden turmoil disorder: Jiexi ST-41, Yinlingquan SP-9, Chengshan BL-57 and Taibai SP-3 (*Great Compendium*).
- Fright palpitations and pounding of the Heart: Jiexi ST-41 and Yangjiao GB-35 (*One Hundred Symptoms*).
- Madness: Jiexi ST-41 and Shenmai BL-62 (*Thousand Ducat Formulas*).
- Weeping with grief: Jiexi ST-41, Xinshu BL-15, Shenmen HE-7 and Daling P-7 (*Supplementing Life*).
- Rebellious qi cough: Jiexi ST-41, Tianchi P-1, Tiantu REN-22, Shanzhong REN-17 and Jianzhongshu SI-15 (*Supplementing Life*).

CHONGYANG ST-42

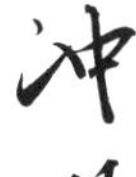
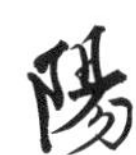

Rushing Yang

Yuan-Source point of the Stomach channel

LOCATION

On the dorsum of the foot, in the depression formed by the junction of the second and third metatarsal bones and the cuneiform bones (second and third), 1.5 cun distal to Jiexi ST-41, on the line drawn between Jiexi ST-41 and Xiangu ST-43, at the point where the pulsation of the dorsalis pedis artery may be palpated.

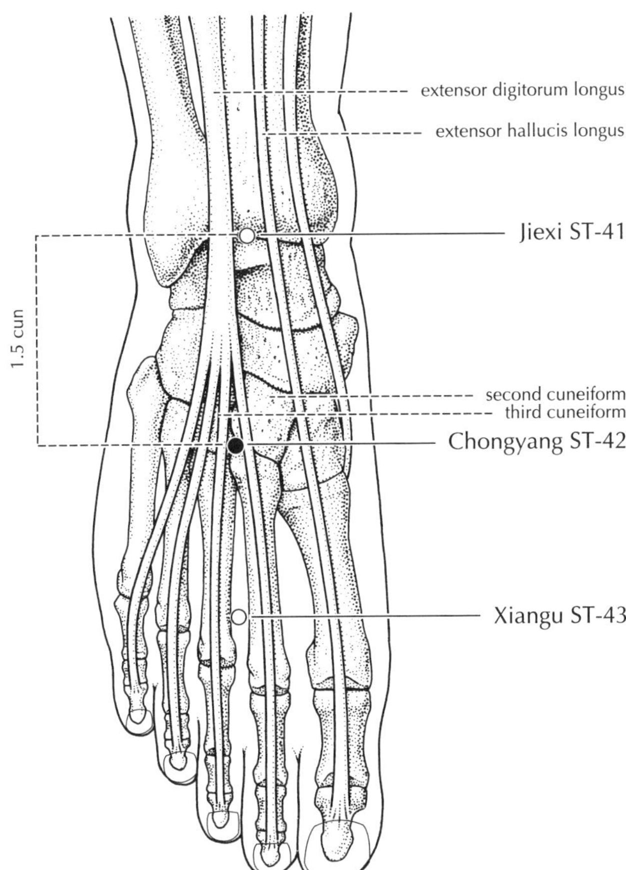

LOCATION NOTE

i. Run the finger proximally from Xiangu ST-43 towards Jiexi ST-41; the point is located in a depression approximately halfway between these two points; ii. This point may lie either side of the medial slip of the extensor digitorum longus tendon, which runs to the second toe.

NEEDLING

Oblique or perpendicular insertion 0.3 to 0.5 cun.

Caution: care should be taken not to puncture the dorsalis pedis artery which lies beneath this point.

ACTIONS

Clears heat from the Stomach channel
Harmonises the Stomach fu
Calms the spirit
Activates the channel and alleviates pain

INDICATIONS

- Deviation of the mouth and eye, swelling and pain of the face, swelling of the face, toothache, tooth decay, heat and pain of the inside of the mouth.
- Abdominal distention with no pleasure in eating, epigastric pain, vomiting.
- Fever with absence of sweating, chills and fever with malarial disorder.
- Mania-depression, desires to ascend to high places and sing, discards clothing and runs around.
- Swelling and pain of the dorsum of the foot, atrophy disorder of the foot.

COMMENTARY

In terms of its actions and indications Chongyang ST-42, the yuan-source point of the Stomach channel, is similar to Jiexi ST-41, although less commonly used in current-day clinical practice.

Chongyang ST-42 is located over the pulsation of the dorsalis pedis artery, and the *Essential Questions* suggests that the knee be raised in order to allow the artery to pulsate more clearly and thus assist in locating this point. This advice is echoed by the traditional observation that if the point Zusanli ST-36 is obstructed, the beating of the artery will be diminished, and in fact if the point Zusanli ST-36 is pressed firmly, the pulsation will disappear entirely.

COMBINATIONS

- Facial swelling: Chongyang ST-42, Tianshu ST-25, Fenglong ST-40, Lidui ST-45 and Xiangu ST-43 (*Thousand Ducat Formulas*).
- Tooth decay: Chongyang ST-42 and Qubin GB-7 (*Thousand Ducat Formulas*).
- Mania, desires to ascend to high places and sing, discards clothing and runs around: Chongyang ST-42, Shenmen HE-7 and Houxi SI-3 (*Great Compendium*).
- Mania disorder with rash behaviour, desires to ascend to high places and sing, discards clothing and runs around: Chongyang ST-42 and Fenglong ST-40 (*Thousand Ducat Formulas*).
- Flaccidity of the legs: Chongyang ST-42, Yanglingquan GB-34, Taichong LIV-3 and Qiuxu GB-40 (*Great Compendium*).
- One-sided wind (hemiplegia): Chongyang ST-42 and Lieque LU-7 (*Great Compendium*).

XIANGU ST-43

Sunken Valley

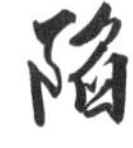

Shu-Stream and Wood point of the Stomach channel

LOCATION

On the dorsum of the foot, between the second and third metatarsal bones, in a depression 1 cun proximal to Neiting ST-44.

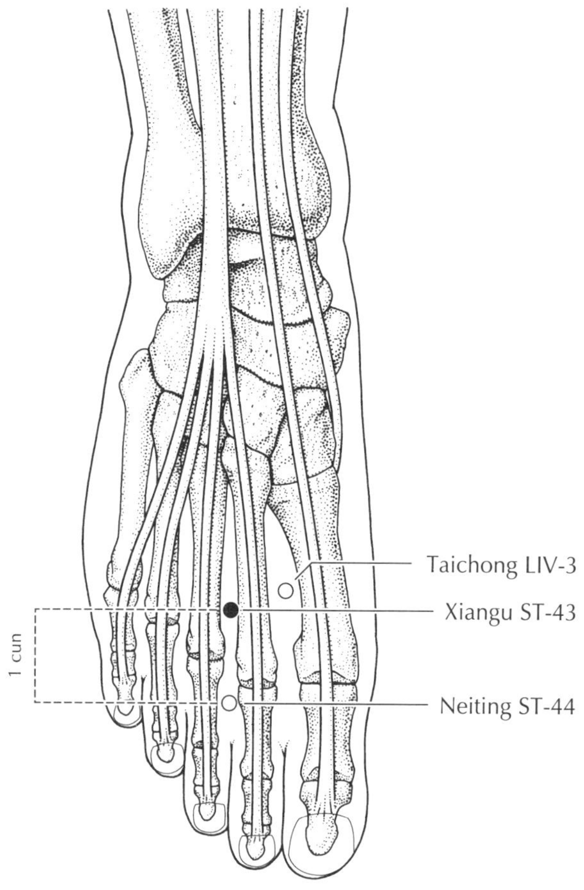

NEEDLING

Perpendicular or oblique insertion 0.5 to 1 cun.

ACTIONS

Regulates the Spleen and dispels oedema
Regulates and harmonises the Stomach and intestines

INDICATIONS

- Oedema, oedema and swelling of the face, pain and swelling of the eyes.
- Abdominal pain, abdominal distention and fullness, borborygmus, fullness of the chest and lateral costal region, belching.
- Fever with absence of sweating, cold shivering with malarial disorders.
- Swelling and pain of the dorsum of the foot, difficulty in flexing and extending the toes.

COMMENTARY

A number of classics cite Xiangu ST-43 for the treatment of oedema, especially of the face and eye region. The name Sunken Valley conjures up the image of a place where water accumulates and gathers, and is considered to reflect this image. Its application in oedema may be explained both by the course of the yangming channel which governs the face, and by the intimate relationship between the Stomach and the Spleen, which plays an important role in the transportation and transformation of fluids. The action of Xiangu ST-43 on regulating the Spleen is further reflected by its use in the treatment of borborygmus and abdominal distention.

Xiangu ST-43 is traditionally indicated for disorders such as swelling and pain of the dorsum of the foot and difficulty in flexing and extending the toes. In more recent times, however, Xiangu ST-43 has been used in combination with Hegu L.I.-4 in the treatment of febrile painful obstruction in any region of the body. Febrile painful obstruction is painful obstruction which manifests with redness, swelling, heat and pain of the joints, aversion to heat in the affected area and systemic signs such as fever, constipation, thirst etc.

COMBINATIONS

- Sudden swelling of the face: Xiangu ST-43, Shangxing DU-23, Xinhui DU-22, Qianding DU-21 and Gongsun SP-4 (*Supplementing Life*).
- Facial swelling: Xiangu ST-43, Tianshu ST-25, Fenglong ST-40, Lidui ST-45 and Chongyang ST-42 (*Thousand Ducat Formulas*).
- Oedema: Xiangu ST-43, Lieque LU-7, Yanggu SI-5, Hegu L.I.-4, Jianshi P-5, Yanglingquan GB-34, Yingu KID-10, Zusanli ST-36, Ququan LIV-8, Jiexi ST-41, Fuliu KID-7, Gongsun SP-4, Lidui ST-45, Chongyang ST-42, Yinlingquan SP-9, Weishu BL-21, Shuifen REN-9 and Shenque REN-8 (*Great Compendium*).
- Post-partum belching: Xiangu ST-43 and Qimen LIV-14 (*Supplementing Life*).
- Borborygmus: Xiangu ST-43 and Xiawan REN-10 (*One Hundred Symptoms*).
- Pain of intestinal abscess: Xiangu ST-43, Taibai SP-3 and Dachangshu BL-25 (*Great Compendium*).

NEITING ST-44

Inner Courtyard

内庭

Ying-Spring and Water point of the Stomach channel
Ma Dan-yang Heavenly Star point

LOCATION

On the dorsum of the foot, between the second and third toes, 0.5 cun proximal to the margin of the web.

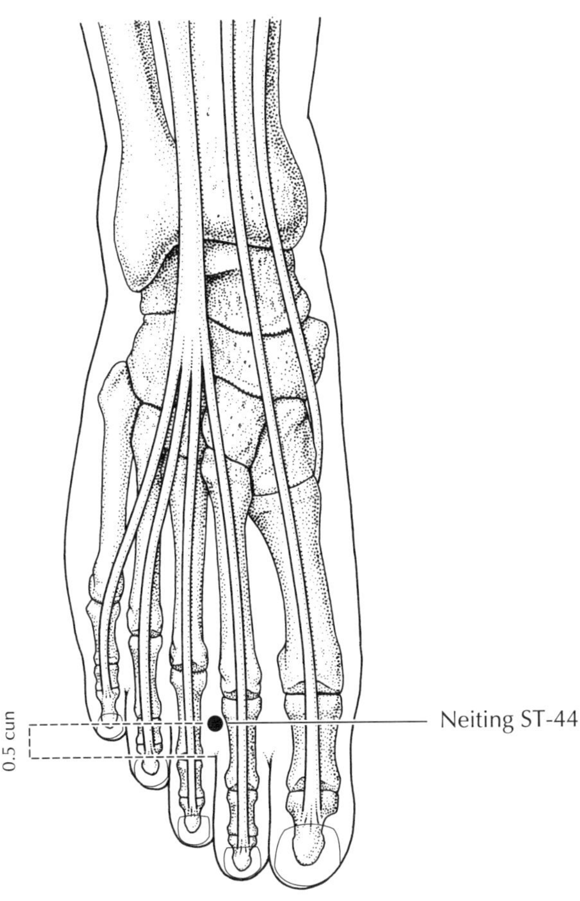

NEEDLING

i. Perpendicular insertion 0.5 cun; ii. Oblique insertion directed proximally, 0.5 to 1 cun.

ACTIONS

Clears heat from the Stomach channel and alleviates pain
Harmonises the intestines and clears damp-heat
Calms the spirit

INDICATIONS

- Toothache, pain of the lower teeth, pain of the upper teeth, pain of the eye, pain of the face, deviation of the mouth and eye, nosebleed, throat painful obstruction, tinnitus, thirst.
- Abdominal pain, distention of the lower abdomen, borborygmus, diarrhoea, dysenteric disorder, blood in the stool, constipation.
- Febrile disease with absence of sweating, malarial disorders with no pleasure in eating, cold shivering, aversion to cold, hands and feet counterflow cold, hot inversion, urticaria, pain of the skin of the chest, blood in the urine.
- Aversion to the sound of people talking, desire for silence, frequent yawning.
- Pain and swelling of the dorsum of the foot.

COMMENTARY

Neiting ST-44, the ying-spring and water point of the Stomach channel, was included by Ma Dan-yang, the great physician of the Jin dynasty, among his 'eleven heavenly star points'[20], his grouping of the most vital acupuncture points of the human body.

According to the *Classic of Difficulties*[41] ying-spring points are indicated for "heat in the body". As a distal point, the principal action of Neiting ST-44 is to clear heat and fire from the Stomach channel, most especially its upper portion. It is a primary point in the treatment of many heat disorders of the head and face such as toothache, pain of the face or eye, nosebleed, throat painful obstruction etc. It is frequently combined for this purpose with Hegu L.I.-4. In the treatment of toothache, some sources recommend the use of Neiting ST-44 for the lower jaw and Hegu L.I.-4 for the upper jaw, whilst others consider Neiting ST-44 equally adept at treating both the upper and lower jaw. This is borne out by the pathway of the Stomach primary channel which descends from the eye region to enter the upper gum, joins the Governing vessel at Renzhong DU-26 and then circles around the lips and descends to meet the Conception vessel at Chengjiang REN-24. Pain of the face almost invariably involves disorder of the Stomach channel, and Neiting ST-44 is an essential point in the treatment of disorders such as trigeminal neuralgia, often in combination with local points such as Dicang ST-4, Jiache ST-6 and Xiaguan ST-7. The Stomach channel also makes various connections with the throat and nose. The primary channel descends alongside the throat, the luo-connecting channel terminates at the throat, the primary channel originates at Yingxiang L.I.-20 and ascends to the root of the nose and the divergent channel passes alongside the nose. Both throat painful obstruction and nosebleed can be due to heat accumulating in the yangming channel, in the latter case causing reckless movement of the blood.

The second important action of Neiting ST-44 is to harmonise the intestines and clear dampness and heat, and it is indicated in the treatment of such disorders as diarrhoea, dysenteric disorder, blood in the stools, constipation and abdominal pain.

One special condition for which Neiting ST-44 is indicated is the symptom of hands and feet counterflow cold, where only the hands and feet are cold but the body is warm. This may occur in the pattern known as 'true heat, false cold', where heat constrained in the interior prevents the yang qi from circulating to the limbs. Despite the apparent cold, the other symptoms, as well as the pulse and the tongue, are indicative of heat and constraint. This condition must be differentiated from 'cold collapse' (cold inversion) where either the whole limb or the areas distal to the elbows and knees are cold.

Finally, like many points of the Stomach channel, Neiting ST-44 has an action on calming the spirit. It is particularly suited to the treatment of depressive type disorders, and is indicated for aversion to the sound of people talking and a desire for silence.

COMBINATIONS

- Pain of the eyeball: Neiting ST-44 and Shangxing DU-23 (*Great Compendium*).
- Throat pain: Neiting ST-44, Zhongzhu SJ-3 and Zhigou SJ-6 (*Thousand Ducat Formulas*).
- Injury by cold with absence of sweating: Neiting ST-44 (reduce), Hegu L.I.-4 (reinforce), Fuliu KID-7 (reduce) and Bailao (M-HN-30) (*Great Compendium*).
- Injury by cold with sweating: Neiting ST-44 (reduce), Hegu L.I.-4 (reduce), Fuliu KID-7 (reinforce) and Bailao (M-HN-30) (*Great Compendium*).
- Loss of consciousness from summerheat stroke: Neiting ST-44, Renzhong DU-26, Hegu L.I-4, Baihui DU-20, Zhongji REN-3 and Qihai REN-6 (*Great Compendium*).
- Red (bloody) dysenteric disorder: Neiting ST-44, Tianshu ST-25, Yinbai SP-1, Qihai REN-6, Zhaohai KID-6 and Neiguan P-6 (*Great Compendium*).
- All types of diarrhoea and abdominal disorders: Neiting ST-44 and Zusanli ST-36 (*Miscellaneous Diseases*).
- Undigested food (in the stool), no pleasure in eating, periumbilical pain: Neiting ST-44, Lidui ST-45 and Tianshu ST-25 (*Supplementing Life*).
- Chronic malaria with no pleasure in eating: Neiting ST-44, Gongsun SP-4 and Lidui ST-45 (*Great Compendium*).
- Oedema of the four limbs: Neiting ST-44, Sanyinjiao SP-6, Zhongdu LIV-6, Hegu L.I.-4, Quchi L.I.-11, Zhongzhu SJ-3, Yemen SJ-2, Xingjian LIV-2 and Yinlingquan SP-9 (*Great Compendium*).
- Fullness and distention of the Heart and abdomen: Neiting ST-44 and Xuanzhong GB-39 (*Great Compendium*).

LIDUI ST-45
Strict Exchange

厲兌

Jing-Well and Metal point of the Stomach channel

LOCATION

On the dorsal aspect of the second toe, at the junction of lines drawn along the lateral border of the nail and the base of the nail, approximately 0.1 cun from the corner of the nail.

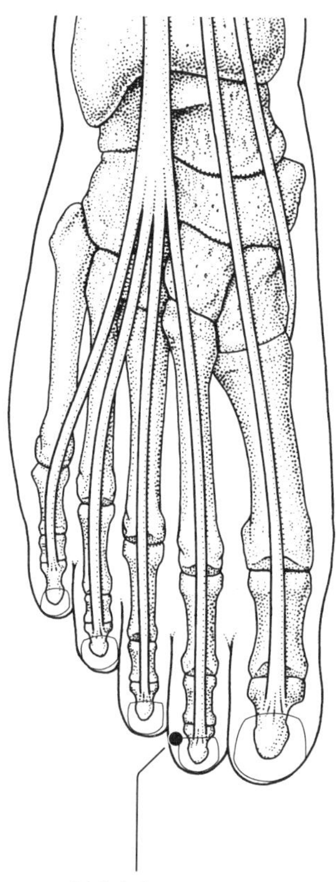

Lidui ST-45

NEEDLING

Perpendicular or oblique insertion directed proximally 0.1 to 0.2 cun, or prick to bleed.

ACTIONS

Clears heat from the Stomach channel
Clears heat, calms the spirit and restores consciousness

INDICATIONS

- Swelling of the face, heat in the head, nosebleed, yellow nasal discharge, rhinitis with nosebleed, toothache, lockjaw, throat painful obstruction, cracked lips, deviation of the mouth.

- Fullness and distention of the chest and abdomen, excessive hunger, lack of appetite, inversion counterflow, malaria, febrile disease, febrile disease with absence of sweating, yellow urine, jaundice.
- Loss of consciousness.
- Excessive dreaming, easily frightened with desire to sleep, insomnia, dizziness, mania-depression, desires to ascend to high places and sing, discards clothing and runs around.
- Sensation of cold in the shin, cold of the lower limbs and feet, swelling and pain of the knee.

COMMENTARY

The two principal actions of Lidui ST-45 are to clear heat from the Stomach channel (and to a certain extent the Stomach fu) and to clear heat and calm the spirit. In addition, in common with all the jing-well points, Lidui ST-45 may be used to restore consciousness.

According to the *Spiritual Pivot*[42] "When the disease is above select [points] from below". This statement emphasises the strong action that the most distal channel points have on treating disorders at the opposite end of the channel. Lidui ST-45 is especially indicated when yangming channel heat rises to the face, nose, teeth and lips, giving rise to such symptoms as swelling of the face, toothache, cracked lips, nosebleed, yellow nasal discharge etc. It is also indicated for heat in the Stomach fu giving rise to excessive hunger.

The action of Lidui ST-45 in clearing heat and calming the spirit is shared by many of the points of the Stomach channel. This is explained both by the pathway of the Stomach divergent channel to the Heart and that of the primary channel which joins with the Governing vessel at Shenting DU-24 and Renzhong DU-26. Lidui ST-45 also shares with the jing-well points as a whole a special ability to calm the spirit, especially in acute situations. It is indicated in the treatment of manic disorders characterised in classical texts by the indications "desires to ascend to high places and sing, discards clothing and runs around", and is especially used for insomnia with excessive dreaming due to fire or phlegm-heat. Its action on insomnia is shared by several of the jing-well points of the feet (Yinbai SP-1, Yongquan KID-1 and Zuqiaoyin GB-44), reflecting the perception that in order to induce sleep, pathologically ascending qi, yang or fire must be drawn downwards. In severe intractable cases of insomnia, moxibustion may be applied to Lidui ST-45. This technique of 'drawing the fire down' is based on the principle 'small fire attracts big fire'. In common with many acupuncture points, Lidui ST-45 has a homeostatic action, and may also be used for depressive disorders characterised by withdrawal and excessive desire to sleep, thus emphasising its ability to calm and regulate the spirit in a variety of situations.

COMBINATIONS

- Facial swelling: Lidui ST-45, Chongyang ST-42, Fenglong ST-40, Tianshu ST-25 and Xiangu ST-43 (*Thousand Ducat Formulas*).
- Nightmares: Lidui ST-45 and Yinbai SP-1 (*One Hundred Symptoms*).
- Somnolence: Lidui ST-45 and Dadun LIV-1 (*Supplementing Life*).
- Somnolence with no desire to move the four limbs: Lidui ST-45, Sanjian L.I.-3, Sanyangluo SJ-8, Tianjing SJ-10 and Zuwuli LIV-10 (*Thousand Ducat Formulas*).
- Somnolence: Lidui ST-45, Taixi KID-3, Zhaohai KID-6, Baihui DU-20, Tianjing GB-21, Erjian L.I.-2, Sanjian L.I.-3 and Ganshu BL-18 (*Great Compendium*).
- Excessive fright: Lidui ST-45, Erjian L.I.-2, Yinxi HE-6 and Jianshi P-5 (*Supplementing Life*).
- Weakness of the legs: Moxa Lidui ST-45, Taichong LIV-3 and Fengshi GB-31 (*Outline of Medicine*).

NOTES

1 *Spiritual Pivot* Chapter 9.
2 *Spiritual Pivot* Chapter 7.
3 *Essential Questions* Chapter 63.
4 *Spiritual Pivot* Chapter 9 and *Essential Questions* Chapter 70.
5 *Spiritual Pivot* Chapter 21.
6 *Spiritual Pivot* Chapter 33.
7 *Essential Questions* Chapter 47.
8 *Essential Questions* Chapter 61.
9 *The Heart & Essence of Dan-xi's Methods of Treatment*, A Translation of Zhu Dan-xi's Dan Xi Zhi Fa Xin Yao, Blue Poppy Press, p. 315.
10 Ibid.
11 *Spiritual Pivot* Chapter 2.
12 The *Ode to Elucidate Mysteries* says that Dabao SP-21 dominates the upper region, Tianshu ST-25 the middle region, and Diji SP-8 the lower region.
13 Quoted in *Grasping the Wind*, by Andrew Ellis, Nigel Wiseman and Ken Boss, Paradigm Publications, 1989, page 79.
14 Many classical texts ascribe these two names to the point Qixue KID-13. The *Supplement to the Thousand Ducat Formulas*, however, is quite clear that the point is Shuidao ST-28, referring to the points located 2 cun either side of Guanyuan REN-4.
15 *Essential Questions* Chapter 62.
16 *Essential Questions* Chapter 61.
17 *Spiritual Pivot* Chapter 33.

18 *Essential Questions* Chapter 61.

19 *Spiritual Pivot* Chapter 78.

20 Ma Dan-yang was the originator of the *Song of the Eleven Heavenly Star Points*. They first appeared in print in the 12th century CE *Classic of the Jade Dragon*. Xu Feng included this text in his work *Complete Collection of Acupuncture and Moxibustion* and added a twelfth point, Taichong LIV-3.

21 *Classic of Difficulties* 68th Difficulty.

22 *Spiritual Pivot* Chapters 4 and 44 respectively.

23 *Spiritual Pivot* Chapter 19.

24 *Classic of Categories*.

25 *Spiritual Pivot* Chapter 56.

26 *Spiritual Pivot* Chapter 60.

27 *Essential Questions* Chapter 18.

28 *Spiritual Pivot* Chapter 33.

29 *Spiritual Pivot* Chapter 78.

30 i. Heart taxation: principally involving damage to Heart blood, ii. Spleen taxation: overeating or excessive worry and pensiveness injure the Spleen qi, iii. Lung taxation: depletion of Lung qi or yin iv. Kidney taxation: damage to Kidney qi from excessive sex, v. Liver taxation: injury to Liver qi by mental excitement with such signs as unclear vision, pain of the chest and hypochondrium, flaccid muscles and tendons and difficulty of movement.

31 *Essential Questions* Chapter 29.

32 *Spiritual Pivot* Chapter 19.

33 *Essential Questions* Chapter 61.

34 *Spiritual Pivot* Chapter 2.

35 *Essential Questions* Chapter 61.

36 *Essential Questions* Chapter 61.

37 *Spiritual Pivot* Chapter 2.

38 *Essential Questions* Chapter 61.

39 *Essential Questions* Chapter 74.

40 Quoted in *Chinese Acupuncture and Moxibustion*, Foreign Languages Press, Beijing.

41 *Classic of Difficulties* 68th Difficulty.

42 *Spiritual Pivot* Chapter 9.

足太陰脾經

THE SPLEEN CHANNEL OF FOOT TAIYIN

THE SPLEEN CHANNEL OF FOOT TAIYIN

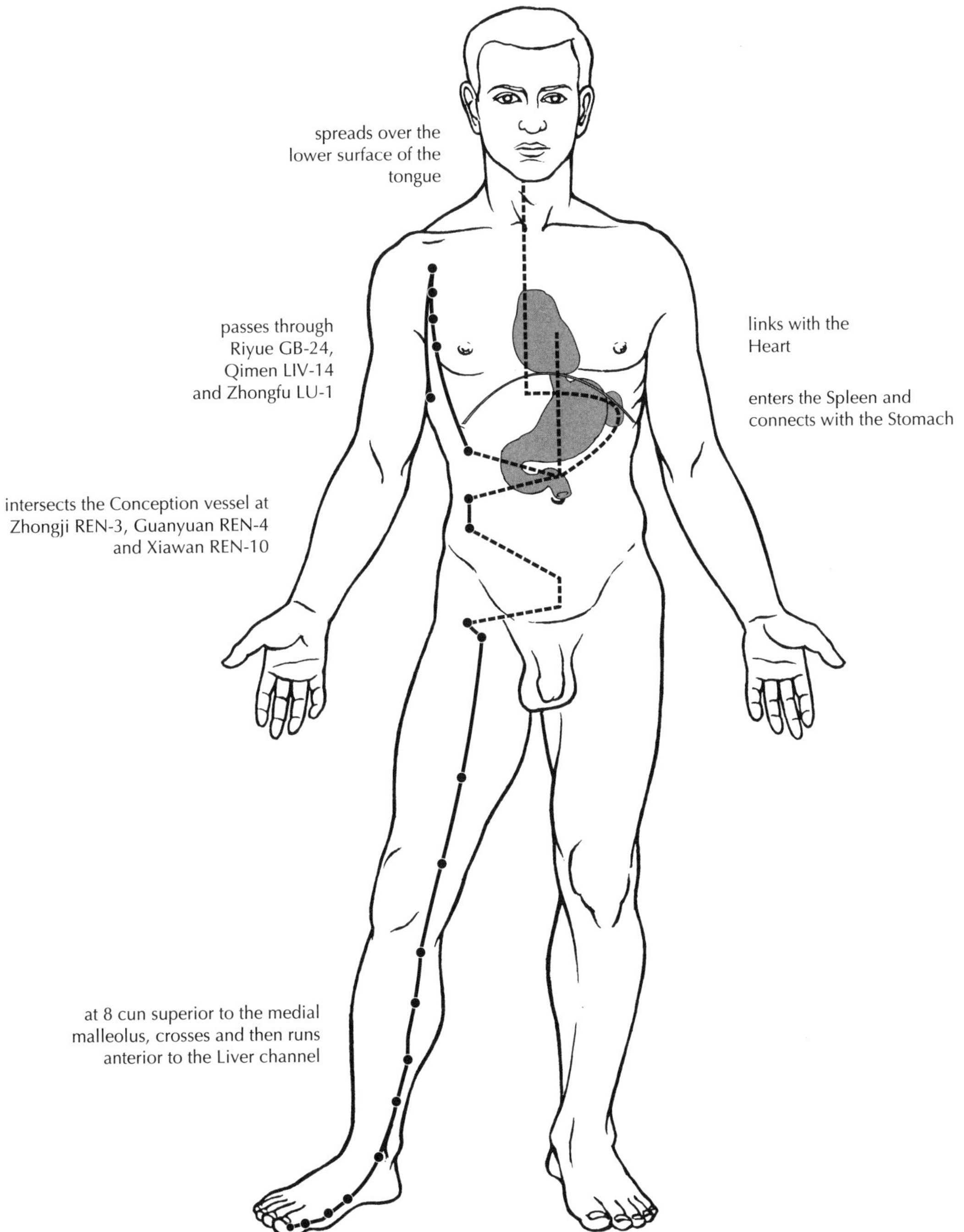
spreads over the lower surface of the tongue
passes through Riyue GB-24, Qimen LIV-14 and Zhongfu LU-1
links with the Heart
enters the Spleen and connects with the Stomach
intersects the Conception vessel at Zhongji REN-3, Guanyuan REN-4 and Xiawan REN-10
at 8 cun superior to the medial malleolus, crosses and then runs anterior to the Liver channel

THE SPLEEN PRIMARY CHANNEL

- begins at the medial side of the tip of the big toe at Yinbai SP-1,
- runs along the medial aspect of the foot, following the border where the skin changes colour,
- ascends in front of the medial malleolus at Shangqiu SP-5,
- follows the posterior border of the tibia up the medial aspect of the leg to a point 8 cun superior to the medial malleolus where it crosses (and then travels anterior to) the Liver channel,
- ascends along the medial aspect of the knee and the antero-medial aspect of the thigh to the lower abdomen where it intersects the Conception vessel at Zhongji REN-3, Guanyuan REN-4 and Xiawan REN-10 before entering the Spleen and connecting with the Stomach,

- emerges in the region of the Stomach and ascends first at 4 cun lateral to the midline then at 6 cun lateral to the midline, passing through Riyue GB-24, Qimen LIV-14 and Zhongfu LU-1, and descends to terminate in the seventh intercostal space on the mid-axillary line at Dabao SP-21.

A branch

- ascends through the diaphragm, runs alongside the oesophagus and spreads over the lower surface of the tongue.

A further branch

- ascends from the Stomach, passes through the diaphragm and flows to link with the Heart.

The Spleen primary channel connects with the following zangfu: Spleen, Stomach, Heart.

The Spleen primary channel meets with other channels at the following points: Zhongfu LU-1, Riyue GB-24, Qimen LIV-14, Zhongji REN-3, Guanyuan REN-4, Xiawan REN-10.

Note: Shanzhong REN-17 is classified as a meeting point of the Spleen primary channel with the Conception vessel, but descriptions of the Spleen channel pathway do not conventionally mention this point.

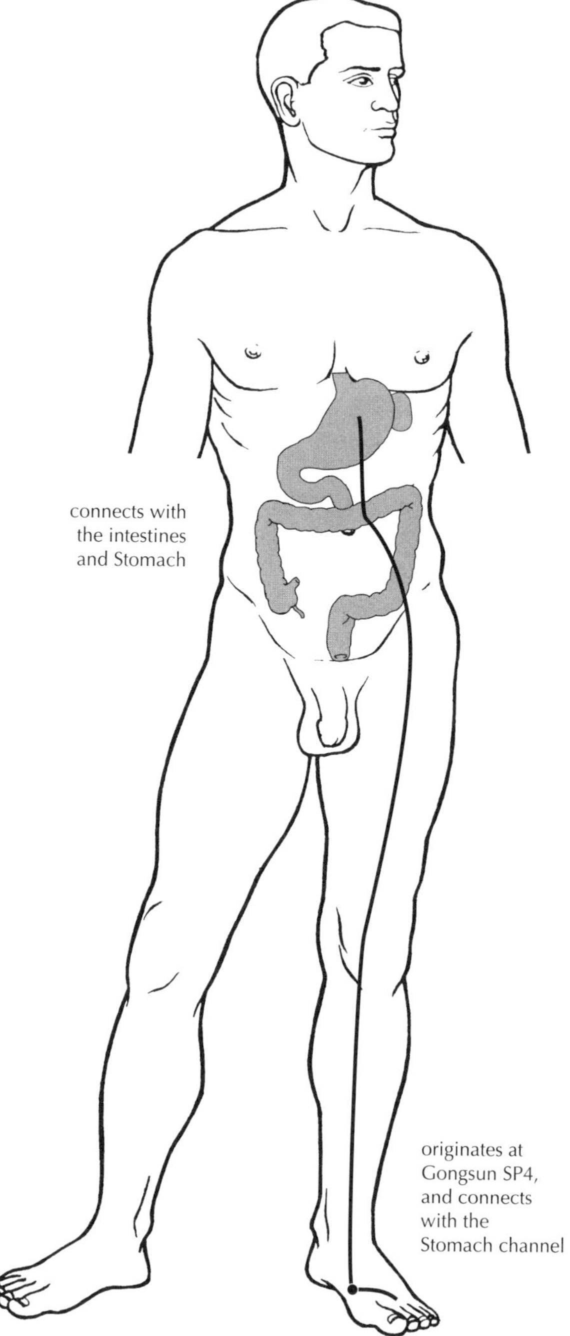

The luo-connecting channel of the Spleen

THE SPLEEN LUO-CONNECTING CHANNEL

- originates at Gongsun SP-4,
- connects with the Stomach channel,
- enters the abdomen and connects with the intestines and Stomach.

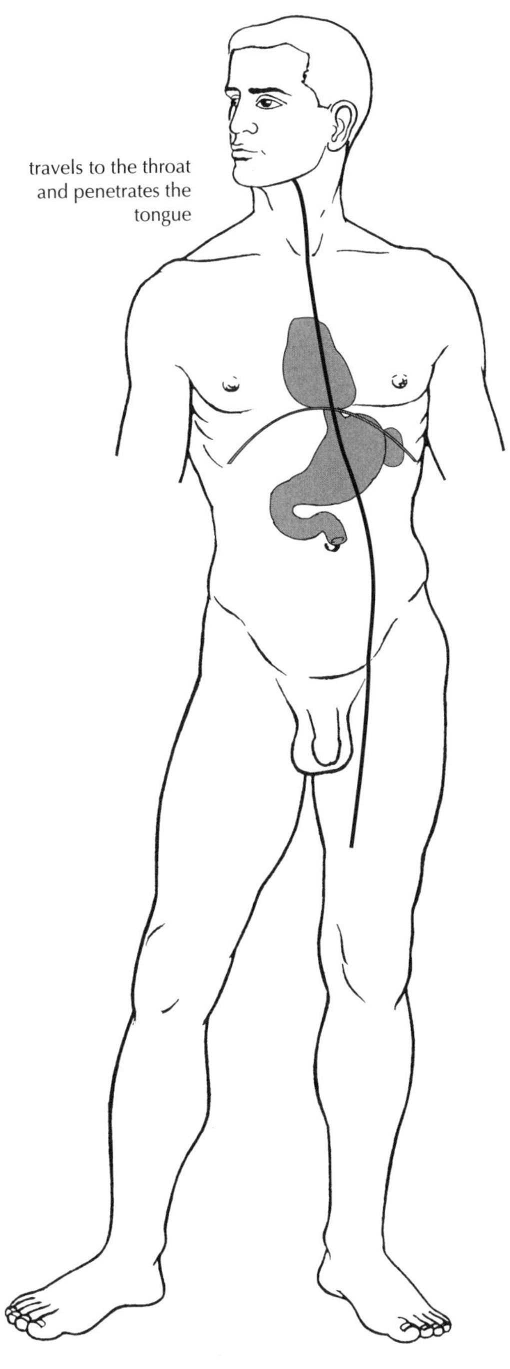

The divergent channel of the Spleen

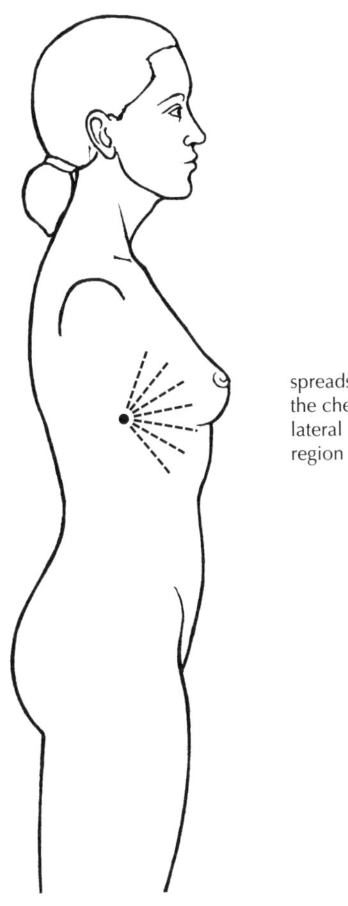

The great luo-connecting channel of the Spleen

THE SPLEEN DIVERGENT CHANNEL

- branches from the primary channel in the middle of the anterior thigh,
- follows the Stomach divergent channel to the throat where it penetrates the tongue.

THE GREAT LUO-CONNECTING CHANNEL OF THE SPLEEN

- separates from the primary channel at Dabao SP-21 on the lateral aspect of the chest,
- spreads through the chest and lateral costal region, gathering the blood of the luo-connecting channels of the whole body.

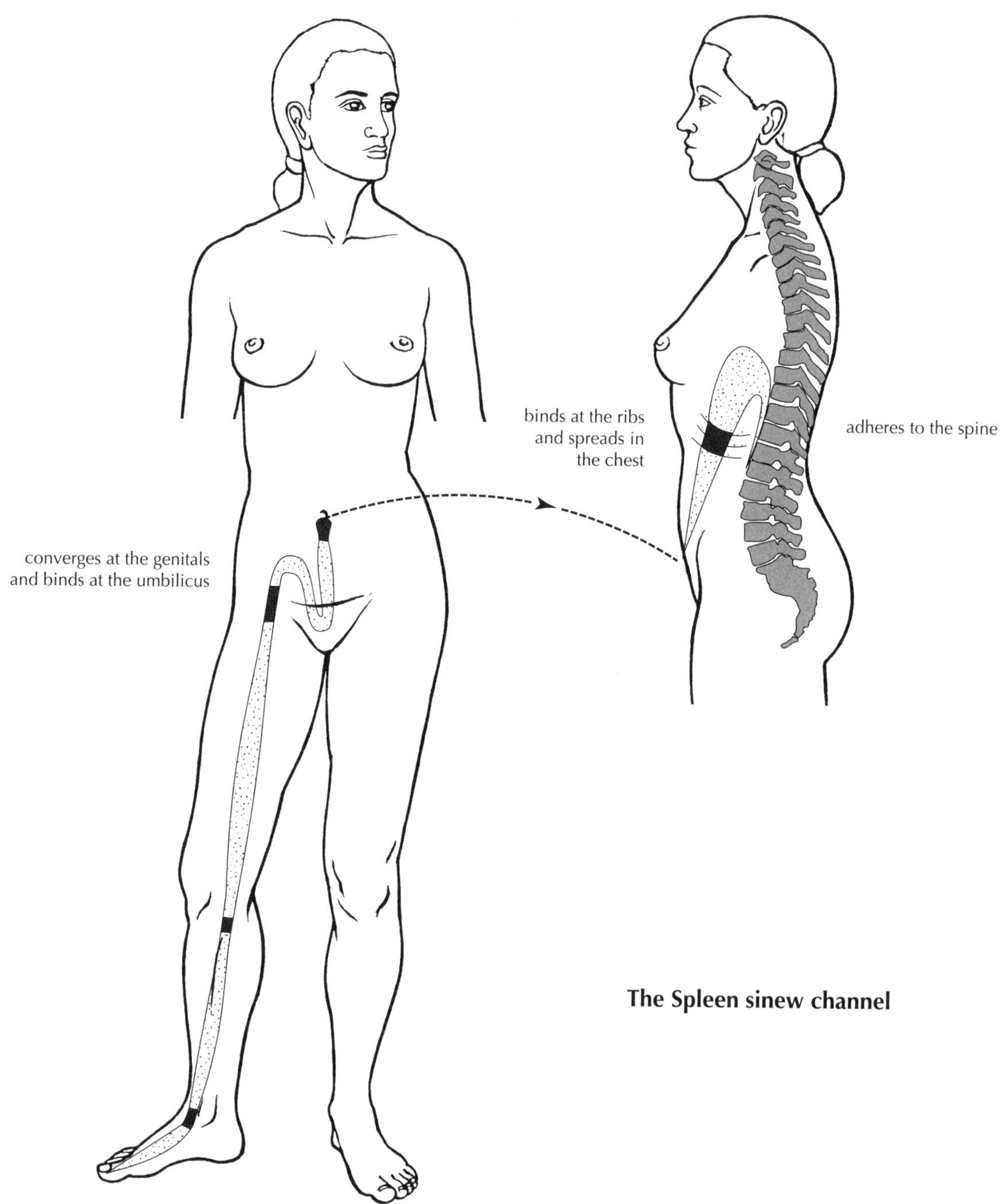

The Spleen sinew channel

THE SPLEEN SINEW CHANNEL

- begins at the medial side of the big toe at Yinbai SP-1 and ascends the foot to bind at the medial malleolus at Shangqiu SP-5,
- ascends the medial aspect of the tibia to bind at the medial side of the knee at Yinlingquan SP-9,
- follows the medial face of the thigh to bind in the groin before converging at the external genitalia,
- ascends the abdomen to bind at the umbilicus,
- enters the abdomen, binds at the ribs and spreads in the chest,
- from the inside of the chest a branch adheres to the spine.

Pathological Symptoms of the Spleen sinew channel
Strained big toe, pain of the medial malleolus, pain and cramping (along the course of the channel), pain of the medial aspect of the knee, pain of the medial thigh that reaches the inguinal region, twisting pain of the genitals that may reach the navel and the lateral costal region or lead to pain of the chest and interior spine.

DISCUSSION

The Spleen channel of foot taiyin is interiorly-exteriorly coupled with the Stomach channel, and paired with the Lung channel of hand taiyin according to six channel theory. The Spleen-Stomach relationship is further strengthened by the fact that:

- the interior pathway of the Spleen primary channel connects with the Stomach fu.
- the Spleen luo-connecting channel connects with both the Stomach channel and the Stomach fu.
- the Spleen divergent channel connects with the Stomach divergent channel.

In addition, it is important to note that:

- the Spleen primary channel joins with the Conception vessel below the umbilicus at Zhongji REN-3 and Guanyuan REN-4 and above the umbilicus at Xiawan REN-10.
- the Spleen primary channel passes through the hypochondrium (meeting with the Gall Bladder and Liver channels at Riyue GB-24 and Qimen LIV-14).
- the Spleen primary channel ascends along the chest to meet with the Lung channel at Zhongfu LU-1, whilst the sinew channel spreads in the chest.
- the Spleen primary channel passes through the lateral costal region at points Shidou SP-17, Tianxi SP-18, Xiongxiang SP-19, Zhourong SP-20 and Dabao SP-21.
- both the Spleen primary and divergent channels connect with the tongue.
- the Spleen primary channel connects with the Heart zang.
- the Spleen luo-connecting channel connects with the intestines.
- the Spleen sinew channel converges at the external genitalia.

The Spleen has five principal functions:

- Dominating the transportation and transformation of the liquid and solid products of digestion after they have been 'rotted and ripened' by the Stomach. It therefore plays a major role in the digestive process, the production of qi and blood, the function of the intestines and the proper discharge of fluid.
- Controlling the blood, dominating the first stage of its formation and holding it in its proper place and preventing haemorrhage.
- Dominating the muscles and the four limbs, providing vigour and bulk.
- Opening into the mouth and dominating the sense of taste.
- Controlling the raising of qi to counteract sinking and prolapse.

It is by virtue of these functions as well as the channel pathways discussed above, that many of the actions and indications of the points of the Spleen channel can be explained. These can be summarised as:

- treating failure of the transportation and transformation function, resulting in borborygmus, loose stools, undigested food in the stool, poor appetite etc.
- treating disorders of the intestines such as dysenteric disorder, diarrhoea and constipation.
- treating retention of dampness and consequent qi stagnation resulting in distention and pain of the abdomen, oedema, heaviness of the body, soreness of the muscles and joints, swelling of the four limbs, difficult urination, leucorrhoea, somnolence, lethargy etc.
- tonifying qi and blood.
- resolving blood stasis, especially in the uterus, and cooling the blood.
- reinforcing the Spleen function of holding blood in its proper place.
- raising qi and treating prolapse.
- treating dyspnoea, fullness and distention of the chest and lateral costal region, sighing etc.
- calming and regulating the spirit.
- treating disorders of the genitals.

YINBAI SP-1

Hidden White

隱白

Jing-Well and Wood point of the Spleen channel
Sun Si-miao Ghost point

LOCATION

On the dorsal aspect of the big toe, at the junction of lines drawn along the medial border of the nail and the base of the nail, approximately 0.1 cun from the corner of the nail.

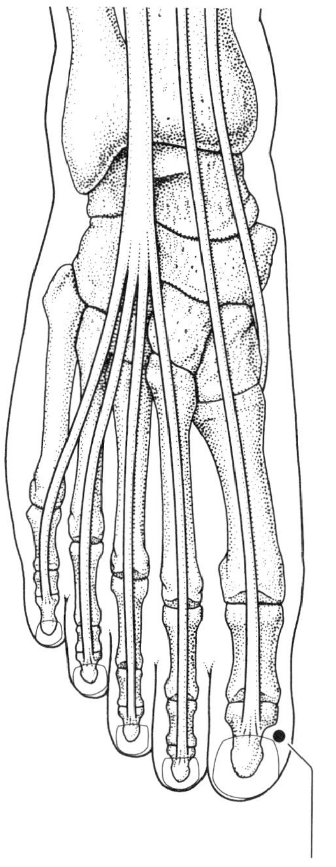

Yinbai SP-1

NEEDLING

Perpendicular or oblique insertion directed proximally 0.1 to 0.2 cun, or prick to bleed.

ACTIONS

Stops bleeding
Regulates the Spleen
Unbinds the chest
Calms the Heart and spirit and restores consciousness

INDICATIONS

- Uterine bleeding, menorrhagia, blood in the urine, blood in the stool, vomiting blood, nosebleed, febrile disease with nosebleed.
- Abdominal distention, sudden swelling of the four limbs, sudden diarrhoea, vomiting, no desire to eat or drink, difficult ingestion.
- Agitation, heat in the chest, fullness of the chest, dyspnoea, sighing, propensity to sadness, mania-depression, excessive dreaming, insomnia, chronic childhood fright wind, loss of consciousness.
- Fever with absence of sweating, cold feet, cold sensation in the lower leg.

COMMENTARY

According to the *Supplement to the Thousand Ducat Formulas* "The Spleen gathers the blood; when the Spleen is deficient it is unable to unite the blood", whilst the *Treatise on Disorders of Blood* states "When Spleen yang is deficient it is unable to gather the blood". Yinbai SP-1, the jing-well point of the Spleen channel, is one of the foremost acupuncture points for strengthening the Spleen's function of holding blood in its proper place. When this function is impaired there will be haemorrhage, usually chronic in nature, and occurring in any part of the body but most commonly in the lower jiao, whether as uterine bleeding or as bleeding into the urine or stools. In such cases moxibustion (either by moxa stick or direct cones) at Yinbai SP-1 is frequently employed, and it is particularly helpful to instruct the patient in the daily use of moxibustion at home. The action of Yinbai SP-1 on stopping bleeding, however, is not confined to cases of Spleen deficiency, but may also be applied where heat enters the blood level giving rise to reckless bleeding. This may manifest either in the lower or the upper part of the body (for example nosebleed or vomiting of blood). In these cases, needling or pricking to bleed is the usual method employed, although some physicians prefer to use moxibustion, despite the presence of heat.

The *Essential Questions*[1] states "Dampness, swelling and fullness all pertain to the Spleen". Yinbai SP-1 is able to regulate the Spleen in the treatment of disorders such as abdominal distention, swelling of the limbs, diarrhoea etc., but as the jing-well and therefore most dynamic point of the Spleen channel, is principally indicated when these disorders are acute and of sudden onset.

According to the *Classic of Difficulties*[2] jing-well points are indicated for "fullness below the Heart". Whilst the region 'below the Heart' specifically refers to the upper epigastrium, like many of the jing-well points Yinbai SP-1 treats fullness in the chest region as a whole. The Spleen primary channel ascends through the chest and lateral costal regions, connecting with points Riyue GB-24, Qimen LIV-14 and Zhongfu LU-1, and terminates at Dabao SP-21 from where the great luo-connecting channel of the Spleen, like the Spleen sinew channel, spreads into the chest, ribs and lateral costal region. Yinbai SP-1, as the starting point of the channel, is especially effective at treating the opposite end of the channel and is indicated for a variety of disorders such as heat in the chest, fullness of the chest, dyspnoea and sighing.

The Spleen channel links with the Heart, reinforcing the close physiological relationship between the two zang. Yinbai SP-1, like many of the jing-well points, is indicated for disorders of the Heart and spirit, in this case agitation of the Heart, mania-depression and propensity to sadness. Like Lidui ST-45, it is especially used for insomnia with excessive or restless dreaming and nightmares, and in clinical practice these two points may be combined for this purpose. Such is its action on the spirit that it was included by Sun Si-miao under its alternative name of Guilei (Ghost Fortress) among the 'thirteen ghost points' for the treatment of mania-depression and epilepsy.

Finally, Yinbai SP-1 shares with most of the other jing-well points the action of reviving and restoring the senses and is indicated for loss of consciousness.

COMBINATIONS

- Haemorrhage: needle Yinbai SP-1 and moxa Zusanli ST-36 (*Glorious Anthology*).
- Red (bloody) dysenteric disorder: Yinbai SP-1, Tianshu ST-25, Neiting ST-44, Qihai REN-6, Zhaohai KID-6 and Neiguan P-6 (*Great Compendium*).
- Vomiting blood and spontaneous external bleeding: Yinbai SP-1, Pishu BL-20, Ganshu BL-18 and Shangwan REN-13 (*Great Compendium*).
- Severe and ceaseless nosebleed: Yinbai SP-1 and Weizhong BL-40 (*Supplementing Life*).
- Heat in the head and rhinitis with nosebleed: Yinbai SP-1, Chengshan BL-57, Feiyang BL-58, Kunlun BL-60 and Jinggu BL-64, (*Thousand Ducat Formulas*).
- Chest pain: Yinbai SP-1, Zhongfu LU-1, Yunmen LU-2, Qimen LIV-14, Feishu BL-13, Hunmen BL-47 and Daling P-7 (*Supplementing Life*).
- Agitation and oppression with inability to lie down: Yinbai SP-1, Taiyuan LU-9, Gongsun SP-4, Feishu BL-13, Yinlingquan SP-9 and Sanyinjiao SP-6 (*Great Compendium*).
- Epilepsy: Yinbai SP-1, Shenmen HE-7, Neiguan P-6, Houxi SI-3 and Xinshu BL-15 (*Complete Collection*).
- Nightmares: Yinbai SP-1 and Lidui ST-45 (*One Hundred Symptoms*).
- Loss of consciousness: Yinbai SP-1 and Dadun LIV-1 (*Systematic Classic*).

DADU SP-2

Great Metropolis

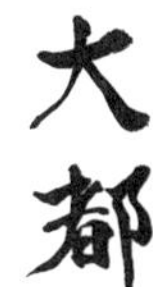

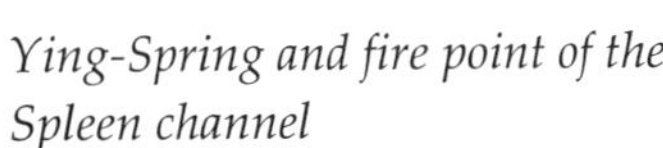
Ying-Spring and fire point of the Spleen channel

LOCATION

On the medial side of the big toe, in the depression distal and inferior to the first metatarso-phalangeal joint.

LOCATION NOTE

In the depression located by sliding the fingertip distally over the side of the ball of the foot.

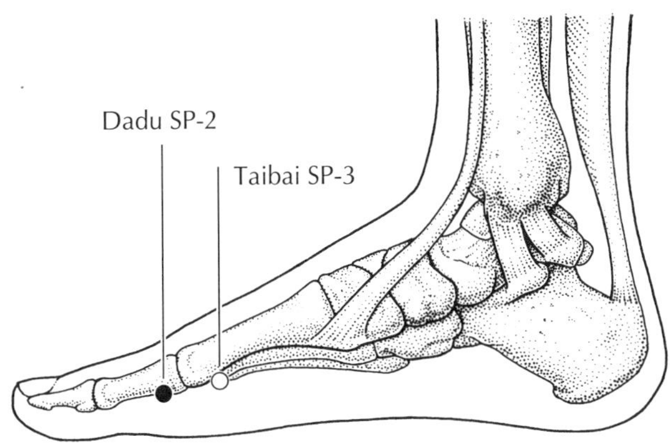

NEEDLING

Oblique inferior insertion 0.3 to 0.5 cun.

ACTIONS

Regulates the Spleen
Resolves dampness and damp-heat
Harmonises the middle jiao and clears heat

INDICATIONS

- Sudden swelling of the four limbs, heaviness of the body with pain of the bones, swelling of the limbs, oppression of the chest.
- Abdominal distention, epigastric pain, vomiting, diarrhoea, constipation, agitation when hungry and dizziness when full, sudden turmoil disorder.
- Agitation, insomnia, Heart pain, febrile disease with absence of sweating, febrile disease that does not disperse, injury by cold leading to hands and feet counterflow cold, visual dizziness.
- Lumbar pain with inability to turn, disorders of the big toe, heat sensation in the soles of the feet.

COMMENTARY

Dadu SP-2 is the ying-spring and fire point of the Spleen channel and the subject of somewhat contradictory statements in different classics. The *Classic of Difficulties*[3] says that the ying-spring points are indicated for "heat in the body", and indeed the ying-spring points of the twelve channels are usually the principal points to clear heat of excess or deficiency type from their respective zangfu or channel. The *Illustrated Classic of Acupuncture Points on the Bronze Man* says "when the Spleen is deficient, reinforce Dadu SP-2", reflecting the status of Dadu SP-2 as the 'mother' point of the Spleen channel (fire is the mother of earth), according to the principle of tonifying the mother to nourish the child. The *Classic of the Jade Dragon* simply states that Dadu SP-2 can treat disharmony of the Spleen and Stomach.

The Spleen dominates the function of the digestive system as a whole, including the Stomach and intestines. Its transportation and transformation function places great demands on the Spleen's qi, and in disharmony the Spleen tends to deficiency, which is why most of the Spleen channel points distal to the knee have some effect on tonifying the Spleen. This deficiency may underlie the patterns of Spleen dampness or damp-heat, either because impaired transportation and transformation leads to the generation of these pathogens inside the body, or because when the Spleen is deficient, the body is especially vulnerable to attack by exterior dampness and damp-heat. It is this picture of Spleen deficiency combined with dampness or damp-heat that is able to reconcile the different statements made in the classics concerning Dadu SP-2. It should be emphasised however, that among the more distal points of the Spleen channel, the Spleen tonifying action of Dadu SP-2 is relatively minor, and its primary action is in reducing excess patterns.

Dadu SP-2 is indicated for excess dampness or damp-heat manifesting as sudden swelling of the four limbs, heaviness of the body with pain of the bones, swelling of the limbs and oppression of the chest. These indications reflect attack by exterior dampness or damp-heat, often as a consequence of underlying Spleen deficiency. Dadu SP-2 is also indicated for heat patterns of the Stomach and intestines such as abdominal distention, epigastric pain, vomiting, diarrhoea or constipation, and sudden turmoil disorder. The indication 'agitation when hungry and dizziness when full' reflects a pattern of phlegm-heat in the Stomach. The heat clearing action of Dadu SP-2 extends to the treatment of febrile diseases, and it is especially indicated when fevers are accompanied by absence of sweating.

Finally, Dadu SP-2 may be used as a local point for disorders of the big toe in combination with points such as Taibai SP-3 and Xingjian LIV-2.

COMBINATIONS

- Vomiting: Dadu SP-2 and Chengguang BL-6 (*Supplementing Life*).
- Febrile disease with absence of sweating: Dadu SP-2 and Jingqu LU-8 (*One Hundred Symptoms*).
- Pain of the Heart and epigastrium: Dadu SP-2 and Taibai SP-3 (*Spiritual Pivot*).
- Stagnation of qi, lumbar pain with inability to stand: Dadu SP-2 and Henggu KID-11 (*Ode of Xi-hong*).

TAIBAI SP-3

Supreme White

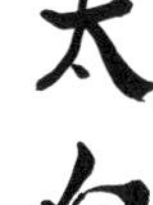

Shu-Stream, Yuan-Source and Earth point of the Spleen channel

LOCATION

On the medial side of the foot in the depression proximal and inferior to the head of the first metatarsal bone.

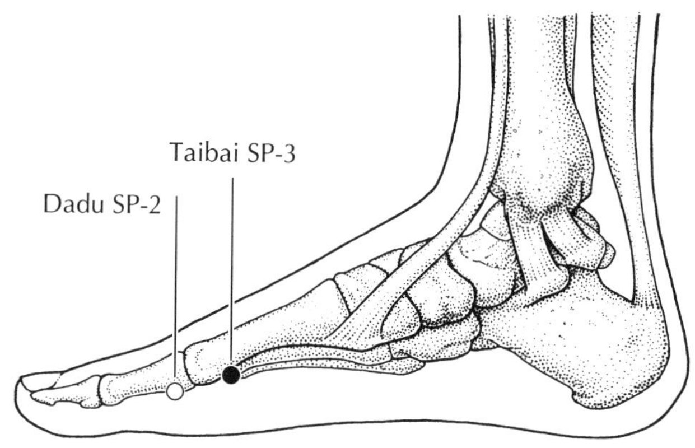

LOCATION NOTE

In the depression located by sliding the fingertip proximally over the side of the ball of the foot.

NEEDLING

Perpendicular insertion 0.5 to 1 cun.

ACTIONS

Tonifies the Spleen and resolves dampness and damp-heat
Harmonises the Spleen and Stomach
Regulates qi

INDICATIONS

- Deficiency of the Spleen and Stomach, heaviness of the body with pain of the bones, oppressive sensation of the four limbs, leg qi, borborygmus, borborygmus with stabbing pain, diarrhoea, undigested food (in the stool), diarrhoea with pus and blood, dysenteric disorder, constipation, haemorrhoids.
- Cutting pain of the abdomen, pain of the abdomen, distention of the abdomen, distention of the epigastrium, pain of the epigastrium, pain of the epigastrium and Heart, distention of the chest and lateral costal region, vomiting, hunger with no pleasure in eating, sudden turmoil disorder with hands and feet counterflow cold.
- Febrile disease with fullness and oppression and inability to lie down, febrile disease that begins with heaviness of the head, pain of the forehead, heat in the body with agitation and fullness.
- Pain of the knee and thigh, joint pains, lumbar pain, atrophy disorder.

COMMENTARY

Taibai SP-3 is the shu-stream, yuan-source and earth point of the Spleen earth channel, and has a powerful action on strengthening and regulating the qi of the Spleen and Stomach. The *Spiritual Pivot* in Chapter 6 recommends the use of the shu-stream points in the treatment of disorders of the zang, whilst in Chapter 1 it says "When the five zang are diseased, select [from] the twelve yuan-source [points]". The *Classic of the Jade Dragon* clearly states that Taibai SP-3 is indicated for "deficiency and feebleness of the Spleen and Stomach". Since deficiency of these zangfu easily leads to excess dampness and consequent obstruction of qi, Taibai SP-3 is an important point for treating both the primary deficiency and the subsequent excess that is often generated.

The *Essential Questions*[4] states "Damp, swelling and fullness all pertain to the Spleen" and "When the Spleen is diseased, damp is generated". The Stomach and Spleen together dominate the transformation of both the solid and liquid parts of food and drink, and the transportation throughout the body of the qi and body fluids transformed from them. When the Stomach and Spleen are deficient these functions of transportation and transformation are impaired, leading to the accumulation of dampness. Taibai SP-3 is indicated for a range of symptoms reflecting this combination of deficiency and excess such as borborygmus and diarrhoea, undigested food in the stool, heaviness of the body, oppressive sensation of the four limbs etc. Although Spleen deficiency most commonly gives rise to diarrhoea and loose stools, Taibai SP-3 is included in several classical combinations for constipation and difficult defecation. This kind of constipation may arise when there is insufficient qi to move and activate the bowels.

Exterior dampness or damp-heat, which most easily penetrate when there is underlying Spleen deficiency or interior dampness, may injure the body in three main ways, for all of which Taibai SP-3 is indicated. Firstly they may combine with wind-cold or wind-heat, giving rise to symptoms such as febrile disease with fullness and oppression and inability to lie down, and febrile disease that begins with heaviness of the head. Secondly, they may directly attack the Spleen and Stomach giving rise to symptoms such as dysenteric disorder, diarrhoea containing pus and blood, vomiting, and heat in the body with agitation and fullness. Thirdly, in the form of wind-damp, they may enter the channels and give rise to painful obstruction manifesting as heaviness of the body with pain of the bones, joint pains, pain of the knee and thigh or lumbar pain. The use of Taibai SP-3 in this latter pattern reflects the statement in the *Classic of Difficulties*[5] that shu-stream points are indicated for "heaviness of the body and pain of the joints". In addition to treating these patterns of exterior dampness, Taibai SP-3 may also be used for leg qi due to damp-heat pouring downwards, and atrophy disorder due either to dampness or to Spleen deficiency. This pattern is discussed in the *Essential Questions* which says "With exposure to dampness over a period of time, the muscles and flesh will be invaded; this will lead to insensitivity and flesh atrophy"[6] and "When there is illness in the Spleen it fails to transport body fluids for the Stomach. The four limbs do not receive the nourishment of water and grain and therefore become weak. There is no free flow through the vessel-pathways and there is no qi to engender the sinews, bones and muscles which therefore cannot function"[7].

It should be noted that Taibai SP-3 is also strongly indicated for various symptoms characterised by distention and pain in the abdomen, epigastrium, chest, Heart and lateral costal region. These are due to stagnation of qi which may arise either due to qi deficiency, in other words when there is insufficient qi to maintain smooth circulation, or when accumulation of turbid dampness obstructs the smooth movement of qi. In the former case the pulse and tongue will reflect deficiency only and the treatment principle is to reinforce Taibai SP-3, according to the theory of 'treating by opposition', in this case 'to treat fullness by filling'. In the latter case the pulse and tongue will show signs of excess and the treatment principle is to reduce Taibai SP-3.

Finally, Taibai SP-3 is frequently used for disorders of the joints of the big toe and the head of the first metatarsal bone.

COMBINATIONS

- Undigested food (in the stool): Taibai SP-3 and Fuai SP-16 (*Supplementing Life*).
- Borborygmus: Taibai SP-3, Gongsun SP-4, Dachangshu BL-25 and Sanjiaoshu BL-22 (*Supplementing Life*).
- Sudden turmoil disorder: Taibai SP-3, Yinlingquan SP-9, Chengshan BL-57 and Jiexi ST-41 (*Great Compendium*).
- Diarrhoea and dysenteric disorder with pus and blood: Taibai SP-3, Xiajuxu ST-39 and Youmen KID-21 (*Supplementing Life*).
- Blood in the stool: Taibai SP-3, Chengshan BL-57, Fuliu KID-7 and Taichong LIV-3 (*Great Compendium*).
- Constipation: Taibai SP-3, Zhaohai KID-6 and Zhangmen LIV-13 (*Great Compendium*).
- Constipation: Taibai SP-3, Zhaohai KID-6, Zhangmen LIV-13 and Zhigou SJ-6 (*Great Compendium*).
- Difficult defecation: Taibai SP-3 and Zhongzhu KID-15 (*Systematic Classic*).
- Pain of intestinal abscess: Taibai SP-3, Xiangu ST-43 and Dachangshu BL-25 (*Great Compendium*).
- Abdominal distention, undigested food (in the stool) and drum distention with great fullness: Taibai SP-3 and Gongsun SP-4 (*Thousand Ducat Formulas*).
- Abdominal distention leading to back pain: Taibai SP-3 and Taichong LIV-3 (*Great Compendium*).
- Drum distention: Taibai SP-3, Fuliu KID-7, Gongsun SP-4, Zhongfeng LIV-4 and Shuifen REN-9 (*Bronze Man*).
- Lumbar pain with inability to bend and extend: Taibai SP-3, Weiyang BL-39, Yinmen BL-37, Yinlingquan SP-9 and Xingjian LIV-2 (*Thousand Ducat Formulas*).

GONGSUN SP-4

Grandfather Grandson

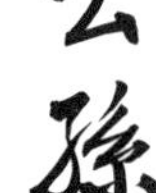

Luo-Connecting point of the Spleen channel
Confluent point of the Penetrating vessel

LOCATION

On the medial side of the foot, in the depression distal and inferior to the base of the first metatarsal bone.

LOCATION NOTE

First locate Taibai SP-3, then slide the finger proximally along the shaft of the first metatarsal bone until it reaches the depression at the base of the bone (approximately 1 cun).

NEEDLING

Perpendicular insertion 0.5 to 1 cun.

ACTIONS

Fortifies the Spleen and harmonises the middle jiao
Regulates qi and resolves dampness
Calms the spirit
Benefits the Heart and chest
Regulates the Penetrating vessel

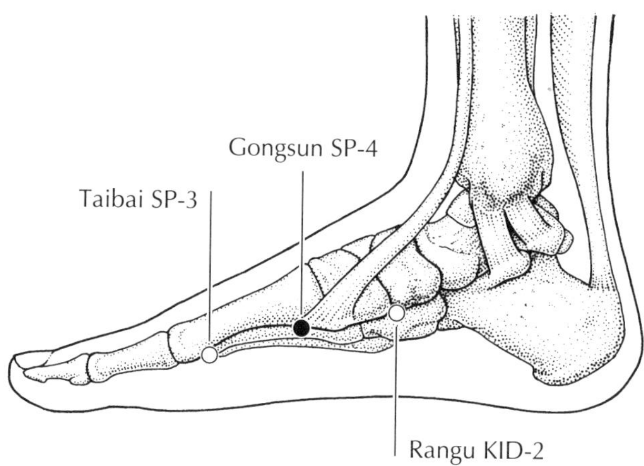

INDICATIONS

- Epigastric pain, vomiting, cold in the Stomach, no pleasure in eating, oesophageal constriction, distention and pain of the abdomen, distention and pain of the umbilical region, cutting pain of the intestines, drum distention, borborygmus, diarrhoea, undigested food (in the stool), dysenteric disorder, blood in the stool, tenesmus, sudden turmoil disorder.
- Mania-depression, manic raving, insomnia and restlessness, epilepsy, Heart pain, Gall Bladder deficiency, much sighing.
- Irregular menstruation, gynaecological disorders, retention of the placenta and lochia.
- Swelling of the head and face, oedema, leg qi, jaundice, malaria, cold malaria.
- Pain of the heel, heat in the soles of the feet.

COMMENTARY

Gongsun SP-4 is the luo-connecting point of the Spleen channel and the confluent point of the Penetrating vessel. Its principal actions are to harmonise the middle jiao, fortify the Spleen, regulate stagnant qi and transform dampness. One explanation of the name 'Grandfather Grandson' refers to its status as the luo-connecting point, the Spleen channel being the grandfather and the Stomach channel the grandson. An alternative explanation is that it refers to the Yellow Emperor, whose family name was Gongsun and who ruled under the earth phase, emphasising the significant action of this point on both the Spleen and the Stomach.

The Stomach and Spleen (which together comprise the middle jiao) are intimately related and their functions and nature complement each other. The 'rotting and ripening' of food and drink in the Stomach, the first stage of the digestive process, is ultimately governed by the Spleen. The Spleen ascends whilst the Stomach descends; the Spleen abhors dampness whilst the Stomach abhors dryness. Gongsun SP-4 connects with the Stomach channel (via the luo-connecting channel) and with the Stomach and intestines themselves (via the primary and luo-connecting channels). It is ideally suited, therefore, to harmonise the relationship between this paired zang and fu, and is indicated on the one hand for vomiting, cold in the Stomach, no pleasure in eating and oesophageal constriction, and on the other hand for borborygmus, diarrhoea, dysenteric disorder, tenesmus etc. It is also indicated for sudden turmoil disorder - the sudden and acute onset of simultaneous diarrhoea, vomiting and abdominal discomfort or pain. This disease is associated with eating unclean food, or with attack of cold, summer-heat, dampness or epidemic qi.

The Spleen channel meets with the Conception vessel on the abdomen both below and above the umbilicus (Zhongji REN-3, Guanyuan REN-4 and Xiawan REN-10), whilst the Penetrating vessel passes through all the Kidney channel points of the lower and upper abdomen. In clinical practice, Gongsun SP-4 is an important point to treat upper and lower abdominal distention or pain due to qi stagnation, blood stasis or obstruction by dampness. According to the discussion of the 'eight therapeutic methods' in the *Ode of the Obstructed River*, Gongsun SP-4 is particularly indicated for abdominal pain below the umbilicus. Other sources emphasise its effectiveness for both epigastric pain and periumbilical pain. Whilst all sources therefore agree on its ability to treat abdominal pain, the variance in opinion on its precise sphere of action reflects both its effect on the Stomach in the upper abdomen and the intestines (via the Spleen) in the lower abdomen, and the pathways of the channels which it influences.

In common with the other luo-connecting points of the yin channels (Lieque LU-7, Tongli HE-5, Dazhong KID-4, Neiguan P-6 and Ligou LIV-5) Gongsun SP-4 has a pronounced effect on emotional disorders. The Spleen channel connects with the Heart, and when phlegm and dampness accumulate and transform into phlegm-heat, this may be carried upwards to obstruct the Heart and agitate the spirit giving rise to mania-depression, manic raving, insomnia, restlessness and epilepsy. Alternatively, if Spleen qi is deficient, the source of blood will be weak and the Heart and spirit will lack nourishment resulting in insomnia and restlessness. Unusually for a Spleen channel point, Gongsun SP-4 is also indicated for Gall Bladder deficiency and much sighing. For a fuller discussion of this pattern, see Danshu BL-19.

The Penetrating vessel disperses in the chest, whilst the Spleen channel connects with the Heart, chest and lateral costal region. The *Complete Collection of Acupuncture and Moxibustion* recommends Gongsun SP-4 for the 'nine types of Heart pain' as well as for low-grade pain of the chest. Neiguan P-6, the confluent point of the Yin Linking vessel is frequently combined with Gongsun SP-4, the confluent point of the Penetrating vessel, to enhance the latter's ability to treat Heart and chest pain, as well as to calm the spirit and regulate qi in the middle jiao and hence treat pain, distention and nausea.

The Penetrating vessel (known as the sea of blood) originates in the lower abdomen and has a specific effect on the uterus. The *Classic of the Jade Dragon* states that Gongsun SP-4 may be used for 'all gynaecological disorders'. Despite this recommendation, however, it is notable that other gynaecological indications in both classical and modern texts are relatively few.

One pathway of the Penetrating vessel ascends to the face, and Gongsun SP-4 is indicated (and included in various classical combinations) for oedema, especially swelling of the face.

Finally the *Great Compendium of Acupuncture and Moxibustion* gives specific indications for excess and deficiency of the luo-connecting points. In the case of Gongsun SP-4, these are cutting pain of the intestines (excess); drum distention (deficiency).

COMBINATIONS

- Abdominal pain: Gongsun SP-4 and Neiguan P-6 (*Ode of Xi-hong*).
- Stagnation of food in the mid-abdomen, stabbing pain that does not cease: Gongsun SP-4, Jiexi ST-41, Zhongwan REN-12 and Zusanli ST-36 (*Complete Collection*).
- Borborygmus: Gongsun SP-4, Taibai SP-3, Dachangshu BL-25 and Sanjiaoshu BL-22 (*Supplementing Life*).
- Vomiting phlegm and watery saliva, dizziness that does not cease: Gongsun SP-4, Fenglong ST-40, Yangxi L.I.-5 and Shanzhong REN-17 (*Complete Collection*).
- Sudden turmoil disorder: Gongsun SP-4, Juque REN-14, Guanchong SJ-1, Zhigou SJ-6 and Jiexi ST-41 (*Systematic Classic*).
- Chronic malaria with no pleasure in eating: Gongsun SP-4, Neiting ST-44 and Lidui ST-45 (*Great Compendium*).
- Pain of the lateral costal region: Gongsun SP-4, Zhigou SJ-6, Yanglingquan GB-34 and Zhangmen LIV-13 (*Complete Collection*).
- Swelling of the face and head: Gongsun SP-4 and Yanglingquan GB-34 (*Supplementing Life*).

SHANGQIU SP-5

Shang Mound

商丘

Jing-River and Metal point of the Spleen channel

LOCATION

On the medial side of the ankle, in the depression which lies at the junction of straight lines drawn along the anterior and inferior borders of the medial malleolus.

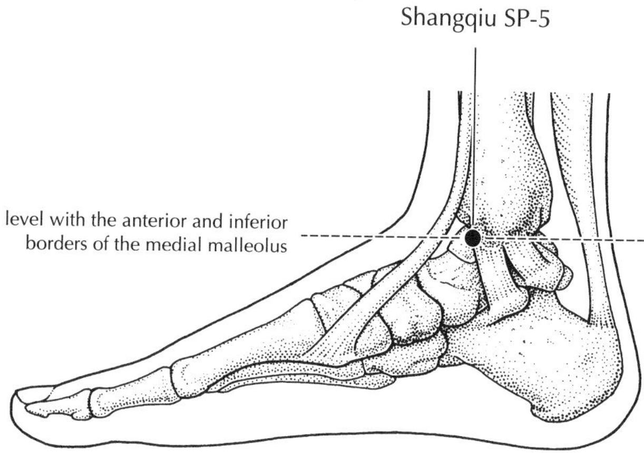

NEEDLING

i. Perpendicular insertion 0.2 to 0.3 cun; ii. Transverse insertion beneath the tendons towards, or to join with, Jiexi ST-41.

ACTIONS

Fortifies the Spleen and resolves dampness
Benefits the sinews and bones
Calms the spirit

INDICATIONS

- Spleen deficiency, indolence, somnolence, lethargy with desire to lie down, abdominal distention, borborygmus, watery diarrhoea, undigested food (in the stool), constipation, cold pain in the epigastrium, excessive eating, chills and fever with vomiting, coughing and diarrhoea in children with no desire to eat, swelling of the face, jaundice, yellow face.
- Stiffness and pain of the root of the tongue, impaired speech, cough, infertility, haemorrhoids, shan disorder.
- Mania-depression, agitation with thirst, excessive thinking, propensity to laughter, nightmares, melancholy Heart, cold body with much sighing, chronic childhood fright wind, childhood fright epilepsy.
- Pain and contraction of the sinews, lockjaw, ankle pain, pain of the inner thigh, bone painful obstruction, heavy body with painful joints, hemiplegia.

COMMENTARY

The term 'Shang' in this point's name refers to the note associated with metal in the theory of five phase correspondences, and Shangqiu SP-5 is the metal and jing-river point of the Spleen channel. According to five phase theory, therefore, it is the child point of the Spleen earth channel, suitable for reducing excess conditions. The *Illustrated Classic of Acupuncture Points on the Bronze Man* says "when the Spleen is excess, reduce Shangqiu SP-5".

The Spleen, dominating the ceaseless yang functions of transportation and transformation, easily becomes deficient in qi and yang, and therefore most of its patterns of disharmony involve deficiency. There are two meanings, however, to the pattern of Spleen excess in relation to the actions of Shangqiu SP-5. Firstly, if exterior pathogenic dampness or damp-heat attack the body, they may disrupt the function of the middle jiao giving rise to acute onset of symptoms such as chills and fever with vomiting, abdominal pain, diarrhoea, coughing and diarrhoea in children with loss of appetite, heaviness of the body and lethargy. Secondly, deficiency of Spleen qi and yang may lead to excess of yin in the form of accumulation of interior dampness, giving rise to chronic lethargy, indolence, somnolence, swelling of the face, diarrhoea and digestive difficulty. In both cases, there will be a thick and greasy tongue coating and a slippery pulse, indicating an excess pattern. Like many points of the Spleen channel, for example Taibai SP-3, Shangqiu SP-5 is able to address both the deficient and excess aspects of Spleen disharmony.

According to the *Spiritual Pivot*[8] "When the disease is at the yin within yang (sinews and bones), needle the jing-river points of the yin channels". Shangqiu SP-5, the jing-river point of the Spleen channel, is an important point in the treatment of disorders of the sinews, muscles and bones due to invasion and retention of pathogenic dampness. Damp painful obstruction, also known as fixed painful obstruction, is characterised by stiffness, swelling and heaviness of the joints and a tendency to worsen during humid weather. Since Spleen deficiency may predispose to or result from damp painful obstruction, points of the Spleen channel such as Shangqiu SP-5 which both tonify the Spleen and resolve dampness are most often employed in the treatment of damp painful obstruction anywhere in the body, in combination with local points. Shangqiu SP-5 is also mentioned in various classics for the treatment of bone painful obstruction, the development of painful obstruction where deformity of the joints occurs. Shangqiu SP-5 is of course especially effective in treating disorders of the ankle joint and its surrounding soft tissue, whether due to painful obstruction or traumatic injury. In such disorders the needle may be directed to join with Jiexi ST-41 at the anterior of the ankle joint.

According to the *Spiritual Pivot*[9] "When the disease manifests itself in the voice, the jing-river point should be selected". Both the Spleen primary and divergent channels rise to the tongue and Shangqiu SP-5 is indicated for stiffness and pain at the root of the tongue as well as for impaired speech.

The Spleen channel links with the Heart, and like several other points of the channel Shangqiu SP-5 has many indications for disturbance of the spirit, for example mania-depression, agitation, melancholia, propensity to laughter, nightmares etc. This can be explained by the ability of Shangqiu SP-5 both to tonify the Spleen and to clear dampness. If Spleen qi is deficient, the source of blood will be weak and the Heart and spirit will lack nourishment. Alternatively when dampness accumulates and transforms into phlegm it may be carried upwards to obstruct the Heart and cloud the spirit, whilst if phlegm transforms to phlegm-heat there will be agitation of the spirit. The *Spiritual Pivot*[10] says "The Spleen stores the nutritive qi; nutritive qi is the residence of thought" whilst the *Systematic Classic of Acupuncture and Moxibustion* says "Thought has its origins in the Spleen but takes shape in the Heart". Shangqiu SP-5 is one of the few points indicated for excessive thinking, the mental activity which both results from Spleen disharmony and leads to injury of the Spleen.

COMBINATIONS

- Vomiting: Shangqiu SP-5, Youmen KID-21 and Zutonggu BL-66 (*Thousand Ducat Formulas*).
- Spleen deficiency constipation: Shangqiu SP-5 and Sanyinjiao SP-6 (*Great Compendium*).
- Infertility: Shangqiu SP-5 and Zhongji REN-3 (*Great Compendium*).
- Infertility: Shangqiu SP-5, Ciliao BL-32 and Yongquan KID-1 (*Supplementing Life*).
- Hypogastric pain radiating to the genitals: Shangqiu SP-5 and Shimen REN-5 (*Thousand Ducat Formulas*).
- Contraction of the legs: Shangqiu SP-5, Chengjin BL-56, Chengshan BL-57 and Jinggu BL-64 (*Thousand Ducat Formulas*).
- Sighing with propensity to sadness: Shangqiu SP-5 and Riyue GB-24 (*Supplementing Life*).
- Wasting and thirsting disorder: Shangqiu SP-5, Chengjiang REN-24, Jinjin (M-HN-20), Yuye (M-HN-20), Renzhong DU-26, Lianquan REN-23, Quchi L.I-11, Laogong P-8, Taichong LIV-3, Xingjian LIV-2, Ranggu KID-2 and Yinbai SP-1 (*Great Compendium*).

SANYINJIAO SP-6

Three Yin Intersection

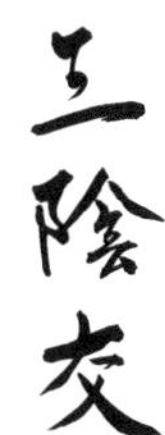

Meeting point of the Spleen, Liver and Kidney channels

LOCATION

On the medial side of the lower leg, 3 cun superior to the prominence of the medial malleolus, in a depression close to the medial crest of the tibia.

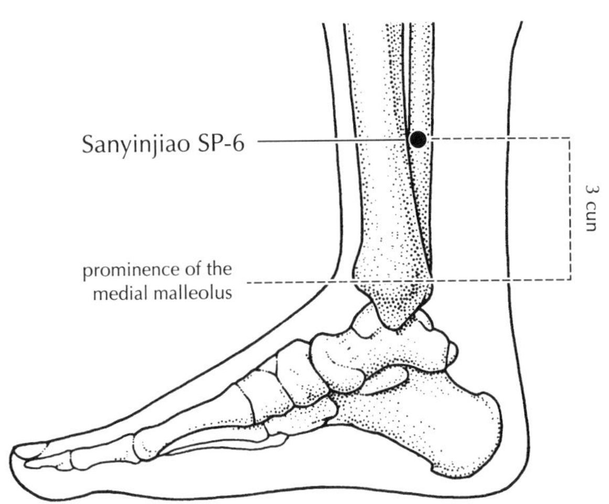

LOCATION NOTE

This point is most readily located one handbreadth superior to the prominence of the medial malleolus.

NEEDLING

Perpendicular or oblique proximal insertion, 1 to 1.5 cun.
Caution: contraindicated in pregnancy.

ACTIONS

Tonifies the Spleen and Stomach
Resolves dampness
Harmonises the Liver and tonifies the Kidneys
Regulates menstruation and induces labour
Harmonises the lower jiao
Regulates urination and benefits the genitals
Calms the spirit
Invigorates blood
Activates the channel and alleviates pain

INDICATIONS

- Spleen and Stomach deficiency, Spleen deficiency with heavy body, heavy body with heaviness of the four limbs, oedema, borborygmus, diarrhoea, undigested food (in the stool), abdominal distention, cold abdomen, unbearable pain below the umbilicus, pain of the Spleen, fullness and distention of the Heart and abdomen, no desire to eat and drink, vomiting of fluid after eating, sudden turmoil disorder.
- Irregular menstruation, uterine bleeding, uterine bleeding with dizziness, menorrhagia, amenorrhoea, dysmenorrhoea, abdominal (zheng jia) masses in women, leucorrhoea, uterine prolapse.
- Infertility, restless foetus syndrome, transverse presentation, delayed labour, prolonged or difficult labour, retention of lochia, retention of dead foetus, post-partum dizziness.
- Seminal emission, seminal emission with dreaming, sexual hyperactivity in men, impotence, pain of the genitals, pain of the penis, contracted testicles, shan disorder, pain due to shan disorder.
- Difficult urination, enuresis, the five types of painful urinary dysfunction, cloudy urine, white turbidity.
- Palpitations, insomnia, Gall Bladder deficiency, sudden fright disorder in children.
- Dizziness, blurred vision, tinnitus, yawning, hypertension.
- Leg pain, crane's knee, damp painful obstruction, atrophy disorder and painful obstruction of the lower limbs, hemiplegia, heat in the soles of the feet, shin pain, eczema, urticaria, counterflow cold of the foot and hand.

COMMENTARY

Sanyinjiao SP-6 (Three Yin Intersection) is the meeting point of the three yin channels of the leg (Spleen, Liver and Kidney) and is one of the most important and widely used of the acupuncture points. Its actions and indications are extraordinarily broad, and it is a primary point in the treatment of many digestive, gynaecological, sexual, urinary and emotional disorders.

Located on the Spleen channel, its strongest action is on harmonising all the functions of the Spleen. The Spleen dominates transportation and transformation and is thus the primary zang responsible for the formation of qi and blood. When Spleen qi or yang is deficient there may be: i. impairment of the transportation and transformation function (undigested food in the stool, diarrhoea, abdominal distention and fullness, borborygmus etc.) ii. inadequate formation of blood (palpitations, blurred vision, amenorrhoea, post-partum dizziness, dizziness associated with uterine bleeding etc.), iii. failure of the Spleen to hold the blood (uterine bleeding, menorrhagia), and iv. sinking of central qi (uterine prolapse). Furthermore, deficiency of Spleen qi and incomplete transportation and transformation may lead to the formation of excess dampness. According to the *Essential Questions*[11] "The lower is the first to suffer from dampness". Dampness, whether damp-heat or cold damp, may lead to heaviness of the body and limbs and oedema, or pour down to the lower jiao giving rise to such symptoms as diarrhoea or leucorrhoea. Sanyinjiao SP-6, exceptionally balanced in its action, is unique among points of the Spleen channel in being able to treat all these different manifestations of Spleen disharmony.

Although its primary action is on the Spleen, Sanyinjiao SP-6 is also an important point to treat disorders of the Liver and Kidneys. It is able to soften and harmonise the Liver, by both spreading the Liver qi and nourishing Liver blood, and at the same time to benefit the Kidney qi. This threefold action of harmonising the Spleen, Liver and Kidneys finds expression in the forte of Sanyinjiao SP-6 in treating all disorders of the lower jiao.

The three leg yin channels dominate menstruation, conception, pregnancy, leucorrhoea and the external genitalia. Sanyinjiao SP-6 is the single most important distal point in the treatment of any gynaecological, obstetrical or post-partum disorder whether characterised by deficiency of qi, blood, yin, yang or Kidney essence, failure of Spleen qi to hold the blood, or stagnation of qi, blood, dampness, damp-heat or phlegm. So wide is its range of action, and so universal its indications, that Sanyinjiao SP-6 appears in classical combinations for the treatment of virtually any disorder of the reproductive system. Sanyinjiao SP-6 is also an essential point to induce labour, assist in transverse presentation and alleviate the pain of childbirth. Despite its indication for restless foetus syndrome, however, its ability to expedite delivery of the live or dead foetus, and the lochia, means that Sanyinjiao SP-6 is generally contraindicated in pregnancy.

According to the *Essential Questions*[12] "The genitals are the gathering place of the sinews". The Spleen sinew channel binds at the genitals and Sanyinjiao SP-6 is an essential point in the treatment of sexual and genital disorders in both men and women, including pain and contraction, seminal emission, impotence, and excessive sexual drive in men. Although impotence is generally related to deficiency of Kidney fire, two classics help to explain its relationship to the Spleen. The *Complete Works of Jing-yue* says "Ming men [the fire of the gate of life stored in the Kidneys] is the sea of the essence and blood, the Spleen is the sea of water and grain; the two together form the foundation of the five zang and six fu", whilst the *Essential Questions*[13] explains "The Kidneys dominate water; they receive essence from the five zang and six fu and store it, therefore only when the five zang are flourishing is ejaculation possible".

Disharmony of the Liver, Spleen or Kidneys is responsible for the majority of urinary disorders, and the principal patterns are accumulation of damp-heat or cold damp, Kidney deficiency, qi deficiency, stagnation of Liver qi or Liver fire. Due to its ability to treat all these pathologies, Sanyinjiao SP-6 is an essential point for the treatment of urinary disorders, including difficult urination, retention of urine, enuresis, painful urinary dysfunction and cloudy urine.

The actions of Sanyinjiao SP-6 are not, however, confined to the middle and lower jiao. Its inclusion in many prescriptions for the treatment of any kind of insomnia (usually in combination with Shenmen HE-7) dramatically illustrates its wide-ranging actions. Insomnia is normally differentiated into five main patterns: i. deficiency of Heart and Spleen (qi and blood deficiency), ii. disharmony of Heart and Kidneys (yin deficiency), iii. disharmony of Heart and Liver (Liver blood and yin deficiency or Liver fire), iv. deficiency of Heart and Gall Bladder (qi deficiency), v. disharmony of Heart and Stomach (accumulation of food or retention of phlegm-heat). Since Sanyinjiao SP-6 is able to fortify the Spleen, tonify qi and blood, nourish Liver and Kidney yin, spread the Liver qi and harmonise the digestion it may be used in any of these patterns.

The especial importance of treating the Spleen in cases of disharmony of the Heart and Kidneys is emphasised in a number of classics. The *Standards of Patterns and Treatments* says "In order to tonify the Kidneys it is best to

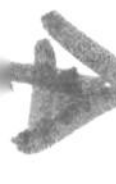

tonify the Spleen; use the Spleen to connect with the Heart in the upper and with the Kidneys in the lower ..." and "The essence of the five zang is all transported from the Spleen; when the Spleen is flourishing then the Heart and Kidneys are in communication". The *Helpful Questions in Medical Cases* says "If you desire to establish communication between the Heart and the Kidneys it is necessary to use the Spleen earth as an intermediary".

Along with Geshu BL-17, Xuehai SP-10 and Diji SP-8, Sanyinjiao SP-6 is considered one of the most important acupuncture points to harmonise and cool blood and to promote and invigorate its circulation. This action finds its most important application in the treatment of gynaecological disorders, but extends to other disorders where blood disharmony plays an important role, for example skin diseases such as eczema and urticaria.

Finally Sanyinjiao SP-6 is cited in the *Song of the Nine Needles for Returning the Yang*, for the treatment of collapse of yang characterised by loss of consciousness, aversion to cold, cold counterflow of the limbs, purple lips etc.

COMBINATIONS

- Diarrhoea containing undigested food: reinforce Sanyinjiao SP-6 and Yinlingquan SP-9 (*Spiritual Pivot*).
- Diarrhoea with thin stools: Sanyinjiao SP-6, Shenque REN-8 and Taichong LIV-3 (*Great Compendium*).
- Undigested food (in the stool): Sanyinjiao SP-6 and Zhongwan REN-12 (*Supplementing Life*).
- Undigested food (in the stool): Sanyinjiao SP-6, Liangmen ST-21, Zusanli ST-36, Dachangshu BL-25, Xiawan REN-10, Sanjiaoshu BL-22 and Xuanshu DU-5 (*Supplementing Life*).
- Sudden turmoil disorder, headache, chest pain and dyspnoeic rales: Sanyinjiao SP-6, Renying ST-9, Neiguan P-6, Guanchong SJ-1 and Zusanli ST-36 (*Compilation*).
- Spleen deficiency constipation: Sanyinjiao SP-6 and Shangqiu SP-5 (*Great Compendium*).
- Irregular menstruation: Sanyinjiao SP-6, Daimai GB-26, Qihai REN-6, Zhongji REN-3 and Shenshu BL-23 (*Great Compendium*).
- Inhibited menstruation: Sanyinjiao SP-6, Zulinqi GB-41 and Zhongji REN-3 (*Great Compendium*).
- Profuse and ceaseless uterine bleeding: Sanyinjiao SP-6, Jiaoxin KID-8, Yingu KID-10 and Taichong LIV-3 (*Supplementing Life*).
- Profuse and ceaseless uterine bleeding: Sanyinjiao SP-6 and Taichong LIV-3 (*Great Compendium*).
- Women who have had too many children: Sanyinjiao SP-6 and Shimen REN-5 (*Great Compendium*).
- Difficult delivery: reduce Sanyinjiao SP-6 and Taichong LIV-3, reinforce Hegu L.I.-4 (*Great Compendium*).
- Retention of the placenta: reduce Sanyinjiao SP-6 and Zhongji REN-3 (*Great Compendium*).
- Retention of the placenta: Sanyinjiao SP-6, Jianjing GB-21 and Zhongji REN-3 (*Meeting the Source*).
- Post-partum dizziness: Sanyinjiao SP-6, Zusanli ST-36 and Zhigou SJ-6 (*Great Compendium*).
- Post-partum blood clot pain: Sanyinjiao SP-6 and Qihai REN-6 (*Great Compendium*).
- Sudden swelling, redness and pain of the vagina: Sanyinjiao SP-6, Huiyin REN-1 and Zhongji REN-3 (*Great Compendium*).
- Red and white leucorrhoea: Sanyinjiao SP-6, Baihuanshu BL-30, Daimai GB-26, Guanyuan REN-4, Qihai REN-6 and Jianshi P-5 (*Great Compendium*).
- Pain of the penis: Sanyinjiao SP-6, Yuji LU-10, Taixi KID-3 and Zhongji REN-3 (*Great Compendium*).
- Sagging and swollen testicle without pain: Sanyinjiao SP-6, Guilai ST-29 and Dadun LIV-1 (*Great Compendium*).
- White turbidity and chronic seminal emission: Sanyinjiao SP-6 and Qihai REN-6 (*One Hundred Symptoms*).

- Lower abdominal pain from the seven kinds of shan disorder: Sanyinjiao SP-6, Zhaohai KID-6 and Ququan LIV-8 (*Ode of Xi-hong*).
- Obstructed urination: Sanyinjiao SP-6, Yinlingquan SP-9 and Qihai REN-6, followed by Yingu KID-10 and Daling P-7 (*Great Compendium*).
- Inability to urinate: Sanyinjiao SP-6, Shimen REN-5, Guanyuan REN-4, Zhongji REN-3 and Qugu REN-2 (*Supplementing Life*).
- Oedema of the four limbs: Sanyinjiao SP-6, Zhongdu LIV-6, Hegu L.I.-4, Quchi L.I.-11, Zhongzhu SJ-3, Yemen SJ-2, Xingjian LIV-2, Neiting ST-44 and Yinlingquan SP-9 (*Great Compendium*).
- Running piglet qi in women: Sanyinjiao SP-6, Qimen LIV-14, Guanyuan REN-4, Zhongji REN-3, Shimen REN-5 and Xuehai SP-10 (*Supplementing Life*).
- Running piglet qi: Sanyinjiao SP-6, Zhangmen LIV-13 and Shimen REN-5 (*Thousand Ducat Formulas*).
- Palpitations and insomnia: Sanyinjiao SP-6, Daju ST-27 and Qihai REN-6 (*Supplementing Life*).
- Insomnia: Sanyinjiao SP-6, Yinlingquan SP-9, Yinbai SP-1, Gongsun SP-4, Feishu BL-13 and Taiyuan LU-9 (*Great Compendium*).
- Cold damp leg qi: Sanyinjiao SP-6 and Zusanli ST-36 (*Song of the Jade Dragon*).
- Hip pain: Sanyinjiao SP-6, Huantiao GB-30, Shugu BL-65, Jiaoxin KID-8 and Yingu KID-10 (*Thousand Ducat Formulas*).
- Pain of the hip with difficulty in walking and pain of the skin of the lateral aspect of the leg: Sanyinjiao SP-6 and Zulinqi GB-41 (*Thousand Ducat Formulas*).
- Leg qi: Sanyinjiao SP-6, Zusanli ST-36 and Xuanzhong GB-39 (*Ode of the Jade Dragon*).
- Insomnia due to Heart and Spleen deficiency: Sanyinjiao SP-6, Shenmen HE-7, Zusanli ST-36 and Yintang (M-HN-3).
- Insomnia due to disharmony of Heart and Kidneys: Sanyinjiao SP-6, Shenmen HE-7, Taixi KID-3 and Zhaohai KID-6.
- Insomnia due to Liver fire: Sanyinjiao SP-6, Shenmen HE-7, Anmian (M-HN-34), Ganshu BL-18 and Danshu BL-19.

LOUGU SP-7

Dripping Valley

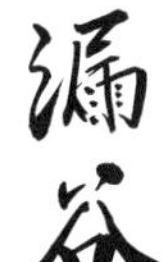

LOCATION

On the medial side of the lower leg, 3 cun superior to Sanyinjiao SP-6, in a depression just posterior to the medial crest of the tibia.

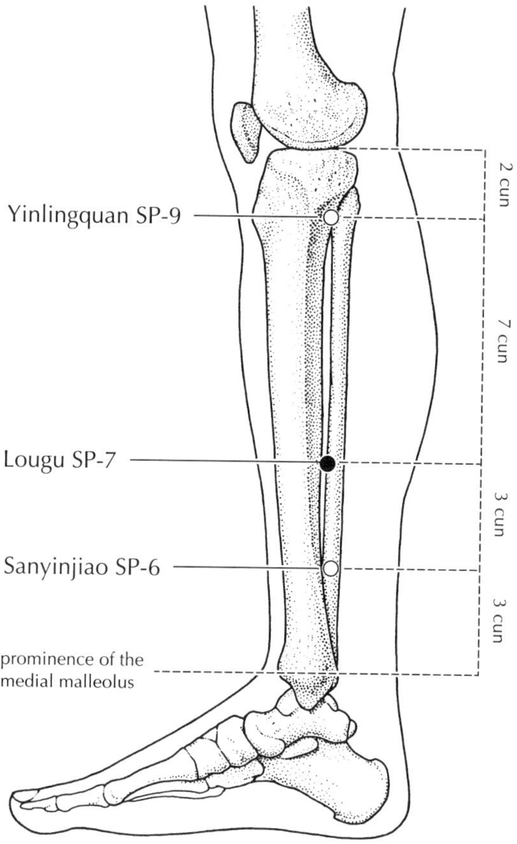

LOCATION NOTE

This point is most readily located one handbreadth superior to Sanyinjiao SP-6.

NEEDLING

Perpendicular or oblique insertion, 1 to 1.5 cun. **Note**: according to several classical texts, this point is contraindicated to moxibustion.

ACTIONS

Fortifies the Spleen and resolves dampness
Promotes urination and disperses swelling

INDICATIONS

- Abdominal fullness, borborygmus, diarrhoea, painful belching, wasting of the muscles and flesh despite normal eating and drinking.
- Oedema, difficult urination, swelling of the ankle.
- Sadness with counterflow qi, seminal emission.
- Paralysis of the legs, leg qi, inversion counterflow of the legs and knees, painful obstruction of the knees.

COMMENTARY

Although not a commonly used point clinically, Lougu SP-7 is indicated for "wasting of the muscles and flesh despite normal eating and drinking". This condition is referred to by Li Dong-yuan in the *Treatise on the Spleen and Stomach* which said "There are also cases of thinness despite eating well. [This is due to] hidden Stomach fire at the qi level resulting in large food intake; Spleen deficiency leads to withered flesh"[14].

COMBINATIONS

- Cold abdomen: Lougu SP-7 and Huiyang BL-35 (*Supplementing Life*).
- Difficult urination and seminal emission: Lougu SP-7, Zhongji REN-3, Ligou LIV-5, Chengfu BL-36 and Zhiyin BL-67 (*Supplementing Life*).

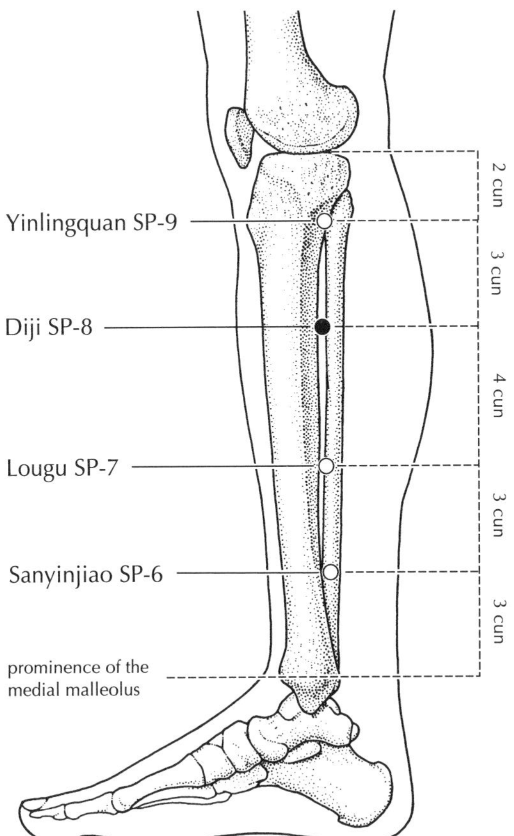

DIJI SP-8

Earth Pivot

地機

Xi-Cleft point of the Spleen channel

LOCATION

On the medial side of the lower leg, 3 cun inferior to Yinlingquan SP-9, in a depression just posterior to the medial crest of the tibia.

LOCATION NOTE

i. This point is most readily located one handbreadth inferior to Yinlingquan SP-9; ii. Alternatively, it may be located at the junction of the upper third and the lower two thirds of a line drawn between the popliteal crease and the prominence of the medial malleolus.

NEEDLING

Perpendicular or oblique insertion, 1 to 1.5 cun.

ACTIONS

Regulates menstruation and invigorates blood
Harmonises the Spleen and resolves dampness
Moderates acute conditions

INDICATIONS

- Irregular menstruation, dysmenorrhoea, abdominal (zheng jia) masses in women.
- Distention of the abdomen and lateral costal region, pain of the abdomen, poor appetite, diarrhoea with thin stools, dysenteric disorder, difficult urination, oedema, leucorrhoea, seminal emission, lumbar pain, insufficiency of essence.

COMMENTARY

Diji SP-8 is the xi-cleft point of the Spleen channel. The xi-cleft points are where the qi and blood, which flow relatively superficially along the channels from the jing-well points, gather and plunge more deeply. The xi-cleft points in general are indicated in the treatment of acute conditions and pain, whilst the xi-cleft points of the yin channels have an additional action of treating disorders of blood.

The Spleen controls blood and its channel enters the lower abdomen, joining with the Conception vessel at Zhongji REN-3 and Guanyuan REN-4. Diji SP-8 has a specific and important action on resolving blood stasis in the uterus and lower abdomen, being indicated in the treatment of dysmenorrhoea, irregular menstruation, and abdominal masses in women due to either blood stasis or qi stagnation. A specific indication for this point mentioned in the *Illustrated Classic of Acupuncture Points on the Bronze Man* is a hot flowing sensation spreading down the inner thigh to the knee when pressure is applied to abdominal masses in women. As the xi-cleft point, Diji SP-8 is especially suited to treating acute conditions, and it is often combined with Hegu L.I.-4 in the treatment of acute dysmenorrhoea, both points being strongly reduced, often with the addition of electro-acupuncture.

Diji SP-8 has a secondary action of harmonising the Spleen and resolving damp, being indicated in the treatment of abdominal distention, poor appetite, difficult urination, oedema and leucorrhoea, especially when these symptoms accompany disorders of menstruation.

The affinity of Diji SP-8 for disorders of the lower abdomen is emphasised in various classics. The *Investigation Into Points Along the Channels* by Yan Zhen-shi of the Ming dynasty goes as far as to say "there is no disorder of the lower region that cannot be treated with Diji SP-8", whilst according to the *Ode to Elucidate Mysteries* Diji SP-8 dominates the lower region (Dabao SP-21 dominates the upper region and Tianshu ST-25 the middle region). In the correspondence system of early Chinese thought, the upper region is heaven, the middle region is man and the lower region is earth, hence the name of this point 'Earth Pivot'.

COMBINATIONS

- Irregular menstruation: Diji SP-8 and Xuehai SP-10 (*One Hundred Patterns*).
- Cold-damp shan disorder: Diji SP-8, Daju ST-27 and Zhongdu LIV-6 (*Systematic Classic*).
- No pleasure in eating: Diji SP-8, Yinlingquan SP-9, Shuifen REN-9, Youmen KID-21 and Xiaochangshu BL-27 (*Supplementing Life*).
- Acute dysmenorrhoea: Diji SP-8 and Hegu L.I.-4.

YINLINGQUAN SP-9

Yin Mound Spring

陰陵泉

He-Sea and Water point of the Spleen channel

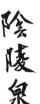

LOCATION

On the medial side of the lower leg, in a depression in the angle formed by the medial condyle of the tibia and the posterior border of the tibia.

LOCATION NOTE

i. Run the finger in the groove posterior to the medial border of the tibia until it falls into the depression below the tibial condyle; ii. This point lies at the same level as Yanglingquan GB-34.

NEEDLING

Perpendicular insertion, 1 to 1.5 cun.

ACTIONS

Regulates the Spleen and resolves dampness
Opens and moves the water passages
Benefits the lower jiao

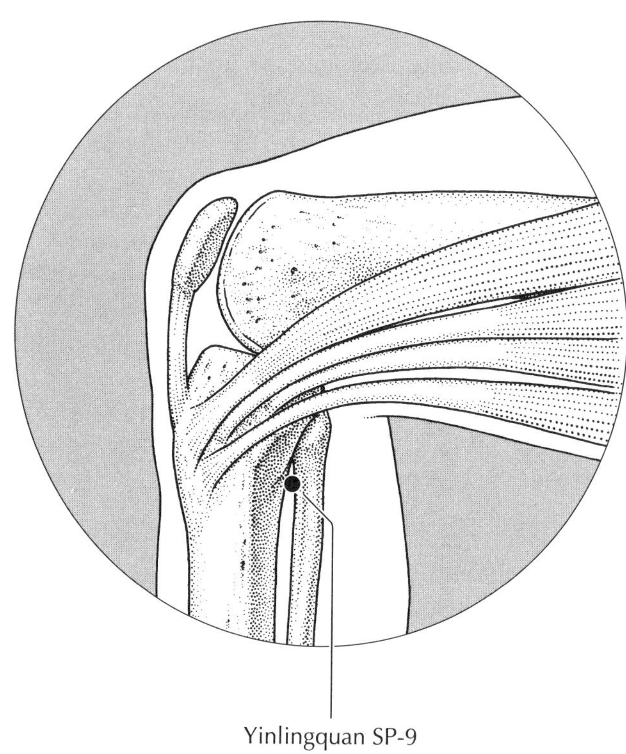

Yinlingquan SP-9

INDICATIONS

- Abdominal distention, cold and pain of the abdomen, pain of the lower abdomen, cutting pain in the middle of the intestines, no desire to eat, jaundice, sudden turmoil disorder, diarrhoea, sudden diarrhoea with undigested food in the stools, dysenteric disorder.
- Oedema, swelling of the lower limbs, retention of urine, difficult urination, enuresis, qi painful urinary dysfunction.
- Seminal emission, leucorrhoea, pain of the genitals, shan disorder.
- Fullness below the Heart, fullness of the lateral costal region, dyspnoea with inability to lie down, heat in the chest, unremitting chills and fever.
- Lumbar pain, pain and swelling of the knee, painful obstruction of the leg.

COMMENTARY

The *Essential Questions* states "When the Spleen is diseased, damp is generated"[15], "Damp, swelling and fullness all pertain to the Spleen"[16], and "The lower is the first to suffer from dampness"[17]. Yinlingquan SP-9, the he-sea and water point of the Spleen channel, is an essential point in the treatment of disorders due to dampness and retention of fluid, especially in the lower jiao.

The *Ode of the Essentials of Understanding* states "Yinlingquan SP-9 opens and moves the water passages". The Spleen dominates the transportation and transformation of food and drink and, along with the Lung and Kidneys, is one of the three zang responsible for the correct distribution of body fluids. When the function of the Spleen is impaired (whether due to deficiency of qi or yang, obstruction by exterior dampness or damp-heat, or transverse invasion by Liver qi) its inability to transform fluids will lead to the accumulation of dampness, resulting in a wide range of symptoms throughout the body. Dampness may combine with pre-existing pathogenic heat, or simply transform to heat over time according to the law of 'similar transformation' expounded by Liu Wan-su. This 'law' describes how a guest will tend to transform according to the nature of the host, and applies equally to political diplomacy, military invasion and medicine. Since the human host is alive and therefore yang and warm, any guest, such as dampness, will over time take on this heat. Yinlingquan SP-9 is the foremost point on the Spleen channel for transforming and draining excess dampness and damp-heat, and compared with points such as Shangqiu SP-5, and especially Taibai SP-3, has relatively little action on tonifying deficiency patterns of the Spleen.

The he-sea points of the three leg yin channels, all water points, share the common property of draining dampness and damp-heat from the lower jiao. Ququan LIV-8 focuses primarily on the genital region (dominated by the Liver channel), and Yingu KID-10 on the urinary system (dominated by the Kidney channel). Because of the close relationship between dampness and the Spleen however, Yinlingquan SP-9 is able to treat all disorders of the lower jiao due to accumulation of dampness and damp-heat. It is indicated when these pathogens afflict the intestines (diarrhoea and dysenteric disorder), urinary system (difficult urination, retention of urine, painful urinary dysfunction) and genitals (leucorrhoea and pain of the genitals), whether acute and due to exterior pathogens or chronic and internally generated.

Despite the tendency of dampness to sink to the lower jiao, it may also affect other regions of the body. In the middle jiao, Yinlingquan SP-9 is able to treat dampness which obstructs the free flow of bile or qi and gives rise to jaundice, abdominal distention, fullness below the Heart (i.e. in the epigastrium) and poor appetite. The *Investigation Into Points Along the Channels* says "There is no pain of the middle and lower regions that cannot be treated with Yinlingquan SP-9".

The Spleen primary and sinew channels and the great luo-connecting channel from Dabao SP-21 all traverse the chest and lateral costal region. The action of Yinlingquan SP-9 on the upper jiao, although clinically less important, includes the treatment of heat in the chest, fullness of the lateral costal region, and dyspnoea with inability to lie down due to fluids overflowing into the Lung. Throughout the body as a whole, Yinlingquan SP-9 is able to treat oedema, and it is a widely used and important point for this purpose.

Finally, Yinlingquan SP-9 is an important point to treat disorders of the knee, particularly those accompanied by swelling. Indeed, because of its wide-ranging ability to resolve dampness, some practitioners use it to treat damp painful obstruction anywhere in the body.

COMBINATIONS

- Oedema around the umbilical region: Yinlingquan SP-9 and Shuifen REN-9 (*One Hundred Symptoms*).
- Oedema of the four limbs: Yinlingquan SP-9, Sanyinjiao SP-6, Zhongdu LIV-6, Hegu L.I.-4, Quchi L.I.-11, Zhongzhu SJ-3, Yemen SJ-2, Xingjian LIV-2 and Neiting ST-44 (*Great Compendium*).
- Enuresis: Yinlingquan SP-9 and Yanglingquan GB-34 (*Thousand Ducat Formulas*).
- Obstructed urination: Yinlingquan SP-9, Qihai REN-6 and Sanyinjiao SP-6, followed by Yingu KID-10 and Daling P-7 (*Great Compendium*).
- Diarrhoea containing undigested food: reinforce Yinlingquan SP-9 and Sanyinjiao SP-6 (*Spiritual Pivot*).
- Cold or damp (dong) diarrhoea with undigested food: Yinlingquan SP-9, Rangu KID-2 and Jingmen GB-25 (*Thousand Ducat Formulas*).
- Heat in the chest with sudden diarrhoea: Yinlingquan SP-9 and Yinbai SP-1 (*Thousand Ducat Formulas*).
- Sudden turmoil disorder: Yinlingquan SP-9, Chengshan BL-57, Jiexi ST-41 and Taibai SP-3 (*Great Compendium*).
- No pleasure in eating: Yinlingquan SP-9, Diji SP-8, Shuifen REN-9, Youmen KID-21 and Xiaochangshu BL-27 (*Supplementing Life*).
- Pain of the Small Intestine that radiates to the umbilicus: Yinlingquan SP-9 and Yongquan KID-1 (*Heavenly Star Points*).
- Swelling of the knee that is difficult to endure: Yinlingquan SP-9 and Yanglingquan GB-34 (*Ode of the Jade Dragon*).
- Paralysis of the lower extremity: Yinlingquan SP-9, Huantiao GB-30, Yangfu GB-38, Taixi KID-3 and Zhiyin BL-67 (*Great Compendium*).

XUEHAI SP-10

Sea of Blood

血海

LOCATION

2 cun proximal to the superior border of the patella, in the tender depression on the bulge of the vastus medialis muscle, directly above Yinlingquan SP-9.

LOCATION NOTE

i. Place the heel of your right palm on the inferior border of the patient's left patella, with the fingers and thumb fully extended and the thumb at 45° to the index finger. This point is found beneath the tip of the thumb, directly above Yinlingquan SP-9; ii. Locate one patella's height (2 cun) above the superior border of the patella, in the tender depression directly above Yinlingquan SP-9.

NEEDLING

Perpendicular or oblique insertion 1 to 1.5 cun.

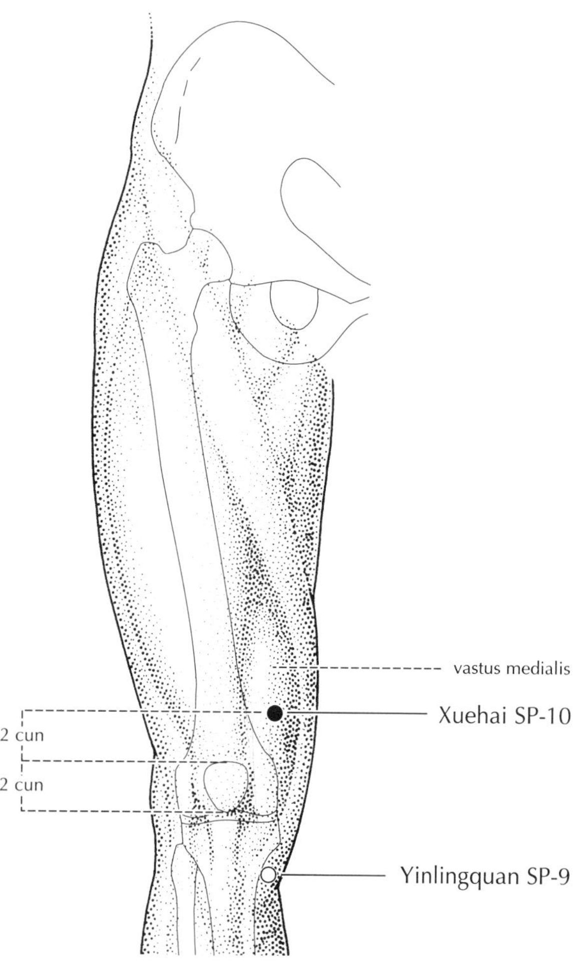

ACTIONS

Invigorates the blood and dispels stasis
Cools blood
Harmonises menstruation
Benefits the skin

INDICATIONS

- Irregular menstruation, dysmenorrhoea, amenorrhoea, uterine bleeding, uterine bleeding containing clots, sudden uterine bleeding, post-partum qi and blood deficiency.
- Urticaria, eczema, erysipelas (cinnabar toxin), herpes zoster, painful hot sores, ulceration and itching of the scrotum, pain and itching of the genitals.
- Leucorrhoea, the five types of painful urinary dysfunction, qi painful urinary dysfunction, blood painful urinary dysfunction, pain of the inner aspect of the thigh.

COMMENTARY

The name of Xuehai SP-10 (Sea of Blood) reflects its pre-eminent role in treating various disorders at the blood level. It is generally recognised as having two principal actions: i. invigorating the blood and dispelling stasis, and ii. cooling the blood. These two actions find their expression in its ability to treat a wide range of gynaecological and dermatological disorders due either to blood stasis or to heat in the blood.

As far as gynaecology is concerned, normal menstruation depends on a number of factors including the smooth circulation of blood. Impairment of blood circulation and consequent stasis may be due to a variety of causes including stagnation or deficiency of qi, traumatic injury, haemorrhage, penetration of cold or heat, chronic disease or emotional factors, and may give rise to many different disorders of menstruation. These include dysmenorrhoea and uterine bleeding characterised by severe fixed pain and the discharge of dark or clotted blood, and amenorrhoea accompanied by distention and pain, a purple coloured tongue and a choppy pulse. By contrast, if heat enters the blood level, most frequently due to internally generated heat from the Liver or Heart or overconsumption of excessively heating foods, then two principal conditions may arise: i. the movement of blood may become reckless and overflow its bounds leading to profuse uterine bleeding, or less commonly, the heat may dessicate the blood leading to amenorrhoea. In both cases there will be signs of heat such as a red dry tongue and a rapid pulse. In fact, both the blood cooling and blood invigorating properties of Xuehai SP-10 come together in its ability to treat uterine bleeding. Blood heat is the most commonly seen pattern of uterine bleeding, but as well as cooling blood, treatment must emphasise resolving stasis, since any pathological bleeding may lead to pooling and stagnation of extravasated blood. This is expressed in the Chinese medicine saying "where there is haemorrhage there is stasis". The close inter-relationship between blood heat and blood stasis is further illustrated by the fact that blood heat may condense and dry the blood giving rise to stasis, as stated in the *Treatise on Epidemic Warm Febrile Disease*[18] "Because latent stagnant fire evaporates the blood's fluid, the blood simmers and forms stasis".

Some authorities further attribute blood nourishing properties to Xuehai SP-10 and incorporate it into prescriptions for the treatment of blood deficiency. In the light of Xuehai SP-10's pre-eminence in invigorating blood, this action reflects the saying in Chinese medicine "if blood stasis is not transformed, new blood cannot be generated". This refers to situations where blood stasis has pooled outside the channels, leading directly to blood deficiency as sufficient blood is no longer available to nourish the body. This complex pattern of haemorrhage with both consequent blood stasis and blood deficiency is commonly encountered after childbirth and profuse uterine bleeding.

As far as dermatology is concerned, blood disharmony often plays a central role. The main dermatological patterns treated by Xuehai SP-10 are heat in the blood level characterised by red lesions, and blood stasis characterised by purple lesions. Xuehai SP-10 may also be used for the concomitant blood deficiency and stasis seen for example in eczema with thickening of the skin (lichenification) or post-herpetic neuralgia. Xuehai SP-10 may also be used to treat the manifestations of wind in skin diseases, the most important of which is intolerable itching. This illustrates the Chinese medicine saying "to treat wind first treat the blood; once blood moves wind will be dispelled".

Although the action of Xuehai SP-10 on invigorating and cooling blood is classically confined to the two principal areas of gynaecology and dermatology, there are in fact relatively few acupuncture points able to treat the blood directly. For this reason, its application may be extended to any disorder in the body with these pathologies. Thus the *Song of the Primary Points of the Fourteen Channels* says "Xuehai SP-10 can treat all blood diseases".

COMBINATIONS

- Irregular menstruation: Xuehai SP-10 and Diji SP-8 (*One Hundred Patterns*).
- Amenorrhoea: Xuehai SP-10 and Daimai GB-26 (*Supplementing Life*).
- The five types of painful urinary dysfunction: Xuehai SP-10 and Qihai REN-6 (*One Hundred Symptoms*).
- The five types of painful urinary dysfunction: Xuehai SP-10 and Dadun LIV-1 (*Song of Points*).
- Running piglet qi in women: Xuehai SP-10, Sanyinjiao SP-6, Qimen LIV-14, Guanyuan REN-4, Zhongji REN-3 and Shimen REN-5 (*Supplementing Life*).
- Urticaria: Xuehai SP-10, Fengmen BL-12, Quchi L.I.-11 and Weizhong BL-40.

JIMEN SP-11

箕门

Winnowing Gate

LOCATION

On the medial side of the thigh, 6 cun superior to Xuehai SP-10, on a line connecting Xuehai SP-10 with Chongmen SP-12.

LOCATION NOTE

i. Locate two handbreadths superior to Xuehai SP-10; ii. Locate midway between the tibiofemoral joint line and Chongmen SP-12.

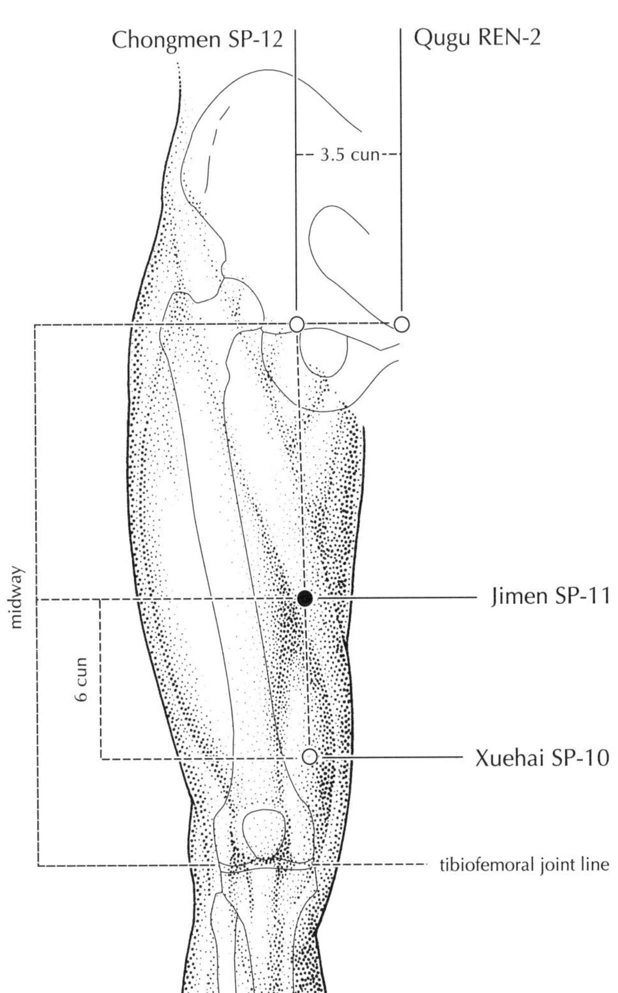

NEEDLING

Perpendicular or oblique insertion 0.5 to 1 cun.

Caution: deep needling may puncture the femoral artery.

ACTIONS

Regulates urination
Drains damp and clears heat

INDICATIONS

- Painful urinary dysfunction, retention of urine, obstructed urination, enuresis.
- Eczema of the scrotum, damp itching of the external genitalia, pain and swelling of the inguinal region, pain of the lower abdomen.

COMBINATIONS

- Enuresis: Jimen SP-11, Tongli HE-5, Dadun LIV-1, Pangguangshu BL-28, Taichong LIV-3, Weizhong BL-40 and Shenmen HE-7 (*Supplementing Life*).

CHONGMEN SP-12

Rushing Gate

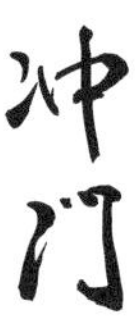

Meeting point of the Spleen and Liver channels with the Yin Linking vessel

LOCATION

3.5 cun lateral to Qugu REN-2, on the lateral side of the femoral artery.

LOCATION NOTE

Palpate to locate the pulsation of the femoral artery, just over one handbreadth lateral to the midline, at the level of the upper border of the pubic symphysis. Locate Chongmen SP-12 in the depression immediately lateral to this pulsation.

NEEDLING

Perpendicular insertion, 0.5 to 1 cun.

Caution: deep needling in a medial direction may puncture the femoral artery, and in a lateral direction, the femoral nerve.

ACTIONS

Invigorates blood, regulates qi and alleviates pain
Drains damp, clears heat and regulates urination

INDICATIONS

- Abdominal pain, cold in the abdomen with fullness, abdominal (ji ju) masses, shan disorder, pain of haemorrhoids, foetal qi rushes upward to the Heart leading to difficulty in breathing, difficult lactation.
- Difficult urination, retention of urine, painful urinary dysfunction, leucorrhoea, sudden turmoil disorder, heat in the body, atrophy disorder and painful obstruction of the lower limb.

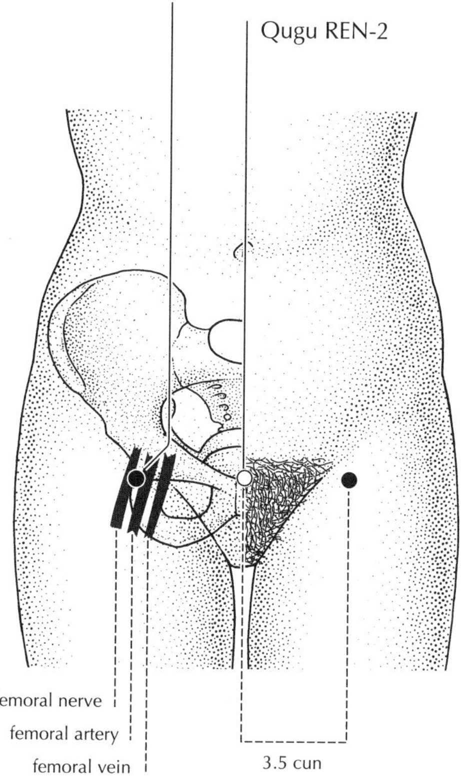

COMMENTARY

Chongmen SP-12 is a coalescent point of the Yin Linking vessel. The *Classic of Difficulties* says "When the Yin Linking vessel is diseased, Heart pain will result"[19]. Chongmen SP-12 (Rushing Gate), like Qichong ST-30 (Rushing Qi), is indicated for foetal qi rushing up to the Heart. This condition, described by Zhu Dan-xi, manifests as distention, fullness and pain of the abdomen and Heart in a pregnant woman, and is common in the later stages of pregnancy.

COMBINATIONS

- Abdominal fullness and abdominal (ji ju) masses: Chongmen SP-12 and Fushe SP-13 (*Supplementing Life*).
- The five types of painful urinary dysfunction with inability to urinate: Chongmen SP-12 and Dadun LIV-1 (*Supplementing Life*).
- Post-partum leucorrhoea and uterine bleeding: Chongmen SP-12 and Qichong ST-30 (*One Hundred Symptoms*).

FUSHE SP-13 府舍

Abode of the Fu

Meeting point of the Spleen and Liver channels with the Yin Linking vessel

LOCATION

On the lower abdomen, 0.7 cun superior and 0.5 cun lateral to Chongmen SP-12, 4 cun lateral to the midline. This point is also defined as lying 4.3 cun inferior to Daheng SP-15.

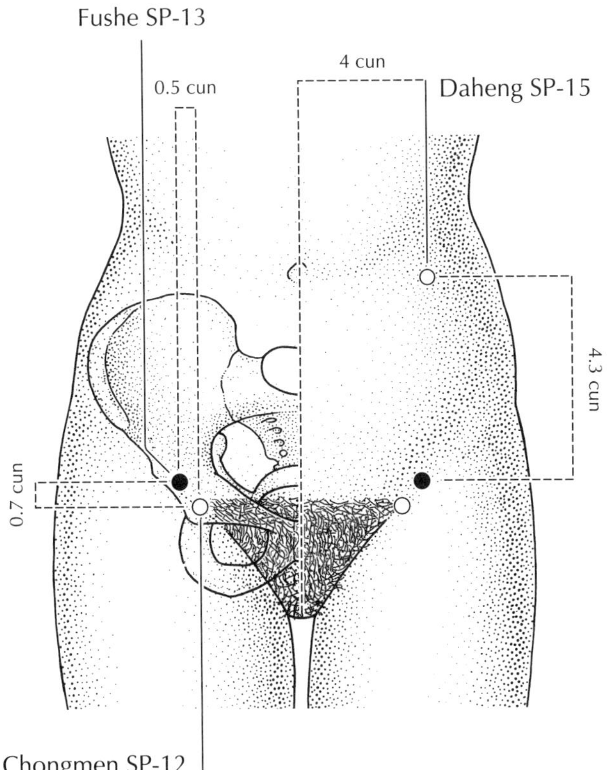

LOCATION NOTE

The 4 cun line is located at the palpable lateral border of the rectus abdominis muscle.

NEEDLING

Perpendicular insertion, 1 to 1.5 cun.
Caution: in thin patients deep needling may penetrate the peritoneal cavity.

ACTIONS

Regulates qi and alleviates pain

INDICATIONS

- Abdominal fullness and pain, painful abdominal (ji ju) masses, shan disorder, constipation, pain of the lateral costal region, sudden turmoil disorder, pain of the thigh.

COMBINATIONS

- Abdominal fullness and abdominal (ji ju) masses: Fushe SP-13 and Chongmen SP-12 (*Supplementing Life*).

FUJIE SP-14

Abdomen Knot

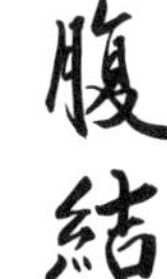

LOCATION

On the lower abdomen, 1.3 cun inferior to Daheng SP-15, 4 cun lateral to the midline.

LOCATION NOTE

The 4 cun line is located at the palpable lateral border of the rectus abdominis muscle.

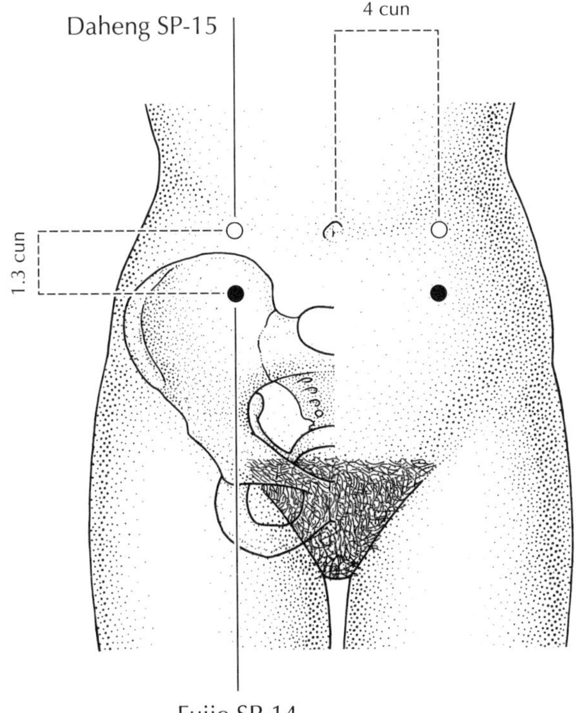

NEEDLING

Perpendicular insertion, 1 to 1.5 cun.
Caution: in thin patients deep needling may penetrate the peritoneal cavity.

ACTIONS

Warms and benefits the lower jiao
Regulates qi and descends rebellion

INDICATIONS

- Periumbilical pain, diarrhoea and dysenteric disorder, diarrhoea due to cold in the abdomen, abdominal distention and constipation, painful shan disorder.
- Qi rushes up to the Heart, Heart pain, cough.

COMMENTARY

The name of Fujie SP-14 (Abdomen Knot) refers to its ability to resolve stagnation of qi in the abdominal region, especially in the area of the umbilicus. It is also able to regulate rebellious qi which either ascends to attack the Heart or which impairs the descending function of the Lung, leading to cough. Interestingly, Heart pain is an indication of disorder in the Yin Linking vessel, and whilst Chongmen SP-12, Fushe SP-13, Daheng SP-15 and Fuai SP-16 are coalescent points of this extraordinary vessel, Fujie SP-14 is not.

Fujie SP-14 also has the function of warming the lower jiao and scattering cold, particularly in the intestinal region, and is indicated for cold diarrhoea and dysenteric disorder.

COMBINATIONS

- Rushing Heart: Fujie SP-14 and Xingjian LIV-2 (*Supplementing Life*).

DAHENG SP-15

Great Horizontal

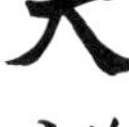

Meeting point of the Spleen channel with the Yin Linking vessel

LOCATION

On the abdomen, in the depression at the lateral border of the rectus abdominis muscle level with the umbilicus.

LOCATION NOTE

This point is normally defined as 4 cun lateral to the midline, and on the abdomen the 4 cun line is located at the lateral border of the rectus abdominis muscle.

NEEDLING

Perpendicular insertion 0.5 to 1 cun.
Caution: i. in thin patients deep needling may penetrate the peritoneal cavity; ii. deep needling at this point may penetrate a substantially enlarged spleen or liver.

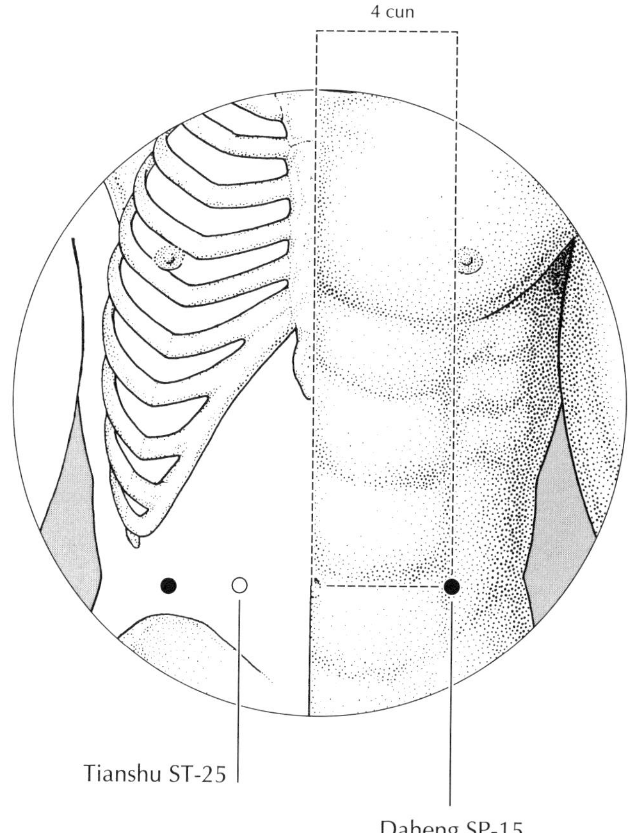

ACTIONS

Moves qi and regulates the intestines

INDICATIONS

- Lower abdominal pain, cold and pain of the lower abdomen, cold or damp (dong) diarrhoea, dysenteric disorder, constipation, sensation of heat in the hypogastrium with sighing.
- Propensity to sadness, sighing, inability to raise and move the four limbs, copious sweating.

COMMENTARY

Daheng SP-15 is an important point for regulating the qi of the Large Intestine. It is indicated for the treatment of diarrhoea, especially of cold or damp type, and due to its ability to move the qi of the Large Intestine is also used in the treatment of constipation due to many different aetiologies. Both Daheng SP-15 and Tianshu ST-25, its neighbouring point, are effective in the treatment of a variety of disorders of the intestines. Clinically, however, Tianshu ST-25 is predominantly used for loose stools, diarrhoea and dysenteric disorder, whilst Daheng SP-15 is favoured for constipation.

Daheng SP-15 is also indicated and included in classical combinations for sadness, weeping and sighing. Whilst there is no special theoretical reason why Daheng SP-15 should have this action, it is interesting to compare it with its neighbouring points Taiyi ST-23 and Huaroumen ST-24 which also have several psycho-emotional indications.

COMBINATIONS
- Arched back with sorrowful weeping: Daheng SP-15 and Tianchong GB-9 (*One Hundred Patterns*).
- Constipation: Daheng SP-15, Dachangshu BL-25 and Zhigou SJ-6.

FUAI SP-16
Abdomen Sorrow

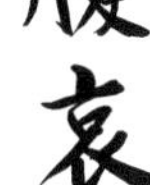

Meeting point of the Spleen channel with the Yin Linking vessel

LOCATION
On the abdomen, in the depression at the lateral border of the rectus abdominis muscle, 3 cun superior to Daheng SP-15. **Note:** in some patients with a narrow subcostal angle, this point may fall on the costal margin; the options then are to i. locate more medially, ii. needle transversely on the costal margin, iii. select a different point.

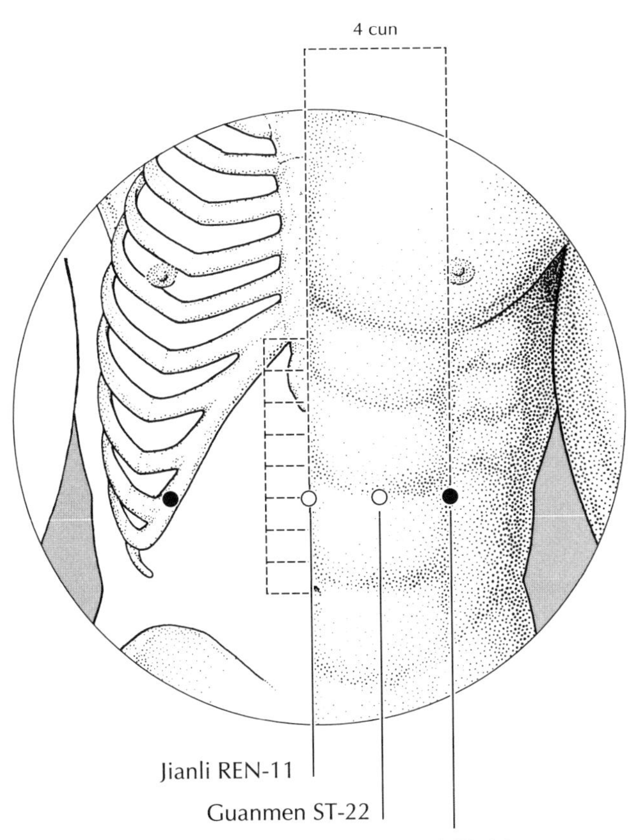

LOCATION NOTE
This point is normally defined as 4 cun lateral to the midline, and on the abdomen the 4 cun line is located at the lateral border of the rectus abdominis muscle.

NEEDLING
Perpendicular insertion 0.5 to 1 cun.
Caution: i. in thin patients deep needling may penetrate the peritoneal cavity; ii. deep needling at this point may penetrate an enlarged spleen.

ACTIONS
Regulates the intestines

INDICATIONS
- Periumbilical pain, cold of the abdomen, undigested food (in the stool), dysenteric disorder, stool containing pus and blood, constipation.

COMBINATIONS
- Undigested food (in the stool): Fuai SP-16 and Taibai SP-3 (*Supplementing Life*).

SHIDOU SP-17
Food Cavity

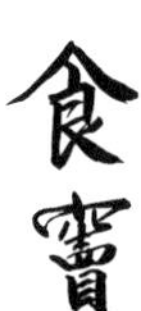

LOCATION
On the lateral side of the chest, in the fifth intercostal space, 6 cun lateral to the midline.

LOCATION NOTE
i. The intercostal spaces are most reliably counted downwards from the second intercostal space which lies immediately below the sternal angle. In males, the nipple almost invariably lies in the fourth intercostal space; ii. The six cun line is located two cun lateral to the mamillary line.

NEEDLING
Transverse-oblique insertion along the intercostal space, 0.5 to 1 cun.
Caution: perpendicular insertion, especially in thin patients, carries a substantial risk of inducing a pneumothorax.

ACTIONS
Dissipates accumulation of food and fluid and promotes digestion

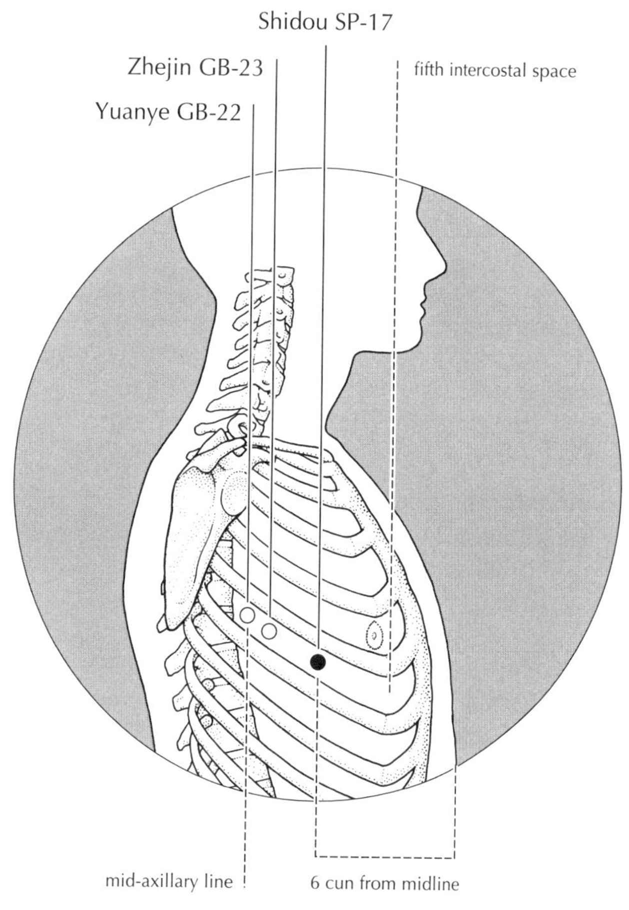

TIANXI SP-18

Heavenly Stream

天溪

LOCATION

On the lateral side of the chest, in the fourth intercostal space, 6 cun lateral to the midline.

LOCATION NOTE

i. The intercostal spaces are most reliably counted downwards from the second intercostal space which lies immediately below the sternal angle. In males, the nipple almost invariably lies in the fourth intercostal space; ii. The six cun line is located two cun lateral to the mamillary line.

NEEDLING

Transverse-oblique insertion along the intercostal space, 0.5 to 1 cun.

Caution: perpendicular insertion, especially in thin patients, carries a substantial risk of inducing a pneumothorax.

ACTIONS

Regulates and descends qi
Benefits the breasts and promotes lactation

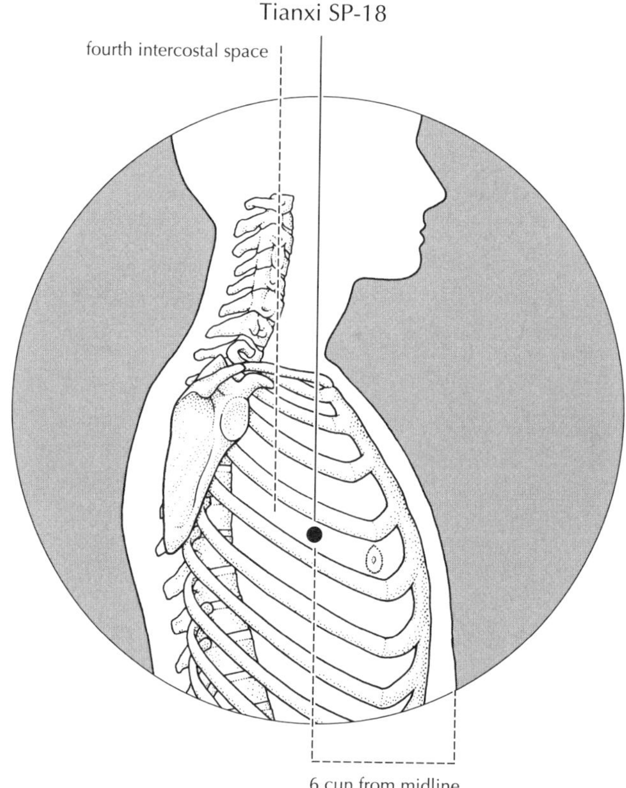

INDICATIONS

- Fullness of the chest and lateral costal region, ceaseless pain of the lateral costal region, abdominal distention, water swelling of the abdomen, oesophageal pain, pain of the diaphragm, belching, vomiting immediately after eating, undigested food (in the stool), borborygmus.
- Cough, swelling of the breasts, chronic Spleen malaria, jaundice.

COMMENTARY

Shidou SP-17 is also known by the alternative name of Mingguan (Gate of Life). According to the *Book of Bian Que's Secrets* Shidou SP-17 "connects the real Spleen qi and cures thirty-six kinds of Spleen disease. In severe disease, when life is hanging by a thread, moxibustion at this point with 200-300 moxa cones will assure the patient's survival. Use this point in any major Spleen disease"[20]. Despite this inspiring quotation, there are few references to this kind of application or combinations which include the point, in other classical texts, and Shidou SP-17 is mainly indicated for pain of the lateral costal region, distention and pain of the abdomen and diaphragm with belching, vomiting and indigested food in the stool, all clear indications of food stagnation.

INDICATIONS
- Fullness and pain of the chest and lateral costal region, shortness of breath, cough, rattling of phlegm in the throat, running piglet qi, hiccup.
- Breast abscess, failure of breast milk to flow, insufficient lactation.

COMBINATIONS
- Abscess, ulceration and swelling of the breast: Tianxi SP-18 and Xiaxi GB-43 (*Thousand Ducat Formulas*).

XIONGXIANG SP-19
Chest Village

胸鄉

LOCATION
On the lateral side of the chest, in the third intercostal space, 6 cun lateral to the midline.

LOCATION NOTE
i. The intercostal spaces are most reliably counted downwards from the second intercostal space which lies immediately below the sternal angle. In males, the nipple almost invariably lies in the fourth intercostal space; ii. The six cun line is located two cun lateral to the mamillary line.

NEEDLING
Transverse-oblique insertion along the intercostal space, 0.5 to 1 cun.
Caution: perpendicular insertion, especially in thin patients, carries a substantial risk of inducing a pneumothorax.

ACTIONS
Regulates and descends qi and unbinds the chest

INDICATIONS
- Fullness of the chest and lateral costal region extending to the back, inability to turn over when lying down, cough, shortness of breath.

COMBINATIONS
- Pain of the chest radiating to the back: Xiongxiang SP-19, Neiguan P-6 and Xinshu BL-15.

ZHOURONG SP-20
Encircling Glory

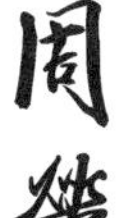
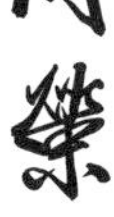

LOCATION
On the lateral side of the chest, in the second intercostal space, 6 cun lateral to the midline.

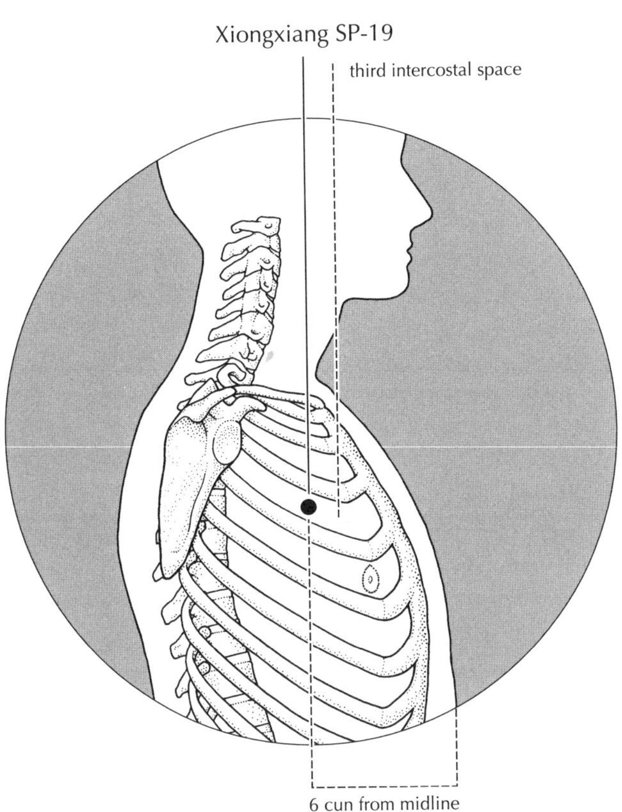

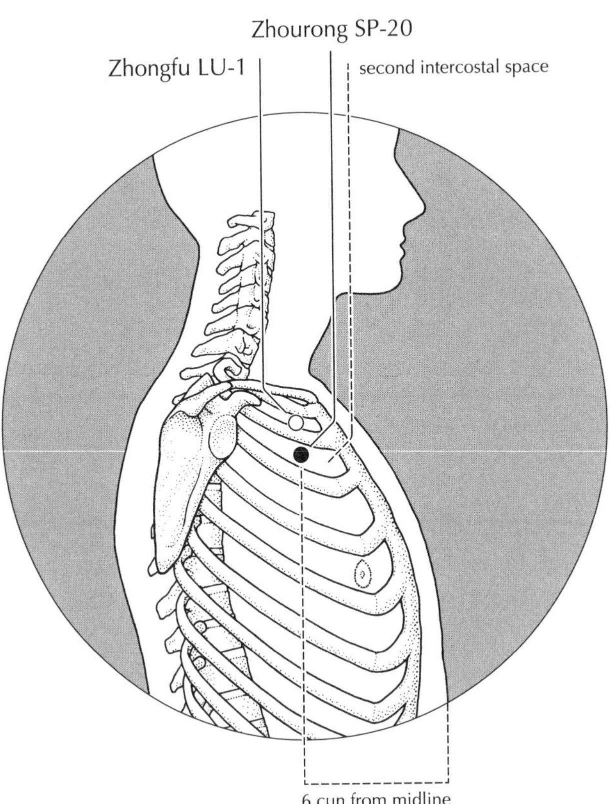

LOCATION NOTE

i. First locate the costal cartilage of the second rib which is level with the sternal angle, then locate the second intercostal space below it; ii. The six cun line is located two cun lateral to the mamillary line; iii. This point lies one intercostal space directly below Zhongfu LU-1.

NEEDLING

Transverse-oblique insertion along the intercostal space, 0.5 to 1 cun.

Caution: perpendicular insertion, especially in thin patients, carries a substantial risk of inducing a pneumothorax.

ACTIONS

Regulates and descends qi and unbinds the chest

INDICATIONS

- Distention and fullness of the chest and lateral costal region, cough, coughing with copious phlegm or pus, shortness of breath, difficult ingestion, desires to drink fluids.

COMBINATIONS

- Difficult ingestion with desire to drink fluids: Zhourong SP-20 and Dachangshu BL-25 (*Thousand Ducat Formulas*).
- Difficult ingestion: Zhourong SP-20, Zhongfu LU-1, Kunlun BL-60, Chengman ST-20 and Yuji LU-10 (*Supplementing Life*).

DABAO SP-21

大包

Great Wrapping

Great Luo-Connecting point of the Spleen

LOCATION

On the mid-axillary line, in the seventh intercostal space. **Note:** some sources locate this point in the sixth intercostal space.

LOCATION NOTE

i. The intercostal spaces are most reliably counted downwards from the second intercostal space which lies immediately below the sternal angle. In males, the nipple almost invariably lies in the fourth intercostal space; ii. the mid-axillary line is drawn vertically down from the apex of the axilla (Jiquan HE-1).

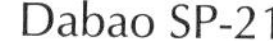

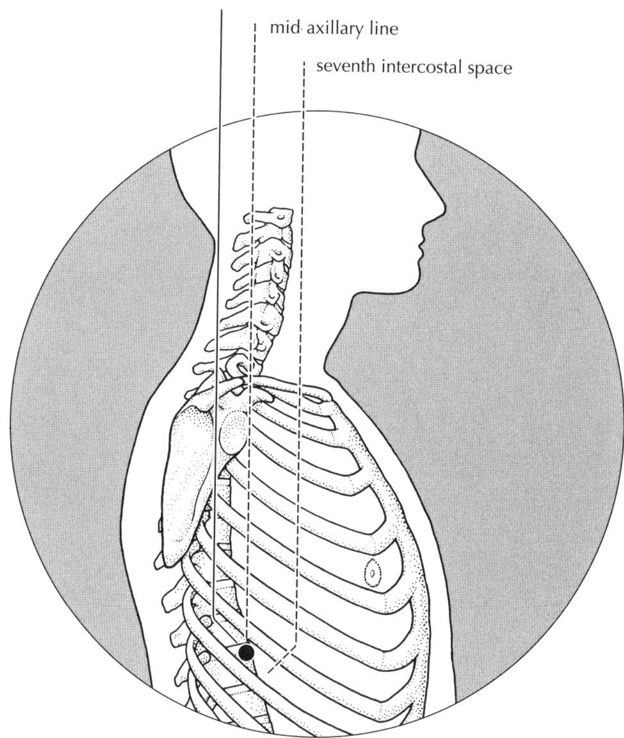

NEEDLING

Transverse-oblique insertion along the intercostal space, 0.5 to 1 cun.

Caution: perpendicular insertion, especially in thin patients, carries a substantial risk of inducing a pneumothorax.

ACTIONS

Regulates qi and blood and firms the sinews and joints

Unbinds the chest and benefits the lateral costal region

INDICATIONS

- Pain of the whole body, weariness of the four limbs, flaccidity of the limbs, flaccidity of the hundred joints.
- Cough, dyspnoea, chest pain, pain in the chest and lateral costal region on respiration, distention and fullness of the lateral costal region.

COMMENTARY

The name of the point Dabao SP-21 is made up of two characters, 'Da' meaning great, and 'Bao' meaning 'to wrap', or 'to envelop'. According to the *Spiritual Pivot*[21] "The great luo of the Spleen is known as Dabao; it emerges at three cun below the axilla spreading in the chest and lateral costal region. When it is excess there is pain of the whole body. When it is deficient the hundred joints are flaccid. This channel embraces the blood of all the luo [connecting channels]".

A possible explanation of this passage from the *Spiritual Pivot* is that one of the functions of the luo-connecting channels in general is to assist in the distribution of qi, and more especially blood, to all the tissues of the body via the network of the minute luo-connecting channels. Since the Spleen controls blood, its great luo-connecting channel dominates this function of blood distribution throughout the body. When blood stagnates "there is pain of the whole body"; when blood is deficient and unable to nourish the tissues "the hundred joints are flaccid".

Dabao SP-21 is also mentioned in the *Ode to Elucidate Mysteries* which says that it dominates the upper region (Tianshu ST-25 dominates the middle region and Diji SP-8 dominates the lower region). Despite these two classical references, Dabao SP-21 appears in no traditional combinations in any of the major classical texts.

COMBINATIONS

- Pain of the whole body and weariness of the four limbs: Dabao SP-21, Yanglingquan GB-34, Quchi L.I.-11 and Tianzhu BL-10.
- Pain of the chest and lateral costal region: Dabao SP-21, Sanyangluo SJ-8, Ximen P-4, Yangfu GB-38 and Zulinqi GB-41.

NOTES

1 *Essential Questions* Chapter 74.
2 *Classic of Difficulties* 68th Difficulty.
3 *Classic of Difficulties* 68th Difficulty.
4 *Essential Questions* Chapter 74.
5 *Classic of Difficulties* 68th Difficulty.
6 *Essential Questions* Chapter 44.
7 *Essential Questions* Chapter 29.
8 *Spiritual Pivot* Chapter 6.
9 *Spiritual Pivot* Chapter 44.
10 *Spiritual Pivot* Chapter 8.
11 *Essential Questions* Chapter 29.
12 *Essential Questions* Chapter 45.
13 *Essential Questions* Chapter 1.
14 *Treatise on the Spleen and Stomach* (Pi Wei Lun) translated by Yang Shou-zhong and Li Jian-yong, Blue Poppy Press, 1993.
15 *Essential Questions* Chapter 74.
16 *Essential Questions* Chapter 23.
17 *Essential Questions* Chapter 29.
18 *Treatise on Epidemic Warm Febrile Disease* by Wu You-ke (1642).
19 *Classic of Difficulties* 29th Difficulty.
20 Quoted in *Acupuncture Cases from China, A Digest of Difficult and Complicated Case Histories* by Zhang Deng-bu, Churchill Livingstone, 1994, p48.
21 *Spiritual Pivot* Chapter 10.

手少陰

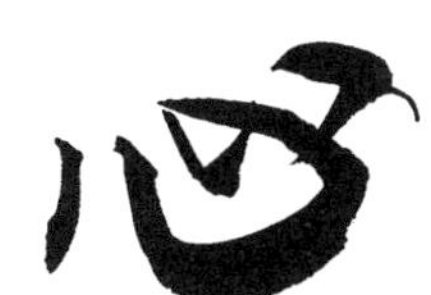

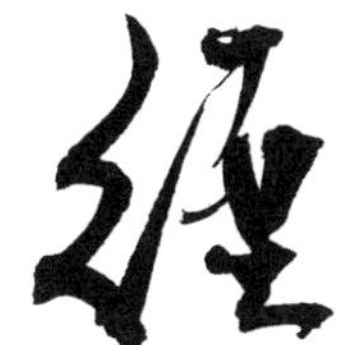

THE HEART CHANNEL OF HAND SHAOYIN

THE HEART CHANNEL OF HAND SHAOYIN

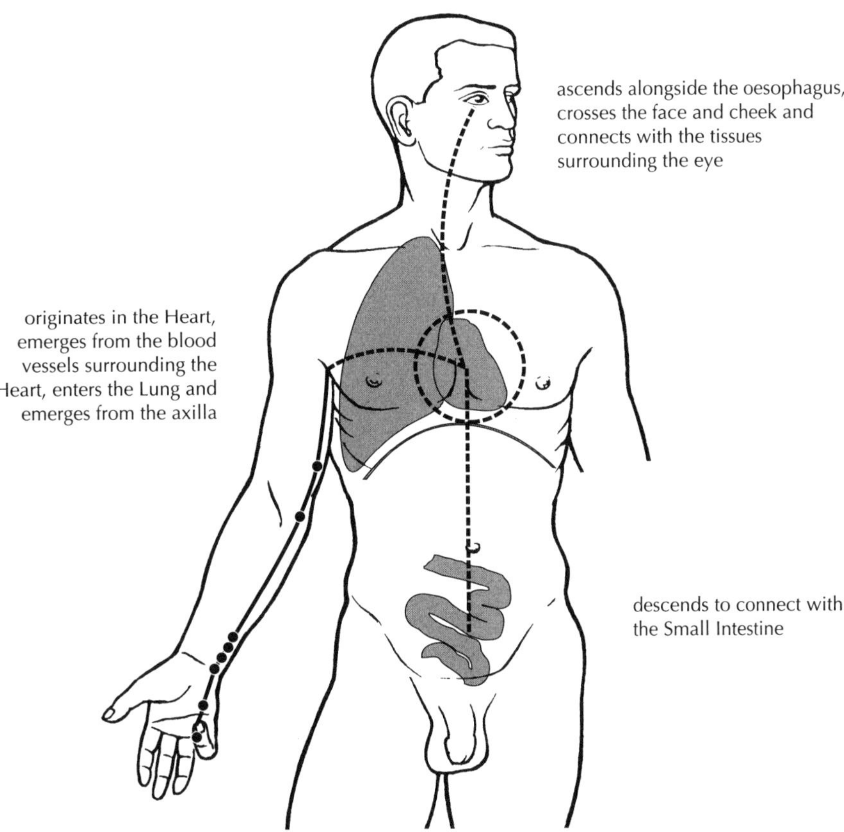

The Heart primary channel

THE HEART PRIMARY CHANNEL

- originates in the Heart,
- emerges from the system of blood vessels surrounding the Heart and descends through the diaphragm to connect with the Small Intestine,
- a branch separates from the Heart, ascends alongside the oesophagus and then across the face and cheek to connect with the tissues surrounding the eye,
- another branch travels directly from the Heart to the Lung and descends to emerge from the axilla at Jiquan HE-1, then
- travels along the medial aspect of the upper arm (medial to the Lung and Pericardium channels) to the elbow at Shaohai HE-3,
- descends along the antero-medial aspect of the lower arm to the pisiform bone of the wrist at Shenmen HE-7,
- travels through the palm and along the radial side of the little finger to terminate at the radial corner of the nail at Shaochong HE-9.

The Heart primary channel connects with the following zangfu: Heart, Lung and Small Intestine.

The Heart primary channel meets with other channels at the following points: None.

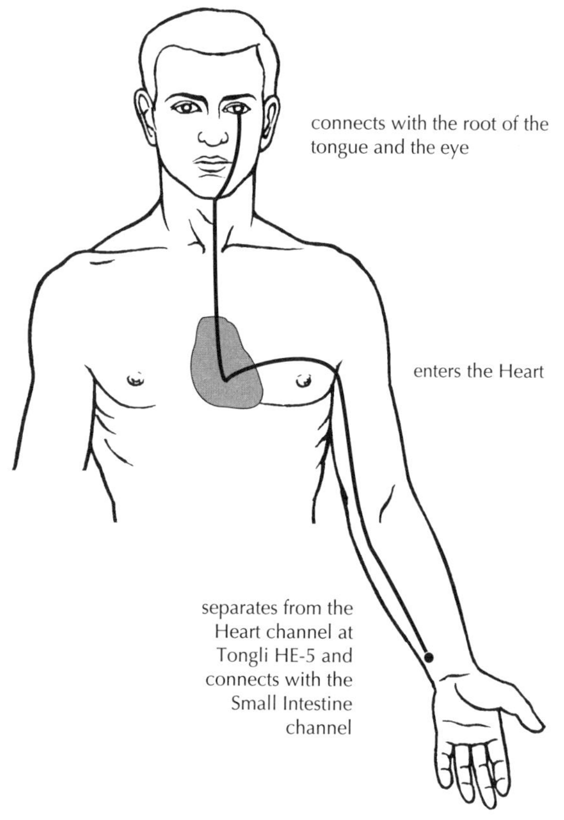

The Heart luo-connecting channel

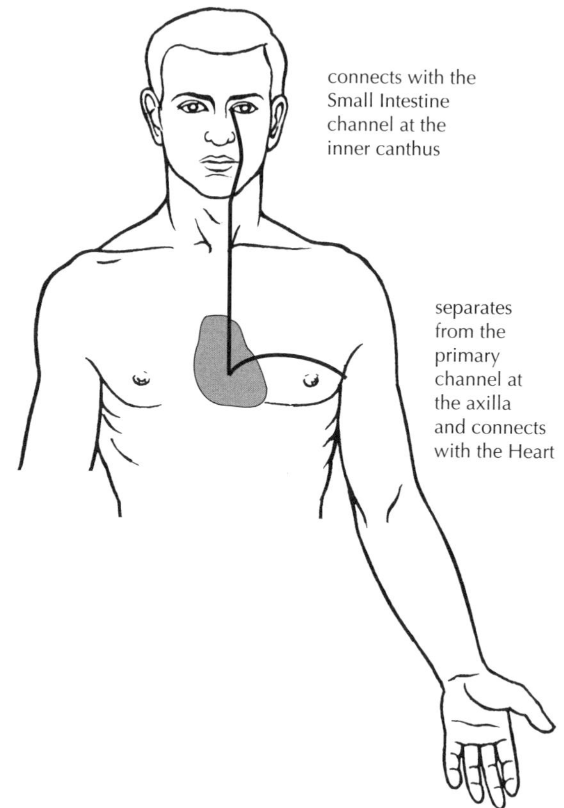

The Heart divergent channel

THE HEART LUO-CONNECTING CHANNEL

- separates from the Heart channel at Tongli HE-5 and connects with the Small Intestine channel,
- follows the Heart channel to the Heart zang then continues to the root of the tongue and the eye.

THE HEART DIVERGENT CHANNEL

- separates from the primary channel at the axillary fossa,
- enters the chest and connects with the Heart,
- ascends along the throat and emerges on the face, connecting with the Small Intestine channel at the inner canthus.

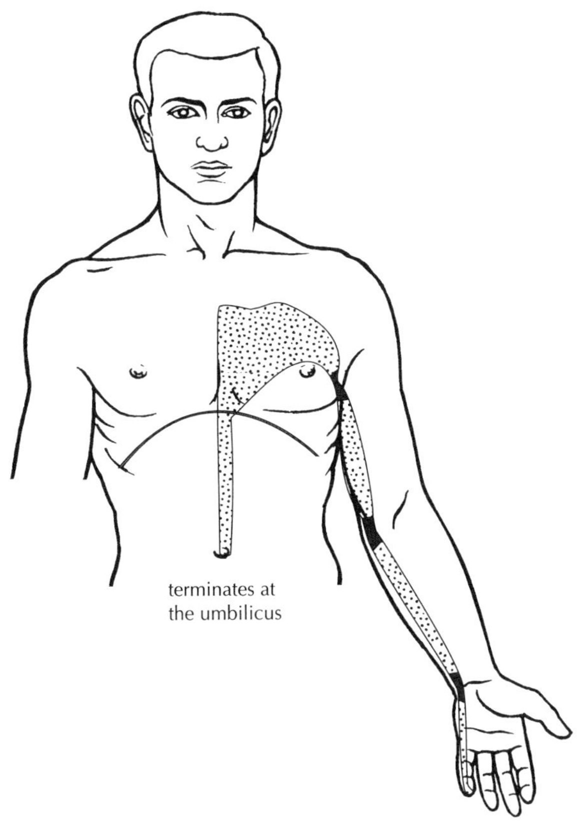

The Heart sinew channel

THE HEART SINEW CHANNEL

- originates at the radial aspect of the little finger and binds at the pisiform bone of the wrist,
- ascends to bind first at the medial aspect of the elbow and then at the axilla,
- enters the axilla, intersects the Lung sinew channel and travels medially across the breast region to the centre of the chest,
- descends across the diaphragm to terminate at the umbilicus.

Pathological symptoms of the Heart sinew channel
Internal tension, accumulation below the Heart, pain, cramping and strain along the course of the channel.

DISCUSSION

The Heart channel of hand shaoyin is interiorly-exteriorly coupled with the Small Intestine channel, and paired with the Kidney channel of foot shaoyin according to six channel theory. The Heart-Small Intestine relationship is further strengthened by the fact that:

- the Heart primary channel connects with the Small Intestine fu.
- the Heart divergent channel conects with the Small Intestine channel at the inner canthus.
- the Heart luo-connecting channel meets with the Small Intestine primary channel.

In addition, it is important to note that:

- a branch of the Heart primary channel ascends alongside the oesophagus.
- a branch of the Heart primary channel connects with the tissues surrounding the eye, the Heart divergent channel ascends to the inner canthus, and the Heart luo-connecting channel ascends to the eye.
- the Heart divergent channel emerges on the face.
- the Heart luo-connecting channel ascends to the root of the tongue.

The Heart has five principal functions:

- governing the blood and blood vessels
- housing the spirit
- opening into the tongue
- governing sweating
- manifesting in the complexion

It is by virtue of these functions, and the channel pathways listed above, that many of the actions and indications of the points of the Heart channel can be explained. These can be summarised as:

- Treating pain of the chest and Heart and disorders of Heart rhythm. According to the *Essential Questions* "All blood pertains to the Heart"[1] and "The Heart dominates the blood vessels of the body"[2]. The qi of the Heart and Lung (with which the Heart channel connects) dominate the gathering qi and thus the circulation of the blood through the chest as well as the rhythmical beating of the heart. All the points of the Heart channel (with the exception of Qingling HE-2) therefore treat either pain of the Heart and chest, or palpitations and other disorders of heart rhythm. Acute pain of the Heart and chest may radiate along the Heart channel in the left arm, down to the abdomen (Heart primary and sinew channels) or up to the throat (Heart primary and divergent channels). In current clinical practice, points of the Pericardium channel are mostly favoured for pain of the chest and Heart, whilst disorders of Heart rhythm are treated by selecting points from both channels.

- Regulating and calming the spirit. According to the *Spiritual Pivot*[3] "The Heart controls the vessels; the vessels are the residence of the spirit", whilst the *Essential Questions*[4] says "The Heart stores the spirit". Points of the Heart channel, especially Tongli HE-5 and Shenmen HE-7, are among the most important of the acupuncture points to harmonise and calm the spirit, whether it loses its harmony due to deficiency and consequent lack of nourishment, to agitation by heat and fire, or to being obscured by phlegm.
- Treating disorders of the tongue and speech, including loss of voice, stiffness of the tongue, and painful and swollen tongue.
- Treating disorders of the throat such as pain, swelling and congestion.
- Treating disorders of the eyes. In addition to the Heart channel connections to the eyes, this may be explained by the fact that the Heart belongs to sovereign fire and the points of the Heart channel may be used to clear heat from any part of the body, in the case of the eyes manifesting as redness, swelling and pain.
- Treating various disorders of the face and complexion, thus for example Ma Dan-yang says of Shenmen HE-7 "when excess ... the head, cheeks and face are red, when deficient there is ... an expressionless face".

JIQUAN HE-1

Summit Spring

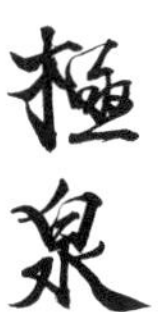

LOCATION

In the depression at the centre of the axilla.

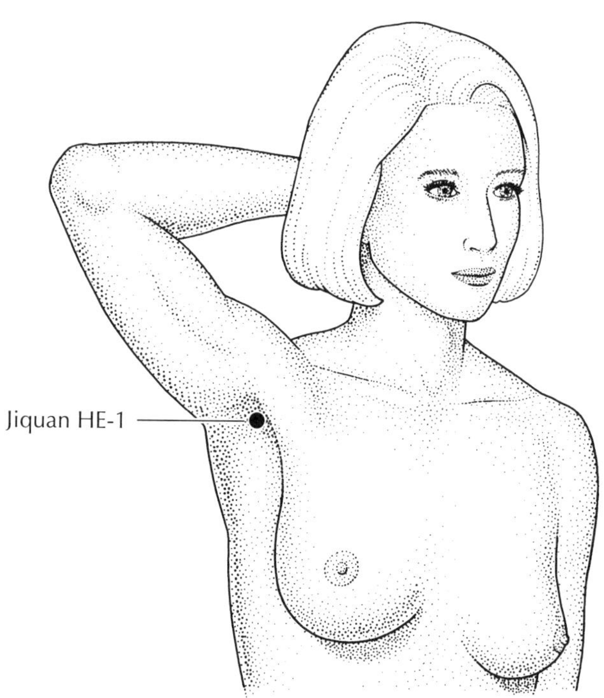

LOCATION NOTE

This point is located with the arm abducted. Slide your finger up the lateral wall of the chest between the two muscle groups (latissimus dorsi posteriorly and pectoralis major anteriorly) into the depression at the highest point of the axillary hollow.

NEEDLING

Perpendicular insertion (in the direction of Jianjing GB-21) 0.5 to 1 cun, avoiding the axillary artery.

Caution: medial insertion towards the chest may puncture the lung.

ACTIONS

Unbinds the chest

Activates the channel and benefits the arm

INDICATIONS

- Heart painful obstruction, Heart pain with retching, chest pain, shortness of breath, distention and fullness of the lateral costal region, sadness and anxiety, palpitations, agitation with thirst and dry throat.

- Inability to raise the shoulder, pain of the axilla, scrofula, numbness and painful obstruction of the upper limb, inversion counterflow of the elbow and arm, cold and pain of the elbow and arm, loss of use of the four limbs, yellow eyes.

COMMENTARY

Jiquan HE-1 is the first point of the Heart channel, where the qi emerges from the Heart and its surrounding blood vessels. Located in the centre of the axilla, it is the point of communication between the Heart and chest on the one hand, and the arm on the other, and has an action on both these regions.

In the chest and lateral costal region it promotes the movement of qi and alleviates pain, being indicated for distention and fullness of the lateral costal region, chest pain and shortness of breath. In the Heart itself it treats pain manifesting as Heart painful obstruction and Heart pain with retching.

When the Heart yang declines, with concomitant blood stasis, qi and blood are unable to maintain their circulation through the channels and vessels of the arm, giving rise to numbness, whilst if the warming function of yang is impaired there will be coldness and pain. By promoting circulation of qi and blood throughout the arm, Jiquan HE-1 is able to treat these disorders.

The axillary region may be viewed as a gateway for the circulation of qi and blood through the arm, implied in the name 'Summit Spring'. In qigong practice and meditation, keeping the axilla slightly open is vital for maintaining the free flow of qi and blood through the upper limb. For this reason it is said that one should stand or sit with enough space in the axilla "to hold an egg". As a result, even in periods of long quiescence the arm and hands will stay warm.

COMBINATIONS

- Heart pain with retching, agitation and fullness: Jiquan HE-1 and Ximen P-4 (*Supplementing Life*).
- Dry throat: Jiquan HE-1, Taiyuan LU-9, Pianli L.I.-6, Taichong LIV-3 and Tiantu REN-22 (*Supplementing Life*).
- Loss of use of the four limbs: Jiquan HE-1, Riyue GB-24 and Pishu BL-20 (*Supplementing Life*).

QINGLING HE-2

Green Spirit

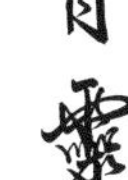

LOCATION

3 cun proximal to the medial end of the transverse cubital crease, on the line connecting Jiquan HE-1 and Shaohai HE-3.

LOCATION NOTE

i. Locate with the elbow flexed; ii. This point is located in the groove medial to the biceps brachii muscle, one handbreadth proximal to Shaohai HE-3.

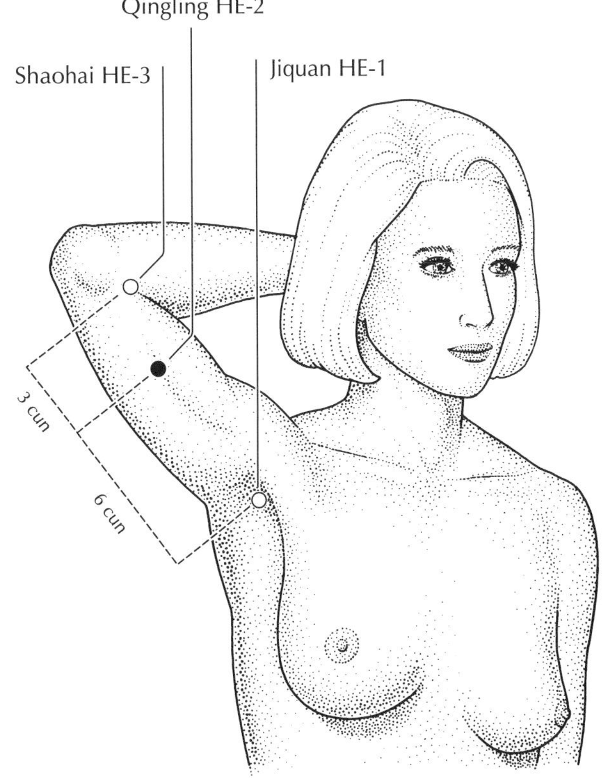

NEEDLING

Oblique distal or proximal insertion, 0.5 to 1 cun, avoiding the brachial artery. **Note:** many early classics only discuss moxibustion in relation to this point, implying that needling was contraindicated, perhaps because of the danger of damaging the brachial artery, whilst the *Introduction to Medicine* specifically contraindicates needling at this point.

ACTIONS

Activates the channel and alleviates pain

INDICATIONS

- Inability to raise the shoulder and arm, swelling, pain and redness of the shoulder, pain of the axilla, headache with cold shivering, yellow eyes, pain of the lateral costal region, scrofula.

COMBINATIONS

- Pain of the shoulder and upper arm: Qingling HE-2, Jianyu L.I.-15 and Quchi L.I.-11.

SHAOHAI HE-3

Lesser Sea

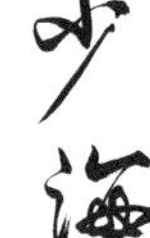

He-Sea and Water point of the Heart channel

LOCATION

Midway between Quze P-3 and the medial epicondyle of the humerus, at the medial end of the transverse cubital crease when the elbow is fully flexed.

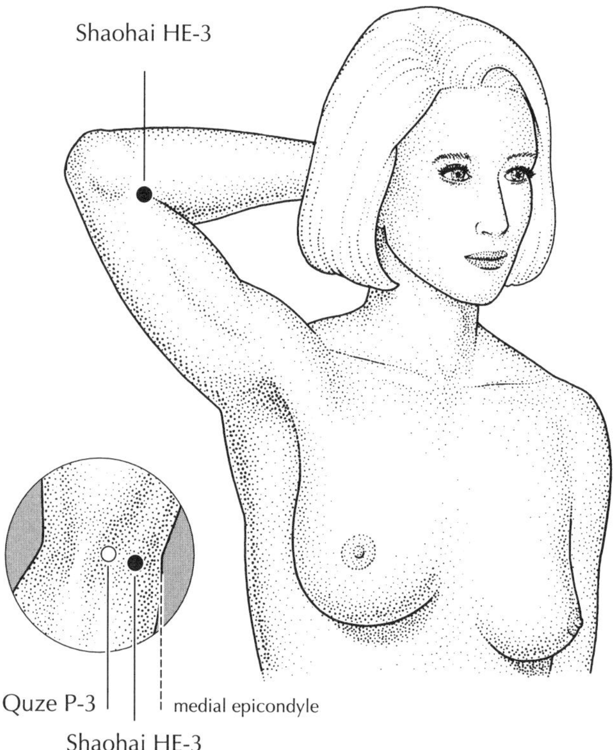

NEEDLING

i. Oblique insertion distally or proximally, or directed towards Quchi L.I.-11, 0.5 to 1.5 cun. **Note**: according to a number of classical sources this point is contraindicated to moxibustion.

ACTIONS

Calms the spirit, transforms phlegm and clears heat
Activates the channel and benefits the arm

INDICATIONS

- Heart pain, fullness of the chest, pain of the axilla and lateral costal region, mania and laughter, epilepsy, tongue thrusting, poor memory, vomiting of foamy (watery) saliva, scrofula.
- Red eyes, headache and wind dizziness, visual dizziness, toothache accompanied by chills and fever, erosion and swelling of the gums.
- Trembling of the hand and arm, numbness of the upper limb, inability to raise the four limbs, swelling and pain of the elbow joint, flaccidity of the elbow, inability to turn the neck, wind painful obstruction.

COMMENTARY

Shaohai HE-3 is the he-sea and water point of the Heart shaoyin (lesser yin) channel, hence the name Shaohai (Lesser Sea). It has three main spheres of action. Firstly it is able to calm the spirit, transform phlegm and clear heat, being indicated in such disorders as mania and laughter, epilepsy, tongue thrusting (where the tongue is repeatedly thrust out of the mouth like a snake's tongue) and poor memory, as well as other manifestations of phlegm such as vomiting of foamy saliva and scrofula. Clinically, however, it is less used for this purpose than points such as Jianshi P-5, Fenglong ST-40 and Tianjing SJ-10.

Secondly, as the water point of the Heart fire channel, Shaohai HE-3 is able to drain heat from the head manifesting as redness of the eyes, erosion and swelling of the gums, and toothache accompanied by chills and fever.

The third and main clinical application of Shaohai HE-3, however, is in the treatment of various disorders of the Heart channel in the upper limb. It is an important point for numbness and trembling of the arm and hand, and disorders of the elbow. According to the *Classic of the Jade Dragon* it is indicated for "fullness of the chest with agitation of the Heart accompanied by numbness and difficulty in raising the shoulder and arm". In the treatment of atrophy disorder and hemiplegia following windstroke, points of yangming channel, which is "abundant in qi and blood" have long been emphasised. Clinical practice has demonstrated, however, that better results are obtained when some points from yin channels are also selected. Due to the important action of Shaohai HE-3 on disorders of the whole arm, it is often stimulated by through needling from Quchi L.I.-11 in the treatment of these disorders.

COMBINATIONS

- Vomiting of foam: Shaohai HE-3, Duiduan DU-27 and Benshen GB-13 (*Supplementing Life*).
- Vomiting of foamy (watery) saliva: Shaohai HE-3 and Zhubin KID-9 (*Supplementing Life*).
- Scrofula: Shaohai HE-3, Tianchi P-1, Zhangmen LIV-13, Zulinqi GB-41, Zhigou SJ-6, Yangfu GB-38, Jianjing GB-21 and Shousanli L.I.-10 (*Great Compendium*).
- Scrofula: Shaohai HE-3 and Tianjing SJ-10 (*Song More Precious Than Jade*).

- Manic raving fear and fright: Shaohai HE-3, Zhizheng SI-7, Yuji LU-10, Hegu L.I.-4, Quchi L.I.-11 and Wangu SI-4 (*Thousand Ducat Formulas*).
- Stiff tongue, tongue thrusting: Shaohai HE-3, Huaroumen ST-24 and Wenliu L.I.-7 (*Supplementing Life*).
- Stubborn numbness of both forearms: Shaohai HE-3 and Shousanli L.I.-10 (*One Hundred Symptoms*).

LINGDAO HE-4

Spirit Path

靈道

Jing-River and Metal point of the Heart channel

LOCATION

On the radial side of the tendon of flexor carpi ulnaris, 1.5 cun proximal to Shenmen HE-7.

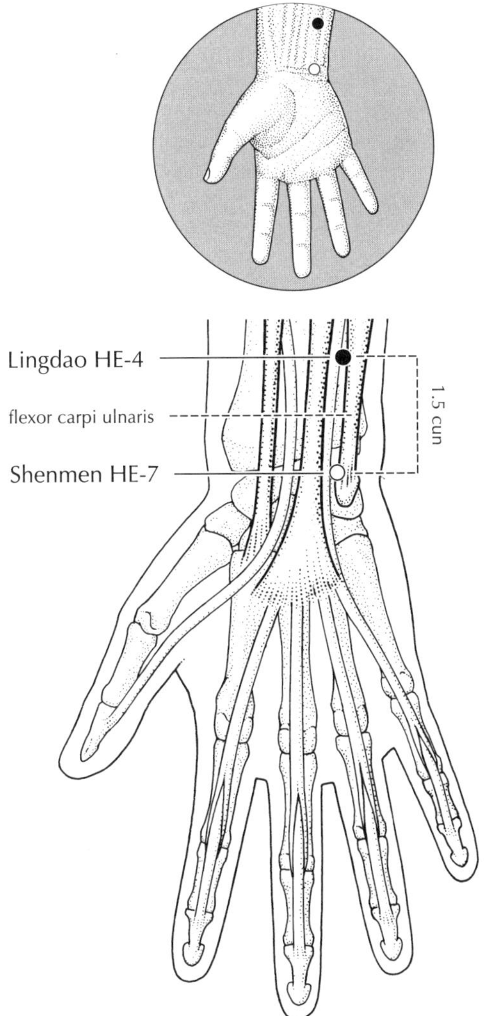

NEEDLING

Perpendicular insertion 0.3 to 0.5 cun, or oblique proximal or distal insertion 0.5 to 1 cun.

ACTIONS

Calms the spirit and benefits the voice
Relaxes the muscles and sinews

INDICATIONS

- Heart pain, sadness and fear, restless zang disorder, sudden loss of voice.
- Retching, throat abscess, redness and swelling of the eyes.
- Cold bones and marrow, clonic spasm, contraction of the elbow and arm, itching of the hand, swelling and pain of the fingers.

COMMENTARY

Lingdao HE-4, as its name 'Spirit Path' implies, has the ability to calm the spirit and is indicated for restless zang disorder and sadness and fear. Restless zang disorder is said to arise due to overthinking, excessive worry and anxiety which injure the Heart, Spleen and Liver. It is characterised by a wide variety of symptoms including unpredictable emotional responses, melancholy, disturbed behaviour, restlessness, insomnia, loss of voice and even mania. In terms of modern medicine it corresponds to hysterical neurosis. The ability of Lingdao HE-4 to treat sudden loss of voice (note combinations below) reflects its status as a jing-river point, since the *Spiritual Pivot*[5] states that the jing-river points should be needled for changes manifesting in the patient's voice.

According to the *Spiritual Pivot*[6] "when the disease is at the yin within yang (sinews and bones), needle the jing-river point of the yin". Lingdao HE-4, the jing-river point of the Heart channel, is indicated for contraction of the elbow and arm and a freezing cold sensation deep within the marrow and bones.

COMBINATIONS

- Sudden loss of voice with lockjaw: Lingdao HE-4, Tiantu REN-22 and Tianchuang SI-16 (*Supplementing Life*).
- Sudden loss of voice: Lingdao HE-4, Zhigou SJ-6, Tianchuang SI-16, Futu L.I.-18 and Qubin GB-7 (*Thousand Ducat Formulas*).
- Loss of voice: Lingdao HE-4, Tiantu REN-22, Yingu KID-10, Fuliu KID-7, Fenglong ST-40 and Rangu KID-2 (*Illustrated Supplement*).

TONGLI HE-5

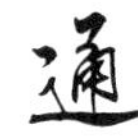
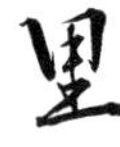

Penetrating the Interior

Luo-Connecting point of the Heart channel
Ma Dan-yang Heavenly Star point

LOCATION

On the radial side of the tendon of flexor carpi ulnaris, 1 cun proximal to Shenmen HE-7.

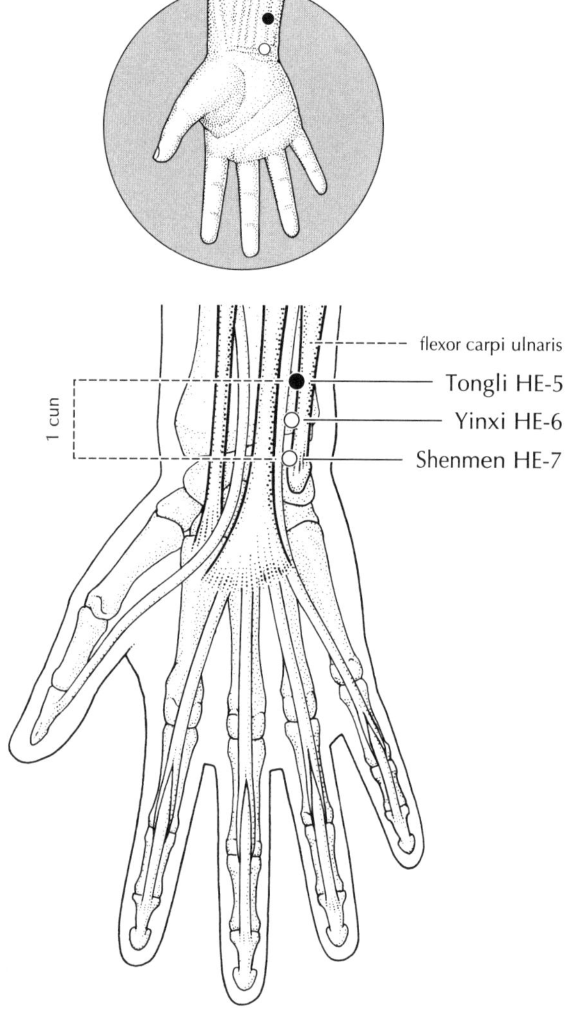

NEEDLING

Perpendicular insertion 0.3 to 0.5 cun, or oblique proximal or distal insertion 0.5 to 1 cun.

ACTIONS

Calms the spirit
Regulates Heart rhythm
Benefits the tongue
Activates the channel and alleviates pain

INDICATIONS

- Frequent yawning and groaning with sadness, restless zang disorder, vexation and anger, sadness and fright, depressive disorder, pain and agitation of the Heart, frequent vexation with burning sensation of the heart, fullness and distention of the chest and diaphragm radiating to the lateral costal region.
- Palpitations, fright palpitations, pounding of the Heart, disorders of Heart rhythm, diminished qi.
- Sudden loss of voice, inability to speak, stuttering, stiffness of the tongue, eye pain, throat painful obstruction, red face with absence of sweating, head wind, headache and dizziness, visual dizziness, bitter vomiting.
- Menorrhagia, profuse uterine bleeding, enuresis.
- Pain and heaviness of the wrist and elbow, contraction of the fingers, pain of the elbow and upper arm, paralysis of the four limbs.

COMMENTARY

Tongli HE-5 was included by Ma Dan-yang, the great physician of the Jin dynasty, among the 'eleven heavenly star points'[7], his grouping of the most vital acupuncture points, and was indicated by him for "inability to speak despite a desire to do so, vexation and anger, pounding of the Heart; when excess there is heaviness of the four limbs, and the head, cheeks and face are red; when deficient there is inability to eat, sudden loss of voice and an expressionless face".

Tongli HE-5 is the luo-connecting point of the Heart channel, from where the luo-connecting channel penetrates deeply into the Heart zang, strengthening the zang-channel relationship, hence the name 'Penetrating the Interior'. It has two principal actions on the Heart: i. to calm the spirit, and ii. to regulate Heart qi.

The *Spiritual Pivot*[8] is the earliest text to record the fundamental principle that "the Heart is the residence of the spirit". The function of housing the spirit in Chinese medicine encompasses mental activity, consciousness, memory, thinking and sleep. At the same time it also refers to the totality of the emotional and spiritual life of a person. According to the *Ode of the Jade Dragon* "Tongli HE-5 treats a frightenable Heart". Tongli HE-5 shares with most of the other luo-connecting points of the yin channels (Lieque LU-7, Gongsun SP-4, Dazhong KID-4, Ligou LIV-5 and Neiguan P-6) the special ability to treat psycho-emotional disorders, but as the luo-connecting point of the Heart zang it is especially suitable for this purpose and is wide-ranging in its effect. Its action on calming the spirit, however, focuses on emotional disorders, rather than disturbances of sleep or memory, for which Shenmen HE-7 is more effective. According to Fei

Bo-xiong[9] "The seven emotions injure the five yin organs selectively but they all affect the Heart". Tongli HE-5 is classically indicated for many different emotional manifestations, not only fright and agitation which are traditionally associated with disharmony of the Heart, but fear, vexation, anger, sadness and depression which are usually considered to injure, or result from injury to, other zangfu. The great doctor Hua Tuo said of the relationship between the Heart and fear "excessive thought gives rise to apprehension, and apprehension injures the Heart; an injured Heart gives rise to loss of spirit, and loss of spirit gives rise to fright and fear"[10].

As for regulating the Heart qi, Tongli HE-5 plays an important role in the treatment of palpitations, fright palpitations, pounding of the Heart and disorders of heart rhythm. In Chinese medicine, palpitations are subdivided into i. simple palpitations which is a general term, ii. fright palpitations which denotes palpitations that are either triggered by or accompanied by feelings of fright, and iii. pounding of the Heart (the most serious kind) which denotes palpitations which may be felt as high up as the heart itself, or as low as the umbilicus (the termination point of the Heart sinew channel). Palpitations may accompany any pattern of the Heart zang, but as a disorder of the rhythmical beating of the heart they always involve the Heart qi.

The pathways of the Heart primary and secondary channels clarify various other classical indications of this point. According to a saying of Chinese medicine "the tongue is the sprouting forth of the Heart", and the Heart luo-connecting channel, after entering the Heart zang, ascends to the root of the tongue. Tongli HE-5 is the primary point to treat loss of voice and stiffness of the tongue which affects the speech, usually resulting from mental disorders or the sequelae of windstroke. It is also indicated for the treatment of stuttering. The Heart channel connects with the tissues surrounding the eye, whilst the luo-connecting channel from Tongli HE-5 both spreads to the Heart's interiorly-exteriorly coupled Small Intestine channel and ascends to the eye. Tongli HE-5 is indicated for (and included in a number of classical combinations for) head wind, headache and dizziness, all of which may be accompanied by redness or pain of the eyes. These symptoms reflect disharmony of both coupled channels.

The Small Intestine channel is paired with the Bladder channel (taiyang) according to six channel theory. This Heart-Small Intestine-Bladder linkage has traditionally been used to explain the relationship between Heart disharmony and urinary disorders, since heat can transmit from the Heart to the Small Intestine and thence to the Bladder, and in the case of Tongli HE-5 its ability to treat enuresis due to accumulation of heat in the Bladder.

The Heart governs blood, whilst according to the *Essential Questions*[11] "The bao mai [uterine channel] pertains to the Heart and is connected with the uterus". If, due to emotional factors, heat accumulates in the Heart and enters the blood, there may be uterine bleeding or menorrhagia due to reckless movement of the blood. Tongli HE-5 is the only point on the Heart channel with such gynaecological indications.

Finally the *Great Compendium of Acupuncture and Moxibustion* gives specific indications for excess and deficiency of the luo-connecting points. In the case of Tongli HE-5 these are: fullness and distention of the chest and diaphragm radiating to the lateral costal region (excess); and inability to speak (deficiency).

COMBINATIONS

- Weary speech and somnolence: Tongli HE-5 and Dazhong KID-4 (*One Hundred Symptoms*).
- Sudden loss of speech: Tongli HE-5 and Yifeng SJ-17 (*Supplementing Life*).
- Head wind, redness of the face and eyes: Tongli HE-5 and Jiexi ST-41 (*Great Compendium*).
- Pain of the head and eyes: Tongli HE-5, Baihui DU-20 and Houding DU-19 (*Supplementing Life*).
- Headache and dizziness: Tongli HE-5, Feiyang BL-58, Kunlun BL-60, Ququan LIV-8, Qiangu SI-2 and Shaoze SI-1 (*Thousand Ducat Formulas*).
- Enuresis: Tongli HE-5, Jimen SP-11, Dadun LIV-1, Pangguangshu BL-28, Taichong LIV-3, Weizhong BL-40 and Shenmen HE-7 (*Supplementing Life*).
- Irregular Heart rhythm: Tongli HE-5, Neiguan P-6, Jueyinshu BL-14 and Xinshu BL-15.

YINXI HE-6

Yin Cleft

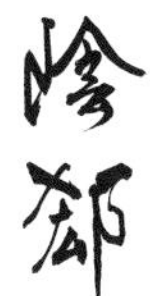

Xi-Cleft point of the Heart channel

LOCATION

On the radial side of the tendon of flexor carpi ulnaris, 0.5 cun proximal to Shenmen HE-7.

NEEDLING

Perpendicular insertion 0.3 to 0.5 cun, or oblique proximal or distal insertion 0.5 to 1 cun.

ACTIONS

Regulates Heart blood
Calms the spirit
Moderates acute conditions
Clears deficiency fire and alleviates night sweating

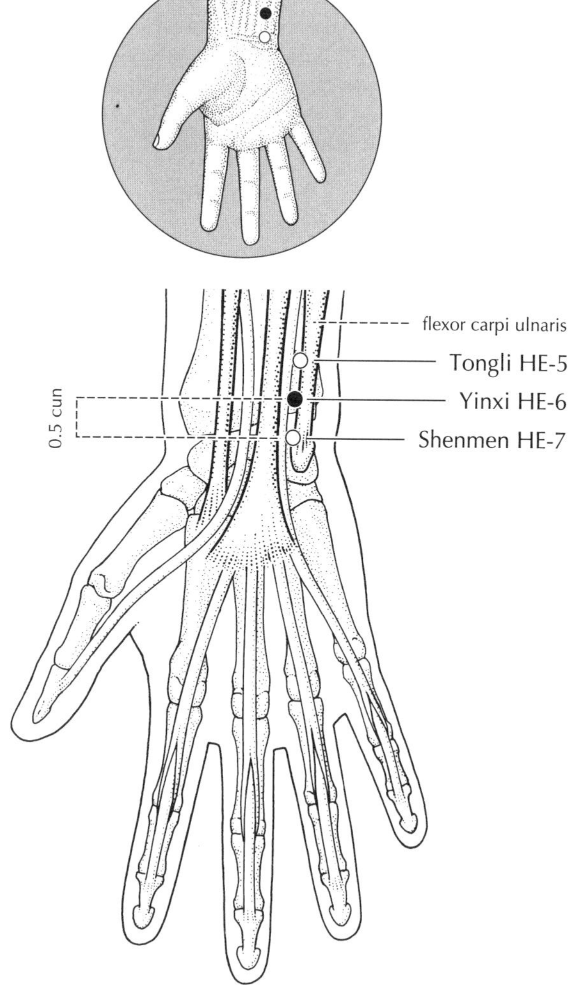

INDICATIONS

- Heart pain, unbearable stabbing pain of the Heart, fullness of the chest, palpitations, fright palpitations, fright, counterflow inversion fright qi, epilepsy, loss of voice, sudden turmoil disorder with cardiac pain.
- Nosebleed, vomiting blood, counterflow qi.
- Night sweating, steaming bone disorder.

COMMENTARY

Yinxi HE-6 is the xi-cleft point of the Heart channel. The xi-cleft points are where the qi and blood, which flow relatively superficially along the channels from the jing-well points, gather and plunge more deeply. The xi-cleft points in general are indicated in the treatment of acute conditions and pain, whilst the xi-cleft points of the yin channels have an additional action of treating disorders of blood. Yinxi HE-6 is indicated for Heart pain due to blood stasis, and bleeding disorders due to excessive heat agitating the blood. However, in terms of both these actions, Ximen P-4 the xi-cleft point of the Pericardium channel, is clinically more important. Acute severe pain from blood stasis which threatens the survival of the Heart zang is therefore primarily treated by using points of the Pericardium channel, the 'protector' of the Heart. This is reflected in the statement in the *Spiritual Pivot*[12] "The Heart is the great master of the five zang and six fu and the residence of the essence-spirit ... If the Heart is injured, the spirit will depart; if the spirit departs, the person will die ... therefore the pathogenic qi that attacks the Heart will be diverted to reside in the Pericardium".

The forte of Yinxi HE-6 lies in its ability to treat the yin fluids of the Heart. According to the *Ode to Elucidate Mysteries* "Reducing Yinxi HE-6 will stop night sweating and treat steaming bone disorder in children". This underlines the primary application of Yinxi HE-6 in clinical practice. According to *Essential Readings from the Medical Tradition* "That which is stored by the Heart internally is blood, externally it is emitted as sweat; sweat is the fluid of the Heart". Owing to this close relationship between the Heart blood and sweating, and the ability of the xi-cleft points to harmonise the blood, Yinxi HE-6 is an essential point in the treatment of night sweating due to deficiency of either yin or Heart blood. Night is the time of maximum yin, and during sleep (when the body is covered and the more yang defensive qi is no longer needed to protect the surface) the defensive qi enters deep within the yin to be nourished. If yin is deficient, it cannot draw and hold the defensive qi inside, and deficiency heat floats to the exterior and forces out the fluids as sweat. Alternatively, when Heart blood is deficient, the balance of qi and blood is disturbed and the qi floats to the surface causing night sweating, characterised by less intense heat sensations than the yin deficiency pattern. Controlling night sweating is always a priority of treatment, since the sweat emitted in this disorder (known in Chinese as 'robbing sweat') contains yin nutrient and its loss further aggravates the deficiency. It should be noted that night sweating, although most often due to the two patterns described above, may also occur as a result of other patterns of disharmony, specifically damp-heat, Spleen deficiency with retention of dampness, half-interior/half-exterior pathogen disorders and disharmony of nutritive qi and defensive qi. Due to its important action in stopping night sweating, Yinxi HE-6 may be used in any of these patterns in combination with appropriate points.

Steaming bone disorder is a form of fever from yin deficiency. It is characterised by a sensation of heat deep within the bones radiating outwards to the skin, and is accompanied by afternoon fever, restless sleep and night sweating. It is a profound form of yin deficiency with raging heat and is usually seen in the context of serious disease. Yinxi HE-6 is one of the principal points used to treat this pattern.

Finally, as the xi-cleft point of the Heart channel, Yinxi HE-6 is able to soothe and calm the Heart in acute situations and is indicated for acute fright - with or without palpitations. It is also specifically indicated for 'counterflow inversion fright qi'. This refers to loss of consciousness (inversion pattern) that arises when severe anger depresses the qi, or fright and fear rapidly and violently descend the qi.

COMBINATIONS

- Profuse night sweating: Yinxi HE-6 and Houxi SI-3 (*One Hundred Symptoms*).
- Excessive fright: Yinxi HE-6, Jianshi P-5, Erjian L.I.-2 and Lidui ST-45 (*Supplementing Life*).
- Heart pain with fullness and agitation and stiff tongue: Yinxi HE-6 and Zhongchong P-9 (*Supplementing Life*).
- Heart pain: Yinxi HE-6 and Xingjian LIV-2 (*Supplementing Life*).

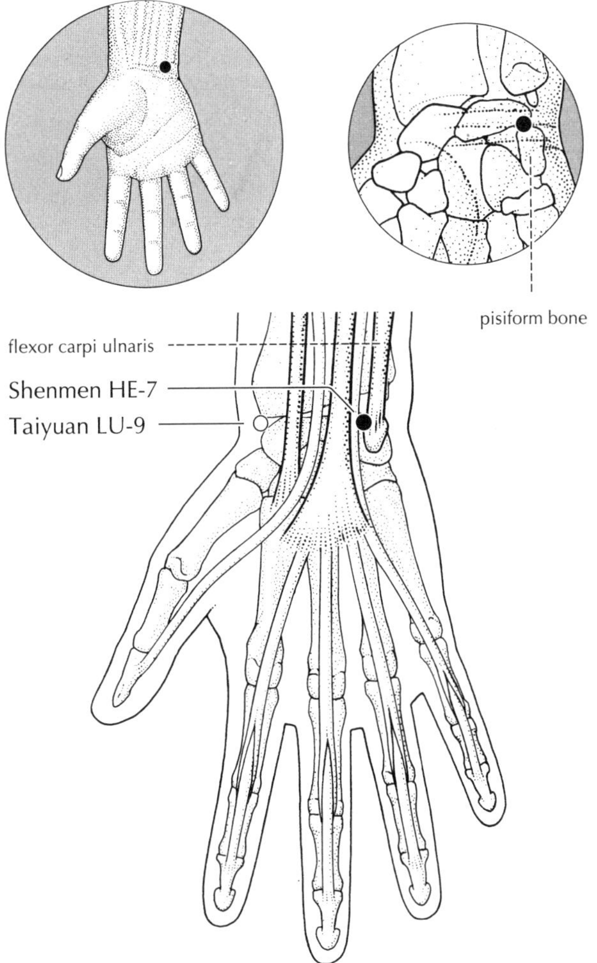

SHENMEN HE-7

Spirit Gate

神門

Shu-Stream, Yuan-Source and Earth point of the Heart channel

LOCATION

At the wrist joint, on the radial side of flexor carpi ulnaris, in the depression at the proximal border of the pisiform bone.

LOCATION NOTE

i. The location of this point is normally given in relation to the crease of the wrist. Since wrist creases are a superficial and variable anatomical feature, it is better to locate this point in relation to the underlying pisiform bone; ii. When it is necessary to needle a patient in the prone position with the arms towards the head, this point may be located and needled on the ulnar side of flexor carpi ulnaris, very close to the tendon insertion; the needle is then directed beneath the tendon towards its radial side.

NEEDLING

Perpendicular insertion 0.3 to 0.5 cun, or oblique insertion proximally, medially or distally 0.5 to 0.8 cun.

Caution: the ulnar artery and ulnar nerve lie adjacent to this point.

ACTIONS

Calms the spirit
Regulates and tonifies the Heart

INDICATIONS

- Insomnia, frequent talking during sleep, poor memory, mania-depression, epilepsy, dementia, desire to laugh, mad laughter, insulting people, sadness, fear and fright, disorientation, restless zang disorder, agitation of the Heart, malaria accompanied by agitation of the Heart, loss of voice.
- Heart pain, palpitations, fright palpitations, pounding of the Heart.
- Throat painful obstruction, dry throat with no desire to drink, vomiting blood, spitting blood, yellow eyes, pain of the lateral costal region, red face, heat of the palms, dyspnoea with heat in the body, shortness of breath, cold shivering, enuresis.

COMMENTARY

Shenmen HE-7 is the shu-stream and yuan-source point of the Heart channel. The *Spiritual Pivot* in Chapter 6 recommends the use of the shu-stream points in the treatment of disorders of the zang, whilst in Chapter 1 it says "When the five zang are diseased, select [from] the twelve yuan-source [points]". Shenmen HE-7 is an essential point to treat i. all disorders of the spirit, and ii. all deficiency disorders of the Heart zang.

Shenmen HE-7 (Spirit Gate) is the foremost acupuncture point to calm and regulate the spirit. According to the *Spiritual Pivot*[13] "the Heart is the residence of the spirit". Disturbance of the spirit may broadly be divided into two main categories: deficiency patterns (mainly of Heart blood or yin) and excess patterns (Heart fire, phlegm or phlegm-fire). When Heart blood or yin are deficient they are no longer able to nourish the Heart and provide the material basis for the Heart to store and anchor the spirit. As a consequence the spirit loses its harmony and becomes restless and unquiet, resulting in such symptoms as anxiety and fearfulness, poor memory, restless zang disorder, insomnia and disturbed sleep. If Heart qi is deficient (especially when accompanied by qi deficiency of the Gall Bladder), a person will be easily frightened and apprehensive. According to the *Spiritual Pivot*[14] "When Heart qi is deficient there is sadness; when excess there is ceaseless laughter". If the Heart loses contact with its associated emotion, joy, a person will be prone to ceaseless and inappropriate laughter. When Heart fire rages out of control it agitates and excites the spirit leading to such symptoms as severe insomnia and mental hyperactivity. When phlegm, or phlegm-fire, obstruct the portals of the Heart, the spirit will be disturbed to varying degrees, ranging from milder manifestations such as insomnia, talking during sleep, disorientation, agitation and restlessness, to the more severe symptoms of dementia, mania, mad laughter, insulting behaviour and epilepsy. Whatever the pattern, Shenmen HE-7 may be used to help restore peace and harmony to the spirit.

The Heart is unique in being susceptible to the four principal kinds of deficiency (qi, blood, yin and yang), Shenmen HE-7, the shu-stream and yuan-source point of the Heart channel, may be used in any of these situations, especially in cases of deficiency of blood and yin. In practice, the tonifying action of Shenmen HE-7 is enhanced and focused through its combination with other suitable points.

Palpitations are a common symptom of Heart disorder. Although fundamentally a disorder of Heart qi (the active, moving aspect of the Heart zang), palpitations may accompany virtually any Heart pattern, whether deficient or excess. Through its action of regulating and tonifying the qi of the Heart, Shenmen HE-7 is indicated for all kinds of palpitations, including fright palpitations and pounding of the Heart (see Tongli HE-5).

The Heart channel ascends to the throat and Shenmen HE-7 is able to clear heat from the channel giving rise to swelling, congestion, dryness and pain of the throat.

Finally, the Heart channel is interiorly-exteriorly coupled with the Small Intestine channel which is paired with the Bladder channel (taiyang) according to six channel theory. This linkage has traditionally been used to explain the relationship between Heart disharmony and urinary disorders, and in the case of Shenmen HE-7 its ability (emphasised in its inclusion in many classical combinations) to treat enuresis due to accumulation of heat in the Bladder.

COMBINATIONS

- Fear and fright with Heart pain: Shenmen HE-7, Shaochong HE-9, Yanglingquan GB-34 and Neiguan P-6 (*Compilation*).
- Fright palpitations with diminished qi: Shenmen HE-7, Ligou LIV-5 and Juque REN-14 (*Supplementing Life*).
- Heart painful obstruction, sadness and fear: Shenmen HE-7, Dadun LIV-1 and Yuji LU-10 (*Great Compendium*).
- Weeping with grief: Shenmen HE-7, Xinshu BL-15, Jiexi ST-41 and Daling P-7 (*Supplementing Life*).
- Dementia: Shenmen HE-7, Shaoshang LU-11, Yongquan KID-1 and Xinshu BL-15 (*Great Compendium*).
- Manic laughter: Shenmen HE-7 and Yanggu SI-5 (*Thousand Ducat Formulas*).
- Mania, desires to ascend to high places and sing, discards clothing and runs around: Shenmen HE-7, Chongyang ST-42 and Houxi SI-3 (*Great Compendium*).
- Manic rushing around: Shenmen HE-7 and Shangwan REN-13 (*One Hundred Symptoms*).
- Epilepsy: Shenmen HE-7, Neiguan P-6, Houxi SI-3, Xinshu BL-15 and Yinbai SP-1 (*Complete Collection*).
- The five types of epilepsy: Shenmen HE-7, Jiuwei REN-15 and Houxi SI-3 (*Song More Precious Than Jade*).
- Heart pain: Shenmen HE-7, Jueyinshu BL-14 and Zulinqi GB-41 (*Supplementing Life*).
- Vomiting blood: Shenmen HE-7, Quze P-3 and Yuji LU-10 (*Great Compendium*).
- Enuresis: Shenmen HE-7, Guanmen ST-22 and Zhongfu LU-1 (*Thousand Ducat Formulas*).
- Enuresis: Shenmen HE-7, Yuji LU-10, Taichong LIV-3, Dadun LIV-1 and Guanyuan REN-4 (*Great Compendium*).
- Enuresis: Shenmen HE-7, Guanmen ST-22 and Weizhong BL-40 (*Systematic Classic*).
- Enuresis: Shenmen HE-7, Pangguangshu BL-28, Tongli HE-5, Dadun LIV-1, Jimen SP-11, Taichong LIV-3 and Weizhong BL-40 (*Supplementing Life*).

SHAOFU HE-8

Lesser Palace

少府

Ying-Spring and Fire point of the Heart channel

LOCATION

On the palm, in the depression between the 4th and 5th metacarpal bones, where the tip of the little finger rests when a fist is made.

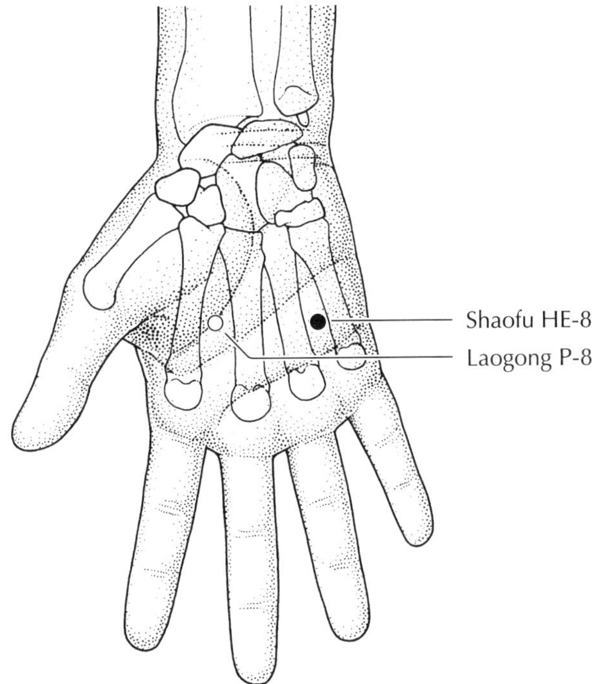

LOCATION NOTE

This point generally lies between the two transverse palmar creases.

NEEDLING

Perpendicular insertion 0.5 cun.

ACTIONS

Clears heat from the Heart and Small Intestine
Calms the spirit
Regulates Heart qi
Activates the channel and alleviates pain

INDICATIONS

- Palpitations, fright palpitations, sadness and worry with diminished qi, fear, fear of people, excessive sighing, plumstone qi (globus hystericus), chest pain, agitation and fullness, epilepsy.
- Itching of the genitals, pain of the genitals, difficult urination, enuresis, prolapse of the uterus.
- Chronic malaria, cold shivering, throat pain, stiffness of the tongue.
- Contraction of the little finger or hand, heat of the palms, pain of the arm, contraction of the elbow and axilla.

COMMENTARY

Shaofu HE-8 is the ying-spring and fire point of the Heart shaoyin (lesser yin) channel, hence the name 'Lesser Palace'. According to the *Classic of Difficulties*[15] ying-spring points are indicated for "heat in the body", whilst a saying of Chinese medicine states "When the Heart is cleared [of heat] the urine will flow". Shaofu HE-8 is a major point for clearing Heart fire which transmits to the hand taiyang Small Intestine channel (its interiorly-exteriorly coupled channel), and thence to the foot taiyang Bladder channel (paired with the Small Intestine according to six channel theory), giving rise to a variety of urogenital symptoms including difficult urination, enuresis, and itching or pain of the genitals. The characteristic accompanying signs of this type of urogenital disorder are insomnia, emotional disturbance, thirst, and sores of the mouth and tongue. Although having some action of clearing Heart fire affecting the upper jiao in this way, Shaofu HE-8 is traditionally less indicated for this purpose than points such as Daling P-7 and Laogong P-8, and its primary application is to clear the lower jiao heat.

The second principal action of Shaofu HE-8 is to regulate the Heart qi in cases both of stagnation and deficiency. Stagnation of qi in the Heart and chest region, principally transmitted from the Liver and due to emotional factors, may present as pain and oppression of the chest accompanied by excessive sighing, fearfulness and even plumstone qi (globus hystericus), all indications classically recorded for this point. Equally, Shaofu HE-8 is indicated for a variety of emotional disorders due to deficiency of Heart qi. This kind of deficiency which often follows severe emotional shock or fright, may give rise to palpitations, sadness and worry (Heart and Lung qi deficiency) or excessive fearfulness (Heart and Gall Bladder qi deficiency), as well as excessive sighing which, although more commonly due to qi stagnation may also result from qi deficiency.

Shaofu HE-8 is indicated for a variety of Heart channel disorders including throat pain, stiff tongue, contracture of the elbow and axilla, and especially heat in the palms and contracture and pain of the little finger.

Finally, according to the *Essential Questions*[11] "The bao mai [uterine channel] pertains to the Heart and is connected with the uterus". Shaofu HE-8 is indicated for (and appears in classical combinations for) uterine prolapse.

COMBINATIONS

- Difficult urination or retention of urine: Shaofu HE-8 and Zusanli ST-36 (*Thousand Ducat Formulas*).
- Uterine prolapse: Shaofu HE-8, Taichong LIV-3, Zhaohai KID-6 and Ququan LIV-8 (*Great Compendium*).
- Qi [stagnation] in the throat as if [obstructed by] a polyp: Shaofu HE-8 and Ligou LIV-5 (*Thousand Ducat Formulas*).
- Diminished qi: Shaofu HE-8, Pangguangshu BL-28, Shaochong HE-9, Bulang KID-22, Xingjian LIV-2 and Dazhong KID-5 (*Supplementing Life*).

SHAOCHONG HE-9

Lesser Rushing

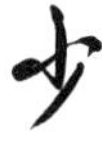

Jing-Well and Wood point of the Heart channel

LOCATION

On the dorsal aspect of the little finger, at the junction of lines drawn along the radial border of the nail and the base of the nail, approximately 0.1 cun from the corner of the nail.

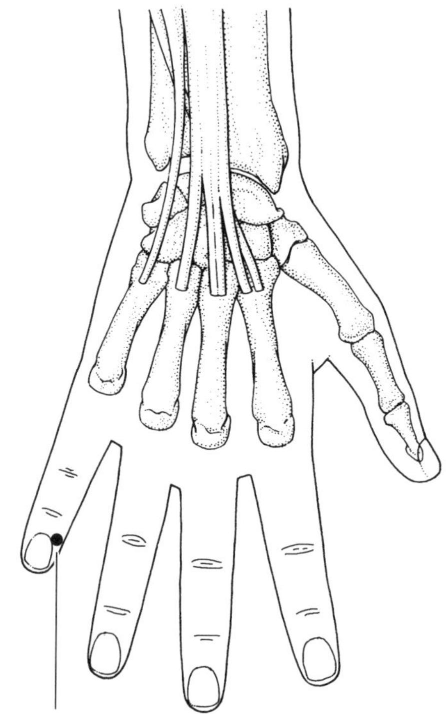

Shaochong HE-9

NEEDLING

Perpendicular or oblique insertion directed proximally 0.1 to 0.2 cun, or prick to bleed.

ACTIONS

Revives consciousness

Clears heat and benefits the tongue, eyes and throat

Regulates Heart qi and calms the spirit

INDICATIONS

- Heart pain, pain of the chest and lateral costal region, palpitations, pounding of the Heart, loss of consciousness from windstroke, loss of consciousness, mania-depression, epilepsy, fright epilepsy, excessive sighing, fright and sadness with diminished qi, febrile disease with agitation and restlessness.
- Pain at the root of the tongue, swollen tongue, tongue thrusting, throat painful obstruction, dry throat, heat in the mouth, pain of the eyes, red eyes, yellow eyes, jaundice, malaria, heat in the body like fire.
- Contraction of the hand, pain of the arm, inability to extend the elbow, pain of the palm that radiates to the elbow, axilla and chest.

COMMENTARY

Shaochong HE-9 is the jing-well point, and thus the terminal and most dynamic point, of the Heart shaoyin (lesser yin) channel, hence the name Lesser Rushing. It shares with the jing-well points of the twelve channels three principal characteristics. Firstly it is able to restore consciousness in cases of collapse, for example from windstroke. Secondly, it has a strong action on clearing heat from the opposite end of the channel. The Heart primary channel ascends alongside the oesophagus and connects with the tissues surrounding the eye, the Heart divergent channel ascends along the throat, and the Heart luo-connecting channel ascends to the root of the tongue and the eye. Shaochong HE-9 is effective to clear heat from the upper reaches of all of these branches of the Heart channel in the tongue (swelling and pain), throat (painful obstruction and dryness), mouth (heat) and eyes (redness and pain), as well as being able to clear febrile heat disturbing the spirit and giving rise to agitation and restlessness. Thirdly the *Classic of Difficulties* states that the jing-well points treat "fullness below the Heart"[16]. The region 'below the Heart' specifically refers to the apex of the epigastrium, but many of the jing-well points in fact treat stagnation and fullness throughout the chest region, and Shaochong HE-9 is indicated for pain of the Heart, chest and lateral costal region.

Whilst its modern clinical use emphasises the treatment of such excess disorders, classical texts place equal weight on its ability to treat Heart qi deficiency. Thus the *Song of the Jade Dragon* states "What of diseases of cold Gall Bladder and Heart deficiency? Bilateral Shaochong HE-9 is the most effective", and the *Song of the Primary Points of the Fourteen Channels* similarly prescribes it for Heart and Gall Bladder qi deficiency. Since Shaochong HE-9 is the wood point of the Heart fire channel, this reflects the principle of treating the mother to nourish the child.

COMBINATIONS

- Heat in the mouth: Shaochong HE-9 and Dazhong KID-4 (*Supplementing Life*).
- Fever: Shaochong HE-9 and Quchi L.I.-11 (*One Hundred Symptoms*).
- Fear and fright with Heart pain: Shaochong HE-9, Shenmen HE-7, Yanglingquan GB-34 and Neiguan P-6 (*Compilation*).

NOTES

1 *Essential Questions* Chapter 10.

2 *Essential Questions* Chapter 44.

3 *Spiritual Pivot* Chapter 8.

4 *Essential Questions* Chapter 62.

5 *Spiritual Pivot* Chapter 44.

6 *Spiritual Pivot* Chapter 6.

7 Ma Dan-yang was the originator of the *Song of the Eleven Heavenly Star Points*. They first appeared in print in the 12th century CE *Classic of the Jade Dragon*. Xu Feng included this text in his work *Complete Collection of Acupuncture and Moxibustion* and added a twelfth point, Taichong LIV-3.

8 *Spiritual Pivot* Chapter 71.

9 Fei Bo Xiong (1800-1879) in Fei Bo Xiong et. al. 1985 *Medical Collection From Four Families from Meng He* (Meng He Si Jia Yi Ji), Jiangsu Science Publishing House, p.40. Quoted in Maciocia, G. *The Practice of Chinese Medicine*, Churchill Livingstone, p. 211.

10 *Master Hua's Classic of the Central Viscera* attributed to Hua Tuo, a translation of the Zong Zang Jing by Yang Shou-zhong, Blue Poppy Press, 1993.

11 *Essential Questions* Chapter 33.

12 *Spiritual Pivot* Chapter 71.

13 *Spiritual Pivot* Chapter 71.

14 *Spiritual Pivot* Chapter 8.

15 *Classic of Difficulties* 68th Difficulty.

16 *Classic of Difficulties* 68th Difficulty.

手太陽小腸經

THE SMALL INTESTINE CHANNEL OF HAND TAIYANG

THE SMALL INTESTINE CHANNEL OF HAND TAIYANG

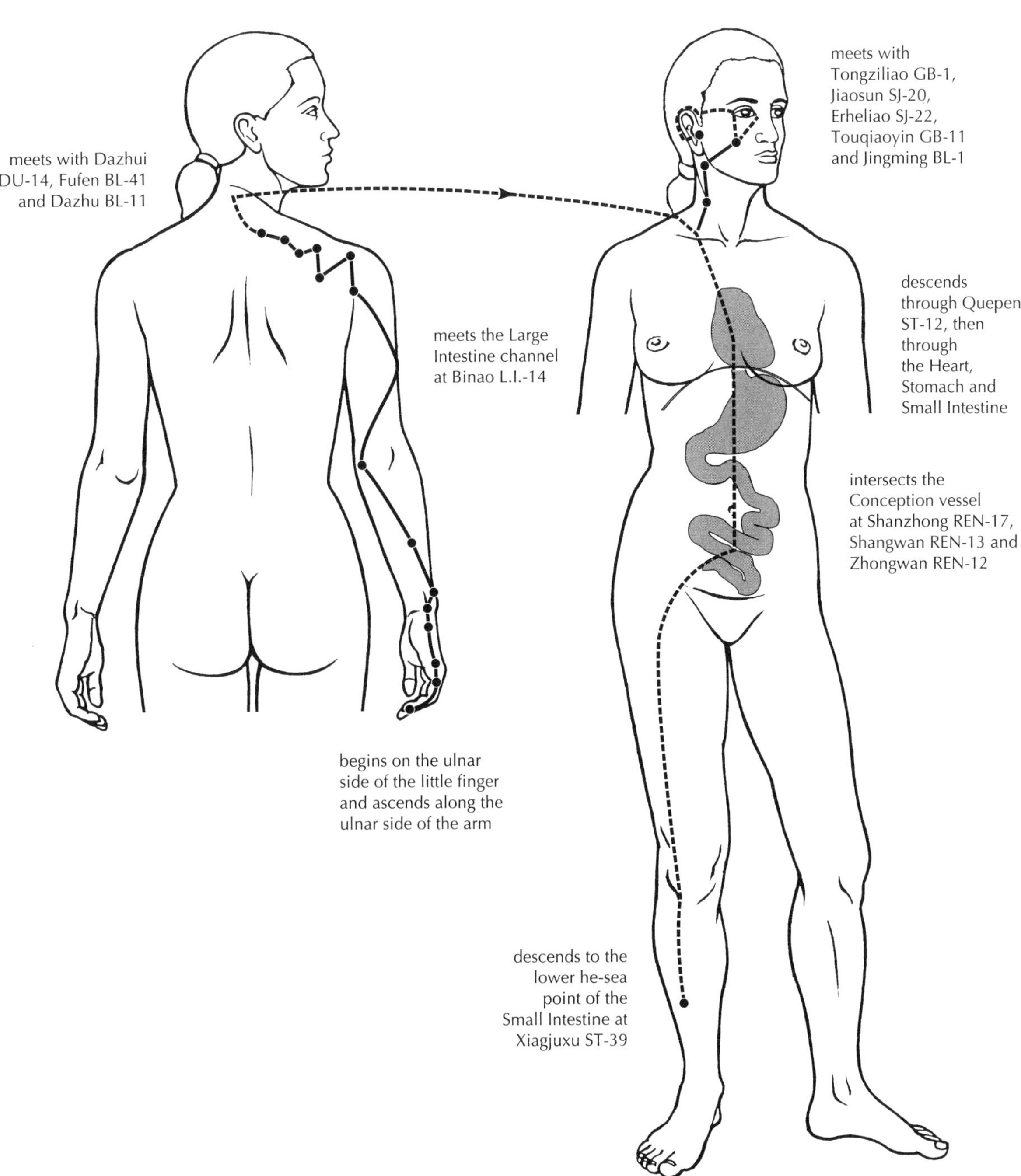
meets with Dazhui DU-14, Fufen BL-41 and Dazhu BL-11
meets with Tongziliao GB-1, Jiaosun SJ-20, Erheliao SJ-22, Touqiaoyin GB-11 and Jingming BL-1
meets the Large Intestine channel at Binao L.I.-14
descends through Quepen ST-12, then through the Heart, Stomach and Small Intestine
intersects the Conception vessel at Shanzhong REN-17, Shangwan REN-13 and Zhongwan REN-12
begins on the ulnar side of the little finger and ascends along the ulnar side of the arm
descends to the lower he-sea point of the Small Intestine at Xiagjuxu ST-39

The Small Intestine primary channel

THE SMALL INTESTINE PRIMARY CHANNEL

- originates at the ulnar side of the tip of the little finger at Shaoze SI-1,
- ascends along the ulnar aspect of the hand to reach the wrist where it emerges at the styloid process of the ulna at Yanglao SI-6,
- follows the ulna to the medial aspect of the elbow, where it passes between the olecranon of the ulna and the medial epicondyle of the humerus at Xiaohai SI-8,
- runs along the posterior aspect of the upper arm (intersecting the Large Intestine channel at Binao L.I-14) to the posterior aspect of the shoulder joint at Naoshu SI-10,
- zig-zags from the inferior fossa to the superior fossa of the scapula through Tianzong SI-11 and Bingfeng SI-12, and then to the medial aspect of the scapular spine at Tianjing SI-13,
- crosses via Jianwaishu SI-14 and Jianzhongshu SI-15 to Dazhui DU-14 at the lower border of the spinous process of C7, intersecting the Bladder channel at Fufen BL-41 and Dazhu BL-11,
- descends into the supraclavicular fossa at Quepen ST-12 and connects with the Heart,
- descends along the oesophagus, intersects the Conception vessel at Shanzhong REN-17 and passes through the diaphragm to the Stomach,
- intersects the Conception vessel at Shangwan REN-13 and Zhongwan REN-12 and enters the Small Intestine.

A branch

- ascends from the supraclavicular fossa to cross the neck and cheek to the outer canthus of the eye, where it meets the Gall Bladder channel at Tongziliao GB-l, then travels posteriorly towards the ear, where it intersects the Gall Bladder channel at Touqiaoyin GB-11 and the Sanjiao channel at Jiaosun SJ-20 and Erheliao SJ-22 and enters the ear at Tinggong SI-19.

Another branch

- separates from the previous branch on the cheek and ascends to the infra-orbital region (Quanliao SI-18) then along the lateral aspect of the nose to the inner canthus where it meets with the Bladder channel at Jingming BL-l.
- According to the *Spiritual Pivot*[1] another branch descends to Xiajuxu ST-39, the lower he-sea point of the Small Intestine.

The Small Intestine primary channel connects with the following zangfu: Heart, Stomach and Small Intestine.

The Small Intestine primary channel meets with other channels at the following points: Binao L.I.-14, Dazhui DU-14, Fufen BL-41, Dazhu BL-11, Quepen ST-12, Shanzhong REN-17, Shangwan REN-13, Zhongwan REN-12, Tongziliao GB-1, Touqiaoyin GB-11, Jiaosun SJ-20, Erheliao SJ-22, Jingming BL-1.

THE SMALL INTESTINE LUO-CONNECTING CHANNEL

- separates from the Small Intestine channel at Zhizheng SI-7 and connects with the Heart channel,
- ascends along the arm and connects with the shoulder at Jianyu L.I.-15.

THE SMALL INTESTINE DIVERGENT CHANNEL

- separates from the primary channel at the shoulder,
- enters the axilla, crosses the Heart and descends to the abdomen where it connects with the Small Intestine.

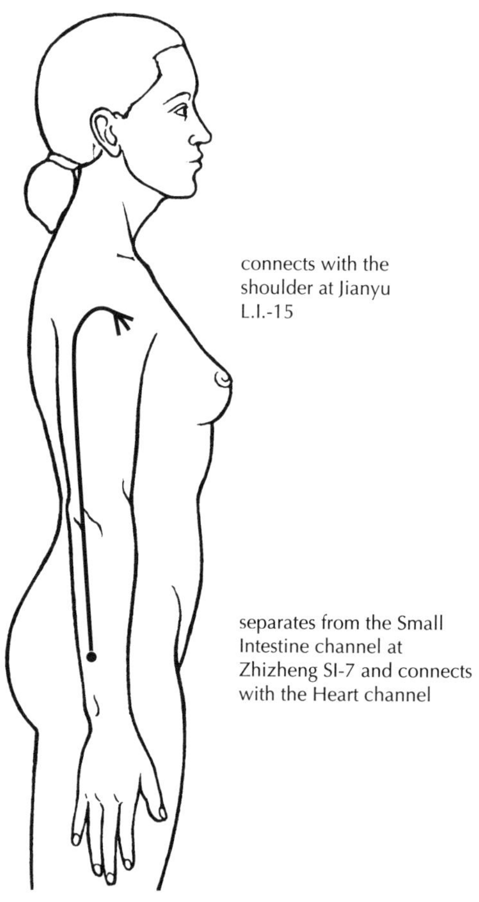

The Small Intestine luo-connecting channel

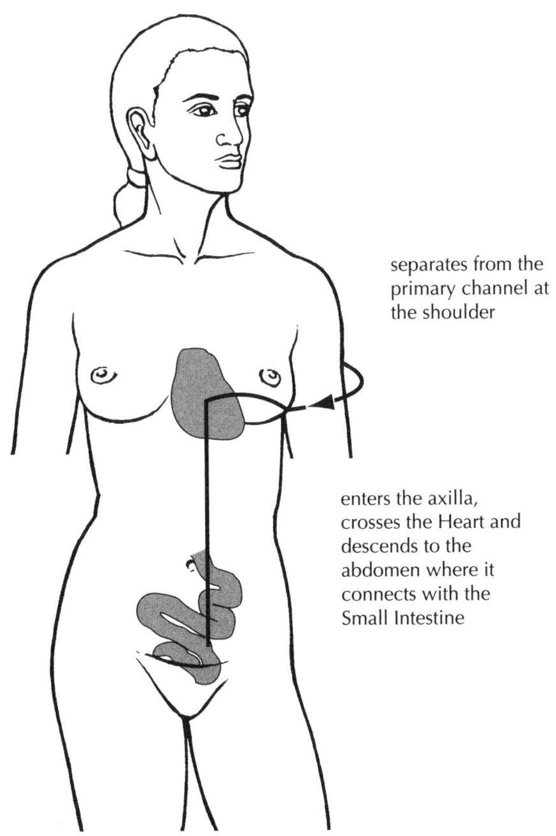
separates from the primary channel at the shoulder
enters the axilla, crosses the Heart and descends to the abdomen where it connects with the Small Intestine

The Small Intestine divergent channel

binds at the mastoid process, the mandible, the outer canthus and corner of the head

a sub-branch enters the ear

surrounds the scapula

The Small Intestine sinew channel

THE SMALL INTESTINE SINEW CHANNEL

- originates on the dorsum of the little finger,
- binds at the wrist,
- ascends the ulnar side of the forearm to the elbow where it binds at the medial condyle of the humerus,
- ascends the arm to bind at the axilla,
- travels behind the axilla and surrounds the scapula,
- ascends the neck, anterior to the Bladder sinew channel, to bind at the mastoid process,
- ascends to behind the ear where a sub-branch enters the ear,
- continues to ascend behind the ear to the region above the ear where it then descends to bind at the mandible,
- ascends across the teeth to bind at the outer canthus,
- ascends to bind at the corner of the head near Touwei ST-8.

Pathological symptoms of the Small Intestine sinew channel
Strained little finger, pain along the medial aspect of the elbow and upper arm, pain below the axilla and on the posterior aspect of the axilla, pain of the scapula that reaches the neck, tinnitus, pain of the ear that may reach the submandibular region, a need to close the eyes for a long period of time before being able to see clearly, tension of the neck sinews that leads to sinew atrophy and swelling of the neck.

DISCUSSION

The Small Intestine channel of hand taiyang is ascribed to fire, and is interiorly-exteriorly coupled with the Heart channel and paired with the Bladder channel of foot taiyang according to six channel theory. As far as the Small Intestine channel pathways are concerned it is worth noting that:

- the primary and divergent channels connect with the Heart.
- the primary and sinew channels travel to the posterior aspect of the shoulder, whilst the luo-connecting channel connects with Jianyu L.I.-15.
- the divergent and sinew channels connect with the axilla.
- the primary channel connects with the scapula, and the sinew channel surrounds the scapula.
- the primary and sinew channels connect with the neck, cheek, outer canthus and ear.
- the primary channel also connects with the inner canthus.
- the sinew channel connects with the mastoid process, the teeth and the corner of the forehead.

It is by virtue of the Small Intestine's status as a fire channel, its links with the Heart and Bladder channels, and the pathways of its primary and secondary channels that many of the actions and indications of the points of the Small Intestine channel can be explained. These can be summarised as:

- clearing heat from the pathways of the channel and reducing fever, especially malarial fever (points Shaoze SI-1 to Wangu SI-4).
- assisting in transforming phlegm and clearing heat from the Heart zang, especially in the treatment of mania disorder (Houxi SI-3, Yanggu SI-5, Zhizheng SI-7 and Xiaohai SI-8).
- cooling heat and fire and alleviating pain along the course of the channel in the arm, axilla, shoulder, scapula, neck (including mumps) and throat, jaw, mouth, teeth, tongue, nose, cheek, eyes and ears. Points of the Small Intestine channel are particularly indicated for swelling (mainly of the neck, throat and cheek).
- treating disorders of the breast (Shaoze SI-1, Qiangu SI-2 and Tianzong SI-11) and lateral costal region (Shaoze SI-1, Wangu SI-4, Yanggu SI-5 and Tianzong SI-11). The meeting of the Small Intestine primary channel with the centre of the chest at Shanzhong REN-17 can in part explain the action of these points on the breast, but there is no obvious reason why points of the Small Intestine channel should influence the lateral costal region.
- Note that even though the principal function of the Small Intestine fu is to receive, transform and separate fluids, the only indications relating to this function are dark and hesitant urination (Qiangu SI-2 and Houxi SI-3). Even more notably, despite the fact that the channel connects with the diaphragm and Stomach, passes through Zhongwan REN-12 and Shangwan REN-13, and descends to the Small Intestine, no points of the Small Intestine channel are indicated for disorders of the digestive system.

SHAOZE SI-1

少澤

Lesser Marsh

Jing-Well and Metal point of the Small Intestine channel

LOCATION

On the dorsal aspect of the little finger, at the junction of lines drawn along the ulnar border of the nail and the base of the nail, approximately 0.1 cun from the corner of the nail.

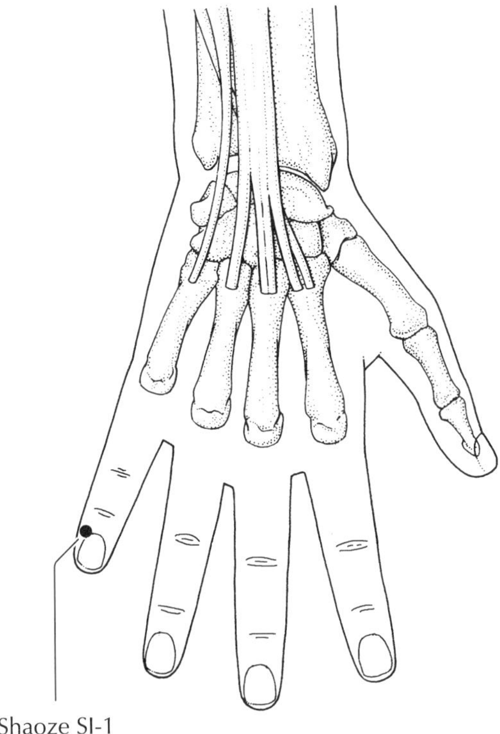

NEEDLING

Perpendicular or oblique insertion directed proximally 0.1 to 0.2 cun, or prick to bleed.

ACTIONS

Clears heat and benefits the sensory orifices
Revives consciousness
Promotes lactation and benefits the breasts

INDICATIONS

- Loss of consciousness from windstroke, cold sensation below the Heart, agitation with Heart pain, oppression and pain of the chest, pain of the lateral costal region, mania disorder, clonic spasm.
- Cold shivering, chills and fever with absence of sweating, febrile disease, malaria, cough.
- Headache, dizziness, superficial visual obstruction, red eyes, nosebleed, deafness, tinnitus, throat painful obstruction, curled tongue, stiff tongue, heat in the mouth, erosion of the mouth, mouth ulcers, drooling.
- Swelling of the breast, breast abscess, absence of lactation.
- Stiff neck, pain of the postero-lateral shoulder and upper arm, pain of the elbow, trembling and numbness of the arm, disorders of the little finger.

COMMENTARY

Shaoze SI-1 is the jing-well point of the Small Intestine channel. In common with all the jing-well points of the yang channels, it has a strong action on clearing heat from the opposite end of the channel in the head. Branches of the Small Intestine channel ascend to the ear, the inner and outer canthus, and alongside the nose, whilst its paired Heart channel opens into the tongue. Shaoze SI-1, therefore, has a strong effect on clearing heat or pathologically ascending yang from the eyes, ears, nose and tongue, as well as the mouth and throat, and is indicated for such excess disorders as red eyes, tinnitus and deafness, erosion and ulceration of the tongue, painful obstruction of the throat, mouth ulcers, drooling and nosebleed.

According to the *Classic of Difficulties*[2] the jing-well points are indicated for fullness below the Heart. Whilst the region 'below the Heart' specifically refers to the upper epigastrium, like many of the jing-well points, Shaoze SI-1 treats fullness in the chest region as a whole and is indicated for oppression and pain of the chest and Heart, cold sensation below the Heart and pain of the lateral costal region.

In clinical practice however, Shaoze SI-1 is principally used for swelling and abscess of the breasts and disorders of lactation. Absence of lactation is primarily differentiated into two types, insufficiency of qi and blood resulting in inadequate production of milk, or stagnation of Liver qi which leads to obstruction and coagulation of milk in the breasts. The Small Intestine primary channel descends to the centre of the chest at Shanzhong REN-17, and these two points are frequently combined to treat insufficiency or total absence of lactation. Breast abscess is usually due to Liver or Stomach fire or transformation of exterior pathogens to heat. In combination with suitable points, Shaoze SI-1 may be used in any of these two patterns.

Finally, in common with the other jing-well points, Shaoze SI-1 is used to revive consciousness and is indicated for loss of consciousness from windstroke.

COMBINATIONS

- Absence of lactation: Shaoze SI-1, Shanzhong REN-17 and Hegu L.I.-4 (*Great Compendium*).

- Absence of lactation: reinforce Shaoze SI-1 and moxa Shanzhong REN-17 (*Great Compendium*).
- Swelling of the breasts: Shaoze SI-1 and Taiyang [M-HN-9] (*Ode of the Jade Dragon*).
- Swelling of the breasts in women: Shaoze SI-1 and Zulinqi GB-41 (*Divine Moxibustion*).
- Swelling of the breasts in women: Shaoze SI-1 and Tongziliao GB-1 (*Illustrated Supplement*).
- Breast abscess: Shaoze SI-1, Xiajuxu ST-39, Zusanli ST-36, Xiaxi GB-43, Yuji LU-10, Weizhong BL-40 and Zulinqi GB-41 (*Great Compendium*).
- Erosion, heat and dryness of the mouth: Shaoze SI-1, Laogong P-8, Sanjian L.I.-3 and Taichong LIV-3 (*Thousand Ducat Formulas*).
- Throat painful obstruction, curled tongue and dry mouth: Shaoze SI-1 Guanchong SJ-1 and Zuqiaoyin GB-44 (*Thousand Ducat Formulas*).

QIANGU SI-2

Front Valley

前谷

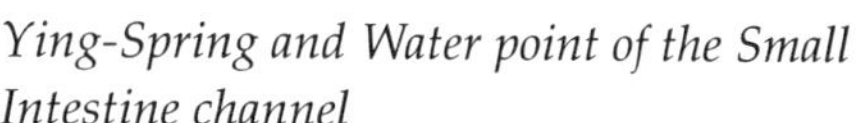

Ying-Spring and Water point of the Small Intestine channel

LOCATION

On the ulnar border of the little finger, in a depression just distal to the metacarpo-phalangeal joint.

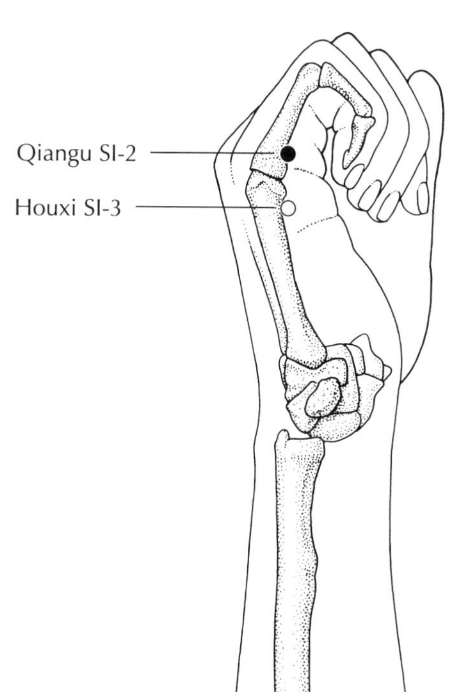

NEEDLING

i. Oblique distal insertion 0.2 to 0.3 cun; ii. Perpendicular-oblique insertion towards the palm, 0.5 cun.

ACTIONS

Clears wind-heat and reduces swelling
Benefits the eyes, ears and throat
Activates the channel and alleviates pain

INDICATIONS

- Mumps, swelling and pain of the neck, swelling of the cheek radiating to the ear, throat painful obstruction, pain of the throat that prevents swallowing.
- Superficial visual obstruction, eye pain with lacrimation, bursting eye pain, red eyes, congested nose, nosebleed, tinnitus.
- Cough with fullness of the chest, coughing blood, febrile disease with absence of sweating, malaria, thirst, difficult urination with dark urine, epilepsy, post-partum absence of lactation.
- Stiffness and pain of the neck and back, pain of the scapula, pain and inability to raise the arm, wrist pain, heat of the palms, heat and pain of the little finger, itching and numbness of the fingers.

COMMENTARY

According to the *Classic of Difficulties* [2] ying-spring points are indicated for "heat in the body", and as the ying-spring and water point of the Small Intestine fire channel, Qiangu SI-2 has an especially strong action on subduing fire. Qiangu SI-2 belongs to taiyang channel, the most exterior of the six channels, and is able to clear heat (especially exterior wind-heat) from the superficial portion of the body, particularly in the eyes, nose and ears. It is indicated for bursting eye pain, redness of the eyes, congested nose, nosebleed and tinnitus. It is also able to clear exterior heat from the Lung and throat (cough, throat painful obstruction, fever and thirst) and to treat malaria.

When heat pathogen is virulent it may give rise to toxic heat characterised by inflammation, pain and swelling. Qiangu SI-2 is indicated for mumps, swelling of the cheek radiating to the ear and swelling and pain of the neck and throat.

Finally, Qiangu SI-2 is indicated for stiffness and pain along the Small Intestine channel from the hand up to the neck, as well as for numbness and heat of the fingers and palms.

COMBINATIONS

- Swelling of the throat with inability to swallow: Qiangu SI-2, Zhaohai KID-6 and Zhongfeng LIV-4 (*Thousand Ducat Formulas*).

- Tired throat, swelling of the neck with inability to turn the head, swelling of the cheek that radiates to the ear: Qiangu SI-2, Wangu GB-12 and Tianyou SJ-16 (*Thousand Ducat Formulas*).
- Deafness: Qiangu SI-2, Houxi SI-3 and Pianli L.I.-6 (*Supplementing Life*).
- Tinnitus: Qiangu SI-2, Pianli L.I.-6, Yangxi L.I.-5, Shangyang L.I.-1, Luoque BL-8 and Wangu SI-4 (*Supplementing Life*).
- Eye pain: Qiangu SI-2, Yangxi L.I.-5, Erjian L.I.-2, Daling P-7, Sanjian L.I.-3 and Shangxing DU-23 (*Great Compendium*).
- Superficial visual obstruction: Qiangu SI-2 and Jinggu BL-64 (*Thousand Ducat Formulas*).
- Malaria with chills and fever: Qiangu SI-2, Lieque LU-7, Houxi SI-3 and Shaoze SI-1 (*Thousand Ducat Formulas*).

HOUXI SI-3

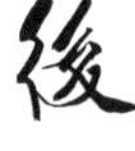

Back Stream

Shu-Stream and Wood point of the Small Intestine channel
Confluent point of the Governing vessel

LOCATION

On the ulnar border of the hand, in the substantial depression proximal to the head of the fifth metacarpal bone.

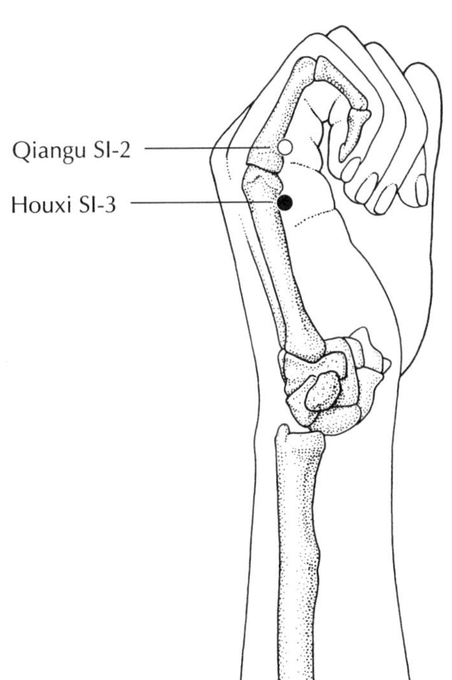

LOCATION NOTE

This point is easier to locate when the hand is made into a loose fist.

NEEDLING

Perpendicular insertion 0.5 to 2 cun, directed towards Sanjian L.I.-3. **Note:** needle with the hand in a loose fist position, i.e. with the metacarpal bones lying in the same plane; this is especially important when needling deeply towards the opposite side of the hand.

ACTIONS

Benefits the occiput, neck and back
Activates the channel and alleviates pain
Clears wind and heat and treats malaria
Calms the spirit and treats epilepsy
Clears heat and benefits the sensory orifices
Regulates the Governing vessel

INDICATIONS

- Stiffness and pain of the neck, difficulty in turning the neck, one-sided headache, bilateral headache, pain of the back and shoulder, pain of the shoulder, elbow and arm, contraction of the elbow, contraction and pain of the fingers, pain of the lumbar region and knees, hemiplegia.
- Malaria, night sweating, cold shivering, chills and fever, febrile disease with absence of sweating, fullness of the chest, jaundice, dark hesitant urination.
- Epilepsy, mania-depression, disorders of the Governing vessel.
- Deafness, tinnitus, superficial visual obstruction, redness and pain of the eyes, swelling of the eyes with lacrimation, nosebleed, toothache, swelling of the throat and cheek, redness, swelling and pain of both cheeks, loss of voice following windstroke.

COMMENTARY

Houxi SI-3 is both the shu-stream point of the Small Intestine channel, which is interiorly-exteriorly coupled with the Heart channel, and the confluent point of the Governing vessel. Most of its actions and indications can be explained by its relationship to these three channels. In clinical practice Houxi SI-3 can be seen to have four main spheres of action.

Firstly it is an important point to treat pain, stiffness and contraction along the course of its related channels. Taiyang (Small Intestine and Bladder) channel traverses the occiput, neck, scapula and paravertebral regions, whilst the Governing vessel ascends along the spinal column from the coccyx to the head. According to the *Classic of Difficulties*[3] the shu-stream points are indicated for "heaviness of the body and pain of the joints". Houxi SI-3 is an essential distal point in the treatment of occipital headache (although also used for one-sided and bilateral headache) and stiffness and pain of the neck, whether acute or chronic and whether due to exterior pathogenic factors or interior disharmony. It has a significant influence on the spine as a whole, and is an important and frequently used distal point for pain of the upper spine and scapula, as well as in the treatment of acute lumbar sprain on the midline or lateral lumbar region. Houxi SI-3 is also important for disorders of the finger joints, especially the little and ring fingers, and may be needled deeply towards Sanjian L.I.-3 when all four fingers are affected. Houxi SI-3 is equally important in the treatment of pain and contraction of the arm, elbow and shoulder.

The second principal action of Houxi SI-3 is to dispel febrile disease. This may be explained by the fact that the taiyang Small Intestine channel belongs to fire, taiyang is the most exterior of the six channels, and the Governing vessel governs all the yang channels and hence the exterior portion of the body as a whole. Houxi SI-3 is especially indicated in the treatment of malaria, and for when attack by exterior pathogenic wind-cold or wind-heat gives rise to chills and fever accompanied by severe neck pain or pain of the spine. A further reflection of its heat clearing action is in the treatment of night sweating, particularly in combination with Yinxi HE-6.

In the *Ode of the Obstructed River* the use of Houxi SI-3 is referred to as one of 'the eight therapeutic methods'. In this description of the application of the eight confluent points of the extraordinary vessels to affect specific symptoms and areas of the body, Houxi SI-3 is indicated for diseases of the Governing vessel and for mania-depression. The third action of Houxi SI-3, therefore, is in calming the spirit and treating both mania-depression and epilepsy. The former is due to phlegm and phlegm-heat which disturb and agitate the spirit, and the latter to disturbance of the spirit and brain by pathogenic wind and phlegm. According to Sun Si-miao, the famous 7th century physician "the head is the supreme leader, the place where man's spirit concentrates"[4], whilst in the 16th century, Li Shi-zhen stated "the brain is the residence of the original spirit". Since the Small Intestine channel is interiorly-exteriorly related to the Heart which stores the spirit, and Houxi SI-3 is the confluent point of the Governing vessel which enters the brain, this point has long been considered important in the treatment of epilepsy. The *Song More Precious Than Jade*, for example, recommends it for the five types of epilepsy.

Fourthly, in common with points Shaoze SI-1 and Qiangu SI-2, Houxi SI-3 is able to clear both exterior and interior heat from the Small Intestine channel in the head (especially the ears and eyes) and to benefit the sensory orifices. It is thus indicated for disorders such as tinnitus and deafness, superficial visual obstruction, redness, pain and swelling of the eyes with lacrimation, nosebleed, and pain and swelling of the cheeks.

COMBINATIONS

- Stiffness of the neck with inability to turn the head: Houxi SI-3 and Tianyou SJ-16 (*Supplementing Life*).
- Headache: Houxi SI-3, Tianzhu BL-10, Taodao DU-13, Dazhu BL-11 and Kongzui LU-6 (*Thousand Ducat Formulas*).
- Pain of the head and eyes: Houxi SI-3 and Waiguan SJ-5 (*Divine Moxibustion*).
- Pain of the forearm: Houxi SI-3, Shousanli LI-10 and Quchi LI-11 (*Supplementing Life*).
- Contraction of the elbow: Houxi SI-3, Chize LU-5, Jianyu L.I.-15, Xiaohai SI-8, Jianshi P-5, Daling P-7 and Yuji LU-10 (*Great Compendium*).
- Pain of the shoulder and back: Houxi SI-3, Wangu SI-4, Fengmen BL-12, Jianjing GB-21, Zhongzhu SJ-3, Zhigou SJ-6 and Weizhong BL-40 (*Great Compendium*).
- Malaria with much heat and little cold: Houxi SI-3, Dazhui DU-14, Jianshi P-5 and Quchi L.I.-11 (*Great Compendium*).
- Malaria with much cold and little heat: Houxi SI-3, Dazhui DU-14 and Quchi L.I.-11 (*Great Compendium*).
- Severe night sweating: Houxi SI-3 and Yinxi HE-6 (*One Hundred Symptoms*).
- The five types of epilepsy: Houxi SI-3, Jiuwei REN-15 and Shenmen HE-7 (*Song More Precious Than Jade*).
- Epilepsy: Houxi SI-3, Neiguan P-6, Shenmen HE-7, Xinshu BL-15 and Yinbai SP-1 (*Complete Collection*).
- Epileptic convulsions, mad walking, inability to sleep, agitation of the Heart: Houxi SI-3, Zanzhu BL-2, Xiaohai SI-8 and Qiangjian DU-18 (*Thousand Ducat Formulas*).
- Mania, desires to ascend to high places and sing, discards clothing and runs around: Houxi SI-3, Shenmen HE-7 and Chongyang ST-42 (*Great Compendium*).
- Sudden mania: Houxi SI-3, Jianshi P-5 and Hegu L.I.-4 (*Great Compendium*).
- Deafness: Houxi SI-3, Qiangu SI-2 and Pianli L.I.-6 (*Supplementing Life*).
- Nosebleed with stifled breathing: Houxi SI-3, Chengling GB-18, Fengchi GB-20, Fengmen BL-12 and Yixi BL-45 (*Thousand Ducat Formulas*).
- Jaundice: Houxi SI-3 and Laogong P-8 (*One Hundred Symptoms*).

WANGU SI-4

Wrist Bone

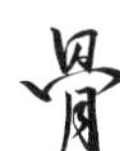

Yuan-Source point of the Small Intestine channel

LOCATION

On the ulnar border of the hand, in the depression between the base of the fifth metacarpal bone and the triquetral bone.

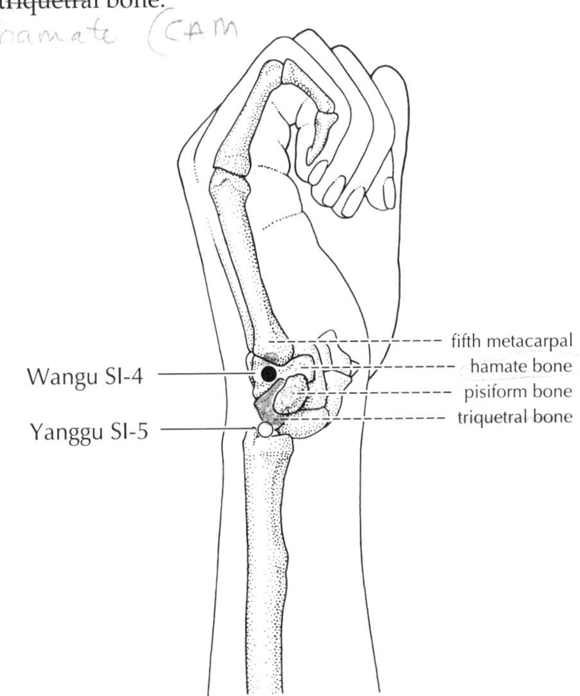

NEEDLING

Perpendicular insertion 0.3 to 0.5 cun.

ACTIONS

Activates the channel and alleviates pain
Clears heat and reduces swelling
Clears damp-heat and treats jaundice

INDICATIONS

- Contraction of the five fingers with difficulty in flexing and extending, weakness and pain of the wrist, contraction of the arm and elbow with difficulty in flexing and extending, stiffness and swelling of the neck, headache, pain of the shoulder, coldness and pain of the shoulder and back, pain of the lateral costal region with inability to catch the breath, lumbar pain radiating to the leg, hemiplegia, clonic spasm.
- Pain and swelling of the cheek radiating to the ear, swelling of the neck, submandibular region and jaw, throat painful obstruction, tinnitus, superficial visual obstruction, lacrimation, loss of sense of taste.
- Jaundice, Spleen deficiency jaundice, febrile disease with absence of sweating, chills and fever, malaria, wasting and thirsting disorder, agitation and fullness.

COMMENTARY

Wangu SI-4 is the yuan-source point of the Small Intestine channel. Its main clinical application is in the treatment of contraction, stiffness and pain along the entire length of the channel including the hand, elbow, arm, shoulder, neck and back. It is one of the main points (along with Yangxi L.I.-5, Zhongzhu SJ-3 and Zhizheng SI-7) to treat disorders of all the five fingers, especially when characterised by contraction and pain.

Wangu SI-4 has a specific effect in the treatment of swelling at the opposite end of the channel, especially the neck, cheek and submandibular region. Like all the previous points of this channel it is also indicated in the treatment of tinnitus, reflecting the pathways of the Small Intestine primary and sinew channels which enter the ear. This is an example of the use of acupuncture points to treat disorders of the channel rather than underlying zangfu disharmony, and Wangu SI-4 may therefore be used in tinnitus due to any aetiology. Wangu SI-4 is specifically indicated in combination (see below) to treat pain and swelling of the submandibular region radiating to the ear and giving rise to tinnitus.

Finally, Wangu SI-4 has been found to be empirically effective in the treatment of different kinds of jaundice, whether due to damp-heat or cold damp, as well as pain of the lateral costal region with inability to catch the breath. This action cannot easily be explained, either by reference to the channel pathway or to the functions of the Small Intestine.

COMBINATIONS

- Contraction of the five fingers with inability to flex and extend: Wangu SI-4 and Zhongzhu SJ-3 (*Thousand Ducat Formulas*).
- Pain of the shoulder and arm: Wangu SI-4 and Tianzong SI-11 (*Supplementing Life*).
- Pain of the submandibular region giving rise to tinnitus and difficult hearing: Wangu SI-4, Yanggu SI-5, Jianzhen SI-9, Xiaxi GB-43 and Zuqiaoyin GB-44 (*Thousand Ducat Formulas*).
- Toothache and tooth decay: Wangu SI-4, Xiaguan ST-7, Daying ST-5 and Yifeng SJ-17 (*Supplementing Life*).
- Pain of the lateral costal region with inability to catch the breath: Wangu SI-4 and Yanggu SI-5 (*Thousand Ducat Formulas*).
- Spleen deficiency jaundice: Wangu SI-4 and Zhongwan REN-12 (*Ode of the Jade Dragon*).

YANGGU SI-5

Yang Valley

陽谷

Jing-River and Fire point of the Small Intestine channel

LOCATION

At the ulnar border of the wrist, in the depression between the head of the ulna and the triquetral bone.

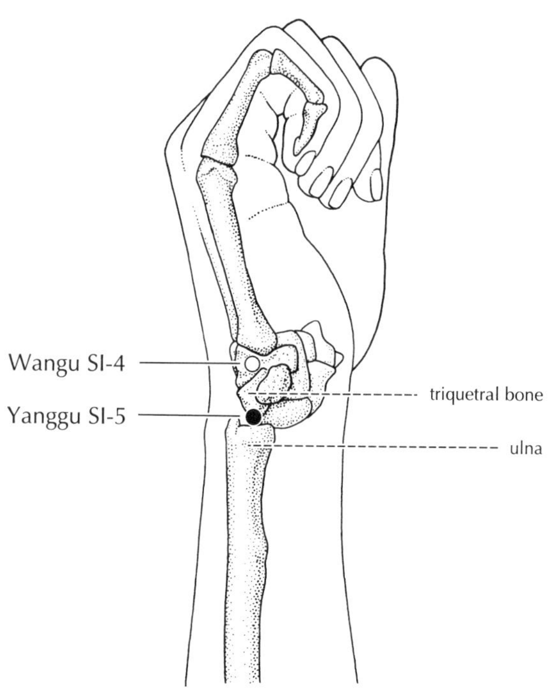

LOCATION NOTE

Most sources locate this point between the styloid process of the ulna and the triquetral bone, but in practice, the styloid process of the ulna may not be palpable and where it is palpable it often lies slightly posterior to Yanggu SI-5.

NEEDLING

Perpendicular insertion 0.3 to 0.5 cun.

ACTIONS

Clears heat and reduces swelling
Calms the spirit

INDICATIONS

- Swelling of the neck and submandibular region, lockjaw, stiffness of the tongue in babies preventing suckling, tongue thrusting, toothache in both the upper and lower jaw, tinnitus and deafness, visual dizziness, redness, swelling and pain of the eye.
- Mania, mad walking, clonic spasm, pain of the chest or lateral costal region with difficulty in breathing, febrile disease with absence of sweating, chills and fever.
- Pain of the wrist and hand, pain of the arm, shoulder pain with inability to dress oneself, painful haemorrhoids.

COMMENTARY

Yanggu SI-5 is the fire and jing-river point of the Small Intestine channel. Unlike the more distal points of the channel, it has relatively less action on the channel as a whole, in other words it is less used to treat disorders of the hand, arm or shoulder, but focuses rather on the eyes, ears and jaw. As a fire point it is able to clear heat and swelling and soothe contraction in these regions. It is specifically indicated for swelling of the neck and submandibular region, lockjaw, contraction of the tongue in babies, tongue thrusting (where the tongue is repeatedly thrust out of the mouth like a snake's tongue) and toothache. Whilst most classical sources recommend this point for toothache of the upper jaw, Sun Si-miao the famous 7th century physician incorporated it in prescriptions for toothache of both the upper and lower jaw.

As the fire point of the Small Intestine channel (interiorly-exteriorly related to the Heart channel) Yanggu SI-5 is able to clear fire from the Heart and calm the spirit and is indicated for mania and 'mad walking'.

Yanggu SI-5 is indicated (and appears in combination with distal points of the Bladder channel) for haemorrhoids.

Finally, in learning the names of the points of the yang channels at the wrist, it is helpful to remember the similarity between their names: Yangxi L.I.-5 (Yang Stream), Yanggu SI-5 (Yang Valley) and Yangchi SJ-4 (Yang Pool).

COMBINATIONS

- Toothache of the upper jaw: Yanggu SI-5 and Zhengying GB-17 (*Thousand Ducat Formulas*).
- Toothache of the lower jaw: Yanggu SI-5, Yemen SJ-2, Shangyang L.I.-1, Erjian L.I.-2 and Sidu SJ-9 (*Thousand Ducat Formulas*).
- Swelling of the submandibular region with lockjaw: Yanggu SI-5 and Xiaxi GB-43 (*One Hundred Symptoms*).
- Tinnitus and deafness: Yanggu SI-5, Xiaguan ST-7, Guanchong SJ-1, Yemen SJ-2 and Yangxi L.I.-5 (*Systematic Classic*).
- Dizziness and eye pain: Yanggu SI-5 and Feiyang BL-58 (*Supplementing Life*).
- Manic laughter: Yanggu SI-5 and Shenmen HE-7 (*Thousand Ducat Formulas*).

- Madness with vomiting: Yanggu SI-5, Zhubin KID-9, Houding DU-19, Qiangjian DU-18, Naohu DU-17, Luoque BL-8 and Yuzhen BL-9 (*Thousand Ducat Formulas*).
- Mad walking: Yanggu SI-5 and Fengfu DU-16 (*Great Compendium*).
- Pain of the elbow, at times cold: Yanggu SI-5, Quchi L.I.-11, Guanchong SJ-1, Shousanli L.I.-10, Zhongzhu SJ-3 and Chize LU-5 (*Thousand Ducat Formulas*).
- Inability to raise the shoulder and put on clothes: Yanggu SI-5 and Qinglengyuan SJ-11 (*Thousand Ducat Formulas*).
- Haemorrhoids, swelling of the axilla: Yanggu SI-5, Chengjin BL-56, Chengfu BL-36 and Weizhong BL-40 (*Thousand Ducat Formulas*).

YANGLAO SI-6

Support the Aged

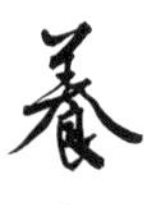

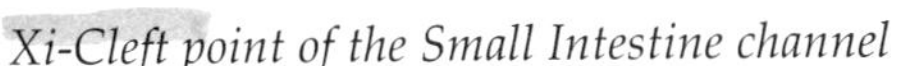

Xi-Cleft point of the Small Intestine channel

LOCATION
When the palm of the hand is placed on the chest, this point is located on the dorsal aspect of the head of the ulna, in a cleft level with and to the radial side of the high point of the styloid process of the ulna.

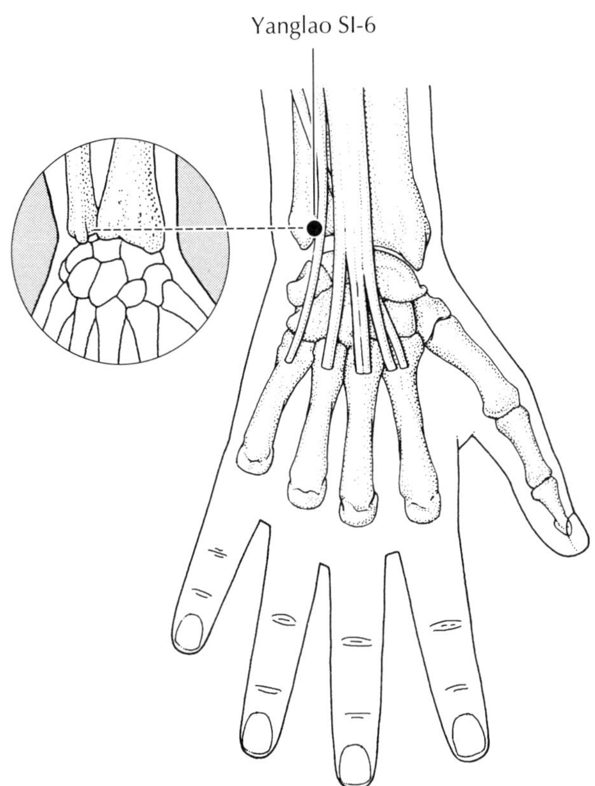

LOCATION NOTE
This point may be located in the following way. Ask the patient to lie with their arm by their side and the hand prone (palm on the couch). If the practitioner places a finger on the high point of the ulnar styloid and asks the patient to place their palm on their chest, the point is found in the cleft where the practitioner's finger then rests.

NEEDLING
Oblique or transverse-oblique insertion distally or proximally, 0.5 to 1 cun.

ACTIONS
Activates the channel and alleviates pain
Benefits the shoulder and arm
Moderates acute conditions
Benefits the eyes

INDICATIONS
- Shoulder pain, pain of the shoulder as if it were broken, pain of the upper arm as if it were dislocated, stiffness and pain of the shoulder and back, numbness of the shoulder and arm, redness and swelling of the exterior aspect of the elbow, heaviness and pain of the lumbar region, difficulty in sitting and rising, contraction of the sinews and painful obstruction of the foot with inability to extend and flex.
- Dimness of vision, blurred vision, eye pain.

COMMENTARY
Yanglao SI-6 is the xi-cleft point of the Small Intestine channel. The xi-cleft points are where the qi and blood, which flow relatively superficially along the channels from the jing-well points, gather and plunge more deeply. The xi-cleft points in general are indicated in the treatment of acute conditions and pain. Yanglao SI-6 is particularly used for pain of the shoulder, scapula and arm that is so severe that it feels as if they are broken or dislocated. This action extends to its paired taiyang foot (Bladder) channel, and thus Yanglao SI-6 is also used as a distal point for acute sprain of the lumbar region and for contraction of the sinews and painful obstruction of the foot.

The Small Intestine primary and sinew channels connect with the outer canthus, and the primary channel also connects with the inner canthus. Yanglao SI-6 is renowned for its use in deficiency-type eye disorders characterised by blurring and dimness of vision, and most authorities explain the name of this point 'Support the Aged' in the light of this action.

COMBINATIONS

- Pain of the shoulder as if it were broken: Yanglao SI-6 and Tianzhu BL-10 (*Thousand Ducat Formulas*).
- Pain of the lumbar region and knee: Yanglao SI-6, Huantiao GB-30, Yanglingquan GB-34, Kunlun BL-60 and Shenmai BL-62 (*Illustrated Supplement*).
- Blurring of vision: Yanglao SI-6 and Tianzhu BL-10 (*One Hundred Symptoms*).
- Dimness of vision: Yanglao SI-6, Hegu LI-4 and Quchai BL-4 (*Supplementing Life*).

ZHIZHENG SI-7

Branch of the Upright

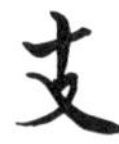

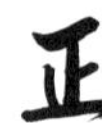

Luo-Connecting point of the Small Intestine channel

LOCATION

On a line connecting Yanggu SI-5 and Xiaohai SI-8, 5 cun proximal to Yanggu SI-5, in the groove between the anterior border of the ulna and the muscle belly of flexor carpi ulnaris.

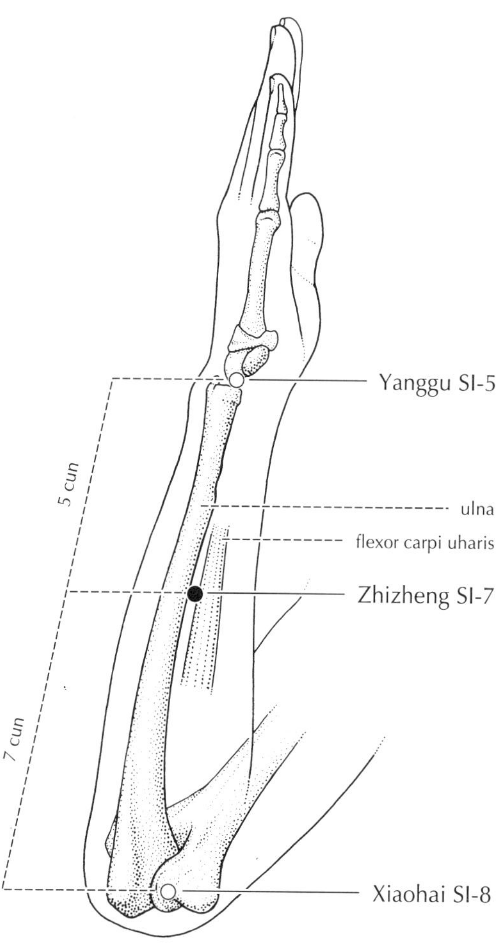

LOCATION NOTE

This point should be located and needled with the patient lying on their back and with their arm either in the supine position or resting on the chest.

NEEDLING

Perpendicular insertion 0.5 to 1 cun.

ACTIONS

Clears heat and releases the exterior
Calms the spirit
Activates the channel and alleviates pain
Benefits the finger joints

INDICATIONS

- Febrile disease, cold shivering and fever, fever with neck and lumbar pain and desire to drink.
- Mania-depression, fear and fright, sadness and anxiety, restless zang disorder.
- Headache, dizziness, visual dizziness, blurred vision, superficial visual obstruction.
- Feebleness of the four limbs, the five taxations, stiffness of the neck, contraction of the elbow, slackness of the joints and inability to move the elbow, severe pain of all the fingers, inability to grip firmly, inability to make a fist, warts.

COMMENTARY

Zhizheng SI-7 has three main actions. Firstly, since the Small Intestine belongs to taiyang channel (the most exterior of the six channels and thus the first to be attacked by exterior pathogenic factors) Zhizheng SI-7 in common with many points of the Small Intestine channel is able to release the exterior. It is primarily used in cases of exterior heat pathogen giving rise to febrile disease, and is especially indicated when the onset is characterised by neck and lumbar pain.

Secondly, Zhizheng SI-7 is the luo-connecting point of the Small Intestine channel from where the Small Intestine luo-connecting channel spreads to join with the Heart channel. This is reflected in the name of this point 'Branch of the Upright', the 'upright' being the Heart channel. The *Guide to the Classics of Acupuncture* states "the luo-connecting points are located between two channels ... if they are punctured, symptoms of the interiorly-exteriorly related channels can be treated"[5]. Zhizheng SI-7 has a pronounced effect on regulating and calming the spirit and is indicated for mania-depression, fear and fright, and sadness and anxiety. The *Methods of Acupuncture and Moxibustion from the Golden Mirror of Medicine* more specifically recommends Zhizheng SI-7 for depression and knotting of all the seven emotions.

Thirdly Zhizheng SI-7 is able to regulate the Small Intestine channel in the region of the head (headache and dizziness), eyes (blurred vision, superficial visual obstruction, visual dizziness), elbow (contraction of the elbow), and especially the fingers (severe pain of all the fingers, inability to grip firmly, inability to make a fist). The principle of selecting distal points to treat disorders of the limbs, trunk and head is fundamental to acupuncture practice, and since the twelve primary channels all flow to or from the hands and feet, there is a profusion of distal points to choose from. In the treatment of disorders of the hands and feet themselves, however, there are by definition no distal points, and there are relatively few proximal points that affect these areas. Zhizheng SI-7 is therefore notable for its action on the fingers and hand.

Finally the *Great Compendium of Acupuncture and Moxibustion* gives specific indications for excess and deficiency of the luo-connecting points. In the case of Zhizheng SI-7, these are slackness of the joints and inability to move the elbow (excess); warts (deficiency).

COMBINATIONS

- Manic raving, fear and fright: Zhizheng SI-7, Yuji LU-10, Hegu L.I.-4, Shaohai HE-3, Quchi L.I.-11 and Wangu SI-4 (*Thousand Ducat Formulas*).
- Visual dizziness and headache: Zhizheng SI-7 and Sanjiaoshu BL-22 (*Supplementing Life*).
- Visual dizziness: Zhizheng SI-7 and Feiyang BL-58 (*One Hundred Symptoms*).

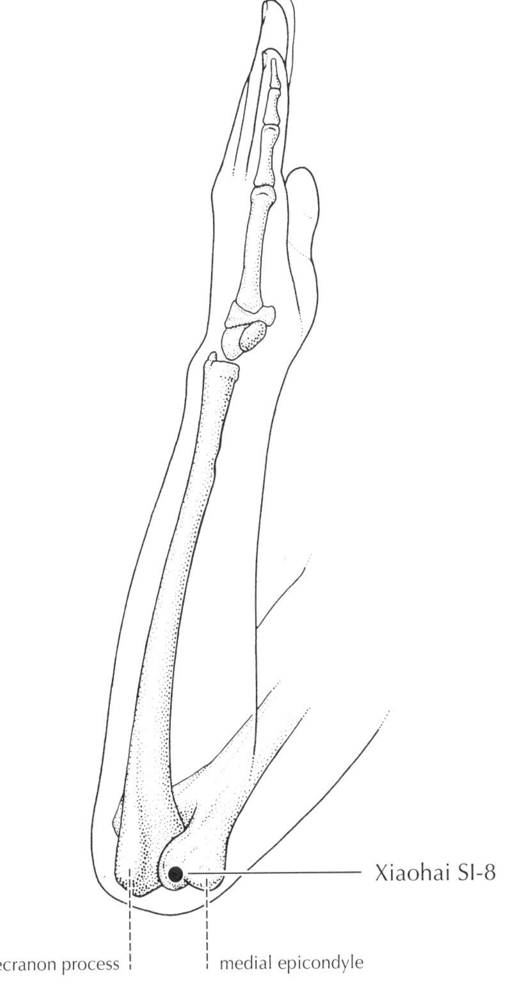

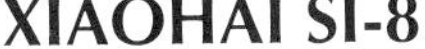

XIAOHAI SI-8

Small Sea

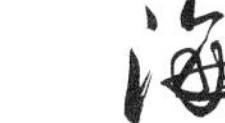

He-Sea and Earth point of the Small Intestine channel

LOCATION

In the depression between the tip of the olecranon process of the ulna and the tip of the medial epicondyle of the humerus.

NEEDLING

i. Oblique distal or proximal insertion 0.5 to 1 cun; ii. Perpendicular insertion 0.3 to 0.5 cun.

Caution: the ulnar nerve lies deep to this point.

ACTIONS

Clears heat and dissipates swelling

Calms the spirit

Activates the channel and alleviates pain

INDICATIONS

- Scrofula, swelling and pain of the throat, swelling of the cheek, swelling of the gums, swelling and pain of the elbow and axilla, toothache, tooth decay, wind dizziness, headache, deafness, yellow eyes, malaria.
- Epilepsy, tongue thrusting, clonic spasm, mad walking, agitation of the Heart.
- Pain of the neck, pain of the neck radiating to the elbow, pain of the scapula, pain of the postero-lateral aspect of the shoulder, pain of the upper arm and elbow, inability to raise the four limbs, lumbar pain radiating to the hypogastrium, lower abdominal pain.

COMMENTARY

Xiaohai SI-8 is the he-sea and earth point of the Small Intestine channel. Despite these important characteristics, it is a relatively infrequently used point, reflected by its appearance in very few classical combinations. It is indicated for many different kinds of swelling involving the gums, throat, cheek, elbow and axilla, as well as scrofula of the neck or axilla. Clinically, however, it is primarily used for pain of the scapula and the posterolateral aspect of the shoulder, arm and elbow. Like Zhizheng SI-7, Xiaohai SI-8 is also able to regulate its coupled Heart zang and is indicated for such disorders as epilepsy, tongue thrusting (where the tongue is repeatedly thrust out of the mouth like a snake's tongue), mad walking and agitation of the Heart.

Finally it is worth noting that despite being the he-sea point of the Small Intestine, Xiaohai SI-8 has no significant action on its respective fu. This reflects the essential contradiction that whilst the Small and Large Intestine fu are located in the lower jiao, their channels run along the upper limb. As a consequence, points of these channels have relatively little action on the fu, and disorders of the Small Intestine are rather treated by points such as Xiajuxu ST-39 or Xiaochangshu BL-27, the lower he-sea and back-shu points of the Small Intestine respectively.

COMBINATIONS

- Contraction of the elbow: Xiaohai SI-8, Chize LU-5, Jianyu L.I.-15, Jianshi P-5, Daling P-7, Houxi SI-3 and Yuji LU-10 (*Great Compendium*).
- Pain of the gums: Xiaohai SI-8 and Jiaosun SJ-20 (*Great Compendium*).
- Epileptic convulsions, mad walking, inability to sleep, agitation of the Heart: Xiaohai SI-8, Houxi SI-3, Zanzhu BL-2 and Qiangjian DU-18 (*Thousand Ducat Formulas*).

JIANZHEN SI-9

True Shoulder

肩貞

LOCATION

On the posterior aspect of the shoulder, 1 cun superior to the posterior axillary crease when the arm hangs in the adducted position.

LOCATION NOTE

This point lies in the depression just below the posterior border of the deltoid.

NEEDLING

Perpendicular insertion 1 to 1.5 cun.

ACTIONS

Expels wind and benefits the shoulder
Activates the channel and alleviates pain

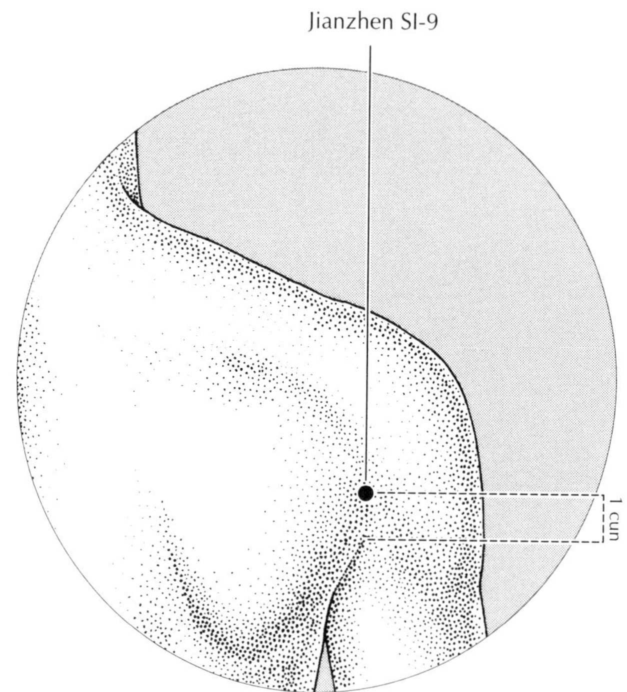

INDICATIONS

- Pain of the shoulder and upper arm, inability to raise the arm, pain of the scapula, heat sensation and pain of the supraclavicular fossa, wind painful obstruction, numbness with inability to raise the hand and foot.
- Chills and fever due to injury by cold, tinnitus and deafness.

COMBINATIONS

- Heat sensation of the shoulder with inability to turn the head: Jianzhen SI-9, Guanchong SJ-1 and Jianyu L.I.-15 (*Thousand Ducat Formulas*).
- Tinnitus and deafness: Jianzhen SI-9 and Wangu SI-4 (*Systematic Classic*).

NAOSHU SI-10

Upper Arm Shu

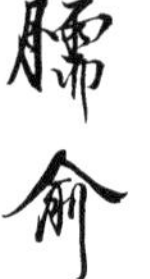

Meeting point of the Small Intestine and Bladder channels with the Yang Linking and Yang Motility vessels

LOCATION

On the posterior aspect of the shoulder, in the depression inferior to the scapular spine, directly superior to the posterior axillary crease when the arm hangs in the adducted position.

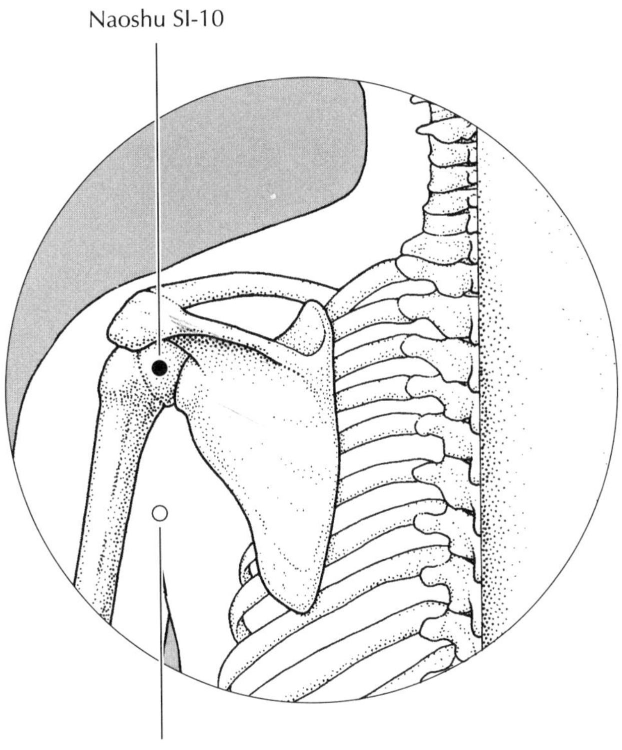

LOCATION NOTE

Slide a finger directly upwards from Jianzhen SI-9 until it falls into the depression just below the scapular spine.

NEEDLING

Perpendicular insertion 1 to 1.5 cun.

ACTIONS

Benefits the shoulder
Activates the channel and alleviates pain

INDICATIONS

- Pain and swelling of the shoulder that radiates to the scapula, weakness and pain of the arm and shoulder, inability to raise the shoulder.
- Chills and fever, scrofula.

COMMENTARY

Naoshu SI-10 is a commonly used point for pain and stiffness of the shoulder, especially its posterior aspect, and allows deep penetration into the joint. Its influence on the shoulder is augmented by the fact that Naoshu SI-10 is also a meeting point of the Yang Motility and Yang Linking vessels, which traverse the posterior (Yang Linking) and the superior and anterior (Yang Motility) portions of the shoulder. In clinical practice Naoshu SI-10 is often used in combination with points such as Jianyu L.I.-15 and Jianliao SJ-14.

COMBINATIONS

- Acute pain of the posterior of the shoulder: Naoshu SI-10 and Yanglao SI-6.
- Immobility and pain of the shoulder joint: First needle Tiaokou ST-38, then Naoshu SI-10, Jianliao SJ-14, Jianyu L.I.-15, Jugu L.I.-16, Quchi L.I.-11 and Yanglao SI-6.

TIANZONG SI-11

Heavenly Gathering

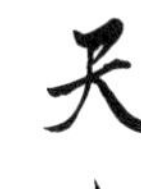

LOCATION

On the scapula, in a tender depression one third of the distance from the midpoint of the inferior border of the scapular spine to the inferior angle of the scapula.

LOCATION NOTE

In practice it may be difficult to palpate the inferior angle of the scapula. An alternative method of location is to draw an equilateral triangle with Jianzhen SI-9 and Naoshu SI-10, after first ensuring that the patient's shoulder is relaxed.

NEEDLING

Perpendicular or oblique insertion 0.5 to 1.5 cun.

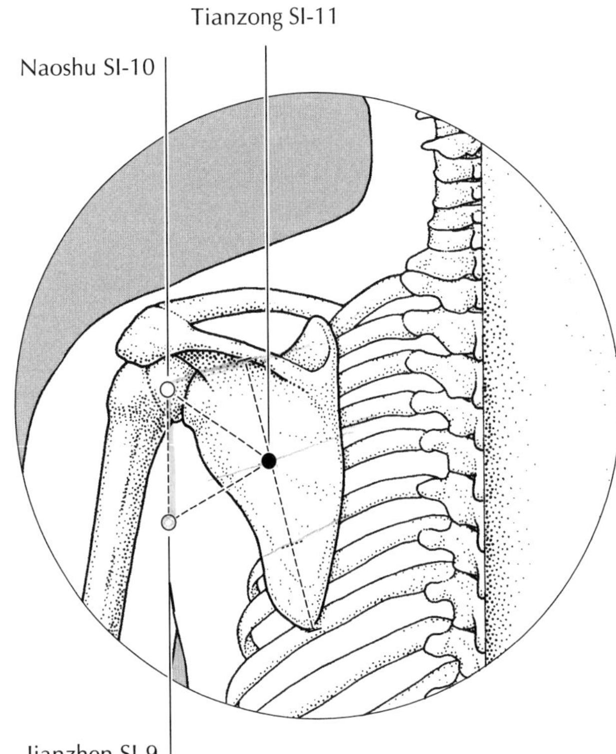

ACTIONS

Activates the channel and alleviates pain
Moves qi and unbinds the chest and lateral costal region
Benefits the breasts

INDICATIONS

- Heaviness and pain of the shoulder, pain of the scapula, pain and inability to raise the elbow and arm, pain of the elbow, swelling of the cheek and submandibular region.
- Fullness of the chest and lateral costal region, cough, pain and swelling of the breast, breast abscess, insufficient lactation.

COMMENTARY

The indications of Tianzong SI-11 reflect both its location and its ability to move qi and unbind the chest. It is an important point for pain of the scapular region whether due to sprain, painful obstruction, overuse, poor posture, Liver qi stagnation or referred pain from Gall Bladder disease, in which cases it is usually found to be acutely tender on palpation. Lying behind the breast, it is also used in combination with points such as Shaoze SI-1 and Shanzhong REN-17 for a wide variety of disorders of the breast including pain, lumps and insufficient lactation.

COMBINATIONS

- Pain of the shoulder and arm: Tianzong SI-11 and Wangu SI-4 (*Supplementing Life*).
- Pain of the arm: Tianzong SI-11, Jianliao SJ-14 and Yanggu SI-5 (*Supplementing Life*).

BINGFENG SI-12

Grasping the Wind

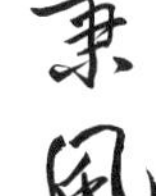

Meeting point of the Small Intestine, Large Intestine, Sanjiao and Gall Bladder channels

LOCATION

In the centre of the suprascapular fossa, directly above Tianzong SI-11, in a depression formed when the arm is raised.

NEEDLING

Oblique medial insertion towards the spine 0.5 to 1 cun. **Caution:** deep perpendicular insertion, especially in thin patients, carries a substantial risk of inducing a pneumothorax.

ACTIONS

Expels wind and benefits the shoulder and scapula

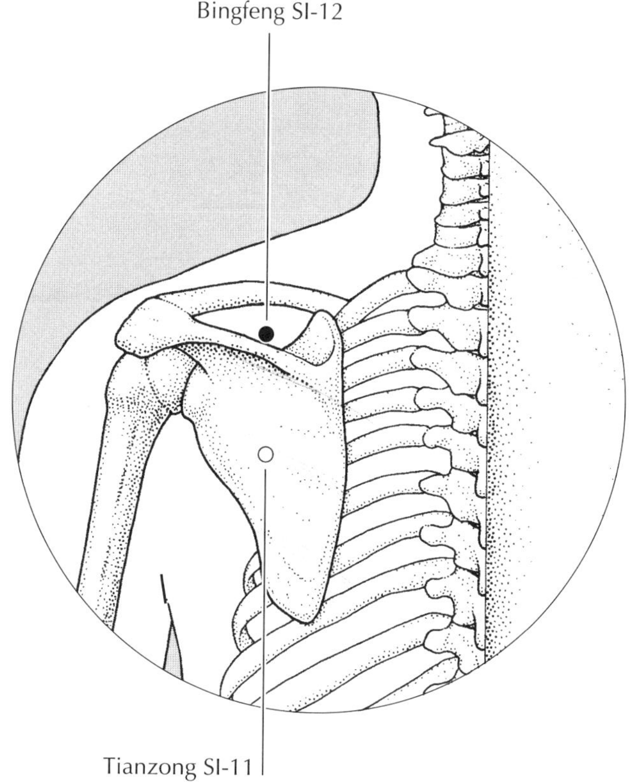

INDICATIONS

- Pain of the shoulder and scapula with inability to raise the arm, stiff neck with inability to turn the head, pain and numbness of the upper arm, cough with stubborn phlegm.

COMMENTARY

Bingfeng SI-12 is a meeting point of the Small Intestine channel with the Large Intestine, Sanjiao and Gall Bladder channels, all of which traverse the scapular and shoulder regions and the neck. As its name 'Grasping Wind' (and by implication controlling wind) implies, Bingfeng SI-12 is a useful local point to invigorate these channels and expel pathogenic wind which has lodged in the muscles of the shoulder and scapula. Although most classical and contemporary sources recommend this point for local disorders only, the Ming dynasty classic *Investigation Into Points Along the Channels* suggests a broader action of expelling wind and recommends the use of Bingfeng SI-12 "when the interstices and pores do not close properly, wind pathogen easily enters [resulting in] cough with stubborn phlegm".

COMBINATIONS

- Pain of the shoulder with inability to raise the arm: Bingfeng SI-12 and Yunmen LU-2 (*Supplementing Life*).
- Pain of the shoulder with inability to raise the arm: Bingfeng SI-12 and Tianrong SI-17 (*Systematic Classic*).

QUYUAN SI-13

Crooked Wall

曲垣

LOCATION

In the tender depression superior to the medial end of the scapular spine, midway between Naoshu SI-10 and the spinous process of T2.

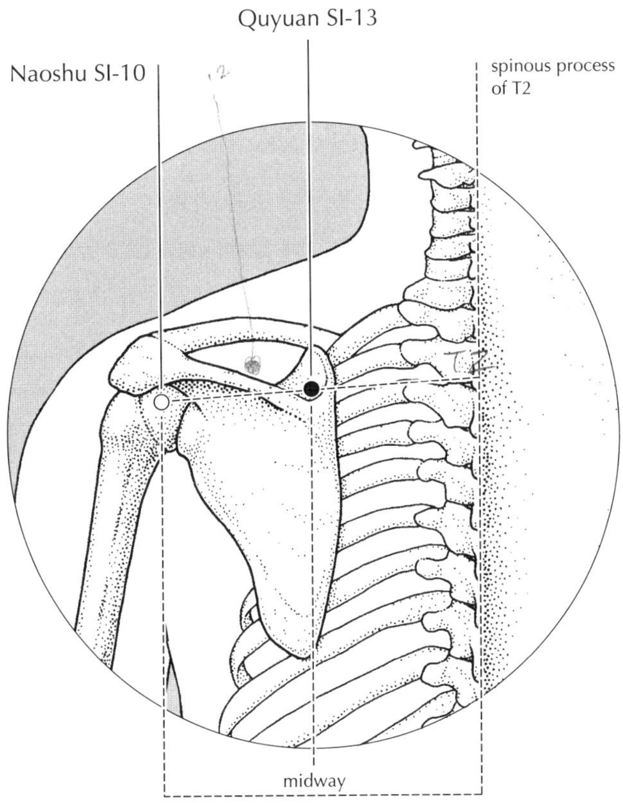

LOCATION NOTE

Slide a fingertip medially along the superior border of the scapular spine until it falls into the tender depression just lateral to the medial border of the scapula.

NEEDLING

i. Perpendicular insertion 0.3 to 0.5 cun; ii. Oblique lateral insertion 0.5 to 1 cun.

Caution: this point is located close to the medial border of the scapula. Too medial an insertion or deep medial-oblique needling may puncture the lungs.

ACTIONS

Benefits the shoulder and scapula

INDICATIONS

- Generalised painful obstruction, painful obstruction of the shoulder and scapula, hot painful obstruction of the shoulder with contraction, pain and an oppressive sensation of the shoulder.

COMMENTARY

The *Great Compendium of Acupuncture and Moxibustion* emphasises the use of Quyuan SI-13 in the treatment of painful obstruction of the shoulder that has persisted and transformed into heat with contraction, pain and oppressive sensation. This transformation of wind, damp or cold into heat is a manifestation of the law of 'similar transformation' expounded by Liu Wan-su (see Yinlingquan SP-9).

COMBINATIONS

- Pain of the shoulder and scapula: Quyuan SI-13, Tianzong SI-11 and Jianzhen SI-9.

JIANWAISHU SI-14

Outer Shoulder Shu

肩外俞

LOCATION

3 cun lateral to the lower border of the spinous process of T1 (Taodao DU-13).

LOCATION NOTE

When the shoulder is relaxed, the three cun line corresponds to the medial border of the scapula.

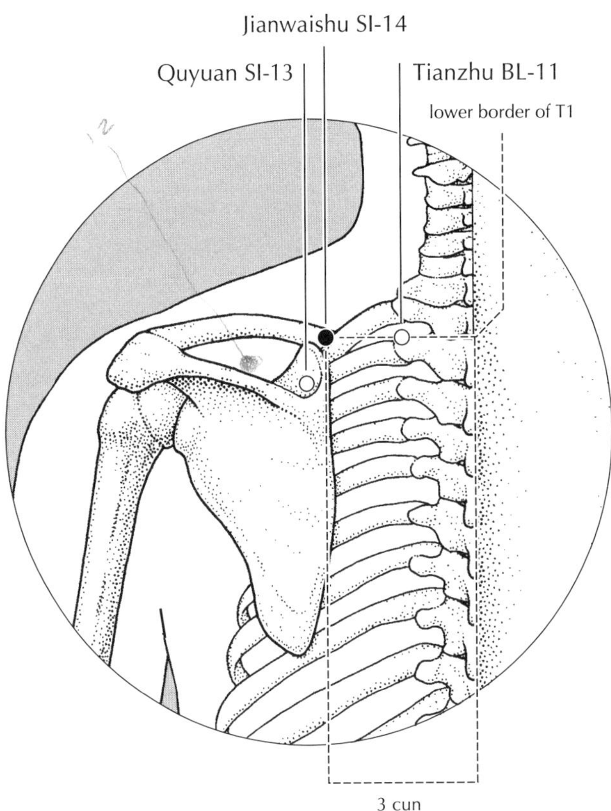

NEEDLING
Oblique medial insertion 0.5 to 1 cun.
Caution: perpendicular insertion, especially in thin patients, carries a substantial risk of inducing a pneumothorax.

ACTIONS
Activates the channel and alleviates pain
Expels wind and cold and benefits the shoulder and scapula

INDICATIONS
- Pain of the shoulder and scapula with cold sensation extending to the elbow, chills and fever accompanied by neck rigidity and inability to turn the head, generalised painful obstruction.

COMBINATIONS
- Pain of the shoulder and back: Jianwaishu SI-14, Kunlun BL-60 and Dazhui DU-14.

JIANZHONGZHU SI-15
Middle Shoulder Shu

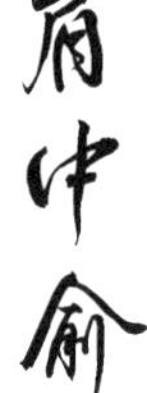

LOCATION
2 cun lateral to the lower border of the spinous process of C7 (Dazhui DU-14).

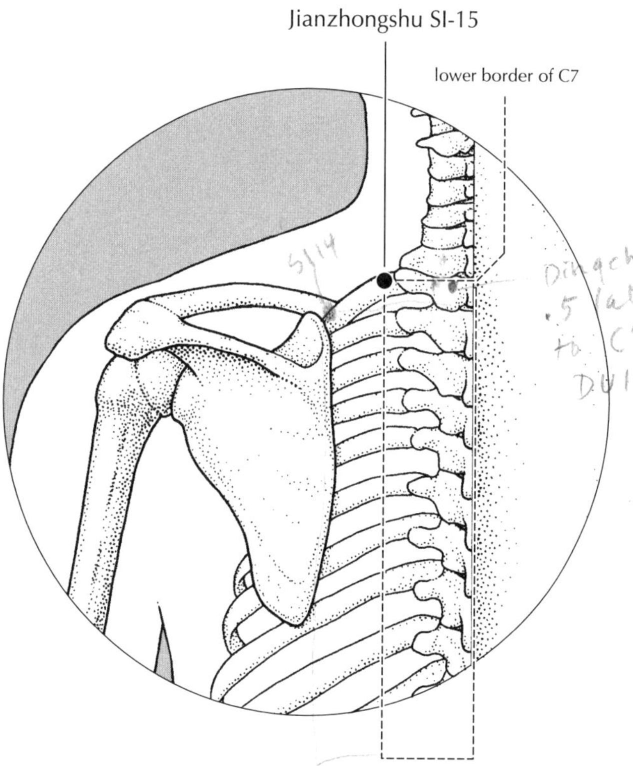

LOCATION NOTE
i. This point may be found two thirds of the distance between the midline and the medial border of the scapula, when the shoulder is in a relaxed position; ii. to locate C7 see page 68.

NEEDLING
Oblique medial insertion towards the spine 0.5 to 1 cun.
Caution: deep insertion inferiorly, especially in thin patients, carries a substantial risk of inducing a pneumothorax.

ACTIONS
Descends Lung qi
Activates the channel and alleviates pain

INDICATIONS
- Cough, spitting blood, chills and fever, dimness of vision, pain of the shoulder and scapula.

COMBINATIONS
- Rebellious qi cough: Jianzhongshu SI-15, Tianchi P-1, Tiantu REN-22, Shanzhong REN-17 and Jiexi ST-41 (*Supplementing Life*).

TIANCHUANG SI-16
Heavenly Window

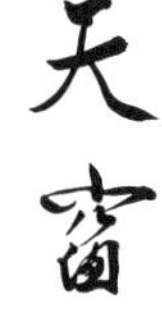

Point of the Window of Heaven

LOCATION
On the posterior border of the sternocleidomastoid muscle, level with the laryngeal prominence.

LOCATION NOTE
i. Palpation of the posterior border of the sternocleidomastoid muscle is made easier if the patient turns their head away from the side to be needled, whilst you apply resistance at the chin; ii. In females the laryngeal prominence is not as pronounced as in males. If it is indistinct, palpate the depression formed by the lower border of the hyoid bone and the upper border of the thyroid cartilage at the midline. The laryngeal prominence lies just below this.

NEEDLING
Perpendicular insertion 0.5 to 0.8 cun.

ACTIONS
Benefits the ears, throat and voice
Regulates qi and calms the spirit
Activates the channel, alleviates pain and clears heat

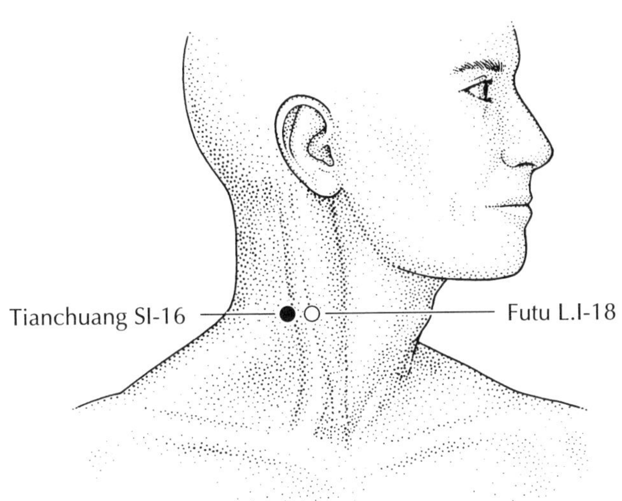

INDICATIONS
- Deafness, tinnitus, ear pain.
- Sudden loss of voice, sudden loss of voice following windstroke, hoarseness due to cold in the throat, lockjaw, clenched teeth from windstroke, headache.
- Throat pain, goitre, swelling and pain of the cheek, heat sensation of the skin of the face, urticaria.
- Manic ghost talk, mania-depression.
- Shoulder pain radiating to the neck, shoulder pain leading to stiffness of the neck with inability to turn the head, neck pain.

COMMENTARY
Tianchuang SI-16 is one of ten points listed in Chapter 2 of the *Spiritual Pivot* that have come to be known as Window of Heaven points. As a group, these ten points have the action of regulating rebellious and chaotic (inversion) qi. Tianchuang SI-16 illustrates many of the characteristic actions of these points in its ability to i. treat goitre and throat disorders, ii. treat headache and heat and swelling of the face and cheek, iii. treat disorders of the sense organs - in this case the ears, iv. treat sudden onset of disorders - in this case loss of voice. In addition, like two other points from this group (Tianzhu BL-10 and Tianfu LU-3) Tianchuang SI-16 treats disorders characterised in the classical texts as seeing or communicating with ghosts and therefore attributed to some form of demonic possession. In terms of modern medicine these indications refer to various forms of severe mental disorder including schizophrenia. For a fuller discussion of the Window of Heaven points see page 48.

Sun Si-miao, the famous 7th century physician, particularly emphasised the use of moxibustion (fifty cones) at this point for loss of speech and hemiplegia.

COMBINATIONS
- Ear pain, deafness and tinnitus: Tianchuang SI-16, Yangxi L.I.-5, Guanchong SJ-1, Yemen SJ-2 and Zhongzhu SJ-3 (*Thousand Ducat Formulas*).
- Deafness and tinnitus: Tianchuang SI-16 and Waiguan SJ-5 (*Supplementing Life*).
- Throat pain: Tianchuang SI-16, Fengfu DU-16 and Laogong P-8 (*Thousand Ducat Formulas*).
- Goitre: Tianchuang SI-16 and Naohui SJ-13 (*Systematic Classic*).
- Sudden loss of voice: Tianchuang SI-16, Zhigou SJ-6, Futu L.I.-18, Qubin GB-7 and Lingdao HE-4 (*Thousand Ducat Formulas*).
- Sudden loss of voice with lockjaw: Tianchuang SI-16, Lingdao HE-4 and Tiantu REN-22 (*Supplementing Life*).
- Lockjaw: Tianchuang SI-16 and Yifeng SJ-17 (*Supplementing Life*).
- Heat sensation of the skin of the face: Tianchuang SI-16 and Tiantu REN-22 (*Supplementing Life*).

TIANRONG SI-17
Heavenly Appearance

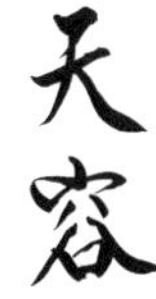

Point of the Window of Heaven

LOCATION
In the depression between the angle of the mandible and the anterior border of the sternocleidomastoid muscle.

LOCATION NOTE
i. Palpation of the anterior border of the sternocleidomastoid muscle is made easier if the patient turns their head away from the side to be needled, whilst you apply resistance at the chin; ii. If the transverse process of C2 is palpable, locate and needle this point anterior to it.

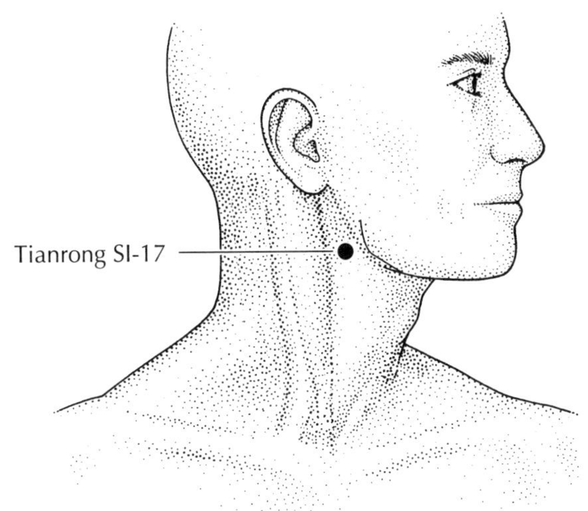

NEEDLING

Directed towards the root of the tongue, anterior to the carotid vessels, 0.5 to 1 cun.

ACTIONS

Benefits the neck and throat and disperses swelling
Descends rebellious qi
Benefits the ears

INDICATIONS

- Throat painful obstruction, obstruction of the throat, goitre, scrofula of the neck, swelling and pain of the neck with inability to speak, clenched teeth, swelling of the cheek, chills and fever.
- Chest fullness with difficulty in breathing, wheezing, asthma, cough, chest pain, vomiting foam.
- Tinnitus and deafness.
- Pain of the shoulder with inability to raise the arm.

COMMENTARY

In the *Spiritual Pivot* Tianrong was classified as a point of the Gall Bladder channel, whilst in the *Systematic Classic of Acupuncture and Moxibustion* it was listed as belonging to the Sanjiao channel. It was not until the 10th century classic *Secrets of a Frontier Official,* that Tianrong was finally ascribed to the Small Intestine channel.

The point Tianrong SI-17 is discussed in the chapter 'Needling Methods and Upright and Pathogenic Qi' in the *Spiritual Pivot*[6]. According to Qi Bo, the Yellow Emperor's adviser, this point should be needled for "great rebellion of yang qi which rises to fill the chest causing congestion of the chest, agitation and raising of the shoulders ... dyspnoea and wheezing with inability to sit or lie down. In such an illness there is aversion to dust and smoke [as it causes] breathing difficulty as if the throat is blocked", a clear reference to an acute attack of asthma. He compares the speed at which needling this point takes effect to "wiping away the dust".

Tianrong SI-17 is one of ten points listed in Chapter Two of the *Spiritual Pivot* that have come to be known as Window of Heaven points. It clearly exemplifies the character and action of these points in its ability to regulate rebellious and chaotic (inversion) qi. Tianrong SI-17 shares with these points the ability to i. treat scrofula and goitre due to stagnation of qi and phlegm in the pivotal neck region, as well as throat disorders, ii. descend rebellious qi, in this case of the Lung and Stomach manifesting as fullness of the chest with difficulty in breathing, cough, asthma, wheezing and vomiting, and iii. treat disorders of the sense organs, in this case the ears (tinnitus and deafness). For a fuller discussion of the Window of Heaven points see page 48.

COMBINATIONS

- Cough with rebellious qi, dyspnoea, vomiting of foam and clenched teeth: Tianrong SI-17, Futu L.I.-18, Lianquan REN-23, Pohu BL-42, Qishe ST-11 and Yixi BL-45 (*Thousand Ducat Formulas*).
- Oppressive sensation of the chest with inability to catch the breath: Tianrong SI-17 and Yangxi L.I.-5 (*Supplementing Life*).
- Deafness and tinnitus: Tianrong SI-17, Tinggong SI-19, Tinghui GB-2 and Zhongzhu SJ-3 (*Thousand Ducat Formulas*).
- Pain of the shoulder with inability to raise the arm: Tianrong SI-17 and Bingfeng SI-12 (*Systematic Classic*).

QUANLIAO SI-18

Cheek Bone Crevice

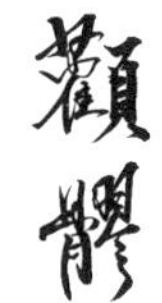

Meeting point of the Small Intestine and Sanjiao channels

LOCATION

Directly below the outer canthus, in the depression at the lower border of the zygomatic bone.

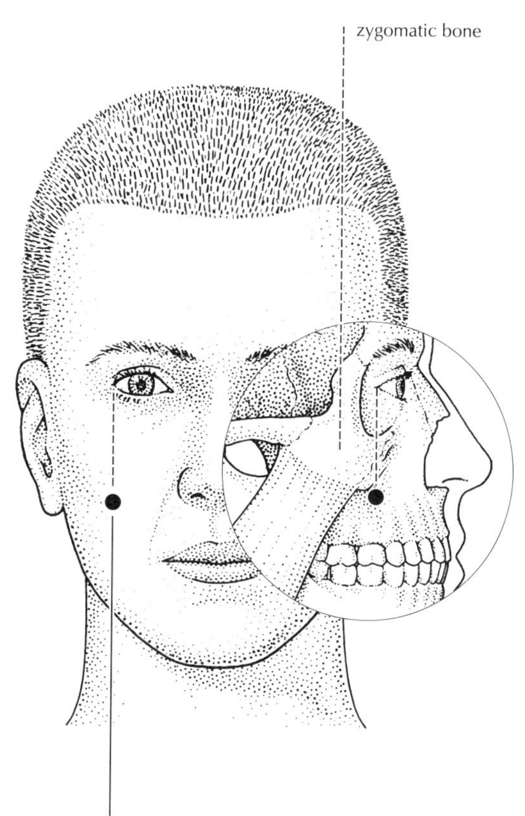

NEEDLING
i. Transverse insertion joined to points such as Dicang ST-4, Xiaguan ST-7, Yingxiang L.I.-20, Jiache ST-6 etc.; ii. Perpendicular insertion 0.5 to 0.7 cun. **Note**: according to the *Illustrated Supplement to the Classic of Categories* and a number of modern texts, this point is contraindicated to moxibustion.

ACTIONS
Eliminates wind and alleviates pain
Clears heat and reduces swelling

INDICATIONS
- Deviation of the mouth and eye, ceaseless twitching of the eyelids, pain of the face, swelling of the cheek with toothache, inability to chew, abscess of the lip, red face, yellow eyes.

COMMENTARY
The location of Quanliao SI-18 renders it an important and commonly-used point in the treatment of facial disorders due to either interior or exterior wind, and it is indicated for facial paralysis, trigeminal neuralgia, twitching of the eyelids and toothache of the upper jaw. In the treatment of the first two conditions it is often joined to points such as Yingxiang L.I.-20, Dicang ST-4 and Jiache ST-6 by transverse needling.

COMBINATIONS
- Toothache: Quanliao SI-18 and Erjian L.I.-2 (*Systematic Classic*).
- Toothache with aversion to cold: Quanliao SI-18, Daying ST-5, Tinghui GB-2 and Quchi L.I.-11 (*Thousand Ducat Formulas*).
- Pain and deviation of the mouth, aversion to wind and cold, inability to chew: Quanliao SI-18 and Jiache ST-6 (*Thousand Ducat Formulas*).
- Red and yellow eyes: Quanliao SI-18 and Neiguan P-6 (*Thousand Ducat Formulas*).

TINGGONG SI-19
Palace of Hearing

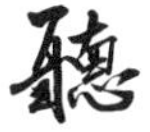

Meeting point of the Small Intestine, Sanjiao and Gall Bladder channels

LOCATION
With the mouth open, this point is located in the depression between the middle of the tragus and the condyloid process of the mandible.

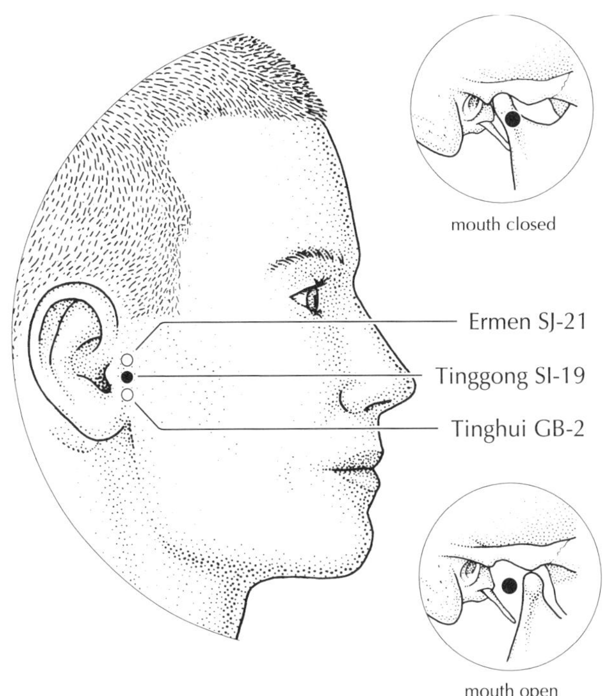

LOCATION NOTE
In order to locate this point, ask the patient to open the mouth so that the condyloid process of the mandible slides forwards to reveal the depression.

NEEDLING
i. Perpendicular insertion 0.5 to 1 cun; ii. Needle with the mouth open; following insertion of the needle the patient may close their mouth.

ACTIONS
Benefits the ears
Calms the spirit

INDICATIONS
- Deafness, tinnitus, purulent discharge from the ear.
- Mania, epilepsy, loss of voice, fullness of the Heart and abdomen, toothache.

COMMENTARY
There are three points anterior to the tragus of the ear, Ermen SJ-21 superiorly, Tinggong SI-19 in the middle, and Tinghui GB-2 inferiorly. All are frequently employed for the treatment of a wide variety of ear disorders, including tinnitus, deafness, pain, itching and discharge. Due to the close proximity of these points and the similar indications for each, it is difficult to distinguish between them clinically. It is worth noting however that Tinggong SI-19 has a secondary action of calming the spirit, whilst

Tinghui GB-2 is the most effective to treat painful disorders of the surrounding area including the jaw and teeth. If it is necessary to needle points around the ear regularly, then these three points should be alternated.

In current practice, where points are numbered, it is easy to remember the relative locations of Ermen SJ-21 (Gate of the Ear), Tinggong SI-19 (Palace of Hearing) and Tinghui GB-2 (Meeting of Hearing), the highest point number being the uppermost point. In China, which has no tradition of numbering the points, one way of recalling the order of their location was by the image of entering through the 'gate' of the 'palace' to convene a 'meeting'.

COMBINATIONS

- Deafness due to qi obstruction: Tinggong SI-19, Tinghui GB-2 and Yifeng SJ-17; then needle Zusanli ST-36 and Hegu L.I.-4 (*Great Compendium*).
- Deafness and tinnitus: Tinggong SI-19, Tianrong SI-17, Tinghui GB-2 and Zhongzhu SJ-3 (*Thousand Ducat Formulas*).
- Deafness: Tinggong SI-19, Zhongzhu SJ-3, Waiguan SJ-5, Erheliao SJ-22, Shangyang L.I.-1, Tinghui GB-2, Hegu L.I.-4 and Zhongchong P-9 (*Precious Mirror*).
- Impaired hearing and deafness: Tinggong SI-19, Ermen SJ-21, Fengchi GB-20, Xiaxi GB-43 and Tinghui GB-2 (*Great Compendium*).
- Sadness below the Heart: Tinggong SI-19 and Pishu BL-20 (*One Hundred Symptoms*).

NOTES

1 *Spiritual Pivot* Chapter 4.

2 *Classic of Difficulties* 68th Difficulty.

3 *Classic of Difficulties* 68th Difficulty.

4 *Thousand Ducat Formulas*.

5 Quoted in *Chinese Acupuncture and Moxibustion*, Foreign Languages Press, Beijing.

6 *Spiritual Pivot* Chapter 75.

足太陽膀胱經

THE BLADDER CHANNEL OF FOOT TAIYANG

THE BLADDER CHANNEL OF FOOT TAIYANG

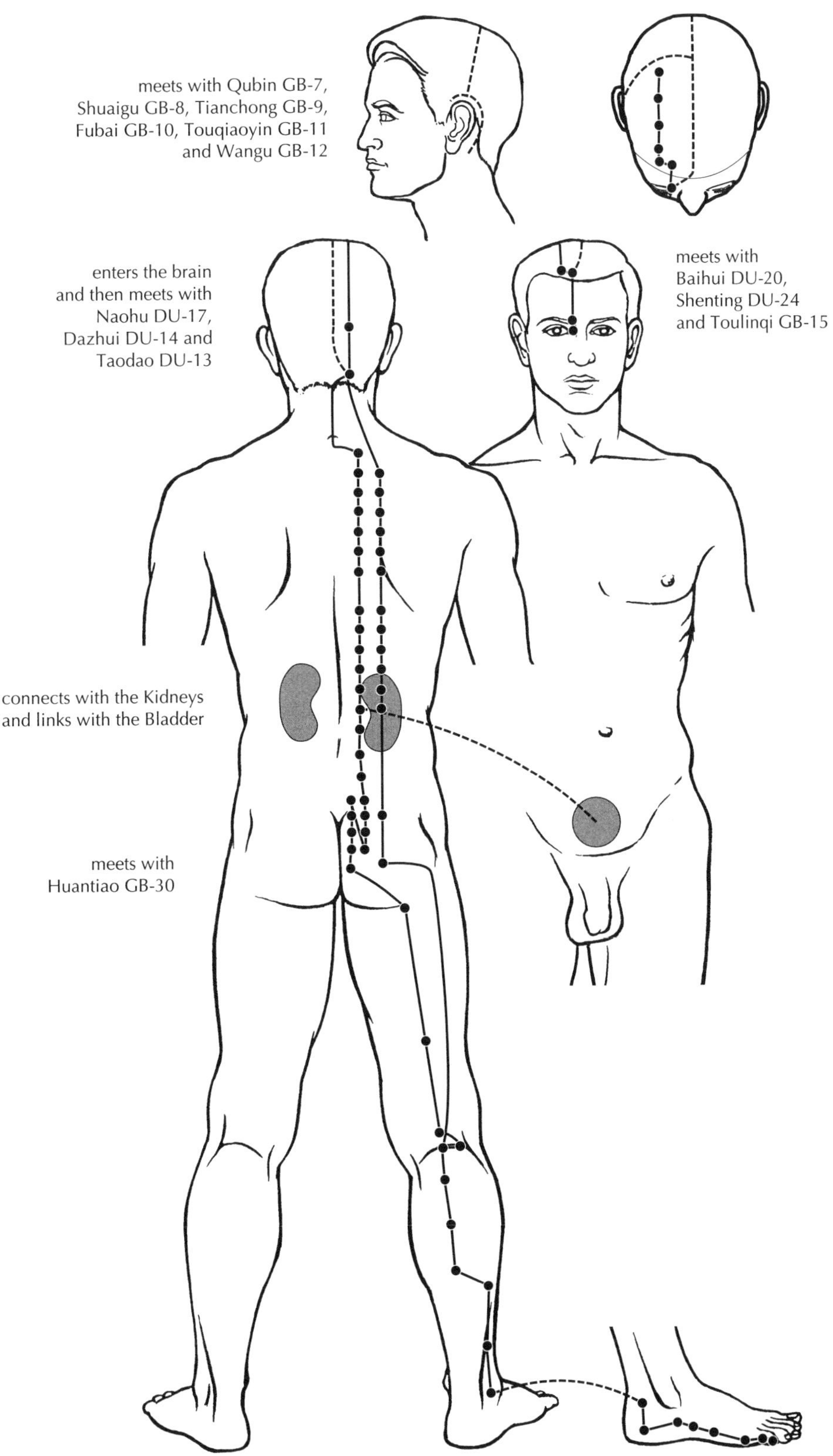
meets with Qubin GB-7,
Shuaigu GB-8, Tianchong GB-9,
Fubai GB-10, Touqiaoyin GB-11
and Wangu GB-12
enters the brain
and then meets with
Naohu DU-17,
Dazhui DU-14 and
Taodao DU-13
meets with
Baihui DU-20,
Shenting DU-24
and Toulinqi GB-15
connects with the Kidneys
and links with the Bladder
meets with
Huantiao GB-30

The Bladder primary channel

THE BLADDER PRIMARY CHANNEL

- begins at the inner canthus of the eye at Jingming BL-1 and ascends along the forehead to the vertex to intersect with Toulinqi GB-15, Shenting DU-24 and Baihui DU-20,
- from the vertex, a branch descends to the temples in the region above the ear, intersecting the Gall Bladder channel at points Qubin GB-7, Shuaigu GB-8, Tianchong GB-9, Fubai GB-10, Touqiaoyin GB-11 and Wangu GB-12,
- from the vertex, another branch enters the brain, meets the Governing channel at Naohu DU-17 and then emerges to descend to the nape of the neck where the channel splits into two branches.

The first (medial) branch

- descends along the posterior aspect of the neck, intersecting Dazhui DU-14 and Taodao DU-13, then descends alongside the spine, 1.5 cun lateral to the midline, to the lumbar region,
- penetrates deep into the interior via the para-vertebral muscles to connect with the Kidneys and link with the Bladder,
- a sub-branch separates in the lumbar region, descends along the sacrum, crosses the buttock and descends to the popliteal fossa of the knee at Weizhong BL-40.

The second (lateral) branch

- separates at the nape of the neck and descends to the medial border of the scapula and then parallel to the spine, 3 cun lateral to the midline, to the gluteal region,
- crosses the buttock to intersect at Huantiao GB-30, then descends along the postero-lateral aspect of the thigh to meet with the previous branch of the channel in the popliteal fossa at Weizhong BL-40,
- descends through the gastrocnemius muscle, emerges posterior to the lateral malleolus at Kunlun BL-60, then follows along the fifth metatarsal bone to terminate at Zhiyin BL-67 at the lateral side of the tip of the fifth toe, where it meets with the Kidney channel.

The Bladder primary channel connects with the following zangfu: Kidneys, Bladder.

The Bladder primary channel meets with other channels at the following points: Baihui DU-20, Shenting DU-24, Toulinqi GB-15, Qubin GB-7, Shuaigu GB-8, Tianchong GB-9, Fubai GB-10, Touqiaoyin GB-11, Wangu GB-12, Naohu DU-17, Dazhui DU-14, Taodao DU-13 and Huantiao GB-30. *Note*: although not mentioned in the classical pathway described above, the following points are also traditionally said to be meeting points with the Bladder channel: Binao L.I.-14, Naoshu SI-10 and Zhejin GB-23.

THE BLADDER LUO-CONNECTING CHANNEL

- separates from the primary channel at Feiyang BL-58 and connects with the Kidney channel.

THE BLADDER DIVERGENT CHANNEL

- diverges from the primary channel in the popliteal fossa and ascends to a point five cun inferior to the sacrum, then winds round the anus, connecting with the Bladder and dispersing in the Kidneys,
- ascends alongside the spine and disperses in the cardiac region, then emerges at the neck to rejoin the Bladder primary channel.

THE BLADDER SINEW CHANNEL

- originates at the little toe and ascends past the lateral malleolus, and then ascends to bind at the (lateral aspect of) the knee,
- another branch separates below the lateral malleolus and binds at the heel, then ascends along the Achilles tendon to the lateral aspect of the popliteal fossa,
- another branch separates from this branch in the calf (at the convergence of the two heads of the gastrocnemius muscle) and ascends to the medial aspect of the popliteal fossa,
- the two branches join in the gluteal region and ascend to bind at the buttock,
- the channel then ascends laterally along the spine to the nape of the neck, where a branch penetrates to bind at the root of the tongue,
- the main ascending branch continues upwards to bind at the occipital bone, and ascends over the crown of the head to bind at the bridge of the nose, then circles the eye and binds at the cheek bone,
- another branch separates on the back and ascends to the medial side of the posterior axillary crease, then binds at Jianyu L.I.-15,
- another branch crosses beneath the axilla and ascends the chest to emerge at the supraclavicular fossa, then ascends to bind at Wangu GB-12 behind the ear, and finally another branch, after emerging from the supraclavicular fossa, rises to the cheek bone alongside the nose.

Pathological symptoms of the Bladder sinew channel
Strain of the little toe, pain and swelling of the heel, spasm of the popliteal region, opisthotonos, spasm and tension of the nape of the neck, inability to raise the shoulder, strain of the axilla, pain and strain of the supraclavicular fossa.

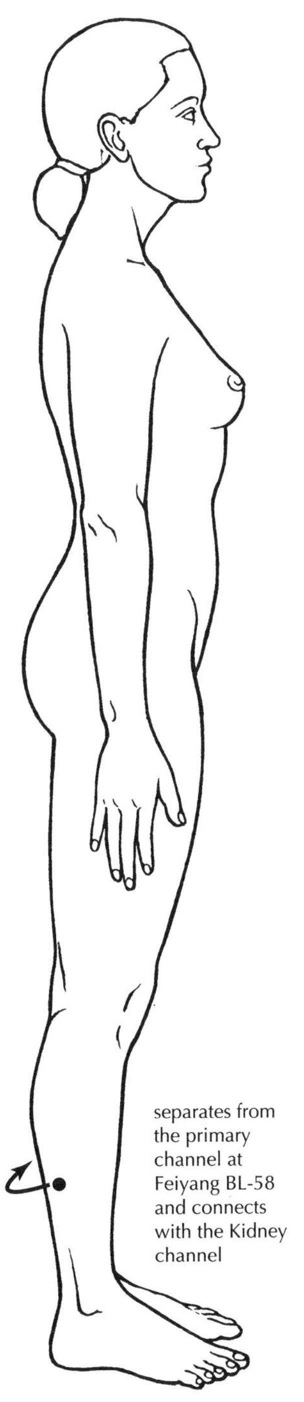
separates from
the primary
channel at
Feiyang BL-58
and connects
with the Kidney
channel

The Bladder luo-connecting channel

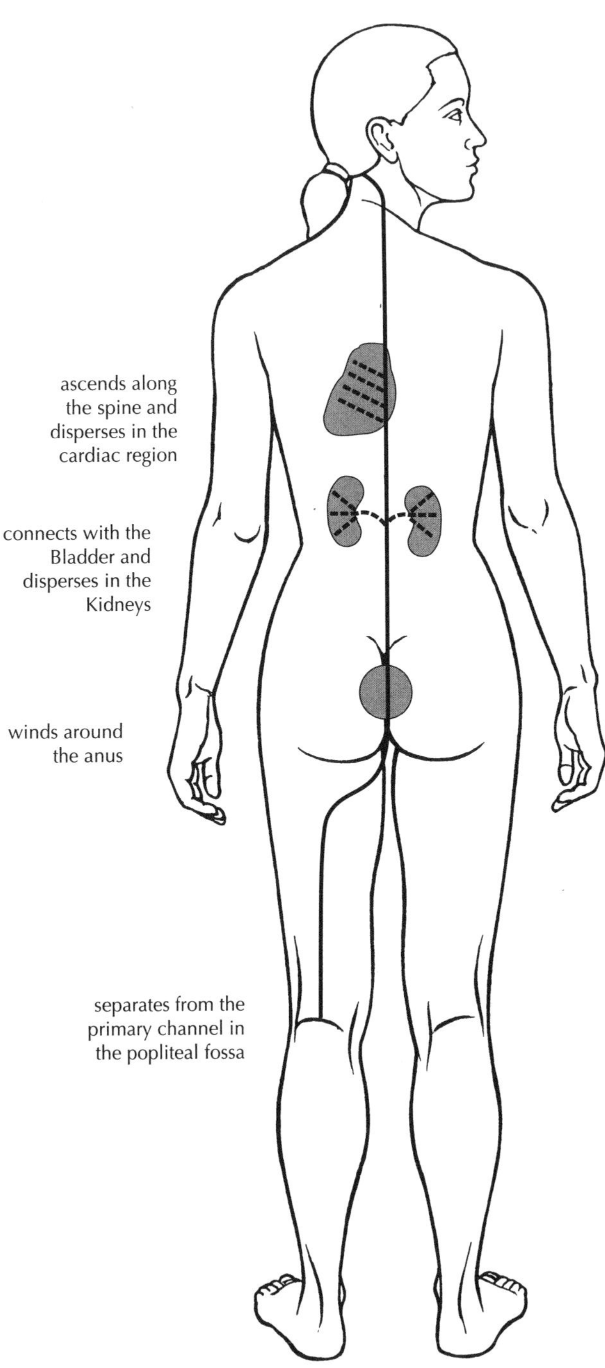
ascends along
the spine and
disperses in the
cardiac region
connects with the
Bladder and
disperses in the
Kidneys
winds around
the anus
separates from the
primary channel in
the popliteal fossa

The Bladder divergent channel

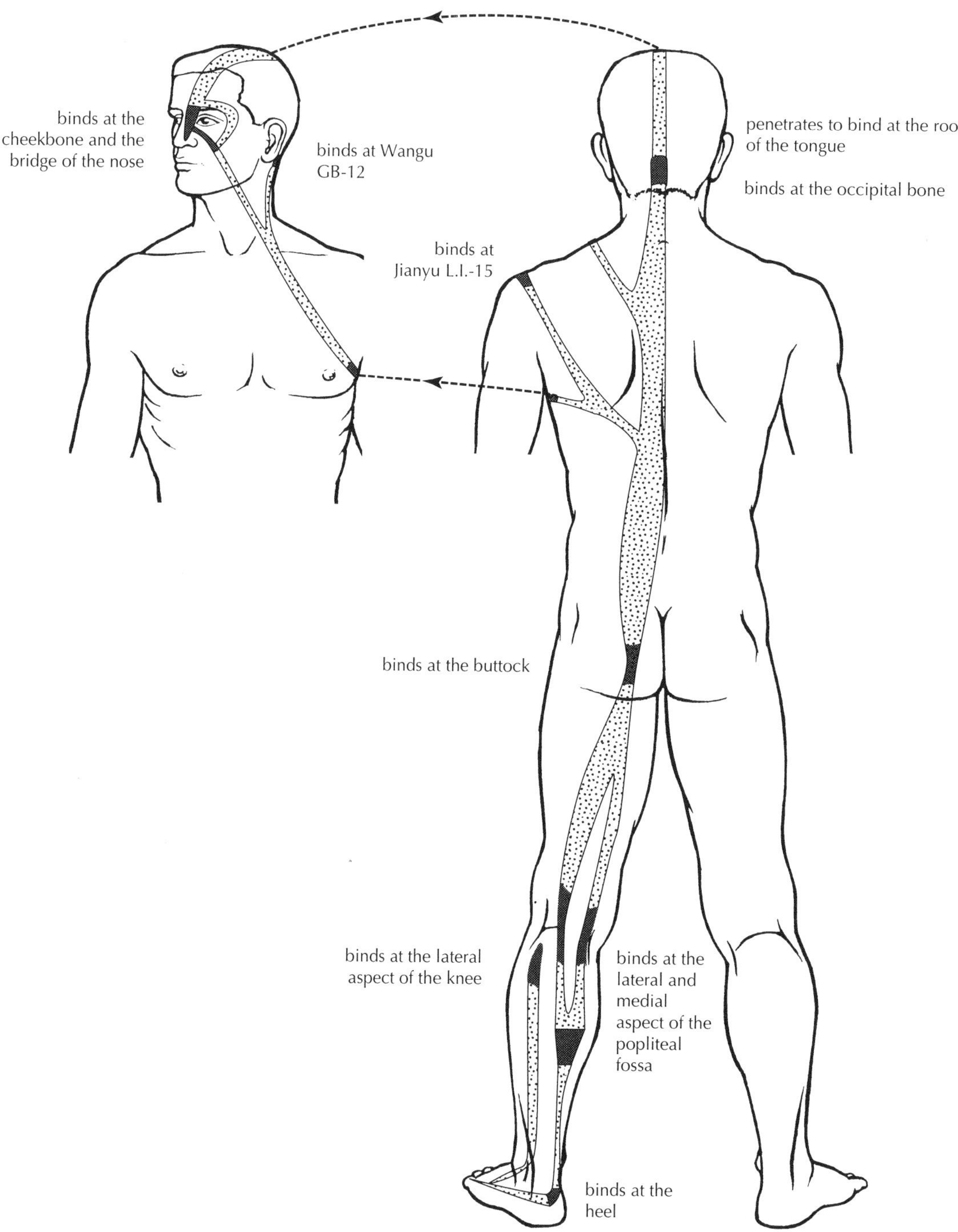
binds at the cheekbone and the bridge of the nose
binds at Wangu GB-12
penetrates to bind at the root of the tongue
binds at the occipital bone
binds at Jianyu L.I.-15
binds at the buttock
binds at the lateral aspect of the knee
binds at the lateral and medial aspect of the popliteal fossa
binds at the heel

The Bladder sinew channel

DISCUSSION

The Bladder channel of foot taiyang channel is interiorly-exteriorly coupled with the Kidney channel, and paired with the Small Intestine channel of hand taiyang according to six channel theory. The Bladder-Kidney relationship is further strengthened by the fact that:

- the Bladder primary channel enters the Kidney zang.
- the Bladder primary channel meets the Kidney channel at Zhiyin BL-67.
- the Bladder divergent channel disperses in the Kidneys.
- the Bladder luo-connecting channel connects with the Kidney channel.

It is also important to note that:

- the Bladder primary channel begins at the inner canthus of the eye.
- the Bladder primary channel intersects the Governing vessel at points Taodao DU-13, Dazhui DU-14, Naohu DU-17 and Baihui DU-20, where it enters the brain.
- the Bladder primary channel descends paravertebrally in two lines, one at 1.5 cun lateral to the midline, the other at 3 cun lateral to the midline; the inner line includes the back-shu points of the twelve zangfu, as well as the hui-meeting points for blood and bones.
- the Bladder divergent channel winds around the anus
- the Bladder divergent channel enters the Heart
- the Bladder sinew channel passes beneath the axilla.

The function of the Bladder is to store fluid and via its qi transformation action to covert the waste into urine for excretion. Like the Small and Large Intestine and Sanjiao channels, however, there is little direct clinical relationship between the Bladder channel and the function of the Bladder fu. It is true that several points of the Bladder channel are important in the treatment of urinary diseases, but this is primarily due to the fact that they are i. back-shu points of the Sanjiao, Kidneys or Bladder (Sanjiaoshu BL-22, Shenshu BL-23 and Pangguangshu BL-28 respectively), ii. local points lying over the region of the Bladder (for example Ciliao BL-32), or iii. distal points with a special relationship to fluid transformation, for example Weiyang BL-39, the lower he-sea point of the Sanjiao.

Due to its length and the different regions of the body it traverses, points of the Bladder channel have a great range of actions and indications:

- The taiyang Bladder channel, with sixty-seven points, is the longest channel in the body. It ascends over the head (yang) and then down the entire posterior, and hence most yang, portion of the body. Taiyang channel is the most superficial of the six channels and is therefore the first to be attacked by exterior wind. Wind is a yang pathogen, and both exterior and interior wind have the tendency to ascend to the head and brain. Many of the points of the Bladder channel, therefore, are important in clinical practice to eliminate both exterior and interior wind from the body.

- The Bladder channel enters the brain, whilst the Bladder divergent channel connects with the Heart. Since the time of the *Essential Questions*, Chinese medicine has recognised that disharmony of the brain or Heart, either singly or together, can give rise to psycho-emotional disorders (for a fuller discussion see the introductory discussion to the Governing vessel). Points of the Bladder channel on the head from Zanzhu BL-2 to BL-10, and on the foot from BL-60 to Zutonggu BL-66 all treat such disorders as mania and epilepsy. In addition certain of the back-shu points such as Feishu BL-13, Xinshu BL-15 and Ganshu BL-18 treat a variety of disorders of the spirit, in this case due to their action on the Lung, Heart and Liver zang as much as their effect on the Bladder channel itself.

- Points Jingming BL-1 (at the inner canthus of the eye) to Tianzhu BL-10 (on the nape of the neck) expel exterior wind from their local area, pacify interior wind and treat disorders of the eyes, nose, head and face.

- The points of the inner, medial portion of the Bladder channel on the back have an enormous variety of actions and indications. Starting with Dazhu BL-11, the hui-meeting point of bone, through to Pangguangshu BL-28, the back-shu point of the Bladder, these points have a profound effect on the zangfu and the various tissues, substances and sense organs of the body. Despite their express action on specific zangfu, however, some generalisations can be made. Points Dazhu BL-11 to Feishu BL-13 are able to expel exterior pathogens and regulate the Lung. Points Jueyinshu BL-14 and Xinshu BL-15 treat the Heart and spirit. Points Geshu BL-17 to Sanjiaoshu BL-22 treat disorders of the middle jiao (Stomach, Spleen, Liver and Gall Bladder). Points Shenshu BL-23 to Huiyang BL-35 and Baohuang BL-53 to Heyang BL-55 treat disorders of the Kidneys, lumbar region and lower jiao (intestines, Bladder, uterus, genitals, anus).

- Points of the outer, lateral, Bladder channel on the back from Fufen BL-41 (level with Fengmen BL-12) through to Zhishi BL-52 (level with Shenshu BL-23) have similar indications to the corresponding points of the inner Bladder channel, although they are generally less extensive in their actions and indications. Exceptions are Pohu BL-42 and Gaohuangshu BL-43 which have a profound effect on tonifying deficiency. It is well-known also that five of these points (Pohu BL-42, Shentang BL-44, Hunmen BL-47, Yishe BL-49 and Zhishi BL-52) are named after the five spiritual aspects. Despite the strong implication that these points may be used to treat disorders of these five aspects of a person's psycho-emotional being, however, there is scanty evidence in classical texts that they have been used for this purpose.

- Points on the posterior portion of the thigh from Chengfu BL-36 to Kunlun BL-60 treat disorders of the lumbar region, anus and leg.

- Feiyang BL-58, located on the calf, is the first distal point of the Bladder channel to have an effect on disorders of the head, and this action becomes more pronounced as the channel travels distally towards Zhiyin BL-67, the terminal point of the channel. The extreme yang nature of the taiyang (supreme yang) Bladder channel, coupled with its penetration of the head and brain, renders these points effective in the treatment of aggressive yang pathogens, whether in the form of exterior wind or heat which injure the upper part of the body, or in the form of interior wind, interior fire and uprising of yang which assault the head and brain. These points, therefore, are indicated in a variety of excess conditions affecting the head, brain and sense organs.

- In keeping with the general characteristics of the channels, especially the yang channels, the more distal the points, the stronger their effect on the channel as a whole rather than simply their local area. This may be observed in the indications for points Kunlun BL-60 to Jinggu BL-64, which treat disorders of the Bladder channel in the head, upper and lower back, upper and lower leg and foot.

JINGMING BL-1

Bright Eyes

睛明

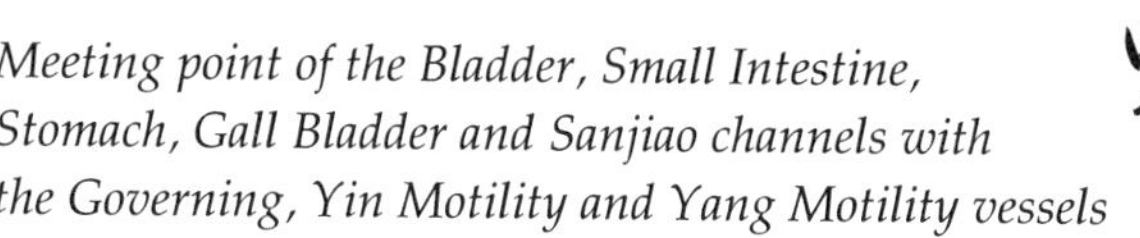

Meeting point of the Bladder, Small Intestine, Stomach, Gall Bladder and Sanjiao channels with the Governing, Yin Motility and Yang Motility vessels

LOCATION

0.1 cun medial and superior to the inner canthus of the eye, near the medial border of the orbit.

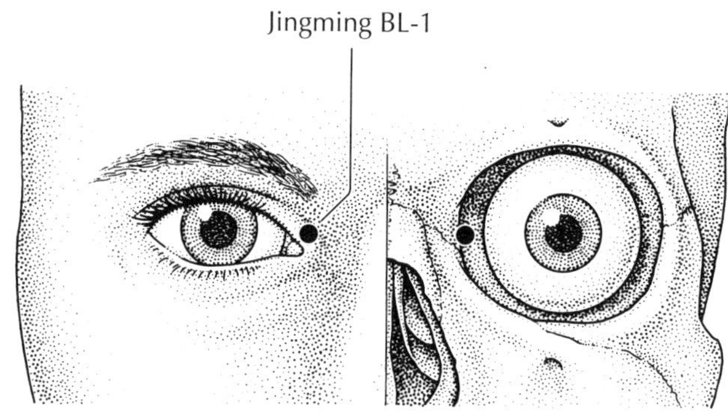

NEEDLING

i. Perpendicular insertion 0.2 to 0.3 cun; ii. **Caution:** the following needling method should not be attempted by those who have not had appropriate clinical supervision: ask the patient to close their eyes and to direct the eyes as far as possible towards the side being needled, i.e. when needling left Jingming BL-1, the patient should look to the left and vice-versa. With the forefinger of one hand, gently push the eyeball to the lateral side and hold it firmly. Insert the needle slowly perpendicularly with the other hand, without lifting, thrusting or rotating to a depth of 0.5 to 1 cun. Immediately on withdrawal of the needle, press firmly with a cotton wool ball for about a minute to prevent haematoma. **Note**: according to several classical and modern texts, this point is contraindicated to moxibustion.

ACTIONS

Benefits the eyes
Expels wind and clears heat

INDICATIONS

- Redness, swelling and pain of the eyes, lacrimation on exposure to wind, redness and itching of the inner canthus, blurred vision, dimness of vision, night blindness, photophobia, colour blindness, visual dizziness, near sightedness, superficial visual obstruction, aversion to cold with headache.

COMMENTARY

Jingming BL-1 (Bright Eyes) is the meeting point of all the yang channels (except the Large Intestine) and the Governing, Yang Motility and Yin Motility vessels. Although the pathology of eye diseases is complex and varied, they may be summarised as due to i. exterior pathogenic factors (mostly wind and heat), or ii. to deficiency or excess patterns of interior disharmony. Yang governs the exterior, and due both to its location and the fact that most of the yang channels meet at this point, Jingming BL-1 is the primary local point for the treatment of virtually any eye disease of exterior origin. It was traditionally indicated for redness, swelling, pain, lacrimation, itching and blurred vision. Equally, Jingming BL-1 is an essential local point for the treatment of eye diseases due to interior disharmony, whatever the pathology, and was traditionally indicated for night blindness, photophobia, blurred vision, visual dizziness etc., and in modern times for glaucoma, optic nerve atrophy, pterygium, astigmatism, optic neuritis, retinal haemorrhage and early cataract.

combinations

- Liver qi night blindness: Jingming BL-1 and Xingjian LIV-2 (*One Hundred Symptoms*).
- Redness, swelling and unbearable pain of both eyes with photophobia: needle Jingming BL-1 and Yuwei (M-HN-7) and bleed Taiyang (M-HN-9) (*Song of the Jade Dragon*).
- When Jingming BL-1 is ineffective in treating diseases of the eye, combine it with Hegu L.I.-4 and Guangming GB-37 (*Ode of Xi-hong*).
- Lacrimation on exposure to wind: Jingming BL-1, Touwei ST-8, Fengchi GB-20 and Toulinqi GB-15 (*Great Compendium*).
- Superficial visual obstruction: Jingming BL-1, Hegu L.I.-4 and Sibai ST-2 (*Great Compendium*).
- Internal eye obstruction: Jingming BL-1, Tongziliao GB-1, Hegu L.I.-4 and Zulinqi GB-41 (*Great Compendium*).

ZANZHU BL-2

Gathered Bamboo

攢竹

LOCATION

Superior to the inner canthus, in a depression on the eyebrow, close to its medial end.

LOCATION NOTE

Palpate laterally along the eyebrow from its medial end and feel for the hollow directly above Jingming BL-1. This point is often found to be tender on palpation.

NEEDLING

i. Transverse-oblique insertion inferiorly towards Jingming BL-1 for eye diseases; ii. Transverse lateral insertion to join with Yuyao (M-HN-6) for supraorbital pain; iii. Prick to bleed for heat disorders. **Note**: according to several classical texts, this point is contraindicated to moxibustion.

ACTIONS

Eliminates wind and clears heat
Benefits the eyes
Clears the head and alleviates pain

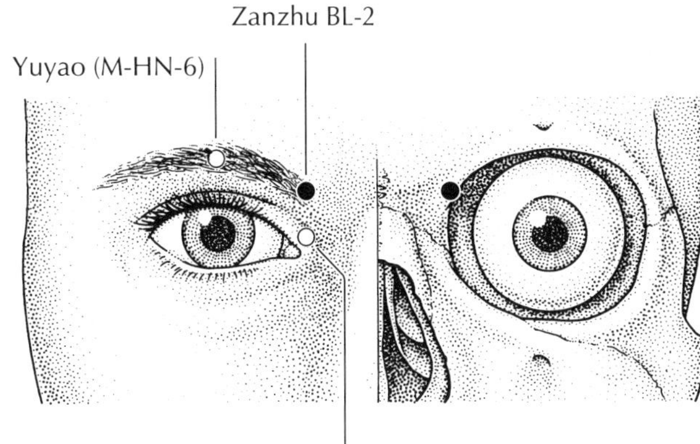

INDICATIONS

- Pain of the eyebrow region, frontal headache, head wind, wind dizziness, nosebleed, rhinitis, sneezing, pain of the face, red face with cheek pain.
- Blurred vision, dimness of vision, visual dizziness, lacrimation on exposure to wind, night blindness, redness, swelling and pain of the eye, itching of the eyes, infantile epilepsy with upward staring eyes, twitching of the eyelids, bursting sensation of the eye.
- Haemorrhoid pain, manic behaviour, loss of consciousness, pain and stiffness of the neck.

COMMENTARY

Zanzhu BL-2 is an important and frequently used local point for the treatment of disorders of the eye and the surrounding region. It may be substituted for Jingming BL-1 in a variety of eye disorders (primarily those due to attack by exterior pathogenic factors), especially by practitioners with insufficient clinical experience in needling points close to the eyeball. For this purpose it may be needled to join with Jingming BL-1, or in the case of heat patterns pricked to bleed. Its effect on redness and itching of the eyes, combined with its ability to treat rhinitis and sneezing, renders it particularly suitable in the treatment of hay fever.

The sphere of action of Zanzhu BL-2 is not confined to the treatment of eye disorders however, and it is frequently used as a local point for frontal headache, pain of the eyebrow region, sinus pain and facial paralysis, and more widely (see combinations below) for one-sided or generalised head wind, and headache following alcohol intoxication. The Bladder divergent channel winds around the anus, and Zanzhu BL-2 is indicated for pain of haemorrhoids, an illustration of the principle of using points above to treat disorders below.

COMBINATIONS

- Wind headache: Zanzhu BL-2, Chengguang BL-6, Shenshu BL-23, Qimai SJ-18, Sizhukong SJ-23 and Erheliao SJ-22 (*Thousand Ducat Formulas*).
- Headache with eye pain: Zanzhu BL-2 and Touwei ST-8 (*Ode of the Jade Dragon*).
- One-sided or generalised head wind: Zanzhu BL-2, Baihui DU-20, Qianding DU-21, Shenting DU-24, Shangxing DU-23, Sizhukong SJ-23, Fengchi GB-20, Hegu L.I.-4 and Touwei ST-8 (*Great Compendium*).
- Head wind following intoxication: Zanzhu BL-2, Yintang (M-HN-3) and Zusanli ST-36 (*Great Compendium*).
- Pain between the eyebrows: Zanzhu BL-2 and Touwei ST-8 (*Song of the Jade Dragon*).
- Twitching of the eyelids: Zanzhu BL-2 and Touwei ST-8 (*Great Compendium*).
- Rhinitis with clear nasal discharge: Zanzhu BL-2, Fengmen BL-12, Shenting DU-24, Hegu L.I.-4, Yingxiang L.I.-20, Zhiyin BL-67 and Futonggu KID-20 (*Thousand Ducat Formulas*).

MEICHONG BL-3

Eyebrows' Pouring

眉冲

LOCATION

Directly superior to Zanzhu BL-2, 0.5 cun within the anterior hairline, level with Shenting DU-24.

LOCATION NOTE

The distance between the anterior and posterior hairlines is measured as 12 cun. If the anterior hairline is indistinct, the distance is measured as 15 cun between the glabella [point Yintang (M-HN-3)] and the posterior hairline; the location of the anterior hairline would thus be defined as one fifth of this distance. If the posterior hairline is indistinct, it can be measured as 1 cun inferior to Fengfu DU-16 which lies immediately below the external occipital protuberance.

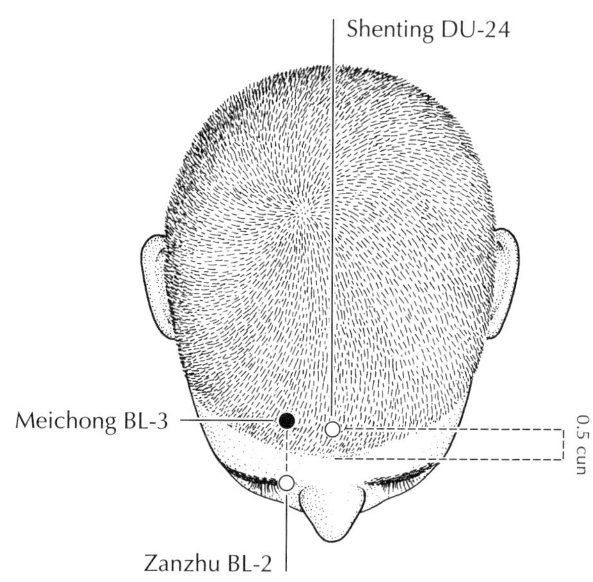

NEEDLING

Transverse insertion 0.5 to 1 cun. **Note**: according to the *Great Compendium of Acupuncture and Moxibustion* this point is contraindicated to moxibustion.

ACTIONS

Expels wind, clears the head and alleviates pain
Benefits the eyes and nose

INDICATIONS

- Headache, vertex headache, dizziness, dimness of vision, nasal congestion, nasal sores, dyspnoea, epilepsy, agitation and fullness of the Heart.

COMBINATIONS

- Headache with nasal congestion: Meichong BL-3, Shangxing DU-23, Yingxiang L.I.-20 and Hegu L.I.-4.

QUCHAI BL-4

Crooked Curve

LOCATION

0.5 cun within the anterior hairline, 1.5 cun lateral to Shenting DU-24 and one third of the distance between Shenting DU-24 and Touwei ST-8.

LOCATION NOTE

To locate the anterior hairline if indistinct, see location note for Meichong BL-3.

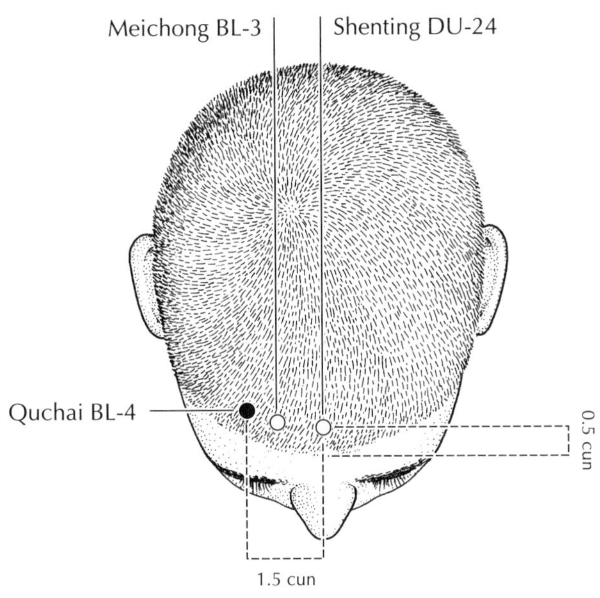

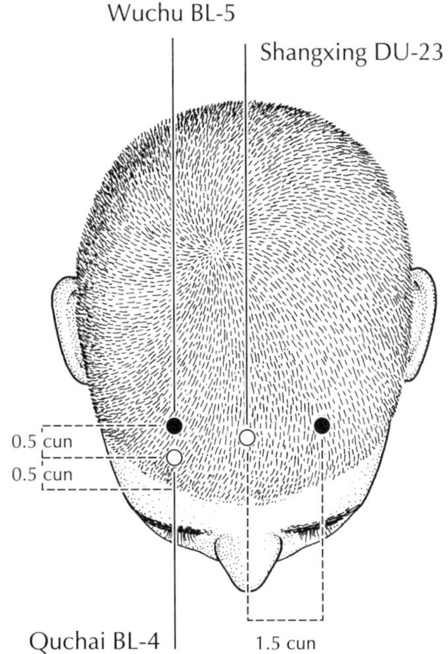

NEEDLING
Transverse insertion 0.5 to 1 cun.

ACTIONS
Expels wind, clears the head and alleviates pain
Benefits the eyes and nose

INDICATIONS
- Headache, vertex headache, swelling of the vertex, blurred vision, eye pain, dimness of vision, nasal congestion, nasal sores, nosebleed, rhinitis.
- Agitation and fullness of the Heart, dyspnoea, absence of sweating, agitation and heat in the body.

COMBINATIONS
- Dimness of vision: Quchai BL-4, Yanglao SI-6 and Hegu LI-4 (*Supplementing Life*).
- Agitation and fullness of the Heart with absence of sweating: Quchai BL-4 and Xinshu BL-15 (*Supplementing Life*).
- Foul-smelling nasal discharge: Quchai BL-4 and Shangxing DU-23 (*Great Compendium*).

WUCHU BL-5
Fifth Place

五處

LOCATION
0.5 cun directly posterior to Quchai BL-4, 1 cun within the anterior hairline, and 1.5 cun lateral to Shangxing DU-23.

LOCATION NOTE
i. To locate the anterior hairline if indistinct, see location note for Meichong BL-3; ii. Note that the distance from the anterior hairline at the midline to Baihui DU-20 is 5 cun.

NEEDLING
Transverse insertion 0.5 to 1 cun. **Note**: according to several classical and modern texts, this point is contraindicated to moxibustion.

ACTIONS
Eliminates wind, descends yang and clears heat
Clears the head and nose

INDICATIONS
- Rigidity of the spine, opisthotonos, upward staring eyes, epilepsy, madness, tetany, clonic spasm, dizziness, visual dizziness, dimness of vision.
- Headache, pain of the head and eye, heaviness of the head, nasal congestion.

COMBINATIONS
- Opisthotonos, clonic spasm, epilepsy and headache: Wuchu BL-5, Shenzhu DU-12, Weizhong BL-40, Weiyang BL-39 and Kunlun BL-60 (*Thousand Ducat Formulas*).
- Constant sneezing: Wuchu BL-5 and Fengmen BL-12 (*Thousand Ducat Formulas*).
- Nasal congestion with inability to distinguish the fragrant from the foul: Wuchu BL-5, Yingxiang L.I.-20, Shangxing DU-23 and Kouheliao L.I.-19 (*Great Compendium*).

CHENGGUANG BL-6 承光

Receiving Light

LOCATION

1.5 cun posterior to Wuchu BL-5, 2.5 cun within the anterior hairline and 1.5 cun lateral to the midline.

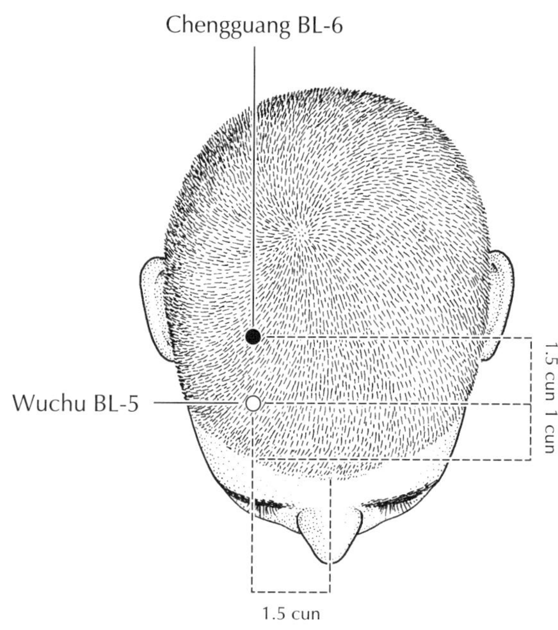

LOCATION NOTE

i. To locate the anterior hairline if indistinct, see location note for Meichong BL-3; ii. Note that the distance from the anterior hairline at the midline to Baihui DU-20 is 5 cun.

NEEDLING

Transverse insertion 0.5 to 1 cun. **Note**: according to several classical and modern texts, this point is contraindicated to moxibustion.

ACTIONS

Eliminates wind and clears heat
Clears the head and benefits the eyes and nose

INDICATIONS

- Vertex headache, wind dizziness, superficial visual obstruction, blurred vision, short sightedness, copious clear nasal discharge, nasal congestion, inability to distinguish the fragrant from the foul, deviation of the mouth.
- Vomiting, agitation of the Heart with vomiting, febrile disease with absence of sweating.

COMBINATIONS

- Wind headache: Chengguang BL-6, Zanzhu BL-2, Shenshu BL-23, Qimai SJ-18, Sizhukong SJ-23 and Erheliao SJ-22 (*Thousand Ducat Formulas*).
- Obstruction of the nose with inability to distinguish the fragrant from the foul: Chengguang BL-6, Shangxing DU-23, Baihui DU-20 and Xinhui DU-22 (*Supplementing Life*).
- Vomiting: Chengguang BL-6 and Dadu SP-2 (*Supplementing Life*).
- Agitation of the Heart: Chengguang BL-6, Baihui DU-20 and Qiangjian DU-18 (*Supplementing Life*).

TONGTIAN BL-7 通天

Heavenly Connection

LOCATION

1.5 cun posterior to Chengguang BL-6 and 4 cun within the anterior hairline, 1.5 cun lateral to the midline.

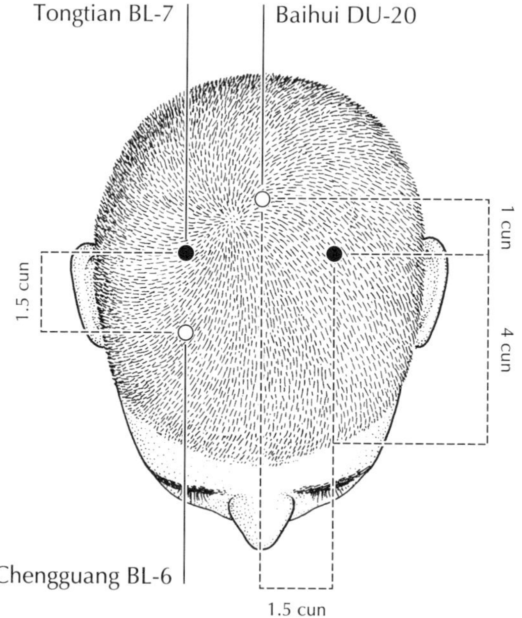

LOCATION NOTE

i. The distance between the glabella (Yintang M-HN-3) and the lower border of the occipital protuberance (Fengfu DU-16) is measured as 14 cun. Tongtian BL-7 is located 1.5 cun lateral to the midpoint of this line; ii. Tongtian BL-7 can also be located 1 cun anterior and 1.5 cun lateral to Baihui DU-20.

NEEDLING

Transverse insertion 0.5 to 1 cun. **Note**: according to several modern texts, this point is contraindicated to moxibustion.

ACTIONS

Benefits and regulates the nose
Clears the head

INDICATIONS

- Nasal congestion and discharge, profuse nasal discharge, rhinitis, loss of sense of smell, nosebleed, nasal sores.
- Vertex headache, heaviness of the head, deviation of the mouth, swollen face, goitre, stiff neck, dyspnoea, collapse on sudden standing, loss of consciousness.

COMMENTARY

The *Essential Questions*[1] says "Heavenly qi connects with the Lung" whilst the *Spiritual Pivot*[2] says "Lung qi connects with the nose". In other words, the heavenly qi of air enters the Lung through its gateway the nose, which plays a part in absorbing the qi. For this reason, in qigong breathing practice, inhaling through the nose is always emphasised, whilst exhaling may be through the nose or mouth. The name Tongtian (Heavenly Connection) refers to the ability of this point to keep the nose free and unobstructed and thus assist in circulating the heavenly qi through the nose and Lung.

Tongtian BL-7 is one of the foremost points on the head to treat all disorders of the nose (including rhinitus, loss of sense of smell, nosebleed and nasal sores), and in such cases is often found to be tender on palpation. According to the *Methods of Acupuncture and Moxibustion from the Golden Mirror of Medicine* by Wu Qian, this point should be combined with Shangxing DU-23 for nasal congestion and discharge and nasal polyps. This text also specifies that moxa should be applied to right Tongtian BL-7 for the left nostril and to left Tongtian BL-7 for the right nostril.

Tongtian BL-7 is also indicated for phlegm obstructing the upper portion of the body and manifesting as profuse nasal discharge, heaviness of the head, swollen face, goitre and dyspnoea.

Finally, Tongtian BL-7 is an important local point in the treatment of vertex headache due to any aetiology.

COMBINATIONS

- Nasal congestion: Tongtian BL-7 and Toulinqi GB-15 (*Supplementing Life*).
- Nasal obstruction and discharge: Tongtian BL-7 and Shangxing DU-23 (*Primary Points of the Fourteen Channels*).
- Deviation of the mouth with profuse clear nasal discharge: Tongtian BL-7 and Chengguang BL-6 (*Supplementing Life*).
- Heaviness of the head: Tongtian BL-7, Yamen DU-15, and Fuyang BL-59 (*Supplementing Life*).
- Pain and heaviness of the head: Tongtian BL-7, Naokong GB-19 and Naohu DU-17 (*Thousand Ducat Formulas*).
- Collapse on sudden standing: Tongtian BL-7 and Luoque BL-8 (*Thousand Ducat Formulas*).

LUOQUE BL-8

Declining Connection

络却

LOCATION

1.5 cun posterior to Tongtian BL-7, and 5.5 cun within the anterior hairline, 1.5 cun lateral to the midline.

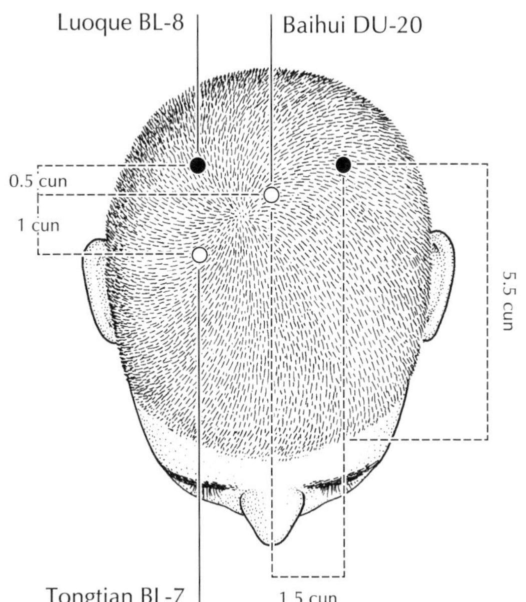

LOCATION NOTE

i. Luoque BL-8 is most easily is located 1.5 cun lateral to and 0.5 cun posterior to Baihui DU-20; ii. To locate the anterior hairline if indistinct, see location note for Meichong BL-3; iii. Note that the distance from the anterior hairline at the midline to Baihui DU-20 is 5 cun.

NEEDLING

Transverse insertion 0.5 to 1 cun.

ACTIONS

Benefits the sense organs
Pacifies wind, transforms phlegm and calms the spirit

INDICATIONS

- Dizziness, tinnitus, nasal congestion, deviation of the mouth, blurred vision.
- Mania-depression, mad walking, epilepsy, disorientation, goitre, vomiting, abdominal distention, collapse.

COMBINATIONS

- Madness with vomiting: Luoque BL-8, Zhubin KID-9, Yanggu SI-5, Houding DU-19, Qiangjian DU-18, Naohu DU-17 and Yuzhen BL-9 (*Thousand Ducat Formulas*).
- Collapse on sudden standing: Luoque BL-8 and Tongtian BL-7 (*Thousand Ducat Formulas*).
- Tinnitus: Luoque BL-8, Tinggong SI-19, Tinghui GB-2, Ermen SJ-21, Baihui DU-20, Yangxi L.I.-5, Qiangu SI-2, Houxi SI-3, Wangu SI-4, Zhongzhu SJ-3, Yemen SJ-2, Shangyang L.I.-1 and Shenshu BL-23 (*Great Compendium*).

YUZHEN BL-9

Jade Pillow

玉枕

LOCATION

1.3 cun lateral to Naohu DU-17 (which is located in the depression superior to the external occipital protuberance, 1.5 cun superior to Fengfu DU-16).

NEEDLING

Transverse insertion 0.5 to 1 cun.

ACTIONS

Expels wind and cold and alleviates pain
Benefits the nose and eyes

INDICATIONS

- Occipital headache, pain from head wind that is difficult to endure, dizziness, pain of the neck with inability to turn the head, pain of the head and neck with aversion to wind and absence of sweating, heaviness of the head and neck, cold sensation in half of the head, cold head with copious sweating, red face, pain of the cheek.
- Eye pain, bursting eye pain, short sightedness, nasal congestion, loss of sense of smell.
- Chills and fever, bone pain with chills and fever, vomiting, madness, mad walking, epilepsy, collapse on sudden standing.

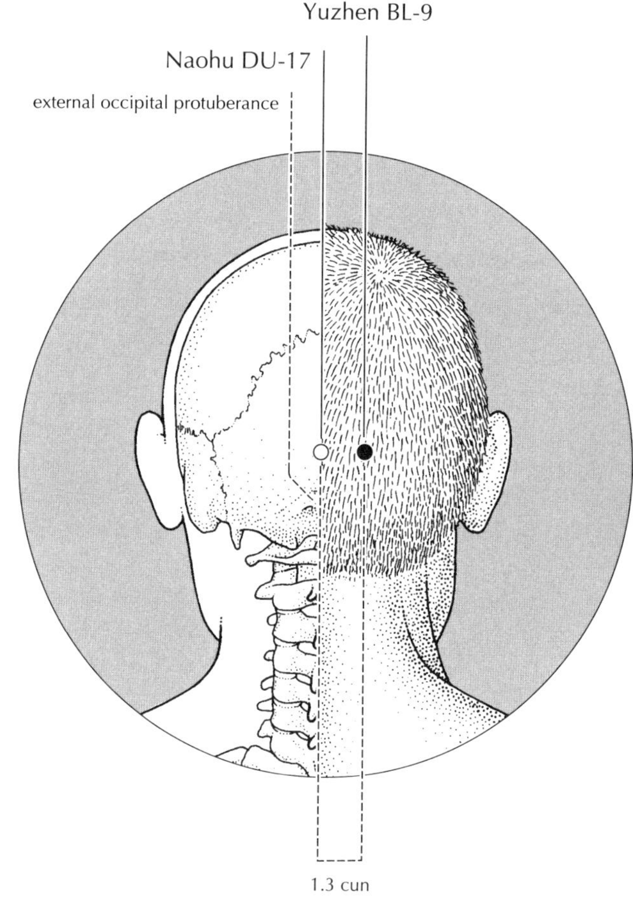

COMMENTARY

The name Yuzhen (Jade Pillow) refers both to the point Yuzhen BL-9 and to the general region around the occipital protuberance. In this latter context, Yuzhen is one of what is known as the three gates (sanguan) through which it may be difficult to circulate the qi in the qigong 'small heavenly circuit' practice; that is the practice of circulating the qi through the Governing and Conception vessels in one continuous circuit using the mind and the breath. The three gates are Yuzhenguan, Jiajiguan (in the region of Mingmen DU-4) and Weiluguan (in the region of Changqiang DU-1).

Yuzhen BL-9 itself is indicated for the treatment of i. occipital headache and severe head wind, stiffness and pain of the neck and coldness and sensitivity to wind in the head and neck region, ii. disorders of the nose and eyes (eye pain, short sightedness, nasal congestion and loss of sense of smell), and iii. madness, mad walking, epilepsy and sudden collapse on standing.

COMBINATIONS

- Pain of the nape of the neck: Yuzhen BL-9 and Wangu GB-12 (*Supplementing Life*).

- Wind dizziness: Yuzhen BL-9, Houding DU-19 and Hanyan GB-4 (*Supplementing Life*).
- Head wind: Yuzhen BL-9 and Xinhui DU-22 (*One Hundred Symptoms*).
- Nasal congestion: Yuzhen BL-9, Baihui DU-20, Toulinqi GB-15, Shangxing DU-23 and Danyang (Extra)[3] (*Supplementing Life*).

TIANZHU BL-10

Celestial Pillar

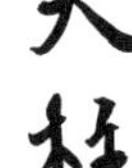

Point of the Window of Heaven

LOCATION

On the lateral aspect of the trapezius muscle, 1.3 cun lateral to Yamen DU-15.

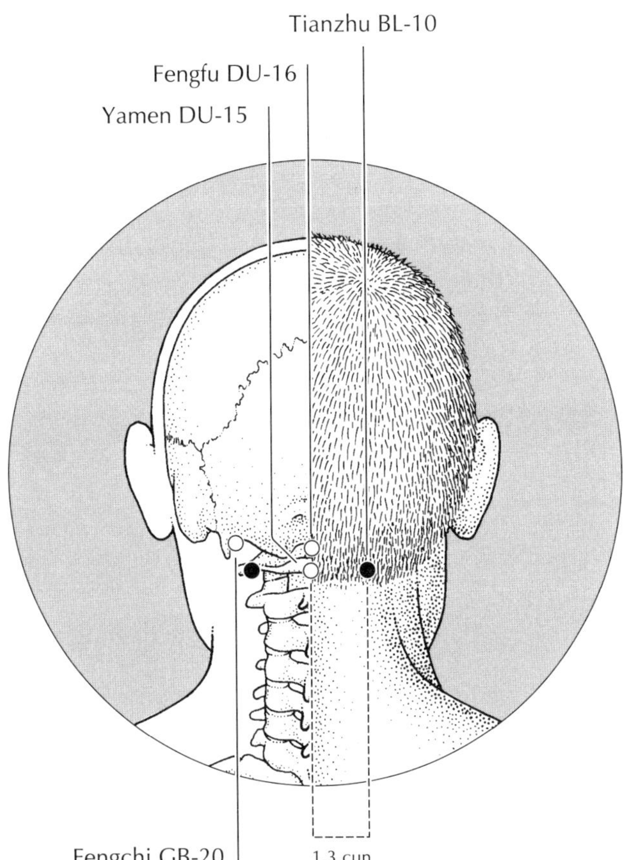

LOCATION NOTE

First locate Fengfu DU-16 directly below the occipital protuberance in a depression between the trapezius on both sides. Then locate Yamen DU-15 which is 0.5 cun below Fengfu DU-16 in the depression 0.5 cun within the hairline. Now locate Tianzhu BL-10, 1.3 cun lateral to Yamen DU-15.

NEEDLING

Perpendicular insertion 0.5 to 0.8 cun.

ACTIONS

Regulates qi and pacifies wind
Benefits the head and sensory orifices
Calms the spirit
Activates the channel and alleviates pain

INDICATIONS

- Dizziness, inability of the legs to support the body, sudden muscular contractions, pain of the body.
- Pain and heaviness of the head, headache, head wind, stiffness of the neck with inability to turn the head, pain of the shoulder and back, bursting eye pain, redness of the eyes, blurred vision, lacrimation, swelling of the throat with difficulty in speaking, nasal congestion, loss of sense of smell, febrile disease with absence of sweating.
- Mania, incessant talking, seeing ghosts, epilepsy, childhood epilepsy, upward staring eyes.

COMMENTARY

Tianzhu BL-10 is one of five points referred to in Chapter 21 of the *Spiritual Pivot* as points of the 'Window of Heaven' (see page 48 for a fuller discussion), and in this passage it is said "Sudden contraction, epilepsy and dizziness, with inability of the legs to support the body, select Tianzhu BL-10". Chapter 24 of the *Spiritual Pivot* says "inversion headache with neck pain followed by lumbar pain select Tianzhu BL-10"

In common with the other Window of Heaven points, Tianzhu BL-10 is indicated when inversion qi (chaotic and rebellious qi) rises to the head. This may give rise to dizziness, headache, heaviness of the head, stiff neck and epilepsy, as well as congestion, pain and swelling of the throat, eyes and nose, whilst at the same time in the lower part the legs are unable to support the body due to unbalanced distribution of qi.

The use of Tianzhu BL-10 for disorders such as inability of the legs to support the body, pain of the body, and headache accompanied by lumbar pain is a reflection of the principle of selecting points above to treat disorders below.

Like Tianfu LU-3 and Tianchuang SI-16 (also points of the Window of Heaven), Tianzhu BL-10 is further indicated for mental disorders characterised by mania and incessant talking, as well as for disorders characterised in the classical texts as seeing or 'communicating with ghosts' and therefore attributed to some form of demonic possession. In terms of modern medicine these indications refer to various forms of severe mental disorder including schizophrenia.

Finally there is some similarity between the indications of Tianzhu BL-10 and Fengchi GB-20, both points being located close to each other. Fengchi GB-20 however is much used clinically both to expel exterior pathogenic wind and to pacify interior wind, whilst the clinical use of Tianzhu BL-10 is primarily confined to pacifying interior wind.

COMBINATIONS

- Headache: Tianzhu BL-10, Taodao DU-13, Dazhu BL-11, Kongzui LU-6 and Houxi SI-3 (*Thousand Ducat Formulas*).
- Head wind: Tianzhu BL-10, Naokong GB-19 and Baihui DU-20 (*Supplementing Life*).
- Dizziness: Tianzhu BL-10, Shangxing DU-23 and Fengchi GB-20 (*Glorious Anthology*).
- Visual dizziness, dimness of vision with bursting eye pain: Tianzhu BL-10, Taodao DU-13 and Kunlun BL-60 (*Supplementing Life*).
- Blurring of vision: Tianzhu BL-10 and Yanglao SI-6 (*One Hundred Symptoms*).
- Stiff neck with great aversion to wind: Tianzhu BL-10 and Shugu BL-65 (*One Hundred Symptoms*).
- Inability of the legs to support the body: Tianzhu BL-10 and Xingjian LIV-2 (*Thousand Ducat Formulas*).
- Childhood fright epilepsy: Tianzhu BL-10, Benshen GB-13, Qianding DU-21 and Xinhui DU-22 (*Thousand Ducat Formulas*).
- Pain of the shoulder as if it were broken: Tianzhu BL-10 and Yanglao SI-6 (*Thousand Ducat Formulas*).

DAZHU BL-11

Great Shuttle

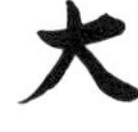

Meeting point of the Bladder, Small Intestine, Sanjiao and Gall Bladder channels and the Governing vessel
Hui-Meeting point of Bones
Point of the Sea of Blood

LOCATION

1.5 cun lateral to the lower border of the spinous process of the first thoracic vertebra (T1).

LOCATION NOTE

Locate at the visible highest point of the paraspinal muscles.

NEEDLING

Oblique insertion towards the spine, 0.5 to 1 cun, or transverse-oblique insertion 1 to 1.5 cun.
Caution: perpendicular needling carries a substantial risk of causing a pneumothorax.

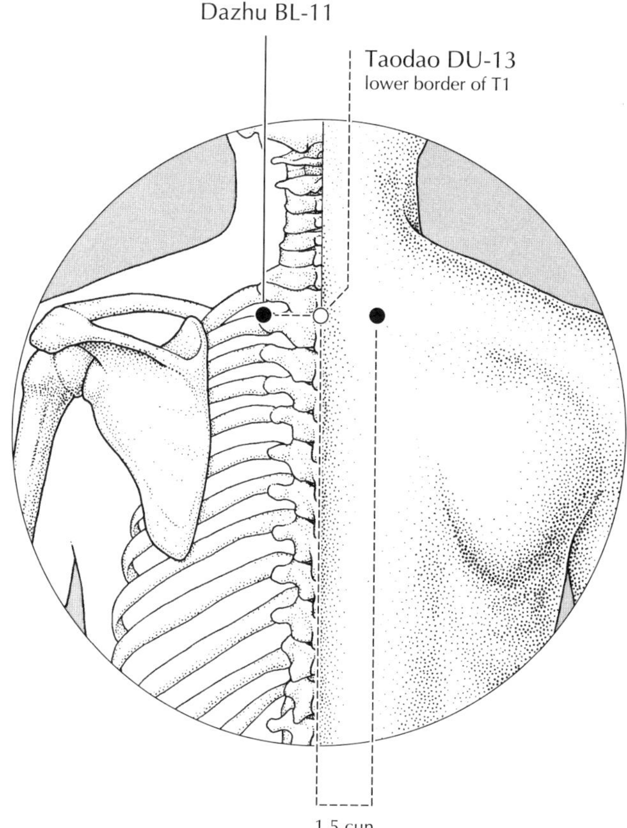

ACTIONS

Benefits the bones and joints
Expels pathogenic factors and firms the exterior
Regulates Lung qi and alleviates cough

INDICATIONS

- Bone diseases, rigidity of the nape of the neck, rigidity of the spine, soreness and pain of the back and scapula, lumbar pain, tetany, clonic spasm, contraction of sinews associated with madness, stiffness and pain of the knee.
- Fever, cold shivering, injury by cold with absence of sweating, injury by wind which does not disperse, failure of the interstices to close, susceptibility to catching wind-cold, malaria, headache, head wind, bursting headache, inversion qi with heavy head, dizziness, blurred vision, collapse, inability to stand for long.
- Cough, fullness of the chest, dyspnoea, cough due to taxation, depression in the chest, heat in the chest, throat painful obstruction, abdominal pain, abdominal urgency with agitation and fullness.

COMMENTARY

Dazhu BL-11 is the hui-meeting point of bones and is indicated for various bone diseases and rigidity and pain of the neck, spine and lumbar region. In modern clinical practice it is used when painful obstruction due to pathogenic wind, cold, damp and heat penetrates deeply into the bones and joints causing deformity (known as bony painful obstruction). Dazhu BL-11 is also indicated for contraction of the sinews, and the *Spiritual Pivot* [4] especially recommends Dazhu BL-11 for treating contraction of the sinews that may accompany madness.

The Ming dynasty classic *Investigation into Points Along the Channels* says that Dazhu BL-11 is indicated "for injury by wind which does not disperse, with bursting headache, soreness and pain of the back and scapula, interstices that are not closed, susceptibility to catching wind-cold". Taiyang channel is the most exterior of the six channels, and therefore most commonly the first to be injured by exterior pathogenic wind-cold. It is for this reason that exterior wind-cold pattern often gives rise to headache and pain of the neck which may extend down the upper back (taiyang channel). At the same time, exterior pathogenic wind-cold which first attacks the surface portion of the body easily penetrates to the Lung, since the Lung controls the skin and body hair. Dazhu BL-11 is a point of taiyang channel and a meeting point of the taiyang Bladder channel with the taiyang Small Intestine channel. Furthermore it is located on the upper back, close to both the neck and the Lung. It therefore has a strong action both on the exterior portion of the body (demonstrated by its ability to expel wind-cold manifesting as stiffness and pain of the neck and scapula, fever, cold shivering and absence of sweating), as well as on the Lung (demonstrated by its ability to relieve coughing, dyspnoea and fullness of the chest). In this respect it is very similar to Fengmen BL-12, especially in its ability both to expel excess pathogenic wind-cold and to firm the exterior in cases of deficiency (e.g. interstices and pores that do not close, susceptibility to catching wind-cold).

According to the *Spiritual Pivot* [5] Dazhu BL-11 is a point of the 'sea of blood'. This passage says "The Penetrating vessel is the sea of the twelve channels (i.e. the sea of blood). In the upper it is conveyed to Dazhu BL-11, and in the lower it emerges at both Shangjuxu ST-37 and Xiajuxu ST-39 ... When the sea of blood is in excess, there is a sensation as if the body were big; one feels disquiet, but does not know what disease there is; when the sea of blood is insufficient, one has the sensation of one's body being small; one feels reduced but does not know what could be the illness". Despite this passage it is worth noting that such indications are not found in later texts. Some commentators however interpret various indications of Dazhu BL-11 as relating to disorder of the Penetrating vessel, especially the signs of qi rebellion in the chest (cough, fullness of the chest, dyspnoea) and head (dizziness). Finally, the *Essential Questions* [6] includes Dazhu BL-11 among the eight points (bilateral Quepen ST-12, Dazhu BL-11, Zhongfu LU-1 and Fengmen BL-12) to clear heat from the chest.

COMBINATIONS

- Coldness and pain of the bone marrow: Dazhu BL-11, Xuanzhong GB-39, Fuliu KID-7, Shenmai BL-62, Lidui ST-45 and Shenshu BL-23 (*Compilation*).
- All wind, painful obstruction, atrophy disorder and inversion diseases: Dazhu BL-11 and Ququan LIV-8 (*Song to Keep Up Your Sleeve*).
- Headache and visual dizziness: Dazhu BL-11, Sibai ST-2 and Yongquan KID-1 (*Supplementing Life*).
- Depression in the chest: Dazhu BL-11 and Xinshu BL-15 (*Thousand Ducat Formulas*).

FENGMEN BL-12

Wind Gate

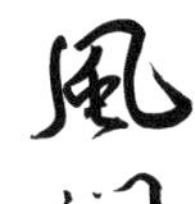

Meeting point of the Bladder channel with the Governing vessel

LOCATION

1.5 cun lateral to the lower border of the spinous process of the second thoracic vertebra (T2).

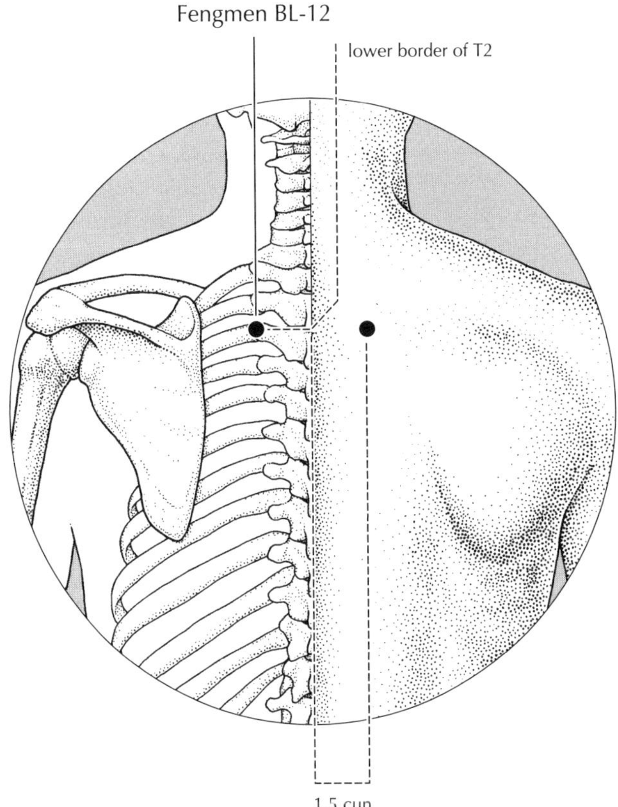

LOCATION NOTE

Locate at the visible highest point of the paraspinal muscles.

NEEDLING

Oblique insertion towards the spine, 0.5 to 1 cun, or transverse-oblique insertion 1 to 1.5 cun.

Caution: perpendicular needling or oblique needling away from the spine carries a substantial risk of causing a pneumothorax.

ACTIONS

Expels wind and releases the exterior
Strengthens the defensive qi and firms the exterior
Disseminates and descends Lung qi
Benefits the nose

INDICATIONS

- Attack by wind with fever, cold shivering, dislike of wind and cold, headache, injury by cold with rigidity of the head and neck, flaccidity of the interstices with frequent coughing and clear watery nasal discharge, flaccidity of the interstices with susceptibility to catching wind-cold, desire to keep the eyes closed, wind dizziness, visual dizziness.
- Cough, cough with chest and back pain, coughing blood, dyspnoea, heat in the chest, wind-taxation coughing, wind-exhaustion vomiting, vomiting.
- Copious nasal discharge, nasal congestion, rhinitis, sneezing, nosebleed.
- Lumbar pain, stiff neck, urticaria, carbuncles of the back, shoulder pain, restless sleep.

COMMENTARY

As its name 'Wind Gate' implies, Fengmen BL-12 is an important point to expel wind and release pathogenic factors from the exterior portion of the body. This action may be explained by three principal factors: i. Fengmen BL-12 belongs to taiyang channel, the most exterior of the six channels, and therefore most commonly the first to be attacked by exterior pathogenic factors; ii. Fengmen BL-12 is located on the upper back, over the upper portion of the Lung which is known as the 'delicate zang' due to its predisposition to be easily injured by exterior pathogens; iii. Fengmen BL-12 is a meeting point of the Bladder channel with the Governing vessel which dominates all the yang channels of the body and hence has a close relationship to the exterior (yang) portion of the body.

When exterior pathogenic wind attacks via the skin, nose or mouth, it may i. obstruct the defensive qi and impair its warming function, giving rise to chills, aversion to wind and cold and headache, whilst fever which accompanies chills is a sign of the struggle between the defensive qi and the pathogen; ii. impair the disseminating and descending function of the Lung, resulting in copious nasal discharge and cough; iii. obstruct taiyang channel giving rise to rigidity and pain of the head and neck. Fengmen BL-12 may be treated by needling or cupping to release the exterior in all cases of attack by wind-cold, wind-heat or wind-dryness which bind the superficial portion of the body and give rise to such excess exterior pathology. In the case of wind-cold, moxibustion may be used. Fengmen BL-12 is also indicated for patterns of exterior deficiency where attack by wind gives rise to disharmony of nutritive qi and defensive qi, characterised by fever and chills unrelieved by sweating, aversion to wind and a weak floating pulse.

The ability of Fengmen BL-12 to firm the exterior and strengthen the defensive qi, thus helping the body to resist attack by exterior pathogenic factors, is discussed in various classics. The *Song of the Jade Dragon* recommends it for "flaccidity of the interstices with frequent coughing and clear watery nasal discharge", whilst *Methods of Acupuncture and Moxibustion from the Golden Mirror of Medicine* recommends it for "flaccidity of the interstices with susceptibility to catching wind-cold". In other words, as well as releasing the exterior and expelling wind, Fengmen BL-12 may be treated by needling or moxibustion to tonify the defensive qi in patients with susceptibility to catching frequent colds.

The nose is the gateway of the Lung. According to the *Spiritual Pivot*[7] "The qi of the Lung opens into the nose; when the Lung is in harmony the nose is able to distinguish the fragrant from the foul". *Methods of Acupuncture and Moxibustion from the Golden Mirror of Medicine* recommends Fengmen BL-12 for "nosebleed and all kinds of nose disorders". Nasal blockage and discharge commonly result from Lung and defensive qi deficiency with concomitant retention of pathogens in the nose and Lung, which render a person liable to frequent nasal stuffiness and discharge, sensitivity to dust and pollen, sneezing etc. The ability of Fengmen BL-12 to firm the defensive qi, expel exterior pathogens and benefit the nose make it especially suitable in the treatment of such cases of perennial and seasonal allergic rhinitis.

It is useful to compare the points Fengmen BL-12 and Feishu BL-13, each reflecting different aspects of the Lung function. Although Fengmen BL-12 is indicated for painful cough and cough with bleeding, this is primarily in the context of exterior disease and its affinity for releasing the exterior and firming the defensive qi underlines its close connection with the more superficial and yang aspect of the Lung. It is significant however, that despite its ability to strengthen the defensive qi which is distributed by the Lung, it is not used to tonify other aspects of Lung deficiency for which the deeper (yin) action of Feishu BL-13 is preferred.

According to the *Illustrated Classic of Acupuncture Points on the Bronze Man* "If Fengmen BL-12 is repeatedly needled it will clear the hot yang qi and the back will always be free of sores and carbuncles". Finally the *Essential Questions*[8] includes Fengmen BL-12 among the eight points (bilateral Quepen ST-12, Dazhu BL-11, Zhongfu LU-1 and Fengmen BL-12) to clear heat from the chest.

COMBINATIONS

- Rhinitis with clear nasal discharge: Fengmen BL-12, Shenting DU-24, Zanzhu BL-2, Yingxiang L.I.-20, Hegu L.I.-4, Zhiyin BL-67 and Futonggu KID-20 (*Thousand Ducat Formulas*).
- Constant sneezing: Fengmen BL-12 and Wuchu BL-5 (*Thousand Ducat Formulas*).
- Nosebleed with stifled breathing: Fengmen BL-12, Chengling GB-18, Fengchi GB-20, Yixi BL-45 and Houxi SI-3 (*Thousand Ducat Formulas*).
- Pain of the shoulder and back: Fengmen BL-12, Jianjing GB-21, Zhongzhu SJ-3, Zhigou SJ-6, Houxi SI-3, Wangu SI-4 and Weizhong BL-40 (*Great Compendium*).
- Injury by cold with fever which clears and then reoccurs: Fengmen BL-12, Hegu L.I.-4, Xingjian LIV-2 and Xuanzhong GB-39 (*Outline of Medicine*).

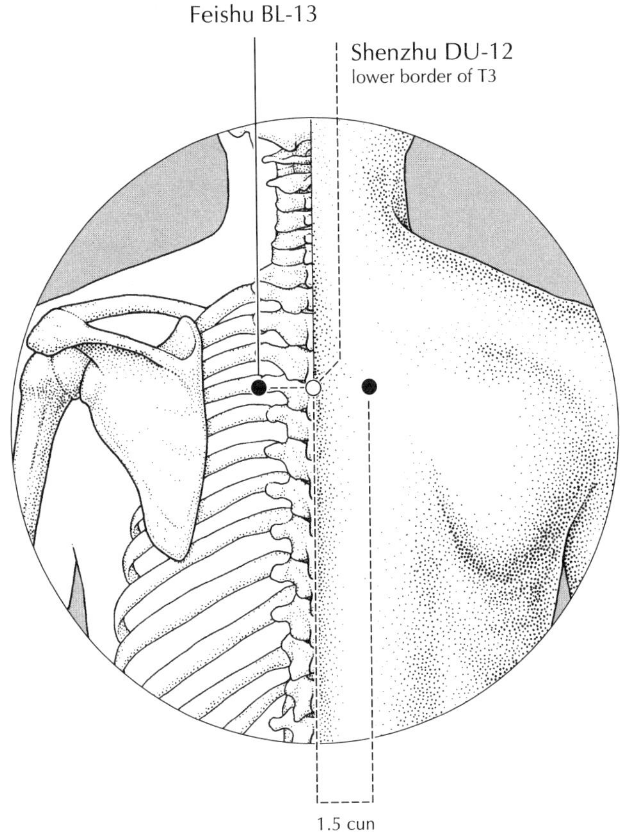

FEISHU BL-13

Lung Shu

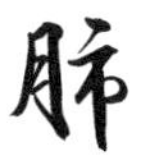

Back-Shu point of the Lung

LOCATION

1.5 cun lateral to the lower border of the spinous process of the third thoracic vertebra (T3).

LOCATION NOTE

Locate at the visible highest point of the paraspinal muscles.

NEEDLING

Oblique insertion towards the spine, 0.5 to 1 cun, or transverse-oblique insertion 1 to 1.5 cun.

Caution: perpendicular needling or oblique needling away from the spine carries a substantial risk of causing a pneumothorax.

ACTIONS

Tonifies Lung qi and nourishes Lung yin
Descends and disseminates Lung qi
Clears heat from the Lung
Releases the exterior

INDICATIONS

- Cough, dyspnoea, asthma, fullness of the chest, shortness of breath with no desire to speak, persistent cough in children, cold Lung, heat sensation in the chest, chest pain, difficult breathing on lying down, coughing of phlegm, Lung abscess, attack of the Lung by wind, rapid pulse, fever, night sweating with chills and fever and aversion to cold, cold shivering, absence of sweating, throat painful obstruction.
- Lung atrophy, consumption, consumption with steaming bone disorder, deficiency-taxation fever, tidal fever, night sweating, spitting blood, wasting and thirsting disorder, dryness of the mouth and tongue, deficiency agitation.
- Mania, heat in the body, mad walking with desire to commit suicide, epilepsy.
- Fullness with no pleasure in eating, vomiting, vomiting fluid after eating, vomiting of foam, goitre, jaundice, pain of the flesh and itching of the skin, urticaria.
- Pain of the upper back and shoulder, crooked spine, turtle back in children, lumbar pain and stiffness.

COMMENTARY

Feishu BL-13 is the back-shu point of the Lung, where the qi of the Lung emanates from the interior to the body surface, and in common with all the back-shu points, especially those of the yin zang, has a strong action on regulating and tonifying its corresponding zangfu at the deepest level. Feishu BL-13 is the pre-eminent acupuncture point to treat all disorders of the Lung zang.

Feishu BL-13 is an essential point to tonify the Lung qi and nourish Lung yin. Lung qi deficiency may derive from constitutional deficiency, previous Lung disease, chronic illness, extreme sadness and grief, excessive desk work (especially with a hunched back), excessive physical labour or lack of exercise. It is characterised by symptoms such as weak cough, dyspnoea and asthma that are worsened by exertion, and shortness of breath with no desire to speak. According to a saying of Chinese medicine "The Lung is the gateway of the voice". When there is insufficiency of Lung qi therefore, there is lack of vigour in the voice, speaking readily tires a person and there is unwillingness to speak. According to the *Essential Questions*[9] "All qi is subordinate to the Lung". Since the Lung dominates the qi of the whole body, there may also be signs of general qi deficiency such as lassitude, facial pallor and a weak pulse. In such cases Feishu BL-13 is often combined with points such as Taiyuan LU-9, Shanzhong REN-17, Zusanli ST-36 and Pishu BL-20. In cases of chronic Lung qi deficiency giving rise to asthma or cough that is worse in winter, intensive moxibustion is often applied to Feishu BL-13 in the summer months.

Lung yin deficiency may derive from prolonged Lung qi deficiency, overwork, febrile disease which consumes yin, or Kidney yin deficiency which fails to nourish and support Lung yin. It is characterised by cough or asthma with dry, stringy or blood-tinged sputum, night sweating and dryness of the mouth, throat and tongue. In more severe cases there may be tidal fever, steaming bone disorder, deficiency agitation and spitting of blood. In such cases Feishu BL-13 is often combined with points such as Gaohuangshu BL-43, Taiyuan LU-9, Guanyuan REN-4 and Shenshu BL-23.

Feishu BL-13 is also classically indicated for Lung atrophy and consumption, both terms denoting conditions of severe exhaustion and depletion. In Lung atrophy, the Lungs are said to wither and shrivel, in the same way that the limbs are seen to wither and shrivel in atrophy disorder, whilst consumption broadly corresponds to pulmonary tuberculosis.

The action of Feishu BL-13 is not restricted to tonifying and nourishing the Lung however, and it is equally important in all excess Lung patterns. Through its actions of regulating Lung qi and clearing heat, it may be used for such patterns as i. excess heat afflicting the Lung, ii. retention of phlegm-damp or phlegm-heat, and iii. toxic heat obstructing the Lung. It is consequently indicated for fullness of the chest, chest pain, Lung abscess, coughing of phlegm and difficult breathing on lying down. In such cases, in addition to other appropriate points, Feishu BL-13 is often combined with Zhongfu LU-1, an example of the principle of combining the back-shu and front-mu points.

Feishu BL-13 is also an important point for the treatment of pathogenic factors lodging at the defensive (or taiyang) level. Combined with points such as Fengmen BL-12, Lieque LU-7 and Hegu L.I.-4 it may be used to release and expel pathogenic factors binding the exterior and giving rise to chills and fever with cough, and to harmonise nutritive qi and defensive qi in cases of night sweating with chills and fever and aversion to cold.

According to *Warp and Woof of Warm Febrile Diseases* "The Lung and Heart are mutually connected, thus when there is Lung heat it most easily enters the Heart". Because of its ability to clear heat of excess or deficiency type from the Lung, and due to its profound effect on the gathering qi and the upper jiao in general, the action of Feishu BL-13 extends to the Heart and various classics mention its use for disorders of the spirit such as mania, mad walking and even desire to commit suicide.

The Lung and Stomach have a particularly close relationship. Both have a strongly descending action, whilst the Lung channel originates in the middle jiao in the region of the Stomach. Failure of the Stomach qi to descend due to deficiency or food stagnation may therefore impair the Lung's descending function leading to coughing and dyspnoea, whilst failure of the Lung qi to descend may injure the Stomach's descending function and lead to rebellion of Stomach qi. Feishu BL-13 is therefore indicated for fullness with no pleasure in eating, vomiting, vomiting of foam and vomiting of fluid after eating, and especially for vomiting accompanied by coughing.

A further important use of Feishu BL-13 is for Lung disorders which give rise to pain of the upper back. In cases of children with severe Lung qi deficiency, there may even be rounding and deformity of the back (turtle back). This condition is referred to in the *Essential Questions*[10] which says "The back is the residence of the chest and when the back is curved and the shoulders are hunched, the residence is about to fall into ruin".

Finally, according to the *Illustrated Appendices to The Classic of Categories*, Feishu BL-13 is one of five points (Feishu BL-13, Xinshu BL-15, Ganshu BL-18, Pishu BL-20 and Shenshu BL-23) which "drain heat from the five zang".

COMBINATIONS

- Cough with phlegm: Feishu BL-13 and Fenglong ST-40 (*Ode of the Jade Dragon*).
- Cough that reaches the voice (hoarse voice): Feishu BL-13 and Tiantu REN-22 (*One Hundred Symptoms*).
- Lung distention: Feishu BL-13 and Taiyuan LU-9 (*Systematic Classic*).
- Chest pain: Feishu BL-13, Yunmen LU-2, Zhongfu LU-1, Yinbai SP-1, Qimen LIV-14, Hunmen BL-47 and Daling P-7 (*Thousand Ducat Formulas*).
- Spitting blood: Feishu BL-13, Kongzui LU-6 and Quze P-3 (*Supplementing Life*).
- Seasonal fever: Feishu BL-13 and Taodao DU-13 (*Glorious Anthology*).
- Mad walking with desire to commit suicide: Feishu BL-13 and Fengfu DU-16 (*Thousand Ducat Formulas*).
- Stiffness of the lumbar region and back with inability to bend to the side: Feishu BL-13 and Yaoshu DU-2 (*Great Compendium*).

JUEYINSHU BL-14

Jueyin Shu

厥陰俞

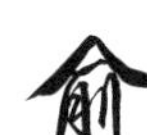

Back-Shu point of the Pericardium

LOCATION

1.5 cun lateral to the lower border of the spinous process of the fourth thoracic vertebra (T4).

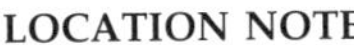

LOCATION NOTE

Locate at the visible highest point of the paraspinal muscles.

NEEDLING

Oblique insertion towards the spine, 0.5 to 1 cun, or transverse-oblique insertion 1 to 1.5 cun.

Caution: perpendicular needling or oblique needling away from the spine carries a substantial risk of causing a pneumothorax.

ACTIONS

Spreads Liver qi and unbinds the chest
Regulates the Heart
Regulates and descends qi

INDICATIONS

- Heart pain, oppression of the chest, pain of the chest and diaphragm due to accumulation of qi, palpitations, agitation and restlessness, agitation and oppression, restless zang disorder.
- Cough, shortness of breath, rebellious qi vomiting, toothache.

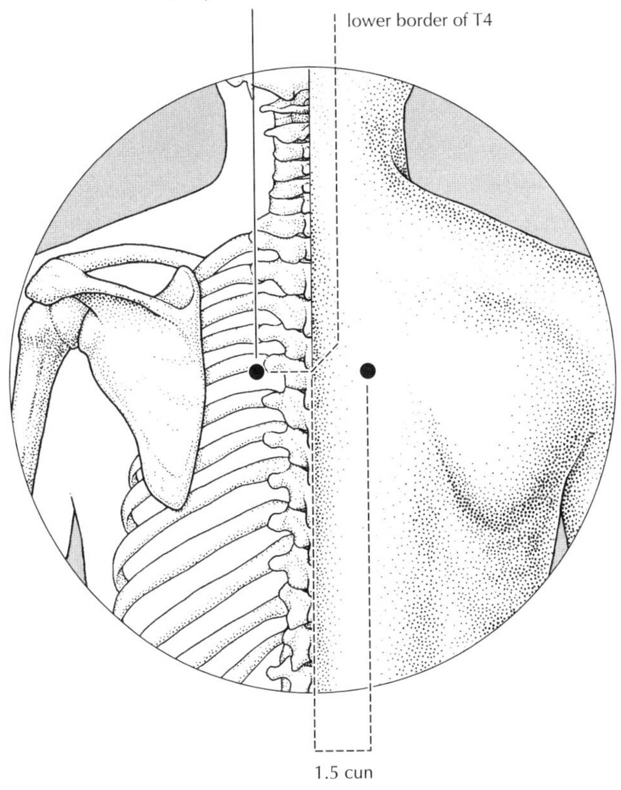

COMMENTARY

Jueyinshu BL-14 is an exception among the back-shu points in that all the others are named after their respective zang or fu. The fact that Jueyinshu BL-14 is named after the jueyin (Pericardium and Liver) channel emphasises its ability to unbind the chest by invigorating the circulation of qi. When Liver qi stagnates, usually as a result of emotional factors, it frequently binds the qi of the upper jiao giving rise to symptoms such as pain and oppression of the Heart, chest and diaphragm, restlessness, agitation and oppression.

As the back-shu point of the Pericardium, Jueyinshu BL-14 is not exclusively reserved for chest and Heart disorders due to qi stagnation, but in combination with Xinshu BL-15 is widely used to regulate the Heart in many kinds of dysfunction.

The descending function of both the Stomach and Lung is assisted by the smooth and unobstructed movement of Liver qi. When Liver qi stagnates and impairs their descent, there may be cough and vomiting respectively.

COMBINATIONS

- Heart pain: Jueyinshu BL-14, Shenmen HE-7 and Zulinqi GB-41 (*Supplementing Life*).

XINSHU BL-15

Heart Shu

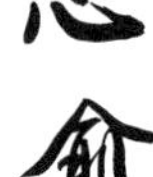

Back-Shu point of the Heart

LOCATION

1.5 cun lateral to the lower border of the spinous process of the fifth thoracic vertebra (T5).

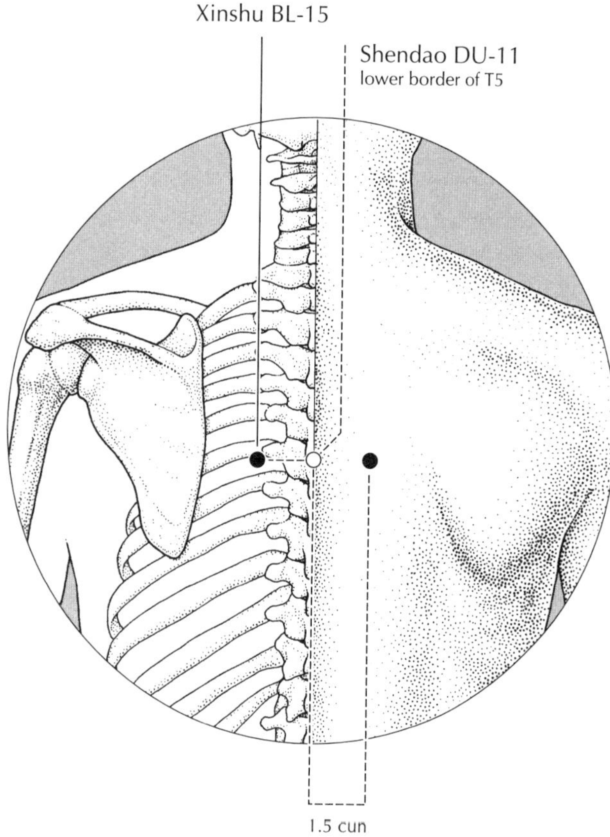

LOCATION NOTE

Locate at the visible highest point of the paraspinal muscles.

NEEDLING

Oblique insertion towards the spine, 0.5 to 1 cun, or transverse-oblique insertion 1 to 1.5 cun.

Caution: perpendicular needling or oblique needling away from the spine carries a substantial risk of causing a pneumothorax.

ACTIONS

Tonifies and nourishes the Heart
Regulates Heart qi
Calms the spirit
Unbinds the chest and resolves blood stasis
Clears Heart fire

INDICATIONS

- Heart pain, oppression of the chest with restlessness, chest pain extending to the back, worried and oppressive sensation of the chest with inability to catch the breath, palpitations, fright palpitations, irregular pulse, Heart qi deficiency in children.
- Poor memory, anxiety, weeping with grief, frightened and cautious with Heart deficiency, insomnia, excessive dreaming, disorientation, delayed speech development, mania-depression, epilepsy, dementia, mad walking, seminal emission.
- Cough, coughing blood, vomiting, vomiting blood, abdominal distention, difficult ingestion, night sweating, redness of the lips accompanied by sweating.
- Lack of strength in the root of the tongue, lacrimation, eye pain, windstroke, hemiplegia, jaundice, nosebleed, white turbidity.

COMMENTARY

Xinshu BL-15 is the back-shu point of the Heart, where the qi of the Heart emanates from the interior to the body surface, and in common with all the back-shu points (especially those of the yin zang) Xinshu BL-15 has a strong action on regulating and tonifying its corresponding zangfu at the deepest level. It is used equally to tonify deficiency (the Heart is unique amongst the zangfu in that it commonly suffers from all the four main kinds of deficiency: blood, yin, qi and yang), and to resolve excess pathogenic factors such as blood stasis, Heart fire and obstruction by phlegm.

According to the *Essential Questions* "The Heart is the monarch from which the spirit emanates"[11] and "The Heart stores the spirit"[12]. Since storage is a yin function, it is primarily the Heart blood and yin that have the function of nourishing the Heart and providing the material basis for the Heart to house the spirit. Blood and yin deficiency of the Heart may originate from physical causes such as loss of blood, chronic illness and overwork or from emotional causes. Fei Bo-xiong[13] said "The seven emotions injure the five yin organs selectively but they all affect the Heart". According to the *Essential Questions*[14] "The Heart stores the spirit ... when the spirit is insufficient there is sadness". When Heart blood or yin are deficient, the malnourished and unrooted spirit loses its harmony and becomes restless and unquiet, resulting in such symptoms as anxiety, poor memory, fearfulness, insomnia, excessive dreaming and weeping with grief. According to *Essential Readings from the Medical Tradition* "That which is stored by the Heart internally is blood, externally it is emitted as sweat; sweat is the fluid of the Heart". Xinshu BL-15 is also indicated for night sweating due to deficiency of either Heart blood or Heart yin, and is therefore ideally suited to treat the commonly encountered pattern of excessive dreaming, or waking with anxiety, accompanied by sweating.

The Heart controls the pulse, and when Heart qi is deficient and is unable to regulate the blood, there may be palpitations or irregular pulse, especially if the Heart blood is also deficient. In the latter case, palpitations will be more likely to be accompanied by anxiety, in contrast to the palpitations caused purely by qi deficiency which are usually unrelated to emotional changes. In fact palpitations may accompany any pattern of Heart disharmony, whether excess or deficient, and in all these cases Xinshu BL-15 may be selected.

References to the relationship between the Heart, the blood and its vessels abound in the classics. The *Essential Questions* says "All blood pertains to the Heart"[15], "The Heart dominates the blood vessels of the entire body"[16] and "The Heart stores the qi of the blood vessels"[17]. The *Classic of Categories* states "The vessels are the pathways of the blood qi, the movement of the vessels is dependent on qi", whilst in the *Spiritual Pivot*[18] it says "When the qi of hand shaoyin channel is exhausted, the vessels are not open, thus the blood will not flow; when the blood does not flow the circulation will eventually stop ... and the blood will die". The above statements all emphasise the close relationship between the circulation of blood, and the qi and yang of the Heart. Clinically this relationship is most clearly manifested in the chest region. When Heart yang is deficient and unable to circulate the blood in the chest and Heart, there may be consequential Heart blood stasis giving rise to pain and oppression. In clinical practice, this pattern is often complicated by deficiency of qi, blood or yin, or stagnation of qi or phlegm. Whatever the pattern, Xinshu BL-15 is an essential point.

The action of Xinshu BL-15 in treating blood stasis reflects its ability to treat both deficiency and excess patterns of the Heart with equal effect. According to a number of classics it is an important point to clear heat of excess or deficiency type from the Heart. The heat-clearing effect of Xinshu BL-15 extends to the treatment of bleeding, and when Heart fire injures the blood vessels of the Lung or Stomach there may be coughing or vomiting of blood. A different explanation of these symptoms is offered by the *Investigation Into Points Along the Channels* which says that Xinshu BL-15 is indicated for "Heart blood unable to enter the Liver; in the upper, there is wild movement, in the lower there is blood in the stools".

The heat-clearing action of Xinshu BL-15 finds its most important expression in the treatment of excess type psycho-emotional disorders. When Heart fire rages out of control it agitates and excites the spirit leading to such symptoms as severe insomnia and excessive dreaming. When Heart fire combines with phlegm and obstructs the portals of the Heart, there will be severe disorders of the spirit such as epilepsy, dementia, mad walking and mania-depression.

The heat clearing action of Xinshu BL-15 extends beyond the Heart itself, and the *Illustrated Supplement to the Classic of Categories* states that Xinshu BL-15 is one of five points (Feishu BL-13, Xinshu BL-15, Ganshu BL-18, Pishu BL-20 and Shenshu BL-23) which "drain heat from the five zang".

Seminal emission may present in a number of different patterns and is broadly differentiated into seminal emission accompanied by dreaming and seminal emission without dreams. Seminal emission with dreams may be due to Heart fire, Heart and Spleen deficiency, Heart and Kidney deficiency, ministerial fire or damp-heat. Even in cases where the Heart is not directly involved, however, if seminal emission is accompanied by erotic dreams, Xinshu BL-15 is indicated.

Finally, in common with most of the yin back-shu points, Xinshu BL-15 is able to treat the tissues and sense organs associated with its corresponding zang. The tongue is the 'sprouting forth' of the Heart and Xinshu BL-15 is indicated for slow speech development in children and lack of strength in the root of the tongue. Xinshu BL-15 is also indicated for lacrimation and eye pain. These indications however, reflect disorder of the Heart channel rather than the Heart zang.

COMBINATIONS

- Weeping with grief: Xinshu BL-15, Shenmen HE-7, Jiexi ST-41 and Daling P-7 (*Supplementing Life*).
- Sadness, anxiety and disorientation: Xinshu BL-15, Tianjing SJ-10 and Shendao DU-11 (*Supplementing Life*).
- Heart disorientation: Xinshu BL-15, Tianjing SJ-10 and Juque REN-14 (*Great Compendium*).
- Dementia: Xinshu BL-15, Shenmen HE-7, Shaoshang LU-11 and Yongquan KID-1 (*Great Compendium*).
- Epilepsy: Xinshu BL-15, Neiguan P-6, Houxi SI-3, Shenmen HE-7 and Yinbai SP-1 (*Complete Collection*).
- Agitation of the Heart: Xinshu BL-15 and Juque REN-14 (*Supplementing Life*).
- Coughing and spitting blood: Xinshu BL-15, Ganshu BL-18, Quepen ST-12, Juque REN-14 and Jiuwei REN-15 (*Supplementing Life*).
- Weakness of the Kidneys and lumbar region accompanied by seminal emission: Xinshu BL-15 and Shenshu BL-23 (*Ode of the Jade Dragon*).
- Depression in the chest: Xinshu BL-15 and Dazhu BL-11 (*Thousand Ducat Formulas*).

DUSHU BL-16

Governor Shu

督俞

LOCATION

1.5 cun lateral to the lower border of the spinous process of the sixth thoracic vertebra (T6).

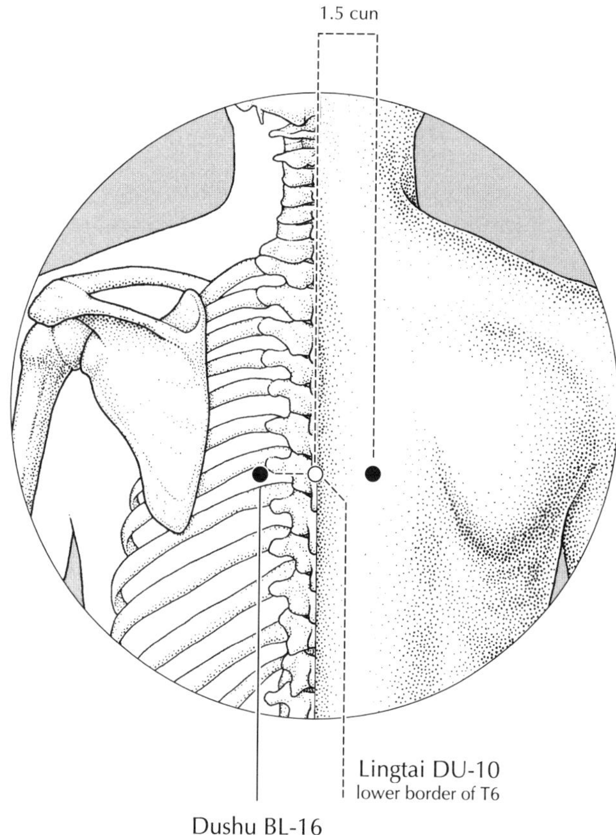

LOCATION NOTE

Locate at the visible highest point of the paraspinal muscles.

NEEDLING

Oblique insertion towards the spine, 0.5 to 1 cun, or transverse-oblique insertion 1 to 1.5 cun.

Caution: perpendicular needling or oblique needling away from the spine carries a substantial risk of causing a pneumothorax.

ACTIONS

Regulates qi in the chest and abdomen

INDICATIONS

- Heart pain, epigastric pain, abdominal distention, borborygmus, chills and fever, breast abscess, itching, psoriasis, alopecia.

COMMENTARY

Although conventionally categorised as the back-shu point of the Governing vessel, it is interesting to note that Dushu BL-16 was not discussed at all in such texts as the *Systematic Classic of Acupuncture and Moxibustion*, the *Illustrated Classic of Acupuncture Points on the Bronze Man* or *Elucidation of the Fourteen Channels*. This downplaying of Dushu BL-16 is reflected in other classics by the absence of any clear indications of disorders of the Governing vessel, and the general paucity of indications and classical combination for this point as a whole. Its modern use is in the treatment of various skin disorders including psoriasis, alopecia and generalised pruritis.

COMBINATIONS

- Psoriasis: Dushu BL-16, Geshu BL-17, Quchi L.I.-11 and Xuehai SP-10.

GESHU BL-17

Diaphragm Shu

膈俞

Hui-Meeting point of Blood

LOCATION

1.5 cun lateral to the lower border of the spinous process of the seventh thoracic vertebra (T7).

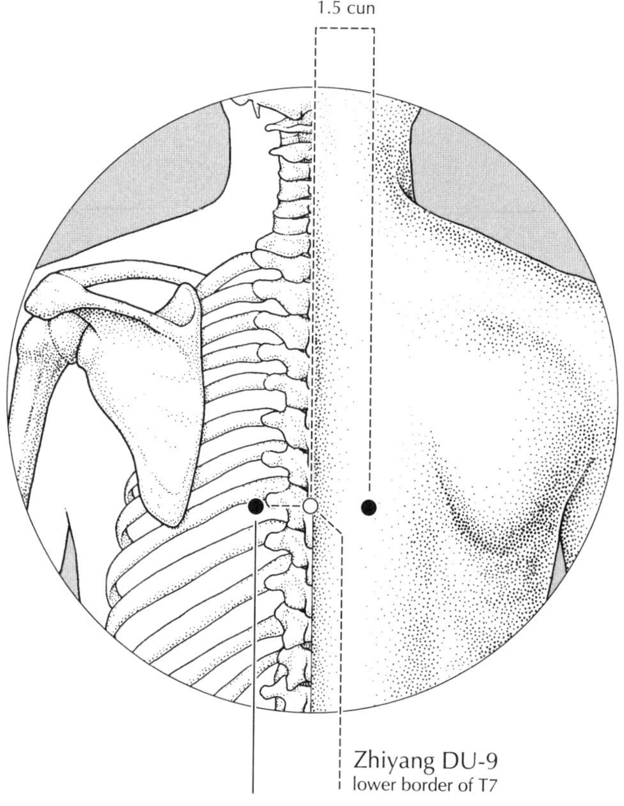

LOCATION NOTE

Locate at the visible highest point of the paraspinal muscles.

NEEDLING

Oblique insertion towards the spine, 0.5 to 1 cun, or transverse-oblique insertion 1 to 1.5 cun.

Caution: perpendicular needling or oblique needling away from the spine carries a substantial risk of causing a pneumothorax.

ACTIONS

Invigorates blood and dispels stasis
Cools blood heat and stops bleeding
Nourishes and harmonises the blood
Harmonises the diaphragm and descends rebellious qi

INDICATIONS

- Oppression of the chest, Heart pain, stabbing pain of the Heart, mania-depression, coughing and dyspnoea, throat painful obstruction.
- Epigastric pain, fullness of the abdomen and lateral costal region, vomiting, vomiting of food eaten the day before, hiccup, oesophageal constriction, difficult ingestion, Stomach reflux, inability to eat, Heart pain on eating, jaundice.
- Coughing blood, vomiting blood, spitting blood, nosebleed, blood in the stool, all blood diseases, urticaria.
- Dizziness, tidal fever, night sweating, steaming bone disorder, spontaneous sweating, fever with absence of sweating, aversion to cold.
- Painful obstruction of the whole body, pain of the whole body, pain of the skin, flesh and bones, frequent stretching and yawning, heaviness of the body, swelling, distention and pain of the body, weariness of the four limbs, lethargy with no desire to move, somnolence, back pain, rigidity of the spine.

COMMENTARY

Geshu BL-17 is the hui-meeting point of blood and, as its name 'Diaphragm Shu' implies, is a kind of honorary back-shu point of the diaphragm, although it is not generally listed as such. These two properties inform its principal actions.

Geshu BL-17 has long been considered a vital point in the treatment of the widest range of blood disorders, indeed many classics simply state that this point can be used for "all blood diseases". Although varied and complex in presentation, disorders of blood may be generalised as being of three main types: blood stasis, blood heat and blood deficiency.

Impairment of blood circulation and consequent blood stasis may be due to stagnation or deficiency of qi, traumatic injury, haemorrhage, penetration of cold, blood deficiency, heat, chronic disease or emotional factors. The variety of symptoms which blood stasis can give rise to is extensive, but of these the principal one is pain. Pain of excess type may be due either to stagnation of qi or stasis of blood, as reflected in the famous adage "without movement there is pain, with movement there is no pain". Pain due to qi stagnation is characterised by a tendency to move and fluctuate, whilst pain due to blood stasis is fixed and stabbing. According to Wang Qing-ren, the Qing dynasty author of *Correcting Errors in Medicine* "whenever there is pain in the abdomen that does not move, it is blood stasis". Tang Rong-chuan in the *Treatise on Disorders of Blood* said "... When blood stasis is between the jingluo and the zangfu the whole body is in pain ... when it is in the upper jiao ... there is stabbing obstinate pain of the arm, chest and diaphragm ... when it is in the middle jiao there is pain of the abdomen and lateral costal region". As is clear from its indications, Geshu BL-17 is applicable in all these cases. It should be noted, however, that due to its location and its special action on the diaphragm which intersects the upper and middle jiao, its main sphere of action is on these two areas and it is less used for blood stasis in the lower jiao. Geshu BL-17 is also an important point to treat various kinds of fever due to blood stasis. The *Treatise on Disorders of Blood* states "when blood stasis is at the level of the pores, the nutritive qi and defensive qi are not harmonised, there is fever accompanied by chills ... when it is half-interior half-exterior ... there is alternating chills and fever ... when it is at the level of the muscles and flesh there will be a burning fever ... when it is in the jingluo and zangfu ... there is necessarily steaming bone consumption fever". Finally, according to Wang Qing-ren in *Correcting Errors in Medicine* "In the pattern of mania-depression, where there is continual crying and laughing, swearing and singing ... then the qi and blood will coagulate in the brain, the qi of the zangfu are disconnected, [the patient] will be as if in a dream". This quotation emphasises the relationship of blood stasis to severe psycho-emotional disorders. Although Wang Qing-ren ascribes the site of the disease to the brain, as discussed elsewhere (see the introductory discussion preceding the Governing vessel points) there is an overlap between the Heart and brain in the various traditions of Chinese medicine. Whatever the location of the disorder, however, the pathology is similar. Blood stasis may directly disturb the spirit, or alternatively blood stasis may both obstruct the blood vessels and transform to heat. The heat agitates the spirit whilst the blood stasis prevents nourishment by fresh blood from reaching the Heart and brain. The combination of heat and Heart blood deficiency leads to a malnourished and restless spirit.

Geshu BL-17 is an important point for many kinds of bleeding disorders, primarily due to blood heat or blood stasis, including coughing blood, vomiting blood, spitting blood, nosebleed and blood in the stool. Heat entering the blood level may be due to a number of causes including constitutional heat, exterior pathogenic heat, overconsumption of excessively heating food or drink, or heat of excess or deficiency type generated by disharmony of the zangfu. When heat agitates the blood it causes it to move recklessly and burst out of the vessels giving rise to haemorrhage that is usually acute and profuse. Geshu BL-17 is able to cool the blood and stop bleeding, primarily from the upper and middle jiao (Lung and Stomach). Another important cause of haemorrhage is blood stasis. When blood is stagnant and does not move, it accumulates and may be forced out of the vessels, giving rise to haemorrhage characterised by its intermittent nature, dark purplish colour and presence of clots. At the same time, haemorrhage due to any aetiology is itself an important cause of blood stasis, as blood that is forced out of the vessels easily pools and stagnates. This is reflected in the saying "where there is haemorrhage there is stasis". The close inter-relationship of blood heat, blood stasis and haemorrhage is further illustrated by the fact that blood heat may condense and dry the blood giving rise to stasis, as stated in the *Treatise on Epidemic Warm Febrile Disease*[19] "Because latent stagnant fire evaporates the blood's fluid, the blood simmers and forms stasis".

The ability of Geshu BL-17 to nourish blood (and yin) is clearly overshadowed in the classical indications by its ability to resolve blood stasis and heat. There are three areas, however, that reflect its nourishing and tonifying properties. The first is its ability to treat disorders such as night sweating and steaming bone disorder due to severe blood and yin deficiency. The second is the combination of Geshu BL-17 with Danshu BL-19 known as the 'four flowers'. The four flowers were first mentioned in *Secrets of a Frontier Official* by Wang Tao in 752 CE, who did not specify the points but described rather a complex location method. He advised tying a piece or string around the neck, with a knot made at the level of Jiuwei REN-15. When the string is allowed to fall down the back, the knot will then lie on the vertebral column at the crossing point of two diagonal lines the end of each of which leads to one of the four points.

The *Classic of Supplementing Life with Acupuncture and Moxibustion* in the 13th century first defined the four flowers by name as Geshu BL-17 and Danshu BL-19 and said that they dominated blood, being indicated (for treatment by moxibustion) for taxation consumption disorder. The third application of the blood nourishing property of Geshu BL-17 is its special ability to treat blood deficiency allied to blood stasis. It has long been understood that following haemorrhage, the consequent blood stasis prevents the formation of new blood. This is reflected in the saying "if blood stasis is not transformed, new blood cannot be generated", and the statement by Tang Rong-chuan in the *Treatise on Disorders of Blood* "In vomiting blood, nosebleeds and blood in the stool, the blood leaves the channels; any blood that has left the channels is separated and no longer connected with the blood that nourishes the entire body ... this blood is unable to augment with good blood, thus the transformation of new blood is hindered". Thus, by pooling outside the channels, blood stasis may lead directly to blood deficiency as sufficient blood is no longer available to nourish the body.

The action of Geshu BL-17 on painful obstruction (commonly referred to as wind-damp in Chinese medicine) which affects the whole body, reflects its action of regulating blood. Prolonged painful obstruction may give rise either to blood stasis or blood deficiency, whilst blood deficiency may render a person prone to invasion by wind-damp. The importance of treating the blood in such cases is reflected in the saying "to treat wind first treat the blood; once blood moves wind will be dispelled".

As its name 'Diaphragm Shu' implies, Geshu BL-17 has an important action on the diaphragm which lies between the upper and middle jiao. By harmonising the diaphragm, Geshu BL-17 is able to descend rebellious qi of both the Lung in the upper jiao (cough and dyspnoea) and the Stomach in the middle jiao (vomiting, Stomach reflux, hiccup and difficult ingestion). Geshu BL-17 is specifically indicated for oesophageal constriction characterised by difficulty in swallowing and, in the latter stages, by vomiting in the evening what was ingested in the morning, and vomiting in the morning what was ingested the evening before.

Finally, due to its action on the diaphragm and Stomach, and by extension the Spleen, Geshu BL-17 is indicated for various kinds of retained fluid giving rise to symptoms such as heaviness, swelling, distention and pain of the body, weariness of the four limbs, somnolence and cold phlegm of the diaphragm and Stomach.

COMBINATIONS

- The hundred syndromes of deficiency-taxation: moxa the four flowers (Geshu BL-17 and Danshu BL-19), Gaohuangshu BL-43 and Huanmen (M-BW-6) (*Compilation*).
- Vomiting: Geshu BL-17 with moxibustion on Zhangmen LIV-13 and Zhongwan REN-12 (*Thousand Ducat Formulas*).
- Cold phlegm in the diaphragm and Stomach: Geshu BL-17 and Shuaigu GB-8 (*Supplementing Life*).

- Contraction and cold of the shoulder and back with pain of the inner aspect of the scapula: Geshu BL-17, Yixi BL-45, Jinmen BL-63 and Chize LU-5 (*Thousand Ducat Formulas*).
- Throat painful obstruction: Geshu BL-17 and Jingqu LU-8 (*Supplementing Life*).
- Bone pain: Geshu BL-17, Zigong REN-19 and Yutang REN-18 (*Supplementing Life*).

GANSHU BL-18

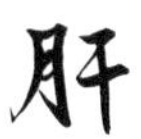
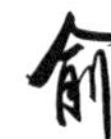

Liver Shu

Back-Shu point of the Liver

LOCATION

1.5 cun lateral to the lower border of the spinous process of the ninth thoracic vertebra (T9).

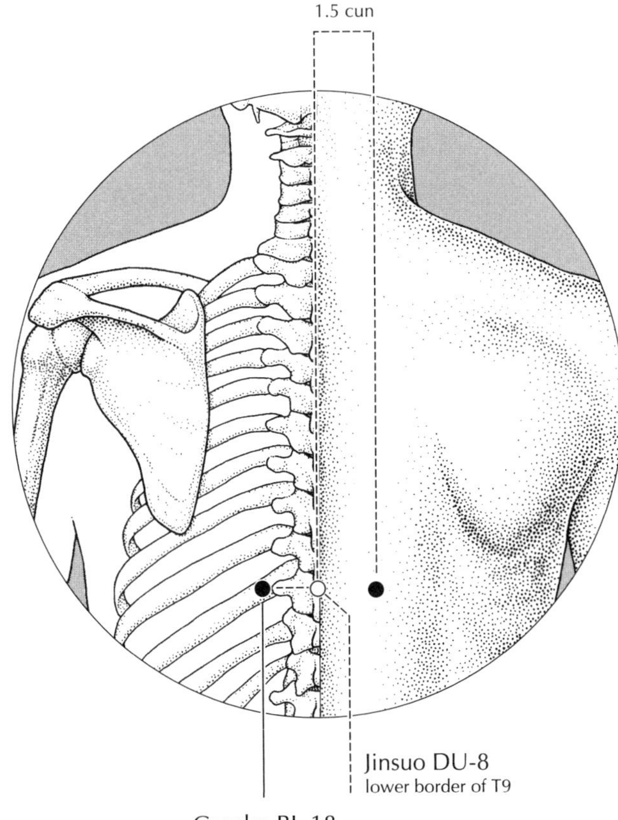

LOCATION NOTE

Locate at the visible highest point of the paraspinal muscles.

NEEDLING

Oblique insertion towards the spine, 0.5 to 1 cun, or transverse-oblique insertion 1 to 1.5 cun.

Caution: perpendicular needling or oblique needling away from the spine carries a substantial risk of causing a pneumothorax.

ACTIONS

Spreads Liver qi
Regulates and nourishes Liver blood
Pacifies wind
Cools fire and clears damp-heat
Benefits the eyes and sinews

INDICATIONS

- Distention and pain of the lateral costal region, epigastric pain, abdominal (ji ju) masses, focal distention, hypogastric fullness and pain, lower abdominal pain, abdominal cramps, shan disorder.
- Fullness of the chest, cough with chest pain, cough with fullness of the lateral costal region and inability to catch the breath, shortness of breath, jaundice, dry mouth.
- Much anger, mania-depression, epilepsy.
- Coughing blood, spitting blood, vomiting blood, nosebleed.
- Blurred vision, redness of the eyes, night blindness, excessive lacrimation, redness pain and itching of the inner canthus, superficial visual obstruction, upward staring eyes, dizziness, visual dizziness, pain of the nose, pain of the supraorbital region.
- Rigidity of the neck and spine, pain of the spine, lumbar pain, pain of the neck and shoulders, lockjaw, opisthotonos, cramps, pain of the sinews, tetany.

COMMENTARY

Ganshu BL-18 is the back-shu point of the Liver, where the qi of the Liver emanates from the interior to the body surface, and like all the back-shu points (especially those of the yin zang) Ganshu BL-18 has a strong action on regulating and tonifying its corresponding zangfu at the deepest level. The principal functions of the Liver are to maintain the free flow of qi, store blood, dominate the sinews and open into the eyes. By spreading Liver qi, nourishing and cooling Liver blood, clearing damp-heat and pacifying wind, Ganshu BL-18 is able to regulate all these aspects of the Liver function.

According to Master Dan-xi of the Jin-Yuan dynasty "The Liver governs spreading". This refers to the Liver's function of ensuring the free and easy flow of qi throughout the body and assisting the normal qi movement of all the zangfu, for example the descending of the Lung and Stomach qi and the ascending of the Spleen qi. Stagnation of Liver qi is considered the pre-eminent pathological pattern of the Liver since it is frequently the starting point of other Liver patterns (for example the transformation of Liver qi into fire) and it commonly accompanies any other pattern of Liver disharmony. The ability of Ganshu BL-18 to promote the free flow of Liver qi is reflected in various ways. Stagnant qi in the upper, middle or lower jiao may give rise to distention and pain of the chest, lateral costal region, epigastrium and hypogastrium as well as to shan disorder. According to the *Spiritual Pivot*[20] "with anger the qi rebels upwards and accumulates in the chest". If Liver qi or Liver fire invade the Lung there will be cough with chest pain, coughing of blood, cough with fullness of the lateral costal region and inability to catch the breath, or shortness of breath. According to *Correcting Errors in Medicine* by Wang Qing-ren of the Qing dynasty "qi is without form and thus unable to congeal into masses; the development of masses requires form in the shape of blood". If stagnation of qi leads to blood stasis, therefore, there will be abdominal masses. If Liver qi stagnation inhibits the function of the Gall Bladder in secreting bile there will be damp-heat of the Liver and Gall Bladder and consequent jaundice. According to the *Spiritual Pivot*[21] "The Liver stores blood, the blood is the residence of the ethereal soul (hun); when Liver qi is deficient there is fear, when excess there is anger". If stagnation of qi is pronounced, and especially if it transforms to fire, there will be emotional manifestations such as anger, mania-depression, and even epilepsy.

The increasing pressure of prolonged qi stagnation may easily transform to fire. According to the *Essential Questions*[22] "Anger will cause the qi to surge upwards; if it is extreme there is vomiting of blood". Since the Liver stores the blood, the heat of Liver fire or Liver yang may easily transmit to the blood and, given the tendency of the Liver qi to rise excessively, cause reckless upward movement of blood leading to symptoms such as vomiting blood, nosebleed, and spitting and coughing blood.

When Liver blood or Liver yin are insufficient, they will be unable to nourish and moisten those regions of the body dominated by the Liver and irrigated by Liver blood, principally the eyes and the sinews. It is a special property of the back-shu points of the zang that they nourish and regulate their corresponding sense organs. According to the *Spiritual Pivot*[23] "Liver qi opens into the eyes; when the Liver is in harmony, the eyes are able to distinguish the five colours", whilst the *Essential Questions*[24] says "The Liver receives blood so there is sight". Insufficiency of Liver blood or Liver yin may lead to disorders such as blurred vision, night blindness, lacrimation and dizziness. If heat from Liver fire or Liver yang rises to disrupt the eyes, there will be redness, itching and pain. If Liver fire leads to the stirring of wind, there will be upward staring of the eyes. The *Investigation into Points Along the Channels* therefore states that Ganshu BL-18 is indicated for "all diseases of the eyes pertaining to the Liver". According to the *Essential Questions* "The Liver dominates the sinews of the entire body"[25], and "When a person sleeps the blood returns to the Liver"[26]. If Liver blood or Liver yin fail to nourish the sinews and thus maintain their softness and flexibility, there may be chronic stiffness and contraction, cramps or pain of the sinews. These symptoms may be especially pronounced both when the body is exhausted and the blood is less effective at nourishing, or during or following sleep or inactivity when the blood returns to the Liver and less is available to circulate throughout the body. This kind of stiffness, contraction, cramping or pain will be even more pronounced when there is concurrent stagnation of Liver qi, or when deficiency of yin or blood leads to stirring up of Liver wind.

According to sayings of Chinese medicine "The Liver governs uprising" and "Anger makes the Liver qi rise to the neck and shoulders". Stagnation of Liver qi or uprising of Liver yang therefore easily lead to stiffness and pain of the neck and shoulders. If Liver fire or high fever consume Liver yin and generate wind there may be such acute spasmodic symptoms as opisthotonos, lockjaw, rigidity of the neck and spine and tetany. Ganshu BL-18 is indicated for all of these symptoms.

Finally the *Illustrated Supplement to the Classic of Categories* states that Ganshu BL-18 is one of five points (Feishu BL-13, Xinshu BL-15, Ganshu BL-18, Pishu BL-20 and Shenshu BL-23) which "drain heat from the five zang".

COMBINATIONS

- Fullness of the hypogastrium: Ganshu BL-18 and Baohuang BL-53 (*Thousand Ducat Formulas*).
- Acute pain of both lateral costal regions: Ganshu BL-18, Pishu BL-20 and Zhishi BL-52 (*Thousand Ducat Formulas*).
- Coughing and spitting blood: Ganshu BL-18, Quepen ST-12, Xinshu BL-15, Juque REN-14 and Jiuwei REN-15 (*Supplementing Life*).
- Vomiting blood and spontaneous external bleeding: Ganshu BL-18, Yinbai SP-1, Pishu BL-20 and Shangwan REN-13 (*Great Compendium*).
- Liver blood deficiency with cloudy vision: reinforce Ganshu BL-18 and reduce Zusanli ST-36 (*Song of the Jade Dragon*).
- Superficial visual obstruction: Ganshu BL-18 and Toulinqi GB-15 (*Great Compendium*).
- Somnolence: Ganshu BL-18, Taixi KID-3, Zhaohai KID-6, Baihui DU-20, Tianjing GB-21, Erjian L.I.-2, Sanjian L.I.-3 and Lidui ST-45 (*Great Compendium*).
- Cold abdominal shan disorder: Ganshu BL-18, Yinshi ST-33 and Taixi KID-3 (*Great Compendium*).

DANSHU BL-19
膽俞

Gall bladder Shu

Back-Shu point of the Gall Bladder

LOCATION

1.5 cun lateral to the lower border of the spinous process of the tenth thoracic vertebra (T10).

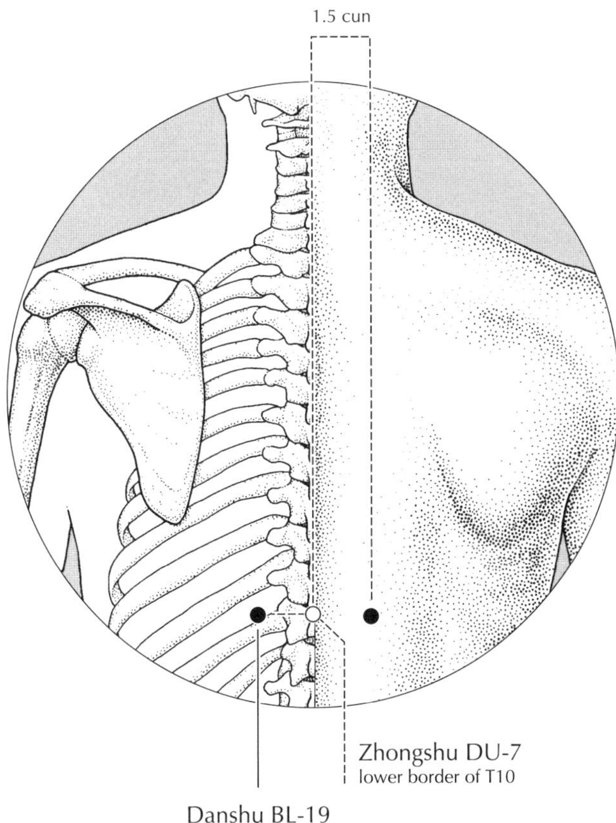

LOCATION NOTE

Locate at the visible highest point of the paraspinal muscles.

NEEDLING

Oblique insertion towards the spine, 0.5 to 1 cun, or transverse-oblique insertion 1 to 1.5 cun.

Caution: perpendicular needling or oblique needling away from the spine carries a substantial risk of causing a pneumothorax.

ACTIONS

Clears damp-heat from the Liver and Gall Bladder
Clears pathogenic factors from the shaoyang
Tonifies and regulates Gall Bladder qi
Tonifies deficiency

INDICATIONS

- Jaundice, yellow eyes, bitter taste in the mouth with a dry tongue, distention and pain of the chest and lateral costal region with inability to turn, vomiting, difficult ingestion, dry retching.
- Fright palpitations with restless sleep, insomnia.
- Steaming bone taxation fever, deficiency-taxation, tidal fever, dryness and pain of the throat, cold shivering with absence of sweating, swelling of the axilla, headache.

COMMENTARY

Danshu BL-19 is the back-shu point of the Gall Bladder fu, where the qi of the Gall Bladder emanates from the interior to the body surface. It is an important point to clear damp-heat from the Gall Bladder and Liver which gives rise to the classic symptoms of jaundice with yellow eyes, vomiting, distention of the lateral costal region and bitter taste in the mouth. Damp-heat in the Gall Bladder and Liver may arise in the following ways: i. stagnation of Liver qi both generates heat and invades the Spleen, suppressing its transportation and transformation function and leading to the formation of dampness, ii. Spleen deficiency leads to failure of its transportation and transformation function and subsequent formation of dampness which either stagnates and ferments over time and transforms to damp-heat or combines with pre-existing Liver stagnant heat, iii. invasion of exterior damp-heat, iv. consumption of contaminated food, or overconsumption of greasy, rich or spicy food and alcohol. In all cases the damp-heat impairs the Gall Bladder function of secreting bile, and whatever the aetiology Danshu BL-19 is indicated.

According to both the *Spiritual Pivot*[27] and the *Essential Questions*[28] "Taiyang is the opening, yangming is the closing and shaoyang is the pivot". In the *Treatise on Injury by Cold* by Zhang Zhong-jing, shaoyang pattern denotes the stage where the pathogen is 'half-exterior, half-interior'. In other words the pathogenic factor resides between the taiyang (exterior) and yangming (interior) levels and in this sense shaoyang is the pivot or hinge between the exterior and interior. When the pathogenic factor disrupts the Gall Bladder function it gives rise to stagnation of qi, impairment of the Stomach descending function and uprising of Gall Bladder heat. The clinical manifestations of shaoyang pattern include alternating fever and chills, dry throat, blurred vision, bitter taste in the mouth, fullness and distention of the chest and lateral costal region, and vomiting and nausea. All but the first of these symptoms are classical indications for Danshu BL-19.

According to five phase theory, wood is the mother of fire, and disorders of either the Liver or Gall Bladder wood may co-exist with or be transmitted to the Heart which belongs to fire. In the case of the Gall Bladder there are two main patterns of disharmony which may give rise to disturbance of the Heart and the spirit: i. Gall Bladder qi deficiency and ii. Gall Bladder damp-heat combined with Stomach phlegm-heat.

According to the *Essential Questions*[29] "the Gallbladder is the upright official from where judgement emanates". If there is sudden fright, unusual or abrupt noise or shock, or continuous fear and fright, whether in the formative years of childhood or as an adult, the qi of the Gall Bladder will be injured, giving rise to palpitations, restless sleep or insomnia, inability to sleep alone, mental restlessness, susceptibility to timidity and fear, and indecisiveness. The Gall Bladder qi can only be injured, however, when the Heart qi is also weak. This was emphasised both in *Achieving Longevity by Guarding the Source*, the 17th Century classic by Gong Ting-xin, which said "Susceptibility to fright ... timidity in which the patient fears being apprehended, all result from deficiency of the qi of Heart and Gall Bladder", and the *Essential Readings from the Medical Tradition* which explained "When the qi of the Heart and Gall Bladder is strong, sudden fright and danger will not cause disease. However, if the qi is deficient, it will be harmful."

In the case of Gall Bladder damp-heat combined with Stomach phlegm-heat, there may be insomnia, palpitations and anxiety accompanied by bitter taste in the mouth, vomiting, and distention and pain of the chest and lateral costal region. In the treatment of both these patterns, Danshu BL-19 forms an important part of the point prescription.

Finally, bilateral Geshu BL-17 and Danshu BL-19 are known as the 'four flowers', indicated for steaming bone taxation fever, deficiency-taxation, tidal fever etc. For a discussion of the history and application of these points see Geshu BL-17.

COMBINATIONS

- Yellow eyes: Danshu BL-19 and Yanggang BL-48 (*One Hundred Symptoms*).
- Yellow eyes: Danshu BL-19, Naohu DU-17, Yishe BL-49 and Yanggang BL-48 (*Supplementing Life*).
- Pain of the lateral costal region: Danshu BL-19 and Zhangmen LIV-13 (*Thousand Ducat Formulas*).
- Difficult ingestion: Danshu BL-19, Zigong REN-19 and Zhongting REN-16 (*Thousand Ducat Formulas*).
- Dry mouth and tongue with difficult ingestion: Danshu BL-19, Shangyang L.I.-1 and Xiaochangshu BL-27 (*Thousand Ducat Formulas*).
- The hundred syndromes of deficiency-taxation: moxa the Four Flowers (Geshu BL-17 and Danshu BL-19), Gaohuangshu BL-43 and Huanmen (M-BW-6) (*Compilation*).
- Fright palpitations: Danshu BL-19 and Yangxi L.I.-5 (*Divine Moxibustion*).
- "When a person is frequently indecisive, the Gall Bladder is deficient. The qi will flow upwards giving rise to a bitter taste in the mouth. To treat this use the front-mu and the back-shu of the Gall Bladder" [i.e. Riyue GB-24 and Danshu BL-19] (*Essential Questions*).

PISHU BL-20

Spleen Shu

Back-Shu point of the Spleen

LOCATION

1.5 cun lateral to the lower border of the spinous process of the eleventh thoracic vertebra (T11).

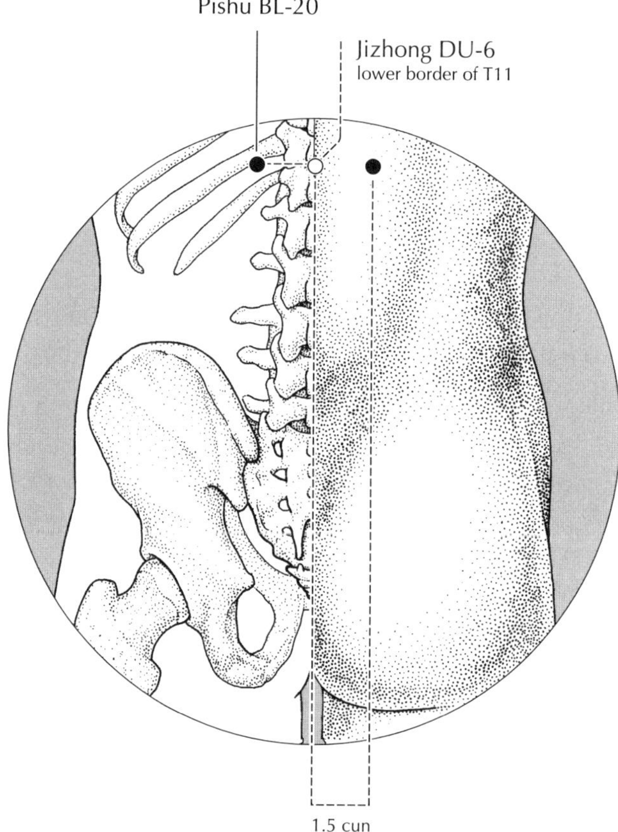

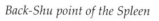

LOCATION NOTE

Locate at the visible highest point of the paraspinal muscles.

NEEDLING

Oblique insertion towards the spine, 0.5 to 1 cun, or transverse-oblique insertion 1 to 1.5 cun.

Caution: perpendicular needling or oblique needling away from the spine carries a substantial risk of causing a pneumothorax.

ACTIONS
Tonifies Spleen qi and yang
Resolves dampness
Raises Spleen qi and holds the blood
Regulates and harmonises the qi of the middle jiao

INDICATIONS
- Distention and pain of the abdomen, focal distention, abdominal (ji ju) masses, lack of appetite, remains thin despite much eating, Spleen qi cold, undigested food (in the stools), diarrhoea, dysenteric disorder, chronic childhood fright wind, childhood nutritional impairment, drum distention, deficiency-taxation, jaundice, yellow body with abdominal fullness and vomiting, pain of the lateral costal region.
- Blood in the stools, blood in the urine, vomiting blood, menorrhagia, chronic haemorrhage, uterine prolapse.
- Oedema, somnolence, lassitude and heaviness of the body with no desire to move, no desire to move the four limbs.
- Malarial diseases with chills and fever, lumbar pain, pain of the shoulder and back, yawning, cough, skin pain, turbid white urine, clonic spasm.

COMMENTARY
Pishu BL-20 is the back-shu point of the Spleen zang, where the qi of the Spleen emanates from the interior to the body surface, and like all the back-shu points (especially those of the zang) has a strong action on regulating and tonifying its corresponding zangfu at the deepest level.

According to the *Complete Works of Jing-yue* "Ming men is the sea of essence [and] blood, the Spleen is the sea of water and grain, together they are the root of the five zang and six fu". The principal function of the Spleen is to dominate the transportation and transformation of the products of food and drink. This vital activity, the basis of the post-natal qi of the body, requires continual yang activity and heat and pathologically therefore, the Spleen suffers mainly from deficiency of qi and yang. This tendency underlies all patterns of disharmony of the Spleen zang.

Spleen qi deficiency may result from constitutional deficiency, irregular diet, excessive thinking or overwork, insufficient or excessive exercise or prolonged illness. Deficiency of Spleen qi and impairment of the transportation and transformation function will give rise to such symptoms as lassitude, lack of appetite, diarrhoea with undigested food in the stools and childhood nutritional impairment, and Pishu BL-20 is an essential point in the treatment of such disorders.

Pishu BL-20 is specifically indicated for the symptom of remaining thin despite much eating. The *Treatise on the Spleen and Stomach* by Li Dong-yuan[30] offers an interesting discussion on the various possible relationships between appetite and obesity or leanness, saying i. that if the Spleen and Stomach are both excess, food intake is large and a person easily becomes fat; ii. if both are deficient there is either inability to eat and a person is thin, or alternatively a person easily becomes fat (yet weak), despite a low food intake, this latter condition being due to accumulation of phlegm-dampness; iii "There are also cases of thinness despite large food intake. [In this case] fire hidden in the qi phase in the Stomach results in large food intake, while Spleen vacuity leads to withered flesh. This is known as food languor. Shu-he has said, 'Large food intake is not incompatible with weak muscles' ". The apparently contradictory condition of Spleen deficiency with a large appetite is often encountered in clinical practice and Li Dong-yuan's explanation of hidden Stomach fire with Spleen qi deficiency explains this well.

The important role that dampness plays in the pathology of the Spleen has been discussed in many classics. According to the *Essential Questions* "The Spleen loathes dampness"[31], "Damp, swelling and fullness all pertain to the Spleen"[32] and "When the Spleen is diseased, damp is generated"[33], whilst the *Case Histories from the Guide to Clinical Patterns* by Ye Tian-shi of the Qing dynasty states "The Spleen likes dryness whilst the Stomach likes moisture". The origin of dampness may be interior or exterior. Interior deficiency of Spleen qi and impairment of the transportation and transformation function may give rise to incomplete separation of the clear and the turbid and the subsequent formation of interior dampness. This dampness may be carried to all parts of the body by virtue of the Spleen's function of distributing qi, but especially to the lower parts since 'the nature of dampness is heavy and turbid'. Alternatively, if exterior dampness or damp-heat attack the body, especially in cases of underlying Spleen deficiency, the function of the Spleen may quickly be compromised. Dampness gives rise to such symptoms as heaviness of the body, lassitude, somnolence, diarrhoea, dysenteric disorder, yin jaundice and oedema. Pishu BL-20 is an essential point both to tonify the Spleen qi and to resolve dampness, whether of internal or external origin.

Two further patterns that may develop from deficiency of Spleen qi are i. failure of the Spleen to hold the blood, and ii. sinking of Spleen qi. According to the *Treatise on Disorders of Blood* "When Spleen yang is deficient it is unable to gather the blood", whilst the *Supplement to The Thousand Ducat Formulas* states "The Spleen gathers the blood, when the Spleen is deficient it is unable to unite the blood". Part of the Spleen's function of controlling the blood is to hold the blood in the vessels. Weakness of this function will lead to haemorrhage in any part of the body, giving rise to such indications as blood in the urine or stools, menorrhagia, vomiting of blood and indeed any kind of chronic haemorrhage. When the Spleen's function of raising the qi is impaired, there may be sinking or prolapse of the uterus. Pishu BL-20, through its action of tonifying and hence raising the Spleen qi, is able to treat both these conditions.

An important further symptom of Spleen disharmony is stagnation in the middle jiao manifesting as abdominal fullness, distention and pain, or pain of the lateral costal region. There are three main causes of this disharmony: i. Spleen qi deficiency leads to impaired circulation of qi, and the treatment principle here is to both tonify and circulate the qi, ii. the formation and retention of dampness in the middle jiao may obstruct the circulation of qi, and the principle of treatment in this case is to resolve damp and circulate qi, iii. Liver-Spleen disharmony, due either to excess of the Liver which overacts on the Spleen, or deficiency of the Spleen which fails to counter the normal aggressive qi of the Liver. The aggressive Liver qi impairs the transportation and transformation function of the Spleen leading to stagnation. The treatment principle in this case is to harmonise the Liver and Spleen. In all these patterns Pishu BL-20 is a primary point.

One particular form of abdominal stagnation for which Pishu BL-20 is indicated is known as focal distention. This is characterised primarily by a sensation of severe blockage and distention, or the appearance of a swelling like an upturned bowl. It is one of what is known as the 'five accumulations' and pertains to the Spleen.

Since Pishu BL-20 tonifies the Spleen and regulates the middle jiao, it may also be used for treating the commonly encountered dual disharmony of the Stomach and Spleen with distention of both the epigastrium and abdomen, nausea and vomiting, and diarrhoea.

Finally the *Illustrated Supplement to the Classic of Categories* states that Pishu BL-20 is one of five points (Feishu BL-13, Xinshu BL-15, Ganshu BL-18, Pishu BL-20 and Shenshu BL-23) which "drain heat from the five zang".

COMBINATIONS

- Spleen deficiency with undigested food (in the stool): Pishu BL-20 and Pangguangshu BL-28 (*One Hundred Symptoms*).
- Much eating but remains thin: Pishu BL-20 and Weishu BL-21 (*Great Compendium*).
- Abdominal pain with no pleasure in eating: Pishu BL-20 and Weishu BL-21 (*Supplementing Life*).
- Sadness below the Heart: Pishu BL-20 and Tinggong SI-19 (*One Hundred Symptoms*).
- Vomiting blood and spontaneous external bleeding: Pishu BL-20, Yinbai SP-1, Ganshu BL-18 and Shangwan REN-13 (*Great Compendium*).
- Loss of use of the four limbs: Pishu BL-20, Jiquan HE-1 and Riyue GB-24 (*Supplementing Life*).
- Acute pain of both lateral costal regions: Pishu BL-20, Ganshu BL-18 and Zhishi BL-52 (*Thousand Ducat Formulas*).

WEISHU BL-21

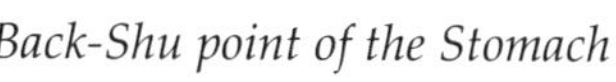

Stomach Shu

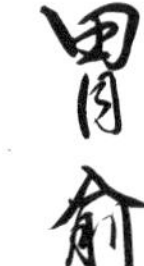

Back-Shu point of the Stomach

LOCATION

1.5 cun lateral to the lower border of the spinous process of the twelfth thoracic vertebra (T12).

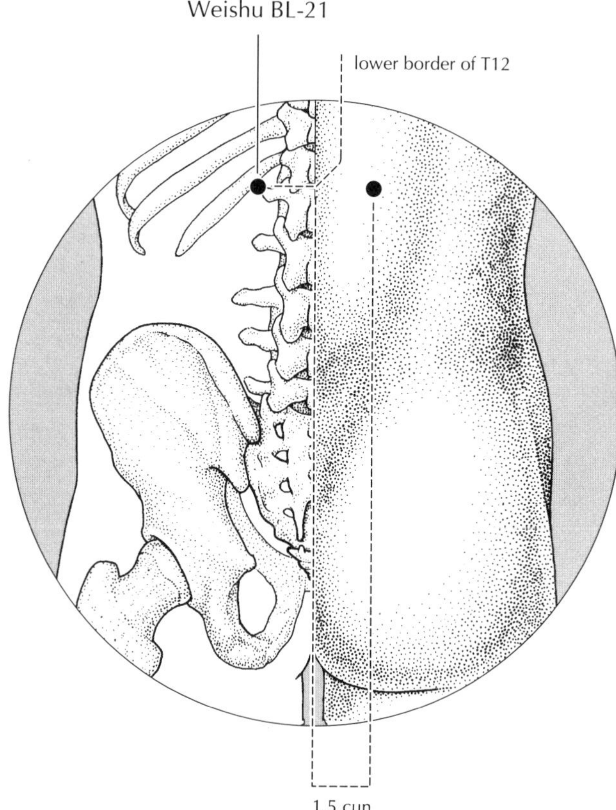

LOCATION NOTE

Locate at the visible highest point of the paraspinal muscles.

NEEDLING

Oblique insertion towards the spine, 0.5 to 1 cun, or transverse-oblique insertion 1 to 1.5 cun.

Caution: perpendicular needling or oblique needling away from the spine carries a substantial risk of causing a pneumothorax.

ACTIONS

Regulates the Stomach and descends rebellion
Harmonises the middle jiao

INDICATIONS

- Epigastric pain, cold and feeble Stomach, distention and cold of the Stomach, distention and fullness of the abdomen and epigastrium, fullness of the lateral costal region, oedema and drum distention.
- Thin body despite much eating, hungry but unable to eat, lack of appetite, difficult ingestion, vomiting, vomiting clear fluid, vomiting in the morning what was eaten the evening before, Stomach reflux, sudden turmoil disorder, contracted sinews, childhood nutritional impairment, regurgitation of milk in children.
- Borborygmus, diarrhoea, undigested food (in the stool).
- Chest pain, contraction and pain of the back, jaundice, malaria, long-term abdominal (ji) masses, dimness of vision, prolapse of the rectum.

COMMENTARY

Weishu BL-21 is the back-shu point of the Stomach fu, where the qi of the Stomach emanates from the interior to the body surface, and is a powerful point to treat all diseases of the Stomach, as well as to regulate the middle jiao as a whole. According to the *Spiritual Pivot*[34] "The Stomach is the sea of water and grain". Its function is to receive food and drink, 'rot and ripen' it and descend it to the Small Intestine. Most pathology of the Stomach, therefore, involves impairment of its descending function. This may be due to deficiency of Stomach qi or Stomach yin, excessive cold, heat or dampness whether of internal or external origin, stasis of blood in the Stomach, stagnation of food, or invasion of the Stomach by Liver or Gall Bladder qi. Failure of the Stomach descending function leads to stagnation of qi and hence distention, fullness and pain of the epigastrium and abdomen, whilst upward rebellion of the Stomach qi leads to Stomach reflux, nausea and vomiting. Whatever the pattern, whether deficient, excess, hot or cold, Weishu BL-21 is a primary point to re-establish harmony of the Stomach.

It is interesting to compare the actions and indications of Weishu BL-21, the back-shu point of the Stomach, with Zusanli ST-36 the he-sea point of the Stomach channel. Both have an equally strong action on regulating disorders of the Stomach fu, but Weishu BL-21 shares none of the ability of Zusanli ST-36 to tonify and nourish the qi and blood of the body as a whole.

The Stomach and Spleen are interiorly-exteriorly related, and the descending of Stomach qi and the ascending of Spleen qi together dominate the whole process of digestion. By virtue of this close relationship, Weishu BL-21 is able to regulate disharmony of both the Stomach and Spleen, giving rise to abnormal ascent of Stomach qi (vomiting), abnormal descent of Spleen qi (diarrhoea) and failure of the Spleen transportation and transformation function (borborygmus and oedema).

A healthy appetite is a sign of the harmonious functioning of both the Spleen and Stomach, and Weishu BL-21 is indicated in various disorders affecting the appetite. Poor appetite may be due either to deficiency of the Stomach and Spleen which lack the force to 'rot and ripen' and transport and transform what is eaten, or to various forms of excess which lead to stagnation of food in the Stomach and hence lack of desire and inability to take in more food. Hunger with inability to eat is due to insufficiency of Stomach yin with consequent deficiency heat, the heat stimulating desire to eat, the yin deficiency and resultant dryness causing inability to digest what is eaten. Excessive eating without gaining weight is a sign of Stomach heat, with or without Spleen deficiency (see commentary on Pishu BL-20). Weishu BL-21 is indicated in all such cases.

COMBINATIONS

- Abdominal pain with no pleasure in eating: Weishu BL-21 and Pishu BL-20 (*Formulas for the Living*).
- Much eating but remains thin: Weishu BL-21 and Pishu BL-20 (*Great Compendium*).
- Vomiting or cold in the Stomach with distention, much eating but remains thin: Weishu BL-21 and Shenshu BL-23 (*Thousand Ducat Formulas*).
- Cold in the stomach with undigested food (in the stool): Weishu BL-21 and Hunmen BL-47 (*One Hundred Symptoms*).

SANJIAOSHU BL-22

Sanjiao Shu

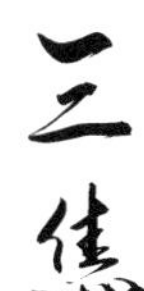

Back-Shu point of the Sanjiao

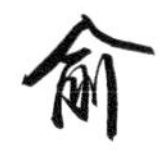

LOCATION

1.5 cun lateral to the lower border of the spinous process of the first lumbar vertebra (L1).

LOCATION NOTE

Locate at the visible highest point of the paraspinal muscles.

NEEDLING

Oblique or perpendicular-oblique insertion towards the spine, 1 to 1.5 cun.

Caution: deep perpendicular needling carries a risk of injuring the kidney.

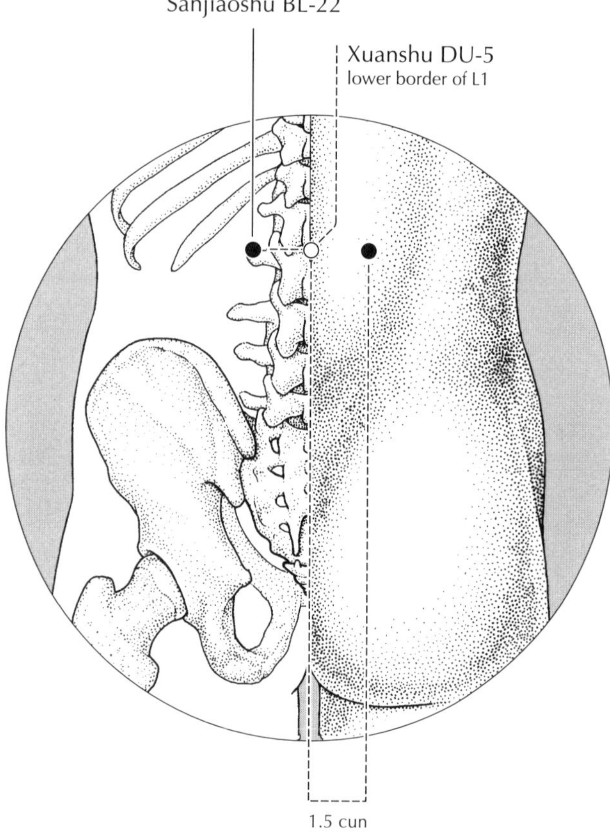

ACTIONS

Moves and regulates the Sanjiao
Regulates the Spleen and Stomach and resolves dampness
Regulates the water passages and promotes urination
Resolves masses

INDICATIONS

- Borborygmus, diarrhoea, undigested food (in the stool), dysenteric disorder, oesophageal constriction, vomiting, difficult ingestion.
- Abdominal distention with emaciation, abdominal (zheng ju) masses and emaciation in women, zangfu (ji ju) masses, large and hard hypogastric (ji ju) masses.
- Oedema, difficult urination, white turbidity, blood in the urine, deficiency-taxation.
- Headache, visual dizziness, alternating chills and fever, heat in the body, bitter taste in the mouth and cracked lips, jaundice.
- Stiffness and pain of the lumbar spine, inflexibility and stiffness of the shoulder and back.

COMMENTARY

Sanjiaoshu BL-22 is the back-shu point of the Sanjiao, where the qi of the Sanjiao emanates from the interior to the body surface. The Sanjiao integrates and harmonises the upper, middle and lower jiao and dominates the free flow of qi and fluids through these three areas. Located between Weishu BL-21 above and Shenshu BL-23 below, Sanjiaoshu BL-22 however has the action of regulating the qi of the middle and lower jiao only. It integrates the activities of the Stomach and Spleen in the middle jiao, and the Kidneys, Bladder and intestines in the lower jiao, and hence the transformation, transportation and excretion of both food and fluid.

The *Classic of Difficulties*[35] states that "the Sanjiao is the pathway of water and grain", the *Essential Questions*[36] says "the Sanjiao is the official in charge of drainage and controls the water passages" and the *Introduction to Medicine* says "The middle jiao dominates transformation of the flavours of water and grain ... therefore it is said the middle jiao is like foam. The lower jiao dominates moving and draining the urine and faeces and at the right time discharging them ... therefore it is said the lower jiao is like a drain".

In cases where there is loss of harmony between the Stomach and Spleen in the middle jiao and the intestines in the lower jiao, there are symptoms such as abdominal distention, borborygmus, diarrhoea or dysenteric disorder, undigested food (in the stool), difficult ingestion, oesophageal constriction and vomiting. In severe cases where there is obstruction and accumulation there may be abdominal masses or hypogastric lumps. Sanjiaoshu BL-22 is especially effective to activate and harmonise the qi of the middle and lower jiao, to resolve damp and to dispel stasis, and is one of the most important classically indicated points for such abdominal masses.

In cases where there is loss of harmony between the Spleen in the middle jiao and the Kidneys and Bladder in the lower jiao there may be oedema with difficult urination, blood in the urine and white turbidity due to deficiency and exhaustion. Sanjiaoshu BL-22 is able to treat such disorders by its ability to move the fluids and activate the qi transformation function of the Bladder.

Finally the Sanjiao channel belongs to shaoyang, and although not a point of the Sanjiao channel, Sanjiaoshu BL-22 is indicated for the treatment of alternating chills and fever, heat in the body, bitter taste in the mouth, headache and visual dizziness, all manifestations of shaoyang pattern.

COMBINATIONS

- Borborygmus, abdominal distention and watery diarrhoea: Sanjiaoshu BL-22, Xiaochangshu BL-27, Xialiao BL-34, Yishe BL-49 and Zhangmen LIV-13 (*Thousand Ducat Formulas*).
- Borborygmus: Sanjiaoshu BL-22, Dachangshu BL-25, Taibai SP-3 and Gongsun SP-4 (*Supplementing Life*).

- Undigested food (in the stool): Sanjiaoshu BL-22, Zusanli ST-36, Dachangshu BL-25, Sanyinjiao SP-6, Xiawan REN-10, Xuanshu DU-5 and Liangmen ST-21 (*Supplementing Life*).
- Hypogastric (ji ju) masses that are hard and big like a plate, with epigastric distention and undigested food (in the stool): Sanjiaoshu BL-22 and Zhongwan REN-12 (*Thousand Ducat Formulas*).

SHENSHU BL-23

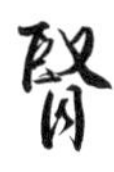
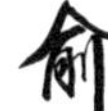

Kidney Shu

Back-Shu point of the Kidneys

LOCATION

1.5 cun lateral to the lower border of the spinous process of the second lumbar vertebra (L2).

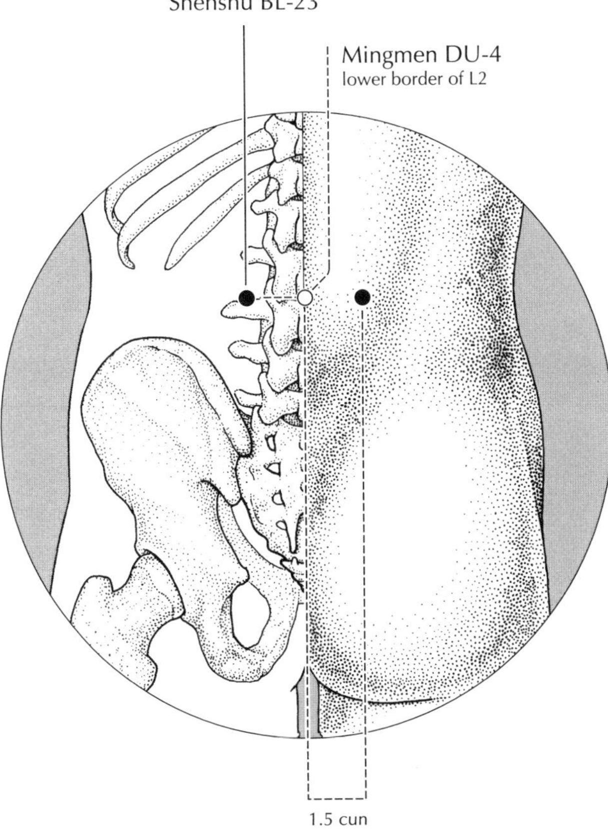

LOCATION NOTE

Locate at the visible highest point of the paraspinal muscles.

NEEDLING

Oblique or perpendicular-oblique insertion towards the spine, 1 to 1.5 cun.

Caution: deep perpendicular needling carries a risk of injuring the kidney.

ACTIONS

Tonifies the Kidneys and fortifies yang
Benefits essence
Nourishes Kidney yin
Firms Kidney qi
Regulates the water passages and benefits urination
Benefits and warms the uterus
Benefits the ears and eyes
Strengthens the lumbar region

INDICATIONS

- Oedema, deficiency-taxation oedema, difficult urination, turbid urine, deficiency-exhaustion white turbidity, enuresis, frequent urination, dripping urination, wasting and thirsting disorder with frequent urination, blood in the urine.
- Seminal emission, seminal emission with dreams, urine containing semen, impotence, premature ejaculation, pain of the genitals, acute hypogastric pain.
- Irregular menstruation, accumulation of cold in women giving rise to taxation, chronic cold of the uterus, emaciation in women due to sexual intercourse during menstruation, leucorrhoea, red and white leucorrhoea.
- Cold or damp (dong) diarrhoea, borborygmus, undigested food in the stools, eats a lot but remains thin, pain of the lateral costal region, cold and distention of the Stomach, cold vomiting.
- Chronic dyspnoea and cough, asthma, diminished qi.
- Kidney deficiency deafness, tinnitus, visual dizziness, night blindness, blurred vision.
- The five taxations and the seven injuries, taxation of the five zang, chronic cold of the water (Kidney) zang, deficiency-taxation emaciation.
- Heavy head with heat in the body, redness and heat of the face, redness of the head and body, yellow-black complexion, wind headache, alternating chills and fever, rebellious qi Heart pain.
- Pain and soreness of the lumbar region and knees, icy-cold sensation of the lumbar region, cold legs, hot and cold sensations of the bones, windstroke, hemiplegia.

COMMENTARY

Shenshu BL-23 is the back-shu point of the Kidney zang where the qi of the Kidneys emanates from the interior to the body surface, and like all the back-shu points (especially those of the zang) has a strong action on regulating and tonifying its corresponding zangfu at the deepest level. Shenshu BL-23 is one of the principal acupuncture points to strengthen the Kidneys, fortify yang, nourish yin, and benefit essence.

According to the *Spiritual Pivot*[37] "The Kidneys store the essence" and "essence is the source of life". The *Essential Questions*[38] states "Essence is the root of the human body", whilst a saying of Chinese medicine emphasises "The Kidney is the root of pre-heaven". Since neither essence nor pre-heaven qi can ever be excessive, the Kidneys can only suffer from deficiency patterns. Kidney deficiency may be congenital in origin, or may develop during the course of a person's life as a result of chronic illness, dissipation, excessive sexual activity, overwork, old age, prolonged fear, or prolonged disharmony of other zangfu which eventually transmits to the Kidneys. Deficiency of the Kidneys is subdivided into the following patterns: i. Kidney qi not firm, ii. Failure of the Kidneys to grasp the qi, iii. deficiency of Kidney essence, iv. deficiency of Kidney yang, v. deficiency of Kidney yin. Shenshu BL-23 is an essential point in the treatment of all these patterns.

The Kidneys dominate the two lower yin (urethra and anus) and control the opening and closing of the Bladder and its qi transformation function. Deficiency of the Kidney qi (Kidney qi not firm) therefore, may impair the Kidneys' ability to firmly hold and astringe the urine resulting in such symptoms of leakage as frequent urination, dripping urination, enuresis, white turbidity due to deficiency and exhaustion etc.

According to the *Master Hua's Classic of the Central Viscera* by the great Han dynasty physician Hua Tuo, the Kidneys "serve the purpose of shutting in the essence in males"[39]. Deficiency of Kidney qi, therefore, may give rise to leakage of essence manifesting as seminal emission, seminal emission with dreams, urine containing semen and premature ejaculation. This kind of leakage may be seen in the context of qi deficiency alone (in other words without accompanying symptoms of cold or heat), or as part of deficiency of either Kidney yang or Kidney yin, more commonly the former since qi belongs to the broad category of yang. Whatever the pattern, Shenshu BL-23 is an important point to firm the holding and astringing action of the Kidneys.

The Kidneys control the movement of water throughout the body, and although the Spleen and Lung also play an important role in the circulation of fluids, their yang qi is ultimately dependent on that of the Kidneys. This is reflected in the statement that 'the Kidneys dominate the yang of the whole body and govern water'. When Kidney yang fails to move the body fluids there may be oedema with difficult urination. The *Supplement to the Thousand Ducat Formulas* says "Shenshu BL-23 treats the hundred oedematous diseases" (i.e. any kind of oedema).

The uterus depends on the Kidney essence for its growth, maturation and nourishment, the Penetrating and Conception vessels are both nourished by and have their root in the Kidneys, and the *Essential Questions* says "the vessel of the uterus connects with the Kidneys"[40]. Shenshu BL-23 is indicated for a variety of disorders of the uterus including irregular menstruation due to Kidney deficiency, chronic cold of the uterus giving rise to taxation, 'emaciation in women due to sexual intercourse during menstruation' and leucorrhoea.

The intimate relationship between the Kidney yang and ming men (the gate of life) has been emphasised in numerous classics. According to the *Classic of Difficulties*[41] "On the left is the Kidney, on the right is ming men", whilst Li Dong-yuan wrote "The dynamic qi that moves between the Kidneys is ming men". Zhang Jing-yue of the Ming dynasty stated "ming men resides between the Kidneys" and "ming men is the root of original qi and the residence of the water and fire; without it the yin qi of the five zang is unable to grow, the yang qi of the five zang is unable to develop". The Kidney yang therefore corresponds to ming men fire and is the source of the fire of the whole body. Failure of Kidney yang to warm the body leads to such symptoms as chronic cold of the uterus, lumbar region, legs and bones. Decline of the Kidney yang and waning of ming men fire may lead to weakness of the sexual function and hence impotence. Kidney yang is also the source of Spleen yang. When Kidney yang is unable to warm Spleen and Stomach earth there may be chronic diarrhoea due to cold or dampness, diarrhoea containing undigested food, cold and distention of the Stomach, and cold vomiting. The diarrhoea associated with this pattern characteristically occurs in the early hours of the morning and is known as fifth-watch (cockcrow) diarrhoea. The *Complete Works of Jing-yue* stated "The opening and closing of the two excretions is dominated by the Kidneys. When the yang qi of the Kidneys is insufficient, then ming men is in decline and yin cold is in abundance; therefore after the fifth watch when the yang qi of the Kidneys is in decline and the yin qi is reaching its zenith there will be ceaseless diarrhoea".

According to the *Complete Works of Jing-yue* "The Lung is the master of qi, the Kidneys are the root of qi. The Lung dominates the exhalation of qi whilst the Kidneys dominate the reception of qi. Only when yin and yang are mutually communicating is respiration harmonious". This quotation emphasises the essential role of the Kidneys in normal respiration. The Lung is the uppermost zang with the function of descending the qi and controlling exhalation, whilst the Kidneys are the bottomost zang with the function of grasping the qi and controlling inhalation. If Kidney qi is deficient and unable to grasp and hold the Lung qi there may be dyspnoea, asthma or cough. This pattern is characterised by its chronic nature and is usually seen with other accompanying signs of Kidney deficiency. As is the case with Kidney qi not firm, this pattern may be seen either without symptoms of cold or heat, or in the context of deficiency of either Kidney yang or Kidney yin.

According to *Essential Readings from the Medical Tradition* "The fire and water of the human body is yin and yang ... without yang, yin cannot engender; without yin, yang cannot transform" whilst in the *Complete Works of Jing-yue* it is said "yin and yang are of the same origin...fire is the ruler of water, water is the source of fire...". These quotations underline the inseparable relationship of the yin and yang of the Kidneys and help explain why all acupuncture points which treat the Kidneys invariably benefit both Kidney yin and Kidney yang. Although the indications for Shenshu BL-23 emphasise deficiency of Kidney qi or Kidney yang, therefore, it also has an action on nourishing Kidney yin.

Like Kidney yang, Kidney yin is the root of the yin of the whole body. Kidney yin deficiency may lead to impaired nourishment of the body and the flaring up of deficiency fire, giving rise to such symptoms as emaciation, wasting and thirsting disorder, and redness and heat of the face and body.

It is a characteristic of the yin back-shu points that they nourish and regulate their corresponding sense organs. According to the *Spiritual Pivot*[42] "The Kidneys open into the ears; if the Kidneys are in harmony, the ears can hear the five sounds". Since the Kidneys store essence, produce marrow which fills up the brain and dominate yin, Shenshu BL-23 is indicated not only for ear disorders such as tinnitus and deafness, but also for blurred vision, night blindness and visual dizziness, all due to deficiency of marrow, essence or yin.

Since the Kidney yin and yang are the root of the yin fluids and the yang qi of the body, this explains the action of Shenshu BL-23 in diseases of chronic deficiency. It is indicated for the five taxations and the seven injuries, taxation of the five zang, and prolonged accumulation of cold leading to taxation. The five taxations as discussed in the *Spiritual Pivot* are i. excessive use of the eyes which injures the blood, ii. excessive lying down which injures the qi, iii. excessive sitting which injures the flesh, iv. excessive standing which injures the bones, and v. excessive walking which injures the sinews. In later texts, the concept of the five taxations was also used to refer to taxation of each of the five zang. Although also referring to a range of male genital disorders (see glossary), the seven injuries in this context are i. overeating which injures the Spleen, ii. great anger which injures the Liver, iii. heavy lifting or prolonged sitting on damp ground which injure the Kidneys, iv. pathogenic cold which injures the Lung, v. worry and anxiety which injure the Heart, vi. wind, rain, cold and summer-heat which injure the body, and vii. excessive fear which injures the emotions.

According to the *Essential Questions* "The Kidneys store the qi of the bone marrow"[43], "The Kidneys reside in the lumbar region"[44], "The Kidneys generate bone marrow"[45] and " ... when there is internal attack, and heat resides in the Kidneys, then the bones will wither and the marrow will be deficient, therefore the legs will not be able to support the body and bone atrophy disorder will develop"[46]. Any Kidney deficiency pattern may give rise to chronic lumbar pain and weakness or soreness of the knees, whilst in cases of Kidney yin deficiency there may be hot sensations in the bones and in case of Kidney yang deficiency, cold sensations of the bones. Located in the lumbar region and having a direct action on the Kidney zang, Shenshu BL-23 is an essential point in the treatment of any kind of lumbar pain which has its root in Kidney deficiency, as well as Kidney deficient atrophy disorder and hemiplegia.

Finally the *Illustrated Supplement to the Classic of Categories* states that Shenshu BL-23 is one of five points (Feishu BL-13, Xinshu BL-15, Ganshu BL-18, Pishu BL-20 and Shenshu BL-23) which "drain heat from the five zang".

COMBINATIONS

- Cold of the lower extremities: Shenshu BL-23, Jinggu BL-64 and Rangu KID-2 (*Supplementing Life*).
- Cold and pain of the bone marrow: Shenshu BL-23, Dazhu BL-11, Xuanzhong GB-39, Fuliu KID-7, Lidui ST-45 and Shenmai BL-62 (*Compilation*).
- Weakness of the Kidneys and lumbar region accompanied by seminal emission: Shenshu BL-23 and Xinshu BL-15 (*Ode of the Jade Dragon*).
- Lumbar pain: Shenshu BL-23, Qihaishu BL-24 and Zhonglushu BL-29 (*Supplementing Life*).
- Lumbar pain due to Kidney deficiency: Shenshu BL-23, Weizhong BL-40, Taixi KID-3 and Baihuanshu BL-30 (*Great Compendium*).
- Lumbar pain in the elderly: Shenshu BL-23 and Mingmen DU-4 (*Compilation*).
- Incontinence of urine and faeces in the elderly: moxa Shenshu BL-23 and Mingmen DU-4 (*Ode of the Jade Dragon*).
- Invasion by cold or damp (dong) diarrhoea containing undigested food: Shenshu BL-23 and Zhangmen LIV-13 (*Thousand Ducat Formulas*).
- Cold or damp (dong) diarrhoea with undigested food: Shenshu BL-23 and Dachangshu BL-25 (*Supplementing Life*).
- Vomiting or cold in the Stomach with distention, much eating but remains thin: Shenshu BL-23 and Weishu BL-21 (*Thousand Ducat Formulas*).

- Deficiency-taxation oedema: moxa Taichong LIV-3 one hundred times, also moxa Shenshu BL-23 (*Thousand Ducat Formulas*).
- Seminal emission, white turbidity: Shenshu BL-23, Guanyuan REN-4 and Sanyinjiao SP-6 (*Great Compendium*).
- Impotence: Shenshu BL-23, Rangu KID-2, Mingmen DU-4 and Qihai REN-6 (*Illustrated Supplement*).
- Pain of the genitals: Shenshu BL-23, Zhishi BL-52, Jinggu BL-64 and Taichong LIV-3 (*Supplementing Life*).
- Irregular menstruation: Shenshu BL-23, Daimai GB-26, Qihai REN-6, Zhongji REN-3 and Sanyinjiao SP-6 (*Great Compendium*).
- Ceaseless uterine bleeding: Shenshu BL-23, Zigong (M-CA-18), Zhongji REN-3 and Shimen REN-5 (*Great Compendium*).
- Deafness due to Kidney deficiency: Shenshu BL-23 and Tinghui GB-2 (*Song of the Jade Dragon*).
- Deafness due to Kidney deficiency: Shenshu BL-23, Pianli L.I.-6 and Tinghui GB-2 (*Illustrated Supplement*).
- Deficiency tinnitus: Shenshu BL-23, Zusanli ST-36 and Hegu L.I.-4 (*Great Compendium*).
- Tinnitus: Shenshu BL-23, Tinggong SI-19, Tinghui GB-2, Ermen SJ-21, Baihui DU-20, Luoque BL-8, Yangxi L.I.-5, Qiangu SI-2, Houxi SI-3, Wangu SI-4, Zhongzhu SJ-3, Yemen SJ-2 and Shangyang L.I.-1 (*Great Compendium*).
- Fullness of the chest and lateral costal region radiating to the abdomen: Shenshu BL-23, Xiajuxu ST-39, Qiuxu GB-40 and Xiaxi GB-43 (*Great Compendium*).
- Chest and diaphragm obstructed by blood stasis: Shenshu BL-23 and Juliao ST-3 (*One Hundred Symptoms*).

QIHAISHU BL-24

Sea of Qi Shu

氣海俞

LOCATION

1.5 cun lateral to the lower border of the spinous process of the third lumbar vertebra (L3).

LOCATION NOTE

Locate at the visible highest point of the paraspinal muscles.

NEEDLING

Perpendicular insertion 1 to 1.5 cun.

ACTIONS

Strengthens the lumbar region and legs
Regulates the lower jiao

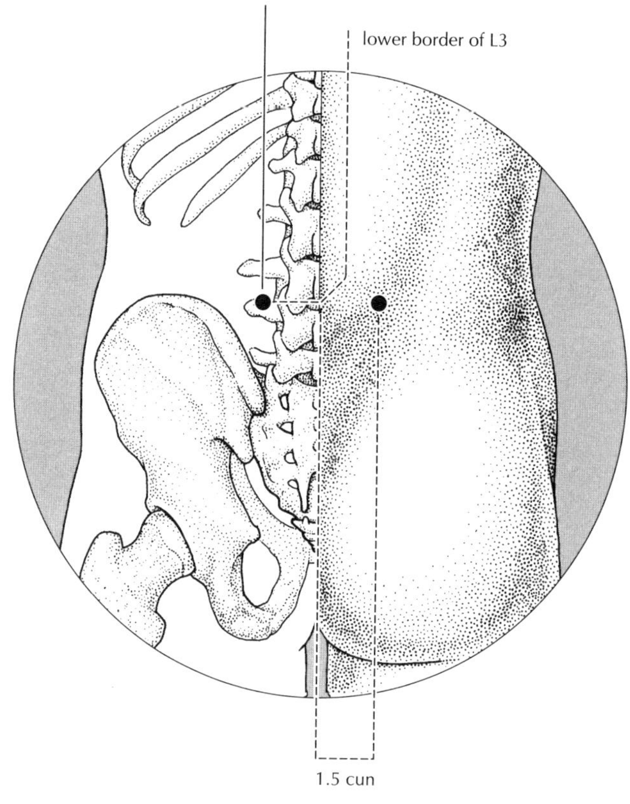

INDICATIONS

- Lumbar pain and stiffness, painful obstruction and pain of the lower limb, atrophy disorder.
- Dysmenorrhoea, irregular menstruation, leucorrhoea.
- Haemorrhoids, bleeding haemorrhoids, diarrhoea, diarrhoea containing blood, abdominal pain.

COMMENTARY

Despite its evocative name 'Sea of Qi Shu', Qihaishu BL-24 is credited with no tonifying or qi regulating properties, and in clinical practice is mostly used (especially when tender) in the treatment of lumbar pain.

COMBINATIONS

- Lumbar pain: Qihaishu BL-24, Shenshu BL-23 and Zhonglushu BL-29 (*Supplementing Life*).

DACHANGSHU BL-25

Large Intestine Shu

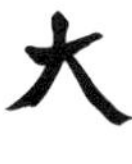
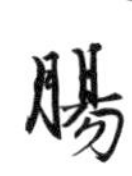
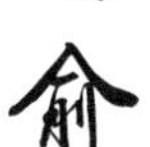

Back-Shu point of the Large Intestine

LOCATION

1.5 cun lateral to the lower border of the spinous process of the fourth lumbar vertebra (L4).

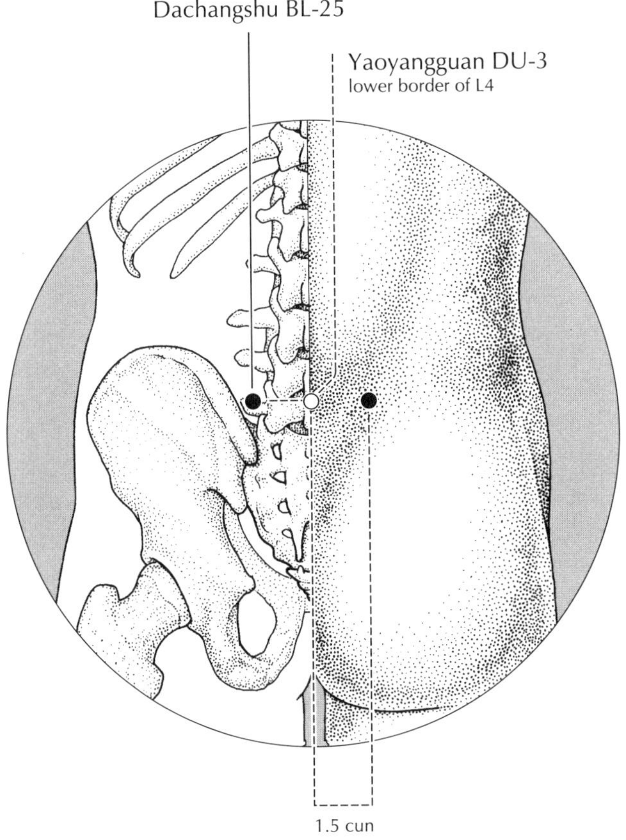

LOCATION NOTE
Locate at the visible highest point of the paraspinal muscles.

NEEDLING
Perpendicular insertion 1 to 1.5 cun.

ACTIONS
Regulates the intestines
Transforms stagnation and alleviates pain
Strengthens the lumbar region and legs

INDICATIONS
- Borborygmus, cold or damp (dong) diarrhoea, undigested food (in the stool), dysenteric disorder, blood in the stool, intestinal abscess, difficulty in urination and defecation, constipation, prolapse of the rectum.
- Distention and pain of the abdomen, hypogastric pain, distention and fullness of the hypogastrium, twisting pain of the lower abdomen, cutting pain of the umbilical region, inability to eat and drink, remains thin despite much eating.
- Lumbar pain, stiffness and rigidity of the lumbar spine, pain and painful obstruction of the lower limbs, atrophy disorder, dysmenorrhoea.

COMMENTARY
Dachangshu BL-25 is the back-shu point of the Large Intestine, where the qi of the Large Intestine emanates from the interior to the body surface. It is an important point to regulate the function of the Large Intestine fu, and its application is very broad.

When the Spleen is deficient or suffers from dampness, there may be loose stools, diarrhoea, undigested food in the stool, blood in the stools, borborygmus and inability to gain weight despite eating copiously. In combination with points that tonify the Spleen and Stomach, Dachangshu BL-25 is an important point to firm and tonify the intestines. When there is stagnation (of qi, blood, damp-heat, toxic heat etc.) in the intestinal region, there will be distention, pain, cutting pain, fullness, constipation, intestinal abscess etc. In combination with other suitable points, Dachangshu BL-25 is able to regulate qi and dissipate stagnation. When the central qi is deficient, or when damp-heat sinks downwards, there may be prolapse of the rectum. Dachangshu BL-25 is a valuable adjacent point used in the treatment of this disorder, in combination with points such as Baihui DU-20 and Chengqiang DU-1, as well as points which treat the underlying disharmony.

Finally Dachangshu BL-25 is an important local point in the treatment of lumbar pain, and like many points of the lower lumbar region is also indicated for painful obstruction and atrophy disorder of the lower limbs.

COMBINATIONS
- Cold or damp (dong) diarrhoea with undigested food: Dachangshu BL-25 and Shenshu BL-23 (*Supplementing Life*).
- Undigested food (in the stool): Dachangshu BL-25, Liangmen ST-21, Zusanli ST-36, Sanyinjiao SP-6, Xiawan REN-10, Sanjiaoshu BL-22 and Xuanshu DU-5 (*Supplementing Life*).
- Incontinence of faeces: Dachangshu BL-25 and Guanyuan REN-4 (*Great Compendium*).
- Borborygmus: Dachangshu BL-25, Taibai SP-3, Gongsun SP-4 and Sanjiaoshu BL-22 (*Supplementing Life*).
- Prolapse of the rectum: Dachangshu BL-25, Baihui DU-20, Changqiang DU-1, Jianjing GB-21, Hegu L.I.-4 and Qichong ST-30 (*Compilation*).
- Prolapse of the rectum in children: Dachangshu BL-25, Baihui DU-20 and Changqiang DU-1 (*Great Compendium*).
- Pain of intestinal abscess: Dachangshu BL-25, Xiangu ST-43 and Taibai SP-3 (*Great Compendium*).
- Difficult ingestion with desire to drink fluids: Dachangshu BL-25 and Zhourong SP-20 (*Thousand Ducat Formulas*).

GUANYUANSHU BL-26

Gate of Origin Shu

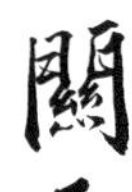
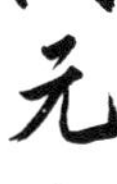
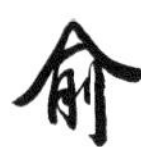

LOCATION

1.5 cun lateral to the lower border of the spinous process of the fifth lumbar vertebra (L5).

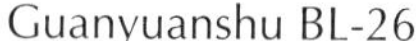

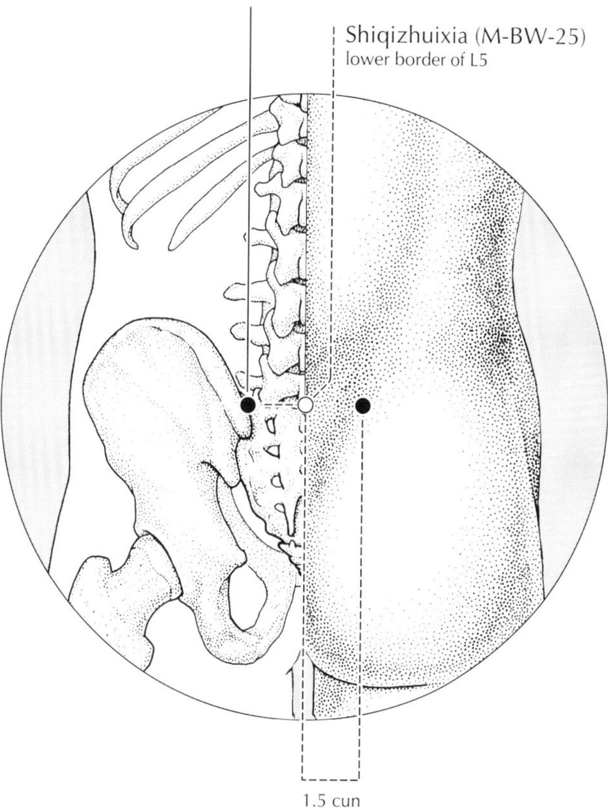

LOCATION NOTE

Locate at the visible highest point of the paraspinal muscles.

NEEDLING

Perpendicular insertion 1 to 1.5 cun.

ACTIONS

Strengthens the lumbar region
Regulates the lower jiao

INDICATIONS

- Lumbar pain, wind-taxation lumbar pain.
- Abdominal distention, deficiency distention, abdominal (jia ju) masses in women, diarrhoea, constipation.
- Enuresis, frequent urination, difficult urination, wasting and thirsting disorder.

COMMENTARY

Guanyuanshu BL-26, due to its proximity to the fifth lumbar vertebra, is much used in the treatment of lumbar pain. Various classics of Chinese medicine have specified the use of this point in the treatment of 'wind-taxation' lumbar pain i.e. lumbar pain due to attack and injury by exterior pathogenic factors which lodge in the back and over time lead to deficiency. This is a common development of back pain due to painful obstruction and reflects the fact that not only can Kidney deficiency lead to weakness of the back and hence invasion of exterior pathogens, but also that prolonged retention of pathogenic factors, especially when the bones are injured, can weaken the Kidneys. Thus *Standards of Patterns and Treatment*[47] said "[In back ache] wind, damp, cold, heat, sprain, blood stasis, stagnation of qi, accumulations are all the manifestation; the root is always Kidney deficiency", whilst the *Essential Questions*[48] stated "In chronic bone painful obstruction where the pathogenic factor repeatedly attacks, it will reach and reside in the Kidneys". The action of Guanyuanshu BL-26 on lumbar pain however, is so valuable that in clinical practice it may be used for any pattern, not solely deficiency, and it is one of the points that should be palpated, and needled if tender, in all cases of backache.

The tonifying action of Guanyuanshu BL-26 is implied in its name 'Gate of Origin Shu'. It is further indicated for such deficiency disorders as wasting and thirsting disorder, deficiency distention, diarrhoea and various urinary disorders, all characterised by deficiency of the Kidneys.

COMBINATIONS

- Wind-taxation lumbar pain: Guanyuanshu BL-26 and Pangguangshu BL-28 (*Supplementing Life*).

XIAOCHANGSHU BL-27

Small Intestine Shu

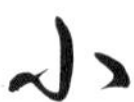
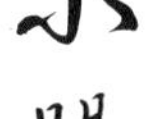
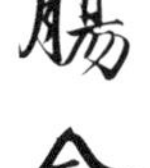
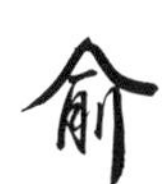

Back-Shu point of the Small Intestine

LOCATION

1.5 cun lateral to the midline, at the level of the first posterior sacral foramen.

LOCATION NOTE

i. As the inner line of the Bladder channel on the back descends towards the sacrum, it runs closer to the midline; the 1.5 cun measurement in this area, therefore, will be relatively shorter; ii. For guidance on locating the sacral foramen see page 69.

NEEDLING

Perpendicular insertion 0.5 to 1 cun.

ACTIONS

Separates the pure from the turbid
Regulates the intestines and Bladder
Drains turbid dampness and clears damp-heat
Regulates Small Intestine qi

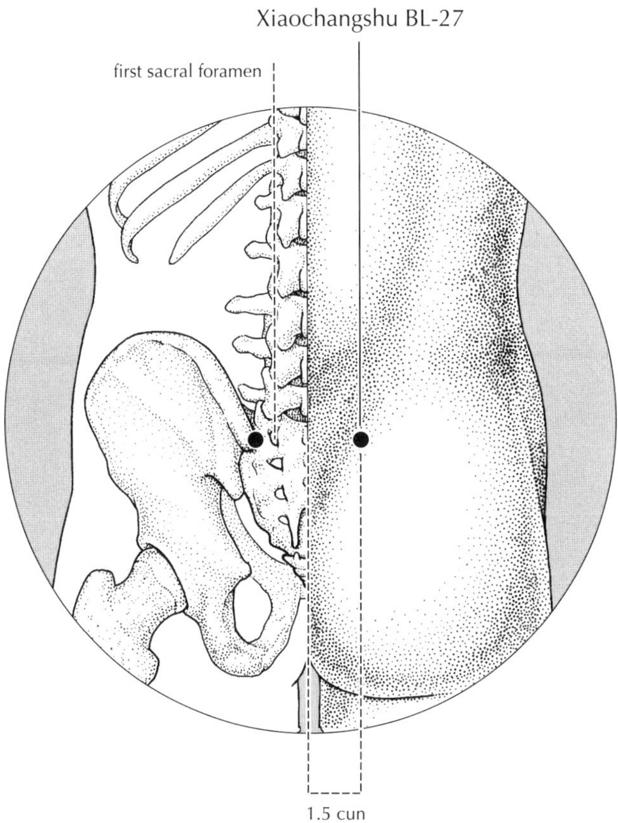

INDICATIONS

- Diarrhoea, dysenteric disorder, blood and mucus in the stools, haemorrhoids, pain of haemorrhoids, constipation.
- Dark yellow urine, enuresis, retention of urine, difficult urination and defecation, blood in the urine, leucorrhoea, seminal emission.
- Lower abdominal pain, painful shan disorder, testicular pain that radiates to the lumbar region.
- Wasting and thirsting disorder, dry mouth that is hard to endure, agitation of the Heart with shortness of breath, swollen feet.

COMMENTARY

Xiaochangshu BL-27 is the back-shu point of the Small Intestine fu, where the qi of the Small Intestine emanates from the interior to the body surface. According to *Introduction to Medicine* by Li Ting of the Ming dynasty "The Small Intestine separates the pure from the turbid; the water enters the upper opening of the Bladder and the dregs enter the upper opening of the Large Intestine". This quotation emphasises the role of the Small Intestine as an intermediary between the Stomach which 'rots and ripens' solid and liquid food, and the Large Intestine and Bladder which eliminate solid and liquid waste respectively. It is the Small Intestine which controls this process of separating the pure from the turbid. Although Xiaochangshu BL-27 is the back-shu point of the Small Intestine fu, therefore, its clinical action extends both to the Large Intestine and the Bladder.

In intestinal disorders it primarily drains turbid dampness and clears damp-heat and can be used in the treatment of diarrhoea, dysenteric disorder and blood and mucus in the stools due to this aetiology. Xiaochangshu BL-27 may also be used for constipation, and for haemorrhoids and accompanying pain.

In disorders of the Bladder it also drains dampness and damp-heat and clears heat transmitted from the Heart (interiorly-exteriorly coupled with the Small Intestine), being indicated in the treatment of dark yellow urine, enuresis, retention of urine, blood in the urine and agitation of the Heart. Following the principle that dampness and damp-heat may be drained from the body via urination, Xiaochangshu BL-27 is also indicated for damp-heat affecting other portions of the lower jiao with symptoms such as leucorrhoea and seminal emission. If damp-heat sinks to the lower limbs there may be swelling of the feet.

Finally, Xiaochangshu BL-27 may be used in the treatment of the pattern of Small Intestine qi pain. This form of painful shan disorder which may arise due to improper diet, stagnation of Liver qi or exposure to cold, leads to obstruction in the circulation of qi in the Small Intestine. Its characteristic symptoms are lower abdominal pain or testicular pain that may radiate to the lumbar region.

COMBINATIONS

- Difficult urination and defecation, dribbling and retention of urine: Xiaochangshu BL-27 and Changqiang DU-1 (*Thousand Ducat Formulas*).
- Dark urine: Xiaochangshu BL-27, Pangguangshu BL-28, Wangu SI-4, Baihuanshu BL-30 and Yanggang BL-48 (*Supplementing Life*).
- Dark urine: Xiaochangshu BL-27, Yanggang BL-48, Wangu GB-12 and Baihuanshu BL-30 (*Thousand Ducat Formulas*).
- Borborygmus, abdominal distention and watery diarrhoea: Xiaochangshu BL-27, Sanjiaoshu BL-22, Xialiao BL-34, Yishe BL-49 and Zhangmen LIV-13 (*Thousand Ducat Formulas*).
- Shan disorder with lumbar pain: Xiaochangshu BL-27, Zhonglushu BL-29 and Baihuanshu BL-30 (*Thousand Ducat Formulas*).

PANGGUANGSHU BL-28

Bladder Shu

膀胱俞

Back-Shu point of the Bladder

LOCATION

1.5 cun lateral to the midline, at the level of the second posterior sacral foramen.

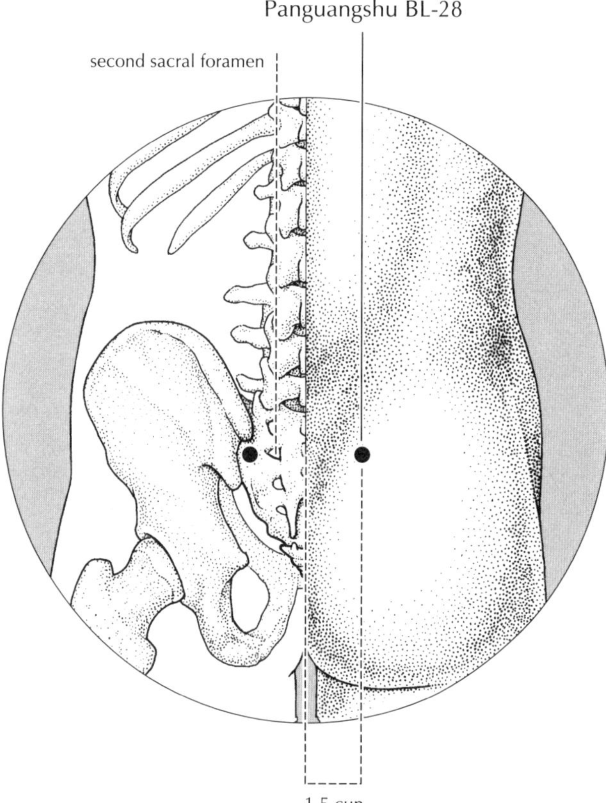

LOCATION NOTE

i. As the inner line of the Bladder channel on the back descends towards the sacrum, it runs closer to the midline; the 1.5 cun measurement in this area, therefore, will be relatively shorter; ii. For guidance on locating the sacral foramen see page 69.

NEEDLING

Perpendicular insertion 0.5 to 1 cun.

ACTIONS

Regulates the Bladder
Clears damp-heat from the lower jiao
Dispels stagnation and resolves masses
Benefits the lumbar region and legs

INDICATIONS

- Difficult urination, dark urination with unsmooth flow, retention of urine, enuresis, turbid painful urinary dysfunction.
- Seminal emission, swelling and pain of the external genitals, genital ulceration, damp itching, swelling and pain of the vagina, deficiency swelling of the penis.
- Diarrhoea, diarrhoea with abdominal pain, difficult defecation, constipation, abdominal fullness, abdominal (jia ju) masses in women, hard abdominal (ji ju) masses, wasting and thirsting disorder, diminished qi.
- Stiffness and pain of the sacrum and coccyx, stiffness and pain of the lumbar spine that radiates to the hypogastrium, difficulty in bending, wind-taxation lumbar stiffness and pain, stiffness and pain of the lower spine and buttock, inability to sit for long, weakness of the leg and knee, cold and contraction of the lower leg, numbness of the leg, atrophy disorder and heaviness of the leg, sciatica.

COMMENTARY

Pangguangshu BL-28 is the back-shu point of the Bladder fu, where the qi of the Bladder emanates from the interior to the body surface. Its principal action is to drain damp-heat excess from the Bladder and genital system. Bladder damp-heat may be due to: i. invasion of exterior pathogenic factors (damp-heat or cold damp which transforms to heat), especially as a result of inadequate clothing or sitting on damp ground; ii. excessive consumption of foods that generate damp-heat (spicy, greasy, sweet, alcohol etc.); iii. Heart fire which transmits downwards via the Small Intestine to the Bladder; iv. Liver damp-heat which pours downwards to the Bladder; or v. excessive sexual activity or inadequate hygiene. Bladder damp-heat typically manifests as painful, difficult, hesitant and frequent urination with scanty dark flow. As the Bladder back-shu point, Pangguangshu BL-28 has a direct action on the Bladder fu and is not only a vital point to drain Bladder damp-heat but is more widely used for any kind of urinary disorder.

The use of Pangguangshu BL-28 is not confined to the Bladder however. It is an important treatment principle of Chinese medicine that damp-heat anywhere in the body, and most especially in the lower jiao, is best eliminated by draining via urination. Pangguangshu BL-28, by its action of promoting urination, is therefore indicated for damp-heat affecting i. the intestinal region giving rise to diarrhoea, and ii. the genital region giving rise to such symptoms as swelling and pain of the external genitals, genital ulceration and damp itching, swelling and pain of the vagina etc.

A second important action of Pangguangshu BL-28 is in

the treatment of a variety of disorders of the lumbar region, sacrum, buttocks, and coccyx as well as the lower limbs, and it may equally be used for excess or deficient disorders of these regions. It is classically indicated for the treatment of 'wind-taxation' lumbar pain (for a fuller discussion see Guanyuanshu BL-26), as well as for weakness of the leg and knee, seminal emission and diminished qi. These indications reflect the fact that as the back-shu point of the Bladder, Pangguangshu BL-28 has some action of strengthening the Kidneys. As far as excess disorders of the lumbar region and legs are concerned, it is especially indicated for back pain, atrophy disorder and heaviness of the legs due to damp-heat.

Finally Pangguangshu BL-28 is able to resolve stagnation in the lower abdomen (abdominal pain, difficult defecation, constipation, abdominal fullness) and to resolve abdominal (jia ju) masses in women as well as hard abdominal (ji ju) masses.

COMBINATIONS

- Enuresis: Pangguangshu BL-28, Tongli HE-5, Dadun LIV-1, Jimen SP-11, Taichong LIV-3, Weizhong BL-40 and Shenmen HE-7 (*Supplementing Life*).
- Dark urine: Pangguangshu BL-28, Wangu GB-12, Xiaochangshu BL-27 and Baihuanshu BL-30 (*Thousand Ducat Formulas*).
- Dark urine: Pangguangshu BL-28, Taixi KID-3, Yingu KID-10, Shenshu BL-23, Qihai REN-6 and Guanyuan REN-4 (*Great Compendium*).
- Spleen deficiency with undigested food (in the stool): Pangguangshu BL-28 and Pishu BL-20 (*One Hundred Symptoms*).
- Difficulty in defecation with abdominal pain: Pangguangshu BL-28 and Shiguan KID-18 (*Supplementing Life*).
- Prolapse of the rectum: Pangguangshu BL-28, Shenque REN-8 and Baihui DU-20 (*Compilation*).
- Wind-taxation lumbar pain: Pangguangshu BL-28 and Guanyuanshu BL-26 (*Supplementing Life*).
- Stiffness and pain of the lumbar region: Pangguangshu BL-28, Xiaochangshu BL-27, Weizhong BL-40, Yaoshu DU-2 and Yongquan KID-1 (*Great Compendium*).

ZHONGLUSHU BL-29

中
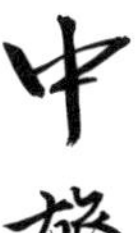
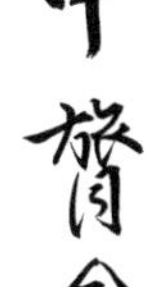

Mid-Spine Shu

LOCATION

1.5 cun lateral to the midline, at the level of the third posterior sacral foramen.

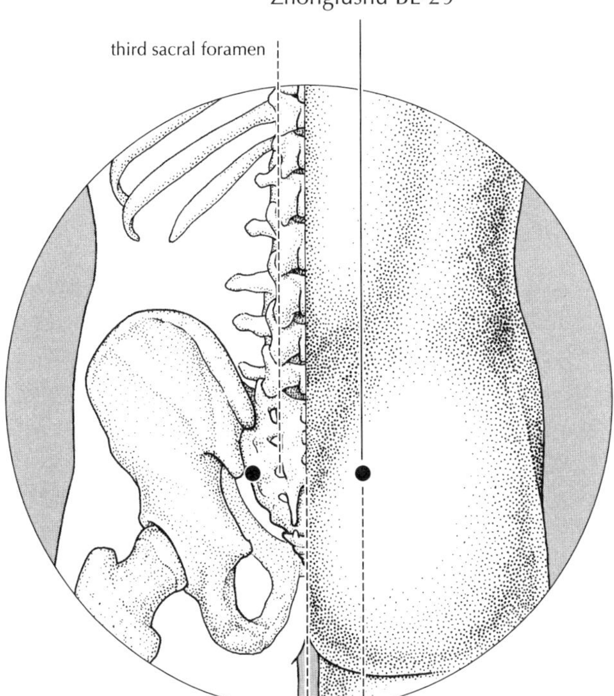

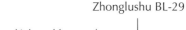

LOCATION NOTE

i. As the inner line of the Bladder channel on the back descends towards the sacrum, it runs closer to the midline; the 1.5 cun measurement in this area, therefore, will be relatively shorter; ii. For guidance on locating the sacral foramen see page 69.

NEEDLING

Perpendicular insertion 0.5 to 1 cun.

ACTIONS

Benefits the lumbar region
Dispels cold and stops diarrhoea

INDICATIONS

- Dysenteric disorder, cold in the intestines, shan disorder, abdominal distention, pain of the lateral costal region, Kidney deficiency wasting and thirsting disorder, absence of sweating.
- Stiffness and pain of the lumbar spine, inability to turn the spine.

COMBINATIONS

- Dysenteric disorder: Hegu L.I.-4 and Zusanli ST-36; if severe add Zhonglushu BL-29 (*Song of Points*).
- Lumbar pain: Zhonglushu BL-29, Shenshu BL-23 and Qihaishu BL-24 (*Supplementing Life*).

BAIHUANSHU BL-30

White Ring Shu

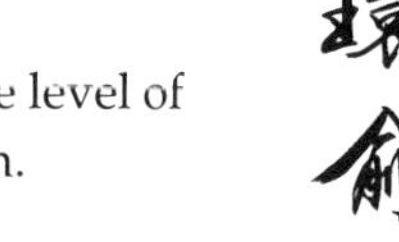

LOCATION

1.5 cun lateral to the midline, at the level of the fourth posterior sacral foramen.

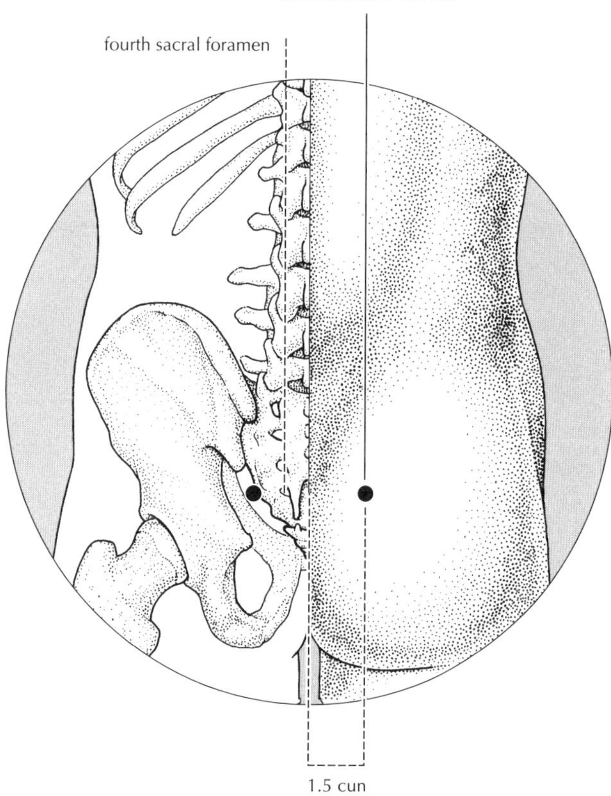

LOCATION NOTE

i. As the inner line of the Bladder channel on the back descends towards the sacrum, it runs closer to the midline; the 1.5 cun measurement in this area, therefore, will be relatively shorter; ii. For guidance on locating the sacral foramen see page 69.

NEEDLING

Perpendicular insertion 0.5 to 1 cun. **Note**: some classical sources forbid moxibustion at this point.

ACTIONS

Benefits the lumbar region and legs
Regulates menstruation
Stops leucorrhoea and seminal emission

INDICATIONS

- Pain of the lumbar spine and sacrum, lumbar pain due to cold, pain of the lumbar region and hip, pain of the coccyx, difficulty in sitting and standing, debility of the leg and knee, contracted sinews associated with painful obstruction.
- Irregular menstruation, dysmenorrhoea, uterine bleeding, infertility.
- Seminal emission, seminal emission with dreams, red and white leucorrhoea, difficult defecation and urination, prolapse of the rectum, dark urine, white turbidity, shan disorder, warm malaria.

COMMENTARY

Baihuanshu BL-30 is primarily used as a local point to activate the circulation of qi and treat pain of the lumbar region and sacrum, pain of the lumbar region and hip, and especially pain of the coccyx.

In common with many points located on the sacrum (see Ciliao BL-32) Baihuanshu BL-30 is also able to regulate the function of the uterus and genito-urinary system. It is specifically indicated for stopping leakage in the form of seminal emission and nocturnal emission, leucorrhoea and white turbid urine.

COMBINATIONS

- Back pain extending to the lumbar region: Baihuanshu BL-30 and Weizhong BL-40 (*One Hundred Symptoms*).
- Lumbar pain due to Kidney deficiency: Baihuanshu BL-30, Shenshu BL-23, Weizhong BL-40 and Taixi KID-3 (*Great Compendium*).
- Red and white leucorrhoea: Baihuanshu BL-30, Daimai GB-26, Guanyuan REN-4, Qihai REN-6, Sanyinjiao SP-6 and Jianshi P-5 (*Great Compendium*).

SHANGLIAO BL-31

Upper Crevice

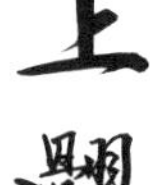

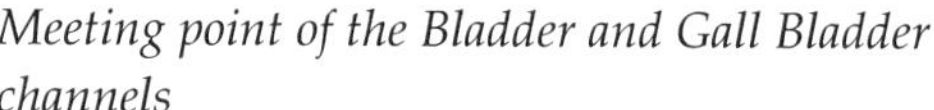

Meeting point of the Bladder and Gall Bladder channels

LOCATION

Over the first posterior sacral foramen.

LOCATION NOTE

For guidance on locating the sacral foramen see page 69.

NEEDLING

Perpendicular insertion 0.5 to 1 cun, or 1.5 to 2 cun through the foramen. Needling through the foramen is facilitated by a slightly oblique medial and inferior insertion.
Note: some classical sources forbid moxibustion at this point.

ACTIONS

Regulates the lower jiao and facilitates urination and defecation
Regulates menstruation and stops leucorrhoea
Benefits the lumbar region and legs

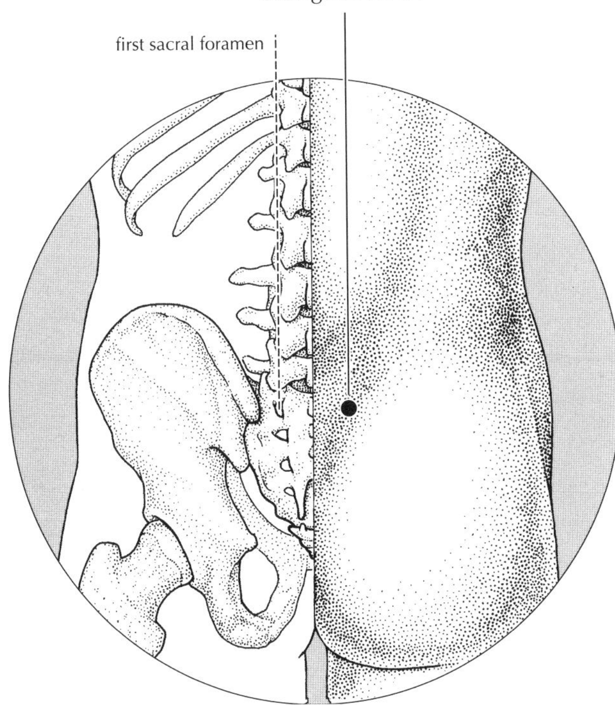

INDICATIONS

- Difficult urination and defecation.
- Irregular menstruation, dysmenorrhoea, infertility, leucorrhoea, incessant white leucorrhoea, red and white leucorrhoea, seminal emission, impotence, itching and pain of the genitals, uterine prolapse.
- Vomiting, nosebleed, malarial chills and fever.
- Lumbar pain, cold and pain of the back and knees.

COMMENTARY

See Ciliao BL-32.

COMBINATIONS

- Difficult urination and defecation: moxa the eight liao (Shangliao BL-31, Ciliao BL-32, Zhongliao BL-33 and Xialiao BL-34 bilaterally) with one hundred cones (*Thousand Ducat Formulas*).
- Febrile disease with absence of sweating: Shangliao BL-31 and Kongzui LU-6 (*Systematic Classic*).

CILIAO BL-32

Second Crevice

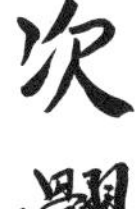

Meeting point of the Bladder and Gall Bladder channels

LOCATION

Over the second posterior sacral foramen.

LOCATION NOTE

For guidance on locating the sacral foramen see page 69.

NEEDLING

Perpendicular insertion 0.5 to 1 cun, or 1.5 to 2 cun through the foramen. Needling through the foramen is facilitated by a slightly oblique medial and inferior insertion.

ACTIONS

Regulates the lower jiao and facilitates urination and defecation
Regulates menstruation and stops leucorrhoea
Benefits the lumbar region and legs

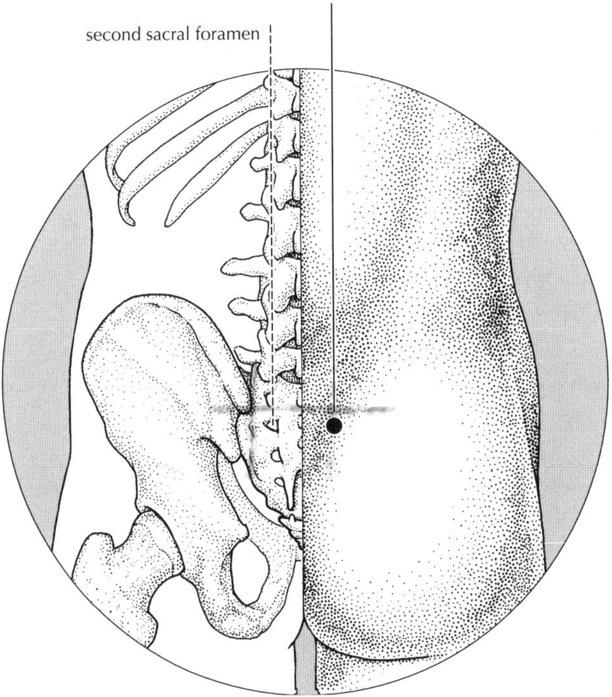

INDICATIONS

- Painful urinary dysfunction, dark urine, retention of urine, enuresis, difficulty in urination and defecation, constipation, borborygmus, watery diarrhoea, shan disorder, hardness and distention below the Heart.

- Red and white leucorrhoea, dysmenorrhoea, irregular menstruation, infertility, pain of childbirth.
- Lumbar pain, sacral pain, numbness of the lumbar region extending down to the feet, cold sensation of the lumbar region, lumbar pain radiating to the genitals, sciatica, pain and painful obstruction of the lower limb, hemiplegia.

COMMENTARY

The points Shangliao BL-31, Ciliao BL-32, Zhongliao BL-33 and Xialiao BL-34 are often considered as a group and are known as Baliao (Eight Crevices). In terms of their actions and indications they are very similar, sharing the common characteristics of regulating various disorders of the lower jiao, specifically: i. The urinary system. Ciliao BL-32 and to a lesser extent Zhongliao BL-33 are the strongest in their action on the urinary system, being indicated for such disorders as painful urinary dysfunction, retention of urine, difficult urination, enuresis etc. ii. The intestines. All four points treat difficult defecation, whilst Xialiao BL-34 has the widest action on the intestines, being indicated in the *Great Compendium of Acupuncture and Moxibustion* for "borborygmus and diarrhoea, internal injury by damp and cold, blood in the stool, iii. Gynaecological disorders such as dysmenorrhoea, infertility, irregular menstruation and leucorrhoea as well as disorders of the genitals for which Xialiao BL-34 is the strongest (swelling and pain, incessant green leucorrhoea with vaginal pain, pain of the testicles); iv. Invigorating the flow of qi and blood in the channels and collaterals of the local area and lower limbs, with Ciliao BL-32 and Zhongliao BL-33 having the strongest action in their ability to treat disorders such as lumbar pain, sacral pain, atrophy disorder and painful obstruction of the lower limbs etc.

Zhongliao BL-33 is indicated for "the five taxations, the seven injuries and the six extremes", all forms of extreme exhaustion. This underlines a further aspect of the actions of the eight liao as a whole, which is to benefit, warm, firm and supplement the Kidneys, having amongst their indications impotence, infertility, seminal emission and incessant white leucorrhoea. All eight liao are specifically indicated for difficulty in urination and/or defecation. Kidney deficiency is an important underlying pattern for this disorder, which is frequently seen in elderly and weak patients. Sun Si-miao, for example, in the *Thousand Ducat Formulas* prescribed moxibustion at all eight liao for difficult urination and defecation.

In clinical practice, Ciliao BL-32 is the most commonly used of the four points, having the most wide-ranging indications. It is frequently used in the treatment of dysmenorrhoea which radiates to the sacral area, as well as for back pain during labour. To relieve labour pain, needling Ciliao BL-32 is often combined with electro-acupuncture. For this purpose the handle of the needle may be bent to 90 degrees and taped to the skin, allowing the woman to lie on her back.

COMBINATIONS

- Difficult urination and defecation: moxa the eight liao (Shangliao BL-31, Ciliao BL-32, Zhongliao BL-33 and Xialiao BL-34 bilaterally) with one hundred cones (*Thousand Ducat Formulas*).
- Infertility: Ciliao BL-32, Yongquan KID-1 and Shangqiu SP-5 (*Supplementing Life*).
- Pain of the lumbar region and aversion to cold: Ciliao BL-32, Baohuang BL-53 and Chengjin BL-56 (*Supplementing Life*).
- Rigidity of the lumbar spine with inability to turn: Ciliao BL-32 and Zhangmen LIV-13 (*Supplementing Life*).
- Sciatica: Ciliao BL-32, Chengfu BL-36, Zhibian BL-54, Weizhong BL-40 and Kunlun BL-60.

ZHONGLIAO BL-33

Middle Crevice

中髎

Meeting point of the Bladder and Gall Bladder channels

LOCATION

Over the third posterior sacral foramen.

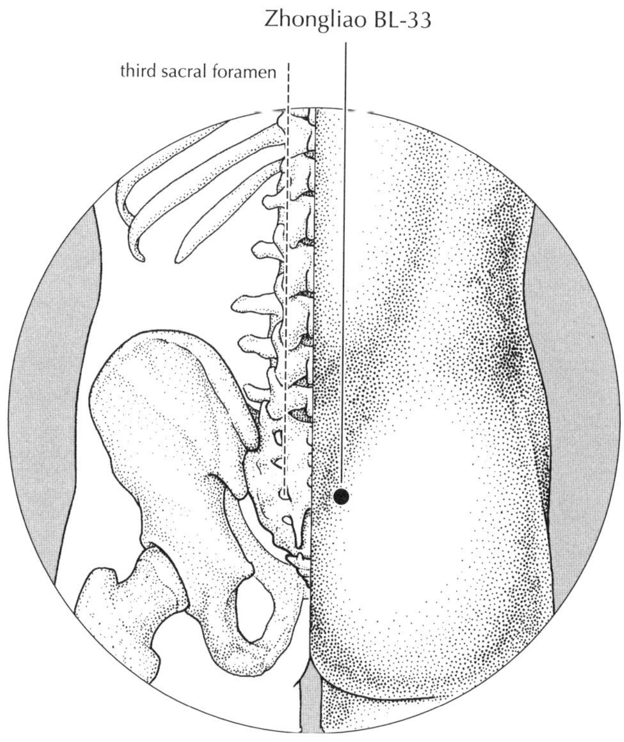

LOCATION NOTE
For guidance on locating the sacral foramen see page 69.

NEEDLING
Perpendicular insertion 0.5 to 1 cun, or 1.5 to 2 cun through the foramen.

ACTIONS
Regulates the lower jiao and facilitates urination and defecation
Regulates menstruation and stops leucorrhoea
Benefits the lumbar region and legs

INDICATIONS
- Difficult urination and defecation, constipation, diarrhoea containing undigested food, retention of urine, painful urinary dysfunction, abdominal distention.
- Leucorrhoea, irregular menstruation, scanty menstruation, infertility.
- Lumbar pain, pain and cold of the sacrum and coccyx, cold sensation of the buttocks, atrophy disorder and painful obstruction of the lower limb.
- The five taxations, the seven injuries and the six extremes.

COMMENTARY
See Ciliao BL-32.

COMBINATIONS
- Difficulty in defecation: Zhongliao BL-33, Shimen REN-5, Chengshan BL-57, Taichong LIV-3, Zhongwan REN-12, Taixi KID-3, Dazhong KID-4 and Chengjin BL-56 (*Thousand Ducat Formulas*).
- Dribbling urination: Zhongliao BL-33, Weiyang BL-39 and Zhishi BL-52 (*Supplementing Life*).

XIALIAO BL-34
下髎
Lower Crevice

Meeting point of the Bladder, and Gall Bladder channels

LOCATION
Over the fourth posterior sacral foramen.

LOCATION NOTE
For guidance on locating the sacral foramen see page 69.

NEEDLING
Perpendicular insertion 0.5 to 1 cun, or 1.5 to 2 cun through the foramen.

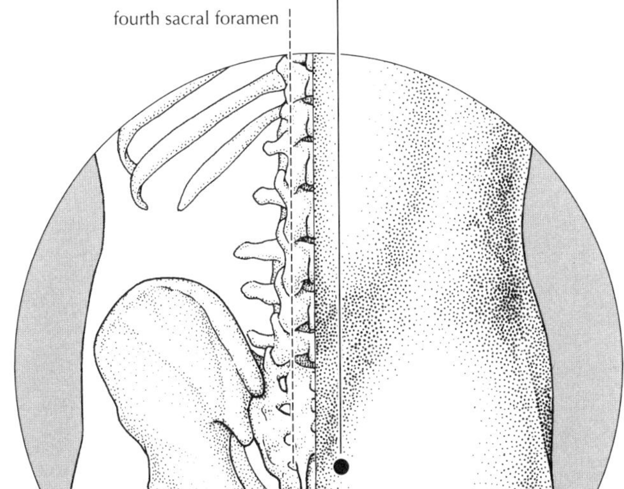

ACTIONS
Regulates the lower jiao and facilitates urination and defecation
Regulates menstruation and stops leucorrhoea
Benefits the lumbar region and legs

INDICATIONS
- Lower abdominal pain, borborygmus, diarrhoea, difficult defecation, constipation, blood in the stool, difficult urination, painful urinary dysfunction, shan disorder.
- Dysmenorrhoea, itching, swelling and pain of the genitals, incessant green leucorrhoea leading to vaginal pain and pain radiating to the lower abdomen.
- Pain of the sacrum and coccyx, lumbar pain, lumbar pain radiating to the testicles.

COMMENTARY
See Ciliao BL-32.

COMBINATIONS
- Borborygmus, abdominal distention and watery diarrhoea: Xialiao BL-34, Sanjiaoshu BL-22, Xiaochangshu BL-27, Yishe BL-49 and Zhangmen LIV-13 (*Thousand Ducat Formulas*).

HUIYANG BL-35

會陽

Meeting of Yang

LOCATION

0.5 cun lateral to the Governing vessel, level with the tip of the coccyx.

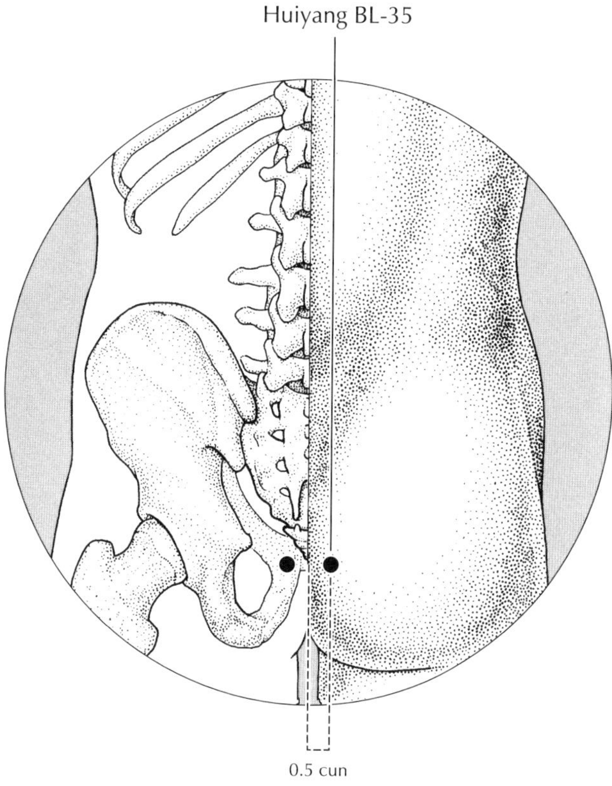

NEEDLING

Perpendicular insertion 1 to 1.5 cun.

ACTIONS

Clears damp-heat and regulates the lower jiao
Benefits the coccyx and treats haemorrhoids

INDICATIONS

- Diarrhoea, dysenteric disorder, blood in the stool, chronic haemorrhoids, prolapse of the rectum, itching of the genitals, sweating of the genitals, leucorrhoea.
- Pain of the coccyx, pain of the lumbar region and leg.
- Yang qi deficiency, impotence, cold abdomen.

COMBINATIONS

- Cold abdomen: Huiyang BL-35 and Lougu SP-7 (*Supplementing Life*).

CHENGFU BL-36

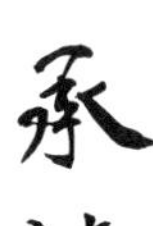

Hold and Support

LOCATION

Just below the buttock, on a line directly superior to Weizhong BL-40, in the centre of the transverse gluteal crease in a depression between the hamstring muscles.

NEEDLING

Perpendicular insertion 1 to 2 cun.

ACTIONS

Activates the channel, relaxes the sinews and alleviates pain
Regulates the lower jiao and alleviates pain
Treats haemorrhoids

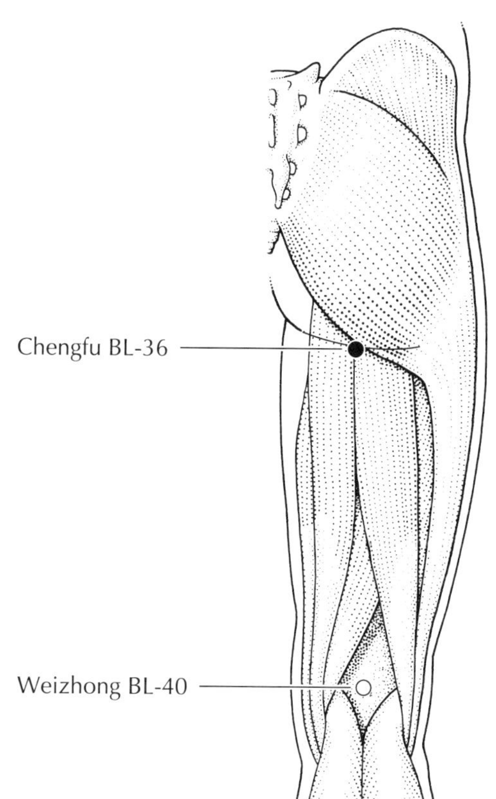

INDICATIONS

- Lumbar pain, pain of the sacrum and coccyx, pain of the buttock, sciatica, painful obstruction and atrophy disorder of the lower limb.
- Difficult defecation, difficult urination, pain of the genitals, seminal emission, cold in the uterus, swelling of the axilla.
- Chronic haemorrhoids, bleeding haemorrhoids.

COMMENTARY

Chengfu BL-36 is much used for pain radiating down the Bladder channel from the lumbar region and buttock. It is especially indicated for pain of the buttocks and sciatic pain that is aggravated by sitting. Its secondary application is as an adjacent point in the treatment of haemorrhoids.

COMBINATIONS

- Difficult urination and seminal emission: Chengfu BL-36, Lougu SP-7, Zhongji REN-3, Ligou LIV-5 and Zhiyin BL-67 (*Supplementing Life*).
- Haemorrhoids, swelling of the axilla: Chengfu BL-36, Chengjin BL-56, Weizhong BL-40 and Yanggu SI-5 (*Thousand Ducat Formulas*).
- Sciatica: Chengfu BL-36, Ciliao BL-32, Zhibian BL-54, Weizhong BL-40 and Kunlun BL-60.

YINMEN BL-37

殷门

Gate of Abundance

LOCATION

On the back of the thigh, in the depression between the hamstring muscles, 6 cun distal to Chengfu BL-36, and 8 cun proximal to Weizhong BL-40, on the line connecting Chengfu BL-36 and Weizhong BL-40.

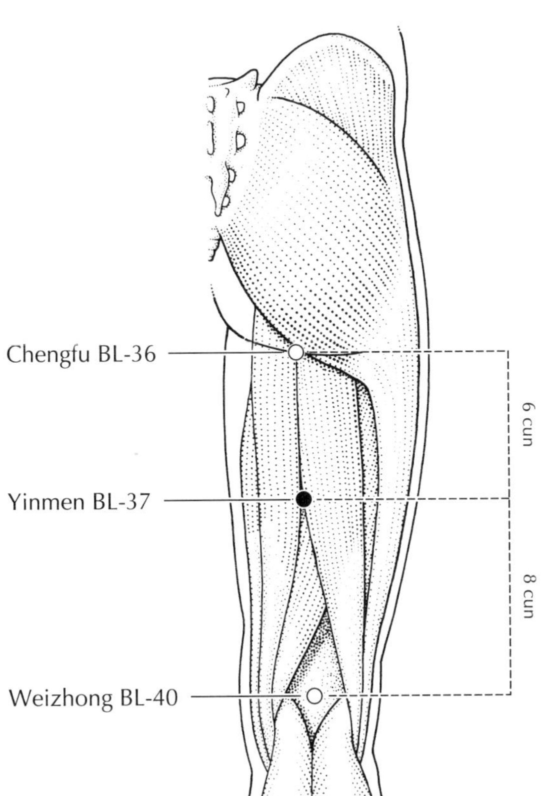

LOCATION NOTE

i. Locate two handbreadths distal to Chengfu BL-36; ii. Find the midpoint between Chengfu BL-36 and Weizhong BL-40 and locate Yinmen BL-37 in the depression 1 cun proximal to this.

NEEDLING

Perpendicular insertion 1 to 2 cun.

ACTIONS

Activates the channel and alleviates pain
Benefits the lumbar spine

INDICATIONS

- Pain and rigidity of the lumbar spine, sciatica, painful obstruction and atrophy disorder of the lower limb, pain of the thigh, swelling of the lateral thigh.
- Watery diarrhoea.

COMMENTARY

The point Yinmen BL-37 is frequently found to be tender on palpation in patients with sciatica, and is therefore commonly needled in the treatment of this condition. It is especially used when more proximal points such as Huantiao GB-30 or Zhibian BL-54 fail to elicit propagated sensation extending down the leg.

COMBINATIONS

- Lumbar pain with inability to bend and extend: Yinmen BL-37, Weiyang BL-39, Taibai SP-3, Yinlingquan SP-9 and Xingjian LIV-2 (*Thousand Ducat Formulas*).
- Sciatica: Yinmen BL-37, Dachangshu BL-25, Huantiao GB-30, Chengshan BL-57, Feiyang BL-58 and Sanyinjiao SP-6.

FUXI BL-38

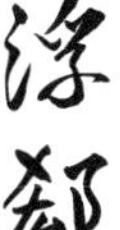
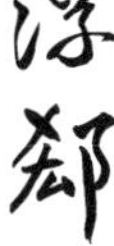

Floating Cleft

LOCATION

On the back of the knee, 1 cun superior to Weiyang BL-39, on the medial side of the tendon of biceps femoris.

LOCATION NOTE

Locate with the knee slightly flexed.

NEEDLING

Perpendicular insertion 1 to 1.5 cun.

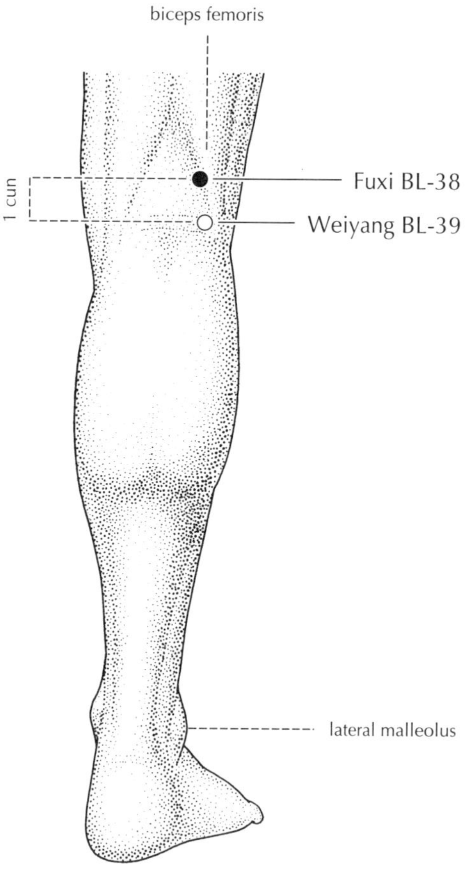

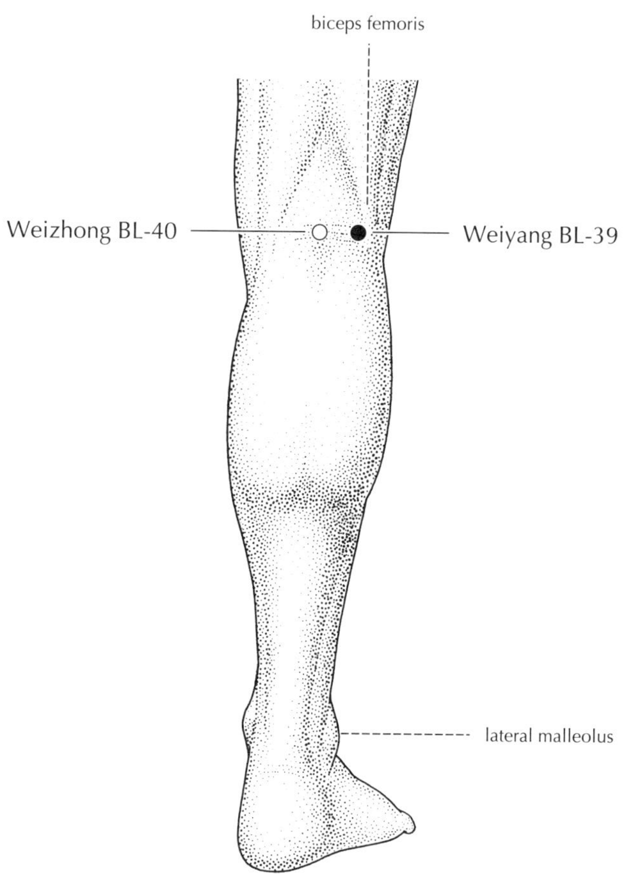

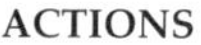

ACTIONS

Relaxes the sinews and alleviates pain
Clears heat and soothes contraction

INDICATIONS

- Numbness of the buttock, contraction of the sinews of the popliteal fossa, contraction and pain of the outer thigh, sudden turmoil disorder with cramps.
- Small Intestine heat, knotting of the Large Intestine, hot urination.

COMBINATIONS

- Heat of the lower abdomen and hard stools: Fuxi BL-38 and Zhongzhu KID-15 (*Great Compendium*).

WEIYANG BL-39

Outside of the Crook

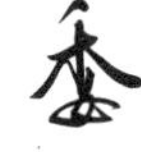

Lower He-Sea point of the Sanjiao

LOCATION

At the back of the knee, on the popliteal crease and towards its lateral end, in the depression medial to the tendon of biceps femoris.

LOCATION NOTE

Locate with the knee slightly flexed.

NEEDLING

Perpendicular insertion 1 to 1.5 cun.

ACTIONS

Harmonises the Sanjiao and regulates urination
Activates the channel and alleviates pain

INDICATIONS

- Difficult urination, retention of urine, painful urinary dysfunction, enuresis.
- Stiffness and pain of the lumbar spine, lumbar pain radiating to the abdomen, contraction and pain of the leg and foot.
- Fullness of the chest, pain and swelling of the axilla, distention and fullness of the lower abdomen, haemorrhoids, constipation.

COMMENTARY

The *Spiritual Pivot*[49] states "The he-sea points treat the internal fu". The three yang channels of the upper limb (Sanjiao, Large Intestine and Small Intestine) each have a he-sea point on their respective channel (Tianjing SJ-10,

Quchi L.I.-11 and Xiaohai SI-8). It is evident however, when one examines the indications for each of these points, that they have relatively little action on their related fu. This is not unexpected in view of the fact that whilst the channels are on the upper limb, in the case of the intestines, their associated fu are in the lower jiao. The same chapter of the *Spiritual Pivot* then goes on to rectify this contradiction by designating a lower he-sea point on the lower limb for each of the yang channels of the arm (Weiyang BL-39, Shangjuxu ST-37 and Xiajuxu ST-39 respectively).

Weiyang BL-39, as the lower he-sea point of the Sanjiao, has a specific action on the treatment of urinary disorders. The *Spiritual Pivot*[50] emphasises the close relationship between the Sanjiao, the Kidneys and the Bladder, and states that there is a direct link between Weiyang BL-39 and the Bladder fu. According to the *Essential Questions* "The Sanjiao is the official in charge of drainage and controls the water passages"[51], whilst the Ming dynasty classic *Introduction to Medicine* elaborated as follows "The lower jiao dominates moving and draining the urine and faeces, and at the right time discharging them ... therefore it is said the lower jiao is like a drain". The *Spiritual Pivot* says of Weiyang BL-39 "When excess there is retention of urine; when deficient there is enuresis; [when there is] enuresis, then reinforce, [when there is] retention then reduce"[52] and "In diseases of the Sanjiao [there will be] fullness of the abdomen, hardness of the lower abdomen with inability to urinate causing extreme anguish, water will overflow and give rise to oedema and abdominal distention ... select Weiyang BL-39"[53]. As the lower he-sea point of the Sanjiao on the Bladder channel, Weiyang BL-39 specifically acts on the qi transforming action of the Bladder (ultimately controlled by the Kidneys) and hence is an important point in the treatment of retention of urine or difficult urination as well as enuresis.

An interesting classical indication for this point is axillary pain and swelling. This may be explained either by the pathway of the Bladder sinew channel, or more pertinently as a symptom of the Sanjiao channel.

COMBINATIONS

- Hardness and pain in the lower abdomen that radiates to the genitals with inability to urinate: Weiyang BL-39, Shimen REN-5 and Yinjiao REN-7 (*Supplementing Life*).
- Dribbling urination: Weiyang BL-39, Zhishi BL-52 and Zhongliao BL-33 (*Supplementing Life*).
- Involuntary erection with difficult urination: Weiyang BL-39, Yingu KID-10, Dadun LIV-1, Qimen LIV-14 and Weizhong BL-40 (*Supplementing Life*).
- Swelling of the axilla: Weiyang BL-39 and Tianchi P-1 (*One Hundred Symptoms*).
- Swelling of the axilla: Weiyang BL-39, Tianchi P-1, Shenmai BL-62, Diwuhui GB-42, Yangfu GB-38 and Zulinqi GB-41 (*Thousand Ducat Formulas*).
- Lumbar pain with inability to bend and extend: Weiyang BL-39, Yinmen BL-37, Taibai SP-3, Yinlingquan SP-9 and Xingjian LIV-2 (*Thousand Ducat Formulas*).

WEIZHONG BL-40

Middle of the Crook

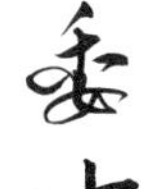

He-Sea and Earth point of the Bladder channel
Gao Wu Command point
Ma Dan-yang Heavenly Star point

LOCATION

At the back of the knee, on the popliteal crease, in a depression midway between the tendons of biceps femoris and semitendinosus.

LOCATION NOTE

Locate with the knee slightly flexed.

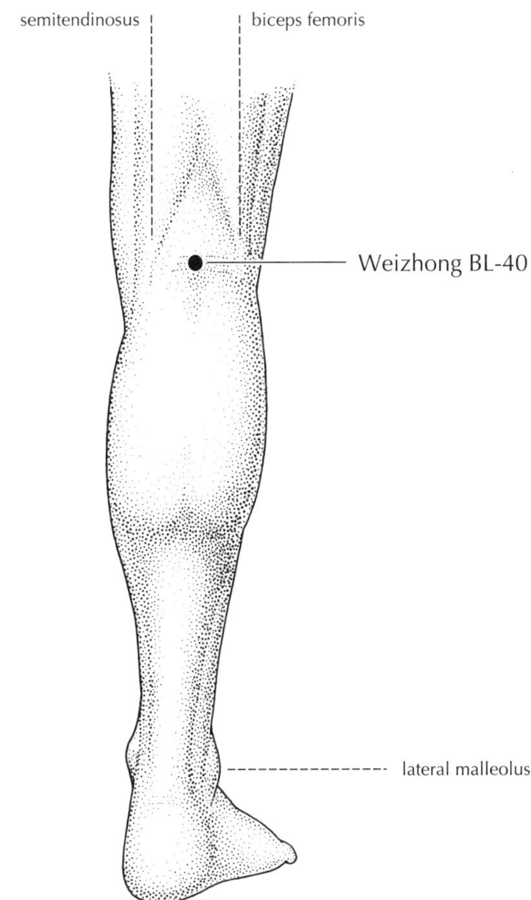

NEEDLING

Perpendicular insertion 1 to 1.5 cun, or prick and bleed the superficial veins.

Caution: the tibial nerve and the popliteal artery and vein lie deep to this point.

ACTIONS

Benefits the lumbar region and knees
Activates the channel and alleviates pain
Cools the blood
Clears summer-heat and stops vomiting and diarrhoea
Benefits the Bladder

INDICATIONS

- Pain and stiffness of the lumbar spine, heaviness of the lumbar region and buttock, cold sensation of the sacrum, coccyx and thigh, knee pain extending to the big toe, difficulty in flexing and extending the hip and knee joints, contraction of the sinews around the popliteal fossa, weakness of the legs, atrophy disorder and painful obstruction of the lower limb, wind painful obstruction, windstroke, hemiplegia.
- Injury by summer-heat, febrile disease with absence of sweating, injury by cold with heat of the four limbs, alternating chills and fever, malaria, ceaseless thirst, sudden turmoil disorder with abdominal pain, fullness of the lower abdomen, vomiting and diarrhoea, dysenteric disorder.
- Enuresis, difficult urination, dark urination, distention and pain of the hypogastrium.
- Nosebleed, pain of the lower teeth, headache, throat painful obstruction, epilepsy, haemorrhoid pain.
- Clove sores, erysipelas (cinnabar toxin), eczema, urticaria.

COMMENTARY

Weizhong BL-40 is the lower he-sea point of the Bladder channel and has long been considered one of the most important of the acupuncture points. According to Ma Dan-yang the great physician of the Jin dynasty, Weizhong BL-40 is one of the 'eleven heavenly star points'[54], indicated for "lumbar pain with inability to straighten up, severe lumbar pain that radiates up the back with pain and stiffness of the sinews and bones, wind painful obstruction that frequently recurs, and difficulty in stretching and bending the knee". The Ming dynasty author Gao Wu in the *Glorious Anthology of Acupuncture and Moxibustion* included it among his 'four command points' with a special action in the treatment of lumbar pain. Sun Si-miao in the *Thousand Ducat Formulas* says of Weizhong BL-40 "pain of the lumbar region and spine that almost reaches the head; in any case of heaviness and pain of the lumbar region and leg, bleed this point".

Weizhong BL-40 is equally effective for acute or chronic lumbar pain, whatever the aetiology, and for sciatic pain radiating down the Bladder channel, and is an important point for atrophy disorder and painful obstruction of the lower limb. In the case of acute lumbar sprain, Weizhong BL-40 may either be needled, or bled by the following method. The region of Weizhong BL-40 is examined (on the affected side if the sprain is unilateral and on both sides if bilateral). If dark and engorged blood vessels are seen at or around this point, the patient is asked to stand (resting their hands on the couch), the blood vessels are slapped to further engorge them and promote the flow of blood, then wiped with alcohol and quickly pricked to induce bleeding.

Weizhong BL-40 is also an important local point in the treatment of knee disorders, whether the location of the discomfort is at the back or the front of the knee, and needling at this point allows deep insertion into the joint.

An alternative name for Weizhong BL-40 used in a number of classics is Xue Xi, (Blood Xi-Cleft). According to the *Spiritual Pivot*[55] "taiyang channel is abundant in blood and limited in qi ... [it is thus suitable to] prick to bleed taiyang and drain blood ...". This not only explains the powerful effect of bleeding Weizhong BL-40 to move blood stasis in acute lumbar sprain, but also its ability to cool the blood in cases of nosebleed and a variety of skin disorders, in which case the point may also be bled. Interestingly, one of the other two channels abundant in blood and limited in qi according to the *Spiritual Pivot*[56] is the jueyin channel, and this may help to explain certain similarities between Weizhong BL-40 and Quze P-3, the he-sea point of the Pericardium jueyin channel. Both points (located in the flexure of the lower and upper limb respectively) are bled to clear heat from the blood level and are used in the treatment of summer-heat stroke, sudden turmoil disorder with heat of the four limbs, ceaseless thirst, vomiting and diarrhoea. As far as Weizhong BL-40 is concerned, not only is it indicated for fever due to summer-heat, but also for febrile disease with absence of sweating, injury by cold with heat of the four limbs, alternating chills and fever and malaria.

The *Spiritual Pivot*[57] states "When the disease is at the yang within yang (skin), needle the he-sea points of the yang channels". Whilst this is not a universally applicable principle, it is Quchi L.I.-11 and Weizhong BL-40, the he-sea points of the Large Intestine and Bladder channels, which are two of the most important points in the treatment of skin diseases. Weizhong BL-40 is indicated for erysipelas (cinnabar toxin), eczema and urticaria.

Relatively few points on the Bladder channel treat their related Bladder fu, notably Pangguangshu BL-28 (the back-shu point of the Bladder), Shenshu BL-23 (the back-shu point of the Kidneys), Weiyang BL-39 (the lower he-sea point of the Sanjiao) and points adjacent to the bladder on the lower back. Weizhong BL-40 itself is indicated for a variety of urinary disorders characterised by enuresis, difficult urination, dark urination, and distention and pain of the hypogastrium, and this may in part be explained by its close proximity to Weiyang BL-39.

The Bladder divergent channel separates from its primary channel at the popliteal fossa and ascends to wind around the anus. Weizhong BL-40 is indicated and included in classical combinations for the treatment of haemorrhoids, often in combination with Chengshan BL-57 which is considered the primary distal point for this purpose.

Finally, according to the *Essential Questions*[58] Weizhong BL-40 is one of the 'eight points for draining heat from the extremities' (although in fact only seven are listed) namely Yunmen LU-2, Jianyu L.I.-15, Weizhong BL-40 and Yaoshu DU-2.

COMBINATIONS

- Pain of the lumbar region and leg: Weizhong BL-40 and Renzhong DU-26 (*Great Compendium*).
- Pain of the lumbar spine: Weizhong BL-40 and Fuliu KID-7 (*Great Compendium*).
- Lumbar pain due to Kidney deficiency: Weizhong BL-40, Shenshu BL-23, Taixi KID-3 and Baihuanshu BL-30 (*Great Compendium*).
- Lumbar pain: Weizhong BL-40, Huantiao GB-30; if the pain radiates up the back add Kunlun BL-60 (*Song of Points*).
- Pain of the legs and lumbar region: Weizhong BL-40, Yinshi ST-33, Huantiao GB-30, Fengshi GB-31, Kunlun BL-60, Chengshan BL-57 and Shenmai BL-62 (*Great Compendium*).
- Lumbar pain with difficulty in moving: Weizhong BL-40, Fengshi GB-31 and Xingjian LIV-2 (*Glorious Anthology*).
- Stiffness and pain of the lumbar region: Weizhong BL-40, Yaoshu DU-2, Yongquan KID-1, Xiaochangshu BL-27 and Pangguangshu BL-28 (*Great Compendium*).
- Back pain extending to the lumbar region: Weizhong BL-40 and Baihuanshu BL-30 (*One Hundred Symptoms*).
- Pain of the lumbar region and lateral costal region due to sprain: Weizhong BL-40, Renzhong DU-26 and Chize LU-5 ... afterwards needle Kunlun BL-60, Shugu BL-65, Zhigou SJ-6 and Yanglingquan GB-34 (*Great Compendium*).
- Pain of the shoulder and back: Weizhong BL-40, Fengmen BL-12, Jianjing GB-21, Zhongzhu SJ-3, Zhigou SJ-6, Houxi SI-3 and Wangu SI-4 (*Great Compendium*).
- Pain of the chest and lateral costal region: Weizhong BL-40 [bleed] and Zhigou SJ-6 [reduce left Zhigou SJ-6 for right-sided pain and vice-versa] (*Classic of the Jade Dragon*).
- Wind damp painful obstruction: Weizhong BL-40 and Xialian L.I.-8 (*Supplementing Life*).
- Feebleness of the legs: Weizhong BL-40, Zusanli ST-36 and Chengshan BL-57 (*Great Compendium*).
- Redness, swelling and pain of the knees: Weizhong BL-40, Xiguan LIV-7, Yinshi ST-33 and Zusanli ST-36 (*Great Compendium*).
- The five types of haemorrhoids: Weizhong BL-40, Chengshan BL-57, Feiyang BL-58, Yangfu GB-38, Fuliu KID-7, Taichong LIV-3, Xiaxi GB-43, Qihai REN-6, Huiyin REN-1 and Changqiang DU-1 (*Great Compendium*).
- Haemorrhoids, swelling of the axilla: Weizhong BL-40, Chengjin BL-56, Chengfu BL-36 and Yanggu SI-5 (*Thousand Ducat Formulas*).
- Enuresis: Weizhong BL-40, Guanmen ST-22 and Shenmen HE-7 (*Systematic Classic*).
- Ceaseless nosebleed: Weizhong BL-40 and Chengjiang REN-24 (*Systematic Classic*).
- Severe and incessant nosebleed: Weizhong BL-40 and Yinbai SP-1 (*Supplementing Life*).

FUFEN BL-41

Attached Branch

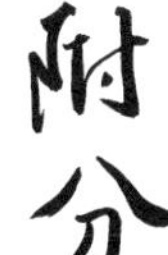

Meeting point of the Bladder and Small Intestine channels

LOCATION

3 cun lateral to the midline, level with the lower border of the spinous process of the second thoracic vertebra (T2) and level with Fengmen BL-12.

LOCATION NOTE

When the shoulder is relaxed, the three cun line corresponds to the medial border of the scapula.

NEEDLING

Oblique insertion 0.3 to 0.5 cun.
Caution: deep perpendicular or deep oblique needling in a medial direction carries a substantial risk of causing a pneumothorax.

ACTIONS

Activates the channel and alleviates pain
Expels wind and cold

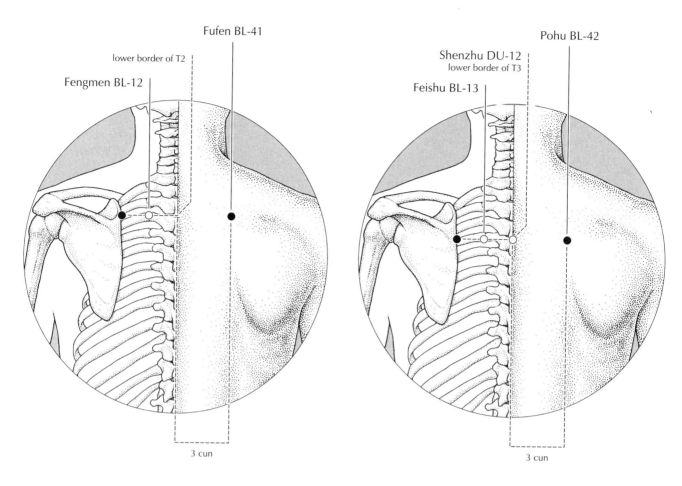

Fufen BL-41
lower border of T2
Fengmen BL-12
3 cun

Pohu BL-42
Shenzhu DU-12
lower border of T3
Feishu BL-13
3 cun

INDICATIONS

- Contraction of the shoulder, scapula and back, pain and stiffness of the neck, back pain radiating to the head, numbness of the elbow and upper arm.
- Wind-cold lodged in the interstices, wind-taxation.

POHU BL-42

Door of the Corporeal Soul

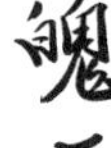

LOCATION

3 cun lateral to the midline, level with the lower border of the spinous process of the third thoracic vertebra (T3) and level with Feishu BL-13.

LOCATION NOTE

When the shoulder is relaxed, the three cun line corresponds to the medial border of the scapula.

NEEDLING

Oblique insertion 0.3 to 0.5 cun.

Caution: deep perpendicular or deep oblique needling in a medial direction carries a substantial risk of causing a pneumothorax.

ACTIONS

Tonifies and nourishes the Lung
Soothes dyspnoea and alleviates cough
Activates the channel and alleviates pain

INDICATIONS

- Lung atrophy, Lung consumption, deficiency-taxation, taxation cough with heat in the body, cough, asthma, dyspnoea, aversion to cold.
- Pain of the shoulder, scapula and back, pain of the chest and back, stiff neck.
- Vomiting with agitation and fullness, three corpse possession disorder, loss of consciousness.

COMMENTARY

Pohu BL-42 is located on the outer portion of the Bladder channel on the back at the level of Feishu BL-13, the back-shu point of the Lung. The name of this point (Door of the Corporeal Soul) suggests that it is effective in treating disorders of the corporeal soul (po) and emotional disorders related to Lung disharmony. In fact, with the exception of 'three corpse possession disorder', the classical indications of this point predominantly reflect its use in nourishing and tonifying the Lung. 'Three corpse possession disorder' is a Daoist concept that refers to some form of 'possession' and is divided into 'upper corpse' which attacks the eyes, 'middle corpse' which attacks the five zang, and 'lower corpse' which attacks human life itself.

The predominant clinical picture expressed by the classical indications for this point is one of severe exhaustion of the Lung. It is indicated for Lung atrophy, Lung consumption, deficiency-taxation, taxation cough with heat in the body etc. In its ability to strengthen the Lung at the deepest level it is similar to Gaohuangshu BL-43, although less renowned.

According to the *Essential Questions*[60] the five outer Bladder points level with the five zang back-shu points (i.e. Pohu BL-42, Shentang BL-44, Hunmen BL-47, Yishe BL-49 and Zhishi BL-52) drain heat from the five zang, an action shared by the back-shu points of the five zang.

COMBINATIONS

- Consumption: Pohu BL-42 and Gaohuangshu BL-43 (*One Hundred Symptoms*).
- Cough with rebellious qi, dyspnoea, vomiting of foam and clenched teeth: Pohu BL-42, Futu L.I.-18, Tianrong SI-17, Lianquan REN-23, Qishe ST-11 and Yixi BL-45 (*Thousand Ducat Formulas*).
- Inability to turn the neck: Pohu BL-42 and Jianjing GB-21 (*Supplementing Life*).

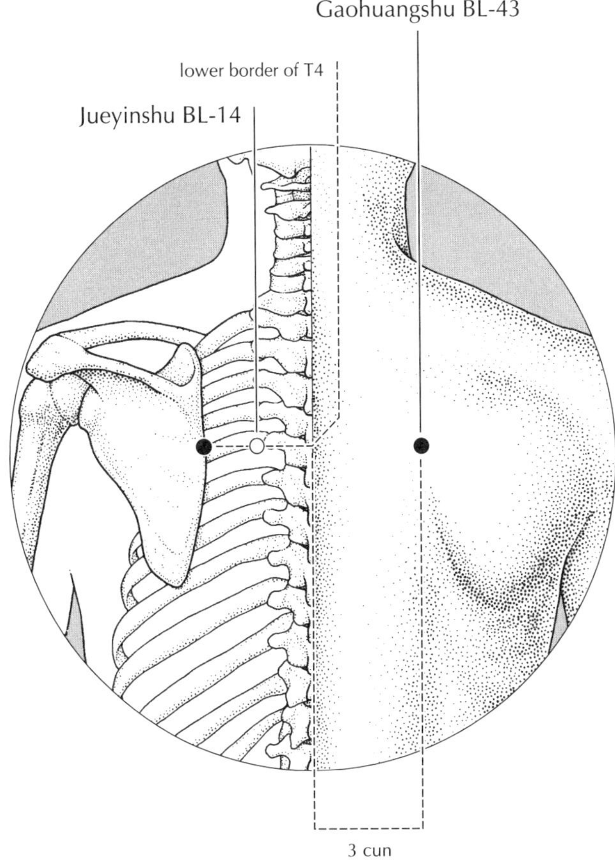

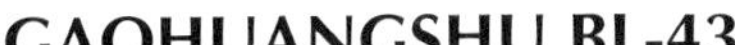

GAOHUANGSHU BL-43

Vital Region Shu

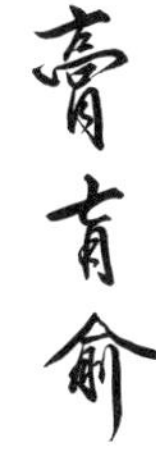

LOCATION

3 cun lateral to the midline, level with the lower border of the spinous process of the fourth thoracic vertebra (T4) and level with Jueyinshu BL-14.

LOCATION NOTE

When the shoulder is relaxed, the three cun line corresponds to the medial border of the scapula.

NEEDLING

Oblique insertion 0.3 to 0.5 cun. **Caution:** deep perpendicular or deep oblique needling in a medial direction carries a substantial risk of causing a pneumothorax.

ACTIONS

Tonifies and nourishes the Lung, Heart, Kidneys, Spleen and Stomach
Nourishes yin and clears heat
Calms the spirit
Fosters the original qi
Resolves phlegm

INDICATIONS

- All kinds of deficiency, Lung deficiency-taxation, deficiency-taxation, the five taxations and the seven injuries, cough, asthma, coughing blood, night sweating, spontaneous sweating, steaming bone disorder, consumption, emaciation.
- Poor memory, pounding of the Heart, insomnia, phlegm-fire mania.
- Seminal emission, seminal emission with dreams, impotence.
- Feebleness and deficiency of the Spleen and Stomach, undigested food (in the stool), oesophageal constriction, weariness of the four limbs, vomiting blood.
- Visual dizziness, dizziness, phlegm disease, pain of the back and shoulder.

COMMENTARY

The name 'Gaohuang' can be translated as 'Vital Region'. This concept, implying one of the deepest and most fundamental regions of the body, is first mentioned in *Master Zuo-jiu's Tradition of the Spring and Autumn Annals* (580 BCE), one of the earliest textual references to acupuncture. The Prince of Jin who was gravely ill sent for the famous Doctor Yi Huan. After examining the patient, Doctor Huan declared that the disease had settled in the gaohuang region (between the Heart and the diaphragm) and hence "it cannot be purged, it cannot be reached (by needling), herbs will not penetrate it, there is nothing to be done"[61].

Gaohuangshu BL-43 was comprehensively discussed in a text called *Method of Moxibustion at Gaohuangshu* by Zhuang Zhuo in 1128. Zhuang was inspired to write this book after being cured of various diseases, including malaria and beri-beri, by three hundred moxa cones burnt on Gaohuangshu BL-43. He measured the location of Gaohuangshu BL-43 on people of various body builds and gave diagrams and specific instructions for locating the point.

In discussing this point, Sun Si-miao in the *Thousand Ducat Formulas* simply states "Gaohuangshu BL-43, there is no [disorder] that it cannot treat" and "once moxibustion is completed, it causes a person's yang qi to be healthy and full". Many classical texts say that Gaohuangshu BL-43 is contraindicated to needling and emphasise its treatment by moxibustion, for example the *Illustrated Classic of Acupuncture Points on the Bronze Man* recommends the application of a hundred or even as many as three hundred moxa cones to Gaohuangshu BL-43. Early texts, however, stress that after moxibustion at Gaohuangshu BL-43, moxibustion should also be applied to points below the umbilicus, e.g. Qihai REN-6 and Guanyuan REN-4, in order to conduct downwards the heat thus generated.

Careful examination of the classical indications of this point demonstrate its actions on the Lung, Heart, Kidneys, Spleen and Stomach. Like Feishu BL-13 and Pohu BL-42, it is able to treat severe deficiency (especially of the yin) of the Lung, and is indicated for consumption, cough, coughing of blood, steaming bone disorder, night sweating and emaciation. By both nourishing and calming the Heart it is applicable in the treatment of poor memory, pounding of the Heart, insomnia and phlegm-fire mania. Acting on the Kidneys, it is able to treat seminal emission, with or without dreams, and impotence. By strengthening the middle jiao it is able to treat feebleness and deficiency of the Spleen and Stomach, undigested food in the stool and weariness of the four limbs. So great was the tonifying action of Gaohuangshu BL-43 considered to be, that it was said to strengthen the original qi and treat every kind of deficiency, the five types of taxation and the seven injuries. Finally, it is interesting to note that Gaohuangshu BL-43 was also indicated for 'phlegm diseases' and Sun Si-miao in his *Supplement to the Thousand Ducat Formulas* says it "stops phlegm in chronic disease". The importance of phlegm as a pathological factor in difficult and chronic diseases is long documented and is reflected in such sayings as "The hundred diseases all pertain to phlegm", "Strange diseases often involve phlegm" and "There is no place that phlegm cannot reach".

COMBINATIONS

- The hundred syndromes of deficiency-taxation: moxa Gaohuangshu BL-43, Huanmen (M-BW-6) and the Four Flowers [Geshu BL-17 and Danshu BL-19] (*Compilation*).
- Consumption: Gaohuangshu BL-43 and Pohu BL-42 (*One Hundred Symptoms*).
- Spontaneous sweating: moxa Gaohuangshu BL-43, Dazhui DU-14 and Fuliu KID-7 (*Divine Moxibustion*).
- Poor memory: Gaohuangshu BL-43, Shendao DU-11, Youmen KID-21 and Lieque LU-7 (*Supplementing Life*).

SHENTANG BL-44

Hall of the Spirit

神堂

LOCATION

3 cun lateral to the midline, level with the lower border of the spinous process of the fifth thoracic vertebra (T5) and level with Xinshu BL-15.

LOCATION NOTE

When the shoulder is relaxed, the three cun line corresponds to the medial border of the scapula.

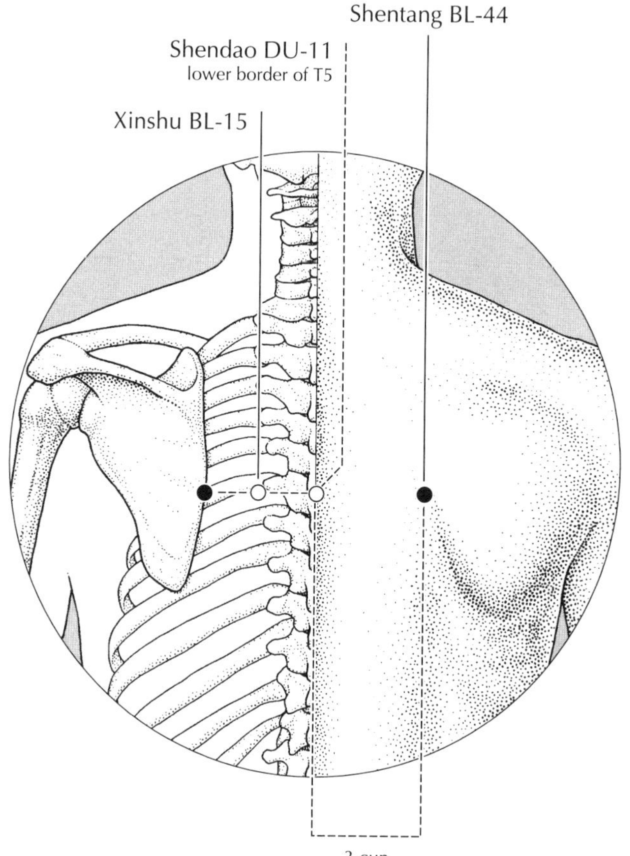

NEEDLING
Oblique insertion 0.3 to 0.5 cun.
Caution: deep perpendicular or deep oblique needling in a medial direction carries a substantial risk of causing a pneumothorax.

ACTIONS
Unbinds the chest and regulates qi
Activates the channel and alleviates pain

INDICATIONS
- Cough, asthma, dyspnoea, fullness of the chest with rebellious qi.
- Stiffness and pain of the back, pain of the shoulder and back that radiates to the chest, oesophageal constriction.

COMMENTARY
Despite the compelling name of this point (Hall of the Spirit) and the fact that Shentang BL-44 lies on the outer Bladder channel at the level of Xinshu BL-15, the back-shu point of the Heart, there are no apparent references in any of the important classics of acupuncture to the use of this point for the treatment of emotional or psychological disorders.

According to the *Essential Questions*[62] the five outer Bladder points level with the five zang back-shu points (i.e. Pohu BL-42, Shentang BL-44, Hunmen BL-47, Yishe BL-49 and Zhishi BL-52) drain heat from the five zang, an action shared by the back-shu points of the five zang.

COMBINATIONS
- Oesophageal constriction: Shentang BL-44 and Zhongfeng LIV-4 (*Supplementing Life*).

YIXI BL-45
Yi Xi

譩譆

LOCATION
3 cun lateral to the midline, level with the lower border of the spinous process of the sixth thoracic vertebra (T6) and level with Dushu BL-16.

LOCATION NOTE
When the shoulder is relaxed, the three cun line corresponds to the medial border of the scapula.

NEEDLING
Oblique insertion 0.3 to 0.5 cun.
Caution: deep perpendicular or deep oblique needling in a medial direction carries a substantial risk of causing a pneumothorax.

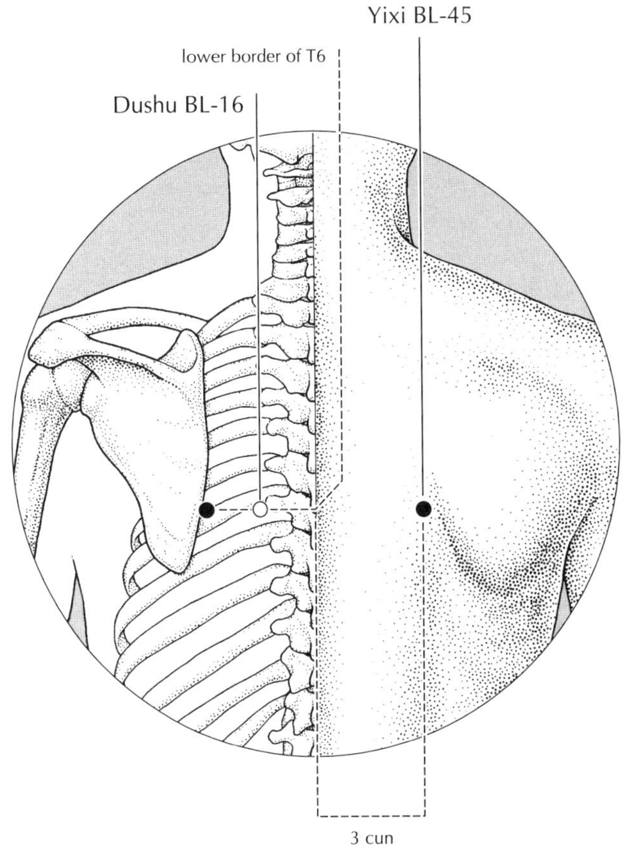

ACTIONS
Expels wind, clears heat and descends Lung qi
Invigorates qi and blood and alleviates pain

INDICATIONS
- Cough, dyspnoea, febrile disease with absence of sweating, attack by wind with absence of sweating, visual dizziness, eye pain, nosebleed, malaria, headache in children whilst eating, five palms agitated and hot.
- Pain of the shoulder, scapula and back, chest pain that radiates to the lumbar region, pain of the lateral costal region accompanied by distention and pain of the hypogastrium, pain of the lateral costal region radiating to the Heart and Lung, abdominal distention, contraction of the axilla.

COMMENTARY
Yixi BL-45 is level with Dushu BL-16 which is listed in some classical texts as the back-shu point of the Governing vessel. Whilst Dushu BL-16 has few indications which reflect disorder of the Governing vessel, some of the indications of Yixi BL-45, for example visual dizziness, eye pain, nosebleed, malaria, headache and chest pain radiating to the lumbar region, may be understood in this way.

COMBINATIONS

- Abdominal fullness: Yixi BL-45 and Zusanli ST-36 (*Supplementing Life*).
- Cough with rebellious qi, dyspnoea, vomiting of foam and clenched teeth: Yixi BL-45, Futu L.I.-18, Tianrong SI-17, Lianquan REN-23, Pohu BL-42 and Qishe ST-11 (*Thousand Ducat Formulas*).
- Swelling of the face: first needle Yixi BL-45, then Tianyou SJ-16 and Fengchi GB-20 (*Systematic Classic*).
- Visual dizziness: Yixi BL-45, Shenting DU-24, Shangxing DU-23, Yongquan KID-1, Yuji LU-10 and Dadu SP-2 (*Supplementing Life*).
- Contraction and cold of the shoulder and back, with pain of the inner aspect of the scapula: Yixi BL-45, Chize LU-5, Geshu BL-17 and Jinmen BL-63 (*Thousand Ducat Formulas*).

GEGUAN BL-46

Diaphragm Gate

膈關

LOCATION

3 cun lateral to the midline, level with the lower border of the spinous process of the seventh thoracic vertebra (T7) and level with Geshu BL-17.

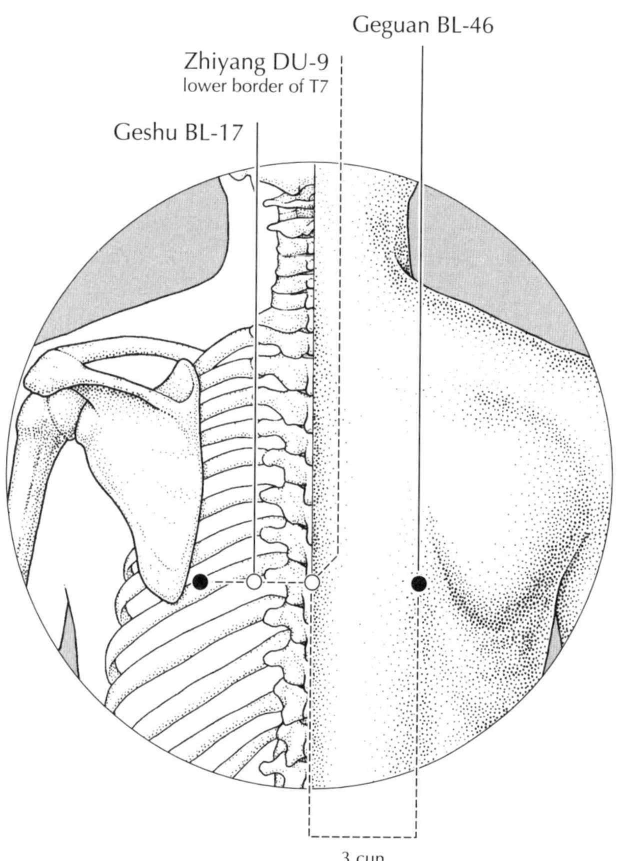

LOCATION NOTE

When the shoulder is relaxed, the three cun line corresponds to the medial border of the scapula.

NEEDLING

Oblique insertion 0.3 to 0.5 cun.

Caution: deep perpendicular or deep oblique needling in a medial direction carries a substantial risk of causing a pneumothorax.

ACTIONS

Regulates the diaphragm, benefits the middle jiao and descends rebellion

Activates the channel and alleviates pain

INDICATIONS

- Belching, sighing, fullness and oppression of the chest and diaphragm, difficult ingestion, vomiting, vomiting blood, drooling, irregular defecation, dark urine.
- Stiffness and pain of the spine, difficulty in bending and extending the spine, back pain with aversion to cold, pain of the body, stiffness of the joints.

COMMENTARY

Geguan BL-46 (Diaphragm Gate) is level with Geshu BL-17 (Diaphragm Shu) the hui-meeting point of blood. Like Geshu BL-17, Geguan BL-46 has an important action on harmonising the diaphragm which lies between the upper and middle jiao and is able to resolve stagnation of qi in the upper jiao (fullness and oppression of the chest and diaphragm, sighing) and descend Stomach qi in the middle jiao (vomiting, difficult ingestion, belching).

COMBINATIONS

- Aversion to cold in the back and stiffness of the spine with difficulty in bending: Geguan BL-46, Zhibian BL-54 and Jinggu BL-64 (*Thousand Ducat Formulas*).

HUNMEN BL-47

Gate of the Ethereal Soul

魂門

LOCATION

3 cun lateral to the midline, level with the lower border of the spinous process of the ninth thoracic vertebra (T9) and level with Ganshu BL-18.

LOCATION NOTE

When the shoulder is relaxed, the three cun line corresponds to the medial border of the scapula.

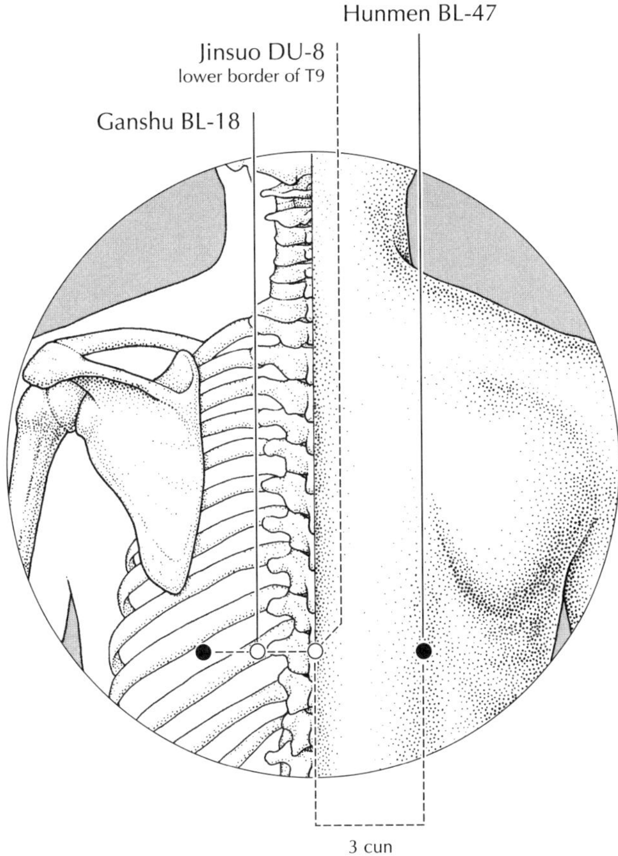

NEEDLING

Oblique insertion 0.3 to 0.5 cun. **Caution:** deep perpendicular or deep oblique needling in a medial direction carries a substantial risk of causing a pneumothorax.

ACTIONS

Spreads Liver qi and relaxes the sinews
Harmonises the middle jiao

INDICATIONS

- Fullness and distention of the chest and lateral costal region, back pain, contraction of the sinews, bone and joint pain of the whole body, corpse collapse walking disorder, aversion to wind and cold.
- Difficult ingestion, vomiting, diarrhoea, borborygmus, irregular defecation, dark urine.

COMMENTARY

Hunmen BL-47 is level with Ganshu BL-18, the back-shu point of the Liver. The Liver stores the ethereal soul (hun), but despite its striking name (Gate of the Ethereal Soul), psychological and emotional indications for this point are notable by their absence in major classical texts[63]. Hunmen BL-47 does, however, have some action on regulating the Liver qi and soothing the sinews, and is indicated for fullness and distention of the chest and lateral costal region, contraction of the sinews, and bone and joint pain of the whole body. It is also able to regulate the middle jiao, treating disharmony of both the Spleen (diarrhoea, borborygmus) and Stomach (difficult ingestion, vomiting).

According to the *Essential Questions*[64], the five outer Bladder points level with the five zang back-shu points (i.e. Pohu BL-42, Shentang BL-44, Hunmen BL-47, Yishe BL-49 and Zhishi BL-52) drain heat from the five zang, an action shared by the back-shu points of the five zang.

COMBINATIONS

- Chest pain: Hunmen BL-47, Feishu BL-13, Yunmen LU-2, Zhongfu LU-1, Yinbai SP-1, Qimen LIV-14 and Daling P-7 (*Thousand Ducat Formulas*).
- Cold Stomach with difficulty in digesting food: Hunmen BL-47 and Weishu BL-21 (*One Hundred Symptoms*).

YANGGANG BL-48

Yang's' Key Link

陽綱

LOCATION

3 cun lateral to the midline, level with the lower border of the spinous process of the tenth thoracic vertebra (T10) and level with Danshu BL-19.

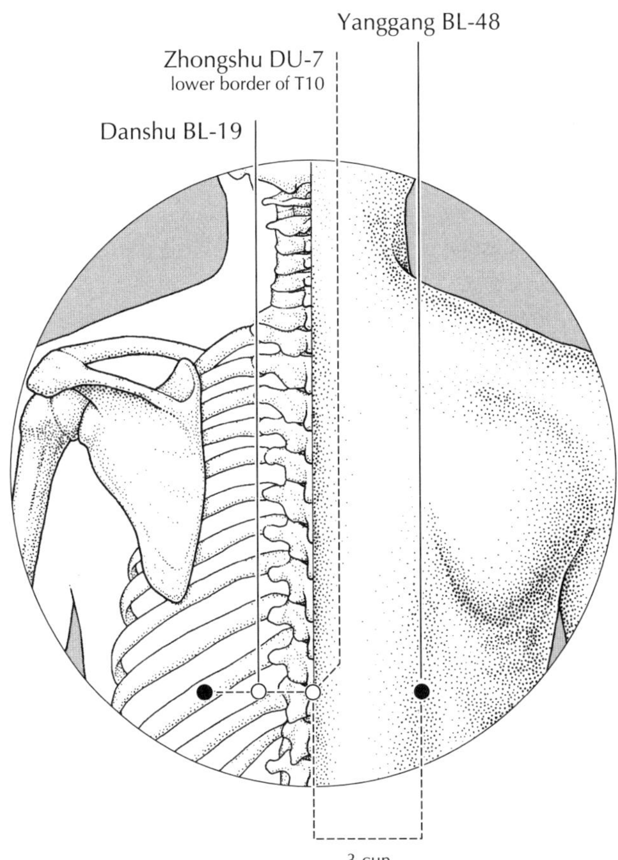

LOCATION NOTE

When the shoulder is relaxed, the three cun line corresponds to the medial border of the scapula.

NEEDLING

Oblique insertion 0.3 to 0.5 cun.
Caution: deep perpendicular or deep oblique needling in a medial direction carries a substantial risk of causing a pneumothorax.

ACTIONS

Regulates the Gall Bladder and clears damp-heat
Harmonises the middle jiao

INDICATIONS

- Heat in the body, yellow eyes and face, pain of the lateral costal region, dark and hesitant urination, indolence.
- Abdominal pain, abdominal distention, borborygmus, diarrhoea, dysenteric disorder with blood, irregular defecation, difficult ingestion, no pleasure in eating.

COMMENTARY

Yanggang BL-48 is level with Danshu BL-19, the back-shu point of the Gall Bladder. Like Danshu BL-19, it is indicated for damp-heat obstructing the Gall Bladder and giving rise to fever, jaundice, pain of the lateral costal region and dark and hesitant urination. At the same time it is able to regulate the middle jiao and clear dampness and heat, being indicated for distention and pain of the abdomen, diarrhoea, dysenteric disorder, irregular defecation and digestive disorders.

COMBINATIONS

- Yellow eyes: Yanggang BL-48 and Danshu BL-19 (*One Hundred Symptoms*).
- Yellow eyes: Yanggang BL-48, Yishe BL-49, Naohu DU-17 and Danshu BL-19 (*Supplementing Life*).
- Difficult ingestion: Yanggang BL-48, Qimen LIV-14, Shaoshang LU-11 and Laogong P-8 (*Thousand Ducat Formulas*).
- Red and hesitant urinary flow: Yanggang BL-48, Guanyuan REN-4, Zhibian BL-54 and Qihai REN-6 (*Supplementing Life*).

YISHE BL-49

Abode of Thought

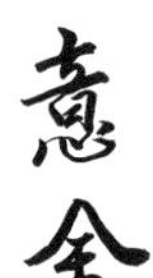

LOCATION

3 cun lateral to the midline, level with the lower border of the spinous process of the eleventh thoracic vertebra (T11) and level with Pishu BL-20.

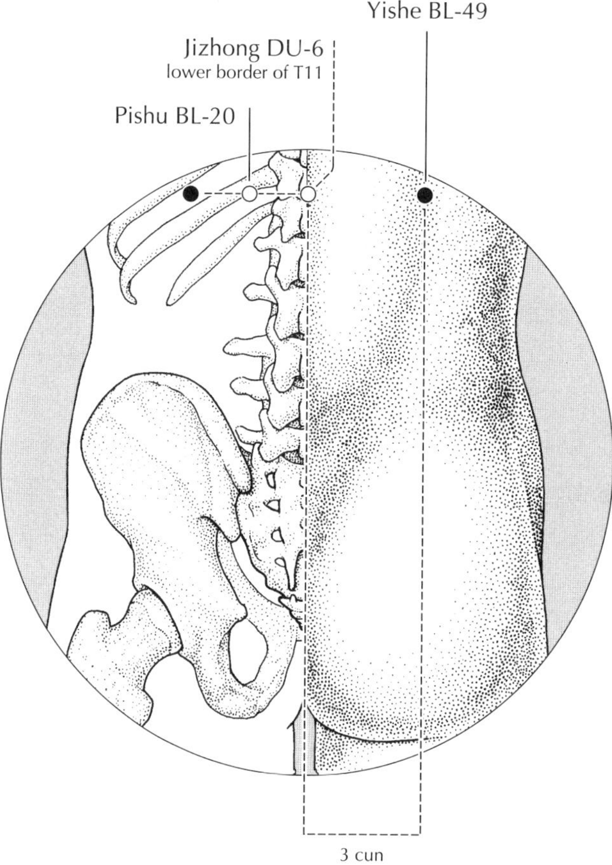

LOCATION NOTE

When the shoulder is relaxed, the three cun line corresponds to the medial border of the scapula.

NEEDLING

Oblique insertion 0.3 to 0.5 cun. **Caution:** deep perpendicular or deep oblique needling in a medial direction carries a substantial risk of causing a pneumothorax.

ACTIONS

Clears damp-heat
Regulates the Spleen and Stomach

INDICATIONS

- Distention and fullness of the abdomen, distention and pain of the chest and lateral costal region, slippery diarrhoea, difficult ingestion, vomiting, reddish-yellow urine, heat in the body with yellow face and eyes.
- Back pain, wasting and thirsting disorder, aversion to wind and cold.

COMMENTARY

Yishe BL-49 is level with Pishu BL-20, the back-shu point of the Spleen. Despite its name (Abode of Thought), psychological and emotional indications are notable by their absence in major classical texts.

Yishe BL-49 is able to clear damp-heat (reddish-yellow urine, heat in the body with yellow face and eyes) and regulate disharmony of the Stomach (vomiting, difficult ingestion) and Spleen (abdominal distention and fullness, slippery diarrhoea).

In the light of its proximity to the pancreas, it is interesting to note the inclusion of this point in a number of classical combinations for wasting and thirsting disorder.

According to the *Essential Questions*[65] the five outer Bladder points level with the five zang back-shu points (i.e. Pohu BL-42, Shentang BL-44, Hunmen BL-47, Yishe BL-49 and Zhishi BL-52) drain heat from the five zang, an action shared by the back-shu points of the five zang.

COMBINATIONS

- Wasting and thirsting disorder with great desire to drink: Yishe BL-49, Guanchong SJ-1 and Rangu KID-2 (*Supplementing Life*).
- Wasting and thirsting disorder with great desire to drink: Yishe BL-49, Chengjiang REN-24, Rangu KID-2 and Guanchong SJ-1 (*Thousand Ducat Formulas*).
- Kidney deficiency wasting and thirsting disorder, absence of sweating, difficulty in moving the lumbar spine, distension of the abdomen and pain of the lateral costal region: Yishe BL-49 and Zhonglushu BL-29 (*Classic of Supplementing Life*)
- Vomiting: Yishe BL-49, Zhongting REN-16 and Shufu KID-27 (*Supplementing Life*).
- Yellow eyes: Yishe BL-49, Yanggang BL-48, Naohu DU-17 and Danshu BL-19 (*Supplementing Life*).

WEICANG BL-50

Stomach Granary

胃倉

LOCATION

3 cun lateral to the midline, level with the lower border of the spinous process of the twelfth thoracic vertebra (T12) and level with Weishu BL-21.

LOCATION NOTE

When the shoulder is relaxed, the three cun line corresponds to the medial border of the scapula.

NEEDLING

Oblique insertion 0.3 to 0.5 cun.
Caution: deep perpendicular or deep oblique needling in a medial direction carries a substantial risk of causing a pneumothorax.

ACTIONS

Harmonises the middle jiao

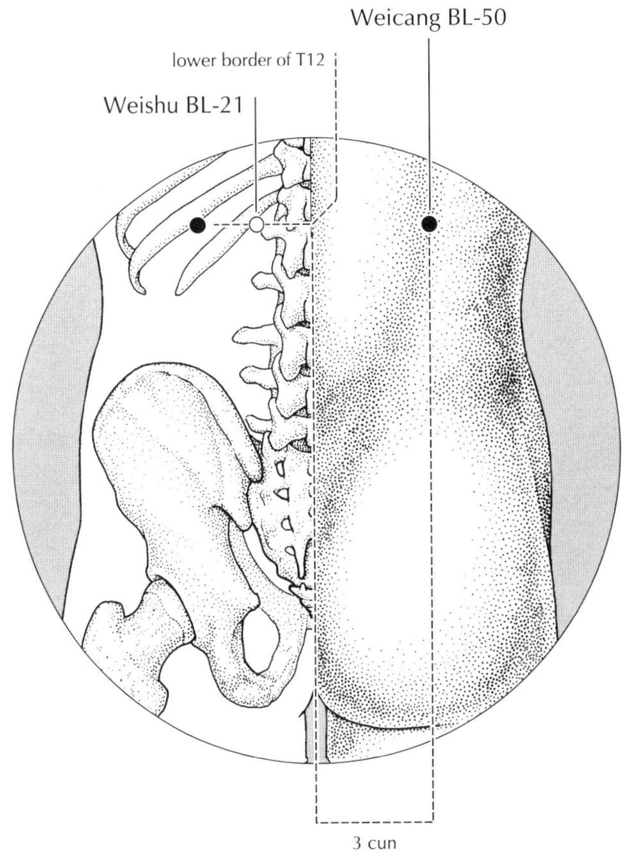

INDICATIONS

- Abdominal fullness, deficiency distention, difficult ingestion, childhood nutritional impairment, sudden turmoil disorder, oedema.
- Aversion to cold, much cold, back pain.

COMBINATIONS

- Difficult ingestion: Weicang BL-50, Yishe BL-49 and Geguan BL-46 (*Supplementing Life*).

HUANGMEN BL-51

Vitals Gate

肓門

LOCATION

3 cun lateral to the midline, level with the lower border of the spinous process of the first lumbar vertebra (L1) and level with Sanjiaoshu BL-22.

LOCATION NOTE

When the shoulder is relaxed, the three cun line corresponds to the medial border of the scapula.

NEEDLING

Oblique insertion 0.5 to 1 cun. **Caution:** deep perpendicular needling carries a risk of injuring the kidney.

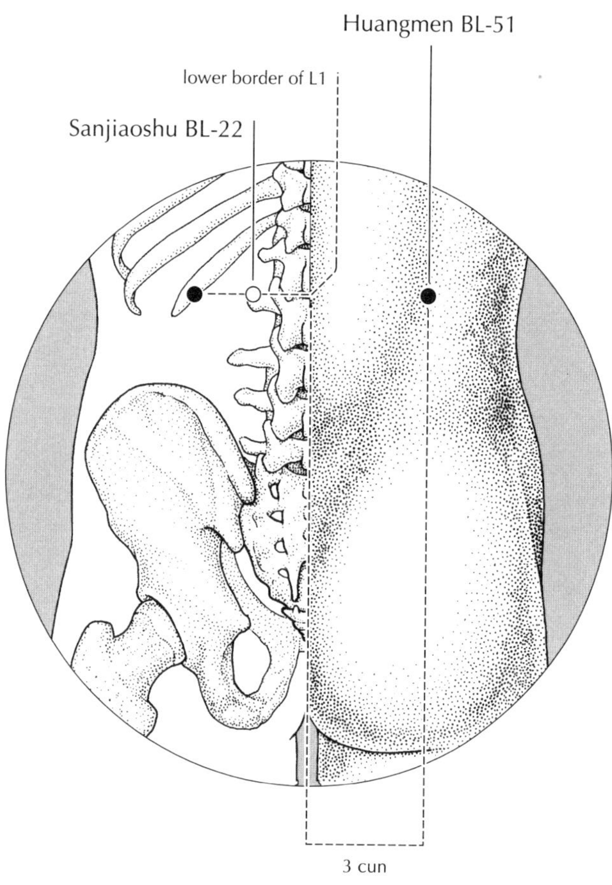

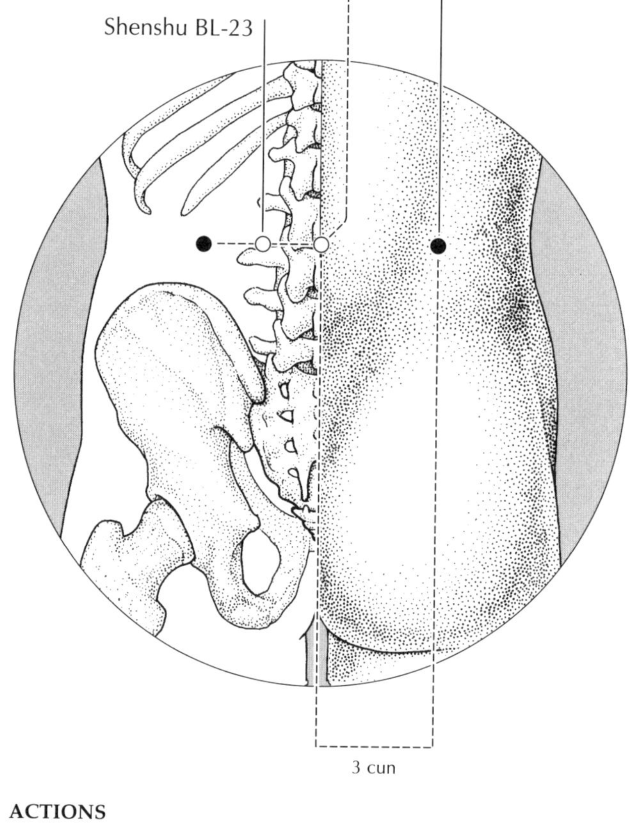

ACTIONS

Dispels stagnation and benefits the breasts

INDICATIONS

- Epigastric pain, great hardness below the Heart, constipation.
- Breast disorders, fullness and pain of the breast.

ZHISHI BL-52

Residence of the Will

志室

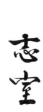

LOCATION

3 cun lateral to the midline, level with the lower border of the spinous process of the second lumbar vertebra (L2) and level with Shenshu BL-23.

LOCATION NOTE

When the shoulder is relaxed, the three cun line corresponds to the medial border of the scapula.

NEEDLING

Oblique insertion 0.5 to 1 cun.

Caution: deep perpendicular needling carries a risk of injuring the kidney.

ACTIONS

Tonifies the Kidneys and benefits the essence
Regulates urination
Strengthens the lumbar region

INDICATIONS

- Lumbar pain and stiffness, back pain, dribbling urination, difficult urination, oedema, impotence, premature ejaculation, seminal emission with dreams, swelling and pain of the genitals.
- Fullness and pain of the lateral costal region, sudden turmoil disorder, vomiting, difficult defecation, hardness of the abdomen and hypogastrium.

COMMENTARY

Zhishi BL-52 is level with Shenshu BL-23, the back-shu point of the Kidneys. Despite its suggestive name 'Residence of the Will', there are no apparent references in any of the important classics of acupuncture to the use of this point for the treatment of emotional or psychological disorders.

Zhishi BL-52 was also known as Jinggong (Palace of Essence), reflecting its ability to fortify the Kidney qi and yang, strengthen the sexual function and control discharge of semen, as evinced by its indications for impotence, premature ejaculation and seminal emission.

It is similarly able to firm the Kidney qi and regulate urination, and is indicated for difficult or dribbling urination and oedema. Zhishi BL-52 is also used clinically in the treatment of pain that spreads widely to the muscles of the lumbar region whether due to sprain, painful obstruction, or deficiency and disease of the Kidneys, for example renal colic. Unlike Shenshu BL-23, however, the application of Zhishi BL-52 is confined to these patterns of Kidney deficiency and it lacks the wider ability of Shenshu BL-23 to deeply nourish and tonify the Kidneys.

According to the *Essential Questions*[66] the five outer Bladder points level with the five zang back-shu points (i.e. Pohu BL-42, Shentang BL-44, Hunmen BL-47, Yishe BL-49 and Zhishi BL-52) drain heat from the five zang, an action shared by the back-shu points of the five zang.

COMBINATIONS

- Lumbar pain with tension of the spine: Zhishi BL-52 and Jingmen GB-25 (*Thousand Ducat Formulas*).
- Acute pain of both lateral costal regions: Zhishi BL-52, Ganshu BL-18, and Pishu BL-20 (*Thousand Ducat Formulas*).
- Pain and swelling of the genitals: Zhishi BL-52 and Baohuang BL-53 (*Supplementing Life*).
- Pain of the genitals: Zhishi BL-52, Shenshu BL-23, Jinggu BL-64 and Taichong LIV-3 (*Supplementing Life*).
- Dribbling urination: Zhishi BL-52, Weiyang BL-39 and Zhongliao BL-33 (*Supplementing Life*).
- Renal colic, blood and stone painful urinary dysfunction with vomiting: Zhishi BL-52, Shenshu BL-23, Dachangshu BL-25, Jingmen GB-25, Tianshu ST-25, Daheng SP-15, Sanyinjiao SP-6 and Neiguan P-6.

BAOHUANG BL-53

Bladder's Vitals

胞肓

LOCATION

3 cun lateral to the midline, at the level of the spinous process of the second sacral vertebra.

LOCATION NOTE

i. For guidance on locating the sacral spinious processes see page 69; ii. When the shoulder is relaxed, the three cun line corresponds to the medial border of the scapula; iii. Alternatively this point may be located midway between the midline and the lateral edge of the buttock, when the lateral edge is firmly pressed in with the palm of the hand.

NEEDLING

Perpendicular insertion 1 to 1.5 cun.

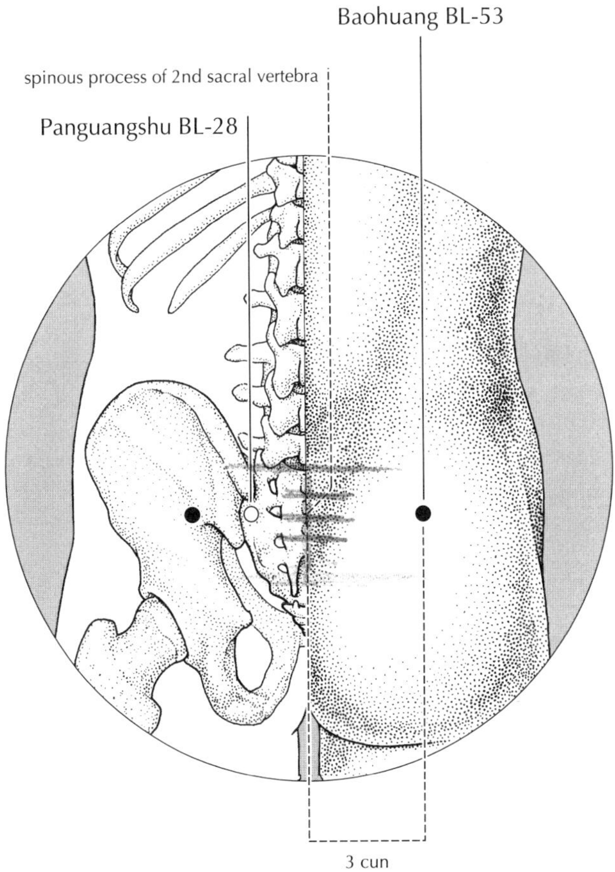

ACTIONS

Benefits the lumbar region, activates the channel and alleviates pain

Regulates the lower jiao and benefits urination

INDICATIONS

- Pain and stiffness of the lumbar region, sciatica.
- Hardness and fullness of the hypogastrium, retention of urine, dribbling urination, oedema, inability to urinate or defecate.
- Borborygmus, abdominal distention, undigested food (in the stool), aversion to wind.

COMMENTARY

Baohuang BL-53 is a commonly used point in the treatment of stiffness and pain of the lumbar region and sciatica. Along with Zhibian BL-54 and Huantiao GB-30, Baohuang BL-53 is one of the points that should be palpated, and needled if tender, in all cases where pain radiates to the buttock and down the leg.

Baohuang BL-53 (Bladder's Vitals) lies lateral to Pangguangshu BL-28, the back-shu point of the Bladder, and in common with many of the points of the sacral region it is able to regulate urination, and to a lesser extent defecation, being indicated for retention of urine, dribbling urination, oedema and inability to urinate or defecate.

COMBINATIONS
- Pain of the lumbar region and aversion to cold: Baohuang BL-53, Ciliao BL-32 and Chengjin BL-56 (*Supplementing Life*).
- Retention of urine: Baohuang BL-53 and Zhibian BL-54 (*Supplementing Life*).
- Fullness of the hypogastrium: Baohuang BL-53 and Ganshu BL-18 (*Thousand Ducat Formulas*).

ZHIBIAN BL-54
Order's Limit

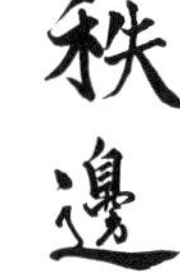

LOCATION
On the buttock, in the depression 3 cun lateral to the sacro-coccygeal hiatus.

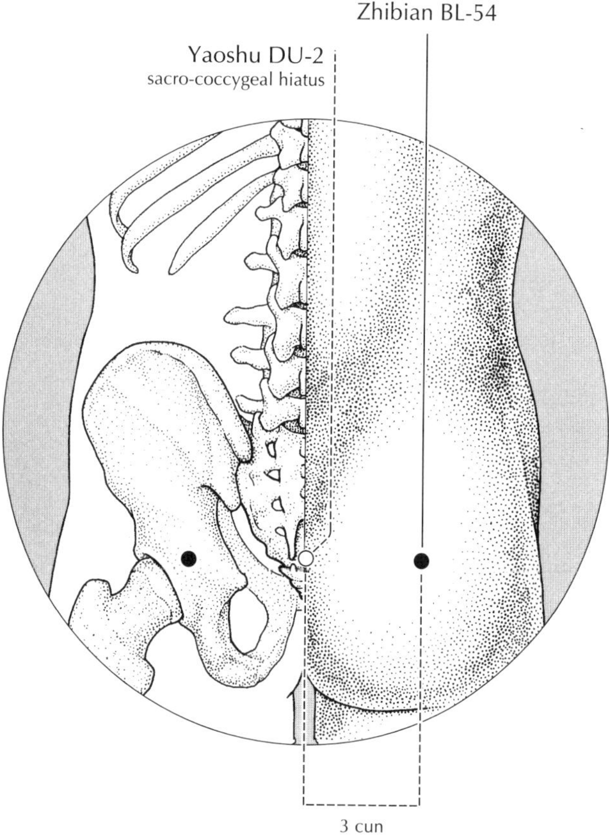

LOCATION NOTE
i. The sacro-coccygeal hiatus is the depression between the bony prominences of the sacral and coccygeal cornua (just below the spinous process of the fourth sacral vertebra if this is palpable); ii. When the shoulder is relaxed, the three cun line corresponds to the medial border of the scapula; iii. Alternatively this point may be located midway between the midline and the lateral edge of the buttock, when the lateral edge is firmly pressed in with the palm of the hand.

NEEDLING
i. Perpendicular insertion 1.5 to 2.5 cun; ii. Slanted towards the anus or the genitalia 2 to 3 cun.

ACTIONS
Benefits the lumbar region, activates the channel and alleviates pain
Regulates urination and treats haemorrhoids

INDICATIONS
- Pain and coldness of the lumbar region and sacrum, Kidney deficiency lumbar pain, pain of the buttock, sciatica, painful obstruction and atrophy disorder of the lower limb.
- Difficult urination, retention of urine, dark urine, difficult defecation, seminal emission, haemorrhoids, turbid leucorrhoea, pain of the genitals.

COMMENTARY
Zhibian BL-54 is an indispensable point in the treatment of pain of the lumbar region, sacrum and buttocks and of sciatica. Along with Baohuang BL-53 and Huantiao GB-30, Zhibian BL-54 is one of the points that should be palpated, and needled if tender, in all cases where pain radiates to the buttock and down the leg.

According to *Investigation Into Points Along the Channels* by Yan Zhen-shi of the Ming dynasty, Zhibian BL-54 is indicated for "Kidney deficiency lumbar pain, seminal emission and turbid leucorrhoea". This quotation emphasises that the use of Zhibian BL-54 in the treatment of lumbar pain is not confined to cases of stagnation (such as painful obstruction), but extends also to aching of the lumbar region due to weakness of the Kidneys.

In common with many points of the sacral region which lies over the Bladder and intestines, Zhibian BL-54 is able to regulate obstructed and difficult urination and defecation. Zhibian BL-54 is also mentioned in a number of classics for the treatment of "the five types of haemorrhoids with swelling".

COMBINATIONS
- Aversion to cold in the back and stiffness of the spine with difficulty in bending: Zhibian BL-54, Geguan BL-46 and Jinggu BL-64 (*Thousand Ducat Formulas*).
- Red and hesitant urinary flow: Zhibian BL-54, Guanyuan REN-4, Qihai REN-6 and Yanggang BL-48 (*Supplementing Life*).
- Retention of urine: Zhibian BL-54 and Baohuang BL-53 (*Supplementing Life*).

HEYANG BL-55

合陽

Confluence of Yang

LOCATION
On the lower leg, 2 cun inferior to Weizhong BL-40, on the line connecting Weizhong BL-40 and Chengshan BL-57, in the depression between the two heads of the gastrocnemius muscle.

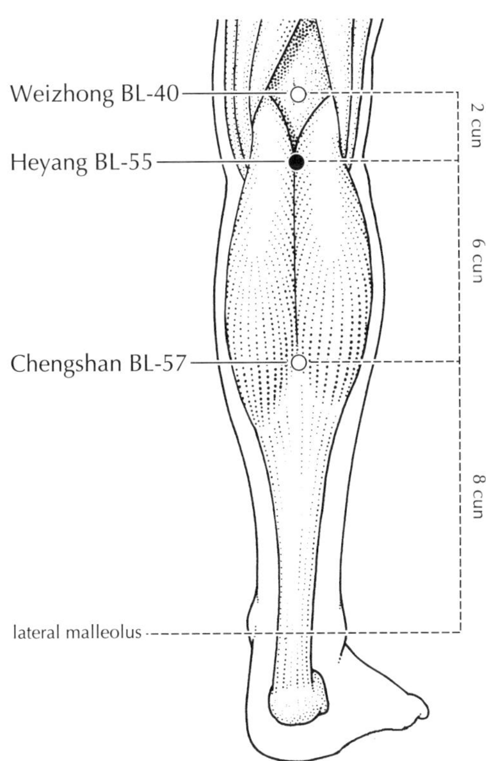

LOCATION NOTE
First locate Chengshan BL-57. Then locate Heyang BL-55 at one quarter of the distance between Weizhong BL-40 and Chengshan BL-57.

NEEDLING
Perpendicular insertion 1 to 1.5 cun.

ACTIONS
Activates the channel and alleviates pain
Stops uterine bleeding and treats pain of the genitals

INDICATIONS
- Lumbar pain radiating to the abdomen, heat sensation of the inner thigh, pain, heat and heaviness of the knees, difficulty in walking.
- Uterine bleeding, leucorrhoea, pain of the genitals, sudden violent pain of the genitals, cold shan disorder.

COMBINATIONS
- Diminished qi uterine bleeding: Heyang BL-55 and Jiaoxin KID-8 (*One Hundred Symptoms*).

CHENGJIN BL-56

承筋

Support the Sinews

LOCATION
On the lower leg, 5 cun below Weizhong BL-40 and midway between Heyang BL-55 and Chengshan BL-57, in the centre of the belly of the gastrocnemius muscle.

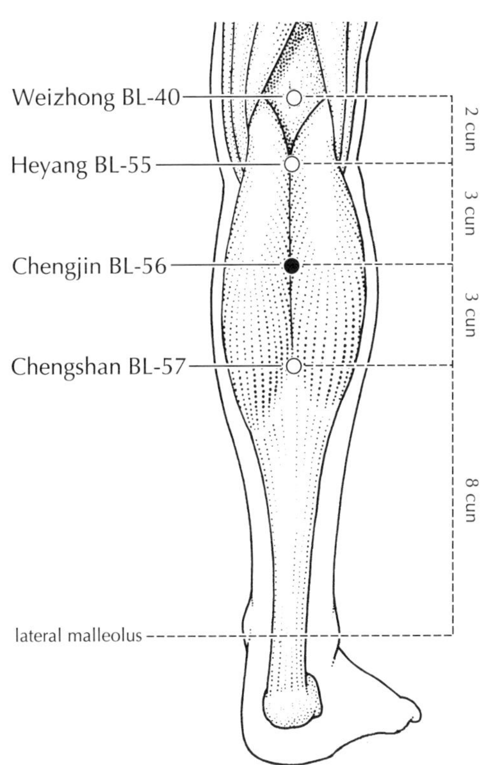

LOCATION NOTE
First locate Chengshan BL-57 then Heyang BL-55. Chengjin BL-56 is located midway between these two points.

NEEDLING
Perpendicular insertion 1 to 1.5 cun. **Note**: according to several classical texts, this point is contraindicated to needling.

ACTIONS
Relaxes the sinews, activates the channel and alleviates pain
Benefits the foot and heel

INDICATIONS

- Contraction and pain of the lumbar spine, painful obstruction of the lower leg, shivering with inability to stand for long, heat sensation in the soles with inability to stand for long, pain and contraction of the foot and heel, swelling of the axilla.
- Haemorrhoids, constipation, incontinence of both urine and faeces.
- Nosebleed, rhinitis, heat in the head, dizziness and headache, sudden turmoil disorder with cramps, clonic spasm, urticaria.

COMMENTARY

As its name 'Support the Sinews' implies, Chengjin BL-56 is indicated for pain and contraction of the muscles and sinews, especially in the lumbar region and calf.

It is one of the attributes of the channels that as they travel distally towards the hand or foot, their points have an increasingly pronounced action on the whole length of the channel. Although not a major point, Chengjin BL-56 is characterised by its ability to treat disorders of the whole Bladder channel in the head (dizziness, headache, heat in the head, nosebleed, rhinitis), the lumbar region, the lower leg and calf, and the foot and heel.

Heel pain is often a difficult disorder to treat, and requires not only local points on the heel itself, but also proximal points. Chengjin BL-56 and Chengshan BL-57 are the two principal proximal points that affect this region of the foot.

Finally, like several distal points of the Bladder channel, Chengjin BL-56 treats both swelling of the axilla and haemorrhoids. This may be explained by the pathways of the Bladder sinew channel to the axilla and the Bladder divergent channel which winds around the anus.

COMBINATIONS

- Haemorrhoids, swelling of the axilla: Chengjin BL-56, Chengfu BL-36, Weizhong BL-40 and Yanggu SI-5 (*Thousand Ducat Formulas*).
- Difficulty in defecation: Chengjin BL-56, Chengshan BL-57, Dazhong KID-4, Zhongliao BL-33, Guanyuan REN-4, Taichong LIV-3, Taixi KID-3 and Zhongwan REN-12 (*Supplementing Life*).
- Pain of the lumbar region and aversion to cold: Chengjin BL-56, Ciliao BL-32 and Baohuang BL-53 (*Supplementing Life*).
- Lumbar pain as if broken: Chengjin BL-56, Shugu BL-65 and Feiyang BL-58 (*Thousand Ducat Formulas*).
- Contraction of the legs: Chengjin BL-56, Chengshan BL-57, Jinggu BL-64 and Shangqiu SP-5 (*Thousand Ducat Formulas*).
- Numbness of the lower leg: Chengjin BL-56, Xiyangguan GB-33 and Huantiao GB-30 (*Thousand Ducat Formulas*).
- Heel pain: Chengjin BL-56, Chengshan BL-57, Kunlun BL-60 and Ahshi points.

CHENGSHAN BL-57

Support the Mountain

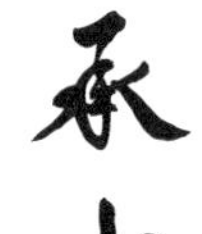

Ma Dan-yang Heavenly Star point

LOCATION

On the lower leg, in the depression formed below the bellies of the gastrocnemius muscle when the muscle is flexed, approximately 8 cun distal to Weizhong BL-40, i.e. midway between Weizhong BL-40 and Kunlun BL-60.

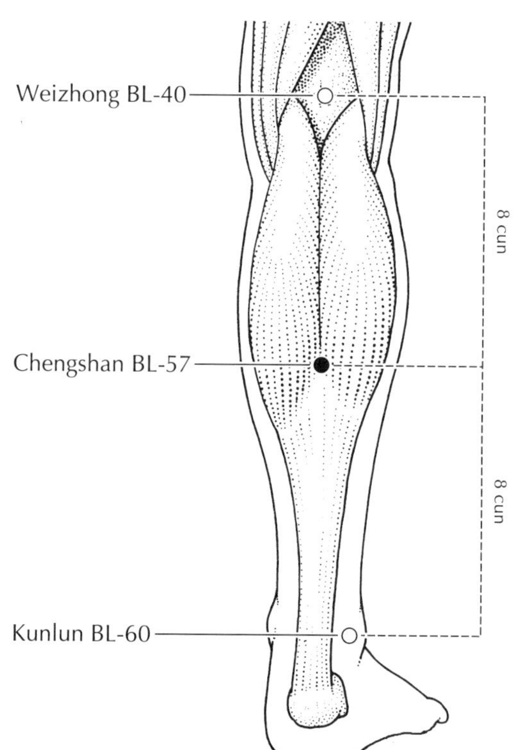

LOCATION NOTE

Run your finger upwards from the Achilles tendon along the midline until it falls into the depression formed between the two origins of the gastrocnemius muscle bellies; this depression may be easier to palpate if you ask the patient to press the ball of their foot against the resistance of your hand.

NEEDLING

Perpendicular or oblique insertion directed proximally or distally, 1 to 1.5 cun.

ACTIONS

Relaxes the sinews, activates the channel and alleviates pain
Benefits the calf and heel
Treats haemorrhoids

INDICATIONS

- Haemorrhoids, bleeding haemorrhoids, swollen and painful haemorrhoids, constipation, prolapse of the rectum.
- Pain and stiffness of the lumbar region, sciatica, difficulty sitting and standing, inability to stand for long, cramps, pain and contraction of the sinews, leg qi with swollen knee, heavy legs, flaccidity and weakness of the leg, pain of the heel, heat sensation in the soles with inability to stand for long.
- Shivering, malaria, sudden turmoil disorder, nosebleed, sore throat, heat in the head.

COMMENTARY

Chengshan BL-57 was included by Ma Dan-yang, the great physician of the Jin dynasty, among the 'eleven heavenly star points'[67], his grouping of the most vital acupuncture points. Clinically, Chengshan BL-57 is used in three principal situations: i. haemorrhoids, ii. contraction and pain of the calf, and iii. heel pain.

The Bladder divergent channel winds around the anal region. Classically, Chengshan BL-57 has been regarded as the primary distal point in the treatment of all kinds of haemorrhoids. For example, the *Song to Keep Up Your Sleeve* says "for the five types of haemorrhoids due to hot blood, select Chengshan BL-57 and await disappearance of the disease without a trace", whilst Ma Dan-yang recommends it for " ... haemorrhoids and difficulty in defecation ... ".

Pain and contraction of the calf may be due to traumatic injury, painful obstruction, or the sequela of sudden turmoil disorder, but is most commonly encountered in the context of deficiency of Liver blood. The *Essential Questions*[68] says "When a person sleeps the blood returns to the Liver". Pain and contraction of the calf therefore tends to occur at night when the body is at rest, the blood returns to the Liver, and the relative insufficiency of circulating blood is unable to nourish and soften the sinews and muscles of the extremities. This symptom is more commonly encountered in those who tend to suffer from blood deficiency, particularly women because of the loss of blood entailed in menstruation, and the elderly because of the inevitable decline of essence and blood inherent in ageing. Although having no action on the Liver blood itself, Chengshan BL-57 is an important local point in the treatment of this disorder.

Heel pain may be due to traumatic injury, painful obstruction or Kidney deficiency. Chengshan BL-57 is an important proximal point for this disorder and may be combined with other suitable points in the treatment of heel pain of whatever aetiology.

Finally, Ma Dan-yang and other classical sources emphasise the use of Chengshan BL-57 in the treatment of lumbar pain. Clinically it is now more commonly used for sciatic pain radiating to the calf region.

COMBINATIONS

- The nine types of haemorrhoids (with bleeding)[59]: Chengshan BL-57 and Changqiang DU-1 (*Song of the Jade Dragon*).
- The five types of haemorrhoids: Chengshan BL-57, Weizhong BL-40, Feiyang BL-58, Yangfu GB-38, Fuliu KID-7, Taichong LIV-3, Xiaxi GB-43, Qihai REN-6, Huiyin REN-1 and Changqiang DU-1 (*Great Compendium*).
- Chronic haemorrhoids: Chengshan BL-57, Erbai (M-UE-29) and Changqiang DU-1 (*Great Compendium*).
- Blood in the stool: Chengshan BL-57, Fuliu KID-7, Taichong LIV-3 and Taibai SP-3 (*Great Compendium*).
- Intestinal wind (blood in the stools): Chengshan BL-57 and Changqiang DU-1 (*One Hundred Symptoms*).
- Difficult defecation: Chengshan BL-57 and Taixi KID-3 (*Supplementing Life*).
- Difficult defecation: Chengshan BL-57, Dazhong KID-4, Zhongliao BL-33, Guanyuan REN-4, Chengjin BL-56, Taichong LIV-3, Taixi KID-3 and Zhongwan REN-12 (*Supplementing Life*).
- Feebleness of the legs: Chengshan BL-57, Weizhong BL-40 and Zusanli ST-36 (*Great Compendium*).
- Pain of the legs and lumbar region: Chengshan BL-57, Yinshi ST-33, Huantiao GB-30, Fengshi GB-31, Weizhong BL-40, Kunlun BL-60 and Shenmai BL-62 (*Great Compendium*).
- Contraction of the legs: Chengshan BL-57, Shangqiu SP-5, Chengjin BL-56 and Jinggu BL-64 (*Thousand Ducat Formulas*).
- Heat in the sole of the foot with inability to stand for long: Chengshan BL-57, Chengjin BL-56, Tiaokou ST-38 and Zusanli ST-36 (*Thousand Ducat Formulas*).

FEIYANG BL-58
Soaring Upwards

飛揚

Luo-Connecting point of the Bladder channel

LOCATION
On the lower leg, 7 cun directly superior to Kunlun BL-60, lateral to and approximately 1 cun inferior to Chengshan BL-57.

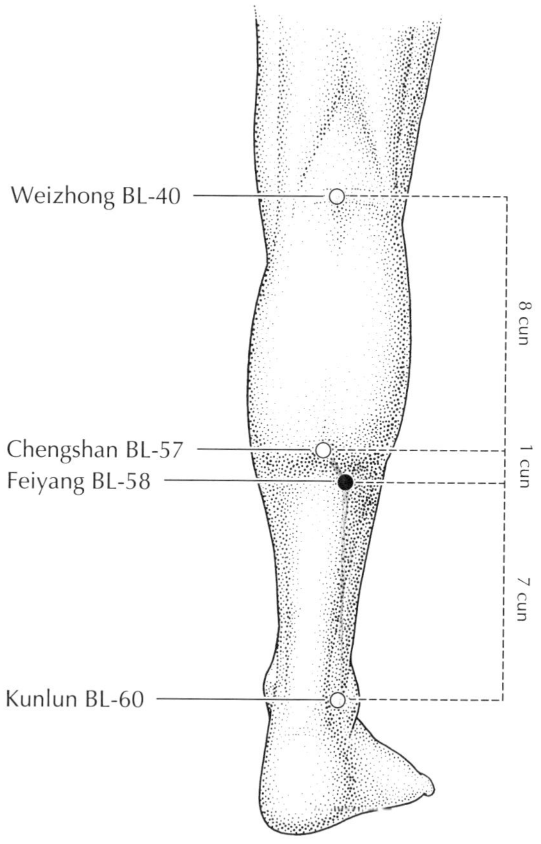

NEEDLING
Perpendicular or oblique insertion directed proximally or distally, 1 to 1.5 cun.

ACTIONS
Harmonises the upper and lower
Expels wind from taiyang channel
Treats haemorrhoids
Activates the channel and alleviates pain

INDICATIONS
- Heat in the head, dizziness, visual dizziness, headache and dizziness, pain of the neck and occiput, pain of the head and back, rhinitis, rhinitis with obstruction and pain of the head and back, nosebleed, nasal congestion, mania, epilepsy.
- Chills and fever, fever with absence of sweating, malaria, malaria with absence of thirst.
- Lumbar pain, heaviness of the body with inability to sit or stand, shivering with inability to sit or stand for long, atrophy disorder of the lower limb, coldness of the lower part of the body, weakness of the legs, difficulty in walking, swelling and pain of the lower limb, sciatica, wind painful obstruction of the joints, inability to flex or extend the toes.
- Haemorrhoids, swollen and painful haemorrhoids, bleeding haemorrhoids.

COMMENTARY
Feiyang BL-58 is the luo-connecting point of the Bladder channel. An examination of its modern application compared with its traditional indications reveals a significant disparity. Clinically it is most commonly used nowadays for disorders of the lower limb and lumbar pain, particularly for sciatic pain which is located either along the course of both the Bladder and Gall Bladder channels, or between these two channels. This reflects the location of Feiyang BL-58 at the place where the Bladder channel, which runs down the back of the leg from Chengfu BL-36, passes laterally towards the Gall Bladder channel on the lower leg.

Its traditional indications however, show a much wider application, characterised by excess in the upper region, sometimes with accompanying deficiency below (a pattern which may explain the name of this point, 'Soaring Upwards' as well as its alternative name 'Flying Yang)'.

From Feiyang BL-58 the luo-connecting channel meets with the Kidney channel, strengthening the relationship between these coupled channels. According to the *Guide to the Classics of Acupuncture* "the luo-connecting points are located between two channels ... if they are punctured, symptoms of the interiorly-exteriorly related channels can be treated"[69]. When the Kidneys are depleted there may be deficiency below manifesting as lumbar pain, coldness of the lower part of the body, inability to stand and weakness of the legs. At the same time there may be excessive yang rising up the coupled Bladder channel to the head and manifesting as dizziness, headache, pain of the neck and occiput, heat in the head and nosebleed.

As the Bladder channel descends towards the foot, its points are increasingly indicated for disorders of the spirit such as mania, and Feiyang BL-58 is the first of these. The Bladder primary channel connects with the Governing vessel at points Taodao DU-13, Dazhui DU-14, Naohu DU-17 and Baihui DU-20, where it enters the brain, whilst the Bladder divergent channel enters the Heart. Since both the brain and the Heart have been cited as the residence of the spirit in different traditions of Chinese medicine, these two channel pathways help explain the ability of points such as Feiyang BL-58 to calm the spirit and treat disorders of the brain such as mania and epilepsy.

When pathogenic factors, principally exterior wind, attack the taiyang channel they may give rise to chills and fever or fever with absence of sweating, as well as various symptoms affecting the head such as pain of the neck and occiput, heat in the head, nasal congestion and rhinitis, nosebleed and dizziness. Feiyang BL-58, a distal point of the foot taiyang channel, is able to expel pathogens from the channel, release the exterior and clear the upper portion of the channel.

The Bladder divergent channel encircles the anal region, and like Chengjin BL-56 and Chengshan BL-57, Feiyang BL-58 is classically indicated for the treatment of haemorrhoids, swollen and painful haemorrhoids and bleeding haemorrhoids.

Finally, the *Great Compendium of Acupuncture and Moxibustion* gives specific indications for excess and deficiency of the luo-connecting points. In the case of Feiyang BL-58, these are rhinitis with obstruction and pain of the head and back (excess); rhinitis with nosebleed (deficiency).

COMBINATIONS
- Dizziness and eye pain: Feiyang BL-58 and Yanggu SI-5 (*Supplementing Life*).
- Headache and dizziness: Feiyang BL-58, Kunlun BL-60, Ququan LIV-8, Qiangu SI-2, Shaoze SI-1 and Tongli HE-5 (*Thousand Ducat Formulas*).
- Heat in the head and rhinitis with nosebleed: Feiyang BL-58, Chengshan BL-57, Kunlun BL-60, Jinggu BL-64 and Yinbai SP-1 (*Thousand Ducat Formulas*).
- Neck pain, joint pain and sweating: Feiyang BL-58, Yongquan KID-1 and Hanyan GB-4 (*Thousand Ducat Formulas*).
- Madness and mania disorder with tongue thrusting: Feiyang BL-58, Taiyi ST-23 and Huaroumen ST-24 (*Thousand Ducat Formulas*).

FUYANG BL-59

Instep Yang

跗陽

Xi-Cleft point of Yang Motility vessel

LOCATION
On the lower leg, 3 cun directly superior to Kunlun BL-60.

LOCATION NOTE
i. Locate one handbreadth proximal to Kunlun BL-60; ii. This point is located in the depression between the Achilles tendon and the peroneal tendons.

NEEDLING
Perpendicular or oblique insertion directed proximally or distally, 1 to 1.5 cun.

ACTIONS
Benefits the lumbar region and legs
Activates the channel and alleviates pain

INDICATIONS
- Lumbar pain with inability to stand for long, inability to stand after sitting, thigh pain, wind painful obstruction with numbness, atrophy disorder of the lower limb, inability to raise the four limbs, heaviness and soreness of the leg and knee, sciatica, cold damp leg qi, ulceration of the leg, redness and swelling of the lateral malleolus.
- Heavy head, chills and fever, pain of the brow, sudden turmoil disorder with cramps, clonic spasm.

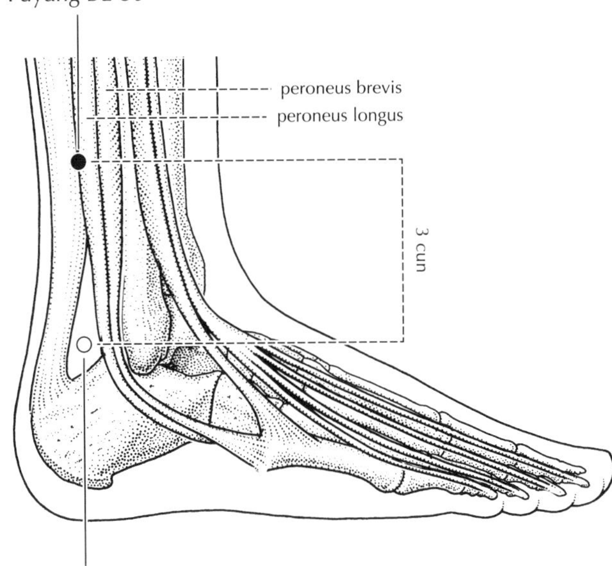

COMBINATIONS
- Clonic spasm: Fuyang BL-59 and Tianjing SJ-10 (*Supplementing Life*).
- Heaviness of the head: Fuyang BL-59 Tongtian BL-7 and Yamen DU-15 (*Supplementing Life*).

KUNLUN BL-60

Kunlun Mountains

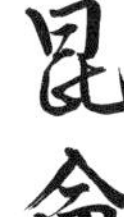

Jing-River and Fire point of the Bladder channel
Ma Dan-yang Heavenly Star point

LOCATION

Behind the ankle joint, in the depression between the prominence of the lateral malleolus and the Achilles tendon.

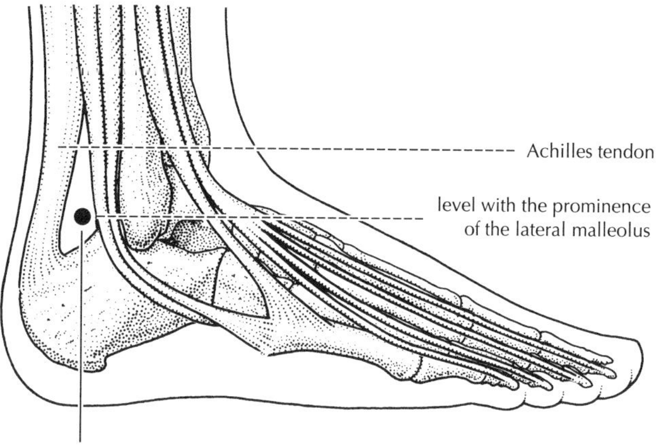

LOCATION NOTE

Locate in the centre of the depression, midway between the prominence of the lateral malleolus and the posterior border of the Achilles tendon.

NEEDLING

Perpendicular insertion 0.5 to 1 cun, or directed superiorly to join with Taixi KID-3, 1.5 to 2 cun.
Caution: contraindicated in pregnancy.

ACTIONS

Clears heat and lowers yang
Pacifies wind and leads down excess
Activates the entire Bladder channel and alleviates pain
Relaxes the sinews and strengthens the lumbar spine
Promotes labour

INDICATIONS

- Childhood epilepsy, epilepsy, madness, lockjaw, headache, heat in the head, visual dizziness, redness pain and swelling of the eyes, bursting eye pain, pain of the upper teeth, rhinitis with nosebleed.
- Stiff neck, contraction of the shoulder and back, Heart pain that radiates to the back, lumbar pain, sacral pain, pain of the coccyx, sciatica, pain behind the knee, ankle pain, heel pain, hemiplegia.
- Fullness of the chest, dyspnoea, cough, malaria, malaria with copious sweating.
- Difficult labour, retention of placenta, difficulty in conceiving, swelling of the genitals, abdominal pain, difficult defecation.

COMMENTARY

Kunlun BL-60 is the fire point of the taiyang Bladder channel and an important point to clear and descend excess wind, fire and yang from the upper part of the body. To best understand the actions of this point, three factors should be taken into account: i. as a fire point, Kunlun BL-60 is able to clear heat, fire and excess yang; ii. taiyang (supreme yang) channel is the most yang of the six channels; iii. Kunlun BL-60 is located on the foot, towards the inferior end of the Bladder channel which traverses the entire posterior (yang) portion of the body.

The principle "for diseases of the head select [points from] the feet" applies well to this point. Kunlun BL-60 is able to clear heat and lead down excess yang from the head in cases of headache, heat in the head, redness, pain and swelling of the eyes, bursting eye pain, nosebleed and toothache, and to extinguish wind from the head in cases of epilepsy and lockjaw. Indeed as long ago as the third century CE the *Systematic Classic of Acupuncture and Moxibustion* stated that Kunlun BL-60 "drains wind from the head to the feet". Although Kunlun BL-60 is principally used clinically in the treatment of occipital headache, it is worth noting that the primary Bladder channel meets the Governing vessel and the Gall Bladder channel at Baihui DU-20 on the vertex, Shenting DU-24 and Toulinqi GB-15 towards the front of the head, and points Qubin GB-7 through to Wangu GB-12 on the side of the head. For this reason, Kunlun BL-60 may be considered for pain in any region of the head.

It is interesting that many of the indications of this point, characterised by uprising of yang, flaring up of fire and stirring of wind, suggest a clinical picture of Liver disharmony. Whilst Kunlun BL-60 has no direct action on the Liver, and is therefore unable to treat the root of such disorders, it has a profound action on subduing the manifestations. At the same time, there is a parallel between Kunlun BL-60, the fire point of the 'supreme yang' channel, and the fierce, indomitable and strong quality of Liver yang.

The ability of Kunlun BL-60 to activate the entire length of the Bladder channel as well as to relax the sinews and strengthen the lumbar spine, renders it an essential point in the treatment of pain and contraction anywhere along the channel. It is the foremost distal point in the treatment of occipital headache and is often combined with Houxi SI-3 for this purpose. It is equally vital in the treatment of disorders of the back and spine from the neck right down to the coccyx. Kunlun BL-60 is one of the few distal points which are able to treat disorders of the middle and upper back, again often combined with Houxi SI-3. It is specifically indicated for Heart pain that radiates from the chest through to the upper back, reflecting the pathway of the Bladder divergent channel to the Heart. In disorders of the lumbar region, in which Kidney deficiency is often the root, Kunlun BL-60 may be joined by through-needling to Taixi KID-3. Ma Dan-yang, the great physician of the Jin dynasty, listed Kunlun BL-60 as one of the 'eleven heavenly star points'[70] "for cramping of the lumbar region and sacrum ... inability to walk or even take a step, as soon as he moves he groans". Kunlun BL-60 is equally valuable in treating obstruction of the Bladder channel in the lower limbs, especially in cases of sciatic pain radiating down the back of the leg, and is often combined with points such as Chengfu BL-36 and Weizhong BL-40 in the 'chain and lock' point association method. In the ankle region, Kunlun BL-60 is an important point for pain and stiffness, and like several distal points of the Bladder channel it is able to treat pain of the heel.

The ability of Kunlun BL-60 to promote labour is another reflection both of the strong descending action of this point, and of the paired relationship of the Bladder and the Kidneys, which dominate the uterus. It may be used, in combination with points such as Hegu L.I.-4, Zhiyin BL-67 and Sanyinjiao SP-6, to induce labour, hasten prolonged labour, control pain and promote the expulsion of the placenta. For this reason Kunlun BL-60 is contraindicated in pregnancy. The *Great Compendium of Acupuncture & Moxibustion* somewhat surprisingly however, also suggests this point for difficult conception.

Finally, it is interesting to note that Kunlun BL-60 is indicated for fullness of the chest, dyspnoea and cough. Whilst these indications have no apparent relationship to the Bladder channel, they do reflect the ability of jing-river points, according to the *Classic of Difficulties*[71], to treat dyspnoea and cough.

COMBINATIONS

- Headache and dizziness: Kunlun BL-60, Ququan LIV-8, Feiyang BL-58, Qiangu SI-2, Shaoze SI-1 and Tongli HE-5 (*Thousand Ducat Formulas*).
- Wind dizziness and headache: Kunlun BL-60, Tianyou SJ-16, Fengmen BL-12, Guanchong SJ-1 and Guanyuan REN-4 (*Thousand Ducat Formulas*).
- Head wind: Kunlun BL-60, Xiaxi GB-43, Shangxing DU-23, Qianding DU-21, Baihui DU-20, Yanggu SI-5, Hegu L.I.-4 and Guanchong SJ-1 (*Great Compendium*).
- Heat in the head and rhinitis with nosebleed: Kunlun BL-60, Chengshan BL-57, Feiyang BL-58, Jinggu BL-64 and Yinbai SP-1 (*Thousand Ducat Formulas*).
- Visual dizziness, dimness of vision with bursting eye pain: Kunlun BL-60, Tianzhu BL-10 and Taodao DU-13 (*Supplementing Life*).
- Opisthotonos, clonic spasm, epilepsy and headache: Kunlun BL-60, Wuchu BL-5, Shenzhu DU-12, Weizhong BL-40 and Weiyang BL-39 (*Thousand Ducat Formulas*).
- Manic raving: Kunlun BL-60, Yangxi L.I.-5, Xialian L.I.-8 and Taiyuan LU-9 (*Great Compendium*).
- Mania, incessant talking without rest: Kunlun BL-60, Shugu BL-65 and Fengfu DU-16 (*Thousand Ducat Formulas*).
- Wind epilepsy with upward staring eyes: Kunlun BL-60, Baihui DU-20 and Sizhukong SJ-23 (*Great Compendium*).
- Lumbar pain: Huantiao GB-30 and Weizhong BL-40; if the pain radiates up the back add Kunlun BL-60 (*Song of Points*).
- Pain of the legs and lumbar region: Kunlun BL-60, Yinshi ST-33, Huantiao GB-30, Fengshi GB-31, Weizhong BL-40, Chengshan BL-57 and Shenmai BL-62 (*Great Compendium*).
- Pain of the lumbar region and knee: Kunlun BL-60, Shenmai BL-62, Yanglao SI-6, Huantiao GB-30 and Yanglingquan GB-34 (*Illustrated Supplement*).
- Straw shoe wind (redness, swelling and pain of the leg and foot): Kunlun BL-60, Shenmai BL-62 and Taixi KID-3 (*Song of the Jade Dragon*).
- Pain of the ankle and heel: Kunlun BL-60, Xuanzhong GB-39 and Qiuxu GB-40 (*Song More Precious Than Jade*).
- Painful obstruction of the calf: Kunlun BL-60 and Fengshi GB-31 (*Compilation*).
- Windstroke with one-sided withering and incessant pain: Kunlun BL-60, Jianyu L.I.-15, Xuanzhong GB-39, Taixi KID-3, Zusanli ST-36 and Quchi L.I.-11 (*Great Compendium*).

PUCAN BL-61

Servant's Respect

僕參

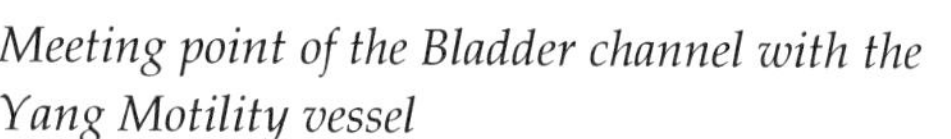

Meeting point of the Bladder channel with the Yang Motility vessel

LOCATION

On the lateral side of the foot, 1.5 cun inferior to Kunlun BL-60, in a tender depression on the calcaneum.

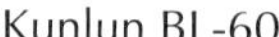

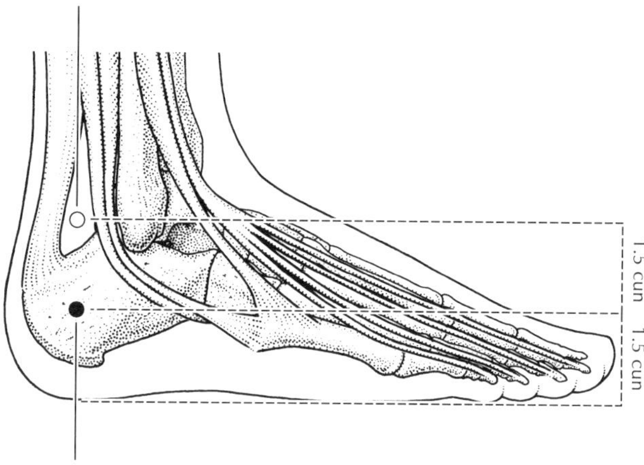

LOCATION NOTE

The distance between the prominence of the lateral malleolus and the sole of the foot is 3 cun; locate Pucan BL-61 directly below Kunlun BL-60 and midway between this point and the sole.

NEEDLING

Transverse insertion 0.3 to 0.5 cun.

ACTIONS

Relaxes the sinews, activates the channel and alleviates pain

INDICATIONS

- Headache, heavy head, heaviness of the head like a stone.
- Mania, manic raving, seeing ghosts, loss of consciousness, childhood epilepsy, vomiting, turbid painful urinary dysfunction.
- Lumbar pain, atrophy disorder of the leg, leg qi, sudden turmoil disorder with cramps, swelling of the knee, heel pain.

COMBINATIONS

- Cramps: Pucan BL-61, Zhiyin BL-67, Jiexi ST-41, Qiuxu GB-40 and Zuqiaoyin GB-44 (*Supplementing Life*).

SHENMAI BL-62

Extending Vessel

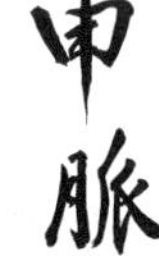

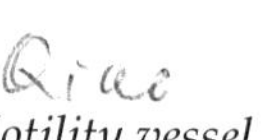

Confluent point of the Yang Motility vessel
Sun Si-miao Ghost point

LOCATION

On the lateral side of the foot, approximately 0.5 cun inferior to the inferior border of the lateral malleolus, in a depression posterior to the peroneal tendons.

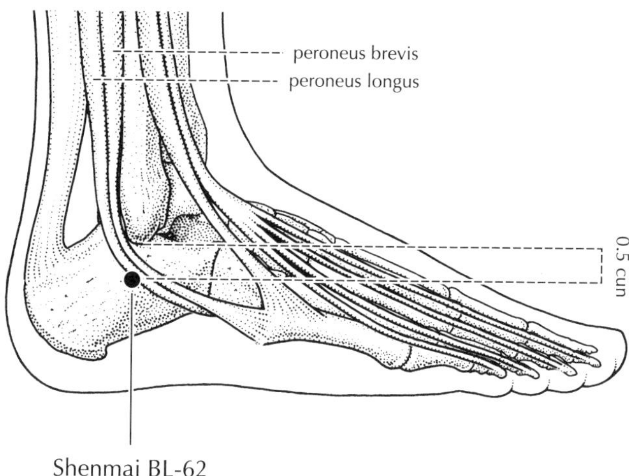

LOCATION NOTE

Locate this point directly inferior to the prominence of the lateral malleolus.

NEEDLING

Oblique insertion directed inferiorly, 0.3 to 0.5 cun.

ACTIONS

Pacifies interior wind and expels exterior wind
Calms the spirit and treats epilepsy
Benefits the head and eyes
Opens and regulates the Yang Motility vessel
Activates the channel and alleviates pain

INDICATIONS

- Chills and fever, aversion to wind with spontaneous sweating and headache.
- Wind dizziness, head wind, headache, lateral and midline headache, thunder head wind, opisthotonos, upward staring eyes, lockjaw, epilepsy, daytime epilepsy, windstroke with inability to speak and hemiplegia, deviation of the mouth, eye and face, counterflow qi.
- Red eyes, eye pain that originates at the inner canthus, nosebleed, deafness, tinnitus.

- Mania-depression, palpitations, Heart fright, insomnia.
- Stiffness of the nape of the neck, stiffness and difficulty in extending the back, cold painful obstruction of the lumbar region and hip, pain of the lumbar region and leg, difficulty in extending and flexing the knee, redness and swelling of the lateral malleolus, straw shoe wind (redness, swelling and pain of the leg and foot).
- Blood and qi pain in women, fullness of the chest, swelling of the neck and axilla.

COMMENTARY

In the *Ode of the Obstructed River* the use of Shenmai BL-62 is referred to as one of 'the eight therapeutic methods'. In this description of the application of the eight confluent points of the extraordinary vessels to affect specific symptoms and areas of the body, Shenmai BL-62 is indicated "to expel cold and heat and [to treat] one-sided and generalised head wind ... ".

Shenmai BL-62 is both a point of the taiyang Bladder channel and the confluent point of the Yang Motility vessel, reflected in its alternative name 'Yang Qiao' (Yang Motility). The taiyang (supreme yang) Bladder channel traverses the head and the entire length of the back, the most yang area of the body. It connects with the Governing vessel at points Taodao DU-13, Dazhui DU-14, Naohu DU-17 and Baihui DU-20, where it enters the brain. The Yang Motility vessel traverses the lateral side of the body and head, connects with the Gall Bladder channel at Fengchi GB-20 and enters the brain at Fengfu DU-16. Furthermore, the Bladder divergent channel enters the Heart. This network of channel pathways helps to explain the principal actions and indications of this point.

Wind is a yang pathogenic factor characterised by sudden onset, rapid changes, constant or abnormal movement and a tendency to attack the head and upper and outer portions of the body. Wind may be of exterior or interior origin. Taiyang channel is the most exterior of the six channels and is generally the first channel to be attacked by exterior pathogenic wind. Shenmai BL-62 is particularly indicated for the commonly-seen pattern of attack of exterior wind (usually in combination with either heat or cold) with chills and fever, aversion to wind, stiff neck and headache. Interior wind, by contrast, arises from interior disharmony, principally of the Liver. It rushes upwards, disturbing the brain and leading to such symptoms as lockjaw, opisthotonos, upward staring eyes, deviation of the mouth and eyes, windstroke and hemiplegia. The ability of Shenmai BL-62 to pacify interior wind and treat such manifestations reflects the extreme yang nature of this point and its channel connections to the head and brain, rather than any action on the Liver zang. In other words Shenmai BL-62 treats the manifestation of wind rather than the root.

Shenmai BL-62 (the confluent point of the Yang Motility vessel) is classically indicated for day-time epilepsy, in contrast to Zhaohai KID-6 (the confluent point of the Yin Motility vessel) which is classically indicated for night-time epilepsy. Epilepsy principally involves three factors, namely stirring of wind, disturbance of the Heart and brain, and phlegm. The fact that the Bladder primary channel enters the brain and the Bladder divergent channel links with the Heart, combined with the ability of Shenmai BL-62 to pacify wind, explains its special effect on epilepsy. Under its alternative name of Guilu (Ghost Path) Shenmai BL-62 was included in a group known as the 'thirteen ghost points' listed by Sun Si-miao for the treatment of epilepsy and mania. Shenmai BL-62 is further indicated for disorders of the Heart and spirit such as palpitations, insomnia and mania-depression.

The *Spiritual Pivot* states "When the taiyang [Bladder] channel enters the brain it is divided into the Yin Motility and the Yang Motility; it is here that the yin and yang meet; yang enters the yin and yin moves outwards to the yang, meeting at the inner corner of the eye. When the yang is abundant, the eyes are staring open; when the yin is abundant, the eyes will be closed shut"[72] and "[When] defensive qi does not enter into the yin it will frequently remain at the yang. [When] it remains at the yang then yang qi will be full, [when] yang qi is full, the Yang Motility vessel [will become] abundant, [when] it does not enter the yin, then yin qi will become deficient and therefore the eyes will not close"[73]. These two quotations have served traditionally to further explain the ability of Shenmai BL-62 to treat insomnia.

Shenmai BL-62 shares with other distal points of the Bladder channel the ability to clear heat and excess from the head, whether due to exterior pathogens, excess fire, uprising of yang or stirring of wind. It is indicated for head wind and headache affecting both the midline (Bladder channel) and lateral (Yang Motility vessel) portions of the head, for dizziness, nosebleed, deafness and tinnitus, and especially for eye disorders, as both the Bladder channel and the Yang Motility vessel link with the inner canthus.

Shenmai BL-62 may be needled for various other disorders affecting both the Bladder channel and the Yang Motility vessel, for example pain of both the lumbar region (Bladder channel) and hip (Yang Motility vessel).

Finally, Shenmai BL-62 is indicated for swelling of the axilla and neck. These indications may be explained by the pathway of the Bladder sinew channel which ascends to the axilla and then emerges at the supraclavicular fossa to cross the neck.

COMBINATIONS

- Head wind and headache: Shenmai BL-62 and Jinmen BL-63 (*Ode to Elucidate Mysteries*).
- Head wind, visual dizziness and stiffness of the nape of the neck: Shenmai BL-62, Shousanli L.I.-10, and Jinmen BL-63 (*Miscellaneous Diseases*).
- Madness: Shenmai BL-62 and Jiexi ST-41 (*Thousand Ducat Formulas*).
- Night-time epilepsy: moxa Shenmai BL-62 and Zhaohai KID-6 (*Glorious Anthology*).
- Coldness and pain of the bone marrow: Shenmai BL-62, Dazhu BL-11, Xuanzhong GB-39, Fuliu KID-7, Lidui ST-45 and Shenshu BL-23 (*Compilation*).
- Pain of the legs and lumbar region: Shenmai BL-62, Fengshi GB-31, Huantiao GB-30, Weizhong BL-40, Kunlun BL-60, Yinshi ST-33 and Chengshan BL-57 (*Great Compendium*).
- Diseases below the ankle: Shenmai BL-62 and Zhaohai KID-6 (*Great Compendium*).
- Swelling of the axilla: Shenmai BL-62, Diwuhui GB-42, Yangfu GB-38, Weiyang BL-39, Tianchi P-1 and Zulinqi GB-41 (*Thousand Ducat Formulas*).

JINMEN BL-63

Golden Gate

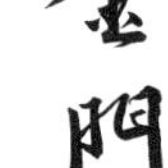

Xi-Cleft point of the Bladder channel
Meeting point of the Bladder channel with the Yang Linking vessel

LOCATION

On the lateral side of the foot, in the depression posterior to the tuberosity of the fifth metatarsal bone.

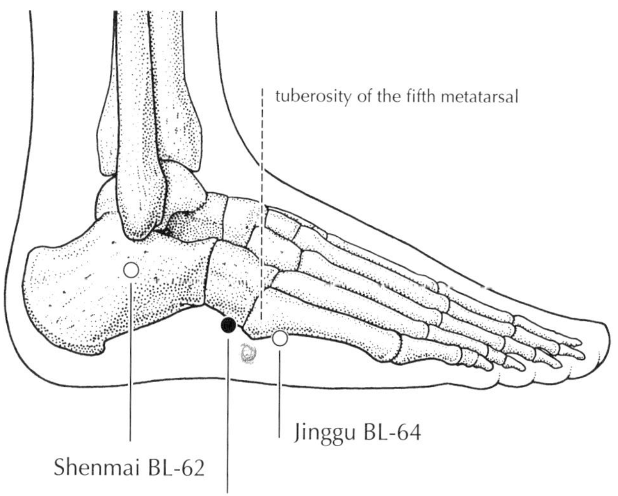

LOCATION NOTE

The tuberosity of the fifth metatarsal bone is the most palpable landmark on the lateral side of the foot.

NEEDLING

Perpendicular insertion 0.3 to 0.5 cun.

ACTIONS

Pacifies wind
Moderates acute conditions
Relaxes the sinews, activates the channel and alleviates pain

INDICATIONS

- Epilepsy, childhood fright wind, toothache, loss of consciousness.
- Sudden and violent shan disorder, sudden turmoil disorder with cramps, malaria, shivering with inability to stand for long.
- Lumbar pain, knee pain, painful obstruction of the lower limb, white tiger joint wind, pain of the external malleolus.

COMMENTARY

Jinmen BL-63 is the xi-cleft point of the Bladder channel. The xi-cleft points, where the qi and blood which flow relatively superficially along the channels from the jing-well points gather and plunge more deeply, are applicable in the treatment of acute conditions and pain. Jinmen BL-63 is indicated for sudden onset of severe shan disorder, sudden turmoil disorder with cramps, epilepsy and white tiger joint pain, a manifestation of painful obstruction characterised by the great severity of the pain which is likened to the bite of a tiger.

Despite its status as the xi-cleft point of the Bladder channel, Jinmen BL-63 (like most of the distal points of the channel) was traditionally ascribed no action on disorders of urination. In this respect, the Bladder channel points are similar to those of the Small and Large Intestine and Sanjiao channels whose points also have little action on their related fu.

COMBINATIONS

- Cramping of the sinews: Jinmen BL-63 and Qiuxu GB-40 (*One Hundred Symptoms*).
- Contraction and cold of the shoulder and back with pain of the inner aspect of the scapula: Jinmen BL-63, Geshu BL-17, Yixi BL-45 and Chize LU-5 (*Thousand Ducat Formulas*).
- Bilateral deafness due to injury by cold: Jinmen BL-63 and Tinghui GB-2 (*Ode of Xi-hong*).
- Deafness: Jinmen BL-63, Zulinqi GB-41 and Hegu L.I.-4 (*Song of Points*).

JINGGU BL-64

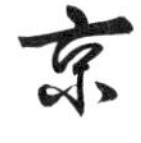
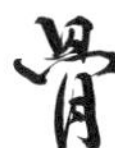

Capital Bone

Yuan-Source point of the Bladder channel

LOCATION

On the lateral side of the foot, in the depression anterior and inferior to the tuberosity of the fifth metatarsal bone.

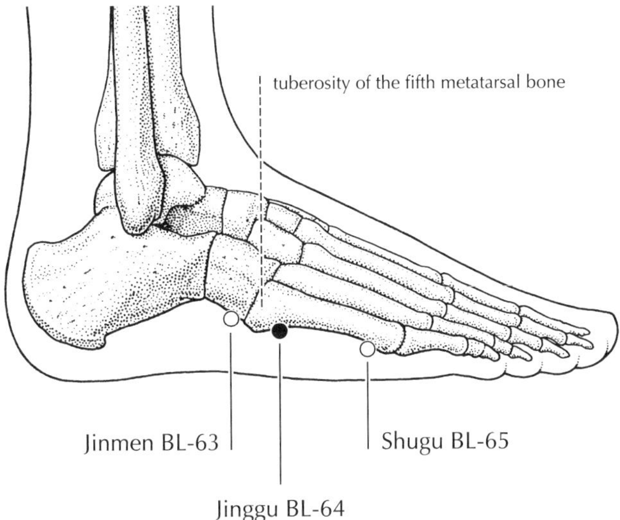

LOCATION NOTE

The tuberosity of the fifth metatarsal bone is the most palpable landmark on the lateral side of the foot.

NEEDLING

Perpendicular insertion 0.3 to 0.5 cun.

ACTIONS

Clears the head and eyes and eliminates wind
Calms the spirit
Relaxes the sinews, activates the channel and alleviates pain

INDICATIONS

- Painful and heavy head with cold feet, splitting headache, heat in the head, shaking of the head, redness of the inner canthus, superficial visual obstruction, visual dizziness, rhinitis with ceaseless nosebleed, chills and fever, malaria, no pleasure in eating.
- Palpitations, Heart pain, mania-depression, propensity to fright, epilepsy.
- Stiff neck, pain of the back and sides of the body, lumbar pain, aversion to cold and pain of the back, cracked and dry feet, cold damp leg qi.

COMMENTARY

Jinggu BL-64 is the yuan-source point of the Bladder channel, and like most of the distal Bladder channel points treats fullness of the head. This fullness may be due to attack of exterior pathogenic wind or wind-heat, to stirring of interior wind, to upsurging of yang due to Kidney deficiency, or simply to disharmony of the upper and lower parts of the body. Excess above manifests as heat, pain and heaviness of the head, splitting headache, shaking of the head, rhinitis with ceaseless nosebleed etc., whilst deficiency below gives rise to cold feet.

The Bladder channel ascends to the inner canthus and Jinggu BL-64 is indicated for various eye disorders such as visual dizziness, redness of the inner canthus and superficial visual obstruction.

The Bladder primary channel enters the brain whilst the Bladder divergent channel enters the Heart, and like several distal Bladder channel points, Jinggu BL-64 is indicated for disorders such as palpitations, Heart pain, epilepsy and mania-depression.

Finally, Jinggu BL-64 is indicated for stiffness, pain and contraction along the course of the Bladder channel from the neck to the feet.

COMBINATIONS

- Heat in the head and rhinitis with nosebleed: Jinggu BL-64, Kunlun BL-60, Feiyang BL-58, Chengshan BL-57 and Yinbai SP-1 (*Thousand Ducat Formulas*).
- Redness and erosion of the inner canthus: Jinggu BL-64 and Shugu BL-65 (*Supplementing Life*).
- Superficial visual obstruction: Jinggu BL-64 and Qiangu SI-2 (*Thousand Ducat Formulas*).
- Cold of the lower extremities: Jinggu BL-64, Rangu KID-2 and Shenshu BL-23 (*Thousand Ducat Formulas*).
- Contraction of the legs: Jinggu BL-64, Chengjin BL-56, Chengshan BL-57 and Shangqiu SP-5 (*Thousand Ducat Formulas*).
- Pain of the genitals: Jinggu BL-64, Shenshu BL-23, Zhishi BL-52 and Taichong LIV-3 (*Supplementing Life*).

SHUGU BL-65

束骨

Restraining Bone

Shu-Stream and Wood point of the Bladder channel

LOCATION

On the lateral side of the foot, in the depression posterior and inferior to the head of the fifth metatarsal bone.

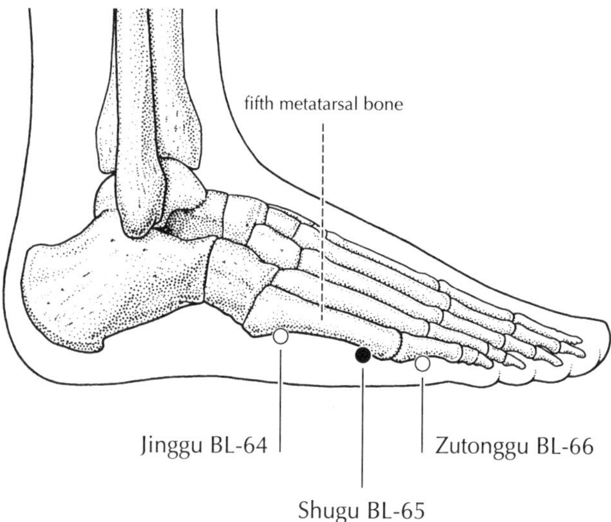

LOCATION NOTE

Run a finger distally along the lateral side of the foot from Jinggu BL-64 until it falls into the depression.

NEEDLING

Perpendicular insertion 0.3 to 0.5 cun.

ACTIONS

Clears the head and eyes
Clears heat and dissipates swelling
Activates the channel and alleviates pain

INDICATIONS

- Headache, occipital headache, stiff neck, deafness, visual dizziness, redness and pain of the eyes, redness and erosion of the inner canthus, yellow eyes.
- Chills and fever, aversion to wind and cold, heat in the body, malaria, mania-depression, carbuncular swellings on the back, clove sores on the back, haemorrhoids, diarrhoea.
- Pain of the lumbar region and back, thigh pain.

COMMENTARY

The *Classic of Difficulties*[74] states "in cases of deficiency reinforce the mother, in cases of excess reduce the child". Shugu BL-65 is the wood point of the Bladder channel, and according to the 'mother-child' theory is able to reduce excess in the Bladder channel (wood is the 'child' of Bladder water), especially fullness and heat in the head region. The Bladder channel ascends from the inner canthus over the vertex, connects with points of the Governing vessel and Gall Bladder channel on the head, and descends through the occipital region and neck. Shugu BL-65, consequently, is indicated for redness and pain of the eyes and inner canthus, headache (especially in the occipital region) and stiff neck.

The heat clearing action of Shugu BL-65 extends to resolving fever, especially due to injury by wind, and to draining heat from the anal region in the treatment of haemorrhoids. Like Weizhong BL-40, Shugu BL-65 is also indicated for carbuncular swellings on the back and for clove sores (small, hard, clove-shaped purulent lesions).

COMBINATIONS

- Stiff neck with great aversion to wind: Shugu BL-65 and Tianzhu BL-10 (*One Hundred Symptoms*).
- Redness and erosion of the inner canthus: Shugu BL-65 and Jinggu BL-64 (*Supplementing Life*).
- Mania, incessant talking without rest: Shugu BL-65, Kunlun BL-60 and Fengfu DU-16 (*Thousand Ducat Formulas*).
- Lumbar pain as if broken: Shugu BL-65, Feiyang BL-58 and Chengjin BL-56 (*Thousand Ducat Formulas*).
- Hip pain: Shugu BL-65, Huantiao GB-30, Jiaoxin KID-8, Sanyinjiao SP-6 and Yingu KID-10 (*Thousand Ducat Formulas*).

ZUTONGGU BL-66

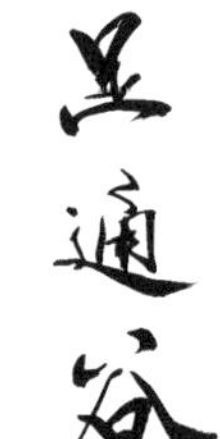

Foot Connecting Valley

Ying-Spring and Water point of the Bladder channel

LOCATION

On the lateral side of the foot, in the depression anterior and inferior to the fifth metatarso-phalangeal joint.

LOCATION NOTE

First locate Shugu BL-65, then run the finger over the prominence of the metatarso-phalangeal joint until it falls into the depression at the base of the little toe.

NEEDLING

Perpendicular-oblique insertion towards the sole 0.2 to 0.3 cun.

ACTIONS
Clears the head
Descends Lung and Stomach qi

INDICATIONS
- Heaviness of the head, neck pain, visual dizziness, redness of the eyes, nosebleed, sweating without aversion to cold, malaria.
- Vomiting, undigested food (in the stool), cough and dyspnoea, fullness of the chest with congested fluids.
- Mania, propensity to fright.

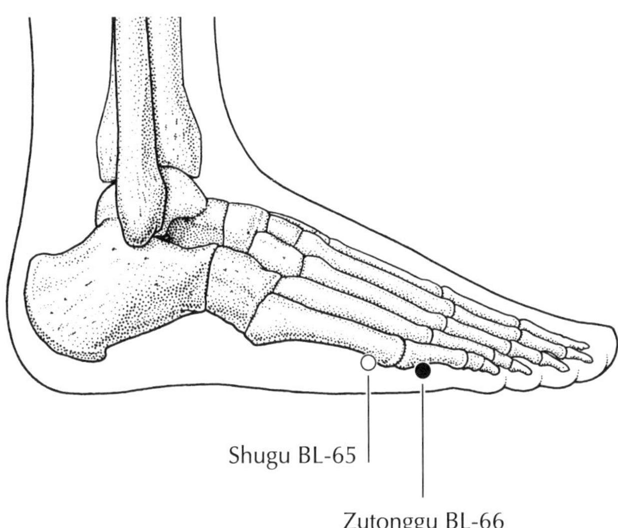

COMMENTARY
Zutonggu BL-66 is the water point of the Bladder water channel. Like all the distal points of the Bladder channel, its principal action is to clear pathologically ascending qi and yang from the head. This was emphasised in the *Spiritual Pivot*[75] which stated "When [chaotic] qi is in the head, select Tianzhu BL-10 and Dazhu BL-11. If needling these fails to work, select the spring and stream points of the foot taiyang" (i.e. Shugu BL-65 and Zutonggu BL-66).

If chaotic qi affects not only the head, but also impairs the descending function of the Lungs and Stomach, the consequent rebellion of qi will give rise to coughing, dyspnoea, fullness of the chest and vomiting.

COMBINATIONS
- Rhinitis with nose bleed: Zutonggu BL-66, Pianli L.I-6, Hegu L.I-4, Sanjian L.I-3 and Kunlun BL-60 (*Supplementing Life*).
- Sudden loss of voice: Zutonggu BL-66, Zhigou SJ-6 and Sanyangluo SJ-8 (*Supplementing Life*).
- Vomiting: Zutonggu BL-66, Shangqiu SP-5 and Youmen KID-21 (*Thousand Ducat Formulas*).

ZHIYIN BL-67
Reaching Yin

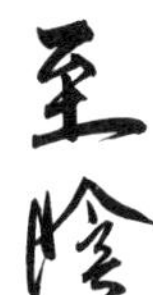

Jing-Well and Metal point of the Bladder channel

LOCATION
On the dorsal aspect of the little toe, at the junction of lines drawn along the lateral border of the nail and the base of the nail, approximately 0.1 cun from the corner of the nail.

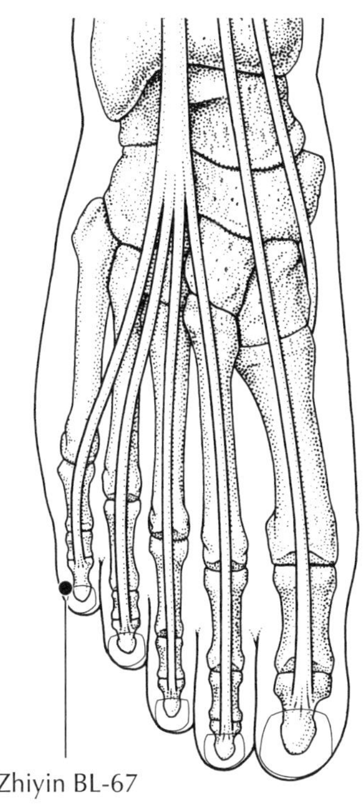

NEEDLING
Perpendicular or oblique insertion directed proximally 0.1 to 0.2 cun, or prick to bleed.

ACTIONS
Expels wind and clears the head and eyes
Turns the foetus and facilitates labour

INDICATIONS
- Vertex headache, occipital headache, heaviness of the head, neck pain, nasal congestion, nosebleed, eye pain, pain of the inner canthus, superficial visual obstruction, deafness and tinnitus, pain of the lateral costal region and chest, agitation of the Heart.
- Retention of placenta, malposition of foetus, delayed labour, prolonged or difficult labour.

- Difficult urination, painful urinary dysfunction, seminal emission, cold malaria, wind cold starting from the little toe, absence of sweating, heat in the soles of the feet, cramps, clonic spasm, swelling of the knees.

COMMENTARY

Zhiyin BL-67 is the jing-well and metal point of the Bladder channel. Unlike most of the other eleven jing-well points, however, it has no apparent classically recorded action of restoring consciousness in case of coma or collapse and its similarity to the other jing-well points is limited to its ability to clear fullness and heat from the opposite end of the channel in the head.

The *Spiritual Pivot*[76] states "for diseases of the head select [points from] the feet", whilst *Song to Keep Up Your Sleeve* says that Zhiyin BL-67 is indicated for "disorders of the face and head". Zhiyin BL-67 is particularly applicable for vertex and occipital headache, whether due to exterior pathogenic wind or to internal disharmony, as well as for disorders of the neck, eyes, nose and ears. As the terminal point of the Bladder channel, Zhiyin BL-67 is especially dynamic in its action, and in clinical practice would be considered when these disorders are acute rather than chronic in nature.

The principal application of Zhiyin BL-67, however, is in the treatment of malposition of the foetus, for which it is renowned. For this purpose it is treated by stick moxibustion for fifteen to twenty minutes bilaterally, or by moxa cones (five to ten cones at each point) once or twice a day. The woman should loosen her clothes and sit in a comfortable semi-reclining position. It is common practice in China to demonstrate this method to the pregnant woman who is then supplied with moxa sticks for self-treatment at home. Best results are achieved if this treatment is started in the 34th week. It is important to note that once the foetus has turned, moxibustion should be discontinued, otherwise further malposition may be induced. The effect of Zhiyin BL-67 on the uterus extends further to inducing delayed labour, hastening delivery once labour has commenced and promoting the expulsion of the placenta after childbirth.

It is interesting to note that despite the intimate relationship between the Kidneys and the uterus, it is points of its coupled Bladder channel, especially Zhiyin BL-67 and Kunlun BL-60, rather than points of the Kidney channel, which have the action of promoting labour. According to yin yang theory "yang is activity, yin is quiescence; yang brings forth and yin develops" and "When yin reaches its maximum it will necessarily transform into yang". The yin of the Kidney nourishes and dominates the development and growth of the foetus through the long months of pregnancy. As the birth date approaches and yin reaches its zenith, yang must begin to grow in order to turn the foetus and prepare for the intense activity of birth. If, towards the time of delivery, there is insufficient yang activity of the uterus, due either to deficiency or stagnation, then yang must be stimulated. Zhiyin BL-67 is the terminal point of the yang Bladder channel, where the qi changes polarity and enters its coupled yin Kidney channel, reflected in its name 'Reaching Yin'. It is the most dynamic point to activate the uterus and hence turn the foetus and promote labour, especially when stimulated by the yang heat of moxibustion.

Finally Zhiyin BL-67 is one of the few distal points on the Bladder channel indicated for disorders of urination, in this case painful urinary dysfunction and difficult urination. Clinically however, distal points of the Bladder channel are rarely used for this purpose.

COMBINATIONS

- To hasten delivery: Zhiyin BL-67 and Zusanli ST-36 (*Song of Points*).
- Seminal emission: Zhiyin BL-67, Ququan LIV-8 and Zhongji REN-3 (*Supplementing Life*).
- Difficult urination and seminal emission: Zhiyin BL-67, Zhongji REN-3, Ligou LIV-5, Chengfu BL-36 and Lougu SP-7 (*Supplementing Life*).
- Itching with much pain: Zhiyin BL-67 and Wuyi ST-15 (*One Hundred Symptoms*).
- Paralysis of the lower extremity: Zhiyin BL-67, Yinlingquan SP-9, Huantiao GB-30, Yangfu GB-38 and Taixi KID-3 (*Great Compendium*).
- Pain of the chest and lateral costal region that changes location: Zhiyin BL-67 and Huantiao GB-30 (*Thousand Ducat Formulas*).
- Vertex headache: Zhiyin BL-67, Baihui DU-20 and Houxi SI-3.

NOTES

1 *Essential Questions* Chapter 5.
2 *Spiritual Pivot* Chapter 17.
3 Danyang (Extra), 0.5 cun posterior to Toulinqi GB-15.
4 *Spiritual Pivot* Chapter 22.
5 *Spiritual Pivot* Chapter 33.
6 *Essential Questions* Chapter 61.
7 *Spiritual Pivot* Chapter 17.
8 *Essential Questions* Chapter 61.
9 *Essential Questions* Chapter 10.
10 *Essential Questions* Chapter 17.
11 *Essential Questions* Chapter 8.
12 *Essential Questions* Chapter 62.

13 Fei Bo Xiong (1800-1879) in Fei Bo Xiong et. al. 1985 *Medical Collection From Four Families from Meng He* (Meng He Si Jia Yi Ji), Jiangsu Science Publishing House, p.40. Quoted in Maciocia, G. *The Practice of Chinese Medicine*, Churchill Livingstone, p. 211.

14 *Essential Questions* Chapter 62.

15 *Essential Questions* Chapter 10.

16 *Essential Questions* Chapter 44.

17 *Essential Questions* Chapter 18.

18 *Spiritual Pivot* Chapter 10.

19 *Treatise on Epidemic Warm Febrile Disease* by Wu You Ke (1642).

20 *Spiritual Pivot* Chapter 6.

21 *Spiritual Pivot* Chapter 8.

22 *Essential Questions* Chapter 39.

23 *Spiritual Pivot* Chapter 17.

24 *Essential Questions* Chapter 10.

25 *Essential Questions* Chapter 44.

26 *Essential Questions* Chapter 10.

27 *Spiritual Pivot* Chapter 5.

28 *Essential Questions* Chapter 6.

29 *Essential Questions* Chapter 8.

30 *Treatise on the Spleen & Stomach by Li Dongyuan*, A Translation of the Pi Wei Lun, by Yang Shou-zhong and Li Jian-yong, Blue Poppy Press, 1993, p. 19.

31 *Essential Questions* Chapter 23.

32 *Essential Questions* Chapter 23.

33 *Essential Questions* Chapter 74.

34 *Spiritual Pivot* Chapter 33.

35 *Classic of Difficulties* 31st Difficulty.

36 *Essential Questions* Chapter 8.

37 *Spiritual Pivot* Chapter 8.

38 *Essential Questions* Chapter 4.

39 *Master Hua's Classic of the Central Viscera* (Zhong Zang Jing) attributed to Hua Tuo, translated by Yang Shou-zhong, Blue Poppy Press, 1993.

40 *Essential Questions* Chapter 47.

41 *Classic of Difficulties* 36th Difficulty.

42 *Spiritual Pivot* Chapter 17.

43 *Essential Questions* Chapter 18.

44 *Essential Questions* Chapter 5.

45 *Essential Questions* Chapter 5.

46 *Essential Questions* Chapter 44.

47 *Standards of Patterns and Treatment* by Wang Ken-tang, 1602, quoted by Maciocia, M., *The Practice of Chinese Medicine*, Churchill Livingstone, p609.

48 *Essential Questions* Chapter 43.

49 *Spiritual Pivot* Chapter 4.

50 *Spiritual Pivot* Chapter 2.

51 *Essential Questions* Chapter 8.

52 *Spiritual Pivot* Chapter 2.

53 *Spiritual Pivot* Chapter 4.

54 Ma Dan-yang was the originator of the *Song of the Eleven Heavenly Star Points*. They first appeared in print in the 12th century CE *Classic of the Jade Dragon*. Xu Feng included this text in his work *Complete Collection of Acupuncture and Moxibustion* and added a twelfth point, Taichong LIV-3.

55 *Spiritual Pivot* Chapter 78.

56 *Spiritual Pivot*, Chapter 9.

57 *Spiritual Pivot* Chapter 6.

58 *Essential Questions* Chapter 61.

59 The nine types of haemorrhoids refer to fleshy growths appearing in any of the nine orifices (eyes, nostrils, ears, mouth, anus and urethra).

60 *Essential Questions* Chapter 61.

61 Cited in *Celestial Lancets* by Lu Gwei-Djen & Joseph Needham, p. 78, Cambridge University Press.

62 *Essential Questions* Chapter 61.

63 Hunmen BL-47 is, however, indicated for 'corpse collapse walking disorder' although it is unclear what this term means, and whether or not it refers to a psycho-emotional or physical disorder.

64 *Essential Questions* Chapter 61.

65 *Essential Questions* Chapter 61.

66 *Essential Questions* Chapter 61.

67 Ma Dan-yang was the originator of the *Song of the Eleven Heavenly Star Points*. They first appeared in print in the 12th century CE *Classic of the Jade Dragon*. Xu Feng included this text in his work *Complete Collection of Acupuncture and Moxibustion* and added a twelfth point, Taichong LIV-3.

68 *Essential Questions* Chapter 10.

69 Quoted in *Chinese Acupuncture and Moxibustion*, Foreign Languages Press, Beijing.

70 Ma Dan-yang was the originator of the *Song of the Eleven Heavenly Star Points*. They first appeared in print in the 12th century CE *Classic of the Jade Dragon*. Xu Feng included this text in his work *Complete Collection of Acupuncture and Moxibustion* and added a twelfth point, Taichong LIV-3.

71 *Classic of Difficulties* 68th Difficulty.

72 *Spiritual Pivot* Chapter 21.

73 *Spiritual Pivot* Chapter 80.

74 *Classic of Difficulties* 69th Difficulty.

75 Quoted in *Treatise on the Spleen & Stomach by Li Dongyuan*, translated by Yang Shou-zhong & Li Jian-yong, Blue Poppy Press, page 140).

76 *Spiritual Pivot* Chapter 9.

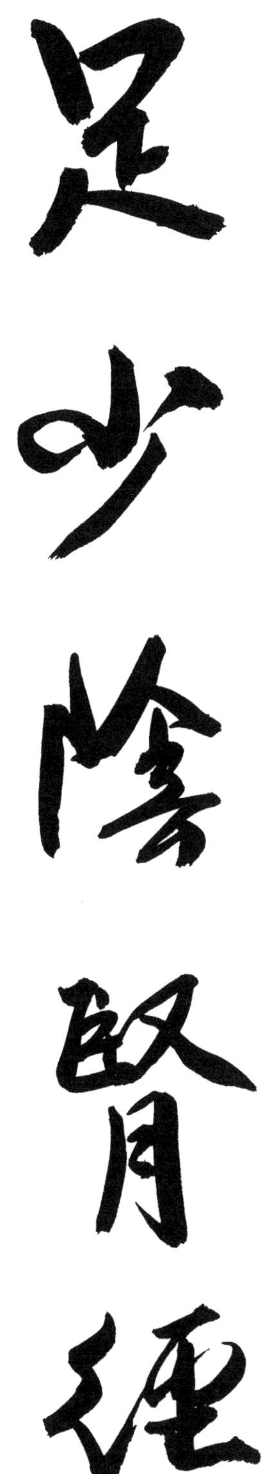

THE KIDNEY CHANNEL OF FOOT SHAOYIN

THE KIDNEY CHANNEL OF FOOT SHAOYIN

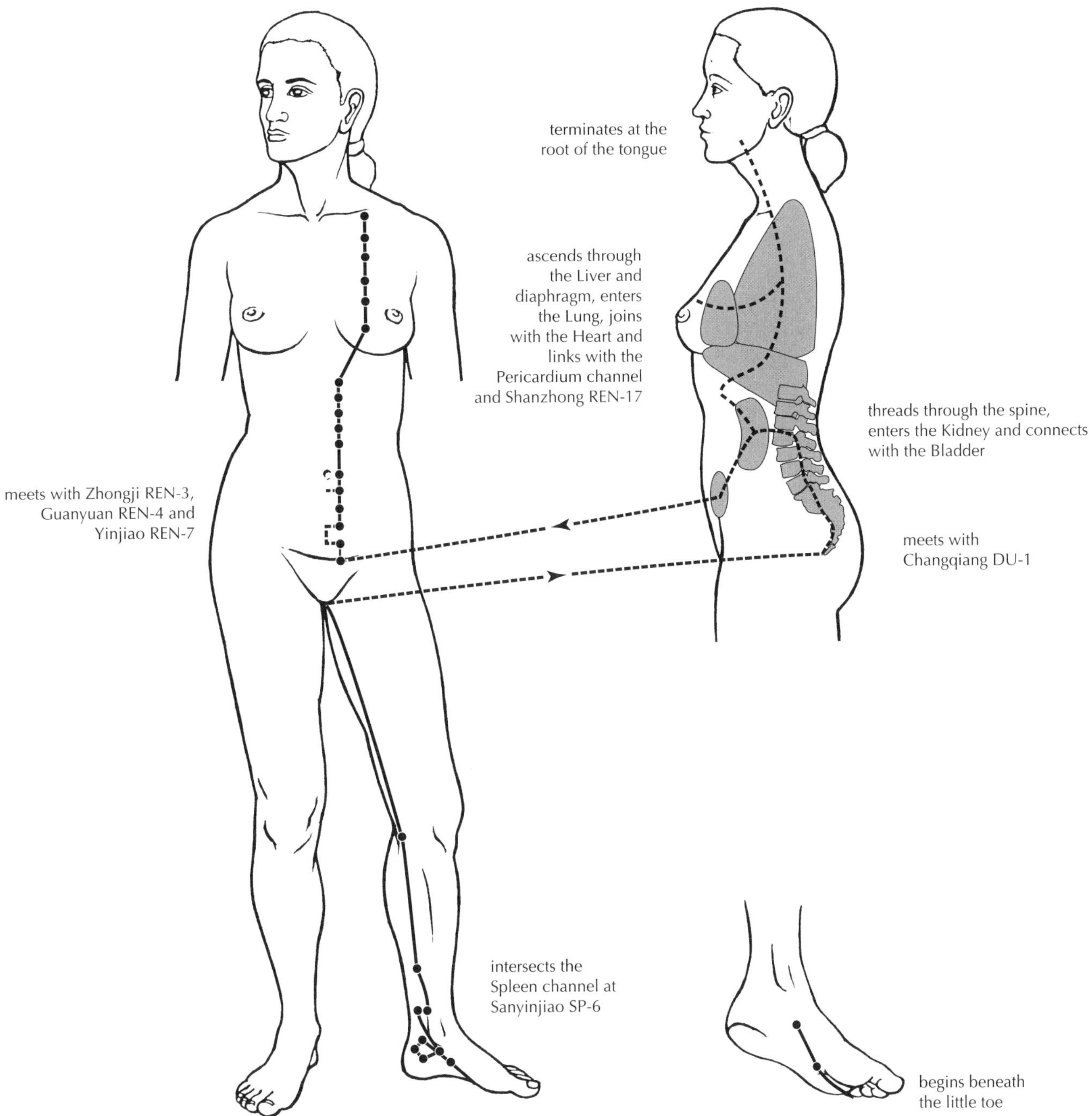
terminates at the
root of the tongue
ascends through
the Liver and
diaphragm, enters
the Lung, joins
with the Heart and
links with the
Pericardium channel
and Shanzhong REN-17
threads through the spine,
enters the Kidney and connects
with the Bladder
meets with Zhongji REN-3,
Guanyuan REN-4 and
Yinjiao REN-7
meets with
Changqiang DU-1
intersects the
Spleen channel at
Sanyinjiao SP-6
begins beneath
the little toe

THE KIDNEY PRIMARY CHANNEL

- begins beneath the little toe,
- crosses the sole of the foot to Yongquan KID-1,
- emerges at Rangu KID-2, anterior and inferior to the navicular tuberosity,
- travels posterior to the medial malleolus at Taixi KID-3 where it descends through the heel and then ascends to below the medial malleolus at Zhaohai KID-6,
- ascends along the medial aspect of the leg, intersecting the Spleen channel at Sanyinjiao SP-6,
- continues up the leg to the medial side of the popliteal fossa at Yingu KID-10 and along the postero-medial aspect of the thigh to the tip of the coccyx where it intersects with the Governing vessel at Changqiang DU-1
- threads its way through the spine, enters the Kidney and connects with the Bladder,
- intersects the Conception vessel at Zhongji REN-3, Guanyuan REN-4 and Yinjiao REN-7,

- one branch emerges from the Kidney, ascends through the Liver and diaphragm, enters the Lung and ascends along the throat to terminate at the root of the tongue,
- another branch separates in the Lung, joins with the Heart and disperses in the chest to link with the Pericardium channel and Shanzhong REN-17.

The Kidney primary channel connects with the following zangfu: Kidney, Bladder, Liver, Lung, Heart.

The Kidney primary channel meets with other channels at the following points: Sanyinjiao SP-6 Changqiang DU-1, Zhongji REN-3, Guanyuan REN-4, Yinjiao REN-7, Shanzhong REN-17.

THE KIDNEY DIVERGENT CHANNEL

- separates from the Kidney primary channel in the popliteal fossa,
- intersects the Bladder divergent channel on the thigh,
- ascends to connect with the Kidneys,
- crosses the Girdling vessel in the region of the second lumbar vertebra,
- ascends to the root of the tongue,
- continues upwards to emerge at the nape of the neck and converge with the Bladder primary channel.

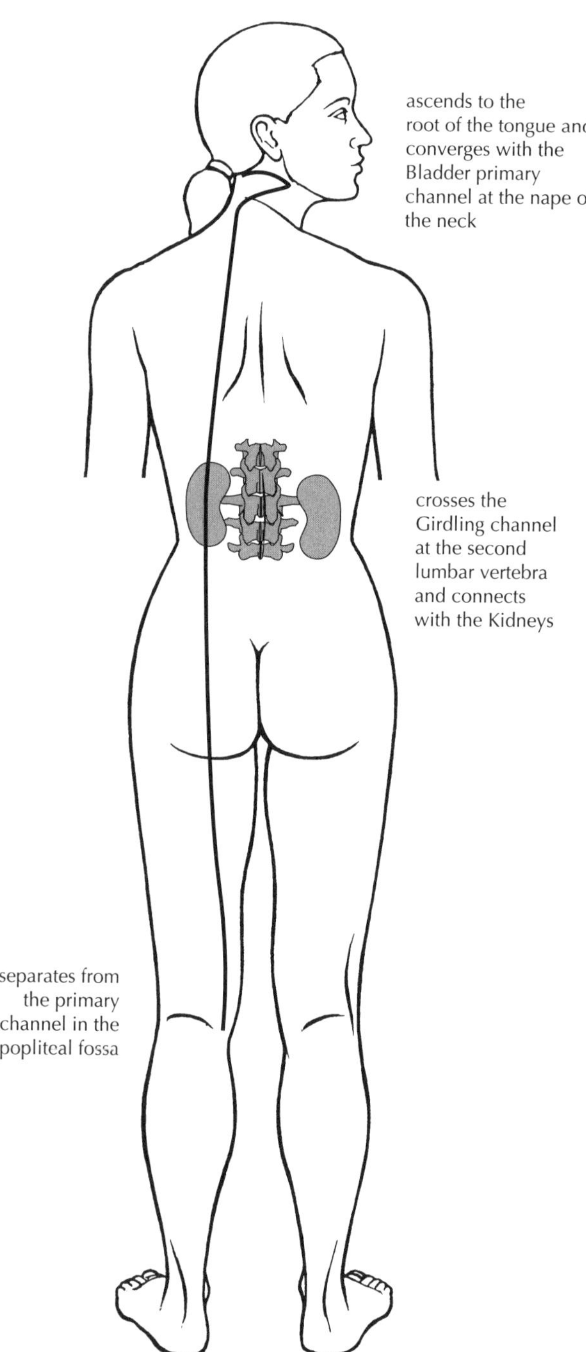

The Kidney divergent channel

THE KIDNEY LUO-CONNECTING CHANNEL

- begins at Dazhong KID-4 on the posterior aspect of the medial malleolus,
- encircles the heel and enters internally to connect with the Bladder channel,
- ascends along with the Kidney primary channel from Dazhong KID-4 to a point below the Pericardium where it travels posteriorly to and spreads into the lumbar vertebrae.

THE KIDNEY SINEW CHANNEL

- begins beneath the little toe and joins the Spleen sinew channel at the inferior aspect of the medial malleolus,
- binds in the heel where it converges with the Bladder sinew channel, then ascends the leg and binds at the medial condyle of the tibia,
- joins with the Spleen sinew channel and follows the medial surface of the thigh to bind at the genitals.

A branch

- travels internally to the spinal vertebrae, ascends the inner aspect of the spine to the nape of the neck where the channel binds to the occipital bone, and converges with the Bladder sinew channel.

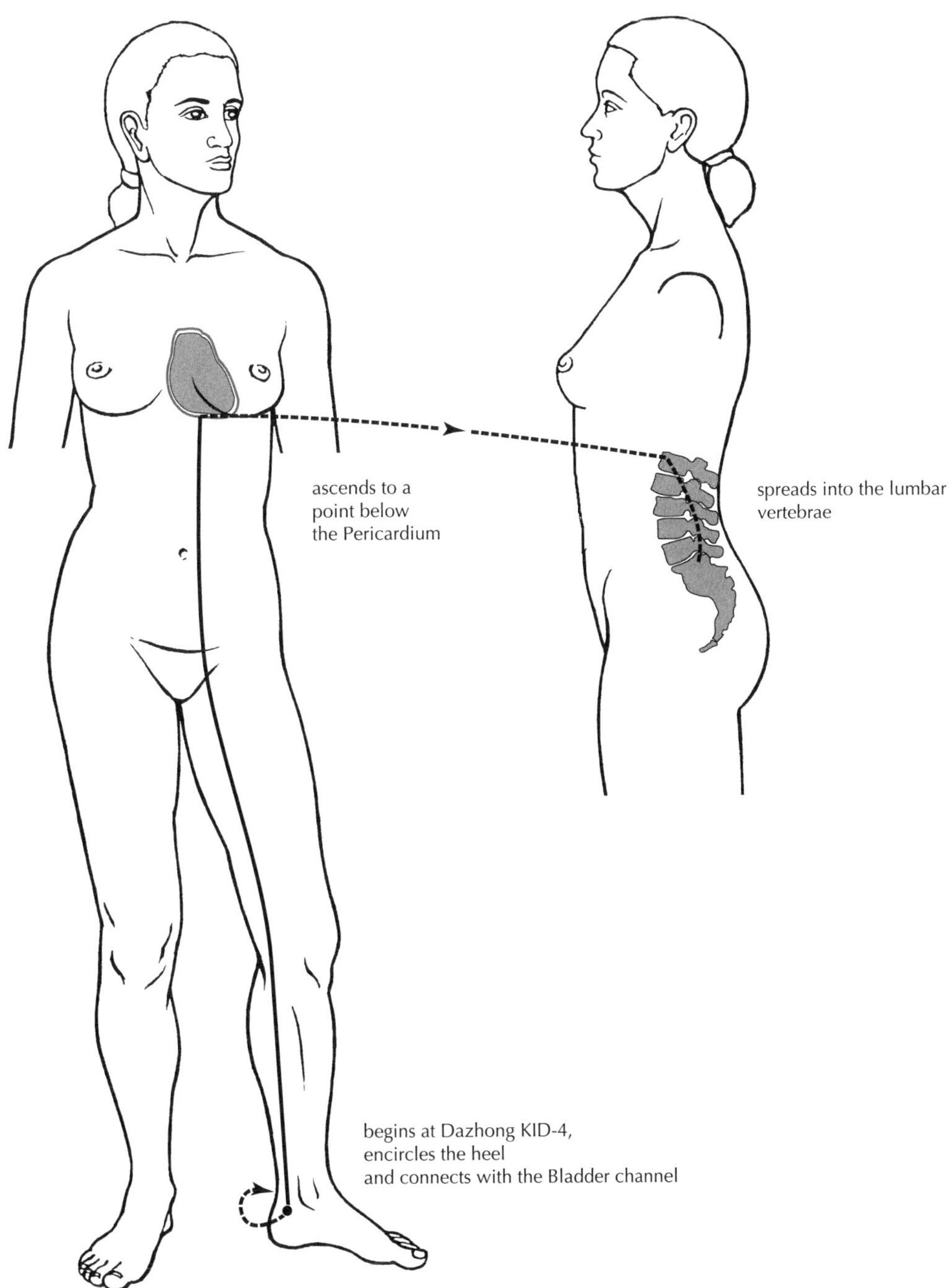
ascends to a
point below
the Pericardium
spreads into the lumbar
vertebrae
begins at Dazhong KID-4,
encircles the heel
and connects with the Bladder channel

The Kidney luo-connecting channel

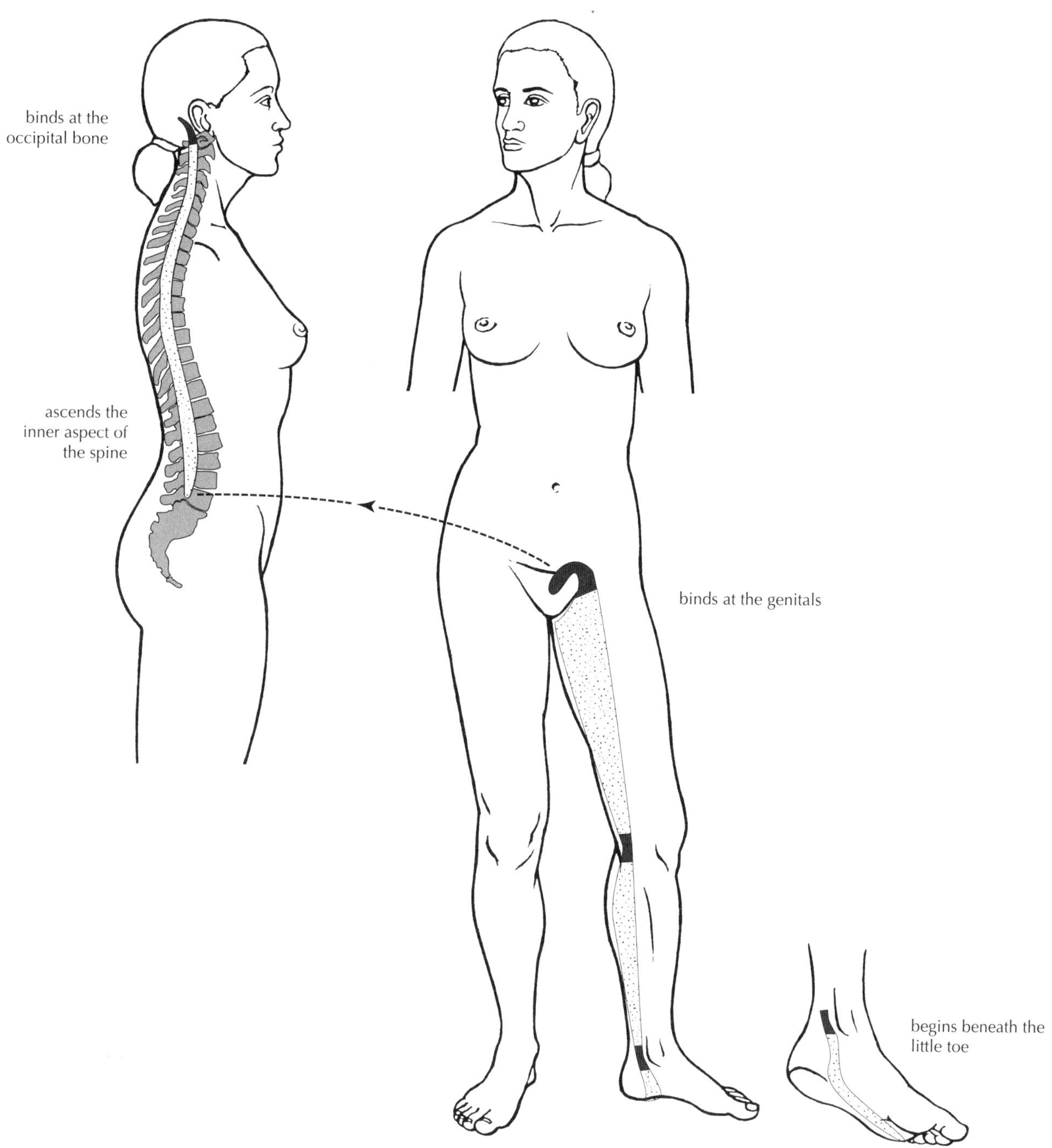
binds at the occipital bone
ascends the inner aspect of the spine
binds at the genitals
begins beneath the little toe

The Kidney sinew channel

Pathological symptoms of the Kidney sinew channel
Cramping of the bottom of the foot, cramping and pain along the course of the channel, convulsion and spasm associated with epilepsy. If the disease is on the exterior the patient cannot bend forward, if the disease is on the interior the patient cannot bend backwards. Thus in a yang disorder there will be inability to bend the lumbar spine forwards, whilst in a yin disorder here will be inability to bend the lumbar spine backwards.

DISCUSSION

The Kidney channel of foot shaoyin is interiorly-exteriorly coupled with the Bladder channel, and paired with the Heart channel of hand shaoyin according to six channel theory. The Kidney-Bladder relationship is further strengthened by the fact that:

- the interior pathway of the Kidney primary channel connects with the Bladder fu.
- the Kidney luo-connecting channel connects with the Bladder channel.
- the Kidney divergent channel intersects the Bladder channel on the thigh.

In addition, it is important to note that:
- the Kidney primary channel intersects the Conception vessel at Zhongji REN-3 and Guanyuan REN-4.
- the Kidney primary channel ascends through the Liver, diaphragm, Lung and Heart.
- the Kidney primary channel ascends through the throat.
- the Kidney primary and divergent channels ascend to the root of the tongue.
- the Kidney primary, luo-connecting and sinew channels spread into the spine.
- the Kidney sinew channel, but not the Kidney primary channel, ascends to the genitals.

The Kidneys have five principal functions:
- storing essence and dominating reproduction, growth and development.
- producing marrow, filling up the brain, dominating bones and assisting in the production of blood.
- dominating water.
- controlling the reception of qi.
- opening into the ears and dominating the two lower yin (the anus and urethra).

In addition, the Kidneys:
- are the lowest zang.
- are the root of the original yin and yang of the body.
- conserve and control the ming men fire.
- house the will.
- are the foundation of the Conception and Penetrating vessels which originate in the uterus, whilst according to the *Essential Questions*[1] "the vessel of the uterus connects with the Kidneys".

It is by virtue of these functions and relationships, as well as the channel pathways discussed above, that many of the actions and indications of the points of the Kidney channel can be explained. These can be summarised as:

- rooting pathologically ascending heat, qi, yang and wind. The Kidneys are the bottomost zang and the root of the yin in the body. When yin is deficient, deficiency heat, or uprising yang or interior wind may ascend to the throat, ears, eyes and head. Points of the Kidney channel are frequently used clinically both to nourish yin (e.g. Taixi KID-3) and to strongly descend pathogens from the head (e.g. Yongquan KID-1).
- nourishing yin and clearing deficiency heat in the treatment of night sweating, wasting and thirsting disorder etc.
- nourishing Liver yin to counteract uprising of Liver yang in the treatment of headache, dizziness etc.
- nourishing Kidney water to balance excessive Heart fire, and harmonising the will and the spirit in the treatment of restlessness, insomnia, poor memory, palpitations, epilepsy, mania, susceptibility to fright etc.
- rooting the qi and harmonising the relationship between the Kidneys and Lung in the treatment of cough, coughing of blood, dyspnoea, asthma, wheezing etc.
- tonifying Kidney yang to strengthen the Kidney function of dominating water in the treatment of oedema and deficiency type urinary disorders.
- tonifying Kidney yang to strengthen the libido in the treatment of impotence, seminal emission etc.
- tonifying Kidney yang to warm the lower body, legs and feet.
- benefiting the throat, especially in the treatment of sore and dry throat or loss of voice due to yin deficiency.
- strengthening the lumbar spine and benefiting the teeth.
- benefiting the ears in the treatment of tinnitus and deafness.
- regulating the Conception and Penetrating vessels and treating diseases of the uterus such as infertility, disordered menstruation, uterine prolapse, postpartum disorders etc.
- draining damp-heat from the lower jiao and regulating the function of the Bladder and intestines in the treatment of difficult urination, retention of urine, painful urinary dysfunction, dark urine, diarrhoea, dysenteric disorder, swelling, itching and pain of the genitals, shan disorder, hypogastric pain etc.
- nourishing Kidney yin in the treatment of constipation due to dryness.

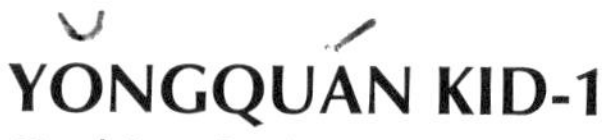

YONGQUAN KID-1

Gushing Spring

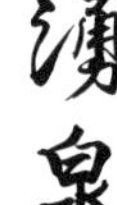

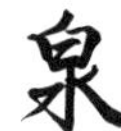

Jing-Well and Wood point of the Kidney channel

LOCATION

On the sole of the foot, between the second and third metatarsal bones, approximately one third of the distance between the base of the second toe and the heel, in a depression formed when the foot is plantar flexed.

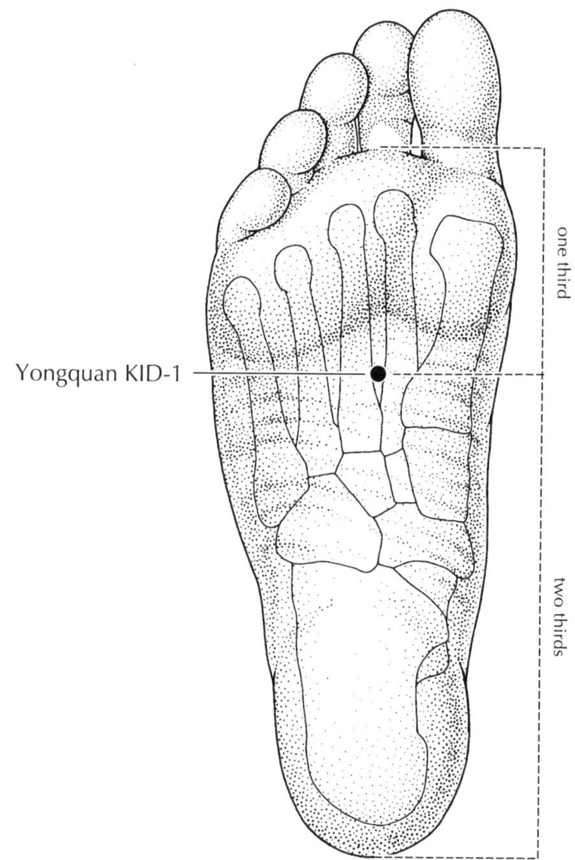

NEEDLING

Perpendicular insertion 0.5 to 1 cun.

ACTIONS

Descends excess from the head
Calms the spirit
Revives consciousness and rescues yang

INDICATIONS

- Loss of consciousness from windstroke, loss of consciousness.
- Epilepsy, childhood fright wind, dizziness, visual dizziness, cloudy vision, vertex headache, hypertension, throat painful obstruction, throat pain with inability to swallow, loss of voice, dry tongue, nosebleed, dark complexion, running piglet qi.
- Agitation, insomnia, poor memory, propensity to fear, rage with desire to kill people, madness, Heart pain.
- Cough, dyspnoea, vomiting and coughing blood.
- Wind rash, sudden turmoil disorder with cramps, contracted sinews.
- Constipation, lumbar pain with difficult defecation, difficult urination, pain in the lower abdomen in pregnant women with inability to urinate, fullness of the lower abdomen, periumbilical pain, shan disorder, infertility, impotence, disorders due to excessive sexual activity, fullness of the lateral costal region, jaundice, diminished qi.
- Lower limb paralysis, chronic leg qi, pain and swelling of the leg, cold sensation of the feet and shins, heat in the soles of the feet, chronic pain and numbness of the foot, pain of the five toes with inability to stand.

COMMENTARY

Yongquan KID-1, the only channel point on the sole of the foot and therefore the lowest point on the body, is the wood point of the Kidney water channel. According to the *Classic of Difficulties*[2] "in cases of deficiency reinforce the mother, in cases of excess reduce the child". As the 'child' point of the Kidney channel, Yongquan KID-1 therefore has a powerful effect on reducing excess above by 'returning the unrooted back to its source', reflected both in the statement in the *Ode to Elucidate Mysteries* that "Yongquan KID-1 echoes the earth"[3], and in alternative names for this point such as 'Earth Surge' (Dichong) and 'Earth Thoroughfare' (Dichong).

When the Kidneys are deficient below, pathologically ascending qi, yang, deficiency heat or wind may rush upwards to harass the head. The powerful effect of Yongquan KID-1 on descending and clearing such excess is recorded in a story about the famous 2nd century physician Hua Tuo who treated General Wei Tai-cu (the posthumously consecrated emperor of the Wei dynasty) for 'head wind, confused mind and visual dizziness'. Following the principle of selecting points below to treat disorders above, Hua Tuo needled Yongquan KID-1 and "the general was immediately cured"[4].

In clinical practice, Yongquan KID-1 is principally used to treat: i. uprising of Liver yang, Liver fire or Liver wind, ii. disharmony of the Heart and Kidneys, and iii. disorders of the throat.

The Kidneys are the root of the yin of all the zangfu. This has especial relevance to the Liver, Heart and Lung, all of which are reached by the Kidney channel. According to a saying of Chinese medicine "the Kidneys and the Liver share the same origin". Kidney water is the mother of Liver wood, and the Kidney yin is the origin and source of Liver yin. When Kidney water fails to nourish Liver wood, the fierce and unrestrained yang of the Liver rushes up to the head giving rise to such symptoms as headache at the vertex, dizziness, visual dizziness, cloudy vision, hypertension and nosebleed. If excess Liver yang generates wind there may be windstroke or epilepsy. Yongquan KID-1 is able both to regulate the Kidneys, the root of these symptoms, and to treat the manifestations by strongly descending the pathological excess.

The Kidneys belong to water and the Heart to fire, and the Kidneys and Heart are said to 'mutually support' each other, the Kidney yin nourishing and moistening Heart yin and restraining Heart fire, and Heart yang descending to warm the Kidneys. Harmony between the Kidneys and Heart is one of the prerequisites for a stable and peaceful spirit. When Kidney yin is deficient and deficiency fire of the Heart blazes, or when the connection is broken and the Kidneys and Heart do not communicate, the spirit becomes agitated, leading to a wide variety of emotional disorders ranging from the relatively mild, (agitation, insomnia, poor memory, propensity to fear) to the severe (madness, rage with desire to kill people). It is recommended (and widely applied in China) for patients suffering from insomnia to massage bilateral Yongquan KID-1 before bedtime, or to steep the feet in a bowl of hot water to draw down the excess yang.

The ability of Yongquan KID-1 to restrain uprising of deficiency heat and Liver yang, and to pacify the spirit, renders it especially suitable to treat menopausal disorder characterised by hot flushes, night sweating, insomnia, agitation, anxiety and headache.

The Kidney channel ascends to the throat and the root of the tongue. When fierce heat from Kidney deficiency rises along the Kidney channel, it scorches the fluids and gives rise to swelling and congestion of the throat, throat pain with inability to swallow and dry tongue. Because of its ability to reduce heat and fire in the throat region, Yongquan KID-1 may also be used in swelling and pain of the throat due to other aetiologies. According to the *Spiritual Pivot*[5] the Kidney channel terminates at Lianquan REN-23, an important point in the treatment of disorders of the tongue, and Yongquan KID-1 is also indicated for loss of voice, whether due to exterior pathogens or to windstroke.

Yongquan KID-1 is secondarily used for: i. disorders of the Lung, ii. running piglet qi, iii. loss of consciousness, and iv. disorders of the two lower yin.

According to a saying of Chinese medicine "The Lung is the canopy and the Kidneys are the root". As the uppermost zang, the Lung receives via respiration the clear qi of heaven (qing qi) in the same way that the canopy of a forest receives the light and air essential for life. Through the grasping and holding function of the Kidneys, the qi is drawn down via inhalation to the root below. If the Kidneys are deficient and fail to grasp the qi, there may be dyspnoea and coughing, both indications for this point.

Running piglet qi primarily arises when stagnant Liver qi transforms to heat, or when Kidney yang deficiency leads to accumulation of cold in the lower jiao. In both cases, qi is violently discharged and rushes upwards along the Penetrating vessel. The action of Yongquan KID-1 in harmonising the Kidneys and Liver and redirecting pathologically ascending qi downwards is reflected in its use in the treatment of this disorder.

Yongquan KID-1 is the jing-well point of the Kidney channel, and like many of the other jing-well points has a powerful action on opening the portals and reviving collapse, whether in windstroke or loss of consciousness. It is cited in the *Song of the Nine Needles for Returning the Yang* for the treatment of collapse of yang characterised by loss of consciousness, aversion to cold, cold counterflow of the limbs, purple lips etc.

The Kidneys rule the two lower yin, the anus and urethra. Yongquan KID-1 may be used in the treatment of constipation, especially when due to yin deficiency and consequent dryness, as well as for difficult urination.

Yongquan KID-1 is an important point in qigong practice. Directing the mind to Yongquan KID-1, or inhaling and exhaling through this point, roots and descends the qi in the lower dantian (cinnabar field) and helps the body absorb the yin energy of the earth. In common with its application in acupuncture, this practice is particularly recommended whenever excessive yang rebels upwards to the Heart, Lung or head.

Finally, Yongquan KID-1 has been the subject of many modern studies into the application of herbal plasters to acupuncture points. A variety of herbal substances are ground, made into a paste and applied to this point for disorders such as mouth ulcers and hypertension.

COMBINATIONS

- Headache and visual dizziness: Yongquan KID-1, Sibai ST-2 and Dazhu BL-11 (*Supplementing Life*).
- Visual dizziness: Yongquan KID-1, Shenting DU-24, Shangxing DU-23, Yixi BL-45, Yuji LU-10 and Dadu SP-2 (*Supplementing Life*).
- The five types of epilepsy: Yongquan KID-1 and Laogong P-8 (*Song of Points*).
- Wind epilepsy: Yongquan KID-1 and Jizhong DU-6 (*Supplementing Life*).

- Wind epilepsy: Yongquan KID-1, Shenting DU-24 and Suliao DU-25 (*Great Compendium*).
- Dementia: Yongquan KID-1, Shenmen HE-7, Shaoshang LU-11 and Xinshu BL-15 (*Great Compendium*).
- Pain of the throat with inability to eat: Yongquan KID-1 and Dazhong KID-4 (*Thousand Ducat Formulas*).
- Throat painful obstruction with chills and fever: Yongquan KID-1 and Rangu KID-2 (*Thousand Ducat Formulas*).
- Loss of voice: Yongquan KID-1, Hegu L.I.-4 and Yangjiao GB-35 (*Systematic Classic*).
- Severe thirst of wasting and thirsting disorder: Yongquan KID-1 and Xingjian LIV-2 (*One Hundred Patterns*).
- Infertility: Yongquan KID-1, Ciliao BL-32 and Shangqiu SP-5 (*Supplementing Life*).
- Pain of the five toes with inability to tread on the ground: Yongquan KID-1 and Rangu KID-2 (*Supplementing Life*).
- Injury by cold with great heat that does not recede: reduce Yongquan KID-1, Hegu L.I.-4, Quchi L.I.-11, Xuanzhong GB-39, Zusanli ST-36 and Dazhui DU-14 (*Great Compendium*).
- Wind rash: Yongquan KID-1 and Huantiao GB-30 (*Supplementing Life*).
- Stiffness and pain of the lumbar region: Yongquan KID-1, Yaoshu DU-2, Weizhong BL-40, Xiaochangshu BL-27 and Pangguangshu BL-28 (*Great Compendium*).
- Menopausal hot flushes: Yongquan KID-1, Taichong LIV-3, Yinxi HE-6 and Guanyuan REN-4.

RANGU KID-2

Blazing Valley

然谷

Ying-Spring and Fire point of the Kidney channel

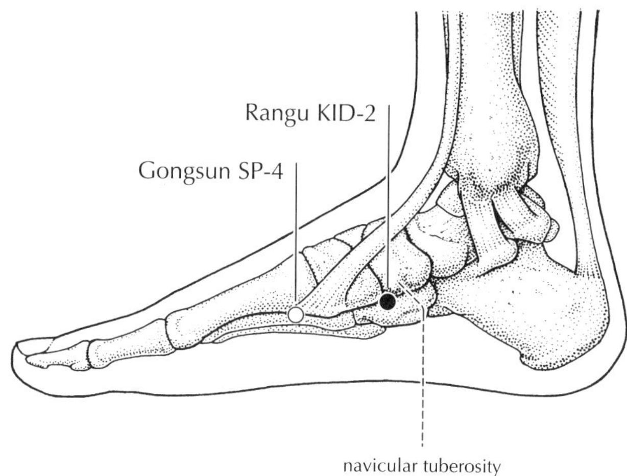

LOCATION

On the medial side of the foot, distal and inferior to the medial malleolus, in the depression distal and inferior to the navicular tuberosity.

LOCATION NOTE

The navicular tuberosity is the prominence found superior to the midpoint between the ball of the foot and the heel.

NEEDLING

Perpendicular insertion 0.5 to 1 cun.

ACTIONS

Clears deficiency heat
Regulates the Kidneys
Regulates the lower jiao

INDICATIONS

- Throat painful obstruction, insufficient saliva to moisten the throat, inability to speak, spontaneous sweating, night sweating, asthma, dyspnoea, diminished qi, coughing blood, wasting and thirsting disorder, jaundice, protrusion of the tongue, fearful as if about to be apprehended, propensity to fear and fright, stabbing Heart pain.
- Itching of the genitals, nocturnal emissions, seminal emission, impotence, infertility, uterine prolapse, irregular menstruation, shan disorder, difficult urination, cold or damp (dong) diarrhoea.
- One foot hot and one foot cold, pain of the lower legs which prevents standing for long, pain and swelling of the instep, restless feet.

COMMENTARY

Rangu KID-2 'Blazing Valley' is the ying-spring and fire point of the Kidney channel. According to the *Classic of Difficulties*[6] ying-spring points are indicated for "heat in the body", and in the case of most ying-spring points the emphasis is on clearing excess heat and fire. The Kidneys are unique, however, in that they do not suffer from excess patterns, since the Kidneys store true yin and true yang which can never be in a state of real excess. Rangu KID-2, therefore, is the principal Kidney channel point to clear heat deriving from Kidney yin deficiency.

The Kidneys are the root of the yin and yang of the body. Kidney yin has the functions of nourishing and moistening as well as balancing and restraining the ming men fire. When Kidney yin is deficient, its nourishing and moistening functions will be impaired and additionally the ming men fire may blaze out of control. The forte of Rangu KID-2, as its name implies, is to clear this deficiency heat, rather than nourish the Kidney yin. It is indicated when such heat: i. ascends along the Kidney channel to the throat giving rise to throat painful obstruction, dry throat with insufficient saliva and inability to speak, ii. floats to the exterior at night giving rise to night sweating, and iii. disrupts the Lung giving rise to dyspnoea and coughing of blood. Heat from yin deficiency may also manifest as wasting and thirsting disorder and hot and restless feet.

Rangu KID-2 has a particular action on the lower jiao. Deficiency of yin and consequent heat may give rise to genital itching. When Kidney yin fails to nourish the Conception and Penetrating vessels there may be irregular menstruation and infertility in women. When deficiency heat agitates the gate of essence in men there may be seminal emission or nocturnal emissions, with or without dreams. In both men and women there may also be excessive sexual desire. If the Kidney qi is deficient, there may be uterine prolapse.

According to the *Complete Works of Jing-yue* "Yin and yang are of the same origin ... fire is the ruler of water, water is the source of fire ...". Neither deficiency of Kidney yin nor Kidney yang exist in isolation, and this is reflected in the fact that Rangu KID-2 also clearly has an action on tonifying Kidney yang. This is partly illustrated by the traditional indications, but is reflected most clearly in a variety of classical combinations (see below). Rangu KID-2 therefore may also be treated by moxibustion in cases of spontaneous sweating, coldness of the feet and legs, cold diarrhoea, oedema and impotence.

Finally, the emotion associated with the Kidneys is fear, and when the Kidneys are deficient there may be propensity to fear and fright and a constant feeling of alarm as though one were "about to be apprehended". Rangu KID-2 is indicated for these various feelings of foreboding.

COMBINATIONS

- Swelling of the inside of the throat: Rangu KID-2 and Taixi KID-3 (*Supplementing Life*).
- Throat painful obstruction with chills and fever: Rangu KID-2 and Yongquan KID-1 (*Thousand Ducat Formulas*).
- Loss of voice: Rangu KID-2, Tiantu REN-22, Lingdao HE-4, Yingu KID-10, Fuliu KID-7 and Fenglong ST-40 (*Illustrated Supplement*).
- Stiffness of the tongue: Rangu KID-2, Yingu KID-10, Yamen DU-15, Shaoshang LU-11, Yuji LU-10, Erjian L.I.-2 and Zhongchong P-9 (*Great Compendium*).
- Drooling: Rangu KID-2 and Fuliu KID-7 (*Supplementing Life*).
- Wasting and thirsting disorder with great desire to drink: Rangu KID-2, Yishe BL-49 and Guanchong SJ-1 (*Supplementing Life*).
- Wasting and thirsting disorder with great desire to drink: Rangu KID-2, Yishe BL-49, Chengjiang REN-24 and Guanchong SJ-1 (*Thousand Ducat Formulas*).
- Wasting and thirsting disorder: Rangu KID-2, Chengjiang REN-24, Jinjin (M-HN-20), Yuye (M-HN-20), Renzhong DU-26, Lianquan REN-23, Quchi L.I-11, Laogong P-8, Taichong LIV-3, Xingjian LIV-2, Shangqiu SP-5 and Yinbai SP-1 (*Great Compendium*).
- Febrile disease with agitation, cold feet and profuse sweating: first needle Rangu KID-2, then Taixi KID-3 (*Systematic Classic*).
- Stabbing Heart pain: Rangu KID-2, Zhigou SJ-6 and Taixi KID-3 (*Thousand Ducat Formulas*).
- Apprehension and fear as if about to be apprehended: Rangu KID-2 and Yanglingquan GB-34 (*Thousand Ducat Formulas*).
- Stone oedema of the upper abdomen: moxa Rangu KID-2, Qichong ST-30, Siman KID-14 and Zhangmen LIV-13 (*Thousand Ducat Formulas*).
- Seminal emission and retraction of the penis: Rangu KID-2 and Dahe KID-12 (*Supplementing Life*).
- Impotence: Rangu KID-2, Mingmen DU-4, Shenshu BL-23 and Qihai REN-6 (*Illustrated Supplement*).
- Cold or damp (dong) diarrhoea with undigested food: Rangu KID-2, Jingmen GB-25 and Yinlingquan SP-9 (*Thousand Ducat Formulas*).
- Cold of the lower extremities: Rangu KID-2, Shenshu BL-23 and Jinggu BL-64 (*Supplementing Life*).

TAIXI KID-3

Supreme Stream

太溪

Shu-Stream, Yuan-Source and Earth point of the Kidney channel

LOCATION

In the depression between the medial malleolus and the Achilles tendon, level with the prominence of the medial malleolus.

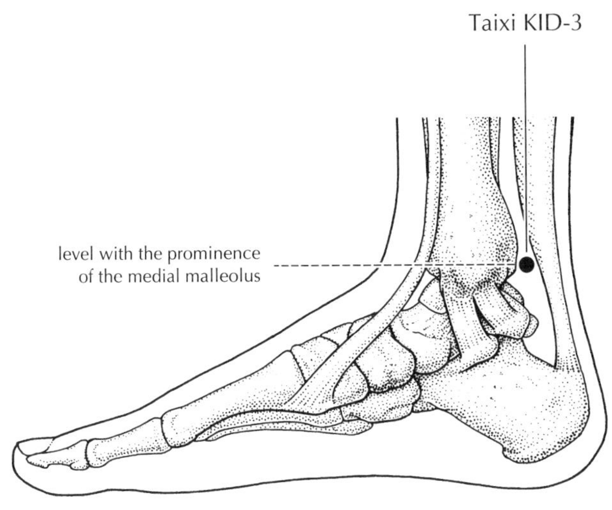

LOCATION NOTE

Locate in the centre of the depression, midway between the prominence of the medial malleolus and the posterior border of the Achilles tendon.

NEEDLING

Perpendicular insertion 0.5 to 1 cun or join to Kunlun BL-60.

ACTIONS

Nourishes Kidney yin and clears deficiency heat
Tonifies Kidney yang
Anchors the qi and benefits the Lung
Strengthens the lumbar spine

INDICATIONS

- Deafness, tinnitus, headache and dizziness, toothache, nosebleed, sore throat, heat sensation in the mouth, phlegm in the mouth that feels like glue, wasting and thirsting disorder, hot disease with copious sweating, chronic malaria, emaciation.
- Cough, coughing blood, cough with no pleasure in eating, wheezing, dyspnoea, asthma, chest pain.
- Insomnia, excessive dreaming, poor memory, heat sensation in the palms, stabbing pain in the Heart.
- Seminal emission, impotence, premature ejaculation, sexual taxation, irregular menstruation.
- Frequent and copious urination, enuresis, heat in the hypogastrium with yellow urine, abdominal distention, difficult defecation, cold shan disorder, damp itchy skin lesions on the inner thigh.
- Lumbar pain, pain of the abdomen and lateral costal region, injury by cold with inversion counterflow of the hands and feet, coldness of the lower limbs, numbness and pain of the legs, swelling and pain of the ankle, swelling and pain of the heel.

COMMENTARY

The Kidneys occupy a unique position among the zangfu, both storing the yin essence and conserving and controlling the ming men fire. The Kidneys are thus the root of the yin and yang of the whole body. Because of this fundamental role, deficiency of the Kidneys may both cause and result from disharmony of any of the other zangfu.

The *Spiritual Pivot* in Chapter 6 recommends the use of the shu-stream points in the treatment of disorders of the zang, whilst in Chapter 1 it says "When the five zang are diseased, select [from] the twelve yuan-source [points]". Taixi KID-3, the shu-stream and yuan-source point, is therefore the principal point on the Kidney channel to treat disharmony of the Kidney zang, which due to the unique nature of the Kidneys always involves deficiency, principally of Kidney yin or Kidney yang.

Kidney yin deficiency may affect the Kidneys alone, or by failing to nourish the Liver, Heart or Lung, all of which are reached by the Kidney channel, affect these zang also. Yin deficiency may manifest in two main ways: failure to nourish and moisten, or failure to restrain fire. The art of treating yin deficiency lies in carefully assessing the relative importance of these two aspects, and placing appropriate emphasis on nourishing yin and cooling fire.

Taixi KID-3 is the foremost point to treat yin deficiency affecting those areas of the body either reached by the Kidney channel or dominated by the Kidneys, specifically the throat, intestines, brain, teeth and ears. The Kidney primary channel ascends to the throat, and if heat from deficiency scorches and dries this region there may be chronic low-grade sore throat which is typically worse with tiredness, at the end of the day and at night. The Kidneys dominate the two lower yin (anus and urethra), and if deficient fluids and deficiency heat dessicate the intestines, there will be difficult defecation, illustrated by Wu Ju-tong's graphic image in the *Systematic Differentiation of Warm Diseases* "When the fluids are deficient there is not enough water to make the boat move". The *Spiritual Pivot*[7] states "The brain is the sea of marrow". Kidney essence produces marrow to fill the brain and spinal cord, and in cases where the sea of marrow is deficient there will be headache and dizziness. According to a saying of Chinese medicine "The teeth are the surplus of the bones". If the Kidneys fail to nourish the teeth, and heat from deficiency rises to this area, there will be chronic toothache accompanied by looseness of the teeth. The *Spiritual Pivot*[8] says "Kidney qi opens into the ears, when the Kidney is in harmony the ears can hear the five sounds". Deficiency of the Kidneys, therefore, can result in tinnitus and deafness. In all these cases, Taixi KID-3 is the primary point to tonify and nourish the Kidneys.

The intimate relationship between the Kidney yin and Liver yin, and the Kidney essence and Liver blood, is emphasised in the saying "the Kidneys and the Liver share the same origin", and the statement in *Comprehensive Medicine According to Master Zhang* "[When] the essence is not discharged it will return to the Liver and transform into clear blood". Taixi KID-3 is commonly used in prescriptions to treat Kidney-Liver disharmony (whether due to failure of water to nourish wood, or to injury to the Kidneys from prolonged Liver disease) giving rise to such symptoms as headache, dizziness, tinnitus and deafness.

The Kidneys pertain to water and the Heart to fire, and both belong to shaoyin. The Heart stores the spirit and the Kidneys store the will. When the Kidneys and the Heart function harmoniously, Heart fire and Kidney water, the spirit and the will, mutually support each other. When the

Heart and Kidneys lose harmony, Heart yang is unable to descend to warm the Kidneys, and Kidney yin is unable to nourish Heart yin and restrain Heart fire. This loss of contact between water and fire disturbs the spirit and gives rise to insomnia, excessive dreaming and poor memory, usually of the severe and chronic kind. Taixi KID-3 is an important point to bolster the Kidneys and enable them to support the Heart.

The Lung is the 'canopy' and the Kidneys are the root. The Lung descends qi and fluids to the Kidneys below, the Kidneys anchor the qi and steam the fluids to moisten the Lung above. Kidney-Lung disharmony commonly manifests in two main ways, i. Kidney yin deficiency fails to moisten and cool the Lung giving rise to symptoms such as wheezing, dry cough and blood-streaked sputum, and ii. the Kidneys fail to receive and anchor the qi from the Lung giving rise to such symptoms as dyspnoea, coughing and asthma. Taixi KID-3 is indicated in both these patterns of "excess above and deficiency below" and was specifically recommended by Sun Si-miao in the *Supplement to the Thousand Ducat Formulas* for Kidney cough.

Although subdivided into Kidney yin and Kidney yang, the Kidneys are of course one zang. Even though in clinical practice deficiency of either yin or yang will usually predominate, when one aspect of the Kidneys is deficient, it is frequently the case that the other will also become deficient. This is clearly spelt out both by the *Essential Questions*[9] which states "Injury to yin will reach the yang, injury to yang will reach the yin", and by the *Essential Readings in Medicine* which says "Without yang, yin cannot engender; without yin, yang cannot transform". It is a long-standing principle of tonifying the Kidneys that in Kidney yang deficiency one should also nourish Kidney yin, and that in nourishing Kidney yin one should also pay attention to the Kidney yang. Thus the *Essential Questions*[10] says "[For] yang diseases treat the yin, [for] yin diseases treat the yang", and Zhang Jing-yue echoes this in his statement "Nourishing yin to help yang is a skilful way to strengthen yang". For this reason, almost all acupuncture points that tonify the Kidneys will benefit both Kidney yin and Kidney yang. Taixi KID-3, the principal point on the Kidney channel to tonify the Kidneys, exemplifies this principle.

When Kidney yang fails to warm the body and transform fluids, there may be coldness of the lower limbs, backache, and urinary symptoms such as frequent and copious urination and incontinence. The close relationship between the Kidneys and the libido and sexual function is underscored by the application of Taixi KID-3 in the treatment of impotence, seminal emission and sexual taxation (depletion and exhaustion due to excessive sexual activity).

According to the *Essential Questions*[11] "The Kidneys dominate hibernation and are the root of sealed storage and the residence of essence; their radiance manifests in the hair and fills the bones". The Kidney primary, luo-connecting and sinew channels all ascend through the spine, and any pattern of Kidney deficiency may lead to malnourishment of the sinews, muscles and bones, especially in the lumbar region, the 'residence' of the Kidneys. Taixi KID-3 has long been used for the treatment of Kidney deficiency lumbar pain, and is also indicated for heel pain, which may be due to Kidney deficiency, traumatic injury or painful obstruction. In the treatment of heel pain, Taixi KID-3 should be needled to obtain sensation radiating strongly to the heel region.

The Penetrating and Conception vessels are both nourished by and have their root in the Kidneys, and the *Essential Questions* says "the vessel of the uterus connects with the Kidneys"[12]. Taixi KID-3 may be used when Kidney deficiency leads to disharmony of these extraordinary vessels resulting in irregular menstruation, although it is interesting to note that this is a modern indication and that no gynaecological indications or combinations appear in any major classical texts.

Finally Taixi KID-3 is cited in the *Song of the Nine Needles for Returning the Yang* for the treatment of collapse of yang characterised by loss of consciousness, aversion to cold, cold counterflow of the limbs, purple lips etc.

COMBINATIONS

- Dry throat and heat in the mouth with saliva like glue: Taixi KID-3 and Shaoze SI-1 (*Thousand Ducat Formulas*).
- Swelling of the inside of the throat: Taixi KID-3 and Rangu KID-2 (*Supplementing Life*).
- Swelling of the throat: Taixi KID-3 and Zhongzhu SJ-3 (*Supplementing Life*).
- Cough with rebellious qi and agitation: Taixi KID-3, Zigong REN-19 and Yutang REN-18 (*Thousand Ducat Formulas*).
- Lumbar pain due to Kidney deficiency: Taixi KID-3, Shenshu BL-23, Weizhong BL-40 and Baihuanshu BL-30 (*Great Compendium*).
- Somnolence: Taixi KID-3, Dazhong KID-4, Shouwuli L.I.-13, Zhaohai KID-6 and Erjian L.I.-2 (*Supplementing Life*).
- Somnolence: Taixi KID-3, Zhaohai KID-6, Baihui DU-20, Tianjing GB-21, Erjian L.I.-2, Sanjian L.I.-3, Lidui ST-45 and Ganshu BL-18 (*Great Compendium*).
- Ceaseless diarrhoea and dysenteric disorder: Taixi KID-3 and Guanyuan REN-4 (*Thousand Ducat Formulas*).
- Difficult defecation: Taixi KID-3 and Chengshan BL-57 (*Supplementing Life*).

- Dark urine: Taixi KID-3, Yingu KID-10, Shenshu BL-23, Qihai REN-6, Pangguangshu BL-28 and Guanyuan REN-4 (*Great Compendium*).
- Pain of the penis: Taixi KID-3, Yuji LU-10, Zhongji REN-3 and Sanyinjiao SP-6 (*Great Compendium*).
- Pain of the inner and outer ankle: Taixi KID-3 and Kunlun BL-60 (*Song to Keep Up Your Sleeve*).
- Paralysis of the lower extremity: Taixi KID-3, Yinlingquan SP-9, Huantiao GB-30, Yangfu GB-38 and Zhiyin BL-67 (*Great Compendium*).
- Straw shoe wind (redness, swelling and pain of the leg and foot): Taixi KID-3, Kunlun BL-60 and Shenmai BL-62 (*Song of the Jade Dragon*).

DAZHONG KID-4

Great Bell

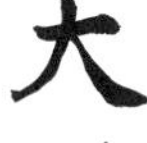
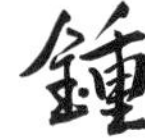

Luo-Connecting point of the Kidney channel

LOCATION

Approximately 0.5 cun posterior to the midpoint of the line drawn between Taixi KID-3 and Shuiquan KID-5, on the anterior border of the Achilles tendon.

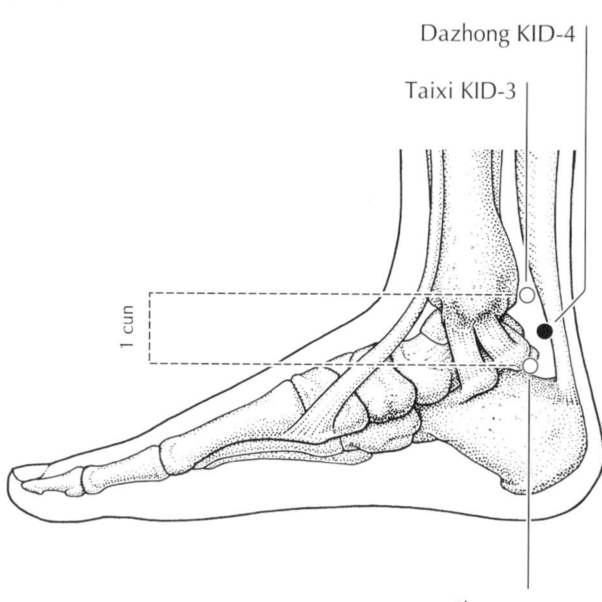

LOCATION NOTE

First locate Shuiquan KID-5, 1 cun directly inferior to Taixi KID-3, then locate Dazhong KID-4 halfway between and 0.5 cun posterior to these two points.

NEEDLING

Oblique-perpendicular insertion directed anteriorly 0.5 cun.

ACTIONS

Reinforces the Kidneys
Anchors the qi and benefits the Lung
Strengthens the will and dispels fear

INDICATIONS

- Coughing blood, dyspnoea due to diminished qi, asthma, wheezing, rattling sound in the throat, cough, shortness of breath, distention and oppression of the chest and abdomen, vomiting.
- Heat in the mouth, dry tongue, painful throat with difficulty in swallowing.
- Palpitations, agitation of the Heart with fullness and vomiting, agitation, dementia, mental retardation, somnolence, propensity to anger, fright, fear and unhappiness, desire to close the door and remain at home.
- Constipation with distended abdomen, difficult urination, dribbling and retention of urine, malaria with much cold and little heat, irregular menstruation.
- Stiffness and pain of the lumbar region, pain and swelling of the heel.

COMMENTARY

Dazhong KID-4, the luo-connecting point of the Kidney channel, regulates the Kidney function in two main ways. Firstly it reinforces and regulates the relationship between the Kidneys and the Lung, and secondly it has a strong effect on stabilising the emotions.

According to the *Complete Works of Jing-yue* "The Lung is the master of qi, the Kidneys are the root of qi. The Lung dominates exhalation of qi, whilst the Kidneys dominate the reception of qi. Only when yin and yang are mutually communicating is respiration in harmony". In discussing dyspnoea, the *Case Histories from the Guide to Clinical Patterns* by Ye Tian-shi states "When it is in the Lung it is excess, when in the Kidneys it is deficient". This latter statement, although something of an over-simplification, nevertheless emphasises that when a respiratory disorder is acute and of excess type, it is the Lung that must be emphasised in treatment, and when it is chronic and deficient in nature, treatment of the Kidneys takes priority. In its action on harmonising the relationship between the Lung and the Kidneys, Dazhong KID-4 is indicated either when the Kidney qi is insufficient to receive and anchor the qi from the Lung resulting in coughing, wheezing, asthma, shortness of breath etc., or when Kidney yin is deficient and unable to moisten and cool the Lung, mouth and throat, resulting in wheezing, coughing of blood, dry and painful throat etc. Both these situations are referred to as "excess above and deficiency below". Compared to Taixi KID-3, Dazhong KID-4 has a relatively stronger effect on addressing the fullness above, and a lesser action on nourishing the Kidneys.

In common with many of the luo-connecting points Dazhong KID-4 has a strong action on the emotions. According to the *Spiritual Pivot* "Deficiency of qi in the Kidney Channel of foot shaoyin may give rise to susceptibility to fear." When the Kidney qi is not animated, the will is deficient and a person easily suffers from fear and lack of confidence, which may be so severe that they withdraw and are unwilling or unable to leave the safety of their home. When congenital essence is deficient, or essence is consumed in old age, there may be a susceptibility to fearfulness, poor mental function or development, and a decline of mental faculties. Susceptibility to fear may not only be due to deficiency of the Kidneys, especially Kidney essence, but also to feebleness and deficiency of qi and blood which fail to nourish and support the spirit, or to deficiency of the Liver and Gall Bladder. Dazhong KID-4, an essential point in the treatment of fear due to Kidney deficiency, also plays an important role in the treatment of any of these patterns because of the close relationship of the Kidneys to fear.

Severe excessive desire to sleep may result either from Spleen deficiency with accumulation of phlegm and dampness, or from Kidney yang or Kidney essence deficiency. Dazhong KID-4 is an important point for somnolence due to Kidney deficiency.

The Kidney luo-connecting channel rises from Dazhong KID-4 to the lumbar spine, accentuating the close relationship of the Kidneys to this region, and this point is therefore indicated for stiffness and pain of the lumbar region. Like Taixi KID-3, Dazhong KID-4 is also used for heel pain.

Finally the *Great Compendium of Acupuncture and Moxibustion* gives specific indications for excess and deficiency of the luo-connecting points. In the case of Dazhong KID-4, these are retention of urine (excess); lumbar pain (deficiency).

COMBINATIONS

- Heat in the mouth: Dazhong KID-4 and Shaochong HE-9 (*Supplementing Life*).
- Fright and fear of people, spirit qi insufficient: Dazhong KID-4 and Ximen P-4 (*Thousand Ducat Formulas*).
- Weary speech and somnolence: Dazhong KID-4 and Tongli HE-5 (*One Hundred Patterns*).
- Somnolence: Dazhong KID-4, Taixi KID-3, Shouwuli L.I.-13, Zhaohai KID-6 and Erjian L.I.-2 (*Supplementing Life*).
- Agitation of the Heart with fullness and vomiting: Dazhong KID-4 and Taixi KID-3 (*Thousand Ducat Formulas*).
- Difficulty in defecation: Dazhong KID-4 and Shiguan KID-18 (*Supplementing Life*).
- Difficulty in defecation: Dazhong KID-4, Zhongliao BL-33, Guanyuan REN-4, Chengjin BL-56, Taichong LIV-3, Chengshan BL-57, Taixi KID-3 and Zhongwan REN-12 (*Supplementing Life*).

SHUIQUAN KID-5

Water Spring

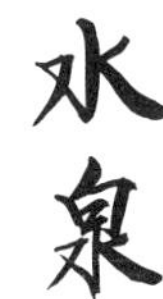

Xi-Cleft point of the Kidney channel

LOCATION

1 cun inferior to Taixi KID-3 in a depression anterior and superior to the calcaneal tuberosity (the site of insertion of the Achilles tendon into the calcaneum).

NEEDLING

Oblique-perpendicular insertion directed away from the bone, 0.3 to 0.5 cun.

ACTIONS

Regulates the Penetrating and Conception vessels and benefits menstruation

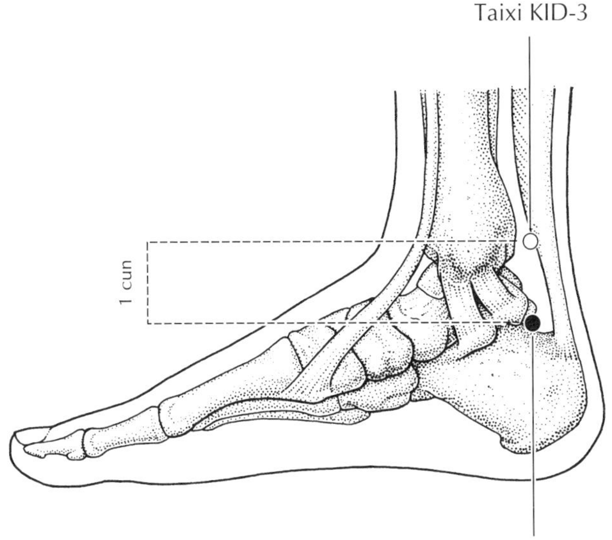

INDICATIONS

- Amenorrhoea, irregular menstruation, dysmenorrhoea, delayed menstruation with oppression and pain below the Heart on onset of menstruation, prolapse of the uterus.
- Cloudy vision, short sightedness, abdominal pain, difficult urination, dribbling urination.

COMMENTARY

Shuiquan KID-5 is the xi-cleft point of the Kidney channel. The xi-cleft points are where the qi and blood, which flow relatively superficially along the channels from the jing-well points, gather and plunge more deeply. The xi-cleft points in general are indicated in the treatment of acute conditions and pain, whilst the xi-cleft points of the yin channels have an additional action of treating disorders of blood.

There is an intimate relationship between the Kidneys, the uterus, blood and menstruation. The *Essential Questions* says "The vessel of the uterus connects with the Kidneys"[13] and "At the age of fourteen, the tian gui[14] matures, the Conception vessel flows and the Penetrating vessel fills, the menses come according to their times, thus conception is possible"[15]. Normal development of the uterus and the Conception and Penetrating vessels depend on healthy functioning of the Kidneys and maturation of the Kidney essence. At the same time, harmonious menstruation depends on adequate formation of blood in the body, especially the Liver blood which flows to the Conception and Penetrating vessels to form menstrual blood. The close relationship between the Kidneys and Liver blood was emphasised in *Comprehensive Medicine According to Master Zhang* which said "[When] the essence is not discharged it will return to the Liver and transform into clear blood", whilst the Kidneys themselves play an important role in the formation of blood, stated unequivocally in *Disease Mechanisms According to Master Sha* "The source of blood is the Kidneys".

If the Kidneys are deficient, then the function of the Conception and Penetrating vessels will be disturbed and the formation of blood impaired. Shuiquan KID-5, the xi-cleft point of the Kidney channel, and thus able to treat disorders of blood, regulates the qi and blood in the Kidney, Conception and Penetrating vessels. It is indicated for a variety of menstrual disorders such as amenorrhoea, irregular menstruation, dysmenorrhoea and delayed menstruation (with oppression and pain below the Heart on onset of menstruation), whether characterised by deficiency (of blood or qi) or excess (stasis of blood).

COMBINATIONS

- Amenorrhoea with much oppression and pain below the Heart: Shuiquan KID-5 and Zhaohai KID-6 (*Thousand Ducat Formulas*).
- Irregular menstruation: Shuiquan KID-5 and Tianshu ST-25 (*One Hundred Symptoms*).
- Uterine prolapse: Shuiquan KID-5, Zhaohai KID-6, Shenmai BL-62 and Ququan LIV-8 (*Supplementing Life*).

ZHAOHAI KID-6

Shining Sea

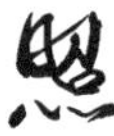

Confluent point of the Yin Motility vessel

LOCATION

1 cun below the prominence of the medial malleolus, in the groove formed by two ligamentous bundles.

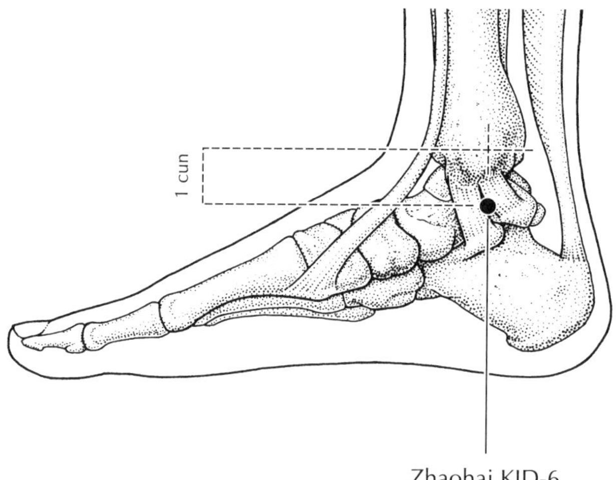

Zhaohai KID-6

LOCATION NOTE

This point lies between the tibialis posterior tendon anteriorly and the flexor digitorum longus tendon posteriorly. These tendons may be highlighted by flexing and inverting the foot.

NEEDLING

Oblique insertion directed superiorly 0.3 to 0.5 cun.

ACTIONS

Benefits the throat
Nourishes the Kidneys and clears deficiency heat
Regulates the Yin Motility vessel
Calms the spirit
Regulates the lower jiao

INDICATIONS

- Swelling and pain of the throat, dry throat, plumstone qi (globus hystericus).
- Redness and pain of the eyes originating at the inner canthus, vision disturbed by seeing spots and stars, head wind, dizziness.
- Insomnia, somnolence, night-time epilepsy, sadness, fright, nightmares, five palms agitated and hot.
- Frequent urination, enuresis, dribbling urination in women, blood painful urinary dysfunction, oedema, constipation.

- Irregular menstruation, amenorrhoea, dysmenorrhoea, chronic cold of the uterus leading to infertility, difficult labour, persistent flow of lochia, post-partum dizziness, post-partum pain in the umbilical region, red and white leucorrhoea, uterine prolapse.
- Itching of the genitals, sudden involuntary erection, seminal emission, shan disorder, hypogastric pain.
- Hot or cold sensation in the lower abdomen, sudden turmoil disorder, distention and fullness of the chest and abdomen, oppressive sensation of the body.
- Tightness and contraction of the inner aspect of the leg, weariness or pain of the four limbs, cold damp leg qi, deficiency in the elderly, cramps of the feet and hands, hemiplegia.

COMMENTARY

Zhaohai KID-6 is the confluent point and according to a passage in the *Great Compendium of Acupuncture and Moxibustion* also the luo-connecting point of the Yin Motility vessel. The Yin Motility vessel traverses the medial aspect of the leg, the perineum, chest and throat, whilst the Kidney primary channel traverses the abdomen, connects with the uterus, joins with the Heart and ascends along the throat. The action of Zhaohai KID-6 can best be understood in relation to three major functions: i. regulating the Yin Motility vessel and the Kidney channel, ii. nourishing yin and clearing deficiency heat from the throat, Heart, intestines, uterus and genitals, and iii. regulating the lower jiao.

In the *Ode of the Obstructed River* the use of Zhaohai KID-6 is referred to as one of the 'eight therapeutic methods'. In this description of the application of the eight confluent points of the extraordinary vessels to affect specific symptoms and areas of the body, Zhaohai KID-6 is indicated for throat wind (swelling and pain with difficulty in swallowing). Both the Yin Motility vessel and the Kidney channel pass through the throat. When heat deriving from yin deficiency scorches the throat, there may be swelling, dryness, redness and pain. This type of sore throat is characterised by its chronic and lingering nature, worsening in the evening and with tiredness, and Zhaohai KID-6 is the main distal point to treat this pattern. Such is its affinity for the throat region, however (due to its ability to clear and regulate both channels), that it may also be selected for any kind of sore throat, whether deficient or excess. It is also indicated for plumstone qi (globus hystericus), a sensation of throat blockage which worsens or ameliorates according to fluctuations in the emotional state and which is normally associated with stagnation of qi and phlegm.

The Yin Motility vessel connects with the Yang Motility vessel at the eyes at Jingming BL-1, and Zhaohai KID-6 is indicated for eye disorders such as redness and pain of the inner canthus and disturbance of the vision by spots and stars. According to the *Spiritual Pivot*[16] "When the [taiyang Bladder] channel enters the brain it is divided into the Yin Motility and the Yang Motility, it is here that the yin and yang meet; yang enters the yin and yin moves outwards to the yang, meeting at the inner corner of the eye. When the yang is abundant, the eyes are staring open; when the yin is abundant, the eyes will be closed shut". This passage has been interpreted to explain the use of Zhaohai KID-6 for both insomnia (excessive opening of the eyes) and somnolence (excessive closing of the eyes). Zhaohai KID-6 is also classically indicated for night-time epilepsy, and Shenmai BL-62, the confluent point of the Yang Motility vessel, is indicated for day-time epilepsy.

The Kidney primary channel enters the Heart which stores the spirit, whilst the Kidneys store the will. When the Kidneys and the Heart function harmoniously, the spirit and the will mutually support each other. As well as being able to treat epilepsy and sleeping disorders, Zhaohai KID-6 is used to restore communication between the Heart and Kidneys (especially when heat deriving from Kidney yin deficiency disrupts the spirit) causing a variety of mental and emotional symptoms such as sadness, fright, insomnia and nightmares.

In the lower jiao Zhaohai KID-6 regulates the functions of the uterus, genitals and the two lower yin (anus and urethra). Its forte is to nourish yin and clear deficiency heat, but like many points of the Kidney channel it is also able to tonify yang and warm cold.

According to the *Essential Questions*[17] "the vessel of the uterus connects with the Kidneys". The Kidneys dominate sexual development and are the origin of the Conception and Penetrating vessels, and normal functioning of the uterus depends in the first instance on a harmonious Kidney function. Zhaohai KID-6 is indicated for a wide variety of disorders of menstruation (irregular menstruation, amenorrhoea, dysmenorrhoea), fertility (chronic cold of the uterus leading to infertility) and childbirth (difficult labour, persistent flow of lochia, post-partum dizziness and pain).

In the treatment of genital disorders, Zhaohai KID-6 is predominantly indicated in heat patterns manifesting as genital itching, sudden involuntary erection, leucorrhoea and seminal emission. In the treatment of urinary disorders Zhaohai KID-6 is indicated for frequent or dribbling urination, enuresis and oedema, all manifestations of deficiency of Kidney qi or Kidney yang. Wang Tao of the Tang dynasty in *Secrets of a Frontier Official* specifically mentioned the use of this point in the treatment of dribbling urination in women.

Another important indication for Zhaohai KID-6 is

constipation. Due to its properties of nourishing the Kidneys and clearing deficiency heat it is predominantly indicated for constipation due either to deficiency of yin or scorching of body fluids from prolonged heat in the intestines. Its frequent inclusion in classical combinations, however, reveal that it has long been considered an important distal point for any kind of constipation.

Finally Zhaohai KID-6 treats disorders along the course of the Kidney channel and the Yin Motility vessel, such as tightness and contraction of the inner aspect of the leg (a traditional indication of disorder of the Yin Motility vessel) and distention and fullness of the chest and abdomen.

COMBINATIONS

- For most types of acute throat pain: first needle Baihui DU-20 then Taichong LIV-3, Zhaohai KID-6 and Sanyinjiao SP-6 (*Ode of Xi-hong*).
- Swelling of the throat with inability to swallow: Zhaohai KID-6, Qiangu SI-2 and Zhongfeng LIV-4 (*Thousand Ducat Formulas*).
- Night-time epilepsy: moxa Zhaohai KID-6 and Shenmai BL-62 (*Glorious Anthology*).
- Somnolence: Zhaohai KID-6, Taixi KID-3, Baihui DU-20, Tianjing GB-21, Erjian L.I.-2, Sanjian L.I.-3, Lidui ST-45 and Ganshu BL-18 (*Great Compendium*).
- Uterine prolapse: Zhaohai KID-6, Shenmai BL-62, Shuiquan KID-5 and Ququan LIV-8 (*Supplementing Life*).
- Uterine prolapse: Zhaohai KID-6, Shaofu HE-8, Taichong LIV-3 and Ququan LIV-8 (*Great Compendium*).
- Uterine prolapse: Zhaohai KID-6, Ququan LIV-8 and Dadun LIV-1 (*Great Compendium*).
- Cold shan disorder: Zhaohai KID-6 and Dadun LIV-1 (*One Hundred Symptoms*).
- Lower abdominal pain from the seven kinds of shan disorder: Zhaohai KID-6, Sanyinjiao SP-6 and Ququan LIV-8 (*Ode of Xi-hong*).
- Dark urine and obstruction of the water pathway: Zhaohai KID-6 and Jingmen GB-25 (*Thousand Ducat Formulas*).
- Heat sensation and pain of the hypogastrium: Zhaohai KID-6, Taixi KID-3, Guanyuan REN-4 and Weizhong BL-40 (*Thousand Ducat Formulas*).
- Constipation: Zhaohai KID-6, Taibai SP-3 and Zhangmen LIV-13 (*Great Compendium*).
- Constipation: Zhaohai KID-6 and Zhigou SJ-6 (*Ode of the Jade Dragon*).
- Constipation: Zhaohai KID-6, Taibai SP-3, Zhangmen LIV-13 and Zhigou SJ-6 (*Great Compendium*).
- Diseases below the ankle: Zhaohai KID-6 and Shenmai BL-62 (*Great Compendium*).

FULIU KID-7

Returning Current

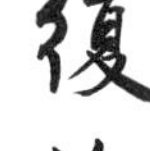
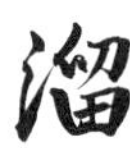

Jing-River and Metal point of the Kidney channel

LOCATION

On the medial aspect of the lower leg, in the depression 2 cun superior to Taixi KID-3, on the anterior border of the Achilles tendon.

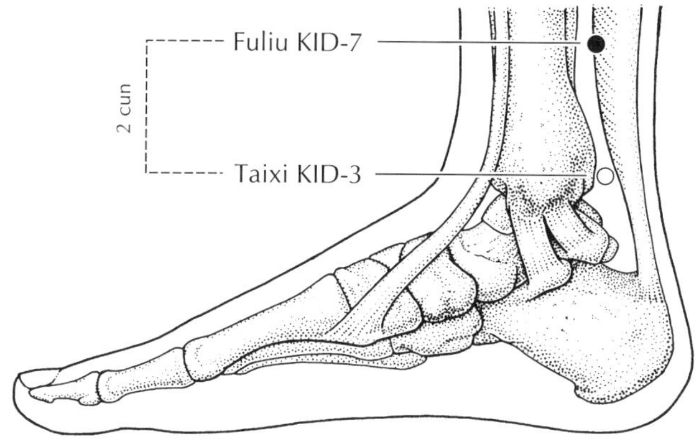

NEEDLING

Perpendicular insertion 0.5 to 1 cun.

ACTIONS

Benefits the Kidneys
Regulates the water passages and treats oedema
Regulates sweating
Drains damp and clears damp-heat
Strengthens the lumbar region

INDICATIONS

- Oedema, the five types of oedema, swelling of the four limbs with drum distention, swelling of the lower limb, difficult urination, dark urine, the five types of painful urinary dysfunction, blood painful urinary dysfunction.
- Spontaneous sweating, night sweating, ceaseless sweating, fever with absence of sweating.
- Diarrhoea, distention of the abdomen with borborygmus, dysenteric disorder, pus and blood in the stool, heavy feeling in the rectum after diarrhoea, bleeding haemorrhoids, constipation.
- Dry tongue and parched mouth, dry tongue with Stomach heat, curled tongue with inability to speak, pain in the nostrils, nosebleed, tooth decay, withered yellow complexion, propensity to anger with incessant talking, propensity to laughter.
- Seminal emission, menorrhagia, uterine bleeding.

- Pain of the lumbar region, lumbar pain due to qi stagnation, atrophy disorder of the leg, cold legs, pulseless syndrome, cold and hot bones.

COMMENTARY

According to the *Classic of Difficulties*[18] "in cases of deficiency reinforce the mother, in cases of excess reduce the child". Fuliu KID-7, the metal and hence 'mother' point of the Kidney water channel, is one of the foremost points to i. strengthen the Kidney function of dominating body fluids and regulating urination, and ii. control sweating.

Oedema has various and complex causes. It may be due to internal or external disharmony and may be acute or chronic. However it predominantly involves disharmony of the Lung, Spleen and Kidneys, the three zang responsible for the movement of fluids. Acute oedema occurs when exterior pathogens lodge in the superficial portion of the body, initially impairing the defensive qi and the Lung function of regulating the water passages. The treatment method is to regulate Lung qi and promote sweating. Alternatively, acute oedema may be due to exterior pathogens which penetrate from the taiyang channel (the most exterior of the six channels) to the taiyang fu, impairing the qi transformation function of the Bladder and leading to difficult urination. Fuliu KID-7 has application in both types of acute oedema by virtue of its dual actions of promoting sweating and urination. Chronic oedema most commonly derives from qi or yang deficiency of the Spleen or Kidneys. Since Kidney yang is the root of Spleen yang, Fuliu KID-7 which is able to tonify Kidney yang and promote urination, may be used in both these types of chronic oedema. In summary, Fuliu KID-7 may be used in any type of oedema but due to its action on the Kidneys, is particularly indicated for chronic lower body oedema.

A special property of Fuliu KID-7 is its ability to control sweating. One explanation of this action is the relationship between the Kidneys and the defensive qi, whose principal functions are to warm and protect the exterior and govern the opening and closing of the pores. There is some disparity in the discussion about the origin of the defensive qi in a variety of classical texts, for example "The Lung controls qi and pertains to defensive qi" (*Warp and Woof of Warm Febrile Diseases*), "Defensive qi is the brave qi of water and grain of yangming, it emanates from the upper jiao" (*Collected Annotations on the Yellow Emperor's Canon of Internal Medicine*), "The Stomach is the source of defensive [qi]" (*Wang Jiu-feng's Medical Records*) and "Defensive qi emanates from the lower jiao" (*Spiritual Pivot*[19]). However a modern Chinese text[20] explains this problem as follows "Defensive qi has its source in the lower jiao, is nourished in the middle jiao and issues from the upper jiao".

Defensive qi is considered to be a part of the original qi which has its origin in the Kidney's pre-heaven qi (lower jiao). It is constantly nourished by the post-heaven essence of water and grain produced by the action of the Stomach and Spleen on food (middle jiao). Finally, it is the Lung which controls the defensive qi and spreads it to the surface of the whole body (upper jiao). It is therefore said that the root of the defensive qi is in the lower jiao, it is nourished by the middle jiao and it spreads in the upper jiao, and this is clarified by the observation that a person's defensive qi may be insufficient due to congenital weakness, inadequate diet or upper jiao deficiency. By virtue of its action on the Kidneys, and hence the source of the defensive qi, Fuliu KID-7 has a wide application in regulating the opening and closing of the pores and treating disorders of sweating (see combinations below). It is able to induce sweating in exterior patterns, stop spontaneous sweating due to qi deficiency, and treat night sweating. Night sweating is most commonly due to fire from yin deficiency. Once again, the ability of Fuliu KID-7 to treat night sweating due to yin deficiency, despite the fact that its primary action is on assisting the Kidney yang function of regulating fluid, demonstrates that all Kidney channel points have some action on both Kidney yin and Kidney yang. In the case of Fuliu KID-7 the ability to nourish yin is further demonstrated by its applicability in the treatment of such symptoms as dry tongue and parched mouth.

It is interesting to note that Fuliu KID-7 is also traditionally indicated for various kinds of bleeding including blood in the urine, blood in the stool, bleeding haemorrhoids, nosebleed, uterine bleeding and menorrhagia. This may reflect the ability of Fuliu KID-7 to astringe blood in the same way that it astringes sweating.

The Kidneys and Bladder are interiorly-exteriorly related. One of the most common pathologies of the Bladder is accumulation of damp-heat giving rise to a variety of urinary symptoms characterised by frequency, urgency, pain, concentrated urine etc. In clinical practice, repeated attacks of Bladder damp-heat often involve underlying Kidney deficiency. By virtue of its dual actions of regulating the Kidneys and draining damp-heat by moving and adjusting the water passages, Fuliu KID-7 is particularly suited to treat these situations.

The damp-heat draining action of Fuliu KID-7 also extends to the intestines, where it is indicated for diarrhoea, dysenteric disorder, pus and blood in the stool, bleeding haemorrhoids etc.

Fuliu KID-7 is commonly used to strengthen the lumbar region in lumbar disorders, particularly when due to Kidney deficiency, although *Methods of Acupuncture and Moxibustion from the Golden Mirror of Medicine* specifically recommends it for lumbar pain due to qi stagnation.

Finally both the Kidney primary and divergent channels ascend to the root of the tongue and the *Spiritual Pivot*[21] states that the jing-river points should be needled for changes manifesting in the patient's voice. Fuliu KID-7, the jing-river point of the Kidney channel, is indicated for dry tongue and parched mouth, dry tongue with Stomach heat, curled tongue with inability to speak, propensity to anger with incessant talking and propensity to laughter.

COMBINATIONS

- Oedema: Fuliu KID-7 and Shuifen REN-9 (*Song of Points*).
- Oedema with qi distention and fullness: Fuliu KID-7 and Shenque REN-8 (*Great Compendium*).
- Drum distention: Fuliu KID-7, Gongsun SP-4, Zhongfeng LIV-4, Taibai SP-3 and Shuifen REN-9 (*Bronze Man*).
- Spontaneous sweating: needle Fuliu KID-7 and Dazhui DU-14 and moxa Gaohuangshu BL-43 (*Divine Moxibustion*).
- Little sweating: reinforce Hegu L.I.-4 and reduce Fuliu KID-7. Copious sweating: first reduce Hegu L.I.-4 then reinforce Fuliu KID-7 (*Great Compendium*).
- Absence of sweating: Fuliu KID-7, Quze P-3, Yuji LU-10, Shaoze SI-1, Shangxing DU-23, Ququan LIV-8, Kunlun BL-60, Xiaxi GB-43 and Zuqiaoyin GB-44 (*Great Compendium*).
- Injury by cold with absence of sweating: Fuliu KID-7 (reduce), Neiting ST-44 (reduce), Hegu L.I.-4 (reinforce) and Bailao (M-HN-30) (*Great Compendium*).
- Injury by cold with sweating: Fuliu KID-7 (reinforce), Neiting ST-44 (reduce), Hegu L.I.-4 (reduce), and Bailao (M-HN-30) (*Great Compendium*).
- Drooling: Fuliu KID-7 and Rangu KID-2 (*Supplementing Life*).
- Blood painful urinary dysfunction: moxa Fuliu KID-7 and the dantian (the area below the umbilicus) (*Thousand Ducat Formulas*).
- Red and white leucorrhoea: Fuliu KID-7, Qugu REN-2 (seven cones of moxa), Taichong LIV-3, Guanyuan REN-4, Sanyinjiao SP-6 and Tianshu ST-25 (one hundred cones of moxa) (*Compilation*).
- Pain of the lumbar spine: Fuliu KID-7 and Weizhong BL-40 (*Great Compendium*).
- Coldness and pain of the bone marrow: Fuliu KID-7, Dazhu BL-11, Xuanzhong GB-39, Shenmai BL-62, Lidui ST-45 and Shenshu BL-23 (*Compilation*).
- Cold sensation of the legs: Fuliu KID-7, Shenmai BL-62 and Lidui ST-45 (*Bronze Man*).
- Breast pain: Fuliu KID-7 and Taichong LIV-3 (*Systematic Classic*).

JIAOXIN KID-8

Exchange Belief

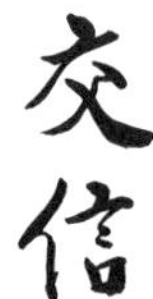

Xi-Cleft point of the Yin Motility vessel

LOCATION

On the medial aspect of the lower leg, 2 cun superior to Taixi KID-3 and 0.5 cun anterior to Fuliu KID-7, posterior to the medial border of the tibia.

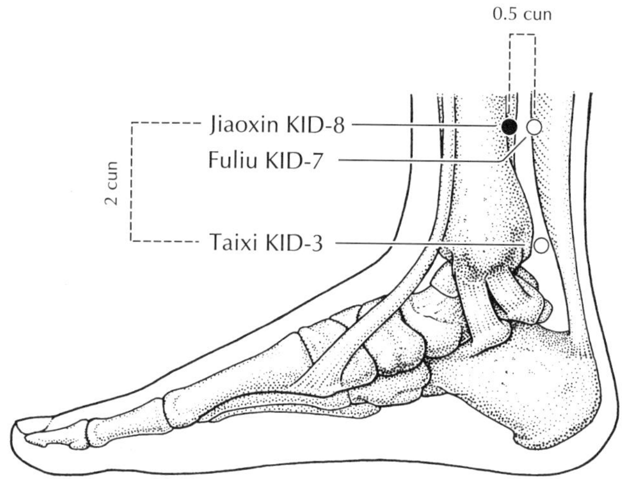

NEEDLING

Perpendicular insertion 0.5 to 1 cun.

ACTIONS

Regulates the Conception and Penetrating vessels and adjusts menstruation
Stops uterine bleeding
Clears heat and drains damp from the lower jiao

INDICATIONS

- Uterine bleeding, irregular menstruation, dysmenorrhoea, amenorrhoea, uterine prolapse.
- Swelling and pain of the testicles, itching of the genitals, sweating of the genitals, shan disorder, night sweating.
- Diarrhoea, dysenteric disorder, difficult defecation or urination, retention of urine, the five types of painful urinary dysfunction, qi painful urinary dysfunction.
- Lumbar pain, pain of the inner aspect of the leg.

COMMENTARY

Jiaoxin KID-8 is the xi-cleft point of the Yin Motility vessel which originates at Zhaohai KID-6. The xi-cleft points of the yin channels have a special action of treating disorders of blood, especially resolving blood stasis, clearing heat from the blood and stopping bleeding. Although the Yin Motility vessel does not enter the uterus, like all the extraordinary vessels it has a close relationship with the

Kidneys, and according to the *Essential Questions*[22] "the vessel of the uterus connects with the Kidneys". The role played by the Kidneys in holding the uterine blood in place was emphasised by the great Han dynasty doctor Hua Tuo who said of the Kidneys "In males they serve the purpose of shutting in the essence, while in females, of wrapping the blood"[23]. Jiaoxin KID-8 is indicated in a variety of menstrual disorders, and most especially uterine bleeding.

Uterine bleeding may be due to a variety of different aetiologies. If the Kidneys are injured by excessively early sexual activity, sexual overindulgence, multiple pregnancies etc. then either the Kidney yin or Kidney yang may become deficient leading to infirmity of the Conception and Penetrating vessels. Jiaoxin KID-8 is predominantly indicated in deficiency patterns of uterine bleeding, particularly in cases of Kidney deficiency, but its status as a xi-cleft point and its secondary action of draining damp-heat renders it suitable in the treatment of uterine bleeding due to blood stasis, reckless movement of hot blood and damp-heat.

Jiaoxin KID-8 has a secondary action of draining damp-heat from the lower jiao. In the genital region it can treat such disorders as itching, swelling, sweating and pain of the genitals. In the urinary system it can promote urination and clear heat in the treatment of retention of urine, difficult urination and painful urinary dysfunction, especially qi painful urinary dysfunction. In the intestines it is indicated in the treatment of diarrhoea, dysenteric disorder and difficult defecation.

COMBINATIONS

- Profuse and ceaseless uterine bleeding: Jiaoxin KID-8, Yingu KID-10, Taichong LIV-3 and Sanyinjiao SP-6 (*Supplementing Life*).
- Diminished qi uterine bleeding: Jiaoxin KID-8 and Heyang BL-55 (*One Hundred Symptoms*).
- Hip pain: Jiaoxin KID-8, Huantiao GB-30, Shugu BL-65, Sanyinjiao SP-6 and Yingu KID-10 (*Thousand Ducat Formulas*).

ZHUBIN KID-9

Guest House

築賓

Xi-Cleft point of the Yin Linking vessel

LOCATION

On the medial aspect of the lower leg, 5 cun superior to Taixi KID-3, on the line drawn between Taixi KID-3 and Yingu KID-10, about 1 cun posterior to the medial border of the tibia.

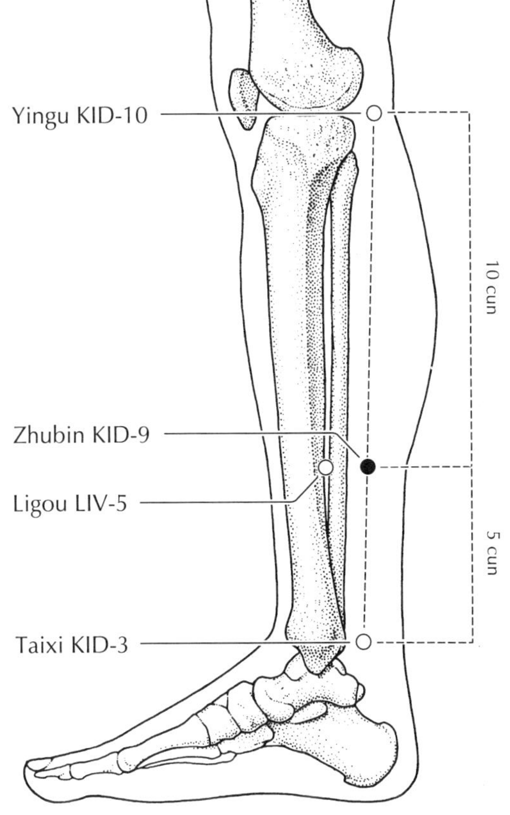

LOCATION NOTE

Locate at the junction of the lower third and upper two thirds of the distance between Taixi KID-3 and Yingu KID-10. Note that this point is on the same level as Ligou LIV-5.

NEEDLING

Perpendicular insertion 1 to 1.5 cun.

ACTIONS

Clears the Heart and transforms phlegm
Regulates qi and alleviates pain

INDICATIONS

- Madness, mania, mania depression disorder, raving, fury and cursing, vomiting of foamy (watery) saliva, tongue thrusting, goitre.
- Shan disorder, umbilical shan disorder in infants.
- Pain of the medial aspect of the leg, contraction of the calf muscle, weakness of the legs.

COMMENTARY

Zhubin KID-9 is the xi-cleft point of the Yin Linking vessel which connects the yin channels of both hand and foot and the Conception vessel. The Yin Linking vessel has a special action on the Heart, thus the *Classic of Difficulties*[24] says "When the Yin Linking vessel is diseased, Heart pain will result". The traditional indications of this point do not include Heart pain, but they do clearly reveal a pattern of phlegm or phlegm-fire obstructing the Heart giving rise to madness, mania, mania depression disorder, raving, fury and cursing and vomiting of foamy (watery) saliva. Phlegm and qi coagulating in the neck region give rise to goitre, whilst tongue thrusting (where the tongue is repeatedly thrust out of the mouth like a snake's tongue) may be due to accumulated heat of the Heart and Spleen.

COMBINATIONS

- Madness with vomiting: Zhubin KID-9, Yanggu SI-5, Houding DU-19, Qiangjian DU-18, Naohu DU-17, Luoque BL-8 and Yuzhen BL-9 (*Thousand Ducat Formulas*).
- Mania disorder, raving, fury and cursing: Zhubin KID-9 and Juque REN-14 (*Thousand Ducat Formulas*).
- Vomiting of foamy (watery) saliva: Zhubin KID-9 and Shaohai HE-3 (*Supplementing Life*).
- Tongue thrusting: Zhubin KID-9 and Taiyi ST-23 (*Supplementing Life*).

YINGU KID-10

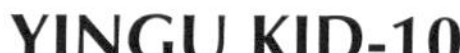

Yin Valley

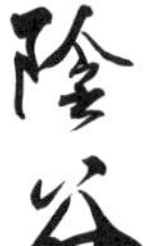

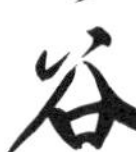

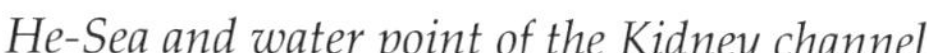

He-Sea and water point of the Kidney channel

LOCATION

At the medial end of the popliteal crease, between the semitendinosus and semimembranosus tendons. Locate and needle with the knee slightly flexed.

LOCATION NOTE

i. In order to accentuate the tendons, ask the patient to tighten the hamstrings; ii. The tendon of semitendinosus, which lies posteriorly to semimembranosus, is the most prominent of the two tendons.

NEEDLING

Perpendicular insertion 1 to 1.5 cun.

ACTIONS

Clears damp-heat from the lower jiao
Benefits the Kidneys
Activates the channel and alleviates pain

INDICATIONS

- Difficult urination, urgency of urination with pain radiating to the thigh, pain on urination, dark urine, diarrhoea.
- Impotence, pain of the genitals, itching of the scrotum.

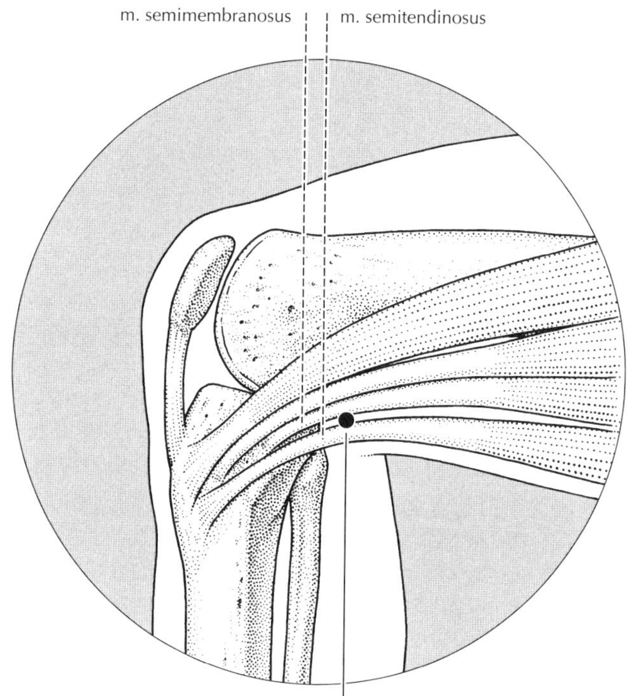

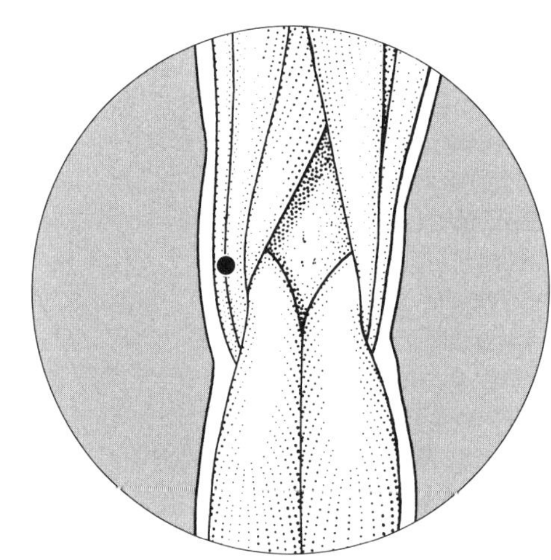

- Shan disorder, hypogastric pain radiating to the genitals and inner thigh, abdominal distention, abdominal pain, periumbilical pain.
- Uterine bleeding, leucorrhoea, difficult conception.
- Manic disorders, mania-depression, protrusion of the tongue with drooling.
- Drilling knee pain with immobility, pain of the inner aspect of the thigh.

COMMENTARY

Yingu KID-10 is the he-sea and water point of the Kidney channel. It shares with the he-sea points of the other leg yin channels the common function of clearing dampness and damp-heat, especially from the lower jiao. Ququan LIV-8 primarily acts on the genital system (dominated by the Liver channel) and Yinlingquan SP-9 by virtue of the intimate relationship between the Spleen and dampness is able to treat all dampness disorders of the lower jiao. Yingu KID-10 predominantly clears damp-heat from the genito-urinary system and is indicated for difficult or urgent urination, dark urine, leucorrhoea and genital itching.

Accumulation of damp-heat may impede the smooth flow of qi and give rise to pain, reflected in the traditional saying "without movement there is pain, with movement there is no pain". Yingu KID-10 is indicated for pain on urination, urgent urination with pain spreading to the thighs, pain of the genitals, periumbilical pain and hypogastric pain radiating to the inner thigh and genitals.

Whilst impotence is most commonly due to decline of ming men fire, it may also be due to accumulation of damp-heat which gives rise to flaccidity. Damp-heat impotence may arise from Liver channel damp-heat or Spleen damp-heat which pour down to the genitals, or from repeated attacks of exterior damp-heat to the Bladder. Yingu KID-10 is primarily indicated for such excess patterns of damp-heat impotence. In females, damp-heat may give rise to uterine bleeding and difficult conception, both indications for Yingu KID-10.

There is a close relationship between lower jiao damp-heat and Kidney deficiency. If Kidney yin deficiency gives rise to heat, this may combine with dampness to form damp-heat, whilst prolonged damp-heat will consume first Kidney yin and then Kidney yang. This dual pattern of Kidney deficiency and damp-heat is commonly encountered in clinical practice, especially in patients with repeated urinary disorders. Due to its secondary action of benefiting the Kidneys, Yingu KID-10 is indicated when these two patterns co-exist.

The degree to which Yingu KID-10 is able to nourish Kidney yin is the subject of frequent discussion. Although ascribed significant yin nourishing properties by some modern authorities, an examination of its classical indications reveals that this does not seem to have been a widely held view historically.

COMBINATIONS

- Involuntary erection with difficult urination: Yingu KID-10, Dadun LIV-1, Qimen LIV-14, Weizhong BL-40 and Weiyang BL-39 (*Supplementing Life*).
- Dark urine: Yingu KID-10, Taixi KID-3, Shenshu BL-23, Qihai REN-6, Pangguangshu BL-28 and Guanyuan REN-4 (*Great Compendium*).
- Profuse and ceaseless uterine bleeding: Yingu KID-10, Jiaoxin KID-8, Sanyinjiao SP-6 and Taichong LIV-3 (*Supplementing Life*).
- Sudden turmoil disorder: Yingu KID-10 and Zusanli ST-36 (*One Hundred Symptoms*).
- Stiffness of the tongue: Yingu KID-10, Rangu KID-2, Yamen DU-15, Shaoshang LU-11, Yuji LU-10, Erjian L.I.-2 and Zhongchong P-9 (*Great Compendium*).
- Swelling below the tongue with difficulty speaking, protrusion of the tongue with drooling: Yingu KID-10, Rangu KID-2 and Lianquan REN-23 (*Thousand Ducat Formulas*).
- Loss of voice: Yingu KID-10, Rangu KID-2, Tiantu REN-22, Lingdao HE-4, Fuliu KID-7 and Fenglong ST-40 (*Illustrated Supplement*).
- Mania: Yingu KID-10, Zusanli ST-36, Jianshi P-5, Baihui DU-20 and Fuliu KID-7 (*Illustrated Supplement*).
- Hip pain: Yingu KID-10, Huantiao GB-30, Shugu BL-65, Jiaoxin KID-8 and Sanyinjiao SP-6 (*Thousand Ducat Formulas*).

HENGGU KID-11

Pubic Bone

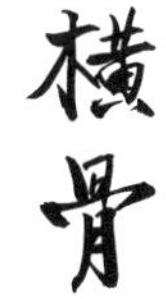

Meeting point of the Kidney channel with the Penetrating vessel

LOCATION

On the lower abdomen, 5 cun below the umbilicus, at the superior border of the symphysis pubis, 0.5 cun lateral to the midline (Qugu REN-2).

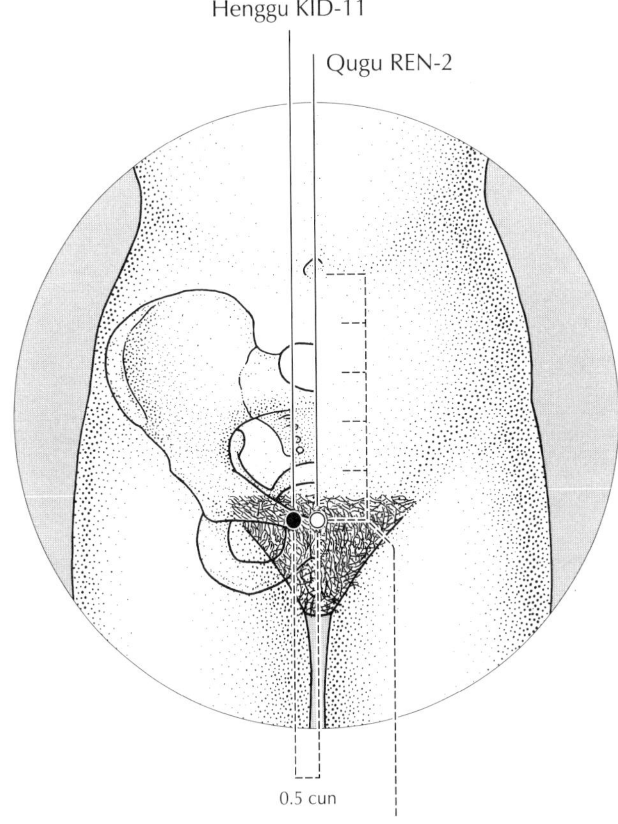

LOCATION NOTE

The *Great Compendium of Acupuncture and Moxibustion* locates the points Henggu KID-11 to Shangqu KID-17 one cun lateral to the midline.

NEEDLING

Perpendicular insertion 0.5 to 1 cun.
Caution: deep insertion will penetrate a full bladder which should therefore be emptied before treatment.

ACTIONS

Benefits the lower jiao

INDICATIONS

- Seminal emission, impotence, deficiency and exhaustion of the five zang with seminal emission, enuresis, retention of urine, the five types of painful urinary dysfunction, pain of the genitals, painful retraction of the genitals, shan disorder, hypogastric pain, redness of the eyes originating at the inner canthus.
- Uterine prolapse, prolapse of the rectum.

COMBINATIONS

- Stagnation of qi, lumbar pain with inability to stand: Henggu KID-11 and Dadu SP-2 (*Ode of Xi-hong*).
- The five types of painful urinary dysfunction from chronic accumulation:: Henggu KID-11 and Huangshu KID-16 (*One Hundred Symptoms*).

DAHE KID-12

Great Luminance

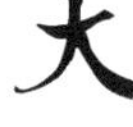

Meeting point of the Kidney channel with the Penetrating vessel

LOCATION

On the lower abdomen, 4 cun below the umbilicus, 1 cun superior to the superior border of the symphysis pubis, 0.5 cun lateral to the midline (Zhongji REN-3). See location note for Henggu KID-11.

NEEDLING

Perpendicular insertion 0.5 to 1 cun.
Caution: deep insertion will penetrate a full bladder which should therefore be emptied before treatment.

ACTIONS

Tonifies the Kidneys and astringes essence

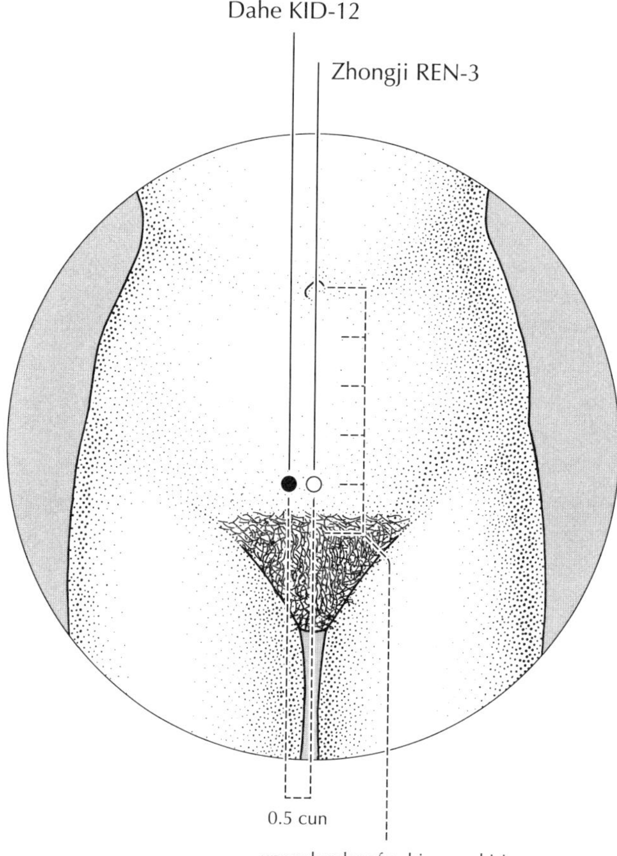

INDICATIONS

- Pain of the genitals, pain of the penis, retraction of the penis, impotence, seminal emission, deficiency-taxation leucorrhoea, red leucorrhoea, uterine prolapse, redness of the eye originating at the inner canthus.

COMMENTARY

The action of Dahe KID-12 in astringing essence is reflected in its application for both seminal emission and leucorrhoea.

Seminal emission (involuntary loss of sperm) may be due to various aetiologies. Ejaculatory function is an aspect of the free and smooth flow of Liver qi, whilst the Kidneys dominate the 'gate of essence'. If there is undue heat (e.g. Liver fire, Heart fire, heat from Kidney yin deficiency) this will force the seminal fluid to burst out recklessly. Alternatively, deficiency of the Kidney astringing function will lead to infirmity of the gate of essence resulting in leakage of seminal fluid. According to Zhu Dan-xi, seminal emission with erotic dreams "is exclusively governed by heat"[25], whilst it is said traditionally that if due to cold and deficiency there will be no such dreaming. Whatever the aetiology, Dahe KID-12 (like a number of other Kidney channel points on the lower abdomen) is an important point in the treatment of seminal emission.

As far as leucorrhoea is concerned, it should be noted that although primarily due to damp, damp-heat or toxic heat, leucorrhoea may also be due to deficiency of Kidney qi or yang, and that this kind of leucorrhoea entails loss of essence and is the female equivalent of loss of seminal fluid.

COMBINATIONS

- Seminal emission and retraction of the penis: Dahe KID-12 and Rangu KID-2 (*Supplementing Life*).

QIXUE KID-13

Qi Cave

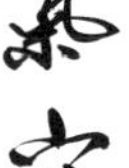

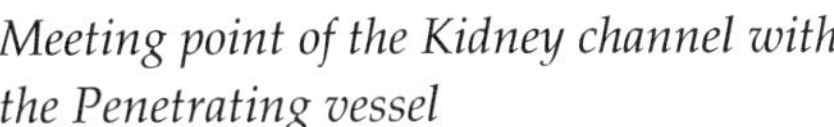

Meeting point of the Kidney channel with the Penetrating vessel

LOCATION

On the lower abdomen, 3 cun below the umbilicus, 2 cun superior to the superior border of the symphysis pubis, 0.5 cun lateral to the midline (Guanyuan REN-4). See location note for Henggu KID-11.

NEEDLING

Perpendicular insertion 0.5 to 1 cun.
Caution: deep insertion will penetrate a full bladder which should therefore be emptied before treatment.

ACTIONS

Regulates the Penetrating and Conception vessels
Regulates the lower jiao

INDICATIONS

- Amenorrhoea, irregular menstruation, uterine bleeding, leucorrhoea, infertility in women.
- Difficult urination, incessant diarrhoea, abdominal pain, running piglet qi, rushing sensation up and down the lumbar spine, lumbar pain, redness of the eye originating at the inner canthus.

COMMENTARY

Qixue KID-13 (like Siman KID-14 and Zhongzhu KID-15) is an important point in the treatment of running piglet qi. According to Zhang Zhong-jing in the *Essentials from the Golden Cabinet* "Running piglet disorder arises from the lower abdomen; it rushes up to the throat with such ferocity that the patient feels he is close to death. It attacks and then remits. It is brought about by fear and fright". In the *Classic of Difficulties*[26] running piglet was classified as one of the 'five accumulations' pertaining to the Kidneys. Running piglet qi primarily arises when stagnant Liver qi transforms to heat, or when Kidney yang deficiency leads to accumulation of cold in the lower jiao. In both cases, qi is violently discharged and rushes upwards along the Penetrating vessel. In clinical practice, running piglet qi may be encountered in a number of variants, all involving a rushing sensation, usually upwards, along the trunk, back or limbs. According to the *Classic of Difficulties*[27] "When the Penetrating vessel is diseased there is counterflow qi". The application of Qixue KID-13, Siman KID-14 and Zhongzhu KID-15 in the treatment of this distressing condition reflects both their location on the Kidney channel and their status as points of the Penetrating vessel, which both ascends through the abdomen to disperse in the chest, and enters the spine and circulates through the back.

Many classical sources list Baomen (Gate of the Uterus) and Zihu (Child's Door) as alternative names for this point. The *Supplement to the Thousand Ducat Formulas*, however, is quite clear that these names correspond to Shuidao ST-28, referring to the points located 2 cun either side of Guanyuan REN-4.

COMBINATIONS

- Irregular menstruation and infertility: Qixue KID-13, Shenshu BL-23, Qihai REN-6, Sanyinjiao SP-6 and Shangqiu SP-5.

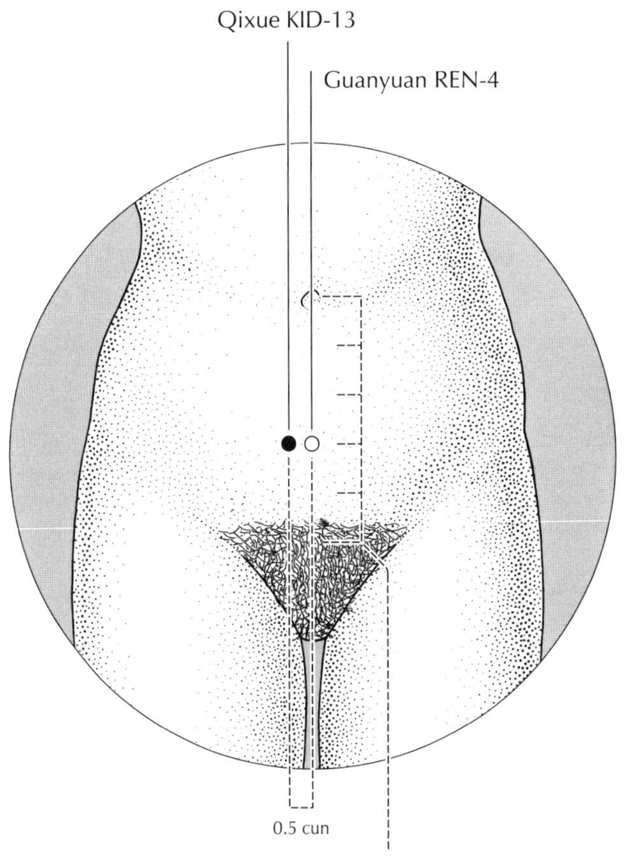

SIMAN KID-14

Four Fullnesses

四滿

Meeting point of the Kidney channel with the Penetrating vessel

LOCATION

On the lower abdomen, 2 cun below the umbilicus, 3 cun superior to the superior border of the symphysis pubis, 0.5 cun lateral to the midline (Shimen REN-5).

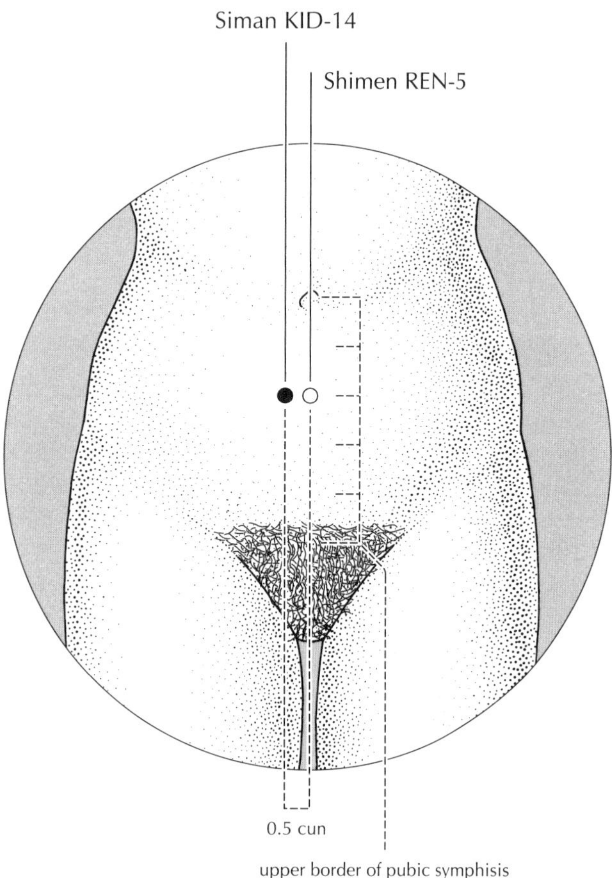

NEEDLING

Perpendicular insertion 1 to 1.5 cun.
Caution: deep needling may penetrate the peritoneal cavity.

ACTIONS

Benefits the lower jiao and alleviates pain
Regulates qi and moves blood stasis
Regulates the water passages and promotes urination

INDICATIONS

- Lower abdominal pain, abdominal distention, shan disorder, cutting pain below the umbilicus, stone oedema of the upper abdomen, oedema, running piglet qi, pain of the Kidneys.
- Irregular menstruation, uterine bleeding, malign blood with acute pain, accumulated cold in the uterus, infertility, leucorrhoea, retention of lochia, seminal emission, white and turbid urethral discharge.
- Dysenteric disorder, diarrhoea, water in the Large Intestine, constipation, cold shivering, pain of both lateral costal regions, redness and pain of the inner canthus.

COMMENTARY

The name of this point (Siman) is translated as 'Four Fullnesses'. Although there are different interpretations of its meaning, one opinion is that it refers to the four kinds of stagnation and accumulation: qi, water, food and blood. There are clear indications that reflect each of these conditions, for example abdominal distention for qi, abdominal oedema for water, and diarrhoea or constipation for food, but overwhelmingly the indications reflect the presence of blood stasis, for example cutting pain below the umbilicus, retention of lochia, and malign blood with acute pain. The term 'malign blood' refers to blood that has left the vessels and which, bereft of the moving force of qi, pools and stagnates.

COMBINATIONS

- Stone oedema of the upper abdomen: moxa Siman KID-14, Rangu KID-2, Qichong ST-30 and Zhangmen LIV-13 (*Thousand Ducat Formulas*).
- Stone oedema of the upper abdomen: Siman KID-14 and Rangu KID-2 (*Supplementing Life*).
- Malign blood in the uterus, internal counterflow fullness and pain: Siman KID-14 and Shiguan KID-18 (*Supplementing Life*).

ZHONGZHU KID-15

Middle Flow

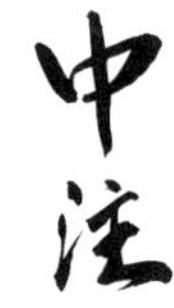

Meeting point of the Kidney channel with the Penetrating vessel

LOCATION

On the lower abdomen, 1 cun below the umbilicus, 4 cun superior to the superior border of the symphysis pubis, 0.5 cun lateral to the midline (Yinjiao REN-7). See location note for Henggu KID-11.

NEEDLING

Perpendicular insertion 1 to 1.5 cun.
Caution: deep needling may penetrate the peritoneal cavity.

ACTIONS
Regulates the intestines
Regulates the lower jiao

INDICATIONS
- Constipation, dry stools, diarrhoea, dysenteric disorder, sensation of heat in the lower abdomen, irregular menstruation, redness and pain of the inner canthus.
- Pain of the lumbar spine and abdomen, rushing sensation up and down the lumbar spine.

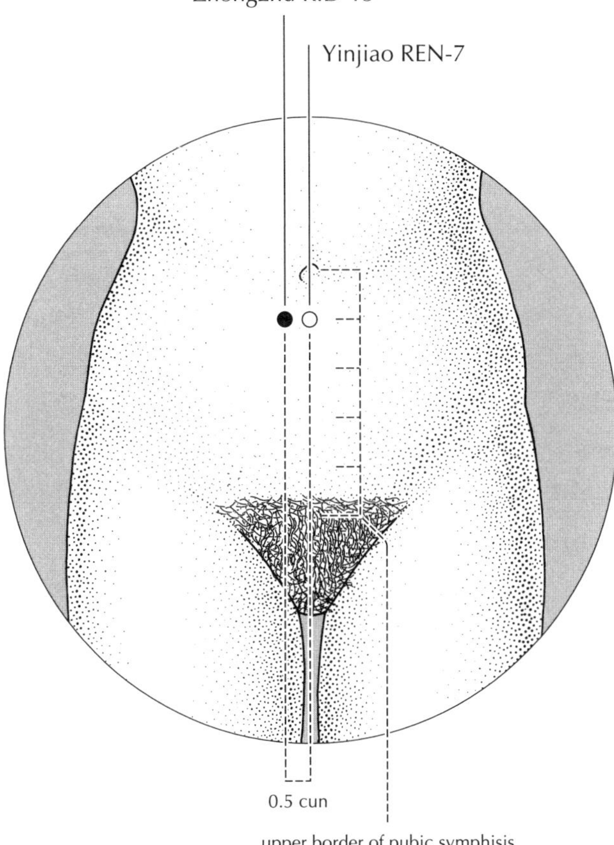

HUANGSHU KID-16

肓俞

Vitals Shu

Meeting point of the Kidney channel with the Penetrating vessel

LOCATION
On the abdomen, 0.5 cun lateral to the centre of the umbilicus. See location note for Henggu KID-11.

NEEDLING
Perpendicular insertion 1 to 1.5 cun.
Caution: deep needling may penetrate the peritoneal cavity.

ACTIONS
Regulates qi and alleviates pain
Regulates and warms the intestines

INDICATIONS
- Constipation, dry stools, borborygmus, diarrhoea, vomiting, the five types of painful urinary dysfunction, redness and pain of the eye originating at the inner canthus.
- Pain of the epigastrium and abdomen, cold in the epigastrium, distention and pain of the abdomen, cutting pain of the abdomen, shan disorder due to cold.

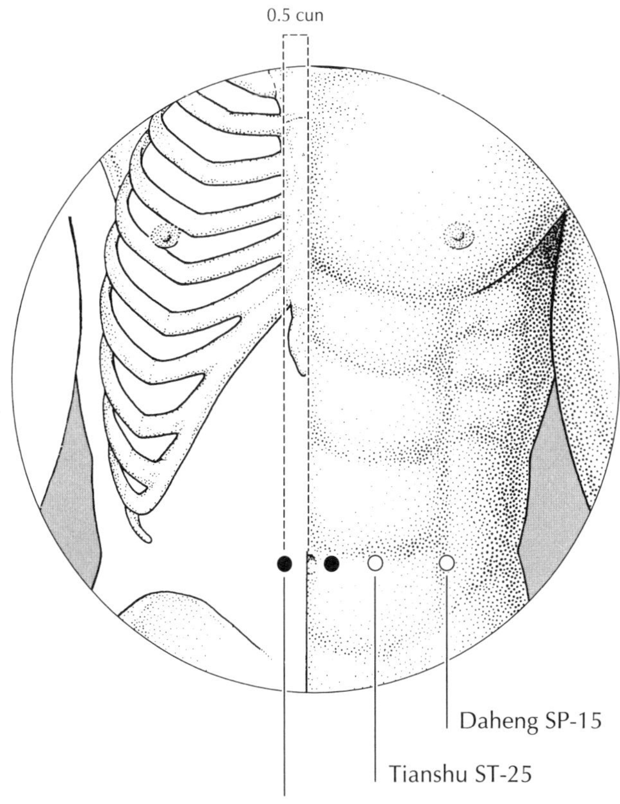

COMMENTARY
Huangshu KID-16 lies on the same level as Shenque REN-8, Tianshu ST-25 and Daheng SP-15, all points with a strong action on the intestines. Various classics recommend Huangshu KID-16 for dry stools, whilst the *Systematic Classic of Acupuncture and Moxibustion* specifically recommended it for accumulation of cold in the Large Intestine giving rise to dry stools and cutting pain of the abdomen. It should be remembered that constipation may be due to accumulation of cold, whether deficiency cold deriving from insufficiency of Kidney yang and usually seen in the elderly or debilitated, or excess cold, usually from dietary factors. In the former case the stool

may be dry, not from the usual causes (heat or deficiency of fluids, blood or yin) but due to Kidney yang deficiency which fails to circulate fluids.

COMBINATIONS

- The five types of painful urinary dysfunction from chronic accumulation: Huangshu KID-16 and Henggu KID-11 (*One Hundred Symptoms*).

SHANGQU KID-17

Shang Bend

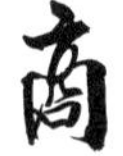
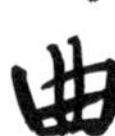

Meeting point of the Kidney channel with the Penetrating vessel

LOCATION

On the upper abdomen, 2 cun above the umbilicus, 0.5 cun lateral to the midline (Xiawan REN-10). See location note for Henggu KID-11.

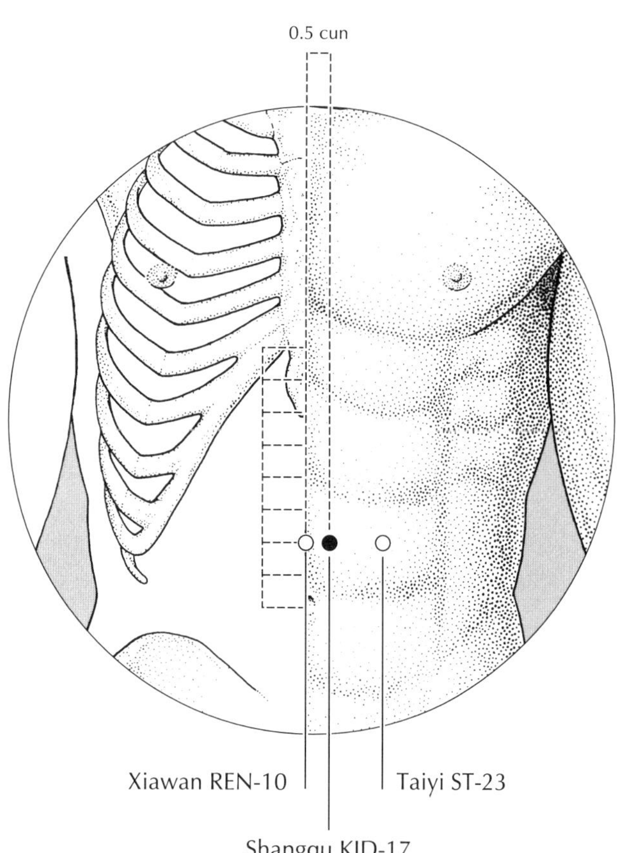

NEEDLING

Perpendicular insertion 1 to 1.5 cun.

Caution: deep needling may penetrate the peritoneal cavity.

ACTIONS

Dispels accumulation and alleviates pain

INDICATIONS

- Abdominal (ji ju) masses with periodic cutting pain, intestinal pain with lack of appetite, redness and pain of the eye originating at the inner canthus.
- Vomiting, diarrhoea, constipation.

SHIGUAN KID-18

Stone Pass

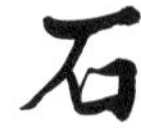
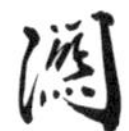

Meeting point of the Kidney channel with the Penetrating vessel

LOCATION

On the upper abdomen, 3 cun above the umbilicus, 0.5 cun lateral to the midline (Jianli REN-11).

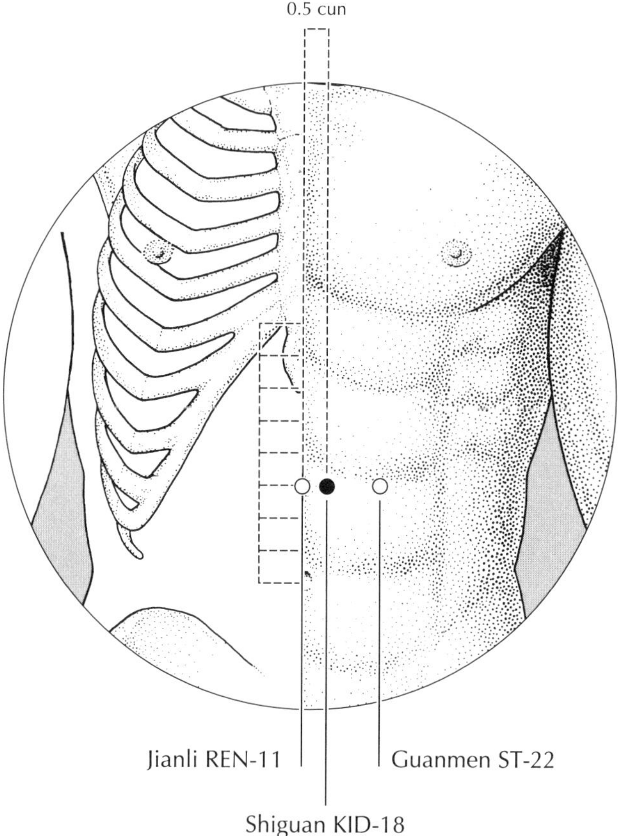

LOCATION NOTE

The *Great Compendium of Acupuncture and Moxibustion* locates the points Shiguan KID-18 to Youmen KID-21, 1.5 cun lateral to the midline.

NEEDLING

Perpendicular insertion 1 to 1.5 cun.

Caution: deep needling may penetrate the peritoneal cavity.

ACTIONS

Regulates the lower jiao and alleviates pain
Regulates qi and moves blood stasis
Harmonises the Stomach

INDICATIONS

- Post-partum abdominal pain, acute pain of the lateral costal region following childbirth, malign blood in the uterus, infertility, unbearable abdominal pain, unendurable stabbing pain of the abdomen, constipation, dark urine, stiffness of the spine, redness and pain of the eye originating at the inner canthus.
- Hiccup, vomiting, retching, much spittle, inability to open the mouth.

COMMENTARY

Unusually for a point located above the umbilicus, Shiguan KID-18 is indicated for a variety of gynaecological disorders including infertility, and especially for severe pain of the abdomen or lateral costal region following childbirth. The indication 'malign blood in the uterus' refers to blood which has left the vessels and which pools and stagnates. All these indications reflect the status of Shiguan KID-18 as a meeting point of the Kidney channel with the Penetrating vessel which originates in the uterus (and is known as the 'sea of blood') and point to a pattern of blood stasis throughout the uterus, the abdomen as a whole and the lateral costal region.

COMBINATIONS

- Difficulty in defecation with abdominal pain: Shiguan KID-18 and Pangguangshu BL-28 (*Supplementing Life*).
- Difficulty in defecation: Shiguan KID-18 and Dazhong KID-4 (*Supplementing Life*).
- Malign blood in the uterus, internal counterflow fullness and pain: Shiguan KID-18 and Siman KID-14 (*Supplementing Life*).
- Infertility: Shiguan KID-18 and Yinjiao REN-7 (*One Hundred Symptoms*).

YINDU KID-19

Yin Metropolis

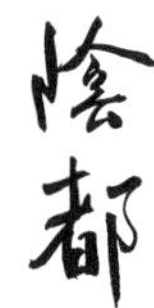

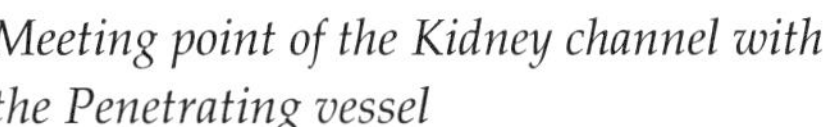
Meeting point of the Kidney channel with the Penetrating vessel

LOCATION

On the upper abdomen, 4 cun above the umbilicus, 0.5 cun lateral to the midline (Zhongwan REN-12).

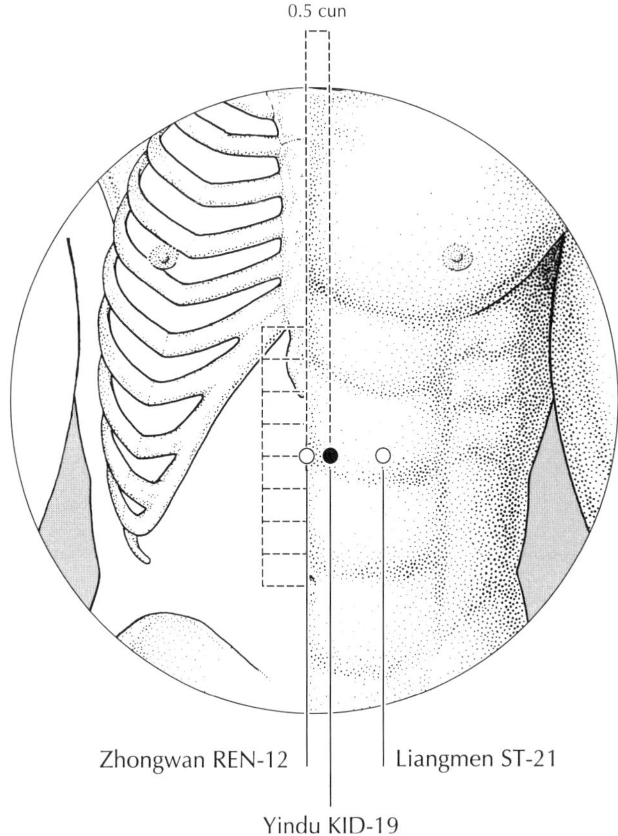

NEEDLING

Perpendicular insertion 0.5 to 1 cun.

Caution: deep needling may penetrate the peritoneal cavity.

ACTIONS

Regulates qi and harmonises the Stomach
Lowers rebellion and alleviates cough and wheezing

INDICATIONS

- Epigastric pain, counterflow qi, vomiting, nausea, fullness and agitation below the Heart, distention and pain of the abdomen, twisting pain in the abdomen, borborygmus, difficult defecation, infertility, malign blood in the uterus.

- Cough, distention of the chest, pain and heat of the lateral costal region, malaria, eye pain, redness and pain of the eye originating at the inner canthus.

COMBINATIONS
- Malaria with generalised fever: Yindu KID-19, Shaohai HE-3, Shangyang L.I.-1, Sanjian L.I.-3 and Zhongzhu SJ-3 (*Supplementing Life*).
- Agitation and fullness of the Heart: Yindu KID-19 and Juque REN-14 (*Supplementing Life*).

FUTONGGU KID-20
Abdomen Connecting Valley

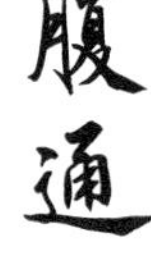

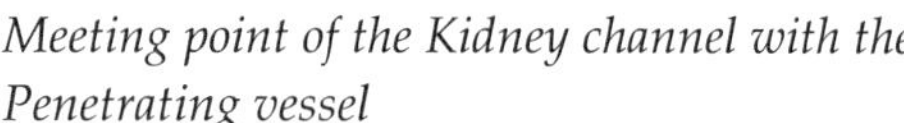

Meeting point of the Kidney channel with the Penetrating vessel

LOCATION
On the upper abdomen, 5 cun above the umbilicus, 0.5 cun lateral to the midline (Shangwan REN-13).

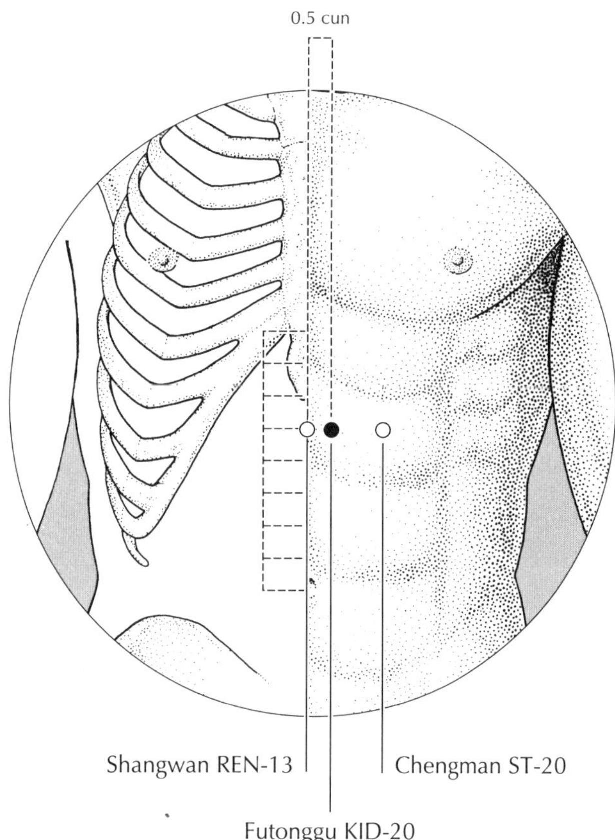

NEEDLING
Perpendicular insertion 1 to 1.5 cun.
Caution: deep needling may penetrate the peritoneal cavity.

ACTIONS
Harmonises the middle jiao
Unbinds the chest and transforms phlegm

INDICATIONS
- Vomiting, undigested food (in the stool), abdominal distention, diarrhoea.
- Fullness of the chest, pain of the lateral costal region, Heart pain, coughing and dyspnoea.
- Palpitations, disorientation, epilepsy, sudden loss of voice, swelling beneath the tongue with difficulty in speaking, protrusion of the tongue, deviation of the mouth.
- Inability to turn the neck, malaria, redness of the eyes originating at the inner canthus.

COMBINATIONS
- Rhinitis with clear nasal discharge: Futonggu KID-20, Hegu L.I.-4, Fengmen BL-12, Shenting DU-24, Zanzhu BL-2, Yingxiang L.I.-20 and Zhiyin BL-67 (*Thousand Ducat Formulas*).

YOUMEN KID-21
Hidden Gate

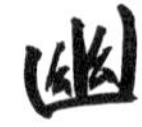

Meeting point of the Kidney channel with the Penetrating vessel

LOCATION
On the upper abdomen, 6 cun above the umbilicus, 0.5 cun lateral to the midline (Juque REN-14).

NEEDLING
Perpendicular insertion 0.5 to 1 cun. **Caution:** deep needling, especially in thin subjects, will puncture the liver on the right side and the peritoneum on the left.

ACTIONS
Fortifies the Spleen, harmonises the Stomach, and lowers rebellion
Spreads Liver qi, benefits the chest and breasts and alleviates pain

INDICATIONS
- Abdominal pain, lower abdominal pain, abdominal urgency, vomiting, nausea and counterflow qi, retching, vomiting of foamy (watery) saliva, much spittle, nausea and vomiting of pregnancy, fullness with no pleasure in eating, difficult ingestion, focal distention below the Heart, fullness and agitation below the Heart, diarrhoea, blood in the stools, dysenteric disorder.

- Chest pain, distention of the lateral costal region, pain of the chest and lateral costal region radiating to the back, cough, coughing blood.
- Breast milk does not flow, breast abscess.
- Heart pain in women, poor memory, redness of the eyes originating at the inner canthus.

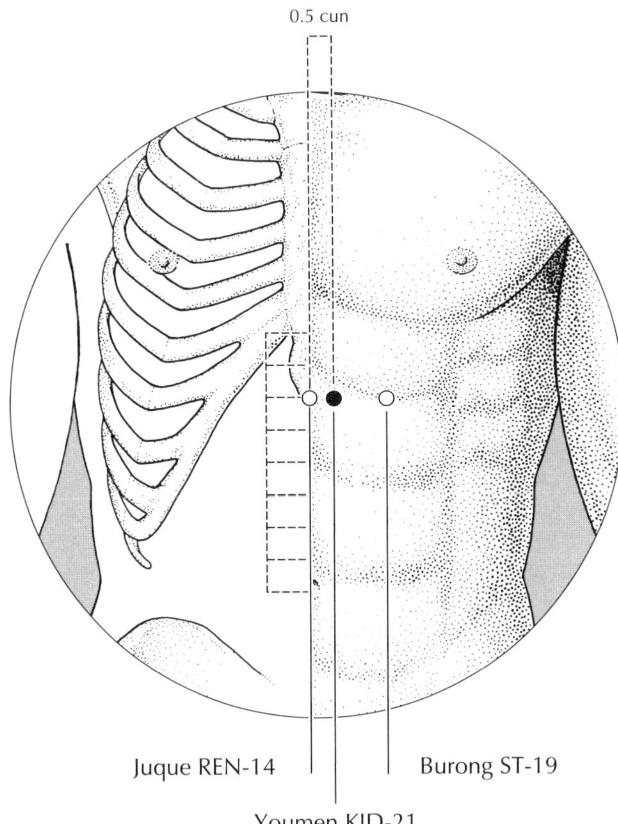

COMMENTARY

According the *Classic of Difficulties*[28] "When the Penetrating vessel is diseased there is counterflow qi and abdominal urgency". Like many of the Kidney channel points on the abdomen, Youmen KID-21 (the final point of the Penetrating vessel on the Kidney channel) is indicated for counterflow qi manifesting as nausea, vomiting, retching and cough. The term abdominal urgency refers to a sensation of acute cramping pain, usually associated with dysenteric disorder.

Like the majority of the Penetrating vessel points on the Kidney channel, Youmen KID-21 is indicated for redness of the eyes originating at the inner canthus. Whilst there is no simple explanation of this symptom, it is worth noting that although some descriptions of the Penetrating vessel suggest that it terminate at the lips, illustrations and other accounts of its pathway usually show it ending at the inner portion of the eyes.

COMBINATIONS

- Agitation of the Heart with vomiting: Youmen KID-21 and Yutang REN-18 (*One Hundred Symptoms*).
- Poor memory: Youmen KID-21, Shendao DU-11, Lieque LU-7 and Gaohuangshu BL-43 (*Supplementing Life*).
- No pleasure in eating: Youmen KID-21, Diji SP-8, Yinlingquan SP-9, Shuifen REN-9 and Xiaochangshu BL-27 (*Supplementing Life*).
- Vomiting: Youmen KID-21, Shangqiu SP-5 and Zutonggu BL-66 (*Thousand Ducat Formulas*).

BULANG KID-22

Walking Corridor

步廊

LOCATION

In the fifth intercostal space, 2 cun lateral to the midline.

LOCATION NOTE

i. First locate the second intercostal space (see Shencang KID-25), then find the fifth intercostal space, three spaces below it; ii. Note that in males the nipple lies in the fourth intercostal space; iii. The 2 cun line is located midway between the midline and the mamillary line.

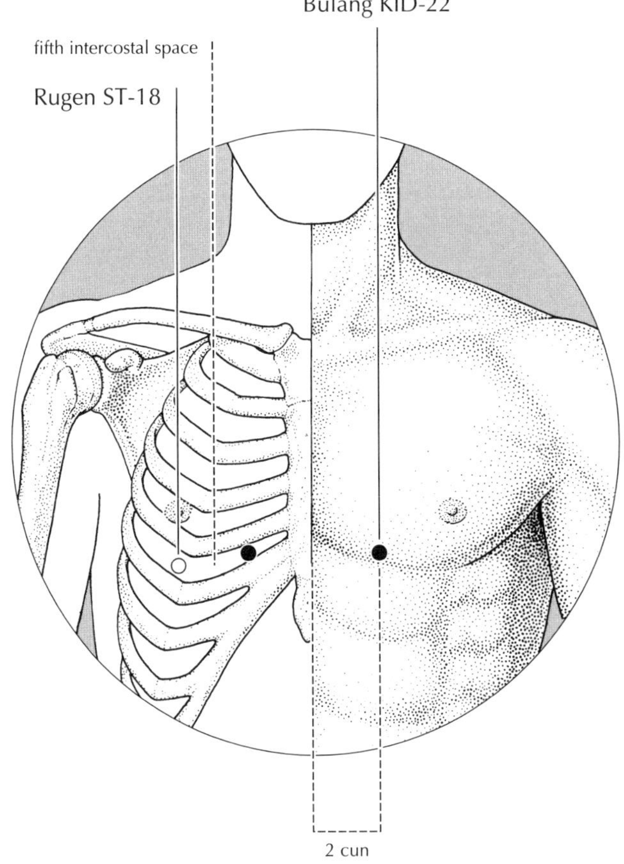

NEEDLING

Transverse-oblique insertion, directed laterally along the intercostal space 0.5 to 1 cun.

Caution: deep perpendicular or oblique needling may puncture the lung and/or liver.

ACTIONS

Unbinds the chest

Lowers rebellious Lung and Stomach qi

INDICATIONS

- Cough, asthma, dyspnoea, wheezing, diminished qi, fullness and pain of the chest and ribs, breast abscess, nasal congestion.
- Vomiting, no pleasure in eating.

COMMENTARY

The points Bulang KID-22, Shenfeng KID-23, Lingxu KID-24, Shencang KID-25, Yuzhong KID-26 and Shufu KID-27 were listed in the *Essential Questions* as the twelve shu points of the chest. They share the common actions of descending rebellious qi of the Lung and Stomach, and are particularly indicated for wheezing, dyspnoea and coughing due to 'fullness above and deficiency below'. This occurs when the Kidney qi is insufficiently strong to grasp the Lung qi.

COMBINATIONS

- Diminished qi: Bulang KID-22, Shaofu HE-8, Pangguangshu BL-28, Shaochong HE-9, Xingjian LIV-2 and Dazhong KID-5 (*Supplementing Life*).

SHENFENG KID-23

Spirit Seal

神封

LOCATION

In the fourth intercostal space, 2 cun lateral to the midline.

LOCATION NOTE

i. First locate the second intercostal space (see Shencang KID-25), then find the fourth intercostal space, two spaces below it; ii. Note that in males the nipple lies in the fourth intercostal space; iii. The 2 cun line is located midway between the midline and the mamillary line.

NEEDLING

Transverse-oblique insertion, directed laterally along the intercostal space 0.5 to 1 cun.

Caution: deep perpendicular or oblique needling may puncture the lung.

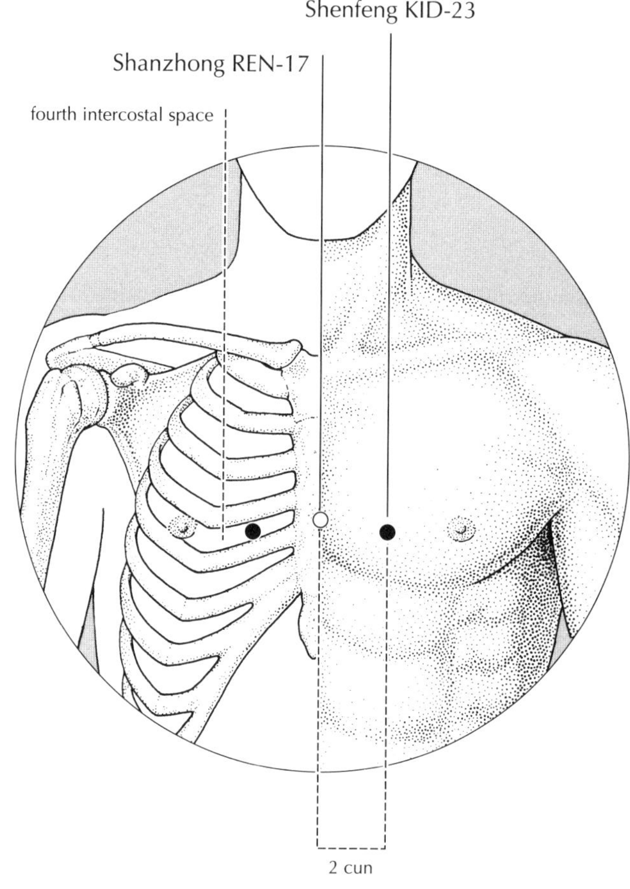

ACTIONS

Unbinds the chest

Lowers rebellious Lung and Stomach qi

Benefits the breasts

INDICATIONS

- Fullness of the chest and lateral costal region with difficulty in breathing, cough, asthma, wheezing, chest painful obstruction, breast abscess.
- Vomiting, no pleasure in eating.

COMBINATIONS

- Breast abscess, chills and fever with shortness of breath, restless sleep: Shenfeng KID-23 and Yingchuang ST-16 (*Supplementing Life*).

LINGXU KID-24

Spirit Ruin

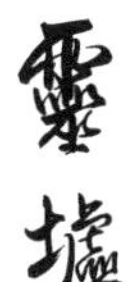

LOCATION

In the third intercostal space, 2 cun lateral to the midline.

LOCATION NOTE

i. First locate the second intercostal space (see Shencang KID-25), then find the third intercostal space, one space below it; ii. Note that in males the nipple lies in the fourth intercostal space; iii. The 2 cun line is located midway between the midline and the mamillary line.

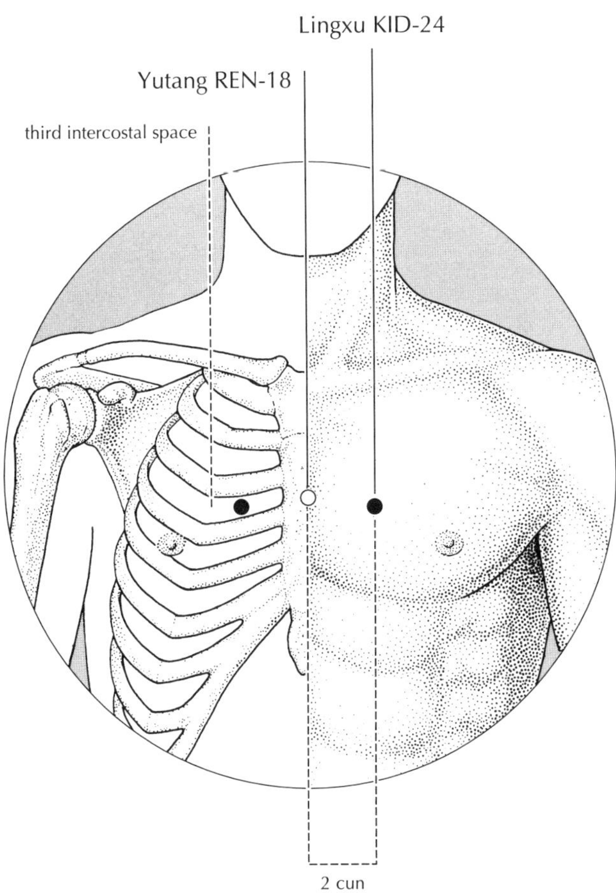

NEEDLING

Transverse-oblique insertion, directed laterally along the intercostal space 0.5 to 1 cun.

Caution: deep perpendicular or oblique needling may puncture the lung.

ACTIONS

Unbinds the chest
Lowers rebellious Lung and Stomach qi
Benefits the breasts

INDICATIONS

- Cough, asthma, wheezing, distention and pain of the chest and lateral costal region with difficulty in breathing, vomiting, inability to eat or drink, no pleasure in eating.
- Breast abscess, palpitations, agitation and fullness.

COMBINATIONS

- Vomiting with fullness of the chest: Lingxu KID-24, Shufu KID-27, Shencang KID-25 and Juque REN-14 (*Thousand Ducat Formulas*).

SHENCANG KID-25

Spirit Storehouse

神藏

LOCATION

In the second intercostal space, 2 cun lateral to the midline.

LOCATION NOTE

i. First locate the costal cartilage of the second rib which is level with the sternal angle, then locate the second intercostal space below it, ii. Note that in males the nipple lies in the fourth intercostal space; iii. The 2 cun line is located midway between the midline and the mamillary line.

NEEDLING

Transverse-oblique insertion, directed laterally along the intercostal space 0.5 to 1 cun.

Caution: deep perpendicular or oblique needling may puncture the lung.

Shencang KID-25
Zigong REN-19
second intercostal space
2 cun

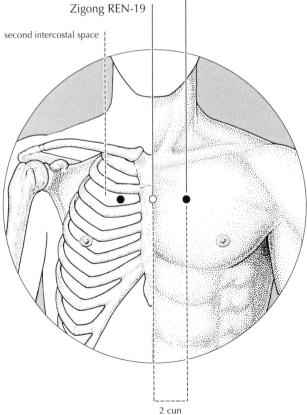

ACTIONS

Unbinds the chest
Lowers rebellious Lung and Stomach qi

INDICATIONS

- Cough, asthma, wheezing, dyspnoea, pain and oppression of the chest, fullness and distention of the chest and lateral costal region.
- Vomiting, agitation and fullness, fullness of the chest with no desire to eat.

COMBINATIONS

- Fullness of the chest with stiffness of the neck: Shencang KID-25 and Xuanji REN-21 (*One Hundred Symptoms*).
- Vomiting with fullness of the chest: Shencang KID-25, Shufu KID-27, Lingxu KID-24 and Juque REN-14 (*Thousand Ducat Formulas*).

YUZHONG KID-26

Comfortable Chest

彧中

LOCATION

In the first intercostal space, 2 cun lateral to the midline.

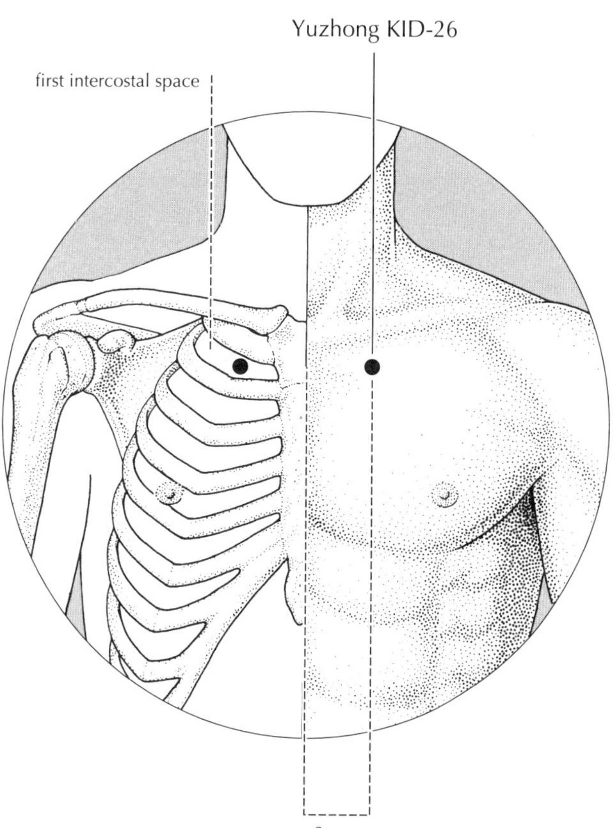

LOCATION NOTE

i. First locate the costal cartilage of the second rib which is level with the sternal angle, then locate the first intercostal space above it; ii. Note that in males the nipple lies in the fourth intercostal space; iii. The 2 cun line is located midway between the midline and the mamillary line.

NEEDLING

Transverse-oblique insertion, directed laterally along the intercostal space 0.5 to 1 cun.
Caution: deep perpendicular or oblique needling may puncture the lung.

ACTIONS

Unbinds the chest and benefits the breasts
Transforms phlegm and lowers rebellious Lung and Stomach qi

INDICATIONS

- Cough, asthma, wheezing, dyspnoea, coughing blood, palpitations, fullness and distention of the chest and lateral costal region.
- Accumulation of phlegm, dyspnoea and cough with inability to eat, vomiting, drooling with much spittle.
- Breast abscess, pityriasis versicolor.

COMBINATIONS

- Drooling with much spittle: Yuzhong KID-26 and Yunmen LU-2 (*Supplementing Life*).

SHUFU KID-27

Shu Mansion

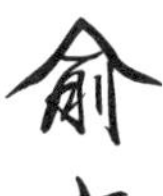
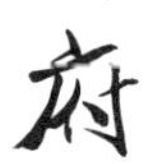

LOCATION

In the depression on the lower border of the clavicle, 2 cun lateral to the midline.

LOCATION NOTE

The 2 cun line is located midway between the midline and the mamillary line.

NEEDLING

Transverse-oblique insertion, directed laterally along the inferior border of the clavicle 0.5 to 1 cun.
Caution: deep perpendicular or oblique needling may puncture the lung.

ACTIONS

Unbinds the chest
Transforms phlegm and alleviates cough and wheezing
Harmonises the Stomach and lowers rebellious qi

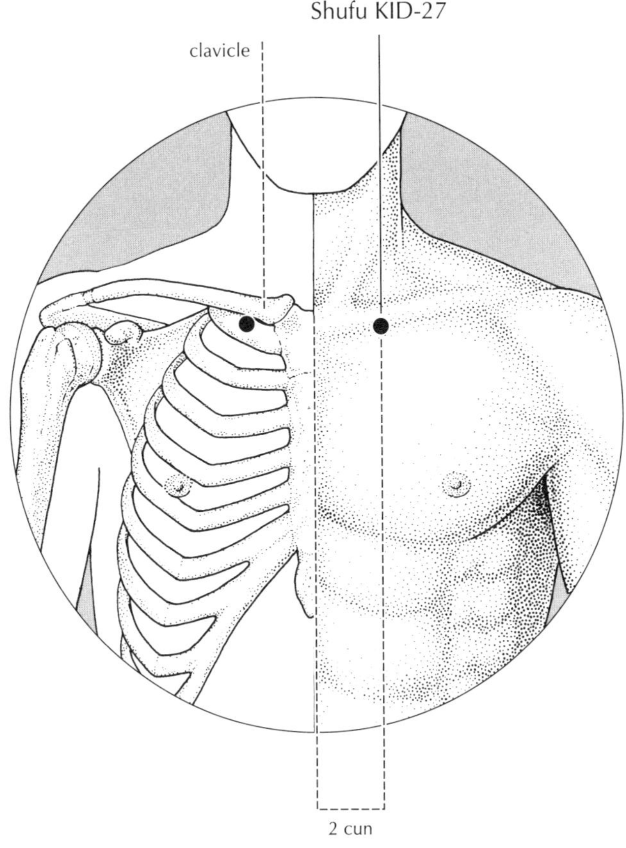

INDICATIONS

- Cough, chronic cough with vomiting of phlegm, wheezing, dyspnoea, chest pain, oppression of the chest with chronic dyspnoea.
- Abdominal distention, nausea, vomiting, inability to eat and drink.
- Reckless movement of hot blood in women, steaming bone disorder.

COMBINATIONS

- Vomiting with fullness of the chest: Shufu KID-27, Lingxu KID-24, Shencang KID-25 and Juque REN-14 (*Thousand Ducat Formulas*).
- Rebellious qi with dyspnoea and inability to catch the breath: Shufu KID-27, Shencang KID-25 and Tianfu LU-3 (*Supplementing Life*).
- Coughing and wheezing with phlegm: Shufu KID-27 and Rugen ST-18 (*Ode of the Jade Dragon*).

NOTES

1 *Essential Questions* Chapter 47.

2 *Classic of Difficulties* 69th Difficulty.

3 The *Ode to Elucidate Mysteries* said "Heaven, earth and man are the three powers. Baihui DU-20 ... echoes Heaven, Xuanji REN-21 ... echoes man and Yongquan KID-1 ... echoes the earth".

4 This story also appears in the *Great Compendium of Acupuncture and Moxibustion* in which the point selected is Naokong GB-19 rather than Yongquan KID-1.

5 *Spiritual Pivot* Chapter 5.

6 *Classic of Difficulties* 68th Difficulty.

7 *Spiritual Pivot* Chapter 33.

8 *Spiritual Pivot* Chapter 17.

9 *Essential Questions* Chapter 5.

10 *Essential Questions* Chapter 5.

11 *Essential Questions* Chapter 9.

12 *Essential Questions* Chapter 47.

13 *Essential Questions* Chapter 47.

14 Tian Gui: i. The essential substance responsible for promoting growth, development and reproductive function as well as the maintenance of the menstrual cycle and pregnancy. It is formed from the combined essence of the parents and slowly develops with constant supplementation from the post-heaven qi; ii. In the *Classic of Categories* tian gui is used as an alternative term for original qi; iii. Occasionally used as an alternative name for menstruation.

15 *Essential Questions* Chapter 1.

16 *Spiritual Pivot* Chapter 21.

17 *Essential Questions* Chapter 47.

18 *Classic of Difficulties* 69th Difficulty.

19 *Spiritual Pivot* Chapter 18.

20 *Fundamentals of Practical Foundations of Chinese Medicine* by Li De Xin, Liaoning Science and Technology Publications, p. 127.

21 *Spiritual Pivot* Chapter 44.

22 *Essential Questions* Chapter 47.

23 *Master Hua's Classic of the Central Viscera* (Zhong Zang Jing) attributed to Hua Tuo, translated by Yang Shou-zhong, Blue Poppy Press.

24 *Classic of Difficulties* 29th Difficulty.

25 *The Heart & Essence of Dan-xi's Methods of Treatment*, A Translation of Zhu Dan-xi's Dan Xi Zhi Fa Xin Yao, Blue Poppy Press, p. 245.

26 *Classic of Difficulties* 56th Difficulty.

27 *Classic of Difficulties* 29th Difficulty.

28 *Classic of Difficulties* 29th Difficulty.

手厥陰心包經

THE PERICARDIUM CHANNEL OF HAND JUEYIN

THE PERICARDIUM CHANNEL OF HAND JUEYIN

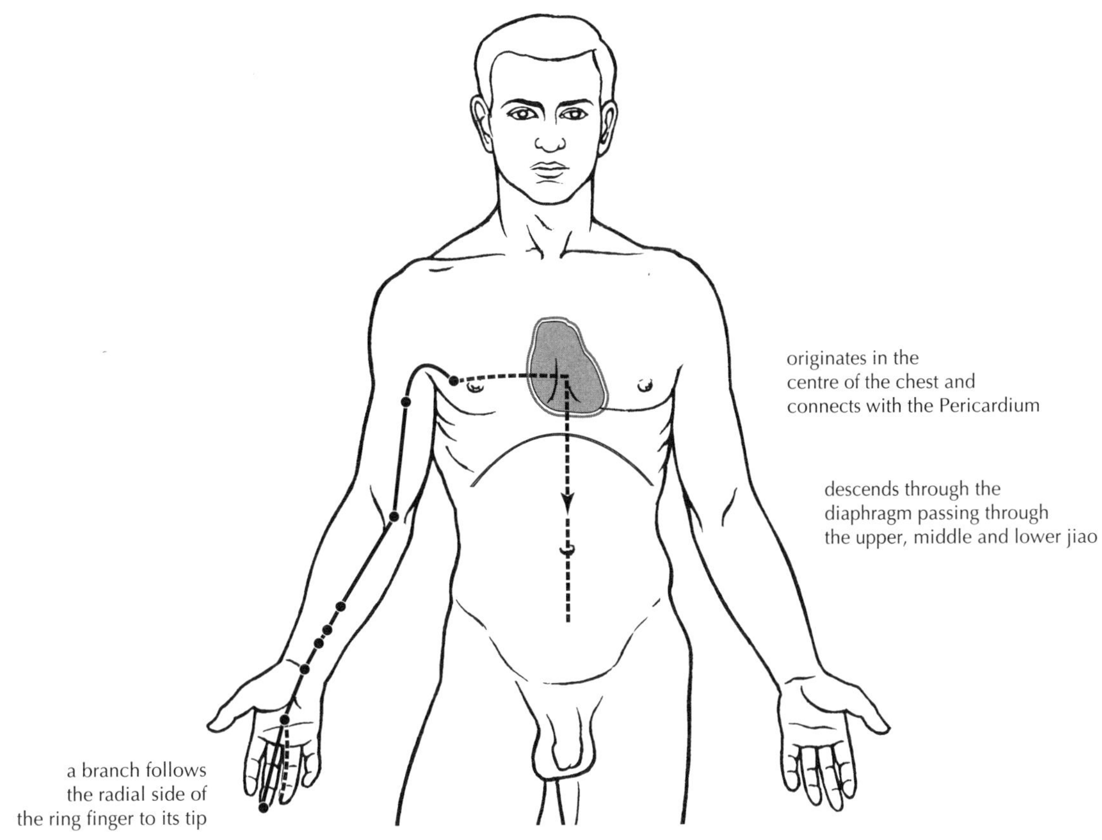

The Pericardium primary channel

THE PERICARDIUM PRIMARY CHANNEL

- originates in the centre of the chest, connects with the Pericardium, and descends through the diaphragm to the abdomen, passing through the upper, middle and lower jiao.

One branch

- runs from inside the chest to emerge in the costal region 3 cun inferior to the anterior axillary fold (near Tianchi P-1),
- arches over the axilla, and follows along the antero-medial aspect of the upper arm, between the Lung and Heart channels to the cubital fossa of the elbow at Quze P-3,
- descends the forearm between the tendons of the palmaris longus and flexor carpi radialis muscles to reach the palm at Laogong P-8,
- travels from the palm along the middle finger to terminate at its tip at Zhongchong P-9.

Another branch

- arises from the palm at Laogong P-8 and follows the radial aspect of the ring finger to its tip .

The Pericardium primary channel connects with the following zangfu: Sanjiao.

The Pericardium primary channel meets with other channels at the following points: None

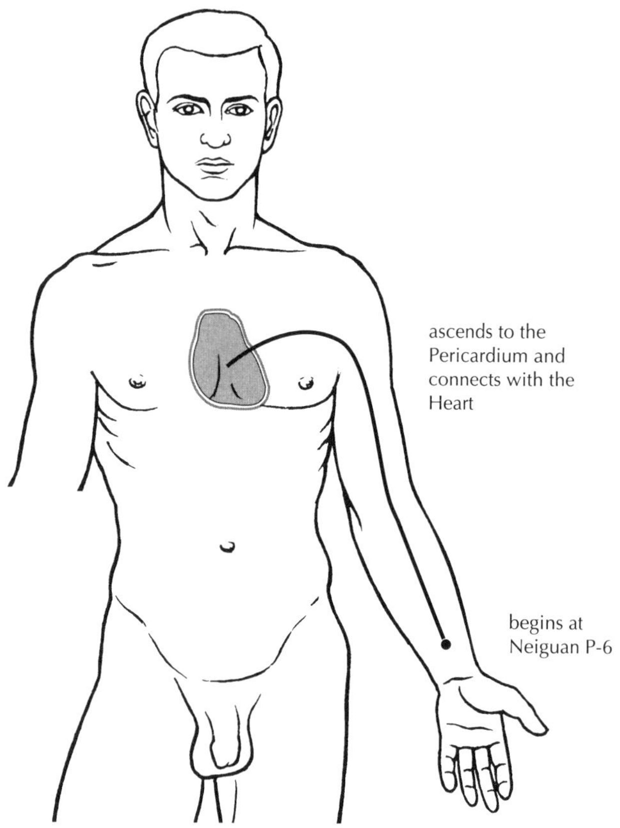

The Pericardium luo-connecting channel

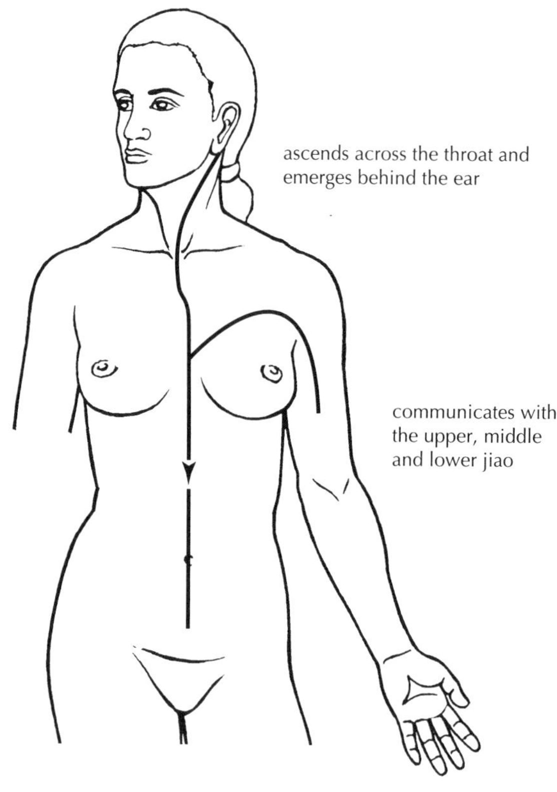

The Pericardium divergent channel

THE PERICARDIUM LUO-CONNECTING CHANNEL

- begins at Neiguan P-6 on the anterior of the forearm,
- ascends along with the Pericardium primary channel to the Pericardium and then connects with the Heart.

THE PERICARDIUM DIVERGENT CHANNEL

- separates from the primary channel on the arm, at the level of a point below the axilla and 3 cun inferior to Yuanye GB-22,
- enters the chest and communicates with the three jiao,
- a branch ascends across the throat and emerges behind the ear to converge with the Sanjiao channel.

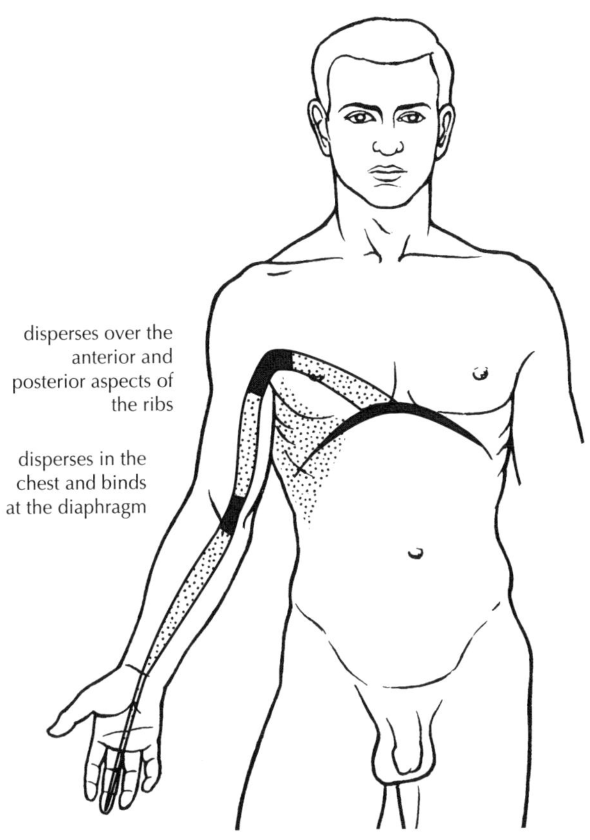

The Pericardium sinew channel

THE PERICARDIUM SINEW CHANNEL

- originates at the tip of the middle finger and runs together with the Lung sinew channel to bind at the medial side of the elbow,
- follows the antero-medial side of the upper arm to below the axilla where it binds before descending to disperse over the anterior and posterior aspects of the ribs,
- a branch enters the chest below the axilla, dispersing in the chest and binding at the diaphragm.

Pathological symptoms of the Pericardium sinew channel
Strained and cramping sensation along the course of the channel, pain of the chest with urgent breathing and an 'inverted cup sensation' below the lower right ribs.

DISCUSSION

The Pericardium channel of hand jueyin originates in the chest and descends through the diaphragm to the middle and lower jiao. It is interiorly-exteriorly coupled with the Sanjiao channel, and with the Liver channel of foot jueyin according to six channel theory. The Pericardium-Sanjiao relationship is strengthened by the fact that:

- a branch of the Pericardium channel separates from Laogong P-8 in the palm of the hand and connects with Guanchong SJ-1 on the ring finger.
- the Pericardium divergent channel connects with the Sanjiao channel behind the ear.
- as far as the Pericardium luo-connecting channel is concerned, in the *Spiritual Pivot* at least there is no reference to it connecting with the Sanjiao channel.

In addition, it is important to note that:

- from Neiguan P-6, the luo-connecting channel travels to the Heart, strengthening the Pericardium-Heart relationship.
- the Pericardium primary channel originates in the chest, its divergent channel enters the chest, and its sinew channel disperses in the chest.
- the primary channel descends through the diaphragm and the sinew channel binds at the diaphragm.
- both the primary and divergent channels connect with the upper, middle and lower jiao.
- the primary channel arches over the axilla and the sinew channel travels inferior to the axilla.
- the sinew channel disperses over the anterior and posterior ribs.

The Pericardium (xin bao/Heart wrapping) is described in Chinese medicine as a membrane surrounding the Heart, and its primary function is to protect the Heart (the Emperor) from attack by exterior pathogenic factors. In the *Yellow Emperor's Inner Classic*, the Pericardium was not accorded independent status as one of the zangfu, and this has been reflected in the Chinese medical tradition ever since in discussion of the 'five zang and six fu'. Although not considered a discrete zang, but rather an appendage of the Heart, the Pericardium channel paradoxically was originally considered the primary channel to treat Heart disorders. Thus in the *Spiritual Pivot*[1] the Yellow Emperor asks Qi Bo "Why does the hand shaoyin channel alone have no shu points"? Qi Bo replies "The shaoyin is the Heart vessel. The Heart is the great master of the five zang and six fu and is the abode of the essence-spirit. It stores so firmly that no pathogen can come to reside. If it does, then the Heart will be injured and the spirit will depart. If the spirit departs there is death. It is for this reason that the pathogens destined to attack the Heart will attack the Pericardium. The Pericardium is the channel that is controlled by the Heart. Therefore the Heart alone has no shu points". In Chapter 2 of the *Spiritual Pivot* Qi Bo describes the Heart channel (rather than the Pericardium channel) as originating at Zhongchong P-9 and travelling to Laogong P-8, Daling P-7 etc. as far as Quze P-3. The *Spiritual Pivot* elsewhere, however, does discuss points of the Heart channel, for example Shenmen HE-7 for Heart disorders, reflecting some of the contradictions inherent in a text written by different authors at different times. It was not until the *Systematic Classic of Acupuncture and Moxibustion*, written in the third century, that the shu points of the Heart channel were first discussed.

In the theory of differentiation of patterns according to the zangfu, the Pericardium has no patterns of disharmony of its own. The only discussion of Pericardium disorders per se follows on from its function as the wrapping or protector of the Heart, and the disturbance of consciousness manifesting as mental confusion and even coma that occurs during the course of febrile diseases is ascribed to the Pericardium rather than to the Heart.

The Pericardium channel pathways, as well as the status of the Pericardium as the protector of the Heart, help explain most of the actions and indications of the points of the Pericardium channel. These can be summarised as:

- treating disorders of the Heart zang such as pain, palpitations, irregular Heart rhythm etc.
- treating disorders of the spirit.
- treating disorders of the chest in general, including disharmony of the Lung.
- treating disorders of the upper or middle jiao due to stagnation of the qi of the foot jueyin Liver channel with which the Pericardium channel is paired according to six channel theory.
- treating disorders of the middle jiao, especially the Stomach.
- treating disorders of the lateral costal region (the Pericardium sinew channel disperses over the anterior and posterior ribs).
- treating febrile diseases: the Pericardium belongs to fire, and takes the brunt of attack by exterior pathogens that might otherwise injure the Heart; the points of the Pericardium channel, therefore, are important in the treatment of febrile diseases, especially at the nutritive and blood levels and when there is disturbance of consciousness.
- treating swelling and pain of the axilla.

TIANCHI P-1

Heavenly Pool

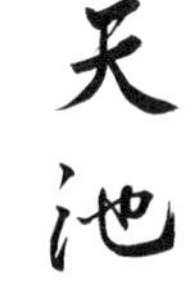

Meeting point of the Pericardium, Gall Bladder, Liver and Sanjiao channels
Point of the Window of Heaven

LOCATION

1 cun lateral and slightly superior to the nipple, in the 4th intercostal space.

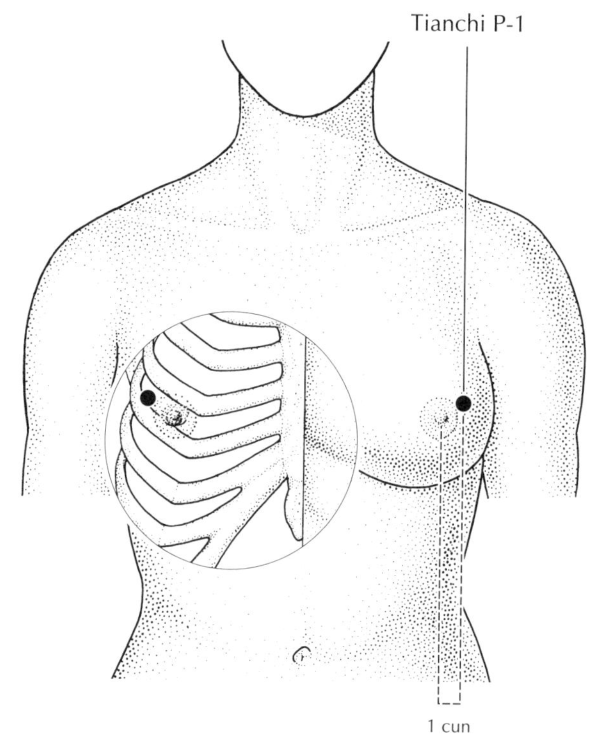

LOCATION NOTE

The level of the fourth intercostal space at this point is more or less the same as that of the fourth intercostal space at its junction with the sternum.

NEEDLING

Transverse-oblique insertion posteriorly along the intercostal space, 0.5 to 1 cun.
Caution: deep needling carries a substantial risk of causing a pneumothorax.

ACTIONS

Unbinds the chest, transforms phlegm and descends rebellion
Regulates qi and dissipates nodules
Benefits the breasts

INDICATIONS

- Cough with copious phlegm, rattling sound in the chest and throat, fullness of the chest, agitation of the chest and diaphragm, shortness of breath, uprising qi, pain of the lateral costal region.
- Swelling and pain of the axilla, scrofula of the neck, breast diseases, breast abscess, insufficient lactation.
- Headache, blurred vision, malaria, fever with absence of sweating, inability to raise the four limbs, pain of the arm.

COMMENTARY

Tianchi P-1 is one of ten points listed in Chapter 2 of the *Spiritual Pivot* that have come to be known as Window of Heaven points. With the exception of Tianchi P-1 and Tianfu LU-3, all are located in the neck region. In common with other points from this group, Tianchi P-1 is indicated for various manifestations of inversion qi (chaotic and rebellious qi), in this case affecting the Lung (uprising qi, cough etc.), head (headache), sense organs (blurred vision) and neck region (scrofula). For a fuller discussion of this point grouping see page 48.

Tianchi P-1 is almost exclusively indicated for excess patterns. Because of its location it is used for disorders of the chest and lateral costal region, especially those characterised by stagnant qi and phlegm. When qi and phlegm stagnate in the chest there is cough with copious sputum, fullness of the chest, agitation of the chest and diaphragm etc. When qi stagnates in the lateral costal region there is pain. When qi and phlegm stagnate in the channels (the Pericardium primary channel arches over the axilla and the sinew channel travels inferior to the axilla) there is axillary swelling and scrofula. Although not classically indicated for breast disorders, modern indications for Tianchi P-1 include breast abscess and insufficient lactation. Both these disorders may be due to stagnation of qi and consequent stagnant heat.

COMBINATIONS

- Swelling of the axilla: Tianchi P-1 and Weiyang BL-39 (*One Hundred Symptoms*).
- Swelling of the axilla: Tianchi P-1, Weiyang BL-39, Shenmai BL-62, Diwuhui GB-42, Yangfu GB-38 and Zulinqi GB-41 (*Thousand Ducat Formulas*).
- Scrofula: Tianchi P-1, Shaohai HE-3, Zhangmen LIV-13, Zulinqi GB-41, Zhigou SJ-6, Yangfu GB-38, Jianjing GB-21 and Shousanli L.I.-10 (*Great Compendium*).
- Rebellious qi cough: Tianchi P-1, Tiantu REN-22, Shanzhong REN-17, Jiexi ST-41 and Jianzhongshu SI-15 (*Supplementing Life*).

TIANQUAN P-2

Heavenly Spring

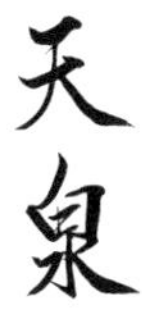

LOCATION

On the anterior aspect of the arm, 2 cun below the anterior axillary fold, between the two heads of the biceps brachii muscle.

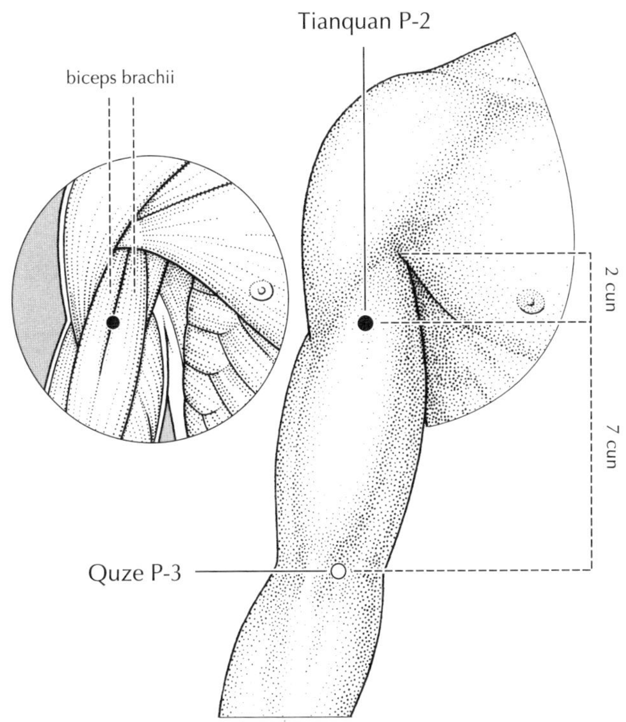

NEEDLING

Oblique insertion distally or proximally along the line of the channel, 1 to 1.5 cun.

ACTIONS

Unbinds the chest, invigorates blood and alleviates pain

INDICATIONS

- Heart pain, disorders of the Heart, pain of the chest, back, shoulder, shoulder blade and arm, fullness of the chest and lateral costal region, palpitations, cough, stone oedema.
- Aversion to wind and cold, blurred vision, pain of the medial aspect of the upper arm.

COMBINATIONS

- Heart pain radiating to the shoulder and arm: Tianquan P-2, Ximen P-4, Neiguan P-6 and Shanzhong REN-17.

QUZE P-3

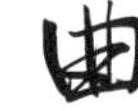

Marsh at the Crook

He-Sea and Water point of the Pericardium channel

LOCATION

On the transverse cubital crease, in the depression immediately to the ulnar side of the aponeurosis of the biceps brachii muscle.

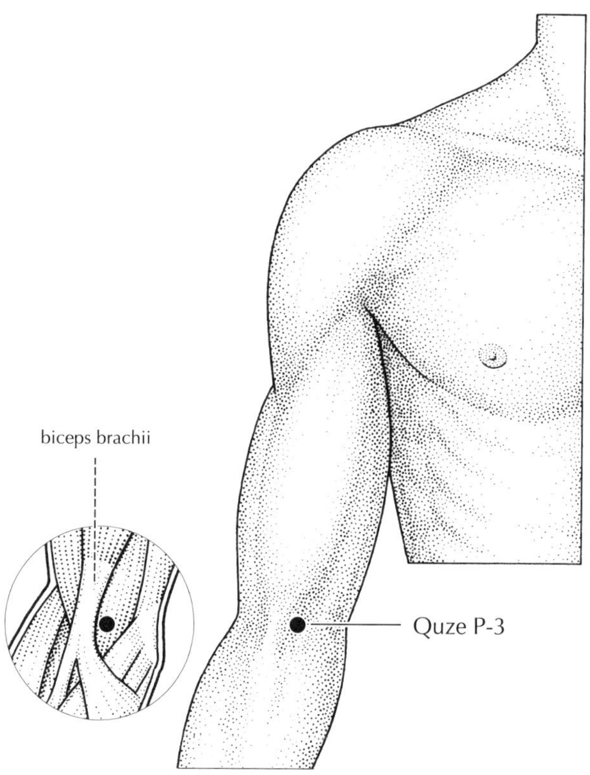

LOCATION NOTE

This point should be located and needled with the elbow slightly bent.

NEEDLING

Perpendicular insertion 0.5 to 1 cun, or prick to bleed. **Caution:** the brachial artery and veins lie deeply, just medial to this point.

ACTIONS

Clears heat from the qi, nutritive and blood levels
Harmonises the Stomach and intestines and stops vomiting
Activates the channel and alleviates pain

INDICATIONS

- Febrile disease, agitation and restlessness, agitation with thirst, dry mouth, dry tongue with pain of the lateral costal region, coughing blood, vomiting blood, summer-heat stroke.
- Vomiting, diarrhoea, dysenteric disorder, sudden turmoil disorder.
- Heart pain, palpitations, pounding sensation below the Heart, propensity to fright, counterflow qi, dyspnoea and cough, wind rash.
- Tremor of the head, tremor of the hand and arm, pain and contraction of the elbow and arm, paralysis of the upper limb.

COMMENTARY

In the 3rd century CE, the *Treatise on Injury by Cold* by Zhang Zhong-jing classified fevers according to their progression through the six channels (taiyang, yangming, shaoyang, taiyin, shaoyin and jueyin). This theory, according to which pathogenic cold attacked and penetrated the body via the skin, dominated Chinese medicine until the early 17th century when the 'wen bing' or 'warm disease' theory was developed (predominantly by Wu You-he, Ye Tian-shi and Wu Ju-tong). The warm disease school placed the emphasis on febrile diseases due to injury by heat which penetrates the body via the nose and mouth, and classified fevers according to four levels of depth: the defensive level (wei), the qi level (qi), the nutritive level (ying) and the blood level (xue). The defensive and qi levels correspond broadly to the taiyang and yangming stages respectively of the *Treatise on Injury by Cold*. When pathogenic heat penetrates further to the deeper levels of the body, it first enters the nutritive level, scorching the body fluids and the yin and disturbing the Pericardium and spirit, and then enters the blood level, giving rise to reckless bleeding. Quze P-3, the water point of the Pericardium fire channel, clears heat and may be needled or bled for heat at the qi level giving rise to high fever, agitation, thirst etc., or for heat which has reached the nutritive and blood levels giving rise to agitation and restlessness, dry mouth and haemorrhage from the Lung and Stomach.

According to the *Classic of Difficulties*[2] the he-sea points treat 'counterflow qi and diarrhoea', whilst the *Spiritual Pivot*[3] says "in disorders of the Stomach and in disorders resulting from irregular eating and drinking, select the he-sea point". These theories are clearly illustrated by Quze P-3 which has the functions of harmonising the Stomach and intestines and stopping vomiting and diarrhoea, especially when these are acute and due to pathogenic heat. It is also worth noting that the interior pathway of the Pericardium channel descends through the diaphragm to the lower abdomen, connecting the upper, middle and lower jiao, which helps to explain the powerful action of this point on these disorders. The dual action of Quze P-3 in harmonising the Stomach and intestines and clearing pathogenic heat, makes it particularly suitable for treating diseases due to summer-heat (heatstroke or sunstroke) characterised by fever, sweating, vomiting and diarrhoea.

According to the *Spiritual Pivot*[4] "jueyin channel is abundant in blood and limited in qi ... [it is thus suitable to] prick to bleed jueyin and drain blood ...". This theory explains the effect of bleeding Quze P-3 on reducing heat in the blood in cases of febrile haemorrhage. Interestingly, one of the two other channels "abundant in blood and limited in qi" according to this passage in the *Spiritual Pivot* is the taiyang channel, and this may help to explain certain similarities between Quze P-3 (the he-sea point of the Pericardium jueyin channel located at the flexure of the elbow) and Weizhong BL-40 (the he-sea point of the Bladder taiyang channel located at the flexure of the knee). Both points may be pricked to bleed to clear heat from the blood level, and are used in the treatment of summer-heat stroke and sudden turmoil disorder with heat of the four limbs, ceaseless thirst, vomiting and diarrhoea.

Finally, Quze P-3 is also widely used for disorders of the Pericardium channel such as pain of the elbow, arm and hand. It is indicated for tremor of the head, and like its close neighbour Shaohai HE-3, for tremor of the hand and arm.

COMBINATIONS

- Vomiting blood: Quze P-3, Shenmen HE-7 and Yuji LU-10 (*Great Compendium*).
- Spitting blood: Quze P-3, Kongzui LU-6 and Feishu BL-13 (*Supplementing Life*).
- Pounding sensation below the Heart and propensity to fright: Quze P-3 and Daling P-7 (*Thousand Ducat Formulas*).
- Pain of the Heart and chest: Quze P-3, Neiguan P-6 and Daling P-7 (*Great Compendium*).
- Heart pain: Quze P-3, Ximen P-4 and Daling P-7 (*Thousand Ducat Formulas*).
- Dry mouth: Quze P-3 and Zhangmen LIV-13 (*Thousand Ducat Formulas*).
- Thirst from blood deficiency: Quze P-3 and Shaoshang LU-11 (*One Hundred Symptoms*).
- Absence of sweating: Quze P-3, Fuliu KID-7, Yuji LU-10, Shaoze SI-1, Shangxing DU-23, Ququan LIV-8, Kunlun BL-60, Xiaxi GB-43 and Zuqiaoyin GB-44 (*Great Compendium*).

XIMEN P-4

Xi-Cleft Gate

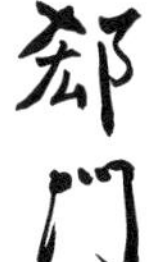

Xi-Cleft point of the Pericardium channel

LOCATION

On the flexor aspect of the forearm, 5 cun proximal to Daling P-7, on the line connecting Daling P-7 and Quze P-3, between the tendons of palmaris longus and flexor carpi radialis.

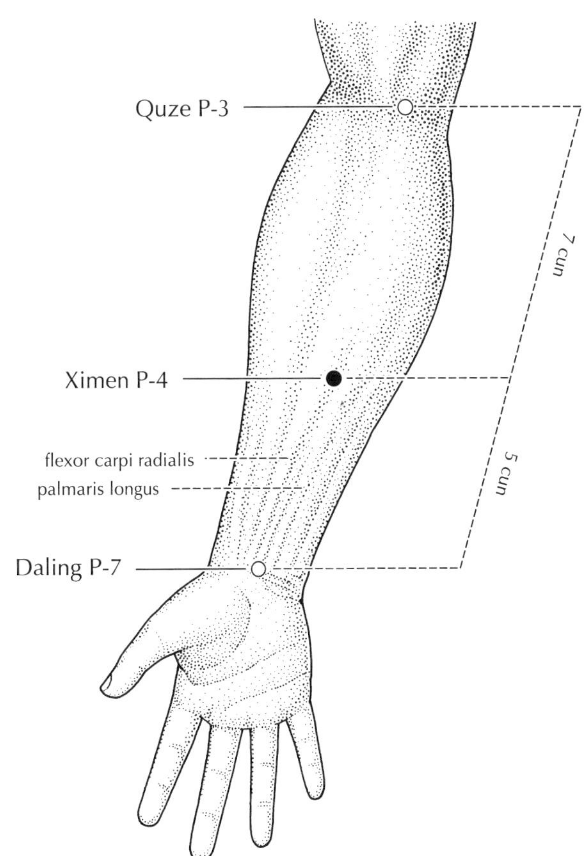

LOCATION NOTE

i. In the absence of the tendon of palmaris longus, locate this point on the ulnar side of the tendon of flexor carpi radialis; ii. Divide the distance between the cubital crease and Daling P-7 into half and locate this point 1 cun distal to this midpoint.

NEEDLING

Perpendicular insertion, 0.5 to 1 cun or oblique proximal insertion 1 to 1.5 cun.

ACTIONS

Invigorates blood and dispels stasis
Cools blood and stops bleeding
Calms the spirit
Moderates acute conditions

INDICATIONS

- Chest pain, Heart pain, Heart pain with vomiting, vomiting blood, coughing blood, nosebleed, five palms agitated and hot.
- Agitation, insomnia, melancholy, fear and fright of people, insufficiency of spirit qi, epilepsy.
- Chronic malaria, chronic haemorrhoids.

COMMENTARY

Ximen P-4 is the xi-cleft point of the Pericardium channel. The xi-cleft points are where the qi and blood, which flow relatively superficially along the channels from the jing-well points, gather and plunge more deeply. The xi-cleft points in general are indicated in the treatment of acute conditions and pain, whilst the xi-cleft points of the yin channels have an additional action of treating disorders of blood. Ximen P-4 is an important point to treat both acute stasis of blood and heat in the blood.

Through its dual actions of invigorating blood and moderating acute conditions, Ximen P-4 is a primary point for treating stagnation of blood in the chest and Heart, giving rise to acute pain which may radiate to the neck, back or left arm, or be accompanied by vomiting. Its important role in the treatment of Heart pain was both emphasised in the classics and is borne out by modern clinical practice and research.

By virtue of its ability to clear heat from the blood and stop bleeding, Ximen P-4 is indicated for hot reckless bleeding in the upper jiao giving rise to nosebleed, and vomiting or coughing of blood.

The second principal group of indications for Ximen P-4 includes a variety of mental and emotional disorders such as agitation of the Heart, insomnia, melancholy, and fear and fright of people. The relationship between Ximen P-4 and emotional disorders is expressed through its effect on the blood and the Heart qi. The Heart rules the blood and houses the spirit, and there is therefore a reciprocal relationship between blood and disturbance of the spirit. On the one hand when the blood is stagnant and does not flow freely, essential nourishment will not reach the Heart and the Heart's function of housing the spirit may be disrupted. On the other hand, emotional disturbance may lead to stagnation of blood. The *Spiritual Pivot*[5] states "... Internally a person may be injured by worry and anger; when this occurs the qi will rebel upwards; when the qi rebels thus the six shu [points of the six channels] will not flow, the warm qi will not circulate and internally the congealed blood will coagulate and not scatter ...". By resolving stasis of blood Ximen P-4 is able both to treat emotional disharmony and to resolve the Heart blood stasis that results from it.

Blood stasis in the Heart most commonly occurs as a result of deficiency of Heart qi and yang. These patterns frequently give rise to feelings of fear, melancholy and a diminished spirit, typically seen in patients after a myocardial infarct or cardiac surgery (the shock of which may further injure the Heart qi). Ximen P-4 is able to regulate the Heart qi, as well as the blood, and is classically indicated for insufficiency of the spirit qi.

Finally there may be symptoms of mental and emotional agitation, as well as haemorrhage, when heat enters the nutritive or blood levels during febrile disease and rises to disturb the spirit. Thus the *Treatise on Epidemic Warm Febrile Disease* stated "When the nutritive system is invaded by heat, the blood is consumed, the spirit is disturbed and there is insomnia". Ximen P-4 is able to calm the spirit in such cases by clearing heat from the nutritive and blood levels.

COMBINATIONS

- Heart pain: Ximen P-4, Quze P-3 and Daling P-7 (*Thousand Ducat Formulas*).
- Heart pain with retching, agitation and fullness: Ximen P-4 and Jiquan HE-1 (*Supplementing Life*).
- Coughing blood: Ximen P-4 and Daling P-7 (*Systematic Classic*).
- Fright and fear of people, spirit qi insufficient: Ximen P-4 and Dazhong KID-4 (*Thousand Ducat Formulas*).
- Pain of the chest and lateral costal region: Ximen P-4, Dabao SP-21, Sanyangluo SJ-8, Yangfu GB-38 and Zulinqi GB-41.

JIANSHI P-5

Intermediate Messenger

間使

Jing-River and Metal point of the Pericardium channel

LOCATION

On the flexor aspect of the forearm, 3 cun proximal to Daling P-7, between the tendons of palmaris longus and flexor carpi radialis.

LOCATION NOTE

i. In the absence of the tendon of palmaris longus, locate this point on the ulnar side of the tendon of flexor carpi radialis; ii. Divide the distance between the cubital crease and Daling P-7 into quarters and locate this point at the junction of the proximal three quarters and the distal quarter.

NEEDLING

Perpendicular insertion, 0.5 to 1 cun or oblique proximal insertion 1 to 1.5 cun.

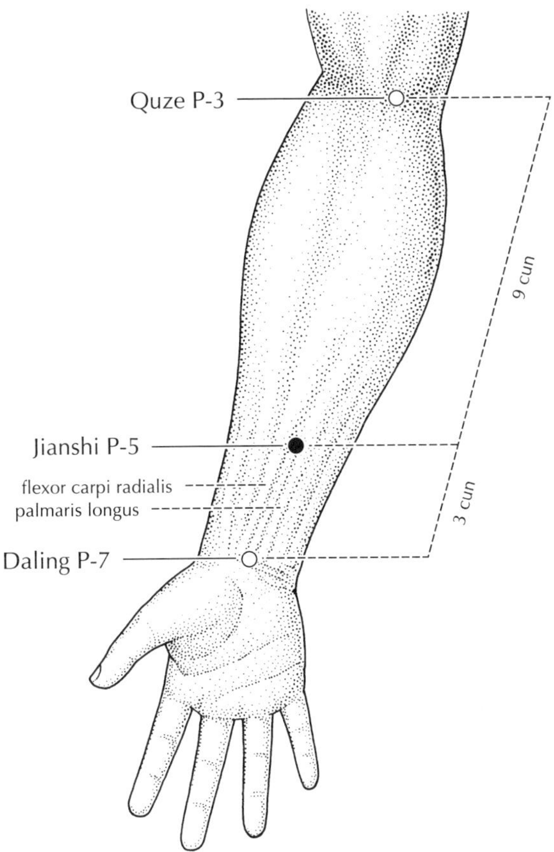

ACTIONS

Transforms phlegm
Settles and calms the spirit
Descends rebellious qi and regulates the Stomach
Regulates menstruation

INDICATIONS

- Sudden Heart pain, palpitations, oppression of the chest, apprehension, propensity to fright, epilepsy, mania, agitation and restlessness, poor memory, loss of voice, halting speech, sudden mania, manic raving as if seeing ghosts, sudden fright disorder in children, ghost evil.
- Plumstone qi (globus hystericus), goitre, scrofula of the neck, drooling following windstroke, obstruction of qi following windstroke leading to impaired breathing.
- Epigastric pain, vomiting, retching, nausea, vomiting and spitting of blood, vomiting of foam, sudden turmoil disorder, abdominal pain, clonic spasm.
- Aversion to wind and cold, febrile disease, malaria, red face and yellow eyes.
- Irregular menstruation, dysmenorrhoea, diseases of menstruation, clotted menstrual flow, leucorrhoea, retention of lochia, painful urinary dysfunction, urethral pain.
- Swelling of the axilla, pain of the inner aspect of the elbow and arm, heat of the palms, weakness of the wrist.

COMMENTARY

The key action of Jianshi P-5 is to transform phlegm in the upper jiao, and predominantly in the Heart. Together with Fenglong ST-40 it is one of the two main acupuncture points to treat phlegm disorders. Phlegm obstructing the Heart may arise in one of the following ways: i. excess of any of the seven emotions results in stagnation of qi which hinders the smooth circulation of body fluids, and by transforming into fire, further condenses the stagnant body fluids to form phlegm; ii. stagnation of Liver qi impairs the Spleen's function of transforming and transporting fluids which form phlegm and rise with stagnant qi to disturb the Heart; iii. high fever condenses the body fluids into phlegm, in which case Chinese medicine convention ascribes the disorder to the Pericardium; iv. fright generates phlegm, a concept expounded by Gong Juzhong in *A Spot of Snow on a Red Hot Stove*[6] "Phlegm is produced by fright. The spirit leaves its residence, and when the residence is empty, the fluids will form phlegm".

When phlegm or phlegm-fire obstruct and agitate the portals of the Heart, the spirit will be disturbed to varying degrees. There may be milder symptoms such as agitation, apprehension, propensity to fright, poor memory, restlessness and being easily startled, or more severe symptoms such as mania, manic raving, epilepsy and what was known as 'ghost evil', a disorder probably attributed to demonic possession. Jianshi P-5 also treats phlegm manifestations such as drooling following windstroke, vomiting of foam, swelling of the axilla, goitre, scrofula, and plumstone qi (globus hystericus), a form of stagnation and obstruction by qi and phlegm characterised by a sensation of throat blockage which worsens or ameliorates according to fluctuations in the emotional state. The importance of Jianshi P-5 in the treatment of mania disorder and epilepsy is reflected by the fact that Sun Si-miao's *Supplement to the Thousand Ducat Formulas* suggested that this point was Guilu (one of the thirteen ghost points), rather than Shenmai BL-62 which was said to correspond to Guilu in the *Thousand Ducat Formulas*.

The Pericardium channel and its interiorly-exteriorly related Sanjiao channel both connect with the upper, middle and lower jiao. The action of Jianshi P-5, therefore, is not confined to the upper jiao. In the middle jiao, like Neiguan P-6, it regulates the function of the Stomach and promotes its descending function, being indicated when Stomach qi stagnates giving rise to pain, and when Stomach qi rebels upwards giving rise to vomiting and nausea. Its ability to regulate the Stomach is considered less powerful than that of Neiguan P-6, but it may be used when nausea and vomiting is due to retention of phlegm in the middle jiao. Jianshi P-5 is also indicated for sudden turmoil disorder characterised by acute vomiting and diarrhoea.

According to the *Essential Questions*[7] "The bao mai (uterine channel) pertains to the Heart and is connected with the uterus". Jianshi P-5 is one of the few points of either the Heart or Pericardium channels that has an action on gynaecological disorders, being indicated for irregular menstruation, dysmenorrhoea, clotted menstrual flow, retention of the lochia and leucorrhoea. Its action on the lower jiao also extends to the treatment of painful urinary dysfunction and urethral pain.

Finally, according to the *Spiritual Pivot*[8] the jing-river points are indicated for 'changes in the patient's voice' and Jianshi P-5 is indicated for halting speech and loss of voice.

COMBINATIONS

- Sudden mania: Jianshi P-5, Hegu L.I.-4 and Houxi SI-3 (*Great Compendium*).
- Mania: Jianshi P-5, Baihui DU-20, Fuliu KID-7, Yingu KID-10 and Zusanli ST-36 (*Illustrated Supplement*).
- Epilepsy: Jianshi P-5 and Renzhong DU-26 (*Ode of Spiritual Brightness*).
- Excessive fright: Jianshi P-5, Yinxi HE-6, Erjian L.I.-2 and Lidui ST-45 (*Supplementing Life*).
- Obstruction of the throat: Jianshi P-5 and Sanjian L.I.-3 (*Great Compendium*).
- Swelling of the face and abdomen: Jianshi P-5, Zhongfu LU-1 and Hegu L.I.-4 (*Thousand Ducat Formulas*).
- Red and white leucorrhoea: Jianshi P-5, Baihuanshu BL-30, Daimai GB-26, Guanyuan REN-4, Qihai REN 6 and Sanyinjiao SP-6 (*Great Compendium*).
- The five types of malaria with severe chills and even more severe fever: Jianshi P-5 and Dazhu BL-11 (*Song More Precious Than Jade*).
- Contraction of the elbow: Jianshi P-5, Xiaohai SI-8, Chize LU-5, Jianyu L.I.-15, Daling P-7, Houxi SI-3 and Yuji LU-10 (*Great Compendium*).

LOCATION NOTE

In the absence of the tendon of palmaris longus, locate this point on the ulnar side of the tendon of flexor carpi radialis.

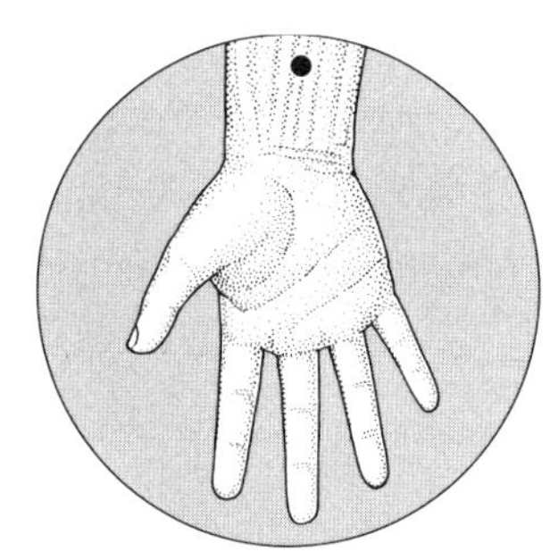

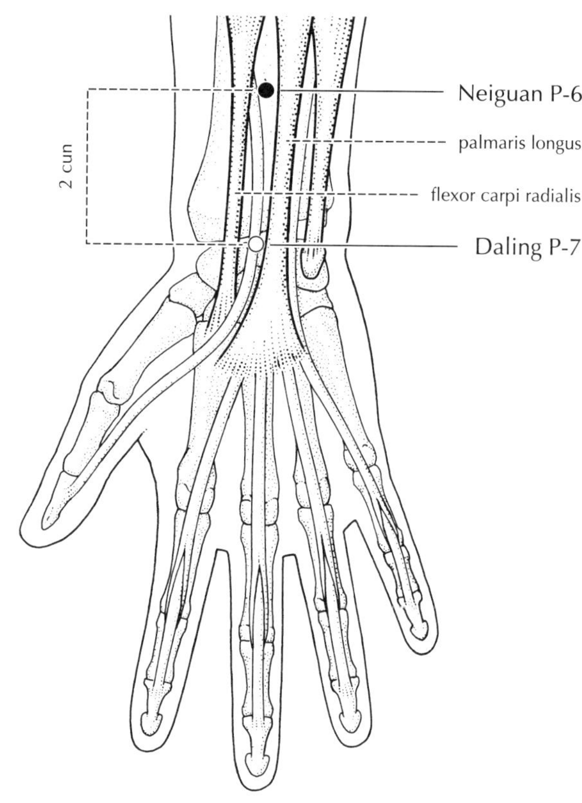

NEIGUAN P-6

Inner Pass

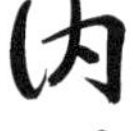

Luo-Connecting point of the Pericardium channel
Confluent point of the Yin Linking vessel

LOCATION

On the flexor aspect of the forearm, 2 cun proximal to Daling P-7, between the tendons of palmaris longus and flexor carpi radialis.

NEEDLING

i. Perpendicular insertion 0.5 to 1 cun, or joined to Waiguan SJ-5; ii. Oblique proximal insertion 1 to 1.5 cun for diseases of the chest; iii. Oblique distal insertion 1 to 1.5 cun for numbness of the fingers.

Caution: the median nerve lies directly under this point and needling commonly induces a significant electric sensation. This is an acceptable manifestation of deqi (arrival of qi), but once elicited, further manipulation is inappropriate and may damage the nerve.

ACTIONS

Unbinds the chest and regulates qi
Regulates the Heart and calms the spirit
Harmonises the Stomach and alleviates nausea and vomiting
Clears heat
Opens the Yin Linking vessel

INDICATIONS

- Heart pain, sudden Heart pain, stuffiness of the chest with agitation of the Heart, palpitations, fright palpitations, pounding sensation of the Heart, disorders of Heart rate and rhythm, pain of the lateral costal region and Heart in women, pain of the lateral costal region, cough, asthma.
- Insomnia, the five types of epilepsy, mania, poor memory, apprehension, fear and fright, sadness, loss of memory following windstroke, inability to speak after windstroke, windstroke, hypertension.
- Nausea, vomiting, hiccup, deficiency and cold of the Spleen and Stomach with incessant vomiting, Spleen and Stomach qi deficiency with distention and fullness, disharmony of the Spleen and Stomach, epigastric pain, stabbing epigastric pain, low-grade abdominal pain, food (ji) masses, blood (jia) masses, focal distention, borborygmus, diarrhoea, blood in the stools, prolapse of the rectum.
- Febrile disease, fever with absence of sweating, headache, stiffness and pain of the head and neck, jaundice, yellow eyes, red eyes, red face with hot skin, malaria, cracked and bleeding tongue, dizziness, post-partum dizziness, irregular menstruation, painful urinary dysfunction.
- Pain and contraction of the elbow and upper arm, swelling of the axilla, stiffness and pain of the head and neck.

COMMENTARY

The Pericardium primary channel originates in the chest, its divergent channel enters the chest, its sinew channel disperses in the chest and over the anterior and posterior ribs and its luo-connecting channel connects with the Heart. Neiguan P-6, a point of the Pericardium channel, is also the confluent point of the Yin Linking vessel which ascends through the chest. According to the *Classic of Difficulties*[9] "When the Yin Linking vessel is diseased, Heart pain will result". In the *Ode of the Obstructed River* the use of Neiguan P-6 is referred to as one of 'the eight therapeutic methods'. In this description of the application of the eight confluent points of the extraordinary vessels to affect specific symptoms and areas of the body, Neiguan P-6 is indicated for disorders of the chest. The *Investigation into Points Along the Channels* by the Ming dynasty author Yan Zhen-shi says "Neiguan P-6 treats all kinds of pain of the zangfu, chest and lateral costal region". Furthermore, Neiguan P-6 was included among the 'six command points' (a grouping derived by later commentators from Gao Wu's 'four command points') for its pre-eminent effect on diseases of the chest and lateral costal region. Neiguan P-6, therefore, has long been considered the single most important distal point for disorders of the chest and it is one of the primary points in acupuncture analgesia for chest surgery. Its range of actions extends not only to the Heart, but also to the Lung.

Pain and stuffiness of the Heart and chest may result from various aetiologies including i. Heart qi and yang deficiency, ii. accumulation of cold, iii. accumulation of phlegm, iv. blood stasis, v. constrained Liver qi, vi. traumatic injury. Whatever the pattern, Neiguan P-6 forms an essential part of any point combination. In the treatment of angina pectoris, however, certain doctors emphasise the use of Ximen P-4 (the xi-cleft point of the Pericardium channel) during acute attacks and Neiguan P-6 during remission. Neiguan P-6 is also effective to treat other disorders of the chest such as asthma and cough, as well as pain in the lateral costal region and hypochondrium. These last two symptoms reflect not only the pathway of the Pericardium sinew channel, but also the relationship of Neiguan P-6 to stagnation of Liver qi, explained by the paired relationship of the Pericardium and Liver jueyin channels. Neiguan P-6, therefore, is especially effective in treating stagnation of Liver qi anywhere in the upper and middle jiao.

The Pericardium is the 'wrapping' of the Heart which stores the spirit, and the Pericardium luo-connecting channel links Neiguan P-6 directly with the Heart. The action of Neiguan P-6 on regulating the Heart zang and calming the spirit emphasises its dual effect on both the physical and emotional aspects of the Heart. It is an important point in the treatment of palpitations, pounding of the Heart and disorders of Heart rhythm, and is also one of the main acupuncture points for regulating and calming the spirit and treating a wide range of emotional disorders whatever the underlying pattern. It is therefore indicated for insomnia, epilepsy, mania, poor memory, loss of memory following windstroke, fright, sadness, fear and apprehension.

The *Investigation into Points Along the Channels*, echoing many other classical texts, states that Neiguan P-6 is indicated "for disharmony of the Stomach and Spleen". The Pericardium primary and divergent channels both descend through the diaphragm to connect with the middle and lower jiao, and this explains the powerful effect of Neiguan P-6 on the function of the middle jiao. Neiguan

P-6 is the pre-eminent point to treat nausea and vomiting due to any aetiology, including vomiting of pregnancy and the side-effects of chemotherapy and radiotherapy. Its considerable effect in the treatment of such side-effects has rendered it the subject of more research in recent years than any other acupuncture point. Neiguan P-6 is further indicated for distention, fullness and pain of the epigastrium and abdomen, and is often combined with Gongsun SP-4, the confluent point of the Penetrating vessel, for this purpose.

The Pericardium channel belongs to fire, and like many other points of the channel Neiguan P-6 is indicated for a variety of manifestations of heat, including fevers, jaundice, red face with hot skin, painful urinary dysfunction, cracked and bleeding tongue etc.

Finally the *Great Compendium of Acupuncture and Moxibustion* gives specific indications for excess and deficiency of the luo-connecting points. In the case of Neiguan P-6 these are sudden Heart pain (excess); stiffness [and pain] of the head [and neck] (deficiency).

COMBINATIONS

- Oppression of the chest: Neiguan P-6 and Jianli REN-11 (*One Hundred Symptoms*).
- Pain of the Heart and chest: Neiguan P-6, Quze P-3 and Daling P-7 (*Great Compendium*).
- Fear and fright with Heart pain: Neiguan P-6, Shenmen HE-7, Shaochong HE-9 and Yanglingquan GB-34 (*Compilation*).
- Epilepsy: Neiguan P-6, Houxi SI-3, Shenmen HE-7, Xinshu BL-15 and Yinbai SP-1 (*Complete Collection*).
- Sudden turmoil disorder, headache, chest pain and dyspnoeic rales: Neiguan P-6, Renying ST-9, Guanchong SJ-1, Sanyinjiao SP-6 and Zusanli ST-36 (*Compilation*).
- Difficult ingestion: Neiguan P-6, Yuji LU-10 and Zusanli ST-36 (*Great Compendium*).
- For quickly treating abdominal disease: Neiguan P-6 and Zhaohai KID-6 (*Ode of the Jade Dragon*).
- Abdominal pain: Neiguan P-6 and Gongsun SP-4 (*Ode of Xi-hong*).
- Abdominal pain: Neiguan P-6, Zusanli ST-36 and Zhongwan REN-12 (*Great Compendium*).
- Cracked and bleeding tongue: Neiguan P-6, Taichong LIV-3 and Yinjiao REN-7 (*Miscellaneous Diseases*).
- Red (bloody) dysenteric disorder: Neiguan P-6, Tianshu ST-25, Neiting ST-44, Yinbai SP-1, Qihai REN-6 and Zhaohai KID-6 (*Great Compendium*).
- Insufficient lactation due to Liver qi stagnation: Neiguan P-6, Rugen ST-18, Shanzhong REN-17, Shaoze SI-1 and Taichong LIV-3.

DALING P-7

Great Mound

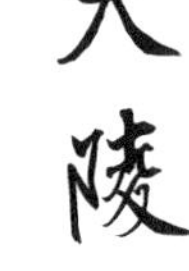

Shu-Stream, Yuan-Source and Earth point of the Pericardium channel
Sun Si-miao Ghost point

LOCATION

At the wrist, between the tendons of palmaris longus and flexor carpi radialis, level with Shenmen HE-7.

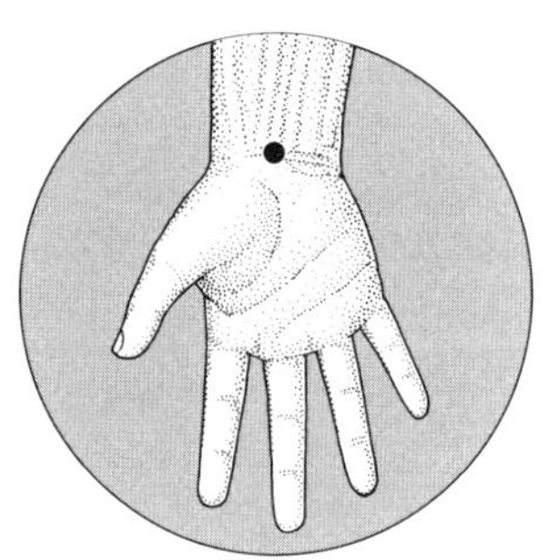

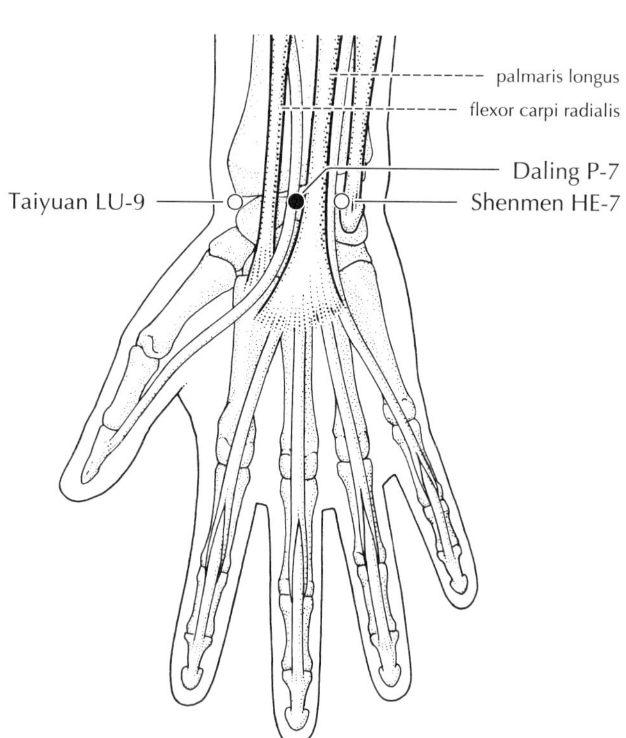

LOCATION NOTE

i. This point is commonly described as being at the wrist crease, which is variable. It is more reliably located level with Shenmen HE-7 which lies at the proximal border of the pisiform bone; ii. In the absence of the tendon of palmaris longus, locate this point on the ulnar side of the tendon of flexor carpi radialis.

NEEDLING

i. Perpendicular insertion 0.3 to 0.5 cun; ii. Oblique distal insertion along the carpal tunnel for carpal tunnel syndrome, 0.5 to 1 cun.

Caution: the median nerve lies directly under this point and needling commonly induces a significant electric sensation. This is an acceptable manifestation of deqi (arrival of qi), but once elicited, further manipulation is inappropriate and may damage the nerve.

ACTIONS

Clears heat from the Heart and calms the spirit
Harmonises the Stomach and intestines
Unbinds the chest
Clears the nutritive level and cools blood

INDICATIONS

- Heart pain, palpitations, pounding sensation of the Heart, insomnia, epilepsy, mania, manic raving, propensity to laugh (without ceasing), agitation, weeping with grief, sadness, fright and fear.
- Fullness of the chest, pain of the chest and lateral costal region, shortness of breath, much sighing, breast abscess, breast pain.
- Stomach pain, vomiting, vomiting blood, sudden turmoil disorder, intestinal abscess, foul breath.
- Fever with agitation and absence of sweating or ceaseless sweating, all wind-heat disorders with absence of sweating, heat in the body like fire.
- Red eyes, yellow eyes, jaundice, throat painful obstruction, dry throat, pain at the root of the tongue, eczema of the hand, wind rash, carbuncles and furuncles, splitting headache.
- Blood in the urine, difficult urination.
- Swelling of the axilla, contraction of the hand, pain and contraction of the elbow, wrist pain, heat in the palms.

COMMENTARY

Daling P-7 is the shu-stream, yuan-source and earth point of the Pericardium channel. The *Classic of Difficulties*[10] states "in cases of deficiency reinforce the mother, in cases of excess reduce the child". The Pericardium channel belongs to fire, and as the earth (child) point of a fire (mother) channel Daling P-7 is able to reduce excess heat or fire from the Pericardium.

The Pericardium is known as the 'wrapping' of the Heart, and like most points of the Pericardium channel, Daling P-7 has a profound action on the Heart and spirit. So close was the relationship between the Pericardium and Heart perceived to be, that the *Spiritual Pivot* listed only five zang (omitting the Pericardium entirely as a discrete zang) whilst describing the Pericardium channel as the channel pertaining to the Heart. Thus, for example, Daling P-7 rather than Shenmen HE-7 was listed as the yuan-source point of the Heart.

Daling P-7 is indicated in a wide variety of emotional disorders and is especially used whenever heat rises to disturb the spirit, whether due to: i. excess of any of the seven emotions transforming into fire; ii. stagnation of qi which both impairs the circulation of body fluids and transforms into fire resulting in phlegm-fire which harasses the Heart; iii. febrile heat collapsing into the Pericardium; iv. blazing heat arising from deficiency of yin. When the spirit is disrupted in this way it will give rise to such symptoms as palpitations, agitation, epilepsy, mania, manic raving, restlessness, insomnia, and anxiety. Under its alternative name of Guixin (Ghost Heart) Daling P-7 was included by Sun Si-miao among his 'thirteen ghost points' for the treatment of mania disorder and epilepsy.

The relationship of excessive laughter to Heart fire has long been recognised, for example Gong Tian-xian in *Achieving Longevity by Guarding the Source* stated "Ceaseless laughter is due to blazing of Heart fire". However as long ago as the *Yellow Emperor's Inner Classic* it was recognised that extravagant joy and deep sadness were equally manifestations of a disordered Heart spirit. Thus the *Spiritual Pivot*[11] says "The Heart rules the vessels, the vessels are the residence of the spirit, when Heart qi is deficient there is sadness, when excess there is ceaseless laughter", whilst the *Essential Questions*[12] states "The Heart stores the spirit ... when the spirit is in excess there is ceaseless laughter, when the spirit is insufficient there is sadness". The fact that Daling P-7 is indicated not only for ceaseless laughter but also for sadness and weeping with grief, reflects its application in both excess and deficiency disorders of the spirit.

If Heart fire transmits to its interiorly-exteriorly coupled Small Intestine channel, and from the Small Intestine (hand taiyang channel) to the Bladder (foot taiyang channel) and thence to the Bladder fu, there may be difficult and bloody urination, both indications for this point.

The Pericardium is interiorly-exteriorly coupled with the Sanjiao channel, whilst the interior pathway of the Pericardium primary and divergent channels pass through the middle and lower jiao. Daling P-7 therefore, like many points of the Pericardium channel, is used to harmonise the Stomach and intestines, especially when fire causes the Stomach qi to rebel upwards with symptoms such as foul breath, epigastric pain, vomiting, vomiting of blood, and sudden turmoil disorder.

The Pericardium (hand jueyin) channel and its coupled Liver (foot jueyin) channel are said to 'share the same qi'. This has special significance in relation to the actions of Daling P-7 in clearing heat from the Heart, calming the spirit and harmonising the Stomach and intestines. Liver qi stagnation may either transform to fire and rise to disturb the Heart and spirit, or transversely invade the Stomach causing Stomach qi to rebel upwards. As a result of the primary focus of Daling P-7 on the upper jiao, its special relationship to the Liver, and the pathway of the Pericardium sinew channel to the anterior ribs, Daling P-7 is also used to unbind the qi of the chest and treat such symptoms as fullness of the chest, shortness of breath, pain of the chest and lateral costal region, sighing and breast pain.

In common with several other points of the channel, Daling P-7 is indicated when febrile disease penetrates to the nutritive and especially the blood levels, agitating the Pericardium and spirit and giving rise to symptoms such as fever with agitation, cracked tongue, insomnia and even mania. This action of Daling P-7 on cooling the blood level further explains its use in the treatment of eczema, wind rash and carbuncles and furuncles. Finally Daling P-7 is the principal point used in the treatment of carpal tunnel syndrome, in which case the needle is inserted obliquely and distally along the carpal tunnel.

COMBINATIONS

- Frequent laughter: Daling P-7, Renzhong DU-26, Lieque LU-7 and Yangxi L.I.-5 (*Great Compendium*).
- Ceaseless laughter: Daling P-7 and Laogong P-8 (*Supplementing Life*).
- Weeping with grief: Daling P-7, Xinshu BL-15, Shenmen HE-7 and Jiexi ST-41 (*Supplementing Life*).
- Pounding sensation below the Heart and propensity to fright: Daling P-7 and Quze P-3 (*Thousand Ducat Formulas*).
- Oppression of the Heart: Daling P-7 and Laogong P-8 (*Ode of the Jade Dragon*).
- Heart pain: Daling P-7, Ximen P-4 and Quze P-3 (*Thousand Ducat Formulas*).
- Unbearable Heart pain: Daling P-7 and Shangwan REN-13 (*Thousand Ducat Formulas*).
- Pain of the Heart and chest: Daling P-7, Neiguan P-6 and Quze P-3 (*Great Compendium*).
- Chest pain: Daling P-7, Yunmen LU-2, Zhongfu LU-1, Yinbai SP-1, Qimen LIV-14, Feishu BL-13 and Hunmen BL-47 (*Thousand Ducat Formulas*).
- Shortness of breath: Daling P-7 and Chize LU-5 (*Great Compendium*).
- Coughing and dyspnoea: Daling P-7 and Shaoshang LU-11 (*Thousand Ducat Formulas*).
- Coughing blood: Daling P-7 and Ximen P-4 (*Systematic Classic*).
- Splitting headache with bursting eye pain: Daling P-7 and Touwei ST-8 (*Thousand Ducat Formulas*).
- Red eyes: Daling P-7 and Muchuang GB-16 (*Supplementing Life*).
- Vomiting clear (watery) saliva: Daling P-7, Shanzhong REN-17, Zhongwan REN-12 and Laogong P-8 (*Great Compendium*).
- Vomiting: Daling P-7, Burong ST-19 and Shangwan REN-13 (*Supplementing Life*).
- Abdominal pain: Daling P-7 and Waiguan SJ-5 (*Song of the Jade Dragon*).
- Abdominal pain and constipation: Daling P-7, Zhigou SJ-6 and Waiguan SJ-5 (*Ode of the Jade Dragon*).
- Obstructed urination: Sanyinjiao SP-6, Yinlingquan SP-9 and Qihai REN-6, followed by Yingu KID-10 and Daling P-7 (*Great Compendium*).

LAOGONG P-8

Palace of Toil

勞宮

Ying-Spring and Fire point of the Pericardium channel
Sun Si-miao Ghost point

LOCATION

Between the second and third metacarpal bones, proximal to the metacarpo-phalangeal joint, in a depression at the radial side of the third metacarpal bone.

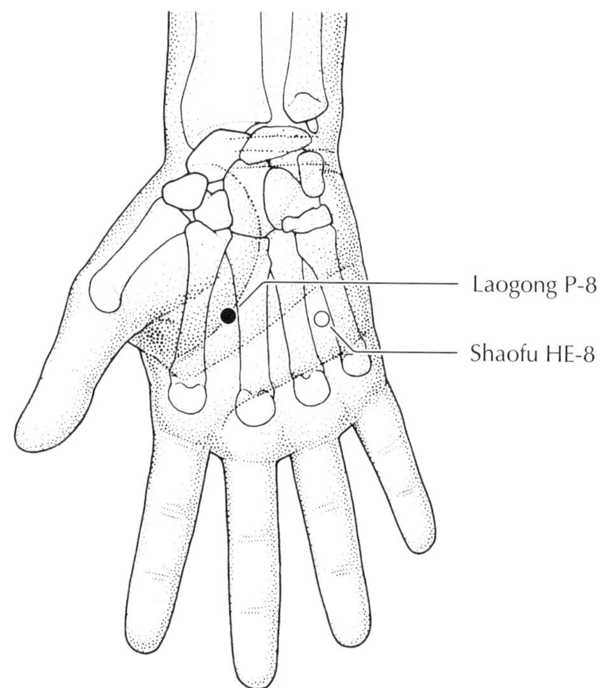

LOCATION NOTE

i. This point may be located at the place where the tip of the middle finger lands when a fist is made; ii. Some classical sources locate this point on the ulnar side of the third metacarpal bone, where the tip of the ring finger lands when a fist is made.

NEEDLING

Perpendicular insertion 0.5 cun.

ACTIONS

Clears heat from the Pericardium and revives consciousness
Clears heat from the Heart and calms the spirit
Harmonises the Stomach and clears heat from the middle jiao
Clears the nutritive level and cools blood

INDICATIONS

- Fever, coma, loss of consciousness, febrile disease accompanied by sweating which continues for days, windstroke, hypertension.
- Epilepsy, mania-depression, fright, sadness, propensity to anger, apprehension, restless zang disorder, ceaseless laughter.
- Heart pain, pain of the chest and lateral costal region, cough.
- Erosion of the mouth and tongue (in children), mouth ulcers, foul breath, difficult ingestion, vomiting, hypogastric (ji ju) masses.
- Vomiting blood, ceaseless nosebleed, blood in the stool, haemorrhoids, dark urine, jaundice, yellow eyes, throat pain.
- Tremor of the hand, eczema and tinea of the hand, scaling of the skin of the hand, heat in the palm of the hand, sweating of the palms, hand painful obstruction.

COMMENTARY

Laogong P-8 is the ying-spring and fire point of the Pericardium channel. According to the *Classic of Difficulties*[13] ying-spring points are indicated for "heat in the body". Laogong P-8 is a powerful point to revive consciousness and calm the spirit in cases where heat 'collapses' into the Pericardium during the course of febrile diseases, leading to disturbance of the emotions, and in severe cases coma.

There are two major discussions on the relationship of the Heart and the Pericardium channel in the *Spiritual Pivot*. At this early date, it is clear that the Pericardium channel was considered to be the main channel that linked with and treated the Heart itself, and indeed it was said that the Heart channel had no shu points of its own, Laogong P-8 being listed as the ying-spring and fire point of the Heart channel. It is therefore not only used to clear febrile heat from the Pericardium, the 'wrapping of the Heart', but is one of the principal points to clear Heart fire generated by internal disharmony. Heart fire may result from a number of different factors (see Daling P-7), but due to the close relationship of the Pericardium and Liver jueyin channels, Laogong P-8 is particularly indicated when stagnant Liver fire transmits to the Heart. If Heart fire agitates the spirit there will be various manifestations of psycho-emotional disharmony such as mania-depression, propensity to anger, ceaseless laughter and epilepsy. Like Daling P-7, Laogong P-8 is also able to bolster the spirit and is indicated for such manifestations of deficiency as fright, sadness and apprehension.

If Heart fire condenses body fluids it may generate phlegm, and when this is combined with wind stirred up by Liver yang, the resultant wind-phlegm may give rise to epilepsy or windstroke. The importance of Laogong P-8 in the treatment of epilepsy and also mania-depression is reflected in its inclusion (under its alternative name of Guicu 'Ghost Cave') by Sun Si-miao in his 'thirteen ghost points' for the treatment of these conditions.

The Heart flowers into the tongue and the Spleen opens into the mouth. Mouth and tongue ulcers are differentiated into six main patterns: i. Heart fire, ii. Spleen and Stomach smouldering heat, iii. Kidney and Heart yin deficiency, iv. Spleen qi deficiency complicated with heat, v. blood deficiency with dry heat, and vi. Kidney yang deficiency. Laogong P-8 is indicated for ulceration or erosion of the mouth and tongue from any of these patterns, especially when heat is involved.

The Pericardium primary and divergent channels pass through the diaphragm to the middle and lower jiao and the Pericardium channel is interiorly-exteriorly coupled with the Sanjiao channel. Like many points of the Pericardium channel, therefore, Laogong P-8 also has a strong action on the middle jiao and is indicated in cases where fire disrupts the descent of Stomach qi resulting in foul breath, vomiting and difficult ingestion.

In common with Quze P-3, Daling P-7 and Zhongchong P-9, Laogong P-8 clears heat from the nutritive and blood levels. It may therefore be used when febrile heat at the blood level leads to reckless bleeding disorders such as vomiting blood, nosebleed, blood in the stool etc. Its ability to clear heat from the blood as well as its location, make it suitable for skin disorders affecting the palm such as eczema, tinea and scaling, as well as for heat and abnormal sweating of the palms. It is also indicated for hand painful obstruction and hand tremors.

In qigong practice, Laogong P-8 can be thought of as mirroring Yongquan KID-1 on the soles of the feet. It is common practice to 'breathe through' either of these points, and focusing on and building the qi at Laogong P-8 is a pre-requisite for emitting qi in the treatment of disease by qigong therapy.

Finally Laogong P-8 is cited in the *Song of the Nine Needles for Returning the Yang* for the treatment of collapse of yang characterised by loss of consciousness, aversion to cold, cold counterflow of the limbs, purple lips etc.

COMBINATIONS

- The five types of epilepsy: Laogong P-8 and Yongquan KID-1 (*Miscellaneous Diseases*).
- Incessant laughter: Laogong P-8 and Daling P-7 (*Supplementing Life*).
- Oppression of the Heart: Laogong P-8 and Daling P-7 (*Ode of the Jade Dragon*).
- Incessant nosebleed: Laogong P-8, Kouheliao L.I.-19 and Duiduan DU-27 (*Supplementing Life*).
- Mouth ulcers: Laogong P-8 and Chengjiang REN-24 (*Compilation*).
- Erosion, heat and dryness of the mouth: Laogong P-8, Shaoze SI-1, Sanjian L.I.-3 and Taichong LIV-3 (*Thousand Ducat Formulas*).
- Throat pain: Laogong P-8, Fengfu DU-16 and Tianchuang SI-16 (*Thousand Ducat Formulas*).
- Difficult ingestion: Laogong P-8, Yanggang BL-48, Qimen LIV-14 and Shaoshang LU-11 (*Thousand Ducat Formulas*).
- Vomiting: Laogong P-8 and Shaoshang LU-11 (*Thousand Ducat Formulas*).

ZHONGCHONG P-9

Middle Rushing

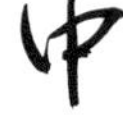

Jing-Well and Wood point of the Pericardium channel

LOCATION

In the centre of the tip of the middle finger. Alternatively, this point is sometimes located at the radial side of the middle finger, at the junction of lines drawn along the radial border of the nail and the base of the nail, approximately 0.1 cun from the corner of the nail.

NEEDLING

Perpendicular or oblique insertion directed proximally 0.1 to 0.2 cun, or prick to bleed.

ACTIONS

Clears heat from the Pericardium and revives consciousness
Clears the Heart and benefits the tongue
Clears summer-heat

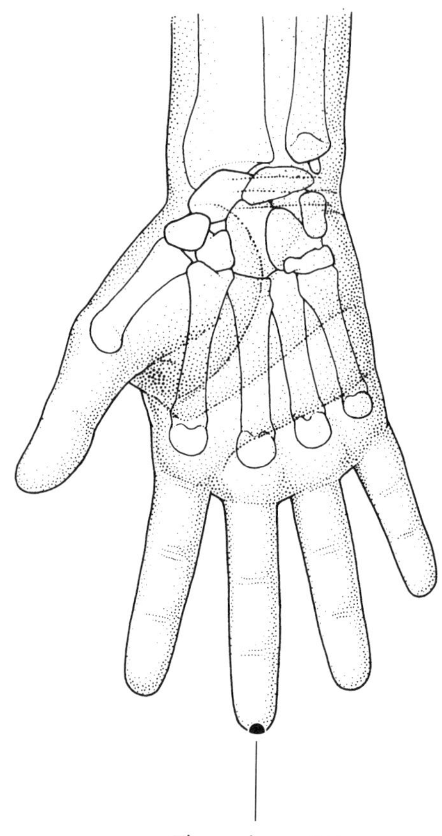

Zhongchong P-9

INDICATIONS

- Windstroke, injury by summer-heat, loss of consciousness, fever, fever with agitation and oppression, heat in the body like fire, headache, hypertension.
- Pain at the root of the tongue, stiffness of the tongue, inability to speak, night-time crying in children.
- Heart pain, agitation of the Heart, oppression of the Heart with absence of sweating, heat of the palms, tinnitus.
- Vomiting and diarrhoea, epigastric pain, sudden turmoil disorder, childhood nutritional impairment.

COMMENTARY

Zhongchong P-9 is the jing-well point of the Pericardium channel, and in common with many of the jing-well points (the terminal and most dynamic point of the channel) has a powerful effect to restore consciousness. There are some particular differences, however, that distinguish Zhongchong P-9 from the other jing-well points. Firstly, located on the middle finger, this is the most distal of all the jing-well points and the only one located in the centre rather than at the corner of the nail. Secondly, as a point of the Pericardium channel, Zhongchong P-9 is especially suitable for restoring consciousness, which occurs when the spirit is dislodged from the Heart.

Loss of consciousness with stiffness of the tongue may occur during the course of febrile diseases when pathogenic heat, complicated with phlegm, collapses into the Pericardium. The affinity of Zhongchong P-9 for the tongue, reflected in such classical indications as pain at the root of the tongue, stiffness of the tongue and inability to speak, underlines the intimate relationship that was held to exist between the Pericardium and the Heart, since it is the Heart which flowers into the tongue and the Heart (luo-connecting) channel rather than the Pericardium channel that travels to the root of the tongue.

Like several points of the Pericardium channel, Zhongchong P-9 also treats injury by summer-heat characterised by fever, agitation, vomiting, diarrhoea and collapse.

The Pericardium primary and divergent channels traverse all three jiao and the Pericardium is interiorly-exteriorly coupled with the Sanjiao channel. Like many points of the Pericardium channel, therefore, Zhongchong P-9 also has a strong action on the middle jiao and is indicated for vomiting and diarrhoea, epigastric pain and sudden turmoil disorder. In the treatment of paediatric disorders, it may be used for night-time crying in children and childhood nutritional impairment. Among other patterns, the former may be due to accumulated heat in the Heart and the latter to heat and blockage in the middle jiao.

COMBINATIONS

- Loss of consciousness from windstroke: Zhongchong P-9, Renzhong DU-26 and Hegu L.I.-4. If this is ineffective, needle Yamen DU-15 and Dadun LIV-1 (*Great Compendium*).
- Swelling and pain below the tongue: Zhongchong P-9 and Lianquan REN-23 (*One Hundred Symptoms*).
- Stiffness of the tongue: Zhongchong P-9, Shaoshang LU-11, Yuji LU-10, Yamen DU-15, Erjian L.I.-2, Yingu KID-10 and Rangu KID-2 (*Great Compendium*).
- Heart pain with fullness and agitation and stiff tongue: Zhongchong P-9 and Yinxi HE-6 (*Supplementing Life*).
- Pain of the Heart with shortness of breath: Zhongchong P-9, Qimen LIV-14, Changqiang DU-1, Tiantu REN-22 and Xiabai LU-4 (*Thousand Ducat Formulas*).
- Heat in the body like fire and splitting headache: Zhongchong P-9 and Mingmen DU-4 (*Supplementing Life*).

NOTES

1 *Spiritual Pivot* Chapter 71.
2 *Classic of Difficulties* 68th Difficulty.
3 *Spiritual Pivot* Chapter 44.
4 *Spiritual Pivot* Chapter 78.
5 *Spiritual Pivot* Chapter 66.
6 *A Spot of Snow on a Red Hot Stove* (Hong Lu Dian Xue) by Gong Ju-zhong 1630.
7 *Essential Questions* Chapter 33.
8 *Spiritual Pivot* Chapter 44.
9 *Classic of Difficulties* 29th Difficulty.
10 *Classic of Difficulties* 69th Difficulty.
11 *Spiritual Pivot* Chapter 8.
12 *Essential Questions* Chapter 62.
13 *Classic of Difficulties* 68th Difficulty.

手少陽三焦經

THE SANJIAO CHANNEL OF HAND SHAOYANG

THE SANJIAO CHANNEL OF HAND SHAOYANG

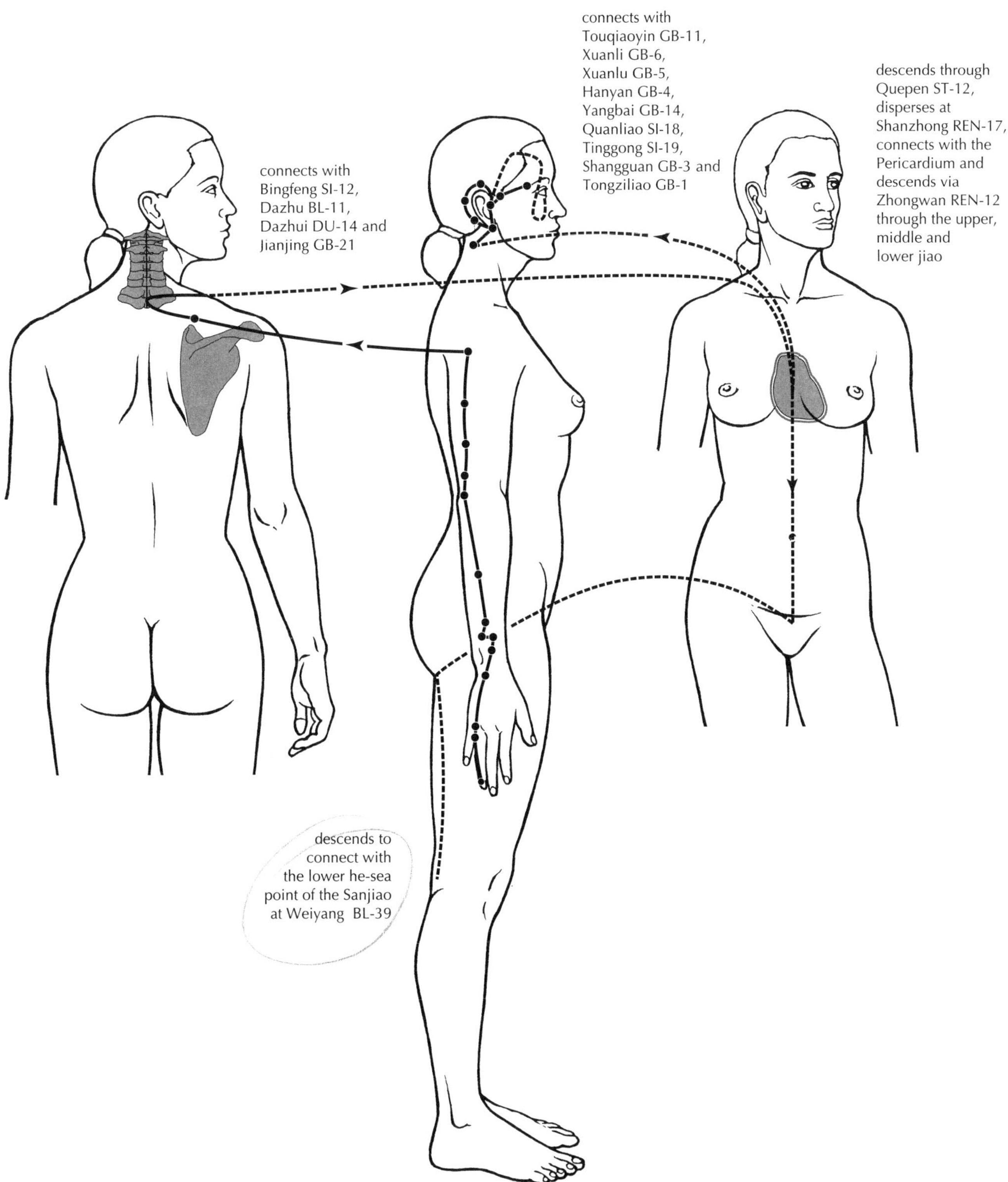
connects with
Touqiaoyin GB-11,
Xuanli GB-6,
Xuanlu GB-5,
Hanyan GB-4,
Yangbai GB-14,
Quanliao SI-18,
Tinggong SI-19,
Shangguan GB-3 and
Tongziliao GB-1
descends through
Quepen ST-12,
disperses at
Shanzhong REN-17,
connects with the
Pericardium and
descends via
Zhongwan REN-12
through the upper,
middle and
lower jiao
connects with
Bingfeng SI-12,
Dazhu BL-11,
Dazhui DU-14 and
Jianjing GB-21
descends to
connect with
the lower he-sea
point of the Sanjiao
at Weiyang BL-39

The Sanjiao primary channel

THE SANJIAO PRIMARY CHANNEL

- begins at the ulnar aspect of the tip of the ring finger and runs between the fourth and fifth metacarpal bones along the dorsum of the hand,
- travels up the posterior aspect of the forearm between the radius and the ulna and between the Large and Small Intestine channels,
- traverses the olecranon of the ulna at Tianjing SJ-10 and continues up the postero-lateral aspect of the upper arm to the shoulder where it intersects the Small Intestine channel at Bingfeng SI-12,
- travels towards the spine via Dazhu BL-11 where it intersects the Governing vessel at Dazhui DU-14,
- ascends laterally to the highest point of the shoulder where it intersects the Gall Bladder channel at Jianjing GB-21,
- descends anteriorly into the supraclavicular fossa at Quepen ST-12, then disperses midway between the breasts at Shanzhong REN-17,
- connects with the Pericardium then descends through the diaphragm to the abdomen via Zhongwan REN-12, linking along its pathway the upper, middle and lower jiao.

A branch of the channel

- separates in the region of Shanzhong REN-17,
- ascends to emerge from the supraclavicular fossa,
- rises along the neck to the posterior aspect of the ear,
- circles behind the ear via Touqiaoyin GB-11 to the temples where it intersects the Gall Bladder channel at Xuanli GB-6, Xuanlu GB-5, Hanyan GB-4 and Yangbai GB-14,
- winds down across the cheek, intersecting the Small Intestine channel at Quanliao SI-18,
- ascends to the inferior aspect of the eye.

Another branch

- separates behind the ear and enters the ear,
- emerges in front of the ear to intersect the Small Intestine and Gall Bladder channels at Tinggong SI-19 and Shangguan GB-3,
- crosses the previous branch on the cheek to terminate at the outer canthus of the eye at Sizhukong SJ-23, linking with Tongziliao GB-1.

According to the *Spiritual Pivot*[1] a branch of the Sanjiao primary channel descends to Weiyang BL-39.

The Sanjiao primary channel connects with the following zangfu: Sanjiao (upper, middle and lower jiao), Pericardium.

The Sanjiao primary channel meets with other channels at the following points: Bingfeng SI-12, Dazhu BL-11, Dazhui DU-14, Jianjing GB-21, Quepen ST-12, Shanzhong REN-17, Zhongwan REN-12, Touqiaoyin GB-11, Xuanli GB-6, Xuanlu GB-5, Hanyan GB-4, Yangbai GB-14, Quanliao SI-18, Tinggong SI-19, Shangguan GB-3, Tongziliao GB-1. *Note*: Jingming BL-1, Tianchi P-1, Baihui DU-20 and Fengchi GB-20 are classified as meeting points of the Sanjiao channel, but illustrations of the channel do not normally show these connections.

THE SANJIAO LUO-CONNECTING CHANNEL

- separates from the Sanjiao primary channel at Waiguan SJ-5,
- proceeds up the posterior aspect of the arm and over the shoulder, converging with the Pericardium channel in the chest.

THE SANJIAO DIVERGENT CHANNEL

- separates from the primary channel on the head and branches to the vertex,
- descends into the supraclavicular fossa and across the three jiao, dispersing in the chest.

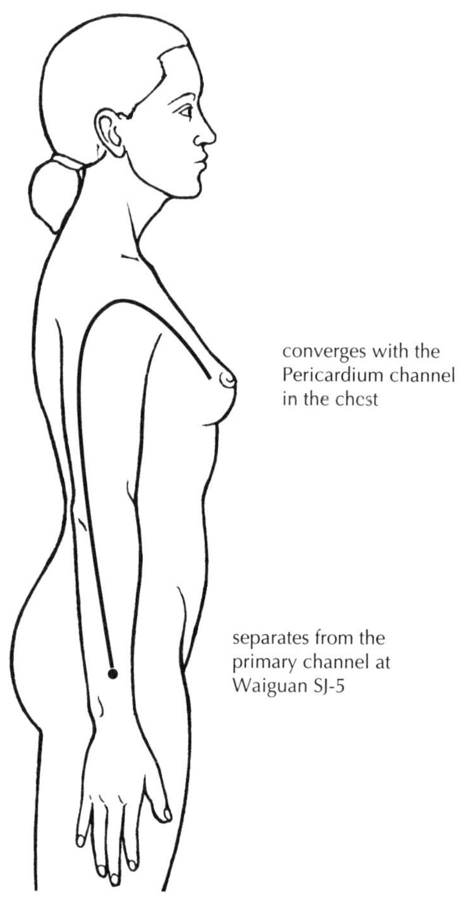

The Sanjiao luo-connecting channel

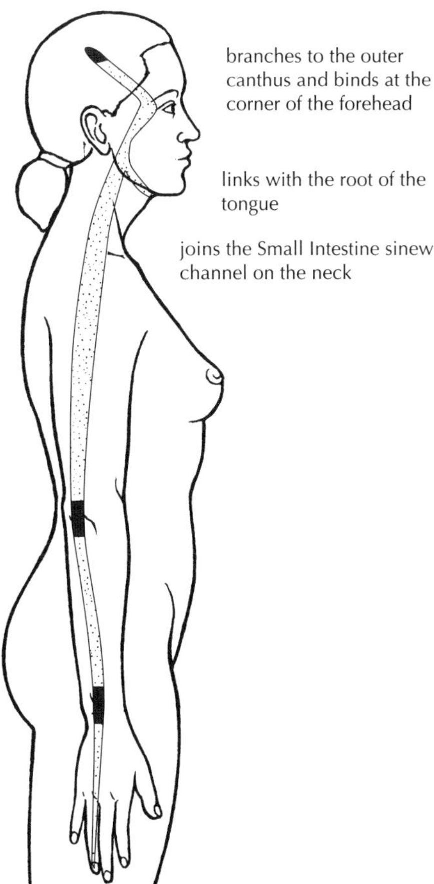
branches to the outer canthus and binds at the corner of the forehead
links with the root of the tongue
joins the Small Intestine sinew channel on the neck

The Sanjiao sinew channel

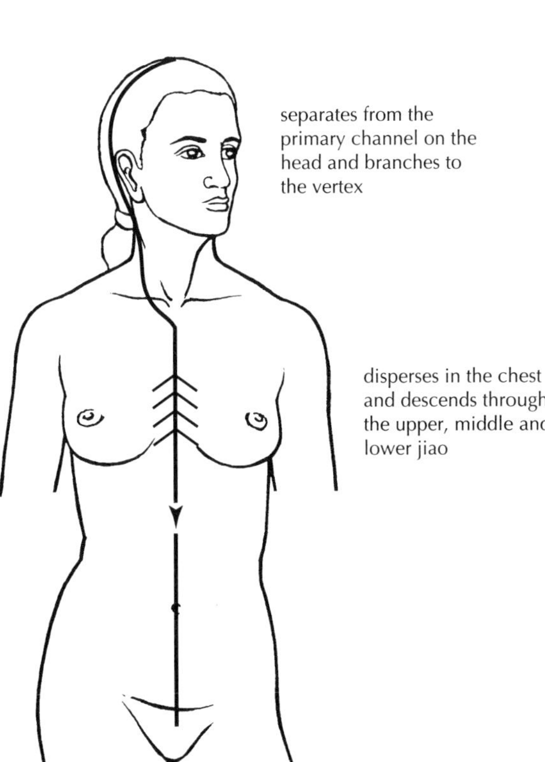
separates from the primary channel on the head and branches to the vertex
disperses in the chest and descends through the upper, middle and lower jiao

The Sanjiao divergent channel

THE SANJIAO SINEW CHANNEL

- begins at the ulnar side of the ring finger and binds at the dorsum of the wrist,
- follows the posterior aspect of the arm and binds at the tip of the elbow,
- ascends the lateral aspect of the upper arm and over the shoulder to the neck where it joins with the Small Intestine sinew channel.

A branch

- separates at the angle of the mandible and enters internally to link with the root of the tongue.

Another branch

- ascends anterior to the ear to join at the outer canthus of the eye,
- then ascends across the temple to bind at the corner of the forehead.

Pathological symptoms

Strained and cramping sensation along the course of the channel, curled tongue.

DISCUSSION

The Sanjiao channel of hand shaoyang belongs to the fire phase, is interiorly-exteriorly coupled with the Pericardium channel, and is paired with the Gall Bladder channel of foot shaoyang according to six channel theory.

The Sanjiao-Pericardium relationship is further strengthened by the fact that:
- the Sanjiao primary channel connects with the Pericardium
- the Sanjiao luo-connecting channel converges with the Pericardium channel in the chest.

The Sanjiao-Gall Bladder relationship is strengthened by the fact that the Sanjiao channel connects with the Gall Bladder channel at the side of the head at points Tongziliao GB-1, Shangguan GB-3 to Xuanli GB-6, Touqiaoyin GB-11, Fengchi GB-20 and at Jianjing GB-21 on the top of the shoulder.

In addition it is important to note that:
- the interior pathway of the Sanjiao primary channel passes through and links the upper, middle and lower jiao.
- the interior pathway of the Sanjiao primary channel descends between the breasts to Shanzhong REN-17.
- the Sanjiao primary channel ascends both posterior and anterior to the ear as well as entering the ear.
- the Sanjiao primary channel ascends to the inferior aspect of the eye and the primary and sinew channels go to the outer canthus of the eye.
- the Sanjiao divergent channel spreads to the vertex.
- the Sanjiao sinew channel connects with the root of the tongue.
- the Sanjiao primary channel ascends through the cheek.

These channel connections, and the status of the Sanjiao as belonging to fire, determine many of the actions and indications of the Sanjiao channel points, which may be summarised as follows:
- Reducing fever. The Sanjiao channel belongs to fire and many of its points are indicated for febrile diseases, especially when due to exterior pathogenic factors. As far as differentiation of fevers according to the four levels is concerned, the Sanjiao channel primarily treats fevers at the defensive and qi levels, whilst the Pericardium channel mainly treats fevers at the nutritive and blood levels, although the most distal points of the Sanjiao channel (where the Pericardium and Sanjiao channels converge) are able to treat both. As far as differentiation of fevers according to the Sanjiao theory is concerned, points of the Sanjiao channel mainly treat febrile diseases affecting the upper jiao Lung pattern, although its most distal points also treat the upper jiao Pericardium pattern. As for fever differentiation according to the six channels, both the *Spiritual Pivot*[2] and the *Essential Questions*[3] state "Taiyang is the opening, yangming is the closing and shaoyang is the pivot". The Sanjiao belongs to shaoyang (the pivot between exterior and interior) and several points of the channel are indicated for alternating chills and fever and malaria, the characteristic indications of shaoyang pattern. The heat-clearing action of the Sanjiao channel points extends to clearing heat from all regions traversed by the channel.
- Benefiting the ears. Various portions of the Sanjiao channel encircle or enter the ear, and many of its points are indicated for disorders of the ear such as tinnitus and deafness, especially when due to heat, uprising of yang or other excess pathogenic factors.
- Clearing heat from the eyes, especially wind-heat and Liver-Gall Bladder heat.
- Clearing heat from the neck, throat and tongue.
- Soothing the Heart and calming the spirit. Due to the close relationship between the Sanjiao and Pericardium channels, many points of the Sanjiao channel are indicated for pain of the chest and Heart as well as agitation, restlessness, mania, epilepsy and other manifestations of disordered spirit.
- Treating headaches. Shaoyang channel traverses the temples and side of the head, and points of the Sanjiao channel are much used in the treatment of headaches affecting this region.
- Harmonising the three jiao. Waiguan SJ-5 and Zhigou SJ-6 especially, are able to regulate the middle and lower jiao in the treatment of vomiting and constipation.

GUANCHONG SJ-1

Rushing Pass

關冲

Jing-Well and Metal point of the Sanjiao channel

LOCATION

On the dorsal aspect of the ring finger, at the junction of lines drawn along the ulnar border of the nail and the base of the nail, approximately 0.1 cun from the corner of the nail.

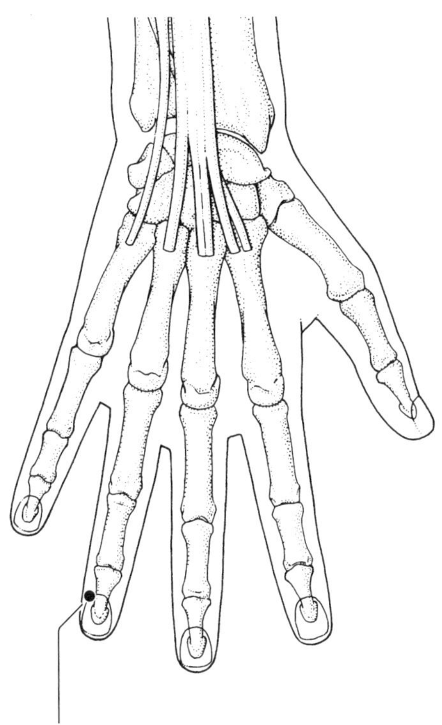

NEEDLING

Perpendicular or oblique insertion directed proximally 0.1 to 0.2 cun, or prick to bleed.

ACTIONS

Clears upper jiao heat
Benefits the ears and tongue
Activates the channel and alleviates pain

INDICATIONS

- Tinnitus, deafness, earache, stiff tongue, curled tongue, pain at the root of the tongue, cracked tongue, dryness of the mouth, dry lips, bitter taste in the mouth, headache, wind dizziness and headache, redness of the eyes, superficial visual obstruction, throat painful obstruction, pain of the submandibular region, dark complexion.
- Febrile disease, congested heat of the Sanjiao, congested heat of the upper jiao, heat in the body like fire, fever, fever with absence of sweating, chills and fever, fever with agitation, oppression of the Heart with absence of sweating, Heart pain.
- Sudden turmoil disorder, vomiting of sour fluid, no pleasure in eating.
- Pain of the elbow and shoulder, pain of the shoulder and back with inability to turn and look backwards.

COMMENTARY

As the jing-well point, Guanchong SJ-1 is the terminal point of the Sanjiao channel, and in common with the other jing-well points has its most powerful influence on the opposite end of the channel. The primary action of Guanchong SJ-1 is in clearing heat affecting the upper jiao, and as a jing-well point it is mainly used for acute symptoms. This action is reflected in two main ways: i. clearing heat from the channel, and ii. treating febrile diseases of external origin.

The *Song of the Jade Dragon* recommends Guanchong SJ-1 for 'congested Sanjiao heat in the upper jiao' and says "bleeding this point will remove toxic blood". The upper portion of the Sanjiao channel originates in the chest and ascends via the neck to the ear, temple, inferior aspect of the eye and outer canthus. If exterior heat (primarily wind-heat) or interior heat (mainly Liver heat which transmits to the foot shaoyang Gall Bladder channel and thence to the hand shaoyang Sanjiao channel) obstruct the Sanjiao channel there may be tinnitus, deafness, earache, headache, dizziness, redness of the eyes, throat painful obstruction etc. The Sanjiao sinew channel ascends to the root of the tongue and Guanchong SJ-1 has a special affinity for this area. It is indicated for stiff tongue (usually due to heat injuring body fluids), curled tongue (usually due to excess or deficiency fire of the Heart) and cracked tongue (usually due to heat scorching body fluids), as well as pain at the root of the tongue.

There are three main systems for differentiating fevers in the corpus of Chinese medicine: i. according to the six channels, ii. according to the four levels, and iii. according to the sanjiao (three jiao). The sanjiao theory divides the body into three portions, the upper, middle and lower jiao. According to this method of differentiating fevers (developed by Wu Ju-tong in the *Systematic Differentiation of Warm Diseases*) the upper jiao corresponds to the Lung and Pericardium. The *Warp and Woof of Warm Febrile Diseases* explains "When a warm pathogen attacks the upper body, first it invades the Lung; it is then transmitted to the Pericardium". As far as exterior pathogenic heat attacking the Lung is concerned, this corresponds to the taiyang channel stage and the defensive level in the differentiations according to the six channels and the four levels respectively, and is the most exterior and superficial stage of fever, manifesting with chills and fever, headache, sore throat, and redness of the eyes. If exterior pathogenic heat penetrates deeper to attack the Pericardium, the heat condenses the body fluids to form phlegm. Phlegm-heat then obstructs the Pericardium and disturbs the spirit, giving rise to such symptoms as high fever with agitation, Heart pain, dry mouth with a bitter taste, and stiff or curled tongue. Since Guanchong SJ-1 is able to dispel pathogenic heat and wind-heat from the upper jiao as a whole and from its interiorly-exteriorly coupled Pericardium channel in particular, it is therefore able to treat both these patterns.

It is interesting to note that in general, points of the Sanjiao channel treat fevers at the defensive and qi levels and the Lung pattern, whilst points of the Pericardium channel treat the nutritive and blood levels and the Pericardium pattern (see Discussion). Since the defensive level, qi level and Lung patterns are relatively more superficial and yang, this reflects the interior-exterior relationship of this yin-yang pair of channels. As the jing-well point of the Sanjiao channel where the qi of the Pericardium enters the Sanjiao, however, Guanchong SJ-1 is ideally suited to treat both the Lung and Pericardium patterns.

Guanchong SJ-1 is indicated in two other conditions. Firstly, acute disharmony of the Stomach and intestines manifesting as sudden turmoil disorder, vomiting of sour fluid and loss of appetite, reflecting the interior pathway of the Sanjiao primary channel to the middle and lower jiao. Secondly, it appears in a number of classical combinations for the treatment of wasting and thirsting disorder, reflecting its ability to clear heat and moisten dryness of the mouth and lips.

COMBINATIONS

- Deafness: Guanchong SJ-1 and Zuqiaoyin GB-44 (*Spiritual Pivot*).
- Tinnitus and deafness: Guanchong SJ-1, Xiaguan ST-7, Yangxi L.I.-5, Yemen SJ-2 and Yanggu SI-5 (*Systematic Classic*).
- Ear pain, deafness and tinnitus: Guanchong SJ-1, Yemen SJ-2, Zhongzhu SJ-3, Tianchuang SI-16 and Yangxi L.I.-5, (*Thousand Ducat Formulas*).
- Wind dizziness and headache: Guanchong SJ-1, Kunlun BL-60, Tianyou SJ-16, Fengmen BL-12 and Guanyuan REN-4 (*Thousand Ducat Formulas*).
- Throat painful obstruction, curled tongue and dry mouth: Guanchong SJ-1, Zuqiaoyin GB-44 and Shaoze SI-1 (*Thousand Ducat Formulas*).
- Flaccid tongue with inability to speak: Guanchong SJ-1 and Yamen DU-15 (*One Hundred Patterns*).
- Wasting and thirsting disorder with great desire to drink: Guanchong SJ-1, Chengjiang REN-24, Rangu KID-2 and Yishe BL-49 (*Thousand Ducat Formulas*).
- Heat sensation of the shoulder with inability to turn the head: Guanchong SJ-1, Jianzhen SI-9 and Jianyu L.I.-15 (*Thousand Ducat Formulas*).

YEMEN SJ-2

Fluid Gate

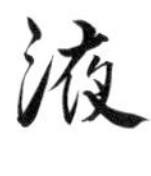

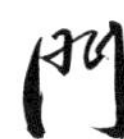

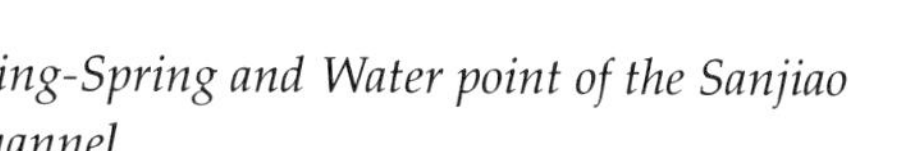

Ying-Spring and Water point of the Sanjiao channel

LOCATION

Between the ring and little fingers, 0.5 cun proximal to the margin of the web.

LOCATION NOTE

This point is usually located and needled with the hand resting in a loose fist; the point may then be located at the proximal end of the visible crease formed by the web space.

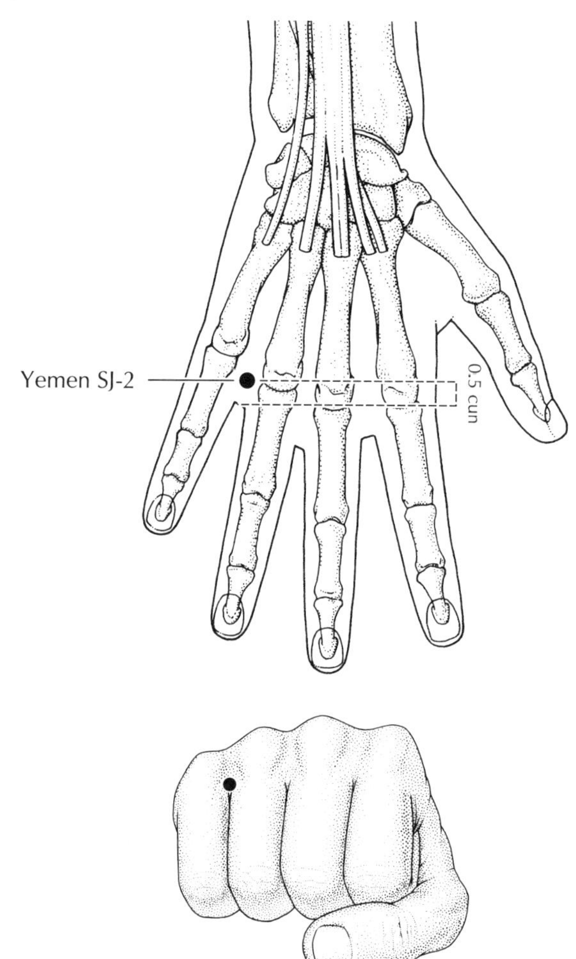

NEEDLING

Perpendicular insertion 0.3 to 0.5 cun.

ACTIONS

Disperses upper jiao heat and benefits the ears
Calms the spirit
Activates the channel and alleviates pain

INDICATIONS

- Deafness, sudden deafness, tinnitus, earache, headache, red eyes, red face with lacrimation, dry eyes, swelling and pain of the throat, toothache, bleeding gums, pain of the gums.
- Fright palpitations, raving, mania, propensity to fright, epilepsy, shortness of breath.
- Malaria, fever with absence of sweating.
- Pain of the arm, inability to raise the arm due to pain, redness and swelling of the back of the hand, contraction of the five fingers, weakness of the wrist, neck pain.

COMMENTARY

According to the *Classic of Difficulties*[4] ying-spring points are indicated for "heat in the body". The Sanjiao primary channel ascends: i. both posterior and anterior to the ear as well as entering the ear, ii. to the inferior aspect of the eye and the outer canthus, and iii. through the cheek. Yemen SJ-2, the ying-spring and water point of the Sanjiao channel, is therefore able to clear heat from the upper reaches of the channel in the ears (deafness, tinnitus, earache), eyes (redness, dryness, lacrimation) and gums and teeth (pain and bleeding).

The Sanjiao is interiorly-exteriorly related to the Pericardium, the 'outer wrapping' of the Heart, and Yemen SJ-2 is able to clear heat from the Heart and spirit manifesting as palpitations, fright, mania, raving and epilepsy.

In comparison with Guanchong SJ-1, it is less effective in the treatment of febrile diseases and distal channel disorders affecting the shoulder and elbow, but more effective in calming the spirit and treating local channel disorders affecting the wrist, hand and fingers.

COMBINATIONS

- Ear pain, deafness and tinnitus: Yemen SJ-2, Tianchuang SI-16, Yangxi L.I.-5, Guanchong SJ-1 and Zhongzhu SJ-3 (*Thousand Ducat Formulas*).
- Tinnitus and deafness: Yemen SJ-2, Guanchong SJ-1, Yangxi L.I.-5, Xiaguan ST-7 and Yanggu SI-5 (*Systematic Classic*).
- Sudden deafness: Yemen SJ-2 and Sanyangluo SJ-8 (*Supplementing Life*).
- Throat pain: Yemen SJ-2 and Yuji LU-10 (*One Hundred Symptoms*).
- Toothache of the lower jaw: Yemen SJ-2, Yanggu SI-5, Shangyang L.I.-1, Erjian L.I.-2 and Sidu SJ-9 (*Thousand Ducat Formulas*).
- Fright palpitations: Yemen SJ-2, Tianjing SJ-10, Baihui DU-20 and Shendao DU-11 (*Supplementing Life*).

ZHONGZHU SJ-3

Central Islet

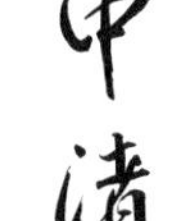

Shu-Stream and Wood point of the Sanjiao channel

LOCATION

On the dorsum of the hand, in the depression just proximal to the fourth and fifth metacarpophalangeal joints.

LOCATION NOTE

i. Locate and needle with the hand resting in a loose fist; ii. This point may be located at the apex of an equilateral triangle formed by this point and the prominences of the metacarpophalangeal joints of the ring and little fingers.

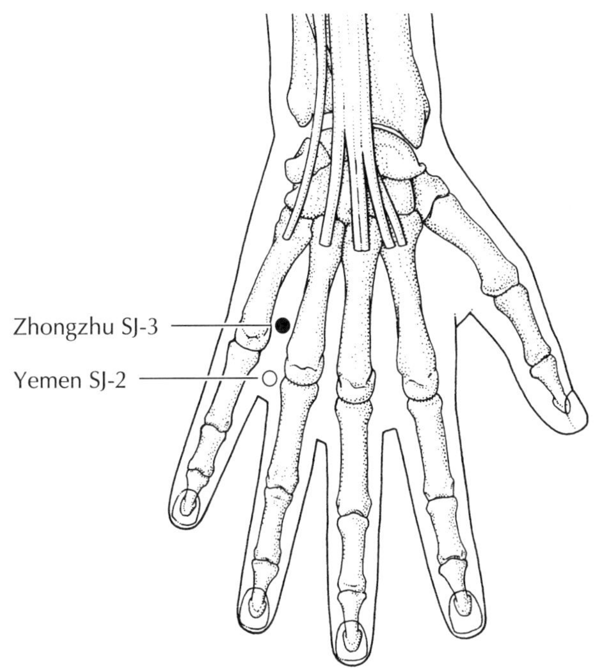

NEEDLING

Perpendicular or oblique insertion directed proximally, 0.5 to 1 cun.

ACTIONS

Clears heat
Benefits the ears
Clears the head and eyes
Activates the channel and alleviates pain

INDICATIONS

- Tinnitus, deafness, earache, one-sided headache, pain of the temples, dizziness, redness and pain of the eyes, superficial visual obstruction, throat painful obstruction.
- Itching of the body and face, red face, red face with absence of sweating, febrile disease, febrile disease with headache, chills and fever, aversion to wind and cold, chronic malaria, mania.
- Inability to flex and extend the fingers, redness, swelling and pain of the elbow and upper arm extending into the shoulder, numbness of the four limbs, pain of the spine at the level of the Heart.

COMMENTARY

The Sanjiao channel both encircles and enters the ear, and Zhongzhu SJ-3 is one of the most important distal points for treating ear disorders due to any pathology. Tinnitus and deafness may be differentiated into six main patterns i. attack by exterior pathogenic wind, ii. uprising of Liver fire or Liver yang, iii. obstruction of the ear by phlegm-damp or phlegm-heat, iv. Kidney deficiency, v. Spleen and Stomach deficiency, and vi. traumatic injury or exposure to sudden or persistent loud noise. Zhongzhu SJ-3 is particularly suited to treating the first two patterns (exterior wind and Liver disharmony). This is because, like most distal points of the Sanjiao channel, it is able to expel exterior pathogens, and also as the wood point of the Sanjiao channel it can assist in descending Liver fire or Liver yang which have transmitted to the shaoyang channel. Due to the intimate relationship of the Sanjiao channel with the ear, however, the application of Zhongzhu SJ-3 extends to the treatment of any pattern of tinnitus and deafness, especially when due to excess. Zhongzhu SJ-3 is equally important as a distal point in the treatment of disorders such as earache, otitis media and blockage of the ears following a head cold. In blockage of the ears during or following flying, Zhongzhu SJ-3 may be massaged or needled whilst the patient pinches their nose shut and attempts to blow through it.

When heat or fire, whether of internal or external origin, harass the Sanjiao channel in the upper body, there may be one-sided headache, pain of the temples, dizziness, redness, swelling and pain of the eyes, throat painful obstruction and red face. In all these situations Zhongzhu SJ-3 will help lower and clear the excess heat.

According to the *Spiritual Pivot* "Taiyang is the opening, yangming is the closing and shaoyang is the pivot". In the six channel differentiation of fevers expounded in the *Treatise on Injury by Cold*, the shaoyang level is the pivot between the interior and the exterior, and shaoyang pattern occurs when the pathogenic factor is trapped between these two levels. The characteristic symptoms of this 'half-interior, half-exterior' pattern are distinct phases of fever alternating with chills (typified by malaria). The Sanjiao shaoyang channel belongs to fire, and many of its points are effective in reducing fever. Zhongzhu SJ-3 is indicated for chills and fever, fever accompanied by headache, and especially for chronic malarial fever.

According to the *Classic of Difficulties*[5] shu-stream points are indicated for heaviness of the body and pain of the joints. Zhongzhu SJ-3 is an important point to circulate the qi of the channel and is indicated in the treatment of pain of the shoulder and elbow, pain of the spine (at the level of the Heart), numbness of the four limbs and inability to flex and extend the fingers.

COMBINATIONS

- Deafness: Zhongzhu SJ-3, Waiguan SJ-5, Erheliao SJ-22, Tinghui GB-2, Tinggong SI-19, Hegu L.I.-4, Shangyang L.I.-1 and Zhongchong P-9 (*Precious Mirror*).
- Deafness and tinnitus: Zhongzhu SJ-3, Tianrong SI-17, Tinggong SI-19 and Tinghui GB-2 (*Thousand Ducat Formulas*).
- Tinnitus: Zhongzhu SJ-3, Tinggong SI-19, Tinghui GB-2, Ermen SJ-21, Baihui DU-20, Luoque BL-8, Yangxi L.I.-5, Qiangu SI-2, Houxi SI-3, Wangu SI-4, Yemen SJ-2, Shangyang L.I.-1 and Shenshu BL-23 (*Great Compendium*).
- Ear pain, deafness and tinnitus: Zhongzhu SJ-3, Guanchong SJ-1, Yemen SJ-2, Tianchuang SI-16 and Yangxi L.I.-5, (*Thousand Ducat Formulas*).
- Visual dizziness: Zhongzhu SJ-3 and Toulinqi GB-15 (*Supplementing Life*).
- Throat pain: Zhongzhu SJ-3, Zhigou SJ-6 and Neiting ST-44 (*Thousand Ducat Formulas*).
- Swelling of the throat: Zhongzhu SJ-3 and Taixi KID-3 (*Supplementing Life*).
- Chronic malaria: Zhongzhu SJ-3, Shangyang L.I.-1 and Qiuxu GB-40 (*Great Compendium*).
- Malaria with generalised fever: Zhongzhu SJ-3, Yindu KID-19, Shaohai HE-3, Shangyang L.I.-1 and Sanjian L.I.-3 (*Supplementing Life*).
- Inability to bend the elbow and fingers: Zhongzhu SJ-3, Quchi L.I.-11, Shousanli L.I.-10 and Waiguan SJ-5 (*Great Compendium*).
- Pain of the elbow, at times cold: Zhongzhu SJ-3, Quchi L.I.-11, Guanchong SJ-1, Shousanli L.I.-10, Yanggu SI-5 and Chize LU-5 (*Thousand Ducat Formulas*).
- Contraction of the five fingers with inability to flex and extend: Zhongzhu SJ-3 and Wangu SI-4 (*Thousand Ducat Formulas*).

YANGCHI SJ-4

Yang Pool

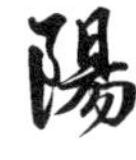
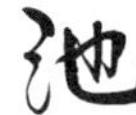

Yuan-Source point of the Sanjiao channel

LOCATION

On the dorsum of the wrist, at the level of the wrist joint, in the depression between the tendons of extensor digitorum communis and extensor digiti minimi.

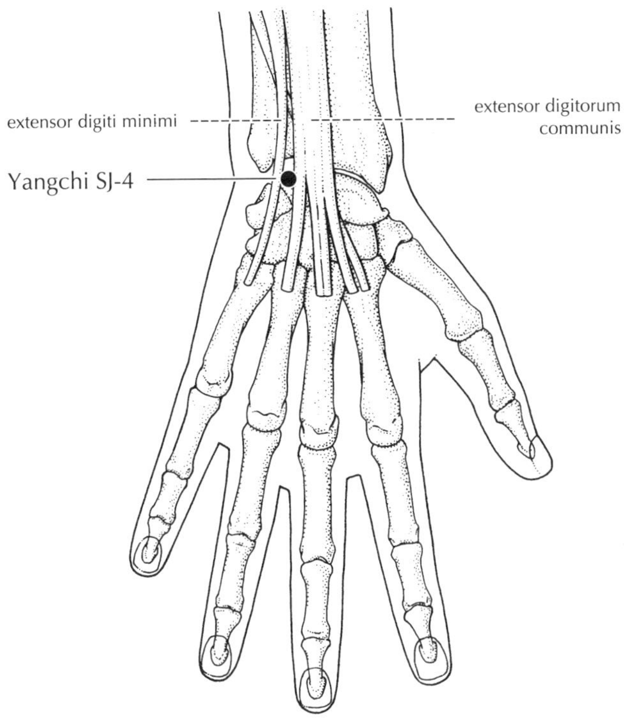

LOCATION NOTE

Follow the interspace between the fourth and fifth metacarpals proximally from Zhongzhu SJ-3 into the depression at the level of the wrist joint. This depression may be more clearly defined by extending the wrist and fingers, but the point should subsequently be needled with the tendons relaxed.

NEEDLING

i. Slightly oblique proximal insertion 0.3 to 0.5 cun; ii. Transverse insertion towards the radial side of the wrist beneath the tendons, 0.5 to 1 cun.

ACTIONS

Relaxes the sinews and alleviates pain
Clears heat

INDICATIONS

- Swelling and pain of the neck, pain of the shoulder and arm, weakness and pain of the wrist, redness and swelling of the wrist.
- Deafness, throat painful obstruction.
- Wasting and thirsting disorder, malaria, febrile disease with absence of sweating.
- Dry mouth with agitation and oppression, Heart pain with fullness of the chest.

COMMENTARY

The *Classic of Difficulties*[6] says " The Sanjiao is the envoy of the original qi ... the places where the original qi resides are known as the yuan source [points]". This passage therefore implies both that the original qi resides at the yuan-source points and that the Sanjiao is the transmitter of the original qi. As the yuan-source point of the Sanjiao channel, therefore, there is every reason to expect that Yangchi SJ-4 would be an important point to strengthen the original qi in the treatment of diseases of deficiency, and Yangchi SJ-4 is used for exactly this purpose in the Japanese tradition of acupuncture. It has also been suggested that Yangchi SJ-4 is effective to regulate the Conception and Penetrating vessels in the treatment of disordered menstruation. Examining the classical Chinese records on the use of Yangchi SJ-4, however, the following observations may be made: i. it appears in very few traditional combinations, ii. there are very few indications or combinations reflecting its effectiveness in tonifying deficiency, and iii. it has no gynaecological indications. It is interesting to note also that Zhigou SJ-6, rather than Yangchi SJ-4, is indicated for 'blockage of the Conception vessel in women'.

In clinical practice, Yangchi SJ-4 is principally used for local disorders of the wrist joint, including redness, swelling, weakness and pain.

Finally, in learning the names of the points of the yang channels at the wrist, it is helpful to remember their similarity: Yangxi L.I.-5 (Yang Stream), Yanggu SI-5 (Yang Valley) and Yangchi SJ-4 (Yang Pool).

COMBINATIONS

- Contraction of the arm with tightness of the sinews of both hands resulting in inability to open the hands: Yangchi SJ-4, Quchi L.I.-11, Chize LU-5, Hegu L.I.-4 and Zhongzhu SJ-3 (*Great Compendium*).

WAIGUAN SJ-5
Outer Pass

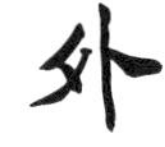

Luo-Connecting point of the Sanjiao channel
Confluent point of the Yang Linking vessel

LOCATION
2 cun proximal to Yangchi SJ-4, in the depression between the radius and the ulna, on the radial side of the extensor digitorum communis tendons.

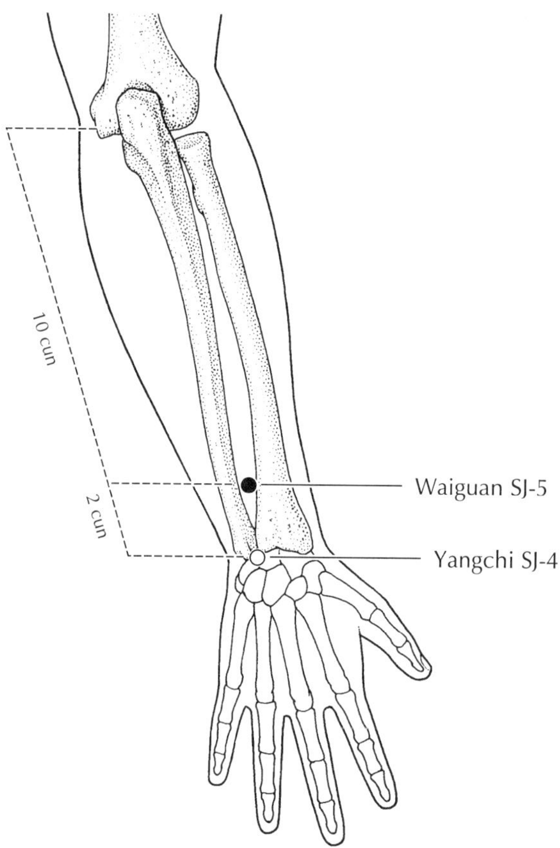

LOCATION NOTE
The point is located between the radius and the extensor digitorum communis tendons, close to the border of the radius.

NEEDLING
i. Slightly oblique insertion towards the ulnar side or oblique proximal or distal insertion towards the elbow or wrist respectively, 0.5 to 1.5 cun, ii. Joined by through-needling to Neiguan P-6.
Caution: movement of the patient's arm or hand after needling this point can result in a bent needle.

ACTIONS
Expels wind and releases the exterior
Benefits the head and ears
Opens the Yang Linking vessel
Clears heat
Activates the channel and alleviates pain

INDICATIONS
- Injury by cold, chills and fever, sweating with heat on the exterior, febrile disease.
- Headache, thunder head wind, head wind, Kidney deficiency headache, one-sided headache, pain of the vertex, frontal headache, pain of the nape, dizziness, phlegm inversion dizziness, wind dizziness, hypertension.
- Deafness, impaired hearing, tinnitus, pain of the ear, itching of the ear, redness, pain and swelling of the root of the ear.
- Redness, pain and swelling of the eyes, cold and pain of the eyes, superficial visual obstruction, lacrimation on exposure to wind, cold lacrimation.
- Swelling and pain of the cheek, stiffness of the tongue with difficulty in speaking, toothache, ulceration of the mouth, cracked lips, nosebleed, scrofula, mumps.
- Constipation, abdominal pain, oppression and tightness of the chest, pain of the lateral costal region, vomiting blood, knotting of heat in the five zang and six fu.
- Pain of the shoulder and back, stiff neck, pain of the ribs and lateral costal region, numbness and pain of the elbow and arm, contraction of the elbow, flaccidity of the elbow, soreness and heaviness of the elbow and wrist, swelling and redness of the arm, paralysis and numbness of the arm, hemiplegia, severe pain of the fingers with inability to grasp objects, coldness, numbness and pain of the hands and feet, tremor of the hand, redness, swelling and pain of the ankle, pain of the toes, pain of the hundred joints.

COMMENTARY
Waiguan SJ-5, the confluent point of the Yang Linking vessel, is the most important and frequently used distal point of the Sanjiao channel with wide clinical application. The Yang Linking vessel, which has no points of its own, links the six yang channels and the Governing vessel. Yang corresponds to the exterior while yin corresponds to the interior, and the yang channels as a whole therefore relate more to the exterior portion of the body. According to the *Classic of Difficulties*[7] "when the Yang Linking vessel is diseased, there will be severe chills and fever", whilst the *Song of Points for Miscellaneous Diseases*

says "use Waiguan SJ-5 for all wind, cold, summer-heat and damp pathogens, headaches and fever". In the *Ode of the Obstructed River* the use of Waiguan SJ-5 is referred to as one of the 'eight therapeutic methods'. In this description of the application of the eight confluent points of the extraordinary vessels to affect specific symptoms and areas of the body, Waiguan SJ-5 is indicated for injury by cold to the exterior accompanied by headache. These classical references emphasise two of the principle applications of Waiguan SJ-5 namely: i. dispelling exterior pathogenic factors, and ii. treating headache.

Exterior pathogenic factors attack the superficial portion of the body first, giving rise to the typical symptoms of chills and fever, and at this stage of progression the treatment principle is to release the exterior. In current clinical practice some authorities emphasise the special ability of Waiguan SJ-5 to resolve wind-heat and Hegu L.I.-4 to resolve wind-cold, whilst others take the opposite view. This inevitably raises the question of when to use Waiguan SJ-5 and when to use Hegu L.I.-4. Although there is no clear-cut answer, it is worth noting that whilst Hegu L.I.-4 is classically indicated for chills and fever accompanied by absence of sweating (characteristic of wind-cold), the only reference to sweating and Waiguan SJ-5 in classical sources is 'sweating with heat on the exterior' (characteristic of wind-heat). Hegu L.I.-4 belongs to yangming channel which dominates the central portion of the face and is strongly indicated for pathogenic factors giving rise to sneezing and nasal discharge, whilst Waiguan SJ-5 belongs to the Sanjiao channel which traverses the lateral portion of the neck and is indicated for swelling of the glands (including scrofula and mumps).

When wind-dampness attacks the body, in addition to chills and fever there is typically pain of the joints, and the *Classic of the Jade Dragon* recommends Waiguan SJ-5 for 'chills and fever and pain of the hundred joints'. In terms of the four levels theory of febrile diseases, Waiguan SJ-5 predominantly treats pathogens at the defensive and qi levels. In terms of the Sanjiao theory of differentiating fevers, it focuses on the more exterior upper jiao Lung pattern, rather than the Pericardium pattern. This is in contrast to points of its coupled Pericardium channel, which predominantly treat pathogens at the nutritive and blood levels according to four level theory, and the Pericardium pattern according to the Sanjiao theory.

As well as chills and fever, Waiguan SJ-5 is indicated for either wind-cold or wind-heat attacking the eyes and ears and giving rise to symptoms such as redness, pain and swelling, lacrimation, deafness and tinnitus etc.

Waiguan SJ-5 is classically indicated for many different kinds of headache, including temporal, vertex, frontal and occipital headaches as well as headache due to Kidney deficiency, head wind and 'thunder head wind' (severe headache with a thundering sound in the head). The widespread action of Waiguan SJ-5 on such varied kinds of headache may be explained by a number of different factors: i. as stated above, Waiguan SJ-5 is an important point to expel pathogenic factors and may be used in the treatment of headache due to penetration by wind-cold, wind-heat or wind-damp; ii. the Yang Linking vessel links all the yang channels (the occipital region is governed by the Governing vessel and taiyang channel, the temporal region by the Yang Linking vessel and shaoyang channel, and the frontal region by yangming channel); iii. the Sanjiao channel specifically connects with such important points for headaches as Benshen GB-13 through to Fengchi GB-20, Touwei ST-8 and Fengfu DU-16; iv. the Sanjiao and Gall Bladder shaoyang channels are linked according to six channel theory, and the Sanjiao channel intersects the Gall Bladder channel at points Tongziliao GB-1, Shangguan GB-3, Hanyan GB-4, Xuanli GB-6 and Jianjing GB-21, whilst the Gall Bladder and Liver channels are interiorly-exteriorly coupled. Waiguan SJ-5 is therefore an especially important point in the treatment of headaches due to Liver disharmony, especially when this gives rise to one-sided temporal headache (shaoyang region). For this purpose Waiguan SJ-5 is often combined with Gall Bladder channel points such as Zulinqi GB-41 (predominantly for headaches due to Liver qi stagnation, including premenstrual headaches), and Yangfu GB-38 and Xiaxi GB-43 (predominantly for headaches due to Liver fire or Liver yang rising).

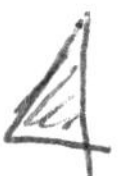

The Yang Linking vessel passes behind the ear whilst the Sanjiao channel both encircles and enters the ear. Waiguan SJ-5 is therefore an important point in the treatment of various ear disorders including tinnitus, deafness, earache and itching of the ear, and along with Zhongzhu SJ-3 is one of the principal distal points in the treatment of disorders of this region.

The Sanjiao channel belongs to fire and its internal pathway passes through all the three jiao. According to *Methods of Acupuncture and Moxibustion from the Golden Mirror of Medicine* Waiguan SJ-5 resolves knotting of heat in the five zang and six fu. Its action on clearing heat from the middle and lower jiao is reflected in its ability to treat constipation, abdominal pain, pain of the lateral costal region and vomiting, but it is especially effective in treating heat disorders of the head (swelling and pain of the cheek, nosebleed, toothache, ulceration of the mouth, cracked lips etc.) and clearing heat and fire poison from the Sanjiao channel in the neck (scrofula and mumps).

Waiguan SJ-5 is also a vital point in the treatment of a wide variety of channel disorders affecting the shoulder, arm, elbow, wrist, hand and fingers. In this respect it acts almost like a point of the hand yangming Large Intestine channel, and is often incorporated with Jianyu L.I.-15, Quchi L.I.-11 and Hegu L.I.-4 in the treatment of painful obstruction, atrophy disorder and hemiplegia of the upper limb. The action of Waiguan SJ-5 on the elbow region is emphasised in the *Great Compendium of Acupuncture and Moxibustion* which gives specific indications for excess and deficiency of the luo-connecting points. In the case of Waiguan SJ-5 these are contraction of the elbow (excess) and flaccidity of the elbow (deficiency).

Finally, Waiguan SJ-5 is the luo-connecting point of the Sanjiao channel from where the luo-connecting channel rises to converge with the Pericardium channel in the chest. Although this strengthens the Sanjiao-Pericardium relationship, with the exception of oppression and tightness of the chest there are no specific indications of this linkage. In clinical practice, however, the points Neiguan P-6 and Waiguan SJ-5 are often joined by through-needling for pain of the chest which radiates to the back.

COMBINATIONS

- Pain of the head and eyes: Waiguan SJ-5 and Houxi SI-3 (*Divine Moxibustion*).
- Impaired hearing and deafness: Waiguan SJ-5 and Huizong SJ-7 (*Thousand Ducat Formulas*).
- Impaired hearing and deafness: Waiguan SJ-5 and Tinghui GB-2 (*Supplementing Life*).
- Deafness: Waiguan SJ-5, Zhongzhu SJ-3, Shangyang L.I.-1, Erheliao SJ-22, Tinghui GB-2, Tinggong SI-19, Hegu L.I.-4 and Zhongchong P-9 (*Precious Mirror*).
- Deafness and tinnitus: Waiguan SJ-5 and Tianchuang SI-16 (*Supplementing Life*).
- Abdominal pain: Waiguan SJ-5 and Daling P-7 (*Song of the Jade Dragon*).
- Abdominal pain and constipation: Waiguan SJ-5, Zhigou SJ-6 and Daling P-7 (*Ode of the Jade Dragon*).
- Pain of the lateral costal region: Waiguan SJ-5, Zhigou SJ-6 and Zhangmen LIV-13 (*Great Compendium*).
- Inability to bend the elbow and fingers: Waiguan SJ-5, Zhongzhu SJ-3, Quchi L.I.-11 and Shousanli L.I.-10 (*Great Compendium*).
- Atrophy disorder and numbness of the arm: Waiguan SJ-5, Tianjing SJ-10 and Quchi L.I.-11 (*Thousand Ducat Formulas*).
- Sabre lumps of the axilla: Waiguan SJ-5, Zhigou SJ-6, Yuanye GB-22 and Zulinqi GB-41 (*Illustrated Supplement*).

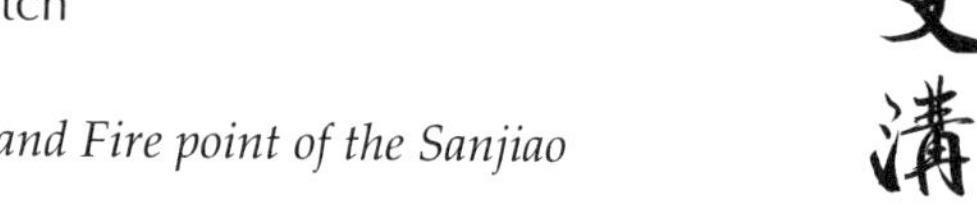

ZHIGOU SJ-6

Branch Ditch

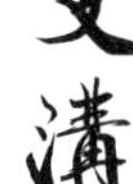

支溝

Jing-River and Fire point of the Sanjiao channel

LOCATION

3 cun proximal to Yangchi SJ-4, in the depression between the radius and the ulna, on the radial side of the extensor digitorum communis muscle.

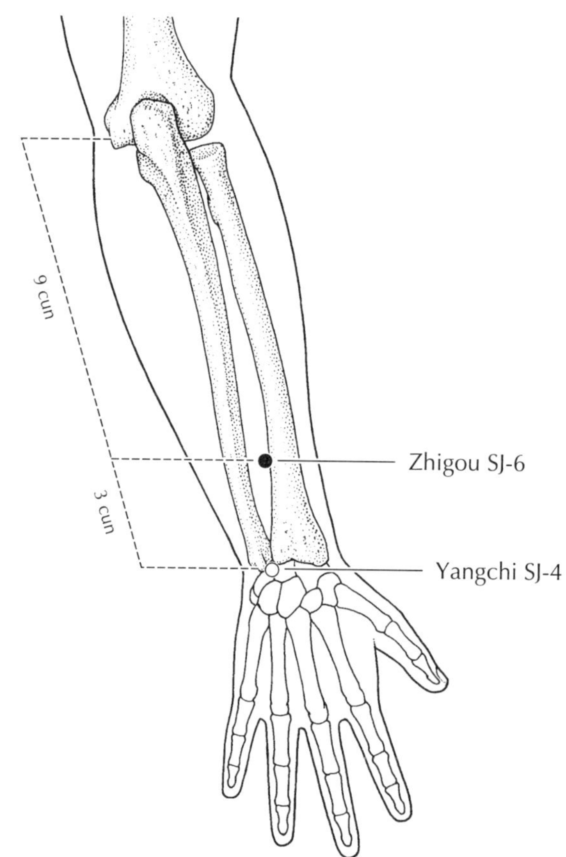

LOCATION NOTE

i. Divide the distance between Yangchi SJ-4 and the lateral epicondyle into half and then halve the distance between this midpoint and Yangchi SJ-4; ii. The point is located between the radius and the extensor digitorum communis muscle, close to the border of the radius.

NEEDLING

i. Slightly oblique insertion towards the ulnar side or oblique proximal or distal insertion towards the elbow or wrist respectively, 0.5 to 1.5 cun; ii. Joined by through-needling to Jianshi P-5.

Caution: movement of the patient's arm or hand after needling this point can result in a bent needle.

ACTIONS

Regulates qi and clears heat in the three jiao
Benefits the chest and lateral costal region
Moves the stool
Benefits the voice
Activates the channel and alleviates pain

INDICATIONS

- Tinnitus, heat-wind tinnitus and deafness, sudden loss of voice, lockjaw, febrile disease with absence of sweating, pain of the eyes, redness, swelling and pain of the eyes, swelling and pain of the throat, scrofula.
- Pain of the lateral costal region, abdominal pain, sudden Heart pain, Heart pain and oppression of the chest, cough, cough with redness and heat of the face.
- Constipation, vomiting, sudden turmoil disorder, post-partum dizziness, blockage of the Conception vessel in women.
- Pain of the axilla, pain of the shoulder, arm and back, painful obstruction of the elbow, tremor of the hand, cold-wind hand trembling, numbness of the hand, hemiplegia.

COMMENTARY

The Sanjiao theory divides the body into three regions, the upper jiao (the area above the diaphragm), the middle jiao (the area between the diaphragm and the umbilicus) and the lower jiao (the area below the umbilicus). Zhigou SJ-6, the jing-river and fire point of the Sanjiao channel, is the most important point on the Sanjiao channel for moving qi and clearing heat in these three areas. According to the *Song of the Primary Points of the Fourteen Channels* Zhigou SJ-6 is able to "drain ministerial fire from the three jiao". Ministerial fire, the primal fire of the body which has its root in the ming men and Kidneys, is 'entrusted' to the Liver, Gall Bladder and Sanjiao. The quotation above emphasises the clinical importance of Zhigou SJ-6 in clearing heat throughout the body, and especially resolving stagnant heat of the Liver and Gall Bladder.

In the upper jiao Zhigou SJ-6 is able to clear heat from the Sanjiao channel, being indicated for febrile diseases, redness, pain and swelling of the eyes, tinnitus and deafness, lockjaw, swollen throat, scrofula etc. It is also able to resolve stagnation of qi in the chest giving rise to oppression of the chest and Heart pain. If stagnant qi transforms into fire and insults the Lung there may be cough with a red face.

In the middle jiao it is an essential point for treating pain of the lateral costal region, and distention due to qi stagnation or any other aetiology. According to the *Ode to Elucidate Mysteries* "For pain of the ribs and lateral costal region needle the Flying Tiger [Feihu, an alternative name for Zhigou SJ-6]" whilst the *Song of the Jade Dragon* says "When there is pain of the lateral costal region with obstruction and knotting, using Zhigou SJ-6 will give extraordinarily wonderful results". Zhigou SJ-6 is also indicated for vomiting and sudden turmoil disorder, and may be used in situations where there is distention and bloating in the upper and lower abdomen, often extending to the chest, with Heart pain, oppression of the chest or cough.

In the lower jiao Zhigou SJ-6 is a major point for moving the qi of the intestines and treating constipation, whether due to stagnation of qi, heat or any other aetiology. In fact Zhigou SJ-6 and Waiguan SJ-5 are the only points on the three arm yang channels indicated for constipation, and of these two Zhigou SJ-6 has always been considered the pre-eminent. According to the *Great Compendium of Acupuncture and Moxibustion* Zhigou SJ-6 is also indicated for blockage of the Conception vessel in women, a further reflection of its ability to move stagnation.

According to the *Spiritual Pivot*[8] the jing-river points should be needled when there are "diseases manifesting in the patient's voice", and Zhigou SJ-6 is an important point (and included in a number of classical combinations) for sudden loss of voice.

Finally, Zhigou SJ-6 is indicated for various channel disorders affecting the whole upper limb, axilla, shoulder and back, including tremors, trembling and numbness of the hand. In current practice it is often combined with Xuanzhong GB-39 in the treatment of wandering painful obstruction.

COMBINATIONS

- Stabbing Heart pain: Zhigou SJ-6, Rangu KID-2 and Taixi KID-3 (*Thousand Ducat Formulas*).
- Pain of the chest and lateral costal region: Zhigou SJ-6 (reduce left Zhigou SJ-6 for right-sided pain and vice-versa) and (bleed) Weizhong BL-40 (*Classic of the Jade Dragon*).
- Pain of the lateral costal region due to injury by cold: Zhigou SJ-6 and Yanglingquan GB-34 (*Outline of Medicine*).
- Pain of the lateral costal region: Zhigou SJ-6, Zhangmen LIV-13 and Waiguan SJ-5 (*Great Compendium*).
- Pain of the lateral costal region: Zhigou SJ-6, Gongsun SP-4, Yanglingquan GB-34 and Zhangmen LIV-13 (*Complete Collection*).
- Sudden loss of voice : Zhigou SJ-6, Tianchuang SI-16, Futu L.I.-18, Qubin GB-7 and Lingdao HE-4 (*Thousand Ducat Formulas*).
- Sudden loss of voice: Zhigou SJ-6, Tonggu BL-66 and Sanyangluo SJ-8 (*Supplementing Life*).

- Vomiting and sudden turmoil disorder: Zhigou SJ-6 and Tianshu ST-25 (*Supplementing Life*).
- Sudden turmoil disorder: Zhigou SJ-6, Guanchong SJ-1, Juque REN-14, Gongsun SP-4 and Jiexi ST-41 (*Systematic Classic*).
- Constipation: Zhigou SJ-6 and Zhaohai KID-6 (*Ode of the Jade Dragon*).
- Deficiency constipation: reinforce Zhigou SJ-6 and reduce Zusanli ST-36 (*Song of Points*).
- Constipation: Zhigou SJ-6, Taibai SP-3, Zhaohai KID-6 and Zhangmen LIV-13 (*Great Compendium*).
- Abdominal pain and constipation: Zhigou SJ-6, Daling P-7 and Waiguan SJ-5 (*Ode of the Jade Dragon*).
- Scrofula: Zhigou SJ-6, Shaohai HE-3, Tianchi P-1, Zhangmen LIV-13, Zulinqi GB-41, Yangfu GB-38, Jianjing GB-21 and Shousanli L.I.-10 (*Great Compendium*).
- Post-partum dizziness: Zhigou SJ-6, Zusanli ST-36 and Sanyinjiao SP-6 (*Great Compendium*).
- Wandering painful obstruction: Zhigou SJ-6 and Xuanzhong GB-39.
- Stagnation of qi in the three jiao leading to distention, oppression and pain in the chest and abdomen: Zhigou SJ-6, Shanzhong REN-17, Zhongwan REN-12, Qihai REN-6 and Taichong LIV-3.
- Pain of the shoulder and back: Zhigou SJ-6, Houxi SI-3, Wangu SI-4, Fengmen BL-12, Jianjing GB-21, Zhongzhu SJ-3 and Weizhong BL-40 (*Great Compendium*).

HUIZONG SJ-7

Ancestral Meeting

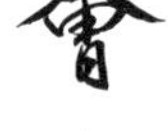
宗

Xi-Cleft point of the Sanjiao channel

LOCATION

3 cun proximal to Yangchi SJ-4, level with and on the ulnar side of Zhigou SJ-6, in the depression between the ulna and the extensor digitorum communis muscle.

LOCATION NOTE

i. Divide the distance between Yangchi SJ-4 and the lateral epicondyle into half and then halve the distance between this midpoint and Yangchi SJ-4; ii. The point lies approximately one fingerbreadth to the ulnar side of Zhigou SJ-6, close to the border of the ulna.

NEEDLING

Slightly oblique insertion towards the ulnar side or oblique proximal or distal insertion towards the elbow or wrist respectively, 0.5 to 1.5 cun.

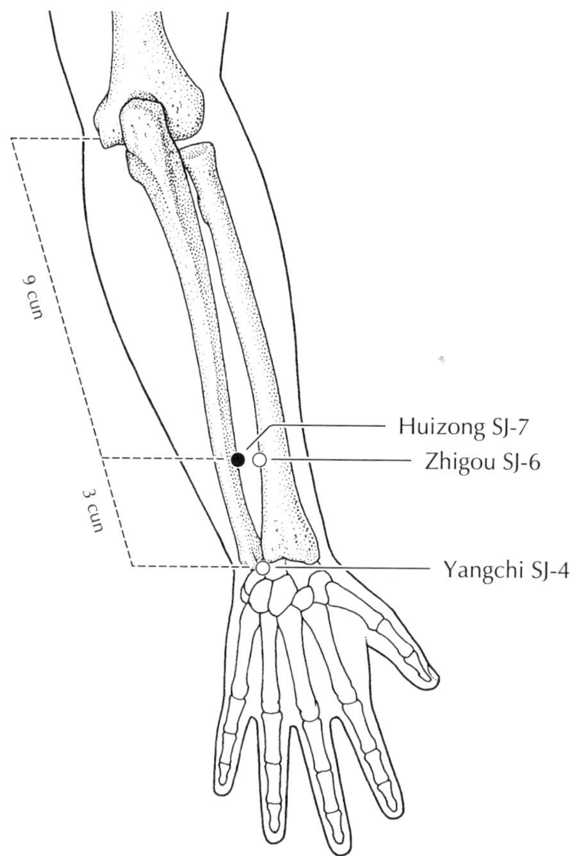

ACTIONS

Clears the Sanjiao channel and benefits the ears

INDICATIONS

- Deafness, tinnitus, epilepsy, pain of the skin and flesh.

COMBINATIONS

- Impaired hearing and deafness: Huizong SJ-7 and Waiguan SJ-5 (*Thousand Ducat Formulas*).
- Deafness: Huizong SJ-7, Yifeng SJ-17 and Xiaguan ST-7 (*Systematic Classic*).

SANYANGLUO SJ-8

Three Yang Luo

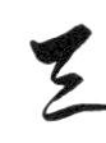
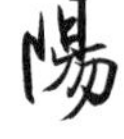
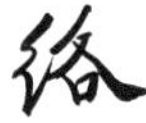

LOCATION

4 cun proximal to Yangchi SJ-4, in the depression between the radius and the ulna, on the radial side of the extensor digitorum communis muscle.

LOCATION NOTE

Divide the distance between Yangchi SJ-4 and the lateral epicondyle into three equal parts. Sanyangluo SJ-8 is located at the junction of the distal third and middle third.

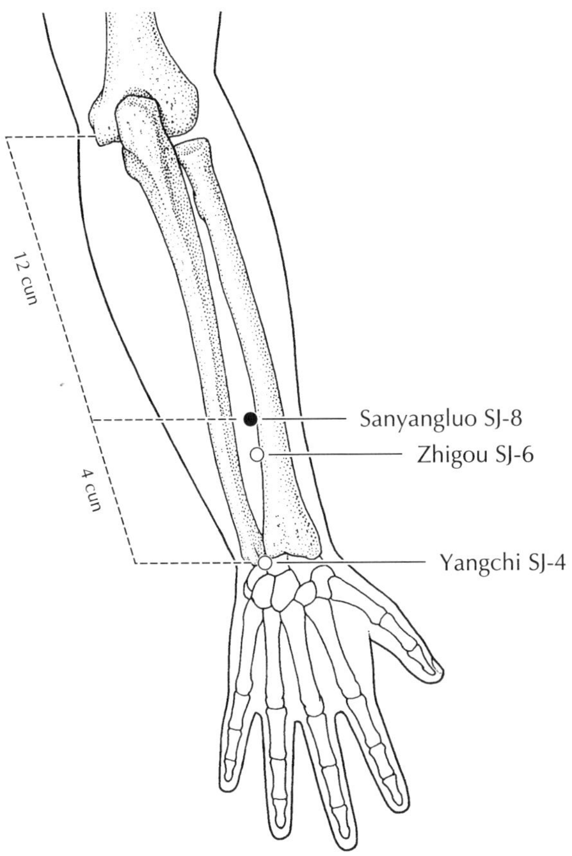

NEEDLING

i. Slightly oblique insertion towards the ulnar side or oblique proximal or distal insertion towards the elbow or wrist respectively, 0.5 to 1.5 cun. **Note:** according to the *Systematic Classic of Acupuncture and Moxibustion* and the *Illustrated Classic of Acupuncture Points on the Bronze Man* this point is contraindicated to needling.

ACTIONS

Clears the Sanjiao channel
Activates the channel and alleviates pain

INDICATIONS

- Sudden deafness, sudden loss of voice, toothache, somnolence, fever, no desire to move the limbs.
- Inability to move the arm, pain of the arm, lumbar pain due to traumatic injury.

COMMENTARY

The name Sanyangluo (Three Yang Luo) implies that this point is a meeting point of the three arm yang channels, in this respect mirroring Sanyinjiao SP-6 on the leg. From an examination of its indications, however, there seems little evidence to justify such a grand name. Sanyangluo SJ-8 does appear in various classical combinations for either sudden deafness or sudden loss of voice.

COMBINATIONS

- Sudden loss of voice: Sanyangluo SJ-8 and Yamen DU-15 (*Supplementing Life*).
- Sudden loss of voice: Sanyangluo SJ-8, Zhigou SJ-6 and Tonggu BL-66 (*Supplementing Life*).
- Sudden deafness: Sanyangluo SJ-8 and Yemen SJ-2 (*Supplementing Life*).
- Somnolence with no desire to move the four limbs: Sanyangluo SJ-8, Tianjing SJ-10, Zuwuli LIV-10, Lidui ST-45 and Sanjian L.I.-3 (*Thousand Ducat Formulas*).
- Pain of the chest and lateral costal region: Sanyangluo SJ-8, Dabao SP-21, Ximen P-4, Yangfu GB-38 and Zulinqi GB-41.

SIDU SJ-9

Four Rivers

四瀆

LOCATION

In the depression between the radius and the ulna, on a line drawn between Yangchi SJ-4 and the lateral epicondyle of the humerus, 7 cun proximal to Yangchi SJ-4.

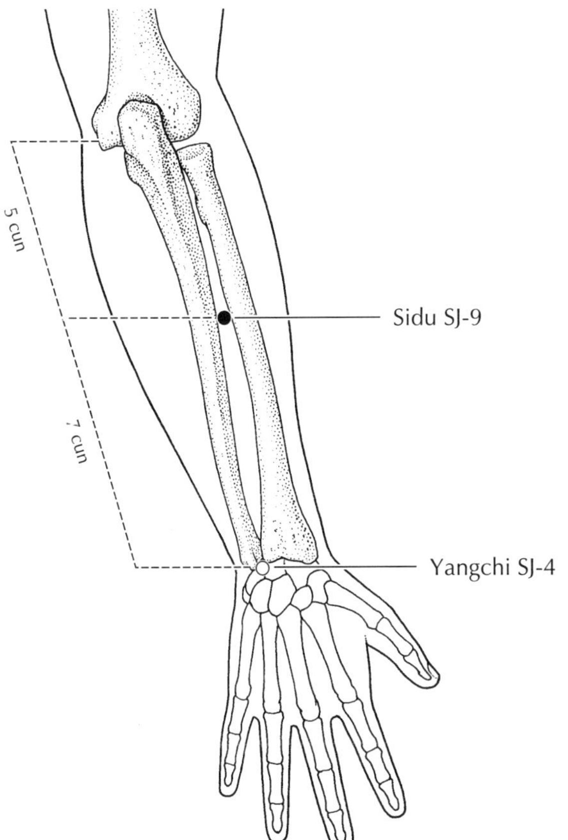

LOCATION NOTE
i. Divide the distance between Yangchi SJ-4 and the lateral epicondyle into half and then locate Sidu SJ-9 1 cun proximal to this midpoint; ii. The point is located in the depression between the muscle bellies of extensor digitorum communis and extensor carpi ulnaris.

NEEDLING
Perpendicular or oblique proximal or distal insertion towards the elbow or wrist respectively, 1 to 2 cun.

ACTIONS
Benefits the throat and ears

INDICATIONS
- Sudden loss of voice, obstruction of the throat, sore throat, sudden deafness, sudden tinnitus, toothache of the lower jaw, shortness of breath, pain of the forearm.

COMBINATIONS
- Sudden deafness: Sidu SJ-9 and Tianyou SJ-16 (*Supplementing Life*).
- Toothache of the lower jaw: Yanggu SI-5, Sidu SJ-9, Yemen SJ-2, Shangyang L.I.-1 and Erjian L.I.-2 (*Thousand Ducat Formulas*).

TIANJING SJ-10
Heavenly Well 天井

He-Sea and Earth point of the Sanjiao channel

LOCATION
With the elbow flexed, this point is located in the depression 1 cun proximal to the olecranon.

NEEDLING
Perpendicular insertion 0.5 to 1 cun.

ACTIONS
Transforms phlegm and dissipates nodules
Regulates qi and descends rebellion
Calms the spirit
Clears heat from the Sanjiao channel
Activates the channel and alleviates pain

INDICATIONS
- Scrofula, coughing phlegm, coughing and vomiting pus and blood, cough with fullness of the abdomen and no pleasure in eating or drinking, chest painful obstruction with Heart pain, pain of the lateral costal region, distention and pain of the lower abdomen.
- Epilepsy, madness, sadness, propensity to fright, fright palpitations, somnolence, leg qi attacking upwards, clonic spasm.
- One-sided headache, tongue thrusting, deafness, swelling and pain of the cheek, swelling and pain of the throat, throat painful obstruction with sweating, eye pain, malaria, alternating chills and fever, urticaria, haemorrhoids.
- Atrophy disorder and numbness of the arm, painful obstruction of the arm, wind painful obstruction with contraction of the sinews and pain of the bones, pain of the neck and upper back, pain of the scapula, numbness of the shoulder, pain of the shoulder and arm, pain of the elbow radiating to the shoulder, pain of the elbow, pain of the lumbar region due to traumatic injury.

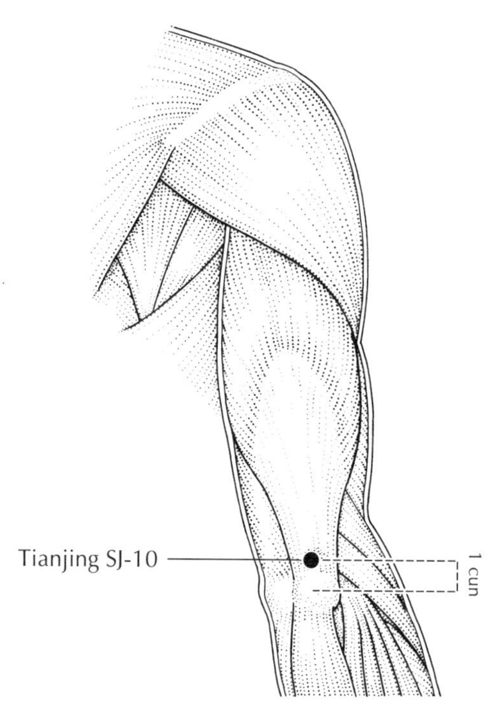

COMMENTARY
According to the *Classic of Difficulties*[9] "The Sanjiao is the pathway of water and grain". The Sanjiao therefore is the passageway for food and fluids throughout the body. When fluids stagnate and condense, whether due to stagnation of Liver qi, the condensing action of heat on the body fluids, or deficiency of any of the three zang responsible for fluid transformation and transportation (the Lung in the upper jiao, the Spleen in the middle jiao and the Kidneys in the lower jiao), phlegm will be generated. Tianjing SJ-10, the he-sea and earth point of the Sanjiao channel, has an important action on transforming phlegm and is indicated for a variety of phlegm patterns

including scrofula, coughing of phlegm and psycho-emotional disorders.

The disease known as scrofula, in which nodules appear on the side of the neck or in the axilla, always involves phlegm combined either with stagnant qi or heat. Tianjing SJ-10 is traditionally indicated and included in various classical combinations for the treatment of this disease.

According to the *Classic of Difficulties*[10] he-sea points are indicated for 'counterflow qi'. The Sanjiao channel enters the chest at Shanzhong REN-17, and Tianjing SJ-10, the he-sea point of the Sanjiao channel, is able to regulate rebellious qi and transform phlegm in the treatment of such disorders as coughing of phlegm, chest painful obstruction with Heart pain, and coughing and vomiting of pus and blood.

As a consequence of its action on transforming phlegm, and the coupled relationship of the Sanjiao and Pericardium channels, Tianjing SJ-10 is also important in the treatment of disturbance of the Heart and spirit by phlegm or phlegm-heat. It is indicated in such disorders as epilepsy, madness, propensity to fright, fright palpitations, sadness and somnolence.

Like many points of the Sanjiao channel, Tianjing SJ-10 is able to clear heat from and invigorate the qi in the upper part of the channel and is indicated for one-sided headache, deafness, swelling and pain of the cheek, obstructed throat, throat painful obstruction with sweating, eye pain etc.

Like Waiguan SJ-5 and Zhigou SJ-6, the action of Tianjing SJ-10 extends throughout the three jiao. As well as treating the head, neck, Lung and Heart in the upper jiao, it is indicated for pain of the lateral costal region in the middle jiao, and haemorrhoids and distention and pain of the abdomen in the lower jiao.

In modern clinical practice the principal application of Tianjing SJ-10 is in the treatment of pain, painful obstruction and atrophy disorder affecting the elbow, arm, shoulder, neck and upper back. There are also clear references in classical sources to its use in the treatment of wind painful obstruction affecting the entire body. This action of resolving painful obstruction is shared to a lesser extent by the two following points on this channel, Qinglengyuan SJ-11 and Xiaoluo SJ-12.

COMBINATIONS

- Scrofula: Tianjing SJ-10 and Shaohai HE-3 (*Song More Precious Than Jade*).
- Scrofula: Tianjing SJ-10 and Shaoze SI-1 (*Great Compendium*).
- Heart disorientation: Tianjing SJ-10, Juque REN-14 and Xinshu BL-15 (*Great Compendium*).
- Sadness, anxiety and disorientation: Tianjing SJ-10, Xinshu BL-15 and Shendao DU-11 (*Supplementing Life*).
- Fright palpitations: Yemen SJ-2, Tianjing SJ-10, Baihui DU-20 and Shendao DU-11 (*Supplementing Life*).
- Somnolence with no desire to move the four limbs: Tianjing SJ-10, Sanyangluo SJ-8, Zuwuli LIV-10, Lidui ST-45 and Sanjian L.I.-3 (*Thousand Ducat Formulas*).
- Chest painful obstruction, Heart pain and fullness of the Heart and abdomen: Tianjing SJ-10 and Shanzhong REN-17 (*Supplementing Life*).
- Chest painful obstruction and Heart pain: Tianjing SJ-10 and Zulinqi GB-41 (*Supplementing Life*).
- Clonic spasm: Tianjing SJ-10 and Fuyang BL-59 (*Supplementing Life*).
- Atrophy disorder and numbness of the arm: Tianjing SJ-10, Waiguan SJ-5 and Quchi L.I.-11 (*Thousand Ducat Formulas*).
- Wind painful obstruction: Tianjing SJ-10, Chize LU-5, Shaohai HE-3, Weizhong BL-40 and Yangfu GB-38 (*Great Compendium*).

QINGLENGYUAN SJ-11

Clear Cold Abyss

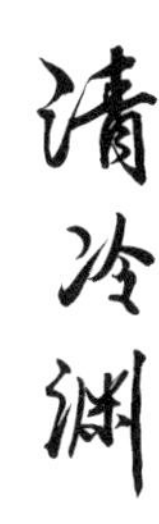

LOCATION

With the elbow flexed, this point is located 1 cun proximal to Tianjing SJ-10.

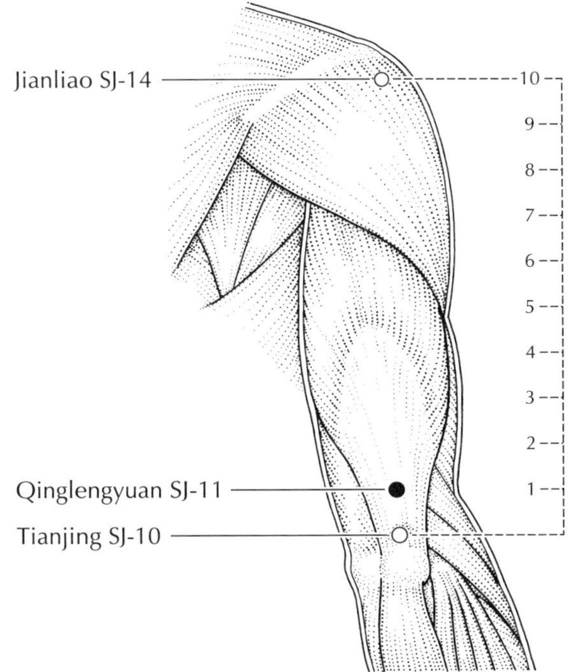

NEEDLING

Perpendicular insertion 0.5 to 1 cun.

ACTIONS

Activates the channel and dispels wind-damp
Clears damp-heat

INDICATIONS

- Headache, heaviness of the head with pain of the submandibular region, pain of the eyes, yellow eyes with pain of the lateral costal region, jaundice.
- Difficulty in raising the shoulder and arm and putting on clothes, painful obstruction of the shoulder and arm, fixed painful obstruction.

COMBINATIONS

- Inability to raise the shoulder and put on clothes: Qinglengyuan SJ-11 and Yanggu SI-5 (*Thousand Ducat Formulas*).

XIAOLUO SJ-12

Dispersing Luo River

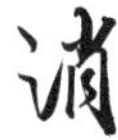

LOCATION

On the upper arm, on a line drawn between Tianjing SJ-10 and Jianliao SJ-14, 4 cun proximal to Tianjing SJ-10 and 6 cun distal to Jianliao SJ-14.

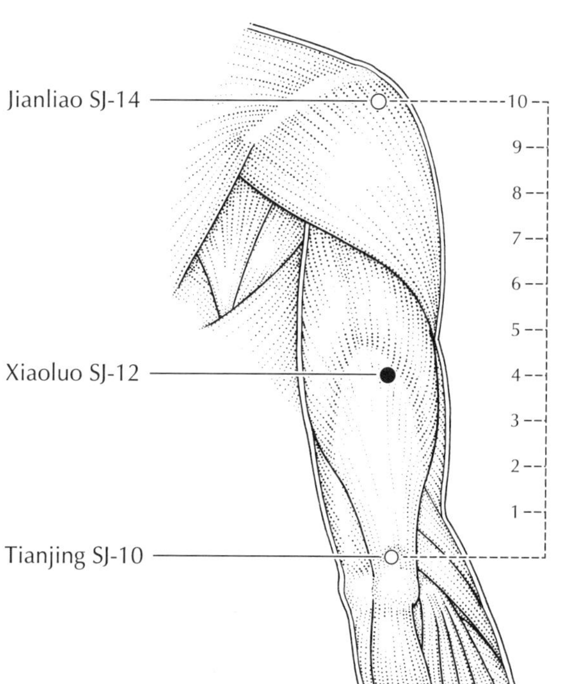

LOCATION NOTE

i. Divide the distance between Tianjing SJ-10 and Jianliao SJ-14 into half and locate this point 1 cun distal to this midpoint; ii. Locate in the depression within the triceps muscle, posterior to the shaft of the humerus (between the muscle bellies of the long and lateral heads of the triceps).

NEEDLING

Perpendicular or oblique insertion 1 to 2 cun.

ACTIONS

Activates the channel and alleviates pain

INDICATIONS

- Stiffness and pain of the nape and back with inability to turn the head, pain of the shoulder and arm, wind painful obstruction.
- Headache, chills and fever, dizziness, toothache, madness.

COMBINATIONS

- Pain of the nape of the neck: Xiaoluo SJ-12 and Touqiaoyin GB-11 (*Supplementing Life*).

NAOHUI SJ-13

Upper Arm Meeting

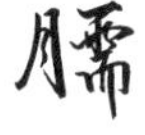

Meeting point of the Sanjiao channel and the Yang Linking vessel

LOCATION

On the upper arm, where the line drawn between Tianjing SJ-10 and Jianliao SJ-14 meets the posterior border of the deltoid muscle, approximately two thirds of the distance between these two points.

LOCATION NOTE

i. Locate in the depression within the triceps muscle, posterior to the shaft of the humerus (between the muscle bellies of the long and lateral heads of the triceps); ii. Although most sources specify both a distance of 3 cun from Jianliao SJ-14 and a location at the posterior border of the deltoid muscle, these do not usually correspond. In practice, palpate the region of this point to find the most tender location.

NEEDLING

Perpendicular or oblique insertion 1 to 2 cun.

ACTIONS

Regulates qi and transforms phlegm
Activates the channel and alleviates pain

INDICATIONS
- Goitre, scrofula, chills and fever, eye diseases, epilepsy, madness.
- Weakness and pain of the shoulder and arm, swelling of the shoulder that leads to pain in the scapula, inability to raise the arm.

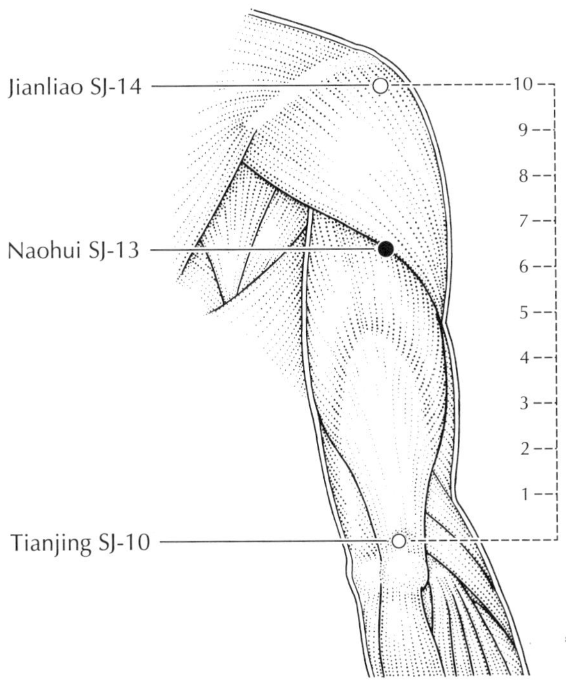

COMMENTARY
Like several of its neighbouring points (e.g. Tianfu LU-3, Shouwuli L.I.-13, Binao L.I.-14, Jianyu L.I.-15, Tianjing SJ-10 and Naohui SJ-13), Naohui SJ-13 is indicated for scrofula and goitre. These two disorders, although different in aetiology, always involve phlegm combined either with stagnant qi or with heat. In the case of Naohui SJ-13, its ability to treat these disorders derives partly from the pathways of the Sanjiao channel and the Yang Linking vessel, which pass through the neck, and partly from the inherent relationship of the Sanjiao to the transformation of fluids and the circulation of qi. Ultimately, however, there is no clear theoretical explanation why points of the upper arm, rather than more distal points, have a special action on these disorders, and this is primarily the fruit of empirical observation and clinical practice. Like Binao L.I.-14, Naohui SJ-13 is also indicated for eye disorders.

The more common clinical application of Naohui SJ-13 is for pain of the upper arm, or for shoulder pain which radiates down the upper arm.

COMBINATIONS
- Goitre: Naohui SJ-13 and Tianchuang SI-16 (*Systematic Classic*).
- Goitre, tumours of the neck and swollen throat: Naohui SJ-13, Tianfu LU-3 and Qishe ST-11 (*Thousand Ducat Formulas*).
- Painful obstruction with difficulty bending and extending the elbow joint, pain and heaviness of the arm with acute pain of the axilla: Naohui SJ-13, Tianfu LU-3 and Qishe ST-11 (*Thousand Ducat Formulas*).

JIANLIAO SJ-14
Shoulder Crevice

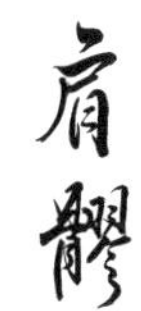

LOCATION
At the origin of the deltoid muscle, in the depression which lies posterior and inferior to the lateral extremity of the acromion.

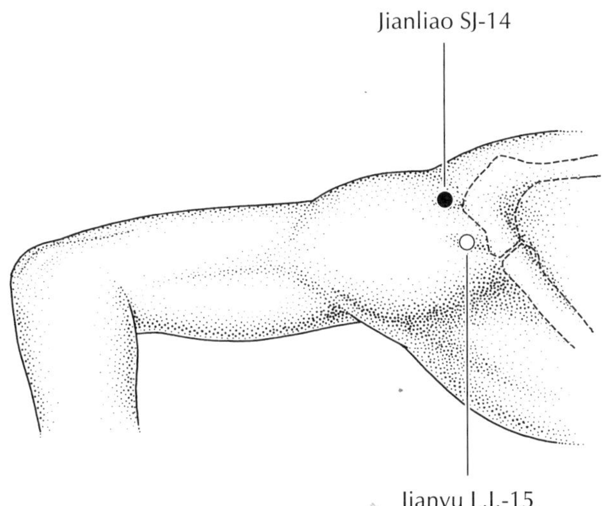

LOCATION NOTE
i. Locate with the arm abducted in order to enhance the depression; ii. Note that Jianyu L.I.-15 is located in the depression which lies anterior and inferior to the lateral extremity of the acromion.

NEEDLING
i. With the arm abducted, perpendicular insertion directed towards the centre of the axilla, 1 to 1.5 cun; ii. Transverse-oblique insertion directed distally towards the elbow, 1.5 to 2 cun.

ACTIONS
Dispels wind-damp
Alleviates pain and benefits the shoulder joint

INDICATIONS
- Shoulder pain, heaviness of the shoulder with inability to raise the arm, numbness, paralysis and pain of the arm.

COMMENTARY
Jianliao SJ-14 is an important point for treating all disorders of the shoulder joint, especially the posterior aspect. Stiffness, pain, immobility and weakness of the shoulder or frozen shoulder may derive from: i. injury by exterior pathogenic wind, cold, damp or heat, ii. stagnation of qi and blood from traumatic injury or overuse, or iii. deficiency of qi and blood from overuse, old age or prolonged obstruction of the channel. In all these cases Jianliao SJ-14 may be used, and in clinical practice is commonly combined with Jianyu L.I.-15.

COMBINATIONS
- Pain of the arm: Jianliao SJ-14, Tianzong SI-11 and Yanggu SI-5 (*Supplementing Life*).
- Frozen shoulder: first needle Tiaokou ST-38 and ask the patient to rotate the shoulder whilst manipulating the needle. Then needle Jianliao SJ-14, Jianyu L.I.-15, Binao L.I.-14, Hegu L.I.-4 and Waiguan SJ-5.

TIANLIAO SJ-15
Heavenly Crevice

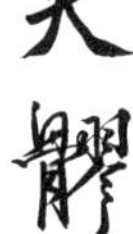

Meeting point of the Sanjiao and Gall Bladder channels and the Yang Linking vessel

LOCATION
In the suprascapular fossa, in the depression midway between Jianjing GB-21 and Quyuan SI-13 (at the medial end of the suprascapular fossa).

LOCATION NOTE
This point may also be located midway between the lateral extremity of the acromion and Dazhui DU-14, and 1 cun posterior to Jianjing GB-21 (the highest point of the trapezius muscle).

NEEDLING
Oblique insertion directed according to the clinical manifestations, 0.5 to 1 cun.
Caution: perpendicular insertion, especially in thin patients, carries a substantial risk of inducing a pneumothorax.

ACTIONS
Dispels wind-damp, activates the channel and alleviates pain
Unbinds the chest and regulates qi

INDICATIONS
- Pain of the shoulder and arm, stiffness and pain of the neck, tension of the nape of the neck, pain in the supraclavicular fossa.
- Agitation and oppression of the chest, heat and fullness of the chest, oppression of the Heart with absence of sweating, heat in the body with absence of sweating, chills and fever, febrile disease.

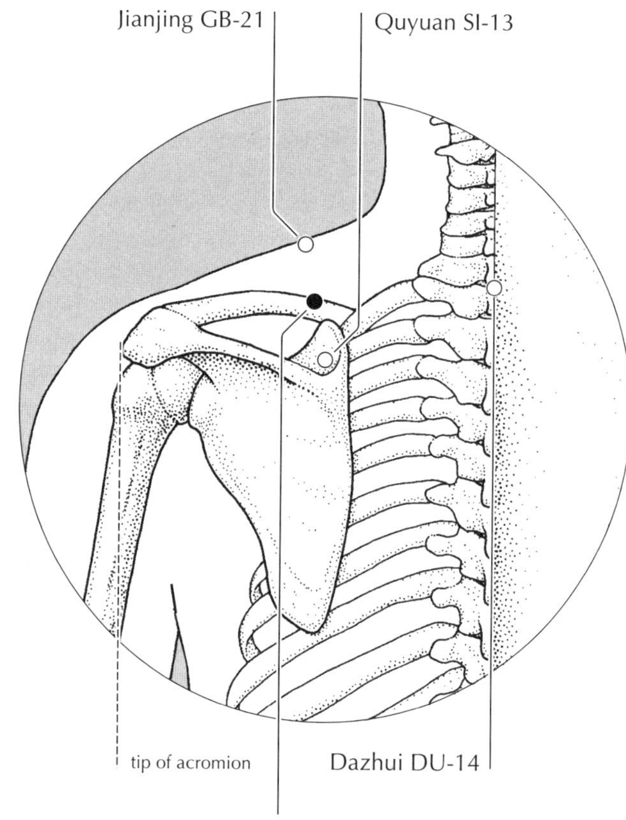

COMMENTARY
Tianliao SJ-15 and Jianjing GB-21 are neighbouring points with a similar effect in the treatment of stiffness, pain and spasm in the area between the shoulder joint and the neck. In such situations they should both be palpated, and the more tender should be needled. Like Jianjing GB-21, the action of Tianliao SJ-15 also extends downwards into the chest, where it is indicated for agitation, oppression, heat and fullness.

COMBINATIONS
- Pain and heaviness of the shoulder with inability to raise the arm: Tianliao SJ-15 and Quchi L.I.-11 (*Supplementing Life*).

TIANYOU SJ-16

Window of Heaven

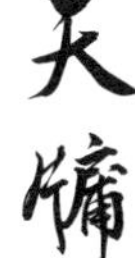

Point of the Window of Heaven

LOCATION

On the posterior border of the sternocleidomastoid muscle, approximately 1 cun inferior to Wangu GB-12, on a line drawn between Tianzhu BL-10 and Tianrong SI-17.

NEEDLING

Perpendicular insertion, 0.5 to 1 cun.

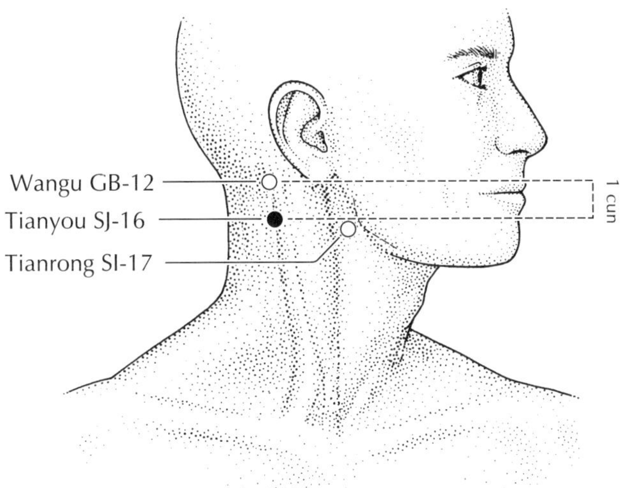

ACTIONS

Benefits the head and sense organs
Regulates and descends qi

INDICATIONS

- Sudden deafness, impaired hearing, dimness of vision, pain of the eyes with inability to see, inability to open the eyes, lacrimation, rhinitis with nosebleed, loss of sense of smell, stuffy nose.
- Wind dizziness, headache, head wind, swollen face, swelling of the submandibular region, throat painful obstruction, scrofula, swelling of the breast, malaria, confused dreaming.
- Stiffness and pain of the neck with inability to turn the head, swelling of the supraclavicular fossa.

COMMENTARY

Tianyou SJ-16 is one of five points referred to in Chapter 21 of the *Spiritual Pivot* as points of the 'Window of Heaven' (see page 48 for a fuller discussion), and in this passage it is said "Sudden deafness with excess of qi, dimness of vision and hearing, select Tianyou SJ-16". Tianyou SJ-16 (Window of Heaven) in fact gave this group of points its name. In his commentary on the above passage, Zhou Zhi-cong said "The points and the orifices of the head and face are like the great windows of a high pavilion by virtue of which qi moves. When there is inversion qi below, then the channels in the upper region do not move and there is lack of clarity of vision and hearing ... ".

In common with the other points of the Window of Heaven, Tianyou SJ-16 is able to regulate and balance the qi between the head and the body, and is indicated when inversion qi (chaotic and rebellious qi) rushes to the head. This gives rise to such symptoms as headache and dizziness, sudden onset of deafness, swelling of the face and disorders of the eyes and nose. Also in common with other Window of Heaven points, Tianyou SJ-16 treats scrofula.

COMBINATIONS

- Sudden deafness: Tianyou SJ-16 and Sidu SJ-9 (*Thousand Ducat Formulas*).
- Wind dizziness and headache: Tianyou SJ-16, Fengmen BL-12, Kunlun BL-60, Guanchong SJ-1 and Guanyuan REN-4 (*Thousand Ducat Formulas*).
- Swelling of the face: first needle Yixi BL-45, then Tianyou SJ-16 and Fengchi GB-20 (*Systematic Classic*).
- Nasal discharge with inability to distinguish the fragrant from the foul: Tianyou SJ-16 and Renzhong DU-26 (*Thousand Ducat Formulas*).
- Lacrimation: Tianyou SJ-16 and Xinshu BL-15 (*Thousand Ducat Formulas*).
- Pain of the shoulder and back: Tianyou SJ-16, Quepen ST-12, Shendao DU-11, Dazhu BL-11, Tiantu REN-22, Shuidao ST-28 and Jugu L.I.-16 (*Thousand Ducat Formulas*).
- Stiffness of the neck with inability to turn the head: Tianyou SJ-16 and Houxi SI-3 (*Supplementing Life*).
- Tired throat, swelling of the neck with inability to turn the head, swelling of the cheek that radiates to the ear: Tianyou SJ-16, Wangu GB-12 and Qiangu SI-2 (*Thousand Ducat Formulas*).

YIFENG SJ-17

Wind Screen

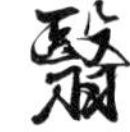
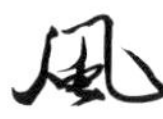

Meeting point of the Sanjiao and Gall Bladder channels

LOCATION

Behind the earlobe, between the ramus of the mandible and the mastoid process, in the depression just superior to the palpable transverse process of the first cervical vertebra.

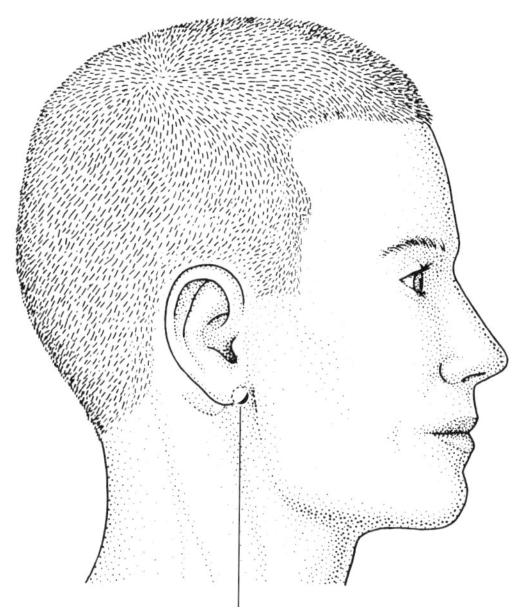

Yifeng SJ-17 (behind earlobe)

LOCATION NOTE

Fold the earlobe forwards to reveal this point.

NEEDLING

Perpendicular insertion, directed towards the opposite ear, 0.5 to 1 cun. **Note**: if the needle is directed too anteriorly or posteriorly, pain will ensue and may cause discomfort on opening and closing the mouth for some while after treatment.

ACTIONS

Benefits the ears
Eliminates wind
Clears heat
Activates the channel and alleviates pain

INDICATIONS

- Deafness, tinnitus, discharge from the ear, damp itching of the inside of the ear, redness pain and swelling of the ear, earache.
- Deviation of the mouth and eye, loss of speech, tetany with inability to speak, lockjaw, pain and swelling of the cheek, toothache of the lower jaw, pain of the teeth and gums, mumps, scrofula, superficial visual obstruction with dimness of vision.
- Mania disorder, clonic spasm.

COMMENTARY

Yifeng SJ-17 is a meeting point of the Sanjiao and Gall Bladder channels, both of which enter the ear, and is an essential local point in the treatment of all ear disorders including tinnitus, deafness, discharge, itching, redness, swelling and pain.

As the name of this point (Wind Screen) indicates, Yifeng SJ-17 has an action on expelling exterior pathogenic wind and treating the manifestations of internal wind, and is used widely for facial paralysis due to windstroke or Bell's palsy, trigeminal neuralgia, spasm and lockjaw.

Through its action of clearing heat and circulating the channel, Yifeng SJ-17 is also indicated for local disorders such as mumps, scrofula, swelling of the cheek and toothache.

COMBINATIONS

- Purulent ear sores with discharge: Yifeng SJ-17, Hegu L.I.-4 and Ermen SJ-21 (*Great Compendium*).
- Deafness: Yifeng SJ-17, Huizong SJ-7 and Xiaguan ST-7 (*Systematic Classic*).
- Deafness due to qi obstruction: Yifeng SJ-17, Tinggong SI-19 and Tinghui GB-2; then needle Zusanli ST-36 and Hegu L.I.-4 (*Great Compendium*).
- Sudden loss of speech: Yifeng SJ-17 and Tongli HE-5 (*Supplementing Life*).
- Toothache and tooth decay: Yifeng SJ-17, Xiaguan ST-7, Daying ST-5 and Wangu SI-4 (*Supplementing Life*).
- Lockjaw: Yifeng SJ-17 and Tianchuang SI-16 (*Supplementing Life*).
- Facial paralysis: Yifeng SJ-17, Dicang ST-4, Jiache ST-6, Xiaguan ST-7, Sibai ST-2 and Hegu L.I.-4.

QIMAI SJ-18

Spasm Vessel

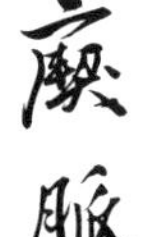

LOCATION

Posterior to the ear, in a small depression on the mastoid bone, one third of the distance along a curved line drawn from Yifeng SJ-17 to Jiaosun SJ-20 following the line of the rim of the ear.

NEEDLING

Subcutaneous insertion along the course of the channel 0.3 to 0.5 cun, or prick to bleed.

ACTIONS
Benefits the ears
Calms fright and pacifies wind

INDICATIONS
- Tinnitus, deafness, pain behind the ear.
- Headache, head wind, vomiting, diarrhoea, seminal emission, discharge from the eye, dimness of vision.
- Infantile fright epilepsy, clonic spasm, fright and fear.

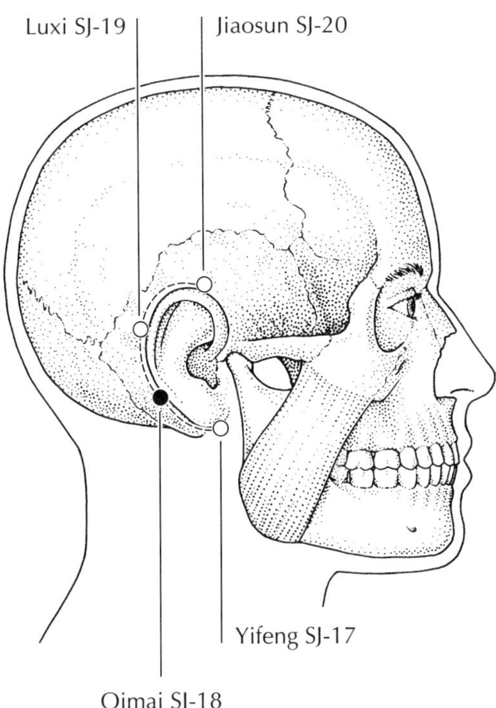

COMBINATIONS
- Childhood epileptic convulsions, vomiting and diarrhoea, fright and fear: Qimai SJ-18 and Changqiang DU-1 (*Systematic Classic*).
- Head wind and pain behind the ear: Qimai SJ-18 and Wangu GB-12 (*Supplementing Life*).
- Wind headache: Qimai SJ-18, Zanzhu BL-2, Chengguang BL-6, Shenshu BL-23, Sizhukong SJ-23 and Erheliao SJ-22 (*Thousand Ducat Formulas*).

LUXI SJ-19
Skull's Rest

顱息

LOCATION
Posterior to the ear, in a small depression two thirds of the distance along a curved line drawn from Yifeng SJ-17 to Jiaosun SJ-20 following the line of the rim of the ear.

NEEDLING
Subcutaneous insertion along the course of the channel 0.3 to 0.5 cun, or prick to bleed. **Note**: according to several classical texts, this point is contraindicated to bleeding.

ACTIONS
Benefits the ears and clears heat
Calms fright and relieves tetany

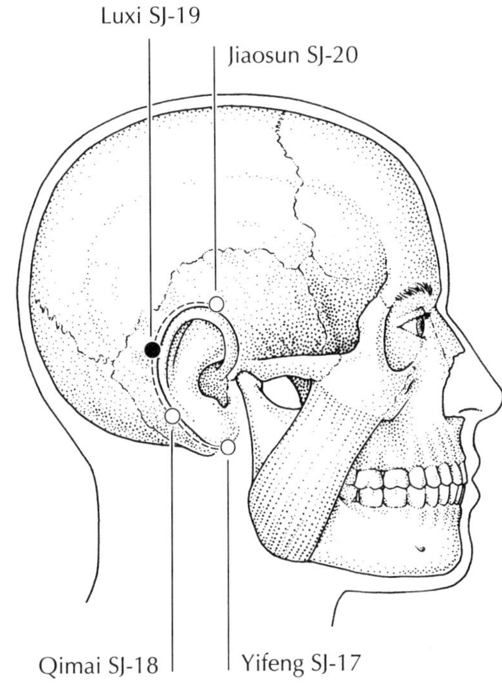

INDICATIONS
- Deafness, tinnitus, ear pain, discharge of pus from the ear, itching of the face, redness and swelling of the corner of the forehead (in the region of Touwei ST-8).
- Headache, heavy head, one-sided headache, heat in the body with headache and inability to sleep, dizziness, childhood epilepsy, tetany, fright and fear, childhood vomiting of foamy (watery) saliva, vomiting and drooling, pain of the chest and lateral costal region, dyspnoea, seminal emission.

COMMENTARY
Although this point is rarely used clinically, the *Ode to the One Hundred Symptoms* stated unequivocally "tetany cannot be treated successfully without Luxi SJ-19". Tetany is a disorder characterised by stiffness and rigidity of the neck and back, lockjaw, twitching of the limbs, opisthotonos etc.

COMBINATIONS

- Pain of the lateral costal region with inability to turn the body: Luxi SJ-19 and Benshen GB-13 (*Thousand Ducat Formulas*).
- One-sided headache: Luxi SJ-19, Fengchi GB-20, Taiyang (M-HN-9), Waiguan SJ-5 and Jianjing GB-21.

JIAOSUN SJ-20

Minute Angle

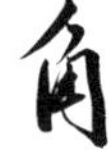
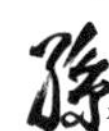

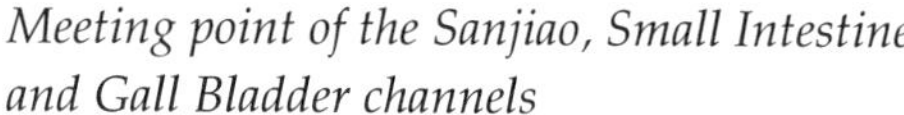
Meeting point of the Sanjiao, Small Intestine and Gall Bladder channels

LOCATION

On the side of the head, directly level with the apex of the ear when the ear is folded forwards.

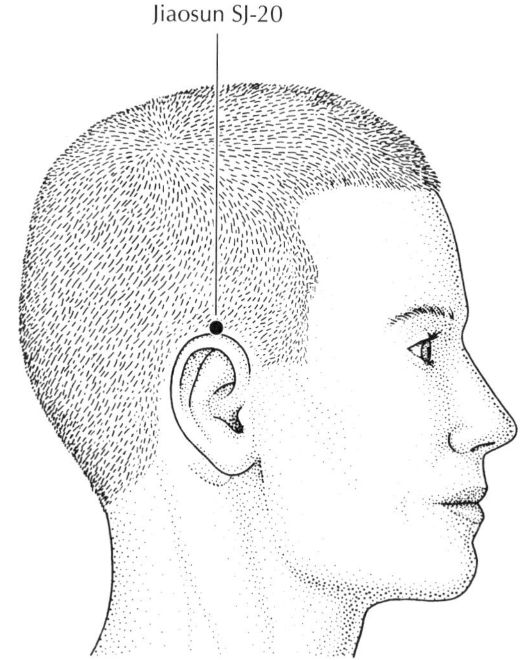

LOCATION NOTE

Fold the ear so that the posterior part of the upper helix directly covers the anterior part of the upper helix. Take care not to push the whole of the ear forwards.

NEEDLING

Transverse insertion 0.5-1.5 cun. **Note:** this point, in common with all points within the hairline, may be needled anteriorly, posteriorly, inferiorly or superiorly. Direction depends on symptomatology, in other words direct needle either towards where the headache or other pain radiates, or join up to connect with other head points. The needle should be inserted within the subcutaneous layers close to the bone of the skull, rather than more shallowly.

ACTIONS

Benefits the ears
Benefits the teeth, gums and lips
Clears heat

INDICATIONS

- Tinnitus, deafness, discharge of pus from the ear, redness and swelling of the back of the ear, redness and swelling of the auricle.
- Toothache, tooth decay, swelling and pain of the gums with inability to masticate, stiffness of the lips, dryness of the lips, superficial visual obstruction, stiffness of the nape of the neck with inability to turn the head.

COMMENTARY

Although rarely used clinically, it is interesting to note that Jiaosun SJ-20 was traditionally indicated, and appeared in combination, for swelling and pain of the gums, dryness of the lips, inability to chew, toothache and tooth decay, and as such may be viewed as a useful adjacent point for such disorders. As far as stiffness of the lips is concerned, it is notable that of the few points that are traditionally said to treat these disorders, the majority (for example Jiaosun SJ-20, Ermen SJ-21, Shangguan GB-3, Zhengying GB-17) are in the region of the ear.

COMBINATIONS

- Pain of the gums: Jiaosun SJ-20 and Xiaohai SI-8 (*Great Compendium*).
- Inability to chew: Jiaosun SJ-20 and Jiache ST-6 (*Thousand Ducat Formulas*).

ERMEN SJ-21

Ear Gate

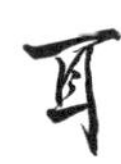
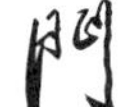

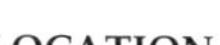
LOCATION

In the depression anterior to the supratragic notch and slightly superior to the condyloid process of the mandible.

LOCATION NOTE

In order to locate this point, ask the patient to open the mouth so that the condyloid process of the mandible slides forwards to reveal the depression. This point is needled with the mouth open. Following needling the mouth can be closed.

NEEDLING

Inferior oblique insertion, slightly posteriorly, 0.5 to 1 cun. **Note**: many classical sources prohibit moxibustion at this point in cases of discharge of pus from the ear.

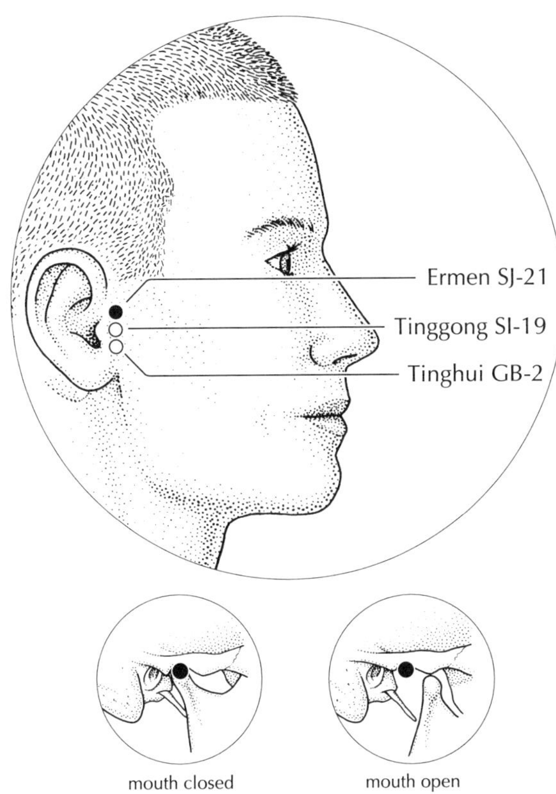

ACTIONS

Benefits the ears
Clears heat

INDICATIONS

- Tinnitus, deafness, impaired hearing, earache, discharge of pus from the ear, swelling of the ear, ear sores.
- Toothache, tooth decay, swelling and pain of the submandibular region, stiffness of the lips, headache, lockjaw, neck pain.

COMMENTARY

Ermen SJ-21 is the uppermost of three points anterior to the ear, the others being Tinggong SI-19 and Tinghui GB-2. All are frequently employed for the treatment of a wide variety of ear disorders including tinnitus, deafness, pain, itching and discharge. Due to the close proximity of these points and the similar indications for each, it is difficult to distinguish between them clinically. If it is necessary to needle points around the ear regularly, then these three points should be alternated.

Like Jiaosun SJ-20, Ermen SJ-21 is also indicated for toothache, tooth decay and stiffness of the lips.

Finally it is interesting to note that according to the arrangement of the Sanjiao channel points in the *Great Compendium of Acupuncture and Moxibustion* Ermen SJ-21 is the last point of the channel.

COMBINATIONS

- Purulent ear sores with discharge: Ermen SJ-21, Yifeng SJ-17 and Hegu L.I.-4 (*Great Compendium*).
- Impaired hearing and deafness: Ermen SJ-21, Fengchi GB-20, Xiaxi GB-43, Tinghui GB-2 and Tinggong SI-19 (*Great Compendium*).
- Tinnitus with lumbar pain: first needle Renying ST-9, then needle Ermen SJ-21 and Zusanli ST-36 (*Secrets of the Celestial Star*).
- Tinnitus: Ermen SJ-21, Tinggong SI-19, Tinghui GB-2, Baihui DU-20, Luoque BL-8, Yangxi L.I.-5, Qiangu SI-2, Houxi SI-3, Wangu SI-4, Zhongzhu SJ-3, Yemen SJ-2, Shangyang L.I.-1 and Shenshu BL-23 (*Great Compendium*).
- Stiffness of the lips and pain from tooth decay of the upper jaw: Ermen SJ-21, Duiduan DU-27, Muchuang GB-16 and Zhengying GB-17 (*Thousand Ducat Formulas*).
- Toothache: Ermen SJ-21 and Sizhukong SJ-23 (*One Hundred Symptoms*).

ERHELIAO SJ-22

Ear Harmony Crevice

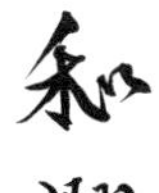

Meeting point of the Sanjiao, Gall Bladder and Small Intestine channels

LOCATION

Approximately 0.5 cun anterior to the upper border of the root of the ear, in a slight depression on the posterior border of the hairline of the temple.

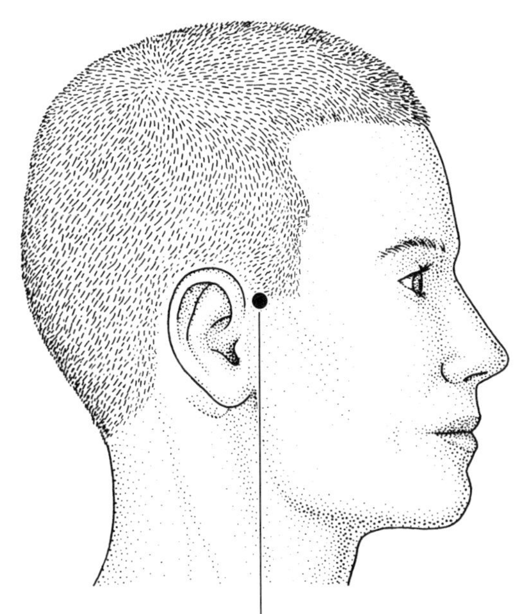

LOCATION NOTE

This point lies just posterior to where the superficial temporal artery can be palpated.

NEEDLING

Transverse insertion 0.3 to 0.5 cun.

ACTIONS

Expels wind and alleviates pain

INDICATIONS

- Tinnitus, pain and heaviness of the head, headache, head wind, swelling and pain of the tip of the nose, nasal discharge, deviation of the mouth, lockjaw, swelling of the submandibular region and neck, clonic spasm.

COMBINATIONS

- Deafness: Erheliao SJ-22, Zhongzhu SJ-3, Waiguan SJ-5, Tinghui GB-2, Tinggong SI-19, Hegu L.I.-4, Shangyang L.I.-1 and Zhongchong P-9 (*Precious Mirror*).
- Wind headache: Erheliao SJ-22, Sizhukong SJ-23, Qimai SJ-18, Zanzhu BL-2, Chengguang BL-6 and Shenshu BL-23, (*Thousand Ducat Formulas*).

SIZHUKONG SJ-23

Silken Bamboo Hollow

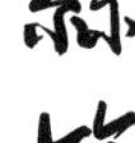
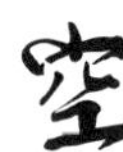
空

LOCATION

In the depression on the supraorbital margin, at the lateral end of the eyebrow.

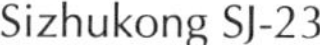

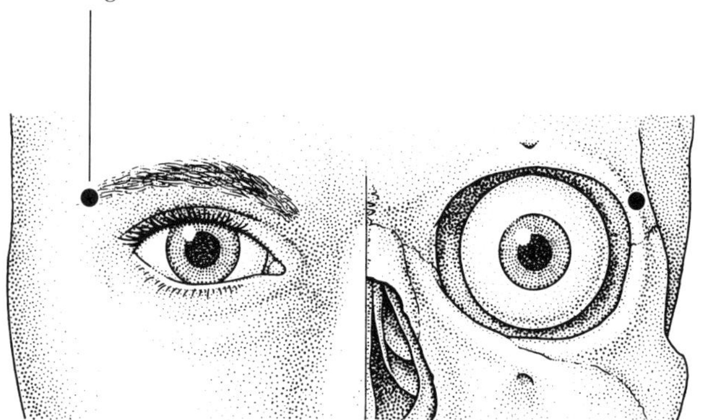

NEEDLING

Transverse insertion, medially along the eyebrow or posteriorly, 0.5 to 1 cun. **Note**: according to several classical texts, this point is contraindicated to moxibustion.

ACTIONS

Eliminates wind and alleviates pain

Benefits the eyes

INDICATIONS

- Headache, one-sided headache, head wind, aversion to wind and cold, dizziness, visual dizziness, tetany, epilepsy with foaming at the mouth, periodic mania with foaming at the mouth, childhood umbilical wind, toothache.
- Upward staring eyes, deviation of the face and eye, blurred vision, pain and redness of the eyes, twitching of the eyelids and eyebrows, ingrown eyelash.

COMMENTARY

Sizhukong SJ-23 is an important local point for the treatment of headache and disorders of the eye, eyelid and eyebrow. According to the *Investigation Into Points Along the Channels* Sizhukong SJ-23 is indicated for "all disorders of the head, face, eyebrows and eyes whether swelling, redness, itching or numbness".

Sizhukong SJ-23 is also able to pacify interior wind and soothe convulsions, and is indicated for dizziness, epilepsy, mania, foaming at the mouth and childhood umbilical wind. Childhood umbilical wind refers to infection of the umbilicus in the new born which gives rise to convulsions, opisthotonos and lockjaw.

COMBINATIONS

- One-sided or generalised wind headache that is difficult to cure: join Sizhukong SJ-23 subcutaneously with Shuaigu GB-8 (*Song of the Jade Dragon*).
- One-sided or generalised headache: Sizhukong SJ-23, Fengchi GB-20 and Hegu L.I.-4 (*Great Compendium*).
- One-sided or generalised head wind: Sizhukong SJ-23, Baihui DU-20, Qianding DU-21, Shenting DU-24, Shangxing DU-23, Fengchi GB-20, Hegu L.I.-4, Zanzhu BL-2 and Touwei ST-8 (*Great Compendium*).
- Wind headache: Sizhukong SJ-23, Erheliao SJ-22, Qimai SJ-18, Zanzhu BL-2, Chengguang BL-6 and Shenshu BL-23 (*Thousand Ducat Formulas*).
- Wind epilepsy with upward staring eyes: Sizhukong SJ-23, Kunlun BL-60 and Baihui DU-20 (*Great Compendium*).
- Toothache: Sizhukong SJ-23 and Ermen SJ-21 (*One Hundred Symptoms*).

NOTES

1 *Spiritual Pivot* Chapter 4.
2 *Spiritual Pivot* Chapter 5.
3 *Essential Questions* Chapter 6.
4 *Classic of Difficulties* 68th Difficulty.
5 *Classic of Difficulties* 68th Difficulty.
6 *Classic of Difficulties* 66th Difficulty.
7 *Classic of Difficulties* 29th Difficulty.
8 *Spiritual Pivot* Chapter 44.
9 *Classic of Difficulties* 31st Difficulty.
10 *Classic of Difficulties* 68th Difficulty.

足少陽膽經

THE GALL BLADDER CHANNEL OF FOOT SHAOYANG

THE GALL BLADDER CHANNEL OF FOOT SHAOYANG

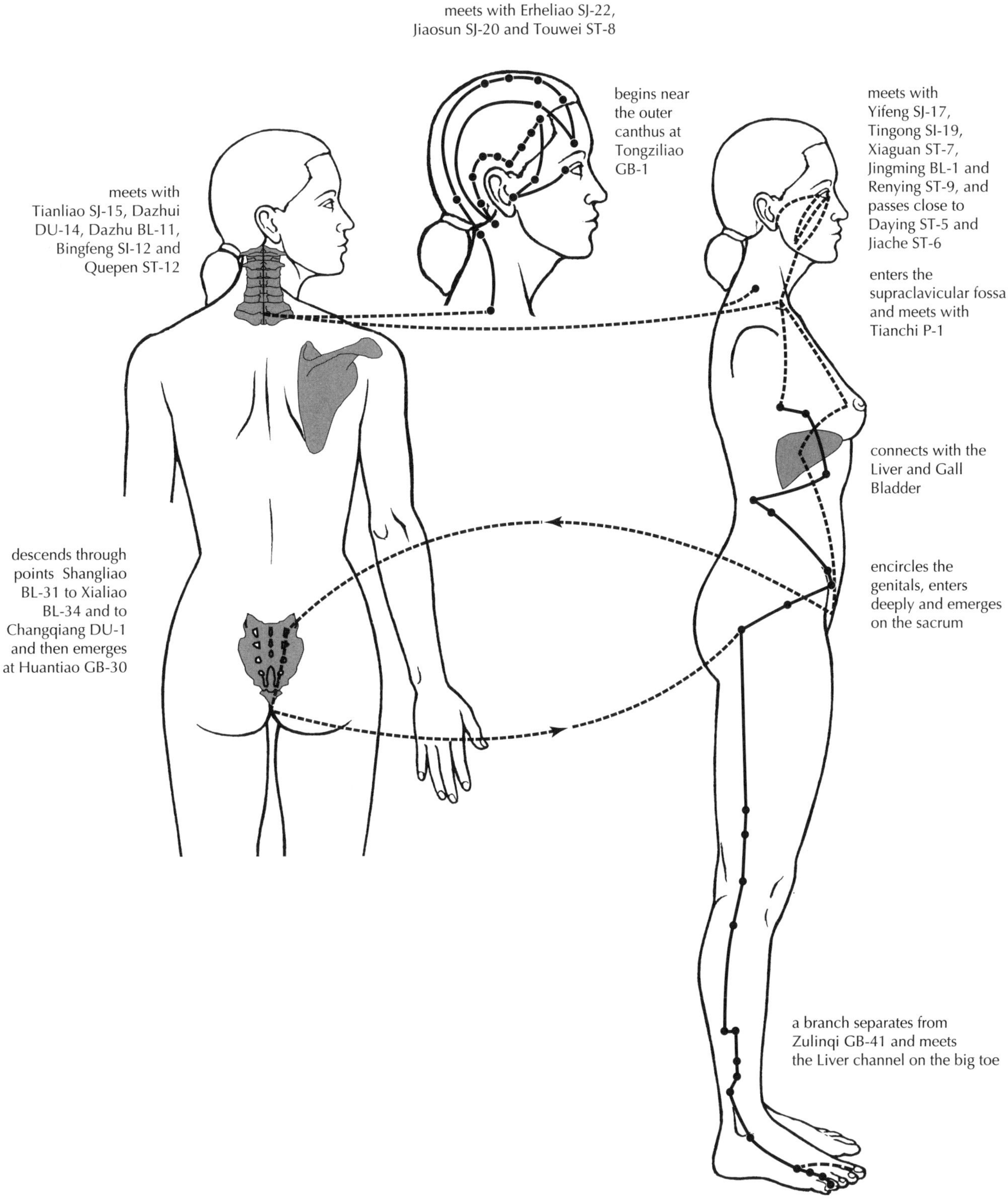

meets with Erheliao SJ-22, Jiaosun SJ-20 and Touwei ST-8

begins near the outer canthus at Tongziliao GB-1

meets with Yifeng SJ-17, Tingong SI-19, Xiaguan ST-7, Jingming BL-1 and Renying ST-9, and passes close to Daying ST-5 and Jiache ST-6

meets with Tianliao SJ-15, Dazhui DU-14, Dazhu BL-11, Bingfeng SI-12 and Quepen ST-12

enters the supraclavicular fossa and meets with Tianchi P-1

connects with the Liver and Gall Bladder

descends through points Shangliao BL-31 to Xialiao BL-34 and to Changqiang DU-1 and then emerges at Huantiao GB-30

encircles the genitals, enters deeply and emerges on the sacrum

a branch separates from Zulinqi GB-41 and meets the Liver channel on the big toe

The Gall Bladder primary channel

THE GALL BLADDER PRIMARY CHANNEL

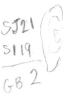

- begins near the outer canthus of the eye at Tongziliao GB-1,
- crosses to the anterior portion of the ear at Tinghui GB-2 then ascends to the upper border of the zygomatic arch at Shangguan GB-3,
- ascends to the corner of the forehead at Hanyan GB-4 and descends via points Xuanlu GB-5, Xuanli GB-6 and Qubin GB-7 to the region above the ear where it meets with Erheliao SJ-22,
- curves posteriorly behind the ear to the mastoid process at Wangu GB-12, meeting with Jiaosun SJ-20 on the way,
- curves upwards across the side of the head to the corner of the forehead at Touwei ST-8 and descends to the supraorbital region at Yangbai GB-14,
- ascends and curves across the side of the head to Fengchi GB-20 below the occiput,
- crosses the top of the shoulder via Jianjing GB-21 and Tianliao SJ-15 to meet with the spine at Dazhui DU-14,
- passes laterally via Dazhu BL-11 to Bingfeng SI-12 then anteriorly to enter the supraclavicular fossa at Quepen ST-12.

A branch

- emerges behind the ear and enters the ear at Yifeng SJ-17,
- emerges in front of the ear and passes via Tinggong SI-19 and Xiaguan ST-7 to the outer canthus,
- descends to the corner of the jaw near Daying ST-5,
- crosses the Sanjiao channel and rises to the infraorbital region, and meets with Jingming BL-1,
- descends to the neck, passing near Jiache ST-6 and intersecting Renying ST-9 to rejoin the main channel in the supraclavicular fossa,
- descends into the chest, meeting with the Pericardium channel at Tianchi P-1,
- crosses the diaphragm, connects with the Liver and unites with the Gall Bladder,
- continues along the inside of the ribs to emerge in the inguinal region,
- encircles the genitals, runs superficially along the margin of the pubic hair then enters deeply to emerge at the sacral region where it meets the Bladder channel at Baliao (the four points of the sacral foramina) and the Governing vessel at Changqiang DU-1,
- emerges on the buttock at Huantiao GB-30.

Another branch

- descends from the supraclavicular fossa to the anterior aspect of the axilla, then passes through Yuanye GB-22, Zhejin GB-23 and Riyue GB-24,
- intersects the Liver channel at Zhangmen LIV-13,
- descends to the hip joint to meet the previous branch at Huantiao GB-30 and continues down the lateral aspect of the thigh and knee,
- descends along the lateral aspect of the lower leg to the anterior aspect of the lateral malleolus,
- follows the dorsal surface of the foot along the groove between the fourth and fifth metatarsals to end on the lateral side of the tip of the fourth toe at Zuqiaoyin GB-44.

Another branch

- separates on the foot at Zulinqi GB-41 and runs between the first and second metatarsal bones to the medial tip of the big toe then through the toenail to link with the Liver channel.

The Gall Bladder primary channel connects with the following zangfu: Gall Bladder and Liver.

The Gall Bladder primary channel meets with other channels at the following points: Xiaguan ST-7, Touwei ST-8, Renying ST-9, Quepen ST-12, Bingfeng SI-12, Tinggong SI-19, Jingming BL-1, Dazhu BL-11, Shangliao BL-31, Ciliao BL-32, Zhongliao BL-33, Xialiao BL-34, Tianchi P-1, Tianliao SJ-15, Yifeng SJ-17, Jiaosun SJ-20, Erheliao SJ-22, Zhangmen LIV-13, Changqiang DU-1, Dazhui DU-14.
Note: Baihui DU-20 is classified as a meeting point of the Gall Bladder channel with the Governing vessel but is not conventionally shown as such on illustrations of the Gall Bladder primary channel.

THE GALL BLADDER LUO-CONNECTING CHANNEL

- separates from the primary channel at Guangming GB-37,
- connects with the Liver channel,
- descends and disperses over the dorsum of the foot.

THE GALL BLADDER DIVERGENT CHANNEL

- diverges from the primary channel on the thigh,
- enters the pubic hairline where it converges with the divergent channel of the Liver,
- enters the flank between the lower ribs,
- connects with the Gall Bladder and spreads upwards through the Liver,
- proceeds upwards across the Heart and oesophagus,
- emerges at the lower jaw, disperses in the face, connects with the eye and rejoins the Gall Bladder primary channel at the outer canthus.

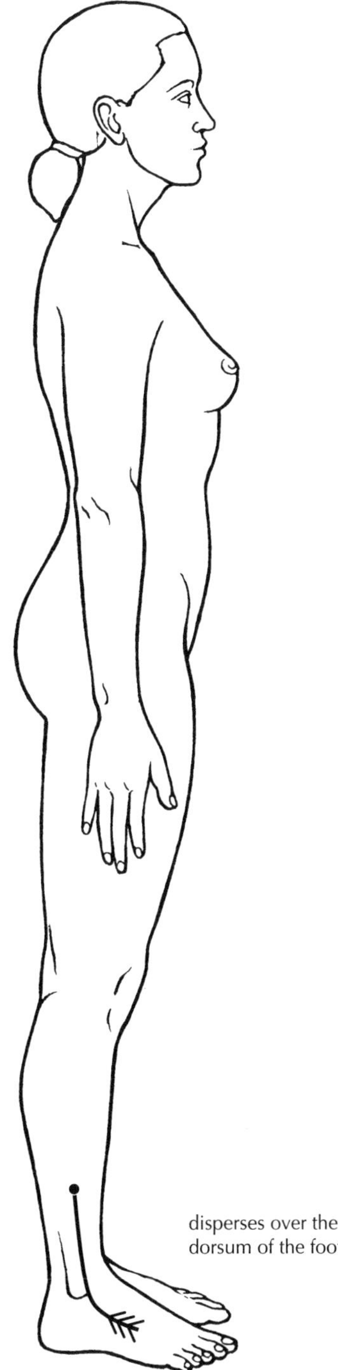
separates from the
primary channel at
Guangming GB-37
and connects with
the Liver channel
disperses over the
dorsum of the foot

The Gall Bladder luo-connecting channel

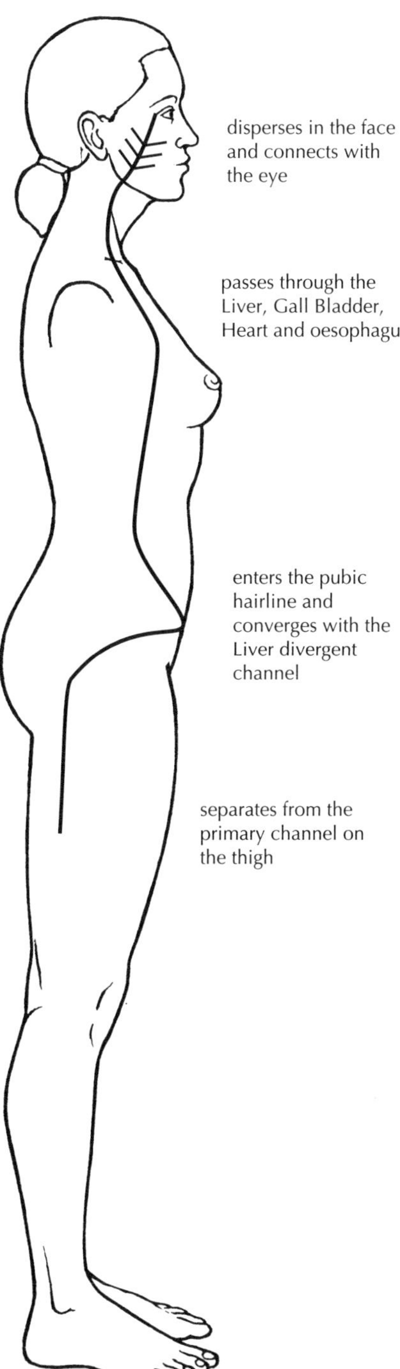
disperses in the face
and connects with
the eye
passes through the
Liver, Gall Bladder,
Heart and oesophagus
enters the pubic
hairline and
converges with the
Liver divergent
channel
separates from the
primary channel on
the thigh

The Gall Bladder divergent channel

THE GALL BLADDER SINEW CHANNEL
- begins at the fourth toe and binds at the lateral malleolus,
- ascends the lateral aspect of the leg to bind at the lateral aspect of the knee,

A branch
- begins in the upper portion of the fibula and ascends along the lateral aspect of the thigh.

A sub-branch
- runs anteriorly to bind in the area above Futu ST-32.

Another sub-branch
- runs posteriorly and binds at the sacrum.

The vertical branch
- ascends across the ribs and travels anteriorly to the axilla, linking first with the breast and then binding at Quepen ST-12.

Another branch
- ascends from the axilla and passes through Quepen ST-12,
- ascends anterior to the Bladder channel, passing behind the ear to the temple,
- continues to the vertex where it meets with its bilateral counterpart.

A branch
- descends from the temple across the cheek and binds at the side of the nose.

A sub-branch
- binds at the outer canthus.

Pathological symptoms of the Gall Bladder sinew channel
Strain and cramping of the fourth toe leading to cramping of the lateral aspect of the knee, inability to extend and bend the knee, spasm of the popliteal region, in the front leading to spasm of the upper thigh, and in the back spasm of the sacrum, radiating to the lateral costal region and the area below the lateral costal region; spasm of the supraclavicular fossa, the sides of the neck and the neck. If one looks to the right, then the right eye will not open and vice versa.

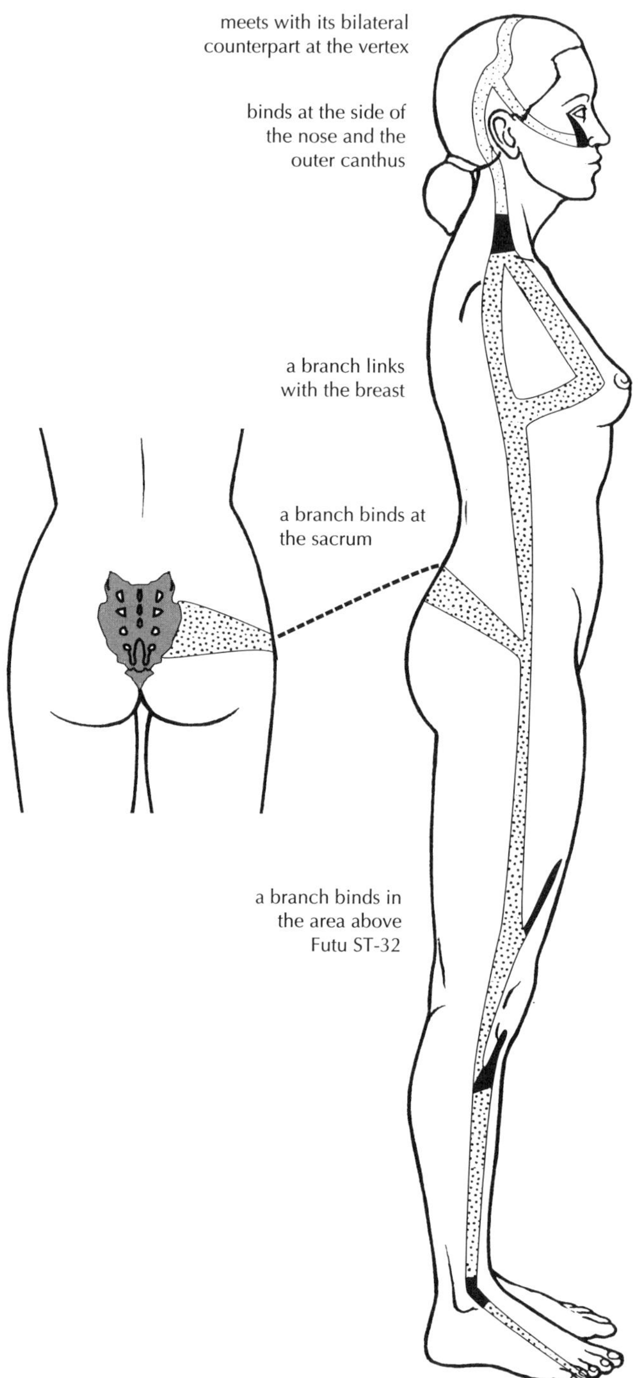

The Gall Bladder sinew channel

DISCUSSION

The Gall Bladder channel of foot shaoyang is interiorly-exteriorly coupled with the Liver channel, and paired with the Sanjiao channel of hand shaoyang according to six channel theory. The Gall Bladder-Liver relationship is further strengthened by the fact that:

- the Gall Bladder primary and divergent channels connect with the Liver.
- the Gall Bladder luo-connecting channel connects with the Liver channel.
- the Gall Bladder divergent channel connects with the Liver divergent channel.

In addition it is important to note that:

- the Gall Bladder primary channel begins at the outer canthus and travels to the infraorbital region, whilst the Gall Bladder divergent channel connects with the eye.
- the Gall Bladder primary channel criss-crosses the side of head as well as meeting with points Erheliao SJ-22, Jiaosun SJ-20 and Touwei ST-8 in this region.
- the Gall Bladder primary channel both passes behind the ear and enters the ear.
- the Gall Bladder primary channel passes through the jaw and throat region.
- the Gall Bladder primary channel descends through the chest and connects with the Pericardium channel at Tianchi P-1.
- the Gall Bladder primary and divergent channels pass anterior to the axilla.
- the Gall Bladder sinew channel links with the breast.
- the Gall Bladder divergent channel connects with the Heart.
- the Gall Bladder primary channel passes through the inguinal region and encircles the genitals.
- the Gall Bladder primary and divergent channels go to the sacrum and the primary channel connects with Changqiang DU-1.

The Gall Bladder belongs to the wood phase and its two principal functions are to store and excrete bile and to rule courage, decision-making and judgement. It is by virtue of these functions as well as the channel pathways discussed above, that many of the actions and indications of the points of the Gall Bladder channel can be explained. These can be summarised as:

- treating disorders of the eyes, especially those due to exterior wind-heat or Liver and Gall Bladder channel heat.
- treating disorders of the ear, especially those due to exterior wind-heat or Liver and Gall Bladder channel heat.
- treating headaches, especially one-sided headaches affecting the shaoyang channel at the temple and side of the head.
- treating disorders of the Liver. The Liver rules the smooth flow of qi, and when this free-flowing function of the Liver is impaired, qi will stagnate. At the same time, the Liver and Gall Bladder are entrusted with the ministerial fire and their stagnant qi readily transforms to fire. If Liver fire consumes yin, it may give rise to the pattern of uprising of Liver yang, whilst either Liver fire or Liver yang may generate interior wind. Liver qi stagnation, Liver fire, Liver yang and Liver wind may all manifest along the course of the Gall Bladder channel in the head, ears, eyes, chest, breast and lateral costal region.
- treating phlegm disorders, scrofula and nodules. The smooth flow of body fluids is in part dependent on the free-flowing of the Liver qi, whilst Liver fire may condense body fluids into phlegm. Points of the Gall Bladder channel are indicated for stagnant qi and phlegm (and the consequent) swelling and nodulation, in the throat, supraclavicular fossa, axilla and breast, all regions traversed by various pathways of the Gall Bladder primary and secondary channels.
- clearing damp-heat from the Gall Bladder fu, manifesting as jaundice, pain of the lateral costal region, nausea and vomiting, fever etc.
- clearing pathogenic factors from shaoyang level giving rise to alternating chills and fever, bitter taste in the mouth, hypochondriac pain, dryness of the mouth and throat, and nausea and vomiting.
- treating disorders of the spirit and ethereal soul (hun): i. the Gall Bladder rules judgement, decisiveness and courage, ii. its divergent channel enters the Heart, and iii. the Gall Bladder (wood) is the 'mother' of Heart (fire). Points of the Gall Bladder channel are therefore able to treat disorder of the spirit and ethereal soul (hun) due principally either to Gall Bladder and Liver fire or Gall Bladder qi deficiency.
- the Girdling vessel only passes through three acupuncture points, Daimai GB-26, Wushu GB-27 and Weidao GB-28, whilst its confluent point is Zulinqi GB-41. This extraordinary vessel is therefore principally influenced by selecting these Gall Bladder channel points.
- the hui-meeting points of the sinews (Yanglingquan GB-34) and the marrow (Xuanzhong GB-39) belong to the Gall Bladder channel which traverses the entire lateral portion of the leg. Many points of the lower portion of this channel, therefore, are important in the treatment of disorders such as atrophy disorder and painful obstruction.

TONGZILIAO GB-1

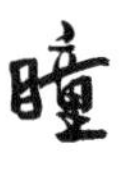
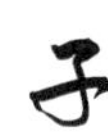
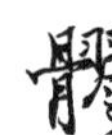

Pupil Crevice

Meeting point of the Gall Bladder, Small Intestine and Sanjiao channels.

LOCATION

In the hollow on the lateral side of the orbital margin, approximately 0.5 cun lateral to the outer canthus.

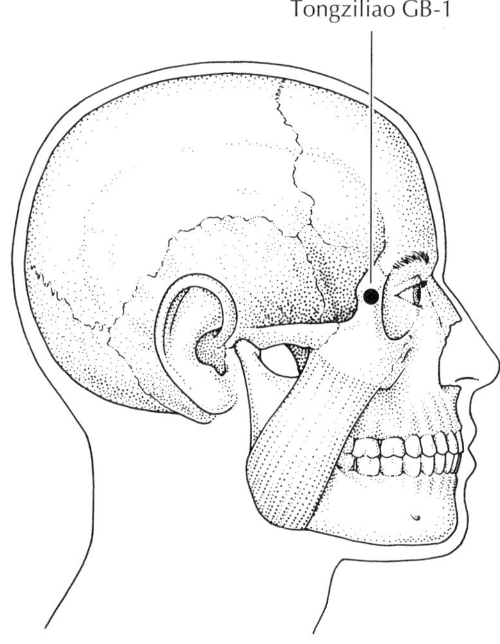

NEEDLING

Transverse insertion posteriorly 0.2 to 0.3 cun, or extend to connect with Taiyang (M-HN-9). **Note**: according to several modern texts, this point is contraindicated to moxibustion.

ACTIONS

Benefits the eyes, eliminates wind and clears heat

INDICATIONS

- Eye pain, redness, swelling and pain of the eyes, lacrimation, lacrimation on exposure to wind, itching of the eyes, redness and itching of the inner or outer canthus, short sightedness, superficial visual obstruction, dimness of vision, night blindness.
- Deviation of the mouth and eye, throat painful obstruction, headache, pain of the supraorbital ridge.

COMMENTARY

The Gall Bladder, Gall Bladder divergent and Liver channels connect with the eye, and the Liver zang (interiorly-exteriorly related to the Gall Bladder) opens into the eyes. Tongziliao GB-1, the first point of the channel and located just lateral to the eye, is used to treat all kinds of eye disorders, especially when due to Liver channel wind-heat. Whilst eye disorders may be due to exterior wind-heat or interior Liver fire, in clinical practice these two patterns are commonly mixed, and a person who suffers from interior Liver fire or Liver yang is prone to attacks of exterior wind or wind-heat. This commonly-seen clinical situation is often referred to as Liver channel wind-heat.

Tongziliao GB-1 is traditionally indicated for pain, swelling, redness and itching of the eyes, lacrimation and disorders of vision, and in modern times for such disorders as glaucoma, photophobia, cataract, nebula, corneal opacity, keratitis, retinal haemorrhage and atrophy of the optic nerve. It is also commonly used for temporal headache and supraorbital pain, especially due to the above aetiologies, as well as for deviation of the mouth and eye due to exterior or interior wind. Interestingly Tongziliao GB-1 is included with Shaoze SI-1 in a classical prescription for breast pain in women. This reflects the pathway of the Gall Bladder sinew channel to the breast.

COMBINATIONS

- Internal eye obstruction: Tongziliao GB-1, Hegu L.I.-4, Zulinqi GB-41 and Jingming BL-1 (*Great Compendium*).
- Superficial visual obstruction: Tongziliao GB-1 and Qiuxu GB-40 (*Supplementing Life*).
- Swelling of the breasts in women: Tongziliao GB-1 and Shaoze SI-1 (*Illustrated Supplement*).

TINGHUI GB-2

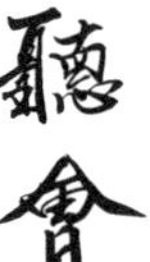

Meeting of Hearing

LOCATION

In the hollow between the intertragic notch posteriorly and the condyloid process of the mandible anteriorly. Locate this point with the mouth wide open.

LOCATION NOTE

In order to locate this point, ask the patient to open the mouth so that the condyloid process of the mandible slides forwards to reveal the depression.

NEEDLING

Slightly posterior insertion 0.5 to 1 cun. This point should be needled with the mouth wide open. The patient may close the mouth after insertion.

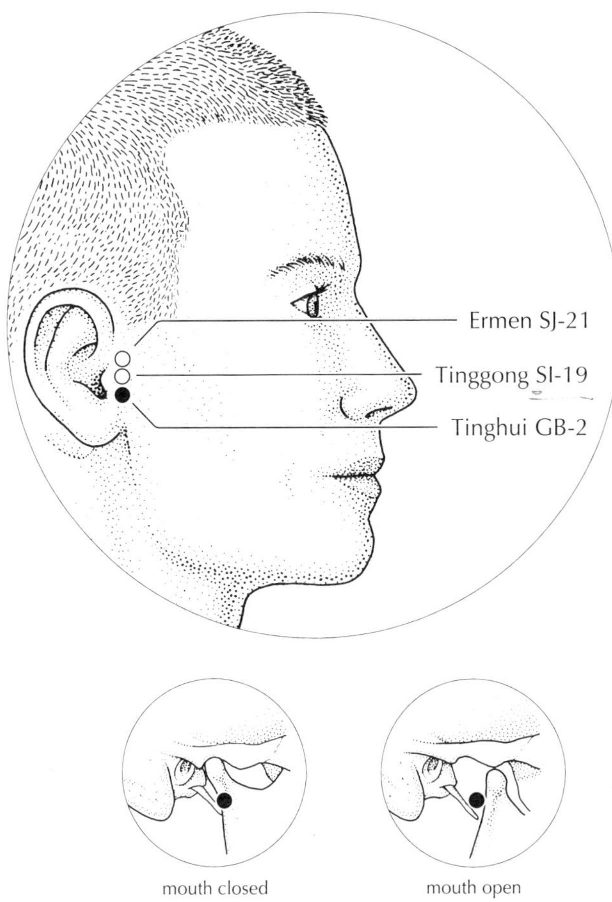

ACTIONS

Benefits the ears, eliminates wind and clears heat
Activates the channel and alleviates pain

INDICATIONS

- Tinnitus, deafness, redness, swelling, pain and purulent discharge from the ear, itching of the ear.
- Mumps, toothache, windstroke, deviation of the mouth and eye, pain of the mandibular joint, dislocation of the jaw, difficulty in masticating, disorientation.

COMMENTARY

There are three points anterior to the tragus of the ear, Tinghui GB-2 inferiorly, Ermen SJ-21 superiorly and Tinggong SI-19 in the centre. All are frequently employed in the treatment of a wide variety of ear disorders, including tinnitus, deafness, pain, itching and discharge. Due to the close proximity of these points and the similar indications for each, it is difficult to distinguish between them clinically, although each practitioner may have their individual preference. If it is necessary to needle points around the ear regularly, then these three points should be alternated.

In addition to its ability to treat ear disorders, Tinghui GB-2 is able to eliminate wind and to activate the channel in the surrounding region, and is indicated for deviation of the mouth and eyes, mumps, toothache, and difficult mastication and other jaw disorders.

COMBINATIONS

- Swelling, pain and redness of the ear: Tinghui GB-2, Hegu L.I.-4 and Jiache ST-6 (*Great Compendium*).
- Deafness due to qi obstruction: Tinghui GB-2, Tinggong SI-19 and Yifeng SJ-17; then needle Zusanli ST-36 and Hegu L.I.-4 (*Great Compendium*).
- Deafness and tinnitus: Tinghui GB-2, Tianrong SI-17, Tinggong SI-19 and Zhongzhu SJ-3 (*Thousand Ducat Formulas*).
- Deafness: Tinghui GB-2, Zhongzhu SJ-3, Waiguan SJ-5, Erheliao SJ-22, Shangyang L.I.-1, Tinggong SI-19, Hegu L.I.-4 and Zhongchong P-9 (*Precious Mirror*).
- Impaired hearing and deafness: Tinghui GB-2, Ermen SJ-21, Fengchi GB-20, Xiaxi GB-43 and Tinggong SI-19 (*Great Compendium*).
- Impaired hearing and deafness: Tinghui GB-2 and Waiguan SJ-5 (*Supplementing Life*).
- Bilateral deafness due to injury by cold: Tinghui GB-2 and Jinmen BL-63 (*Ode of Xi-hong*).
- Tinnitus: Tinghui GB-2, Tinggong SI-19, Ermen SJ-21, Baihui DU-20, Luoque BL-8, Yangxi L.I.-5, Qiangu SI-2, Houxi SI-3, Wangu SI-4, Zhongzhu SJ-3, Yemen SJ-2, Shangyang L.I.-1 and Shenshu BL-23 (*Great Compendium*).
- Toothache with aversion to cold: Tinghui GB-2, Daying ST-5, Quanliao SI-18 and Quchi L.I.-11 (*Thousand Ducat Formulas*).
- Deviation of the mouth and eye: Tinghui GB-2, Jiache ST-6, Dicang ST-4 Renzhong DU-26, Chengjiang REN-24 and Hegu L.I.-4 (*Illustrated Supplement*).

SHANGGUAN GB-3

Above the Joint

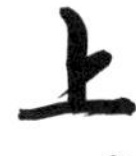

Meeting point of the Gall Bladder, Sanjiao and Stomach channels

LOCATION

Anterior to the ear, in a hollow above the upper border of the zygomatic arch, directly superior to Xiaguan ST-7.

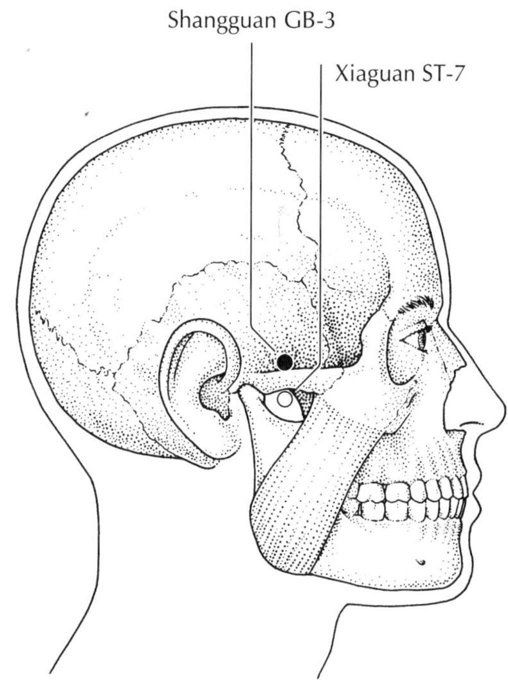

LOCATION NOTE

First locate Xiaguan ST-7 at the lower border of the zygomatic arch, in the depression anterior to the condyloid process of the mandible. Then run the palpating finger superiorly over the zygomatic arch into the hollow.

NEEDLING

Perpendicular insertion 0.3 to 0.5 cun.

Caution: it is traditionally emphasised that deep needling should be avoided at this point.

ACTIONS

Eliminates wind and benefits the ears
Activates the channel and alleviates pain

INDICATIONS

- Deafness, tinnitus, purulent discharge from the ear, dimness of vision, pain of the face, toothache of the upper jaw, stiffness of the lips.
- Headache, aversion to wind and cold, chills and fever, hemiplegia, deviation of the mouth and eye, lockjaw, tetany leading to bone pain, clonic spasm.

COMMENTARY

Although less important than its neighbouring point Xiaguan ST-7, Shangguan GB-3 may be used as a local point in the treatment of disorders of the surrounding region, including the ears, eyes, face, teeth, jaw, lips and head. In the treatment of trigeminal neuralgia it is sometimes needled 0.5 cun anterior to its textbook location.

COMBINATIONS

- Hemiplegia with deviation of the mouth and eye: Shangguan GB-3 and Xiaguan ST-7 (*Supplementing Life*).
- Lockjaw: Shangguan GB-3, Jiache ST-6 and Ahshi points (*Compilation*).

HANYAN GB-4

Jaw Serenity

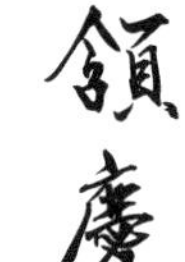

Meeting point of the Gall Bladder, Sanjiao and Stomach channels

LOCATION

In the temporal region, within the hairline, one quarter of the distance between Touwei ST-8 and Qubin GB-7.

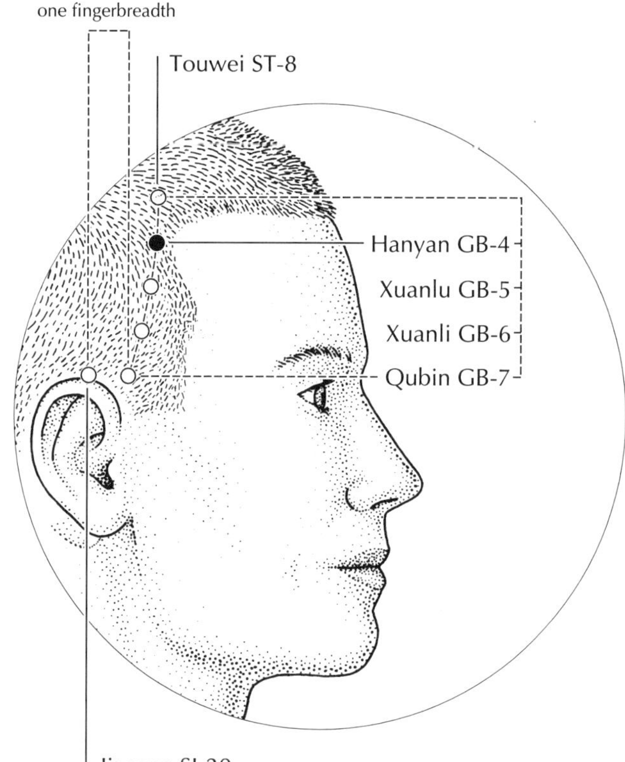

NEEDLING

Transverse insertion 0.5-1.5 cun. **Note:** this point, in common with all points within the hairline, may be needled in any direction. Direction depends on symptomatology, in other words direct the needle either towards where the headache or other pain radiates, or join by through-needling to other head points. The needle should be inserted deep to the subcutaneous layer, into the loose areolar tissue adjacent to the bone of the skull, rather than more shallowly.

ACTIONS

Eliminates wind and clears heat
Activates the channel and alleviates pain

INDICATIONS

- One-sided headache, head wind (with pain at bilateral Taiyang M-HN-9), headache with heat in the body, visual dizziness, pain and redness of the outer canthus.
- Tinnitus, earache.
- Clonic spasm, lockjaw, epilepsy, deviation of the mouth and eye, toothache, sneezing.
- Neck pain, wrist pain, inability to flex the wrist, joint wind with sweating.

COMMENTARY

Yan Zheng-shi of the Ming dynasty, in *Investigation of Points Along the Channels*, recommended Hanyan GB-4 specifically for head wind with pain in the region of both Taiyang (M-HN-9) points. Clinically, Hanyan GB-4 should always be palpated in cases of one-sided headache, and needled if tender. Unusually for a point on the head, Hanyan GB-4 is also indicated in the *Great Compendium of Acupuncture and Moxibustion* for pain and stiffness of the wrist as well as 'joint wind' (i.e. painful obstruction) accompanied by sweating.

COMBINATIONS

- One-sided headache: Hanyan GB-4 and Xuanlu GB-5 (*One Hundred Symptoms*).
- Wind dizziness and one-sided headache: Hanyan GB-4, Qianding DU-21 and Houding DU-19 (*Thousand Ducat Formulas*).
- Wind dizziness: Hanyan GB-4, Houding DU-19 and Yuzhen BL-9 (*Supplementing Life*).
- Neck pain, joint pain and sweating: Hanyan GB-4, Feiyang BL-58 and Yongquan KID-1 (*Thousand Ducat Formulas*).

XUANLU GB-5

Suspended Skull

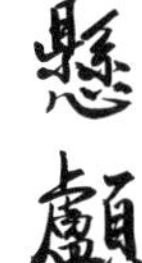

Meeting point of the Gall Bladder, Stomach, Sanjiao and Large Intestine channels

LOCATION

In the temporal region, within the hairline, half the distance between Touwei ST-8 and Qubin GB-7.

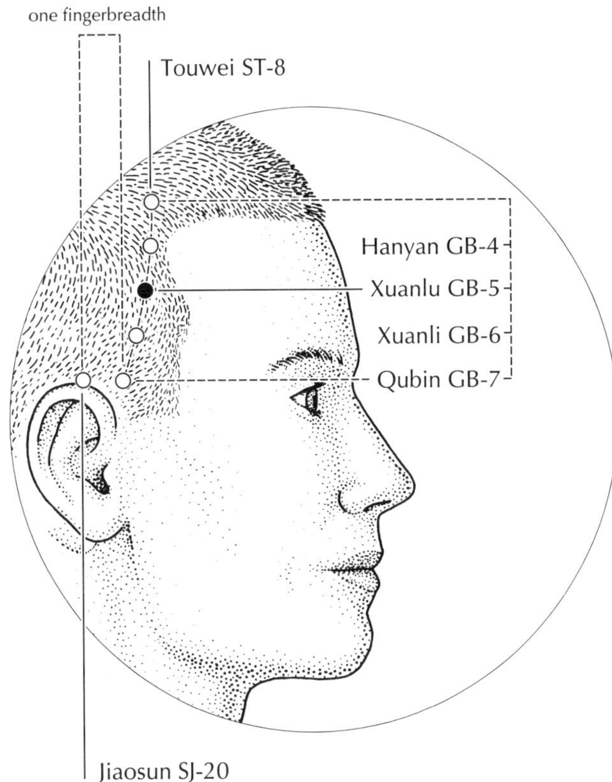

NEEDLING

Transverse insertion 0.5-1.5 cun. See note Hanyan GB-4.

ACTIONS

Expels wind and clears heat
Activates the channel and alleviates pain

INDICATIONS

- One-sided headache extending to the outer canthus, pain of the outer canthus, headache.
- Toothache, pain, swelling and redness of the skin of the face, nosebleed, incessant turbid nasal discharge, rhinitis, febrile disease with agitation and fullness and absence of sweating.

COMBINATIONS

- One-sided headache: Xuanlu GB-5 and Hanyan GB-4 (*One Hundred Symptoms*).

XUANLI GB-6

Suspended Hair

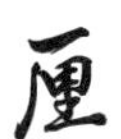

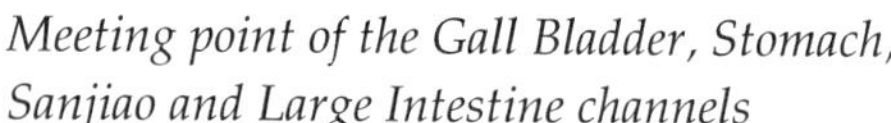

Meeting point of the Gall Bladder, Stomach, Sanjiao and Large Intestine channels

LOCATION

In the temporal region, within the hairline, three quarters of the distance between Touwei ST-8 and Qubin GB-7.

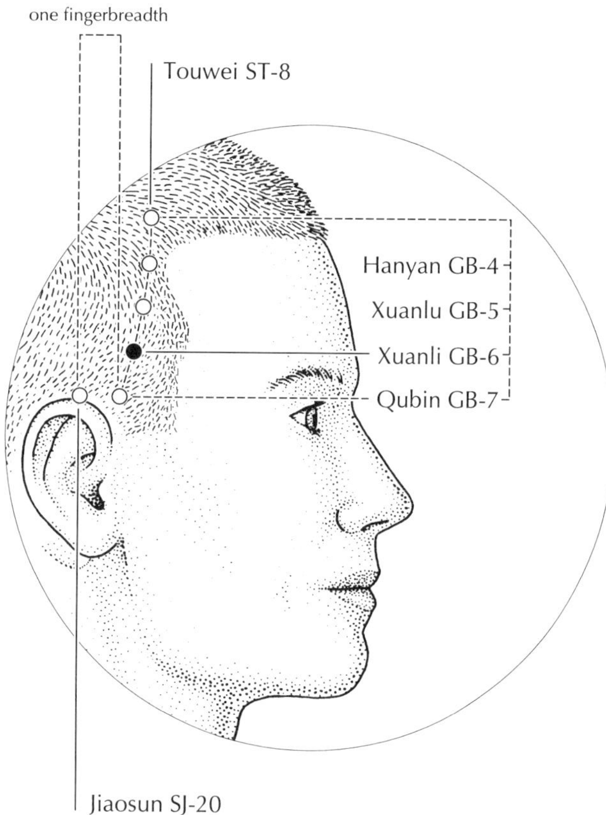

NEEDLING

Transverse insertion 0.5-1.5 cun. See note Hanyan GB-4.

ACTIONS

Expels wind and clears heat

Activates the channel and alleviates pain

INDICATIONS

- One-sided headache, one-sided headache extending to the outer canthus, pain of the outer canthus, sneezing, tinnitus, swelling and redness of the skin of the face.
- Febrile disease with absence of sweating, agitation of the Heart with no desire to eat, heat in the middle jiao.

COMBINATIONS

- Febrile disease with one-sided headache: Xuanli GB-6 and Jiuwei REN-15 (*Thousand Ducat Formulas*).

QUBIN GB-7

Crook of the Temple

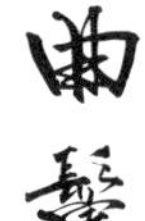

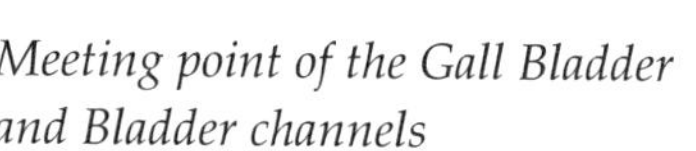

Meeting point of the Gall Bladder and Bladder channels

LOCATION

In the temporal region, within the hairline, level with and one finger-breadth anterior to Jiaosun SJ-20.

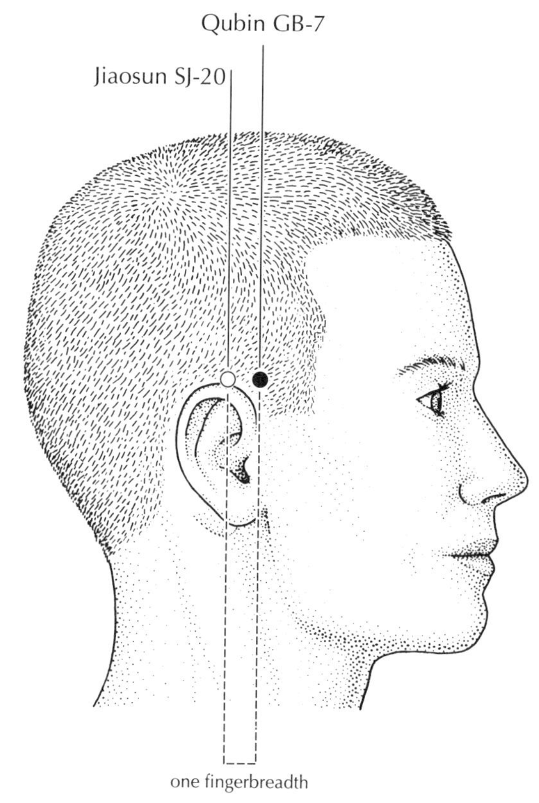

LOCATION NOTE

Jiaosun SJ-20 is located directly level with the apex of the ear, when the ear is folded forwards. Fold the ear so that the posterior part of the upper helix directly covers the anterior part of the upper helix. Take care not to push the whole of the ear forwards.

NEEDLING

Transverse insertion 0.5-1.5 cun. See note Hanyan GB-4.

ACTIONS

Eliminates wind and benefits the mouth and jaw

INDICATIONS

- Headache, swelling of the cheek and submandibular region, lockjaw, loss of speech, deviation of the mouth and eye.
- Vomiting, stiff neck with inability to turn the head.

COMBINATIONS
- Tooth decay: Qubin GB-7 and Chongyang ST-42 (*Thousand Ducat Formulas*).
- Sudden loss of voice: Qubin GB-7, Tianchuang SI-16, Zhigou SJ-6, Futu L.I.-18 and Lingdao HE-4 (*Thousand Ducat Formulas*).

SHUAIGU GB-8

Leading Valley

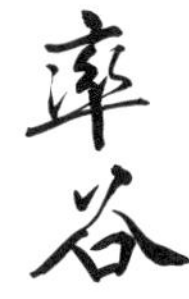

Meeting point of the Gall Bladder and Bladder channels

LOCATION

In the temporal region, in the slight depression 1 cun directly above the apex of the ear.

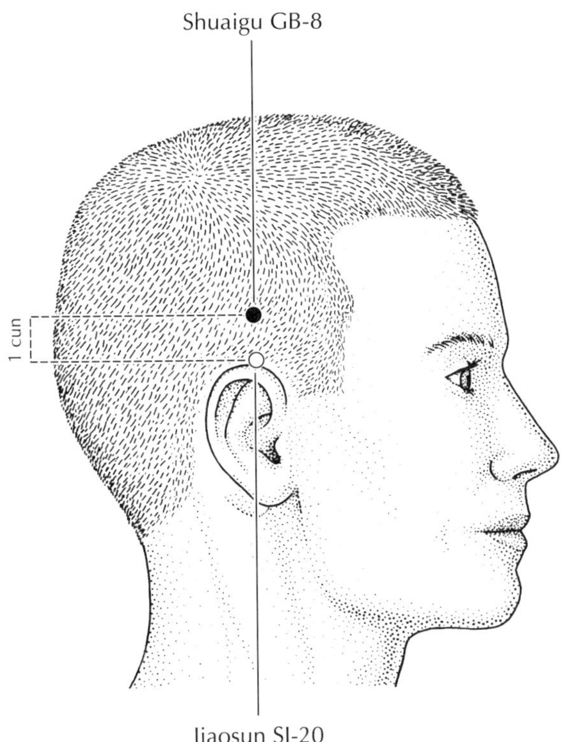

LOCATION NOTE

Fold the ear forward to define the apex. Fold the ear so that the posterior part of the upper helix directly covers the anterior part of the upper helix. Take care not to push the whole of the ear forwards.

NEEDLING

Transverse insertion 0.5-1.5 cun. This point may be joined by through-needling to Taiyang (M-HN-9). See note Hanyan GB-4.

ACTIONS

Eliminates wind, benefits the head and alleviates pain
Harmonises the diaphragm and Stomach and alleviates vomiting
Treats alcohol intoxication

INDICATIONS
- One-sided headache, heaviness of the head, head wind, pain at the corner of the forehead (the area of Touwei ST-8), deviation of the mouth and eye, acute and chronic childhood fright wind, dizziness, eye disorders.
- Incessant vomiting, cold Stomach, phlegm qi diaphragm pain, inability to eat, agitation and fullness on eating or drinking, injury by alcohol with vomiting, phlegm dizziness, oedema.

COMMENTARY

Shuaigu GB-8 is an important point for treating parietal or temporal headache and heaviness, especially when unilateral, and is frequently found to be tender in such cases. The Gall Bladder primary and sinew channels traverse the side of the head, and the Gall Bladder channel is interiorly-exteriorly related to the Liver channel. Shuaigu GB-8 is particularly indicated in cases where exterior wind attacks the head, or Liver fire, Liver yang or Liver wind ascend along the Gall Bladder channel to harass the head causing severe one-sided headache.

According to the *Illustrated Classic of Acupuncture Points on the Bronze Man* Shuaigu GB-8 is especially indicated for "cold and phlegm in the diaphragm and Stomach, injury by alcohol, wind giving rise to severe and stubborn pain at both corners of the brain, inability to eat and drink, agitation and fullness with ceaseless vomiting". This is a clear reference to migrainous headache. Since Shuaigu GB-8 harmonises the diaphragm and Stomach, it is the main point on the head to treat headache accompanied by vomiting due to attack on the Stomach by Liver qi, or to Gall Bladder and Stomach phlegm-heat. Alcohol may induce migraine headache and vomiting by aggravating Liver heat and disrupting the harmony between the Liver and the Stomach, or by inducing or aggravating damp-heat in the Gall Bladder and Stomach. Many classics therefore recommend this point for headache and vomiting induced by alcohol.

Shuaigu GB-8 is also indicated for accumulation of phlegm in the diaphragm and Stomach, giving rise to ceaseless vomiting and 'phlegm qi diaphragm pain'. In clinical practice the pattern of phlegm or phlegm-heat in the Stomach is commonly seen in combination with Gall Bladder stagnation and heat. Shuaigu GB-8 is especially indicated when these symptoms are accompanied by one-sided headache.

COMBINATIONS

- One-sided or generalised wind headache that is difficult to cure: join Sizhukong SJ-23 subcutaneously with Shuaigu GB-8 (*Song of the Jade Dragon*).
- Cold phlegm in the diaphragm and Stomach: Shuaigu GB-8 and Geshu BL-17 (*Supplementing Life*).

TIANCHONG GB-9

Heavenly Rushing

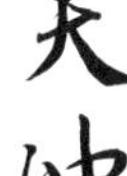

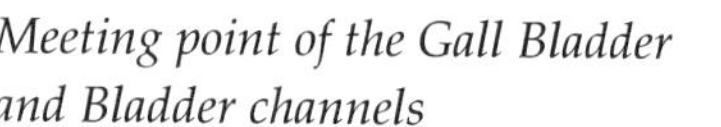

Meeting point of the Gall Bladder and Bladder channels

LOCATION

Above the ear, in the depression 0.5 cun posterior to Shuaigu GB-8.

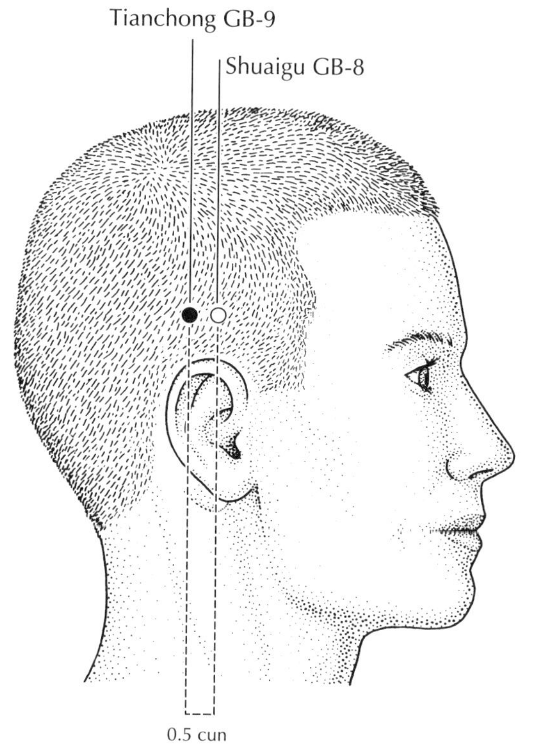

NEEDLING

Transverse insertion 0.5-1.5 cun. See note Hanyan GB-4.

ACTIONS

Clears Gall Bladder channel heat
Calms the spirit and pacifies fright

INDICATIONS

- Headache, tinnitus, damp itching of the ear, toothache, swelling and pain of the gums, goitre.
- Propensity to fear and fright, fright palpitations, epilepsy, tetany, madness.

COMMENTARY

Chapter 21 of the *Spiritual Pivot* lists five points known as the points of the Window of Heaven (Renying ST-9, Futu L.I.-18, Tianyou SJ-16, Tianzhu BL-10 and Tianfu LU-3). Chapter 2 of the same text gives an unnamed list of ten points which includes the five Window of Heaven points and adds the points Tiantu REN-22, Tianchuang SI-16, Tianrong SI-17, Fengfu DU-16 and Tianchi P-1. This passage first discusses Tiantu REN-22, and then the six yang channel points as a sequence of vertical lines spreading from the Conception vessel and ending with Fengfu DU-16 on the Governing vessel, with Tianfu LU-3 and Tianchi P-1 as additional points. Later commentators (particularly Ma Shi, the great physician of the Ming dynasty and expert on the *Yellow Emperor's Inner Classic*) pointed out that this passage discusses Tianrong SI-17 as a point of shaoyang channel whereas in fact it is a point of the hand taiyang channel. They therefore suggested that Tianrong SI-17 should in fact be Tianchong GB-9. If so, all the six yang channels would then be represented.

These ten points have certain common properties, being indicated especially for disharmony between the head and body, disorders of the head and sense organs, goitre and scrofula, rebellion of Lung or Stomach qi and emotional disorders.

Many classics indicate Tianchong GB-9 for a variety of mental and psychological diseases characterised by propensity to fear and fright, fright palpitations, epilepsy, madness etc. According to modern acupuncture research in psychiatric hospitals, many head points are effective in treating disorders of the underlying portion of the brain, and this may help explain these traditional indications.

COMBINATIONS

- Arched back with sorrowful weeping: Tianchong GB-9 and Daheng SP-15 (*One Hundred Patterns*).
- Headache: Tianchong GB-9, Fengchi GB-20 and Muchuang GB-16 (*Systematic Classic*).

FUBAI GB-10

Floating White

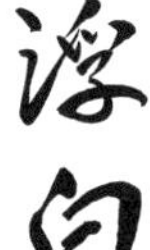

Meeting point of the Gall Bladder and Bladder channels

LOCATION

Posterior to the ear, along a curved line drawn from Tianchong GB-9 to Wangu GB-12 running within the hairline and more or less parallel to the line of the rim of the ear, in a depression about one third of the distance between Tianchong GB-9 and Wangu GB-12.

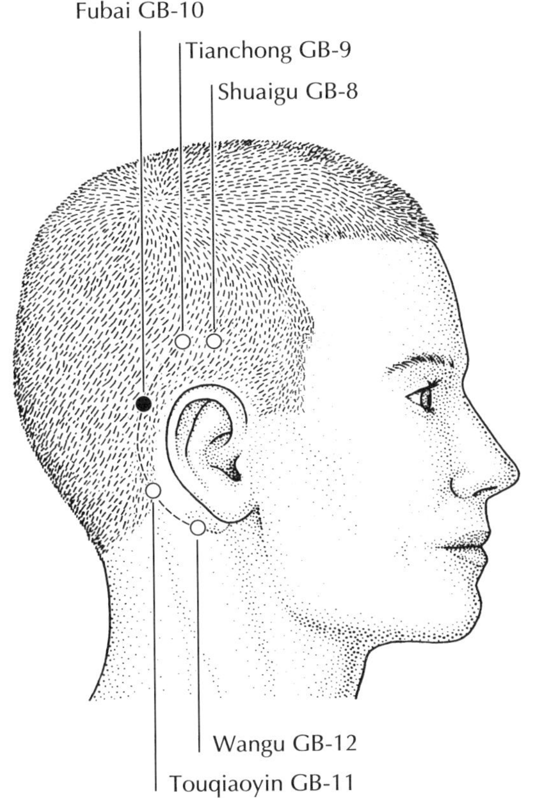

NEEDLING
Transverse insertion 0.5-1.5 cun. See note Hanyan GB-4.

ACTIONS
Clears the head and benefits the neck region
Activates the channel and alleviates pain

INDICATIONS
- Headache, heaviness of the head, chills and fever, toothache, deafness, tinnitus.
- Stiffness and pain of the neck, goitre, swelling and pain of the neck, throat painful obstruction.
- Fullness of the chest with dyspnoea, chest pain, cough with expectoration of phlegm and foam.
- Pain of the shoulder and arm, inability to raise the arm, flaccidity of the legs with inability to walk.

COMMENTARY
The points Fubai GB-10, Touqiaoyin GB-11 and to a certain extent Tianchong GB-9, have certain comparable indications and these are not dissimilar to the indications for the points of the Window of Heaven (See page 49). All are indicated for goitre, and Fubai GB-10 additionally for stiffness, swelling and pain of the neck. Both Fubai GB-10 (headache, toothache, deafness and tinnitus) and Touqiaoyin GB-11 (headache and eye, ear, tongue and mouth disorders) are indicated for disorders of the head and sense organs and for rebellion of Lung qi characterised by cough. Both also treat disorders of the lower body, Fubai GB-10 for flaccidity of the legs with inability to walk, and Touqiaoyin GB-11 for contraction of the sinews of the four limbs, bone consumption, and agitation and heat of the hands and feet. This latter application reflects the principle expounded in the *Yellow Emperor's Inner Classic*[1] "When the disease is below select [points] from above".

COMBINATIONS
- Toothache and tooth decay: Fubai GB-10 and Wangu GB-12 (*Systematic Classic*).

TOUQIAOYIN GB-11

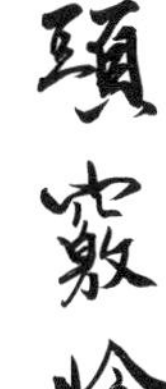

Yin Portals of the Head

Meeting point of the Gall Bladder, Bladder, Small Intestine and Sanjiao channels

LOCATION
Posterior to the ear, along a curved line drawn from Tianchong GB-9 to Wangu GB-12 running within the hairline and more or less parallel to the line of the rim of the ear, in a depression slightly greater than two thirds of the distance between Tianchong GB-9 and Wangu GB-12.

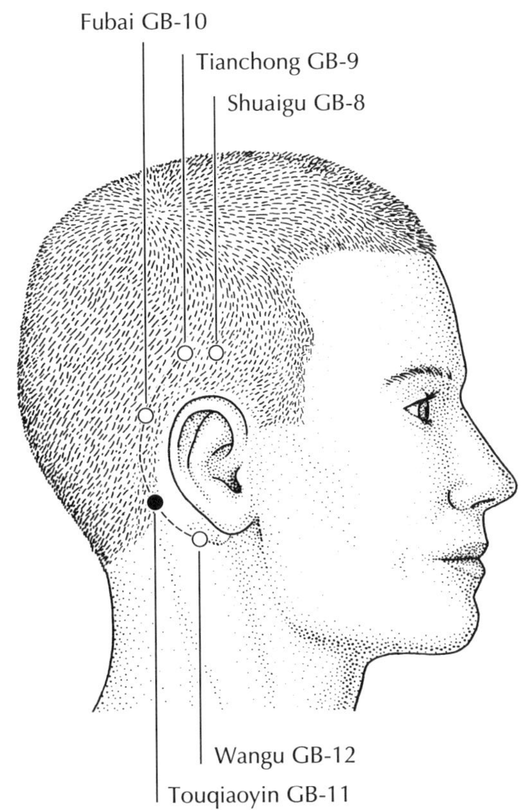

NEEDLING
Transverse insertion 0.5-1.5 cun. See note Hanyan GB-4.

ACTIONS
Clears the head and benefits the sense organs
Activates the channel and alleviates pain

INDICATIONS
- Headache, dizziness, eye pain, ear pain, tinnitus, deafness, stiff tongue, bleeding from the root of the tongue, nauseating bitter taste in the mouth.
- Stiffness and pain of the neck, goitre, throat painful obstruction.
- Pain of the lateral costal region, cough, absence of sweating, contraction of the sinews of the four limbs, bone taxation, agitation and heat of the hands and feet.

COMMENTARY
The name of Touqiaoyin GB-11 (Yin Portals of the Head) is said to refer to its ability to treat diseases of the sense organs associated with the five zang, namely the eyes (Liver), ears (Kidneys), tongue (Heart), mouth (Spleen) and nose (Lung). In fact, classical indications appear for all of these except the nose. In this respect, Touqiaoyin GB-11 in the upper body mirrors Zuqiaoyin GB-44 (Yin Portals of the Foot) in the lower body. For further discussion of Touqiaoyin GB-11 see Fubai GB-10.

COMBINATIONS
- Bleeding from the root of the tongue: Touqiaoyin GB-11, Futu L.I.-18 and Dazhong KID-4 (*Thousand Ducat Formulas*).
- Stabbing pain of the head with inability to move: Touqiaoyin GB-11 and Qiangjian DU-18 (*Supplementing Life*).
- Pain of the nape of the neck: Touqiaoyin GB-11 and Xiaoluo SJ-12 (*Supplementing Life*).

WANGU GB-12
Mastoid Process

完骨

Meeting point of the Gall Bladder and Bladder channels

LOCATION
In the depression just posterior and inferior to the mastoid process.

LOCATION NOTE
Place a finger on the prominence of the mastoid process then slide it posteriorly into the depression.

NEEDLING
Oblique inferior insertion 0.5-1 cun.

ACTIONS
Eliminates wind, benefits the head and alleviates pain
Calms the spirit

INDICATIONS
- Headache, head wind with pain behind the ear, shaking of the head, stiffness and pain of the neck with inability to turn the head.
- Toothache, swelling of the cheek radiating to the ear, pain of the ear, throat painful obstruction.
- Hemiplegia, deviation of the mouth and eye, clenched jaw, withering and contraction of the muscles around the mouth, weakness and flaccidity of the legs, atrophy disorder of the arms and legs, malaria, sweating with no aversion to cold.
- Epilepsy, mania, agitation of the Heart, insomnia, dark urine.

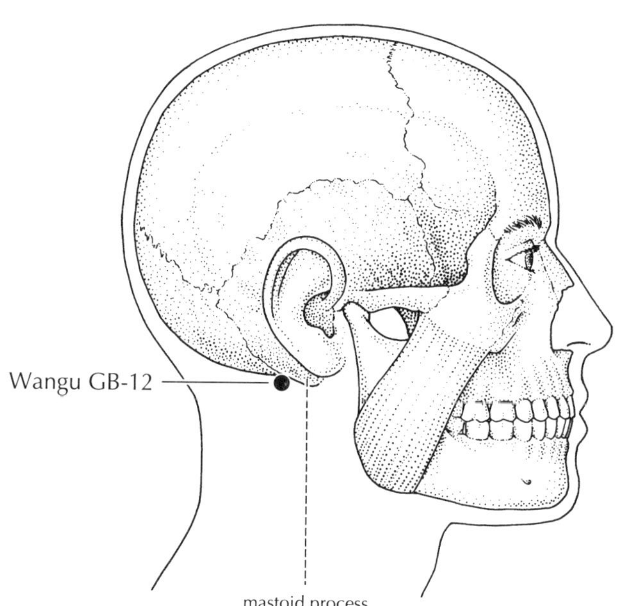

COMMENTARY
Wangu GB-12 is able to benefit the head region and eliminate both exterior and interior wind. It is indicated for i. headache and head wind, especially when there is pain behind the ear, ii. stiffness and pain of the neck, and iii. heat, pain and swelling affecting the teeth, cheek, ear and throat.

Like many points in the neck region, Wangu GB-12 is also able to regulate disharmony between the head and the body. When interior wind stirs and rushes up to the head there may be hemiplegia, deviation of the mouth and eyes, shaking of the head and clenched jaw. At the same time as pathogenic wind rushes up to the head, there may be deficiency in the lower part of the body manifesting as atrophy disorder and weakness and flaccidity of the four limbs. This latter application reflects the principle expounded in the *Yellow Emperor's Inner Classic*[2] "When the disease is below select [points] from above".

Another important action of Wangu GB-12 is to regulate and calm the spirit, and it is indicated in such disorders as mania, agitation of the Heart and insomnia. This is reflected in its close proximity to the extra point Anmian (M-HN-34) 'Peaceful Sleep', located just posterior and slightly superior to Wangu GB-12, which is much used for insomnia.

COMBINATIONS

- Head wind and pain behind the ear: Wangu GB-12 and Qimai SJ-18 (*Supplementing Life*).
- Pain of the nape of the neck: Wangu GB-12 and Yuzhen BL-9 (*Supplementing Life*).
- Tired throat, swelling of the neck with inability to turn the head, swelling of the cheek that radiates to the ear: Wangu GB-12, Tianyou SJ-16 and Qiangu SI-2 (*Thousand Ducat Formulas*).
- Toothache and tooth decay: Wangu GB-12 and Fubai GB-10 (*Systematic Classic*).
- Deviation of the mouth and face: Wangu GB-12 and Lieque LU-7 (*Supplementing Life*).
- Dark urine: Wangu GB-12, Xiaochangshu BL-27, Baihuanshu BL-30 and Yanggang BL-48 (*Thousand Ducat Formulas*).

BENSHEN GB-13

本神

Root of the Spirit

Meeting point of the Gall Bladder channel with the Yang Linking vessel

LOCATION

On the forehead, 0.5 cun within the anterior hairline, two thirds of the distance between Shenting DU-24 and Touwei ST-8.

LOCATION NOTE

Some sources locate this point on the line directly above the outer canthus of the eye.

NEEDLING

Transverse insertion 0.5-1.5 cun. See note Hanyan GB-4.

ACTIONS

Eliminates wind, resolves phlegm and treats epilepsy

INDICATIONS

- Headache, visual dizziness, stiffness and pain of the neck, pain of the chest and lateral costal region with inability to turn the body.
- Epilepsy, childhood fright epilepsy, vomiting of foamy saliva, windstroke, hemiplegia, deviation of the mouth and eyes.

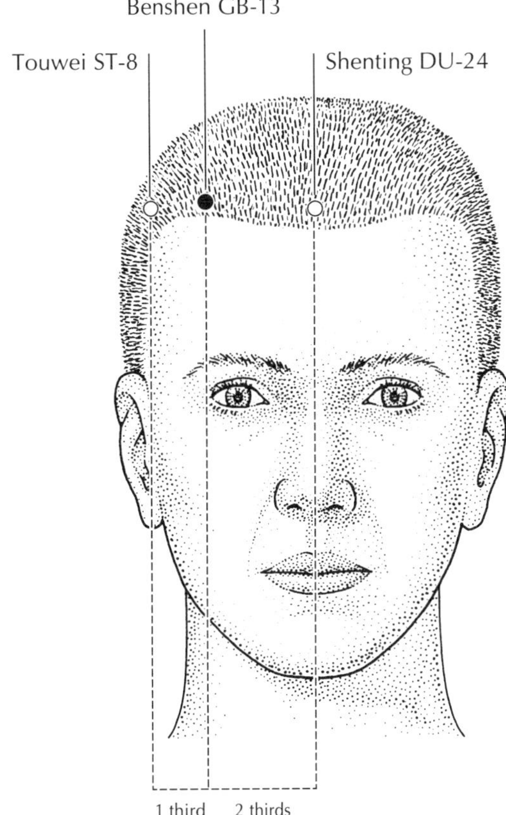

COMBINATIONS

- Madness: Benshen GB-13 and Shenzhu DU-12 (*One Hundred Symptoms*).
- Childhood fright epilepsy: Benshen GB-13, Qianding DU-21, Xinhui DU-22 and Tianzhu BL-10 (*Thousand Ducat Formulas*).
- Vomiting of foam: Benshen GB-13, Shaohai HE-3 and Duiduan DU-27 (*Supplementing Life*).
- Epilepsy with vomiting of foam: Benshen GB-13 and Duiduan DU-27 (*Supplementing Life*).
- Pain of the lateral costal region with inability to turn the body: Benshen GB-13 and Luxi SJ-19 (*Thousand Ducat Formulas*).

YANGBAI GB-14

Yang White

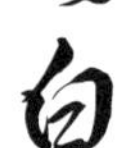

Meeting point of the Gall Bladder with the Yang Linking vessel and the Sanjiao, Stomach and Large Intestine channels

LOCATION

On the forehead, 1 cun superior to the middle of the eyebrow, directly above the pupil when the eyes are looking straight ahead.

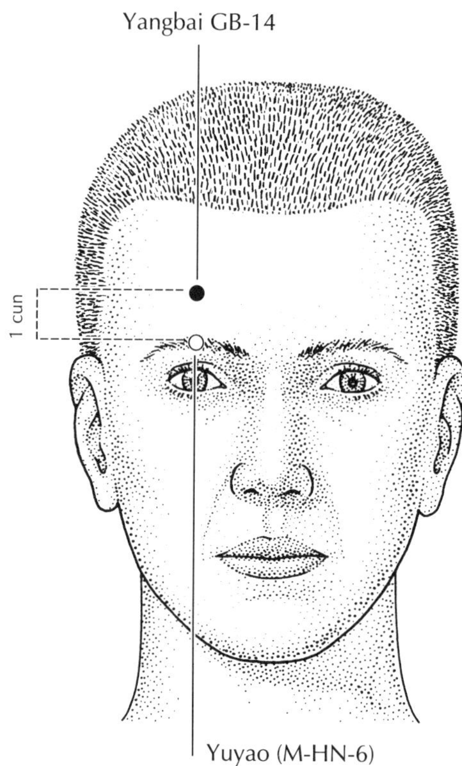

LOCATION NOTE

The distance between the glabella and the anterior hairline at the midline is measured as 3 cun.

NEEDLING

With the fingers of one hand pinch up the skin over the point, and with the other hand needle transversely in an inferior direction, 0.5 to 0.8 cun, or needle to connect with Yuyao (M-HN-6) [the midpoint of the eyebrow].

ACTIONS

Eliminates wind, benefits the head and alleviates pain
Benefits the eyes

INDICATIONS

- Pain of the forehead, pain of the supraorbital ridge, head wind, wind-cold headache, dizziness, pain of the face.
- Eye pain, lacrimation on exposure to wind, night blindness, short sightedness.
- Deviation of the mouth and eye, upward staring eyes, drooping of the eyelid, twitching of the eyelids, itching of the eyelids, pain and itching of the pupils.
- Inability to get warm despite wearing much clothing, shivering and aversion to cold on the back.

COMMENTARY

In theory, the forehead is most closely associated with the yangming channel. In clinical practice pain of the forehead region may be due to involvement either of yangming channel, in which case it is often accompanied by pain of the infraorbital region (often seen in sinusitis), or of shaoyang channel, in which case it is frequently accompanied by pain of the temporal or parietal regions and eye (often seen in migrainous headaches). Yangbai GB-14 is a meeting point of the Gall Bladder shaoyang channel with the Stomach and Large Intestine yangming channels, and is therefore the pre-eminent local point in the treatment of pain of the forehead, whether due to interior disharmony or invasion of exterior pathogenic factors. Some classical sources, for example the *Great Compendium of Acupuncture and Moxibustion*, also imply that Yangbai GB-14 can dispel wind-cold from the body as a whole and recommend it for inability to get warm despite wearing much clothing, and shivering and aversion to cold on the back.

Yangbai GB-14 is also an important local point for the treatment of various diseases of the eyes and eyelids due to a wide range of aetiologies, especially exterior or interior wind, manifesting as lacrimation, deviation of the eye, drooping, twitching or itching of the eyelids, pain and itching of the pupils and night-blindness.

COMBINATIONS

- Head wind with splitting sensation, pain between the eyebrow and the eye: Yangbai GB-14, Jiexi ST-41 and Hegu L.I.-4 (*Classic of the Jade Dragon*).

TOULINQI GB-15

Head Governor of Tears

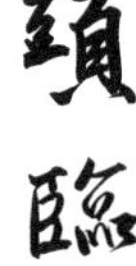

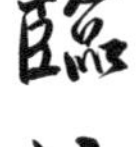

Meeting point of the Gall Bladder and Bladder channels with the Yang Linking vessel

LOCATION

On the forehead, directly above Yangbai GB-14, 0.5 cun within the anterior hairline, midway between Shenting DU-24 and Touwei ST-8.

LOCATION NOTE
The distance between the anterior and posterior hairlines in the midline is measured as 12 cun. If the anterior hairline is indistinct, the distance is measured as 15 cun between the glabella [point Yintang (M-HN-3)] and the posterior hairline; the location of the anterior hairline would thus be defined as one fifth of this distance. If the posterior hairline is indistinct, it can be measured as 1 cun inferior to Fengfu DU-16 which lies immediately below the external occipital protuberance. Note that the line of the anterior hairline away from the midline usually curves somewhat posteriorly, and this should be taken into account when locating the Gall Bladder points on the scalp (Toulinqi GB-15 to Naokong GB-19).

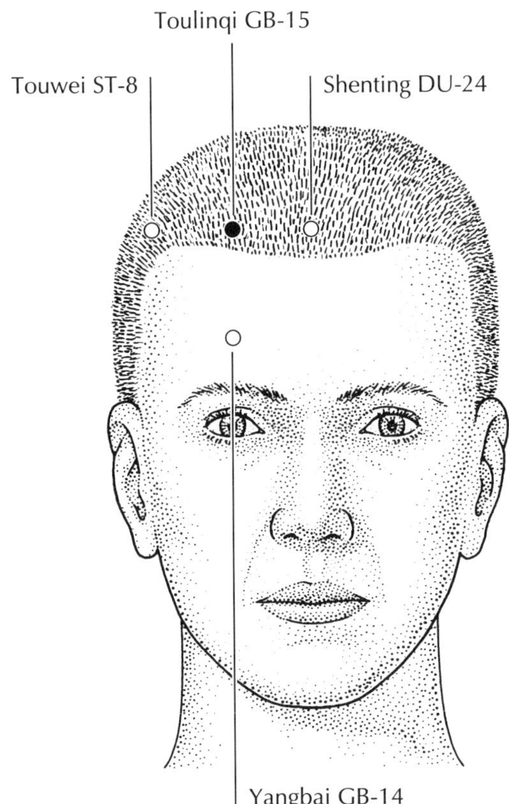

NEEDLING
Transverse insertion 0.5-1.5 cun. See note Hanyan GB-4.

ACTIONS
Eliminates wind, benefits the head and alleviates pain
Benefits the nose and eyes

INDICATIONS
- Nasal congestion, nasal congestion with aversion to cold.
- Headache, head wind, visual dizziness, pain of the occiput and forehead, pain of the supraorbital ridge.
- Redness and pain of the eyes, superficial visual obstruction, lacrimation on exposure to wind, pain at the outer canthus.
- Windstroke, epilepsy, loss of consciousness, malaria, pain of the supraclavicular fossa, swelling of the axilla.

COMMENTARY
As its name (Head Governor of Tears) implies, Toulinqi GB-15 is indicated for lacrimation as well as for redness and pain of the eyes and superficial visual obstruction. In this respect it mirrors Zulinqi (Foot Governor of Tears) towards the distal end of the channel. Like several other points on the crown of the head (e.g. Tongtian BL-7 and Shangxing DU-23) it also has a pronounced action on the nose and is indicated for nasal congestion.

COMBINATIONS
- Lacrimation on exposure to wind: Toulinqi GB-15, Touwei ST-8, Jingming BL-1 and Fengchi GB-20 (*Great Compendium*).
- Lacrimation: Toulinqi GB-15 and Touwei ST-8 (*One Hundred Patterns*).
- Visual dizziness: Toulinqi GB-15 and Zhongzhu SJ-3 (*Supplementing Life*).
- Superficial visual obstruction: Toulinqi GB-15 and Ganshu BL-18 (*Great Compendium*).
- Red eyes and bleeding from Yingxiang L.I.-20 (i.e. nosebleed): Toulinqi GB-15, Taichong LIV-3 and Hegu L.I.-4 (*Song of Points*).
- Nasal congestion: Toulinqi GB-15 and Tongtian BL-7 (*Supplementing Life*).

MUCHUANG GB-16
Window of the Eye

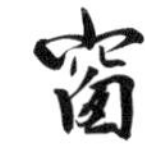

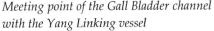

Meeting point of the Gall Bladder channel with the Yang Linking vessel

LOCATION
Above the forehead, on a curved line drawn between Toulinqi GB-15 and Fengchi GB-20, following the contour of the cranium, 1.5 cun posterior to Toulinqi GB-15.

LOCATION NOTE
i. See location note for Toulinqi GB-15; ii. First locate Toulinqi GB-15 0.5 cun posterior to the hairline and then locate Chengling GB-18 directly lateral to Baihui DU-20, on the line of the Gall Bladder channel. Muchuang GB-16 is then located one third of the distance between Toulinqi GB-15 and Chengling GB-18.

NEEDLING

Transverse insertion 0.5-1.5 cun. See note Hanyan GB-4.

ACTIONS

Benefits the eyes
Eliminates wind and alleviates pain

INDICATIONS

- Visual dizziness, superficial visual obstruction, redness, swelling and pain of the eyes, short sightedness, all kinds of eye diseases.
- Headache, swelling of the head and face, toothache of the upper jaw, swelling of the gums, nasal congestion, epilepsy.
- Aversion to cold, chills and fever with absence of sweating.

COMMENTARY

According to *Investigation into Points Along the Channels* by the Ming dynasty author Yan Zhen-shi, Muchuang GB-16 (Window of the Eye) is indicated for all kinds of eye diseases. In modern clinical practice, however, this point is rarely used.

COMBINATIONS

- Red eyes: Muchuang GB-16 and Daling P-7 (*Supplementing Life*).
- Headache: Muchuang GB-16, Tianchong GB-9 and Fengchi GB-20 (*Systematic Classic*).
- Stiffness of the lips and pain from tooth decay of the upper jaw: Muchuang GB-16, Zhengying GB-17, Duiduan DU-27 and Ermen SJ-21 (*Thousand Ducat Formulas*).

ZHENGYING GB-17

Upright Nutrition

正營

Meeting point of the Gall Bladder channel with the Yang Linking vessel

LOCATION

In the parietal region, on a curved line drawn between Toulinqi GB-15 and Fengchi GB-20, following the contour of the cranium, 1.5 cun posterior to Muchuang GB-16.

LOCATION NOTE

i. See location note for Toulinqi GB-15; ii. First locate Toulinqi GB-15, 0.5 cun posterior to the hairline, and then locate Chengling GB-18 directly lateral to Baihui DU-20, on the line of the Gall Bladder channel. Zhengying GB-17 is then located two thirds of the distance between Toulinqi GB-15 and Chengling GB-18.

NEEDLING

Transverse insertion 0.5-1.5 cun. See note Hanyan GB-4.

ACTIONS

Benefits the head and alleviates pain
Pacifies the Stomach

INDICATIONS

- Headache, one-sided headache, toothache of the upper jaw.
- Visual dizziness, dizziness due to phlegm-fluid, ceaseless vomiting, nausea, stiff neck, stiffness of the lips, aversion to wind and cold, aversion to the sound of people talking.

COMBINATIONS

- Toothache of the upper jaw: Zhengying GB-17 and Yanggu SI-5 (*Thousand Ducat Formulas*).
- Pain from tooth decay: Zhengying GB-17, Sanjian L.I.-3 and Daying ST-5 (*Supplementing Life*).
- Stiffness of the lips and pain from tooth decay of the upper jaw: Zhengying GB-17, Duiduan DU-27, Muchuang GB-16 and Ermen SJ-21 (*Thousand Ducat Formulas*).

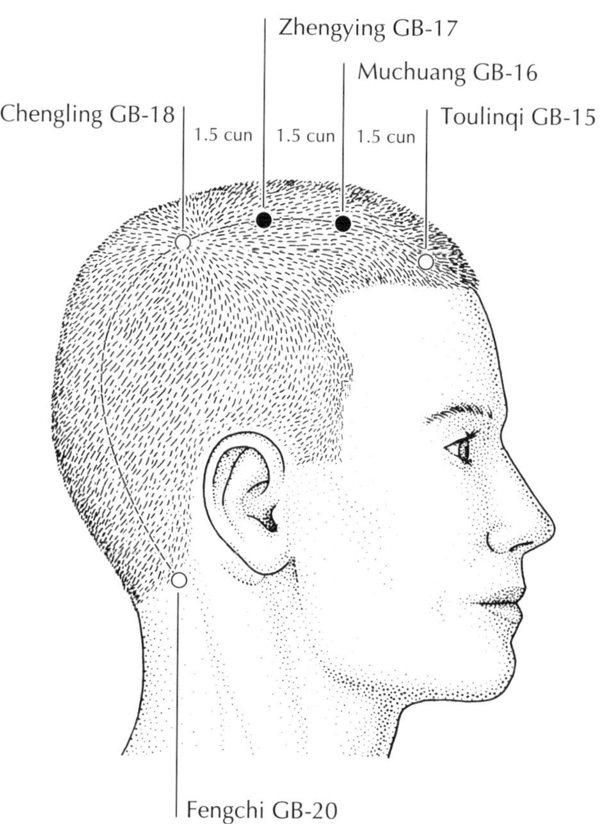

CHENGLING GB-18
Support Spirit

承靈

Meeting point of the Gall Bladder channel with the Yang Linking vessel

LOCATION

In the parietal region, on a curved line drawn between Toulinqi GB-15 and Fengchi GB-20, following the contour of the cranium, 1.5 cun posterior to Zhengying GB-17.

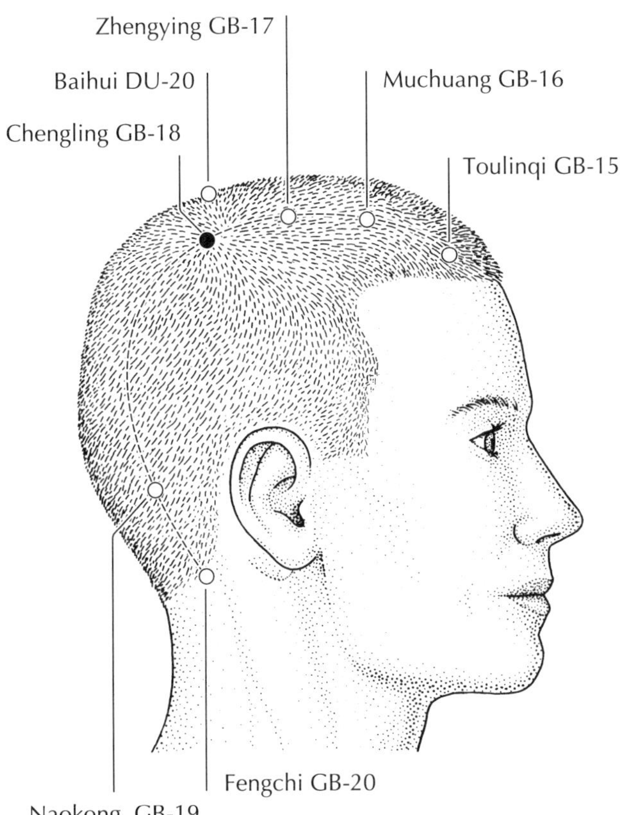

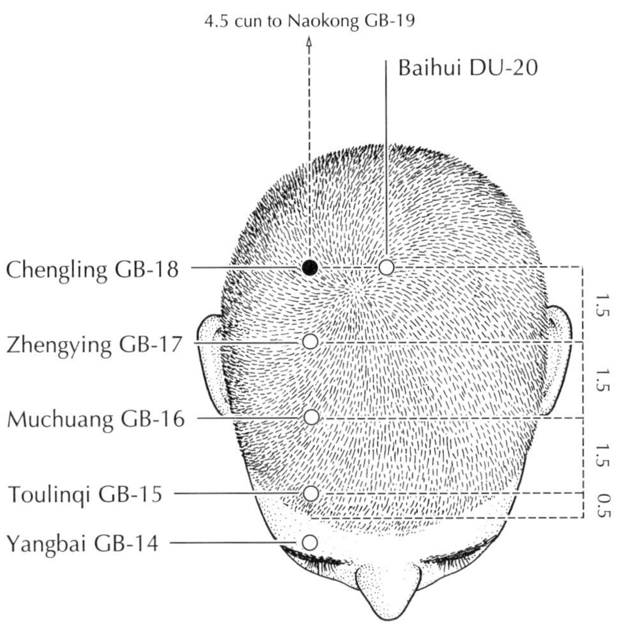

LOCATION NOTE

Locate directly lateral to Baihui DU-20, on the line of the Gall Bladder channel (2.25 cun from the midline).

NEEDLING

Transverse insertion 0.5-1.5 cun. See note Hanyan GB-4.

ACTIONS

Benefits the head and alleviates pain
Benefits the nose and descends Lung qi

INDICATIONS

- Headache, brain wind, dizziness, eye pain.
- Rhinitis and nosebleed, nasal congestion, dyspnoea, cough, aversion to wind and cold.

COMBINATIONS

- Nosebleed with stifled breathing: Chengling GB-18, Fengchi GB-20, Fengmen BL-12, Yixi BL-45 and Houxi SI-3 (*Thousand Ducat Formulas*).

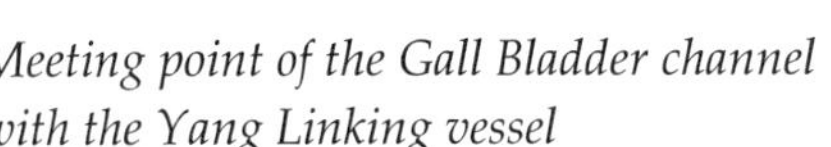

NAOKONG GB-19
Brain Hollow

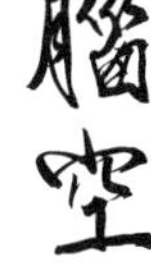

Meeting point of the Gall Bladder channel with the Yang Linking vessel

LOCATION

In the occipital region, directly above Fengchi GB-20, level with Naohu DU-17.

LOCATION NOTE

i. Locate Naohu DU-17 1.5 cun directly above Fengfu DU-16, in the depression directly superior to the external occipital protuberance; ii. Alternatively (if the external occipital protuberance is indistinct) locate Naokong GB-19 one quarter of the distance between Fengchi GB-20 and Chengling GB-18.

NEEDLING

Transverse insertion 0.5-1.5 cun. See note Hanyan GB-4.

ACTIONS

Benefits the head and alleviates pain
Pacifies wind and clears the sense organs

INDICATIONS

- Headache, head wind, brain wind, one-sided headache and heaviness of the head, stiffness and pain of the neck with inability to turn the head, wind dizziness.
- Redness, swelling and pain of the eyes, deafness and tinnitus, pain of the nose, nasal congestion, nosebleed.
- Fright palpitations, mania depression disorder, taxation disorders with emaciation, heat in the body.

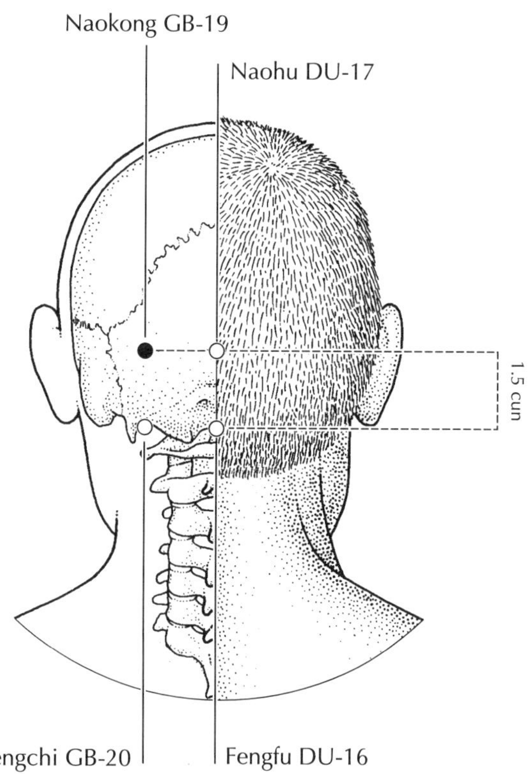

COMMENTARY

The *Great Compendium of Acupuncture and Moxibustion* records how Hua Tuo, the famous 2nd century physician, treated General Wei Tai-cu (the posthumously consecrated emperor of the Wei dynasty) for 'head wind, confused mind and visual dizziness'. After needling Naokong GB-19, the General was cured. This story, however, also appears in an earlier source in which the point needled is Yongquan KID-1.

COMBINATIONS

- Pain and heaviness of the head: Naokong GB-19, Naohu DU-17 and Tongtian BL-7 (*Thousand Ducat Formulas*).
- Head wind: Naokong GB-19, Baihui DU-20 and Tianzhu BL-10 (*Supplementing Life*).

FENGCHI GB-20

Wind Pool

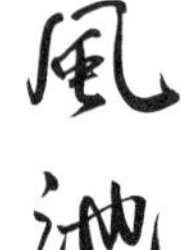

Meeting point of the Gall Bladder and Sanjiao channels with the Yang Motility and Yang Linking vessels

LOCATION

Below the occiput, approximately midway between Fengfu DU-16 and Wangu GB-12, in the hollow between the origins of the sternomastoid and trapezius muscles.

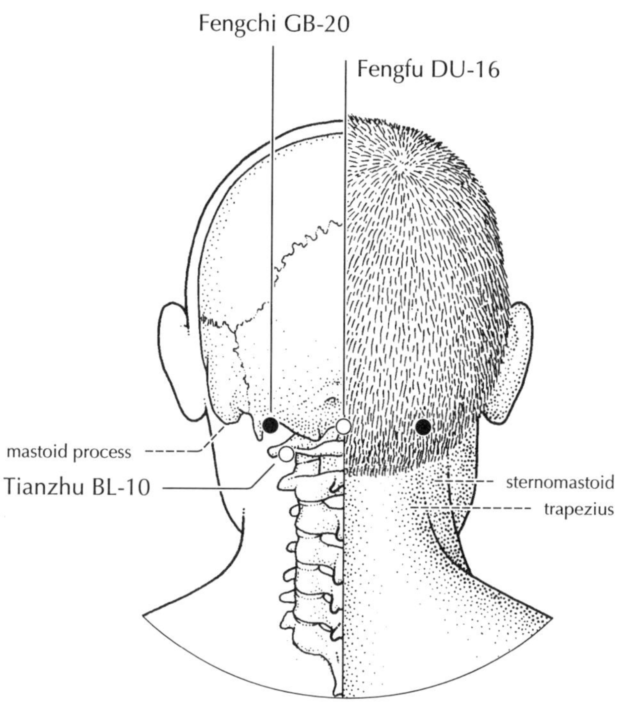

LOCATION NOTE

i. Locate close to the base of the skull; ii. This point is normally located as the most tender point of the hollow.

NEEDLING

i. Slightly oblique inferior insertion in the direction of the channel, 1 to 1.5 cun; ii. Directed towards the tip of the nose, the contralateral eyeball or Yintang (M-HN-3), 0.5 to 1 cun. **Caution:** deeper needling may damage the spinal cord; iii. Joined by through-needling to contralateral Fengchi GB-20, 2 to 3 cun.

ACTIONS

Eliminates wind
Benefits the head and eyes
Clears the sense organs
Activates the channel and alleviates pain

INDICATIONS

- Headache, head wind, one-sided and generalised headache, dizziness, visual dizziness, hypertension, hemiplegia, deviation of the mouth and eye, goitre, lockjaw.
- Insomnia, loss of memory, epilepsy, loss of speech following windstroke.
- Injury by cold, injury by cold with absence of sweating, chills and fever, warm febrile disease with absence of sweating, malaria, throat painful obstruction, swelling of the face, urticaria.
- Redness and pain of the eyes, redness and pain of the inner canthus, blurred vision, lacrimation (especially on exposure to wind), night blindness, dimness of vision.
- Nosebleed, rhinitis, nasal congestion and discharge.
- Deafness, tinnitus, blocked ears.
- Stiffness and pain of the neck with inability to turn the head, pain of the shoulder and upper back, pain of the lumbar spine, crooked lumbar spine leading to flaccidity and lack of strength in the sinews of the neck.

COMMENTARY

Fengchi GB-20, located at the nape of the neck, occupies a pivotal position between the head and the body and is one of the pre-eminent acupuncture points to treat all diseases of the head, brain and sensory organs, especially the eyes.

Wind, a yang pathogenic factor whose nature is to harass the uppermost (and therefore most yang) part of the body, may be of two kinds: i. exterior pathogenic wind which attacks the most superficial portion of the body, and ii. interior wind which has its origin in disharmony of the Liver. As its name (Wind Pool) implies, Fengchi GB-20 is an important local point to treat both kinds of wind disease affecting the head.

Exterior wind is known as the 'spearhead of the hundred diseases' and easily combines with other pathogenic factors and drives them into the body. When exterior pathogenic wind, wind-cold or wind-heat injure the body, the characteristic sign is chills and fever. Fengchi GB-20 is a meeting point of the Gall Bladder channel with both the Yang Motility vessel and the Yang Linking vessel. The Yang Motility vessel is indicated for aversion to wind, whilst the Yang Linking vessel links all the yang channels of the body, including the Governing vessel. Yang corresponds to the exterior while yin corresponds to the interior, and the yang channels as a whole therefore relate more to the exterior portion of the body. According to the *Classic of Difficulties*[3] "when the Yang Linking vessel is diseased, there will be severe chills and fever". Fengchi GB-20 is especially indicated when injury by wind is accompanied by headache or other symptoms of the head region such as lacrimation, red and sore eyes, nasal congestion and discharge, sore throat, swelling of the face etc.

Fengchi GB-20 is equally important to pacify pathologically ascending interior wind and to settle yang and clear fire from the head, and is therefore indicated for such disorders as headache, head wind, dizziness, deviation of the mouth and eyes, hemiplegia and lockjaw as well as for hypertension.

According to a saying of Chinese medicine, "The head is the residence of the yang". The Yang Linking vessel links all the yang channels and connects with the Governing vessel (which enters the brain) at Yamen DU-15 and Fengfu DU-16, and Fengchi GB-20 is the single most important acupuncture point in the treatment of headache, whatever the aetiology and whichever the involved channels. A more specific recommendation is found in the *Ode of the Jade Dragon* which proposes the use of Fengchi GB-20 for 'head wind with phlegm' and Hegu L.I.-4 for 'head wind without phlegm'. In the same way that it treats any variety of headache, Fengchi GB-20 may be used for dizziness due to any pattern of disharmony.

Fengchi GB-20 has a strong action on the eyes and nose, and to a lesser extent the ears, and is indicated for red and painful eyes, visual disorders, lacrimation, nosebleed, rhinitis, nasal congestion and discharge, tinnitus and deafness whether due to interior disharmony or exterior wind. By virtue of its connection with the Yang Linking vessel, and hence the Governing vessel, and of its action of pacifying interior wind, it is also effective in 'awakening' the brain and can be used for such symptoms as the sequelae of windstroke, loss of speech following windstroke, epilepsy and loss of memory.

Fengchi GB-20 has a strong effect on activating the channel and alleviating pain, and is an important point in the treatment of disorders of the neck, shoulders and upper back. It is interesting to note that Fengchi GB-20 is also indicated for lumbar pain and 'crooked lumbar spine leading to flaccidity and lack of strength in the sinews of the neck'.

The wide range of disorders of the head and neck that may be treated by Fengchi GB-20 is reflected in the variety of needle directions that may be employed at this point. In the treatment of neck disorders, Fengchi GB-20 is normally needled either perpendicularly or towards opposite Fengchi GB-20; in the treatment of nose disorders it is needled towards the tip of the nose; in the treatment of eye disorders it is needled towards the opposite eye, and in the treatment of mental disorders towards Yintang (M-HN-3).

COMBINATIONS

- "In taiyang disorder, initially prescribe Gui Zhi Tang (Cinnamon Twig Decoction). If this causes agitation, needle Fengchi GB-20 and Fengfu DU-16, then re-prescribe Gui Zhi Tang. Recovery will follow" (*Treatise on Injury by Cold*).

- The hundred disorders due to injury by cold: Fengchi GB-20 and Fengfu DU-16 (*Ode of Xi-hong*).
- Headache: Fengchi GB-20, Muchuang GB-16 and Tianchong GB-9 (*Systematic Classic*).
- One-sided or generalised headache: Fengchi GB-20, Hegu L.I.-4 and Sizhukong SJ-23 (*Great Compendium*).
- One-sided or generalised head wind: Fengchi GB-20, Baihui DU-20, Qianding DU-21, Shenting DU-24, Shangxing DU-23, Sizhukong SJ-23, Hegu L.I.-4, Zanzhu BL-2 and Touwei ST-8 (*Great Compendium*).
- Head wind and dizziness: Fengchi GB-20, Hegu L.I.-4, Fenglong ST-40 and Jiexi ST-41 (*Great Compendium*).
- Dizziness: Fengchi GB-20, Shangxing DU-23 and Tianzhu BL-10 (*Glorious Anthology*).
- Lacrimation on exposure to wind: Fengchi GB-20, Touwei ST-8, Jingming BL-1 and Toulinqi GB-15 (*Great Compendium*).
- Cold lacrimation: Fengchi GB-20, Zulinqi GB-41, Jingming BL-1 and Wangu SI-4 (*Great Compendium*).
- Pain of the eyes with inability to see: Fengchi GB-20, Naohu DU-17, Yuzhen BL-9, Fengfu DU-16 and Shangxing DU-23 (*Thousand Ducat Formulas*).
- Nosebleed with stifled breathing: Fengchi GB-20, Chengling GB-18, Fengmen BL-12, Yixi BL-45 and Houxi SI-3 (*Thousand Ducat Formulas*).
- Impaired hearing and deafness: Fengchi GB-20, Xiaxi GB-43, Tinghui GB-2, Ermen SJ-21 and Tinggong SI-19 (*Great Compendium*).
- Swelling of the face: first needle Yixi BL-45, then Tianyou SJ-16 and Fengchi GB-20 (*Systematic Classic*).
- Redness and swelling of the face: Fengchi GB-20, Shangxing DU-23, Xinhui DU-22, Qianding DU-21 and Naohu DU-17 (*Thousand Ducat Formulas*).
- Curvature of the lumbar spine: reinforce Fengchi GB-20 and reduce Xuanzhong GB-39 (*Ode of the Jade Dragon*).

JIANJING GB-21

Shoulder Well

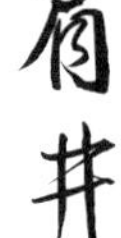

Meeting point of the Gall Bladder, Sanjiao and Stomach channels with the Yang Linking vessel

LOCATION

Midway between Dazhui DU-14 and the tip of the acromion, at the crest of the trapezius muscle.

LOCATION NOTE

i. The crest refers to the highest point of the trapezius muscle on the sagittal (anterior-posterior) plane; ii. This point is normally located at the point of maximum tenderness.

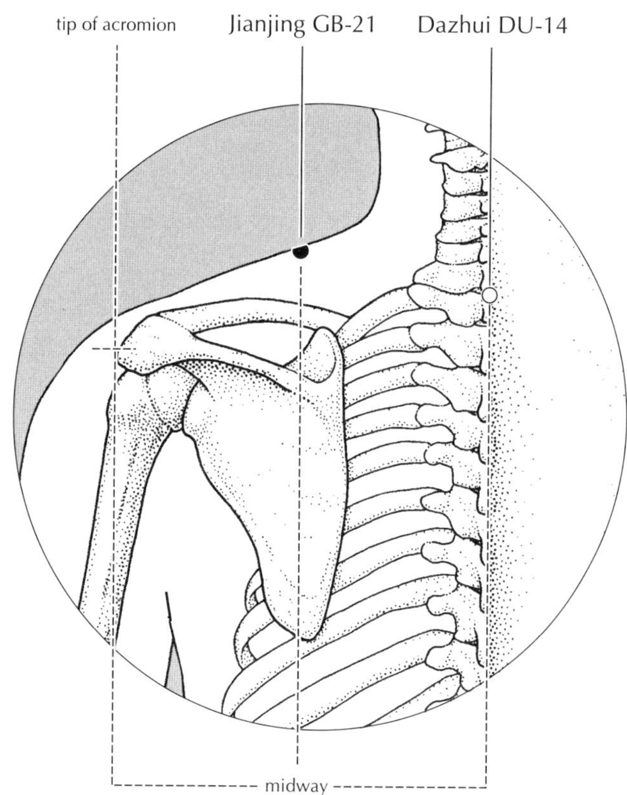

NEEDLING

Posterior oblique insertion, 0.5-1 cun.

Caution: i. perpendicular insertion, especially in thin patients, carries a substantial risk of inducing a pneumothorax; ii. contraindicated in pregnancy.

ACTIONS

Regulates qi, activates the channel and alleviates pain
Transforms and lowers phlegm and dissipates nodules
Benefits the breasts and expedites delivery

INDICATIONS

- Stiffness and pain of the neck, pain of the shoulder and back, inability to raise the hand and arm, hemiplegia.
- Loss of speech following windstroke, windstroke, wind-taxation, the five taxations and the seven injuries, steaming bone disorder, Kidney deficiency lumbar pain.
- Cough and dyspnoea, rebellion of qi, mania-depression, redness of the face.
- Scrofula, goitre, leg qi ascending to attack the Heart, pain of the Spleen.
- Difficult or prolonged labour, inversion counterflow of the arms and legs following miscarriage, retention of the placenta, uterine bleeding.
- Breast pain, breast abscess, breast milk does not flow, furuncles and carbuncles.

COMMENTARY

The region of Jianjing GB-21, at the crest of the trapezius muscle, is particularly prone to symptoms of contraction, tightness and pain due to a variety of aetiologies. The Gall Bladder is interiorly-exteriorly coupled with the Liver. Stagnation of Liver qi or uprising of Liver yang due to anger, frustration, resentment etc. commonly vent upwards along the Gall Bladder channel, and readily accumulate in and below the neck, especially when tightness and restriction in the relatively narrow neck region prevent their upward flow. The close relationship between the upper body and anger was emphasised in many texts, for example the *Essential Questions*[4] which stated "anger will cause the qi to surge upwards". Alternatively, the region of Jianjing GB-21 may be injured by sprain, penetration by wind-cold (especially after sleeping in a cold draught), prolonged poor posture or occupational strain. Jianjing GB-21 may be needled in all such cases of stiffness of the neck and shoulders, which may extend to the back or arm.

Jianjing GB-21 is indicated for a variety of phlegm disorders. Phlegm may involve Liver or Gall Bladder pathology in the following three ways: i. Liver qi stagnation leads to stagnation of fluids which condense into phlegm, summed up in the statement in the *Treatise on Disorders of Blood* "When qi flows, water also flows", ii. Liver wind ascends carrying phlegm with it (this is one of the main pathological features of windstroke), and iii. Liver or Gall Bladder fire steams and condenses fluids into phlegm. By virtue of its actions of regulating qi, lowering and transforming phlegm and dissipating nodules, Jianjing GB-21 is used in the treatment of such phlegm disorders as hemiplegia, loss of speech following windstroke, windstroke, scrofula and goitre

Jianjing GB-21 also has a strong qi descending action and is indicated in various disorders of rebellious qi such as cough and dyspnoea, rebellion of qi, and leg qi ascending to attack the Heart. Leg qi is a disorder characterised by numbness, pain, weakness, spasm, swelling, redness and heat sensations of the feet and legs. In severe cases the pathogen attacks more deeply affecting the abdomen and Heart.

Difficult labour may be due to stagnation or deficiency of qi and blood. In either case, due to its strong descending action, Jianjing GB-21 has long been used to expedite delivery and promote the descent of the placenta, and for this reason is contraindicated in pregnancy. Jianjing GB-21 is also specifically indicated by the *Classic of Supplementing Life with Acupuncture and Moxibustion* for "Inversion counterflow coldness of the arms and legs following miscarriage". A similar condition in post-partum women is described by the famous Qing dynasty gynaecologist Fu Qing-zhu who says "In the course of delivery, some women overexert themselves with taxation and fatigue injuring the Spleen. As a result, there occurs inversion with counterflow chilling of the limbs, qi ascends to fill up the chest, the pulse departs, and form deserts"[5]. The implied ability of Jianjing GB-21 to tonify deficiency following miscarriage, is surprisingly mirrored in its indications for a variety of deficiency patterns including wind-taxation, the five taxations and seven injuries, Kidney deficiency lumbar pain and steaming bone disorder.

So strong is the action of Jianjing GB-21 in descending qi that Gao Wu, in the *Ode of Xi-hong*, says "When you needle Jianjing GB-21 you must needle Zusanli ST-36. If this is not done, the qi will not be regulated". In other words, the action of Zusanli ST-36 on tonifying and raising the qi will help to counter any excessive descent of the qi resulting from needling Jianjing GB-21.

Jianjing GB-21 is also indicated for breast disorders. The Gall Bladder primary channel penetrates the chest and the Gall Bladder sinew channel connects with the breast, whilst Jianjing GB-21 is a meeting point of the Gall Bladder channel with the Stomach channel which descends through the nipple. Excessive worry, anger, frustration, resentment or depression may lead to stagnation and knotting of Liver qi, or accumulated heat in the Stomach channel may gather at the breast, leading to breast pain, breast abscess, and failure of the breast milk to flow. Jianjing GB-21 may be selected in all these situations.

COMBINATIONS

- Inability to turn the neck: Jianjing GB-21 and Pohu BL-42 (*Supplementing Life*).
- Pain of the shoulder and back: Jianjing GB-21, Fengmen BL-12, Zhongzhu SJ-3, Zhigou SJ-6, Houxi SI-3, Wangu SI-4 and Weizhong BL-40 (*Great Compendium*).
- Pain of the forearm: Jianjing GB-21 and Quchi L.I.-11 (*Ode to Elucidate Mysteries*).
- Pain and cold of the arm: Jianjing GB-21, Quchi L.I-11 and Xialian L.I-8 (*Great Compendium*).
- Scrofula: Jianjing GB-21, Shaohai HE-3, Tianchi P-1, Zhangmen LIV-13, Zulinqi GB-41, Zhigou SJ-6, Yangfu GB-38 and Shousanli L.I.-10 (*Great Compendium*).
- Retention of the placenta: Jianjing GB-21 and Zhongji REN-3 (*Great Compendium*).
- Retention of the placenta: Jianjing GB-21, Zhongji REN-3 and Sanyinjiao SP-6 (*Meeting the Source*).
- Pain and soreness of leg qi: first needle Jianjing GB-21, then needle Zusanli ST-36 and Yanglingquan GB-34 (*Celestial Star*).
- Prolapse of the rectum: Jianjing GB-21, Baihui DU-20, Changqiang DU-1, Dachangshu BL-25, Hegu L.I.-4 and Qichong ST-30 (*Compilation*).

YUANYE GB-22

淵腋

Armpit Abyss

LOCATION

On the mid-axillary line, in the fifth intercostal space, approximately 3 cun inferior to the apex of the axilla, at the level of the nipple.

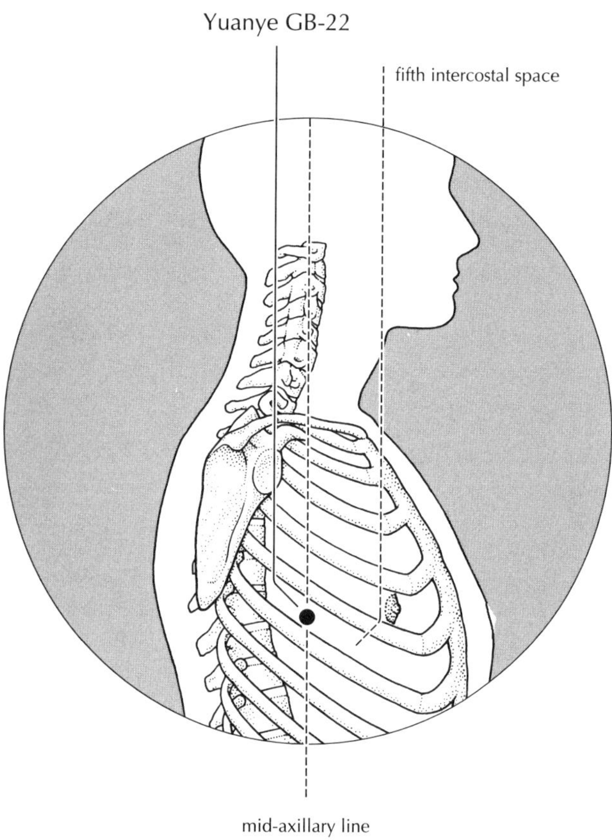

LOCATION NOTE

i. The mid-axillary line is drawn vertically down from the apex of the axilla (Jiquan HE-1); ii. First locate the costal cartilage of the second rib which is level with the sternal angle, locate the second intercostal space below it and then locate the fifth intercostal space, three spaces below that; in males the nipple lies in the fourth intercostal space; iii. Some sources locate this point in the fourth intercostal space.

NEEDLING

Transverse-oblique insertion along the intercostal space, 0.5 to 1 cun.

Caution: deep or perpendicular needling may induce a pneumothorax. **Note**: according to several classical texts, this point is contraindicated to moxibustion.

ACTIONS

Regulates qi and unbinds the chest
Benefits the axilla

INDICATIONS

- Cough, fullness of the chest, chills and fever, pain of the lateral costal region, swelling of the axilla, scrofula of the axilla, sabre lumps.
- Pain of the shoulder and arm, inability to raise the arm.

COMBINATIONS

- Sabre lumps of the axilla: Yuanye GB-22, Zhigou SJ-6, Waiguan SJ-5 and Zulinqi GB-41 (*Illustrated Supplement*).

ZHEJIN GB-23

輒筋

Flank Sinews

Meeting point of the Gall Bladder and Bladder channels

LOCATION

Below the axilla in the fifth intercostal space, 1 cun anterior to Yuanye GB-22, approximately at the level of the nipple.

LOCATION NOTE

See Yuanye GB-22.

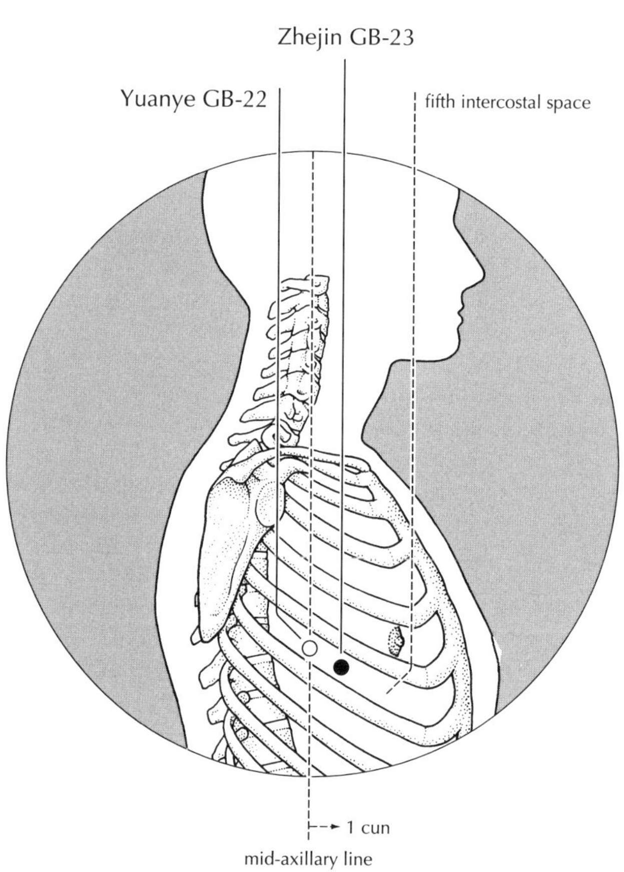

NEEDLING

Transverse-oblique insertion along the intercostal space, 0.5 to 1 cun.

Caution: deep or perpendicular needling may induce a pneumothorax.

ACTIONS

Unbinds the chest and lowers rebellion
Regulates qi in the three jiao

INDICATIONS

- Sudden fullness of the chest, pain of the lateral costal region, dyspnoea, asthma, scrofula, pain of the shoulder and arm.
- Sighing and tendency to sadness, insomnia, heat of the lower abdomen.
- Vomiting, acid regurgitation, much spittle, loss of use of the four limbs.

COMMENTARY

According to the *Great Compendium of Acupuncture and Moxibustion* this point rather than Riyue GB-24 is the front-mu point of the Gall Bladder, and an alternative name for Zhejin GB-23 given in this classic was Danmu i.e. 'Gall Bladder Mu'. In fact the classical indications for Zhejin GB-23 and Riyue GB-24 are very similar, with a greater emphasis on disorders of the chest in the case of Zhejin GB-23 reflecting its higher location.

Excessive anger, frustration and resentment, especially when not spontaneously expressed, will impair the free-flowing function of the Liver. Qi stagnates along the course of the Gall Bladder channel in the lateral costal region, and binds the chest, restricting its smooth expansion and contraction. Breathing is impaired leading to fullness and pain, sighing and sadness. Zhejin GB-23 is an important local point used in the treatment of these conditions. If stagnation of qi transforms to fire it may affect the upper jiao (Heart) giving rise to sleep disturbance, the middle jiao leading to vomiting and acid regurgitation, or the lower jiao giving rise to heat of the lower abdomen.

RIYUE GB-24

Sun and Moon

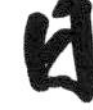

Meeting point of the Gall Bladder and Spleen channels
Front-Mu point of the Gall Bladder

LOCATION

On the anterior chest wall, in the seventh intercostal space, directly below the nipple, 4 cun lateral to the midline.

LOCATION NOTE

First locate the costal cartilage of the second rib which is level with the sternal angle, locate the second intercostal space below it and then locate the seventh intercostal space, five spaces below that. In males the nipple lies in the fourth intercostal space.

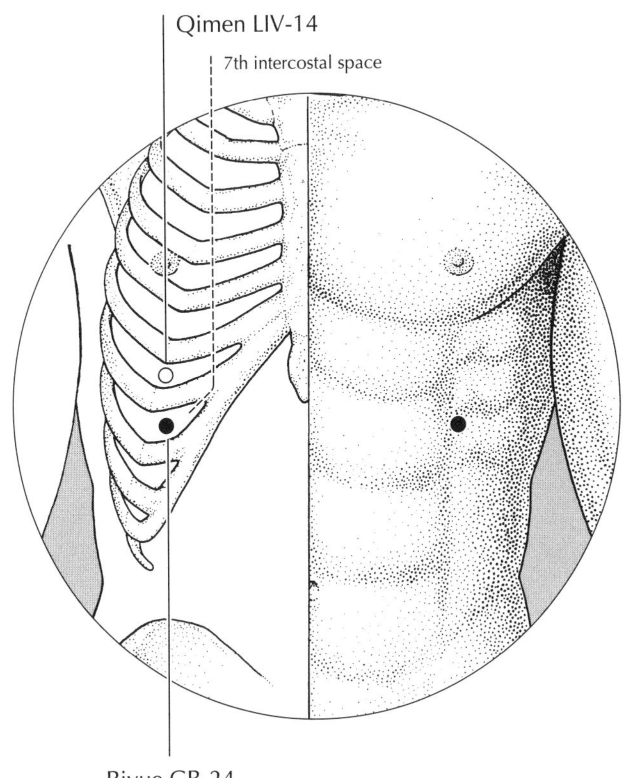

NEEDLING

Transverse-oblique insertion along the intercostal space, 0.5 to 1 cun.

Caution: deep or perpendicular needling may induce a pneumothorax.

ACTIONS

Benefits the Gall Bladder and spreads Liver qi
Lowers rebellious qi and harmonises the middle jiao
Resolves damp-heat

INDICATIONS

- Distention, fullness and pain of the lateral costal region, pain of the ribs, epigastric pain, abdominal distention, jaundice.
- Vomiting, much spittle, acid regurgitation, hiccup.
- Sighing with tendency to sadness, heat of the lower abdomen, heat of the hypogastrium, loss of use of the four limbs.

COMMENTARY

According to the *Essential Questions*[6] "The Gall Bladder is the upright official from where judgement emanates". When the characters for sun and moon (the name of this point) are combined, they form a new character 'ming' which means 'clear', intelligent' or 'to understand'. 'Ming' describes the quality of judgement emanating from a healthy Gall Bladder. Riyue GB-24 has traditionally been ascribed the ability to rectify deficiency patterns of the Gall Bladder and was indicated as early as the *Essential Questions* (with Danshu BL-19) for the treatment of Gall Bladder deficiency giving rise to indecisiveness, and elsewhere for sighing with a tendency to sadness.

Riyue GB-24 was established as the front-mu point of the Gall Bladder by the time of the *Yellow Emperor's Inner Classic*. Although many centuries later the *Great Compendium of Acupuncture and Moxibustion* designated Zhejin GB-23 as the Gall Bladder front-mu point, it is Riyue GB-24 which has retained this status to the present day. The term 'mu' means to gather or to collect, and the front-mu points are where the qi of the zangfu gathers and concentrates on the anterior surface of the body. Riyue GB-24 is an important point to treat diseases of the Gall Bladder fu which may derive from the following three aetologies: i. emotional disharmony results in stagnation of Liver qi which impairs the circulation of qi in its interiorly-exteriorly related Gall Bladder channel, and gives rise to distention, fullness and pain of the lateral costal region, sighing and a sensation of heat in the lower abdomen; ii. disharmony of the Stomach and Spleen transportation and transformation function leads to accumulation of dampness which transforms to damp-heat and ferments in the Liver and Gall Bladder; bile does not flow and seeps into the muscles and skin giving rise to jaundice; iii. Gall Bladder qi invades the Stomach and interferes with its descending function resulting in vomiting, acid regurgitation, hiccup and epigastric pain. All these three patterns may be encountered in diseases such as cholecystitis, cholelithiasis and hepatitis.

COMBINATIONS

- "When a person is frequently indecisive, the Gall Bladder is deficient. The qi will flow upwards giving rise to a bitter taste in the mouth. To treat this use the Mu and the Shu of the Gall Bladder" [Riyue GB-24 and Danshu BL-19] (*Essential Questions*).
- Sighing with propensity to sadness: Riyue GB-24 and Shangqiu SP-5 (*Supplementing Life*).
- Loss of use of the four limbs: Riyue GB-24, Jiquan HE-1 and Pishu BL-20 (*Supplementing Life*).
- Cholecystitis: Riyue GB-24, Burong ST-19, Dannangxue (M-LE-23), Zhigou SJ-6 and Qiuxu GB-40.

JINGMEN GB-25

Capital Gate

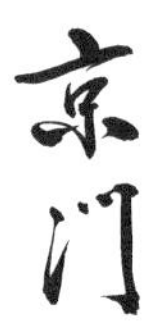

Front-Mu point of the Kidneys

LOCATION

Below the lateral aspect of the ribcage, anterior and inferior to the free end of the 12th rib.

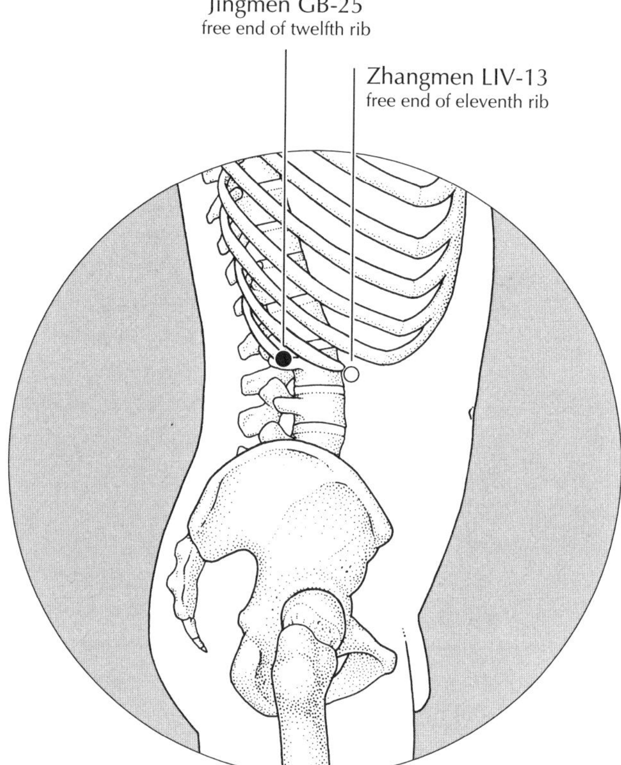

LOCATION NOTE

To locate the free end of the twelfth rib, first place the entire hand on the upper abdomen and with gentle finger pressure palpate downwards along the costal margin, until the end of the eleventh rib is located just above the level of the umbilicus. Then palpate further along the inferior margin of the ribcage until the free end of the twelfth rib is located in the lateral lumbar region.

NEEDLING

Perpendicular insertion 0.5 to 1 cun.
Caution: in thin subjects, deep needling may penetrate the peritoneal cavity.

ACTIONS

Tonifies the Kidneys and regulates the water passages
Fortifies the Spleen and regulates the intestines
Strengthens the lumbar region

INDICATIONS
- Borborygmus, cold or damp (dong) diarrhoea, abdominal distention, vomiting, pain of the lower abdomen, painful shan disorder.
- Difficult urination, dark urine, swelling of the face, failure of the water passages to flow, desire to drink.
- Chills and fever, disgruntled with inability to catch the breath.
- Weakness of the spine, lumbar pain with inability to stand for long, pain of the lateral costal region and back, pain of the inner aspect of the shoulder blade, pain of the hip.

COMMENTARY
Jingmen GB-25 is the front-mu point of the Kidneys. The term 'mu' means to gather or to collect, and the front-mu points are where the qi of the zangfu gathers and concentrates on the anterior surface of the body.

The main action of Jingmen GB-25 is to assist the mutual relationship between the Kidneys and the Spleen. According to the *Complete Works of Jing-yue* "Ming men is the sea of essence [and] blood, the Spleen is the sea of water and grain, together they are the root of the five zang and six fu". The Kidneys are the source of pre-heaven qi and rule the fluids, whilst the Spleen is the source of post-heaven qi, and rules the transportation and transformation of food and water. The Kidney yang is the root of all the yang of the body, and its fire is the source for the vigour of the Spleen's transportation and transformation function. At the same time, it is the Spleen which extracts the essence from food to supplement the Kidney essence. When this mutual support between the Kidneys and Spleen breaks down, there will be impairment of both the Spleen's digestive function, and the Kidneys' function of ruling the fluids. Jingmen GB-25 is indicated for cases of cold or damp (dong) diarrhoea, borborygmus and abdominal distention resulting from Spleen yang deficiency which either derives from Kidney yang deficiency, or due to its prolonged nature has injured the Kidney yang. It is also used to tonify Kidney yang to facilitate the flow of water in urinary diseases and is indicated for difficult urination, concentrated urine, swelling of the face and 'failure of the water passages to flow'.

The Kidneys rule the lumbar region and the bones. The other principal application of Jingmen GB-25 is in the treatment of disorders of the lumbar region and spine, particularly when due to deficiency of the Kidneys. It is therefore indicated for weakness of the spine and for lumbar pain with inability to stand for long. Due to its location on the Gall Bladder channel it is also indicated for combined pain of the back and lateral costal region, for example in renal colic, as well as for pain of the hip.

COMBINATIONS
- Cold or damp (dong) diarrhoea with undigested food: Jingmen GB-25, Rangu KID-2 and Yinlingquan SP-9 (*Thousand Ducat Formulas*).
- Cold or damp (dong) diarrhoea with body pain: Jingmen GB-25 and Kunlun BL-60 (*Thousand Ducat Formulas*).
- Dark urine and obstruction of the water pathway: Jingmen GB-25 and Zhaohai KID-6 (*Thousand Ducat Formulas*).
- Swelling of the lower abdomen: Jingmen GB-25, Ligou LIV-5 and Zhongfeng LIV-4 (*Supplementing Life*).
- Lumbar pain with inability to stand for long or move: Jingmen GB-25 and Xingjian LIV-2 (*Systematic Classic*).
- Lumbar pain with tension of the spine: Jingmen GB-25 and Zhishi BL-52 (*Thousand Ducat Formulas*).

DAIMAI GB-26
Girdling Vessel

帶脈

Meeting point of the Gall Bladder channel with the Girdling vessel

LOCATION
Directly below Zhangmen LIV-13 (anterior and inferior to the free end of the eleventh rib), level with the umbilicus.

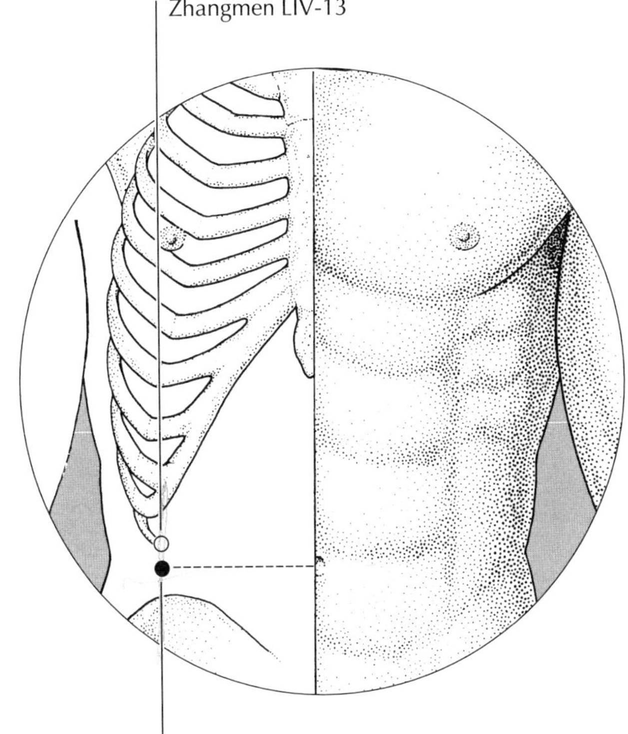

LOCATION NOTE

i. To locate the free end of the eleventh rib, place the entire hand on the upper abdomen and with gentle finger pressure palpate downwards along the costal margin, until the end of the eleventh rib is located just above the level of the umbilicus; ii. The free end of the eleventh rib usually lies on or near the mid-axillary line which is drawn vertically down from the apex of the axilla (Jiquan HE-1).

NEEDLING

Perpendicular insertion, 0.5 to 1 cun. **Caution:** in thin subjects, deep needling may penetrate the peritoneal cavity.

ACTIONS

Regulates the Girdling vessel and drains dampness
Regulates menstruation and stops leucorrhoea
Activates the channel and alleviates pain

INDICATIONS

- Red and white leucorrhoea, disorders of menstruation, irregular menstruation, amenorrhoea, infertility, uterine prolapse, hardness and pain of the hypogastrium in women, lower abdominal pain in women.
- Unendurable pain of the lateral costal region which radiates to the back, pain of the lateral costal region, lumbar pain, shan disorder, tenesmus, clonic spasm.

COMMENTARY

The Girdling vessel, encircling the waist like a belt, is the only major channel that runs horizontally. It passes through the points Daimai GB-26, Wushu GB-27 and Weidao GB-28, and encircles and binds the Penetrating, Conception and Governing vessels and the Kidney, Liver and Spleen channels. The Girdling vessel plays an important role in controlling leucorrhoea and may be damaged by turbid dampness which sinks downwards, deficiency of Kidney yin or Kidney yang, invasion of exterior dampness which transforms into heat, or pouring down of Liver and Gall Bladder channel damp-heat, all of which may result in leucorrhoea. In fact, the term 'dai xia' (leucorrhoea) is made up of the characters 'dai', meaning belt or girdle, and 'xia' meaning downward. As the most important point to regulate the qi of the Girdling vessel, Daimai GB-26 is indispensable in the treatment of leucorrhoea resulting from any of the above patterns.

According to the *Spiritual Pivot*[7] "The Penetrating and Conception vessels both start in the uterus", whilst *Confucians' Duties to Their Parents*, the 13th century classic by Zhang Cong-zheng, states "The Penetrating, Conception and Governing vessels have the same starting point but different circulation, the same source but different branches, each of them connects with the Girdling vessel". The Conception vessel, Penetrating vessel and Governing vessel therefore all originate in the uterus in females and are all bound by the Girdling vessel. Daimai GB-26 is not just an important point to activate the Girdling vessel itself, but has a significant influence on the Conception and Penetrating vessels, and is able to treat disorders of the uterus and menstruation such as infertility, irregular menstruation and amenorrhoea, and sinking of qi giving rise to uterine prolapse.

As well as regulating the qi of the Girdling vessel, Daimai GB-26 is effective as a local point to resolve stagnation of qi deriving from disharmony of the Liver. Disorder of the Girdling vessel and qi stagnation in the lower jiao may lead to pain, distention and hardness of the lower abdomen in women, pain of the lateral costal region, shan disorder and lumbar pain.

COMBINATIONS

- Red and white leucorrhoea: Daimai GB-26, Guanyuan REN-4, Qihai REN-6, Sanyinjiao SP-6, Baihuanshu BL-30 and Jianshi P-5 (*Great Compendium*).
- Amenorrhoea: Daimai GB-26 and Xuehai SP-10 (*Supplementing Life*).
- Irregular menstruation: Daimai GB-26, Qihai REN-6, Zhongji REN-3, Shenshu BL-23 and Sanyinjiao SP-6 (*Great Compendium*).
- Pain and hardness of the hypogastrium: Daimai GB-26 and Xiaxi GB-43 (*Supplementing Life*).

WUSHU GB-27

Five Pivots

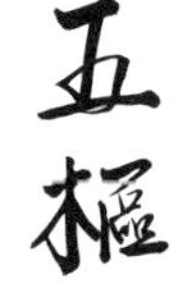

Meeting point of the Gall Bladder channel with the Girdling vessel

LOCATION

In the depression just anterior to the anterior superior iliac spine, approximately level with Guanyuan REN-4 (3 cun below the umbilicus).

LOCATION NOTE

To locate the anterior superior iliac spine (ASIS), place the hand on the lateral part of the lower abdomen, below the level of the umbilicus. The ASIS is then readily palpated as the pronounced bony prominence. Alternatively, follow the ridge of the iliac crest and palpate the ASIS as its anterior prominence.

NEEDLING

Perpendicular insertion 1 to 1.5 cun.

ACTIONS

Regulates the Girdling vessel
Regulates the lower jiao and transforms stagnation

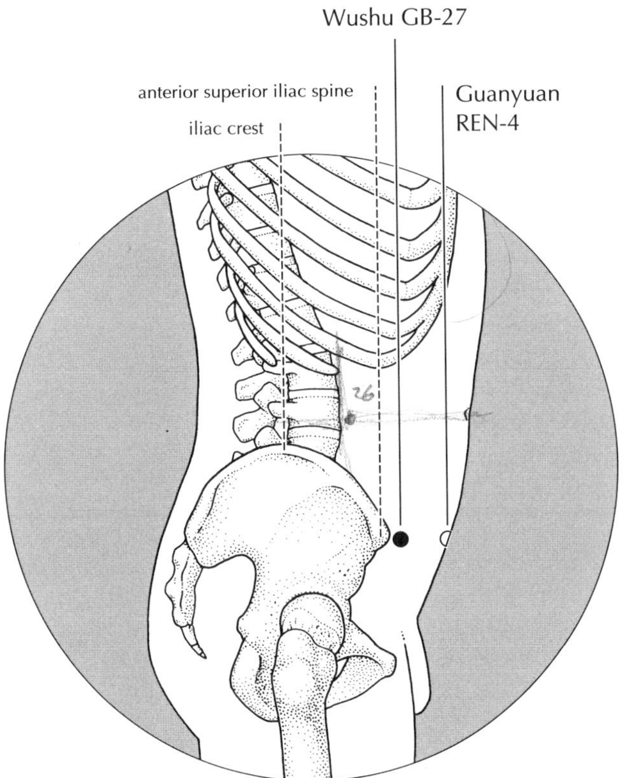

INDICATIONS

- Uterine prolapse, red and white leucorrhoea, irregular menstruation.
- Lower abdominal pain, cold shan disorder in men, abdominal pain due to retraction of the testicles, constipation, tenesmus, pain of the back, lumbar region and ilium, clonic spasm.

COMMENTARY

Like Daimai GB-26, Wushu GB-27 (a coalescent point of the Girdling vessel) regulates the Girdling vessel, treats menstrual disorders and leucorrhoea, and spreads the Liver qi in the lower abdomen (lower abdominal pain and constipation).

In comparing the two points, however, it is interesting to note that the traditional qi moving and pain relieving indications of this point lean more towards male disorders such as cold shan disorder in men and abdominal pain due to retraction of the testicles, whilst those of Daimai GB-26 lean more towards female disorders such as hardness of the hypogastrium in women and lower abdominal pain in women. This is reflected in Zhu Danxi's statement "Serious shan qi is acute pain in the testicles extending to the lower abdomen. The pain may be in the testicles or in the neighbourhood of the point Five Pivots (Wushu GB-27). In either case it involves the foot jueyin channel"[8].

COMBINATIONS

- Retracted testicle: Wushu GB-27 and Guilai ST-29 (*Supplementing Life*).

WEIDAO GB-28

Linking Path

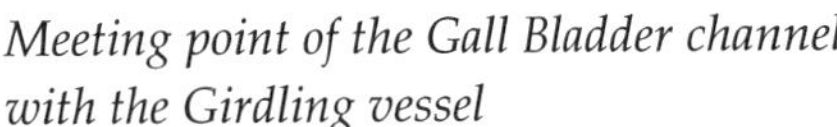

维道

Meeting point of the Gall Bladder channel with the Girdling vessel

LOCATION

0.5 cun anterior and inferior to Wushu GB-27.

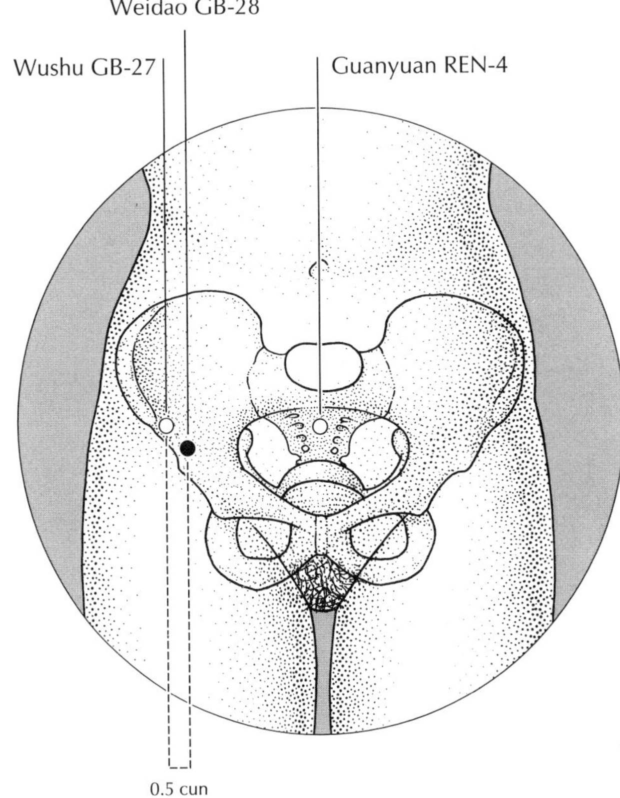

LOCATION NOTE

See Wushu GB-27.

NEEDLING

Perpendicular insertion 1 to 1.5 cun.

ACTIONS

Regulates the Girdling vessel
Regulates the lower jiao and transforms stagnation

INDICATIONS
- Uterine prolapse, irregular menstruation, leucorrhoea.
- Pain of the back and ilium, lower abdominal pain, shan disorder.
- No pleasure in eating, vomiting.

JULIAO GB-29
Stationary Crevice

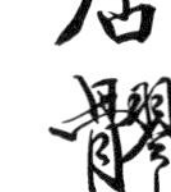

Meeting point of the Gall Bladder channel with the Yang Motility vessel

LOCATION
On the lateral aspect of the hip joint, at the midpoint of a line drawn between the anterior superior iliac spine and the prominence of the greater trochanter.

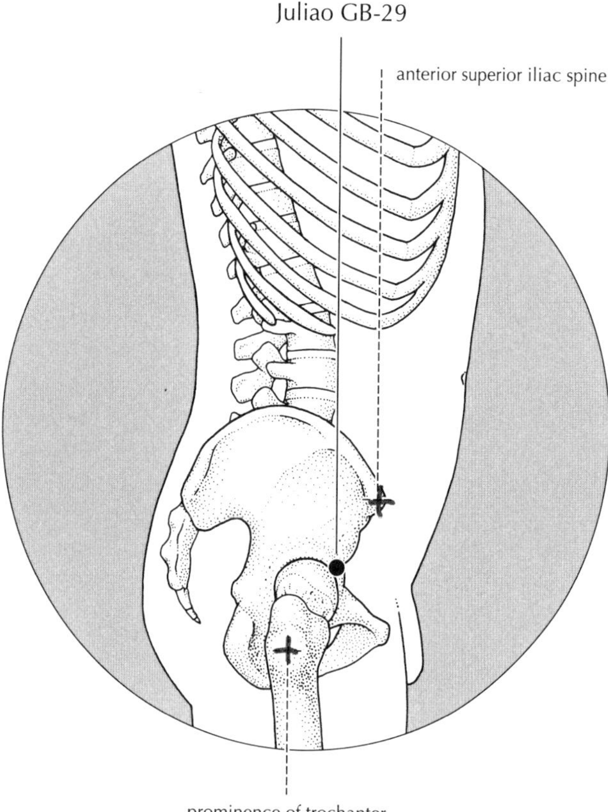

LOCATION NOTE
i. To locate the anterior superior iliac spine see Wushu GB-27; ii. To accurately palpate the prominence of the greater trochanter place one hand over the lateral aspect of the hip joint at the level of the perineum, and with the other hand rotate the foot in order to feel the movement of the prominence of the greater trochanter; iii. Alternatively, flex the hip joint and locate Juliao GB-39 at the lateral end of the crease thus formed.

NEEDLING
Perpendicular insertion 1 to 2 cun, or oblique insertion inferiorly 2 to 3 cun.

ACTIONS
Activates the channel and alleviates pain
Benefits the hip joint

INDICATIONS
- Pain of the back and leg, lumbar pain radiating to the lower abdomen, hip pain radiating to the groin, weakness and paralysis of the leg, sciatica, shan disorder, pain of the front of the shoulder radiating to the chest, inability to raise the arm.
- Oedema, vomiting, diarrhoea.

COMMENTARY
Juliao GB-29 is very commonly used in clinical practice in the treatment of hip disorders, and is especially indicated when pain radiates from the hip to the groin and lower abdomen. Correct needling will ensure radiation of sensation to these areas.

In the cross-needling method of point selection, the shoulder joint in the upper body corresponds to the hip joint in the lower body, and Juliao GB-29 is not only indicated for hip pain radiating forward to the groin, but also for shoulder pain radiating forward to the chest.

COMBINATIONS
- Wind-damp leg pain: Juliao GB-29, Huantiao GB-30 and Weizhong BL-40 (*Song of the Jade Dragon*).
- Sciatica: Juliao GB-29, Huantiao GB-30, Ciliao BL-32 and Weizhong BL-40.

HUANTIAO GB-30
Jumping Circle

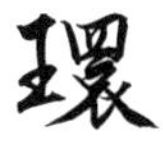
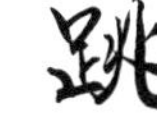

Meeting point of the Gall Bladder and Bladder channels
Ma Dan-yang Heavenly Star point

LOCATION
On the postero-lateral aspect of the hip joint, one third of the distance between the prominence of the greater trochanter and the sacro-coccygeal hiatus (Yaoshu DU-2).

LOCATION NOTE
i. This point may most readily be located (and needled) with the patient lying on their side; ii. To accurately palpate the prominence of the greater trochanter place one hand over the lateral aspect of the hip joint at the level

of the perineum, and with the other hand rotate the foot in order to feel the movement of the prominence of the greater trochanter; iii. The sacro-coccygeal hiatus is located in-between the cornua of the sacrum and coccyx, in the depression inferior to the fourth sacral spinous process if this is palpable. Note, however, that the sacro-coccygeal hiatus may sometimes extend as high as the level of the third sacral foramina.

NEEDLING

Perpendicular insertion, directed towards the genitals, 2 to 3.5 cun. **Note**: a radiating or electric sensation may travel to the foot. Since this manifestation of deqi (arrival of qi) is particularly indicated in cases of sciatica it may be more readily induced by locating Huantiao GB-30 one cun inferior to its normal position.

ACTIONS

Activates the channel and alleviates pain
Benefits the hip joint and leg
Dispels wind-damp

INDICATIONS

- Pain of the buttock, pain or sprain of the hip and leg, sciatica, atrophy disorder and painful obstruction of the lower limb, hemiplegia, cold-wind-damp painful obstruction, numbness of the leg, inability to flex and extend the knee, contraction and pain of the thigh and knee, pain of the lumbar region and lateral costal region, pain of the lumbar region and leg, leg qi.
- Urticaria, eczema.

COMMENTARY

Huantiao GB-30 was included by Ma Dan-yang, the great physician of the Jin dynasty, among the 'eleven heavenly star points'[9], his grouping of the most vital acupuncture points, and was indicated by him for " ... cold wind and damp painful obstruction, pain radiating from the hip to the calf, sighing with pain when turning over". Huantiao GB-30 is unrivalled in importance for the treatment of disorders of the hip joint and buttock, whether due to traumatic injury, painful obstruction, stagnation of qi or deficiency.

Huantiao GB-30 is located at the pivotal hip region, the gate of the lower limb, and as its name 'Jumping Circle' implies, is able to influence the movement of the whole lower limb. It is a vital point to promote circulation of qi and blood in the treatment of all kinds of painful obstruction, atrophy disorder, numbness, stiffness, pain and contraction of the leg. In the treatment of sciatica, it is considered by many practitioners to be the single most important point which may be used whatever the nature and distribution of the pain. Its importance in the treatment of painful obstruction of the lower extremities was emphasised in the *Secrets of the Heavenly Star* which asked "Cold wind damp painful obstruction, where do you needle? First choose Huantiao GB-30, then Yanglingquan GB-34". Its ability to promote circulation throughout the leg also renders it an essential point in the treatment of hemiplegia with an action similar to points of the yangming Stomach channel.

The Bladder channel unites with the Gall Bladder channel at this point, and Huantiao GB-30 can therefore also treat disorders of the lumbar region (through which the Bladder channel courses), whether extending to the hip and buttock, or radiating upwards along the Gall Bladder channel to the lateral costal region.

Finally Huantiao GB-30 is cited in the *Song of the Nine Needles for Returning the Yang* for the treatment of collapse of yang characterised by loss of consciousness, aversion to cold, cold counterflow of the limbs, purple lips etc.

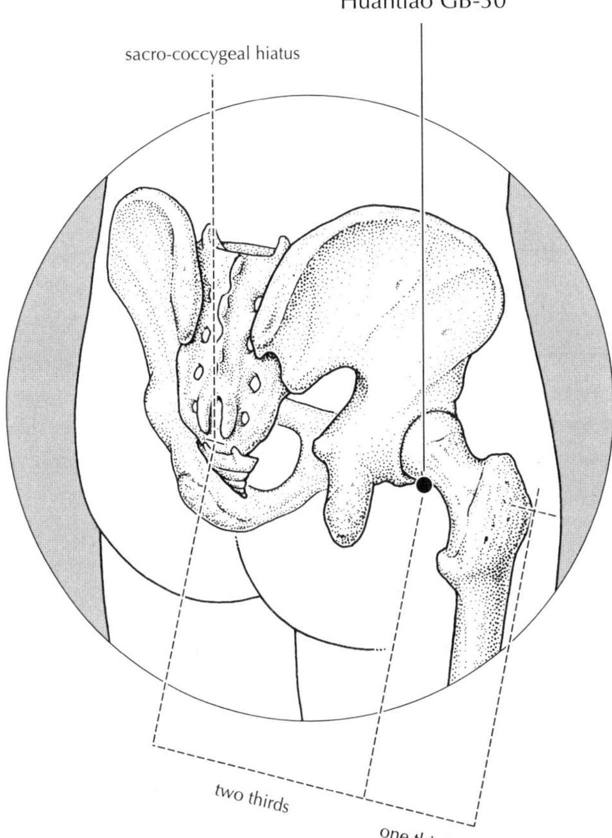

COMBINATIONS

- One-sided wind (hemiplegia): Huantiao GB-30, Yanglingquan GB-34 and Quchi L.I.-11 (*Supplementing Life*).
- Cold-wind-damp painful obstruction: first needle Huantiao GB-30 then Yanglingquan GB-34 (*Secrets of the Heavenly Star*).

- Hip pain: Huantiao GB-30, Shugu BL-65, Jiaoxin KID-8, Sanyinjiao SP-6 and Yingu KID-10 (*Thousand Ducat Formulas*).
- Hip pain: Huantiao GB-30, Yanglingquan GB-34 and Qiuxu GB-40 (*Great Compendium*).
- Pain of the lumbar region and knee: Huantiao GB-30, Yanglingquan GB-34, Yanglao SI-6, Kunlun BL-60 and Shenmai BL-62 (*Illustrated Supplement*).
- Lumbar pain: Huantiao GB-30 and Weizhong BL-40; if the pain radiates up the back add Kunlun BL-60 (*Song of Points*).
- Lumbar pain that radiates down the leg: Huantiao GB-30, Xingjian LIV-2 and Fengshi GB-31 (*Song of Points*).
- Pain of the legs and lumbar region: Huantiao GB-30, Fengshi GB-31, Weizhong BL-40, Kunlun BL-60, Yinshi ST-33, Chengshan BL-57 and Shenmai BL-62 (*Great Compendium*).
- Wind-damp leg pain: Huantiao GB-30, Juliao GB-29 and Weizhong BL-40 (*Song of the Jade Dragon*).
- Cold wind painful obstruction that is difficult to cure: Huantiao GB-30 and Yaoshu DU-2 (*Ode of Xi-hong*).
- Pain of the leg radiating to the lateral costal region and axilla: Huantiao GB-30 and Yanglingquan GB-34 (*Song of Points*).
- Atrophy disorder: needle Huantiao GB-30 and Zhongdu GB-32, moxa Zusanli ST-36 and Feishu BL-13 (*Glorious Anthology*).
- Numbness of the lower leg: Huantiao GB-30, Xiyangguan GB-33 and Chengjin BL-56 (*Thousand Ducat Formulas*).
- Paralysis of the lower extremity: Huantiao GB-30, Yinlingquan SP-9, Yangfu GB-38, Taixi KID-3 and Zhiyin BL-67 (*Great Compendium*).
- Pain of the chest and lateral costal region that changes location: Huantiao GB-30 and Zhiyin BL-67 (*Thousand Ducat Formulas*).
- Disorders of the knee and the region above the knee: moxa Huantiao GB-30 and Yinshi ST-33 (*Great Compendium*).
- Wind rash: Huantiao GB-30 and Yongquan KID-1 (*Supplementing Life*).
- Pain radiating from the hip along the Stomach channel: Huantiao GB-30, Biguan ST-31, Zusanli ST-36 and Jiexi ST-41.
- Pain radiating from the hip along the Gall Bladder channel: Huantiao GB-30, Fengshi GB-31, Yanglingquan GB-34 and Xuanzhong GB-39.
- Pain radiating from the hip along the Bladder channel: Huantiao GB-30, Yinmen BL-37, Weizhong BL-40 and Kunlun BL-60.
- Pain radiating from the hip along the Bladder and Gall Bladder channels: Huantiao GB-30 and Feiyang BL-58.
- Pain radiating to the groin: Huantiao GB-30, Juliao GB-29 and Yinbao LIV-9.

FENGSHI GB-31

Wind Market

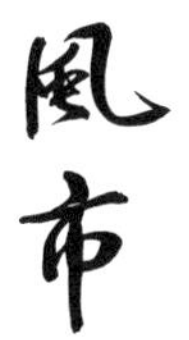

LOCATION

On the lateral aspect of the thigh, directly below the greater trochanter, 7 cun superior to the popliteal crease.

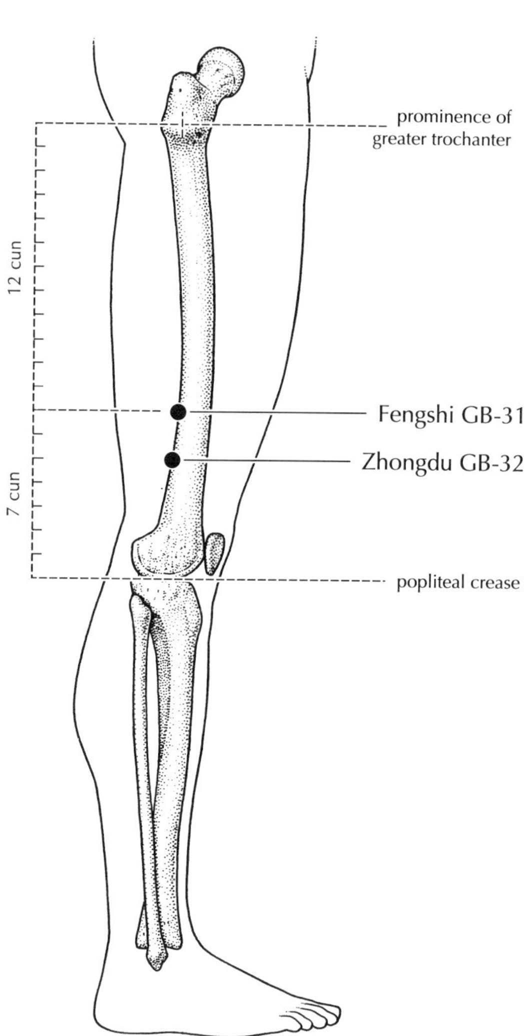

LOCATION NOTE

i. To palpate the prominence of the greater trochanter place a hand over the lateral aspect of the hip joint at the level of the perineum; ii. The distance between the prominence of the greater trochanter and the popliteal crease is 19 cun, thus Fengshi GB-31 is located at the tender point approximately 1 cun proximal to the junction of the upper two thirds and lower third of this line; iii. This point is traditionally described as being located where the tip of the middle finger reaches when a person stands erect with their arms extended by their sides, although the significant differences found in body proportions render this unreliable.

NEEDLING

i. Perpendicular or slightly oblique insertion posteriorly 1 to 2 cun; ii. Oblique insertion, directed proximally or distally, 1.5 to 2.5 cun.

ACTIONS

Eliminates wind
Alleviates itching
Activates the channel and alleviates pain

INDICATIONS

- Hemiplegia, atrophy disorder and painful obstruction of the lower limb, cold painful obstruction, sciatica, leg qi, numbness of the leg, weakness and feebleness of the legs, heavy sensation of the legs with difficulty in sitting, contraction and pain of the knees.
- Itching of the whole body, urticaria.

COMMENTARY

As its name 'Wind Market' implies, Fengshi GB-31 is an important point to treat disorders of wind, with three main spheres of application. Firstly it is indicated for pathogenic wind-damp which attacks the lower limb and gives rise to painful obstruction, especially where wind is the main pathogenic factor and the pain is wandering in nature. The *Complete Works of Jing-yue* stated "Fengshi GB-31 is the essential point for treating wind painful obstruction". Secondly, Fengshi GB-31 is recommended for when pathogenic wind gives rise to skin diseases characterised by rapid onset and itching, for example urticaria. Thirdly Fengshi GB-31 is indicated for hemiplegia following windstroke.

COMBINATIONS

- Windstroke: first needle the healthy arm and leg and then the diseased arm and leg, using Fengshi GB-31, Qiuxu GB-40 and Yanglingquan GB-34 (*Great Compendium*).
- Weakness of the legs: Moxa Fengshi GB-31, Taichong LIV-3 and Lidui ST-45 (*Outline of Medicine*).
- Lack of strength in the legs: Fengshi GB-31 and Yinshi ST-33 (*Ode of the Jade Dragon*).
- Lumbar pain that radiates down the leg: Fengshi GB-31, Huantiao GB-30 and Xingjian LIV-2 (*Song of Points for Miscellaneous Diseases*).
- Lumbar pain with difficulty in moving: Fengshi GB-31, Weizhong BL-40 and Xingjian LIV-2 (*Glorious Anthology*).
- Pain of the legs and lumbar region: Fengshi GB-31, Huantiao GB-30, Weizhong BL-40, Kunlun BL-60, Yinshi ST-33, Chengshan BL-57 and Shenmai BL-62 (*Great Compendium*).
- Painful obstruction of the calf: Fengshi GB-31 and Kunlun BL-60 (*Compilation*).

ZHONGDU GB-32

Middle Ditch

中瀆

LOCATION

On the lateral aspect of the thigh, 2 cun inferior to Fengshi GB-31.

LOCATION NOTE

i. First locate Fengshi GB-31 (see above) and then locate Zhongdu GB-32, 2 cun inferior to it; ii. The distance between the prominence of the greater trochanter and the popliteal crease is 19 cun, thus Zhongdu GB-32 is located at the tender point just proximal to the junction of the upper three quarters and the lower quarter of this line.

NEEDLING

i. Perpendicular or slightly posteriorly oblique insertion 1 to 2 cun; ii. Oblique insertion, directed proximally or distally, 1.5 to 2.5 cun.

ACTIONS

Expels wind, damp and cold
Activates the channel and alleviates pain

INDICATIONS

- Atrophy disorder and painful obstruction of the lower limb, sinew painful obstruction with numbness, numbness, hemiplegia, sciatica, pain of the back and hip, cold qi residing in the muscles and sinews.
- Urticaria.

COMMENTARY

Both the *Systematic Classic of Acupuncture and Moxibustion* and the *Great Compendium of Acupuncture and Moxibustion* recommend Zhongdu GB-32 for cold pathogenic qi which lodges in the muscles and sinews. This indication reflects the two principal ways of understanding and classifying painful obstruction that were discussed in the *Yellow Emperor's Inner Classic*. The first is according to the type of pathogen that predominates, i.e. cold, wind or damp. The second is according to the depth of penetration of the pathogen. In this method of differentiation, the most superficial level of invasion is the skin, followed by the muscles, vessels, sinews and bones. Each of these levels corresponds to one of the zang (the Lung, Spleen, Heart, Liver and Kidneys respectively) and an unresolved pathogen at any level might injure its related zang.

COMBINATIONS

- Atrophy disorder: needle Zhongdu GB-32 and Huantiao GB-30, moxa Zusanli ST-36 and Feishu BL-13 (*Glorious Anthology*).

XIYANGGUAN GB-33

Knee Yang Gate

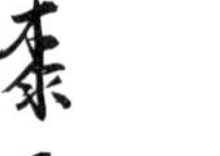
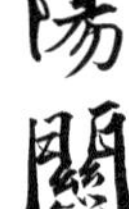

LOCATION

On the lateral side of the knee, in the depression above the lateral epicondyle of the femur, between the femur and tendon of biceps femoris.

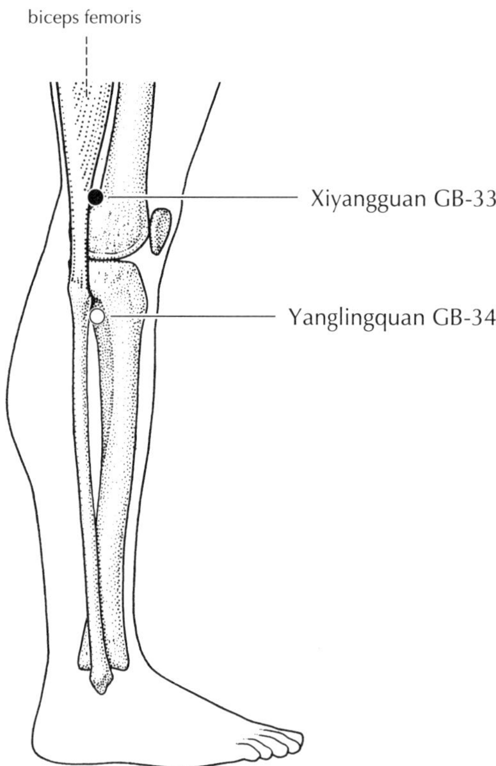

LOCATION NOTE

Starting above the knee joint, run a finger down the lateral aspect of the thigh in the groove between the femur and the tendon of biceps femoris, until the finger falls into the depression just proximal to the lateral epicondyle of the femur.

NEEDLING

Perpendicular insertion 1 to 2 cun. **Note**: according to several classical texts, this point is contraindicated to moxibustion.

ACTIONS

Relaxes the sinews and benefits the joints
Dispels wind-damp

INDICATIONS

- Redness, swelling and pain of the lateral aspect of the knee joint, inability to flex and extend the knee, wind painful obstruction with numbness, painful obstruction and numbness of the lower leg, leg qi.

COMMENTARY

An alternative name for Xiyangguan GB-33 is Hanfu (Mansion of Cold). This name reflects the observation that pathogenic cold tends to concentrate at the lateral side of knee, and that it may be treated by using this point. In clinical practice, Xiyangguan GB-33 is a valuable local point for pain of the lateral side of the knee which extends upwards along the thigh.

COMBINATIONS

- Numbness of the lower leg: Xiyangguan GB-33, Huantiao GB-30 and Chengjin BL-56 (*Thousand Ducat Formulas*).
- Contraction of the sinews and difficulty in flexing and extending the knee, with inability to walk: Xiyangguan GB-33, Liangqiu ST-34 and Ququan LIV-8 (*Thousand Ducat Formulas*).

YANGLINGQUAN GB-34

Yang Mound Spring

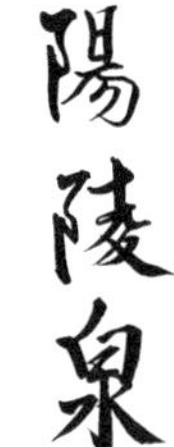

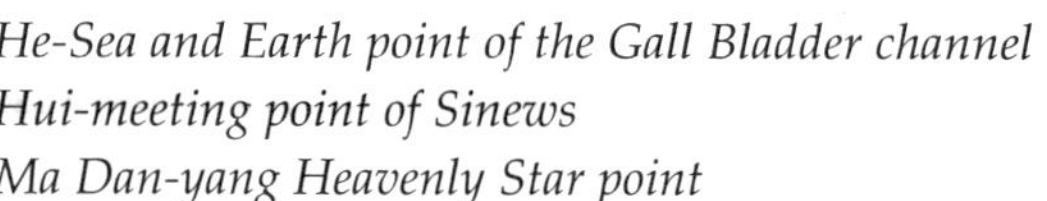
He-Sea and Earth point of the Gall Bladder channel
Hui-meeting point of Sinews
Ma Dan-yang Heavenly Star point

LOCATION

Below the lateral aspect of the knee, in the tender depression approximately 1 cun anterior and inferior to the head of the fibula.

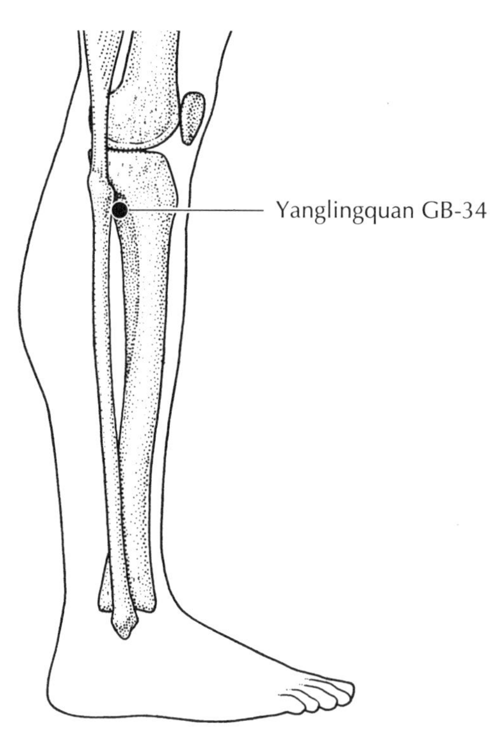

LOCATION NOTE

To avoid confusing the head of the fibula with the tibial condyle, slide your fingers up the lateral aspect of the lower leg until the soft tissue of the musculature gives way to the bony prominence of the head of the fibula.

NEEDLING

Perpendicular or slightly oblique posterior insertion 1 to 1.5 cun. This point is sometimes through-needled to Yinlingquan SP-9, in which case it should be located in a slightly more distal position.

ACTIONS

Benefits the sinews and joints
Activates the channel and alleviates pain
Spreads Liver qi and benefits the lateral costal region
Clears Liver and Gall Bladder damp-heat
Harmonises shaoyang

INDICATIONS

- Disorders of the sinews, contraction of the sinews, contraction and pain of the calf muscles in sudden turmoil disorder, contraction of the sinews of the foot, stiffness and tightness of the muscles and joints, numbness, hemiplegia, stiffness of the neck and shoulders, pain of the elbow, atrophy disorder and painful obstruction of the lower limb, swelling, pain and redness of the knee, cold painful obstruction of the hip and knee, sciatica, numbness and pain of the thigh and knee, coldness and pallor of the feet, leg qi.
- Diseases of the Gall Bladder, fullness and pain of the lateral costal region, frequent sighing, fear of people as if about to be apprehended, constipation, enuresis, epilepsy.
- Bitter taste in the mouth, dry throat, vomiting, jaundice, chills and fever, malaria, swelling of the face and head, hypertension.

COMMENTARY

According to the *Essential Questions*[10] "the knees are the residence of the sinews; when the knees are unable to flex and extend and walking is achieved with a hunched back and the help of a cane, then the sinews are exhausted". Yanglingquan GB-34, located just inferior to the knee joint, is the hui-meeting point of the sinews and has long been considered the main point to influence these tissues throughout the body, for example the *Great Compendium of Acupuncture and Moxibustion* simply stated "for diseases of the sinews select Yanglingquan GB-34".

The Gall Bladder is interiorly-exteriorly related with the Liver which dominates and nourishes the sinews, and Yanglingquan GB-34, the he-sea point of the Gall Bladder channel, is an essential point for contraction of the sinews and stiffness and tightness of the muscles and joints, and most especially for disorders of the leg such as knee pain, hip pain, sciatica, hemiplegia, atrophy disorder and painful obstruction. The importance of Yanglingquan GB-34 in disorders of the lower leg as a whole is further emphasised by its inclusion in Ma Dan-yang's 'eleven heavenly star points'[9], his grouping of the most vital acupuncture points. According to this great physician of the Jin dynasty, Yanglingquan GB-34 was indicated for swelling and numbness of the knee, cold painful obstruction, hemiplegia and inability to raise the leg. The action of Yanglingquan GB-34 is not confined to the lower limb, however, and it may be used in the treatment of stiffness of the neck and shoulders and pain of the sinews in the elbow, for example tennis elbow. In summary, Yanglingquan GB-34 may be used for pain, cramping, contraction, stiffness and sprain of the sinews and muscles in any part of the body.

It is a characteristic of the channels, especially the yang channels, that points located at the extremities tend to influence most strongly the extreme opposite end of the channel (i.e. the head region), whilst points located towards the elbow or knee tend to have their strongest influence on the middle region of the body. Yanglingquan GB-34 clearly demonstrates this principle and is an essential point to treat all disorders of the lateral costal region whether due to stagnation of qi, stasis of blood, accumulation of damp-heat, or deficiency of blood or yin. This is reflected in the unequivocal statements in the *Song of Points for Miscellaneous Diseases* which says "Pain of the lateral costal region, you only need Yanglingquan GB-34", and the *Ode of Essentials of Understanding* which says "when there is pain of the lateral costal region and of the ribs, needling Yanglingquan GB-34 will alleviate the pain promptly". The special affinity of Yanglingquan GB-34 for the lateral costal region reflects both the course of the Gall Bladder channel which traverses this area, and its actions of spreading Liver qi and clearing Liver and Gall Bladder damp-heat, and thus treating two of the main patterns in distention and pain of this region.

Yanglingquan GB-34 is the he-sea point of the Gall Bladder channel. According to the *Spiritual Pivot*[11] "He-sea points treat the internal fu". The primary disharmony of the Gall Bladder is accumulation of damp-heat which may arise from i. failure of the Spleen transportation and transformation function leading to accumulation of either dampness or damp-heat which obstruct the function of the Liver and Gall Bladder, ii. over-consumption of rich greasy food or alcohol, iii. attack of external pathogenic damp-heat, or iv. stagnation of Liver qi which both obstructs the movement of fluids and transforms into heat, giving rise to damp-heat. Whatever the aetiology, Yanglingquan GB-34 can be used to clear damp-heat from the Gall Bladder, manifesting with symptoms such as bitter taste in the mouth, nausea and vomiting, jaundice, cholecystitis etc. Another reflection of the influence of Yanglingquan GB-34 on the fu is its application in the treatment of constipation, particularly when due to qi stagnation or heat.

According to both the *Spiritual Pivot*[12] and the *Essential Questions*[13] "Taiyang is the opening, yangming is the closing and shaoyang is the pivot". In the differentiation of fevers expounded in the *Treatise on Injury by Cold*, the shaoyang level is the pivot between the interior and the exterior, and shaoyang pattern occurs when the pathogenic factor is trapped between these two levels. The characteristic symptoms of this 'half-interior, half-exterior' pattern are distinct phases of fever alternating with chills, bitter taste in the mouth, pain of the lateral costal region, dryness of the mouth and throat, and nausea and vomiting. Yanglingquan GB-34, the he-sea point of the foot shaoyang channel, is one of the main points to treat this pattern and is therefore indicated for any disorder with this presentation including malaria.

According to *Achieving Longevity by Guarding the Source*, the 17th Century classic by Gong Ting-xin, "Susceptibility to fright ... timidity in which the patient fears being apprehended, all result from deficiency of the qi of Heart and Gall Bladder ". Yanglingquan GB-34 is indicated for "fear of people as if about to be apprehended" and frequent sighing, reflecting a pattern of Gall Bladder qi deficiency.

Finally, the *Spiritual Pivot*[14] says "in disorders of the Stomach and in disorders resulting from irregular eating and drinking, select the he-sea point". Yanglingquan GB-34 is indicated in cases where qi stagnation generates phlegm and heat which obstruct the Stomach and impair its descending function. This combined pattern of Gall Bladder and Stomach disharmony manifests with such symptoms as bitter taste in the mouth, nausea and vomiting.

COMBINATIONS

- One-sided wind (hemiplegia): Yanglingquan GB-34, Huantiao GB-30 and Quchi L.I.-11 (*Supplementing Life*).
- Hemiplegia: Yanglingquan GB-34 and Quchi L.I.-11 (*One Hundred Symptoms*).
- Disorders of the knee and below the knee: moxa Yanglingquan GB-34, Dubi ST-35, Xiguan LIV-7 and Zusanli ST-36 (*Supplementing Life*).
- Numbness of the knee: Yanglingquan GB-34, Dubi ST-35 and Biguan ST-31 (*Supplementing Life*).
- Swelling of the knee that is difficult to endure: Yanglingquan GB-34 and Yinlingquan SP-9 (*Ode of the Jade Dragon*).
- Pain of the lateral aspect of the knee: Yanglingquan GB-34 and Xiaxi GB-43 (*Thousand Ducat Formulas*).
- Bone painful obstruction and numbness of the hip joint and knee: Yanglingquan GB-34, Yangjiao GB-35 and Yangfu GB-38 (*Thousand Ducat Formulas*).
- Flaccidity of the legs: Yanglingquan GB-34, Chongyang ST-42, Taichong LIV-3 and Qiuxu GB-40 (*Great Compendium*).
- Pain and soreness of leg qi: first needle Jianjing GB-21, then needle Zusanli ST-36 and Yanglingquan GB-34 (*Celestial Star*).
- Pain of the lumbar region and knee: Yanglingquan GB-34, Huantiao GB-30, Kunlun BL-60, Shenmai BL-62 and Yanglao SI-6 (*Illustrated Supplement*).
- Cold-wind-damp painful obstruction: first needle Huantiao GB-30 then Yanglingquan GB-34 (*Secrets of the Heavenly Star*).
- Hip pain: Yanglingquan GB-34, Huantiao GB-30 and Qiuxu GB-40 (*Great Compendium*).
- Pain of the leg radiating to the lateral costal region and axilla: Yanglingquan GB-34 and Huantiao GB-30 (*Song of Points*).
- Pain of the lateral costal region: Yanglingquan GB-34, Gongsun SP-4, Zhigou SJ-6 and Zhangmen LIV-13 (*Complete Collection*).
- Pain of the lateral costal region due to injury by cold: Yanglingquan GB-34 and Zhigou SJ-6 (*Outline of Medicine*).
- Fullness of the abdomen and lateral costal region: Yanglingquan GB-34, Zulinqi GB-41 and Shanglian L.I.-9 (*Great Compendium*).
- Swelling of the face and head: Yanglingquan GB-34 and Gongsun SP-4 (*Supplementing Life*).
- Hot constipation, qi constipation: First needle Changqiang DU-1 then Dadun LIV-1 and Yanglingquan GB-34 (*Song of Points*).
- Fear and fright with Heart pain: Yanglingquan GB-34, Shenmen HE-7, Shaochong HE-9 and Neiguan P-6 (*Compilation*).
- Apprehension and fear as if about to be apprehended: Yanglingquan GB-34 and Rangu KID-2 (*Thousand Ducat Formulas*).

YANGJIAO GB-35

陽交

Yang Intersection

Xi-Cleft point of the Yang Linking vessel

LOCATION

On the lateral aspect of the lower leg, 7 cun superior to the prominence of the lateral malleolus, in the depression at the posterior border of the fibula.

LOCATION NOTE

i. The distance between the tip of the lateral malleolus and the popliteal crease is 16 cun; locate Yangjiao GB-35 one cun distal to the midpoint of this line; ii. Above the region of Xuanzhong GB-39, the fibula is not easily palpable because it is covered by the peroneus brevis muscle; therefore feel for the posterior border of the fibula above the malleolus where it is easily palpable and extend a line towards the head of the fibula.

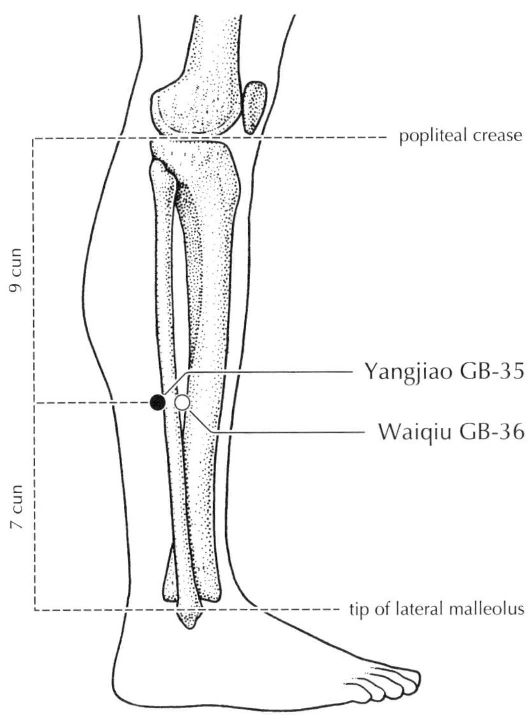

NEEDLING

Perpendicular insertion 1 to 1.5 cun.

ACTIONS

Activates the channel and alleviates pain
Regulates Gall Bladder qi and calms the spirit

INDICATIONS

- Swelling and pain of the knee, atrophy disorder and painful obstruction of the lower limb, cold painful obstruction, contraction of the sinews in sudden turmoil disorder.
- Mania induced by fright, fullness, distention and pain of the chest and lateral costal region, swelling of the face and eyes, throat painful obstruction.

COMBINATIONS

- Fullness of the chest: Yangjiao GB-35 and Zulinqi GB-41 (*Supplementing Life*).
- Fright palpitations and pounding of the Heart: Yangjiao GB-35 and Jiexi ST-41 (*One Hundred Patterns*).
- Loss of voice: Yangjiao GB-35, Hegu L.I.-4 and Yongquan KID-1 (*Systematic Classic*).
- Bone painful obstruction and numbness of the hip joint and knee: Yangjiao GB-35, Yangfu GB-38, and Yanglingquan GB-34 (*Thousand Ducat Formulas*).

WAIQIU GB-36

Outer Hill

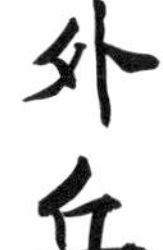

Xi-Cleft point of the Gall Bladder channel

LOCATION

On the lateral aspect of the lower leg, 7 cun superior to the prominence of the lateral malleolus, at the anterior border of the fibula.

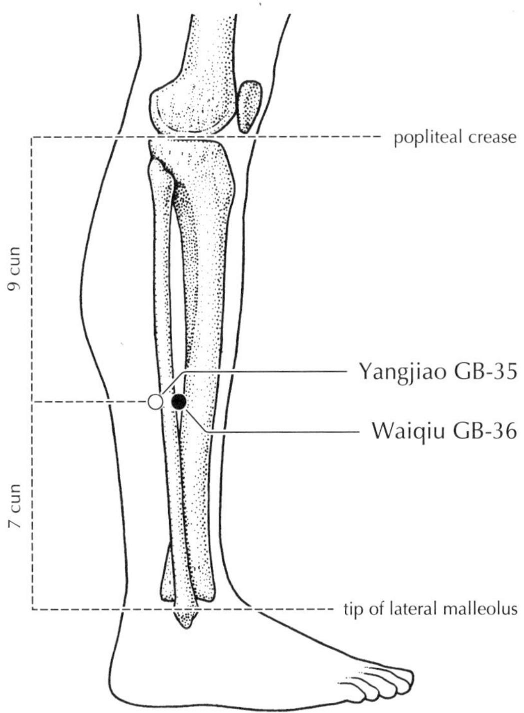

LOCATION NOTE

i. The distance between the tip of the lateral malleolus and the popliteal crease is 16 cun; locate Waiqiu GB-36 one cun distal to the midpoint of this line; ii. Above the region of Xuanzhong GB-39, the fibula is not easily palpable because it is covered by the peroneus brevis muscle; therefore feel for the anterior border of the fibula above the ankle joint where it is easily palpable and extend a line towards the head of the fibula.

NEEDLING
Perpendicular insertion 1 to 1.5 cun.

ACTIONS
Activates the channel and alleviates pain
Clears heat and detoxifies poison

INDICATIONS
- Distention of the chest and lateral costal region, pigeon chest in children, headache, mania, abdominal pain, rabies.
- Atrophy disorder and painful obstruction of the lower limb, pain of the skin, cold damp leg qi, cold sensation and stiffness and pain of the nape and neck, aversion to wind-cold.

COMMENTARY
Waiqiu GB-36 is the xi-cleft point of the Gall Bladder channel. The xi-cleft points are where the qi and blood, which flow relatively superficially along the channels from the jing-well points, gather and plunge more deeply. The xi-cleft points in general are indicated in the treatment of acute conditions and pain, and Waiqiu GB-36 is indicated for pain of the skin. Thus the *Systematic Classic of Acupuncture and Moxibustion* said "Painful skin with atrophy disorder and painful obstruction, principally select Waiqiu GB-36".

Unusually, this point is also indicated for rabies. The *Illustrated Classic of Acupuncture Points on the Bronze Man* said "Rabies with chills and fever, quickly moxa Waiqiu GB-36 three times and then moxa the bitten area".

COMBINATIONS
- Pain of the neck with aversion to wind-cold: Waiqiu GB-36 and Houding DU-19 (*Supplementing Life*).

GUANGMING GB-37

Bright Light

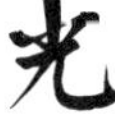
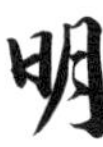

Luo-Connecting point of the Gall Bladder channel

LOCATION
On the lateral aspect of the lower leg, 5 cun superior to the prominence of the lateral malleolus, at the anterior border of the fibula.

LOCATION NOTE
i. The distance between the tip of the lateral malleolus and the popliteal crease is 16 cun; locate Guangming GB-37 just distal to the junction of the upper two thirds and lower third of this line; ii. Above the region of Xuanzhong GB-39, the fibula is not easily palpable because it is covered by the peroneus brevis muscle; therefore feel for the anterior border of the fibula above the ankle joint where it is easily palpable and extend a line towards the head of the fibula.

NEEDLING
Perpendicular insertion 1 to 1.5 cun.

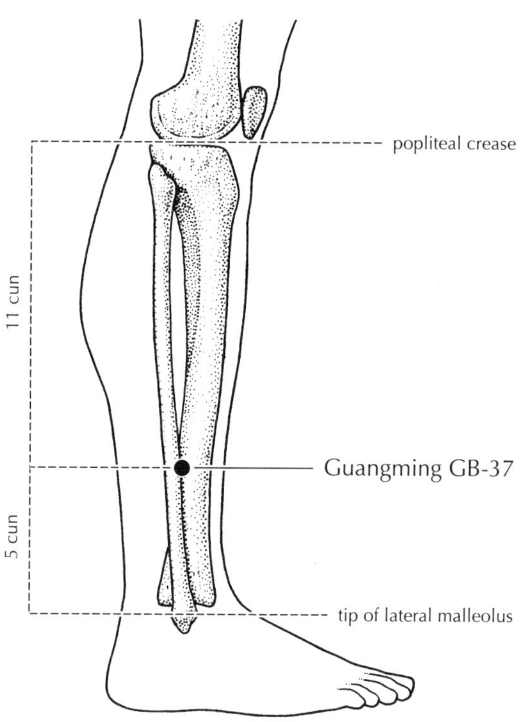

ACTIONS
Benefits the eyes
Dispels wind-damp, activates the channel and alleviates pain

INDICATIONS
- Eye pain, night blindness, itching of the eyes, long sightedness, short sightedness.
- One-sided headache, grinding of the teeth, distention and pain of the breast, febrile disease with absence of sweating, sudden mania.
- Knee pain, pain of the lower legs with inability to stand for long, atrophy disorder of the legs with difficulty in standing after sitting, atrophy disorder and painful obstruction of the lower limb with numbness, numbness of the body, heat and pain of the lower leg.

COMMENTARY

The *Guide to the Classics of Acupuncture* states "the luo-connecting points are located between two channels ... if they are punctured, symptoms of the interiorly-exteriorly related channels can be treated"[15]. The Liver 'opens' into the eyes, and the Liver, Gall Bladder, and Gall Bladder divergent channels connect with the eye. Many eye diseases derive from Liver pathology, and as its name 'Bright Light' suggests, Guangming GB-37, the luo-connecting point of the Gall Bladder channel, is the principal distal point on the channel for the treatment of a wide range of eye disorders, including pain, redness, itching, long and short sightedness and night blindness.

Its second function of activating the channel and alleviating pain is important in two ways. Firstly, by dispelling wind-damp and regulating the circulation of qi in the lower limb, it is effective in treating a wide range of disorders of the lower leg including knee pain, pain of the lower legs with inability to stand for long, atrophy disorder and painful obstruction of lower limb with numbness and heat, and pain of the lower leg. Secondly, the Gall Bladder primary channel passes through the chest whilst its sinew channel links with the breast, and Guangming GB-37 is indicated for distention and pain of the breast due to stagnation of Liver qi.

Finally the *Great Compendium of Acupuncture and Moxibustion* gives specific indications for excess and deficiency of the luo-connecting points. In the case of Guangming GB-37, these are heat sensation of the lower leg, knee pain, numbness of the body and propensity to grind the teeth (excess); atrophy disorder of the legs with difficulty in standing after sitting (deficiency).

COMBINATIONS

- Pain and itching of the eyes: reduce Guangming GB-37 and Diwuhui GB-42 (*Ode to Elucidate Mysteries*).
- When Jingming BL-1 is ineffective in treating diseases of the eye, combine it with Hegu L.I.-4 and Guangming GB-37 (*Ode of Xi-hong*).
- Grinding of the teeth: Guangming GB-37 and Zulinqi GB-41 (*Thousand Ducat Formulas*).
- Headache, swollen cheeks, difficult defecation, painful urinary dysfunction, susceptibility to anger with a blue-green (qing) colour, painful shan disorder and pain of the lateral costal region, hypogastrium and uterus: Guangming GB-37 and Taichong LIV-3 (*Golden Mirror*).
- Short-sightedness: Guangming GB-37, Taichong LIV-3, Chengqi ST-1, Jingming BL-1, Fengchi GB-20 and Hegu L.I.-4.

YANGFU GB-38

Yang Assistance

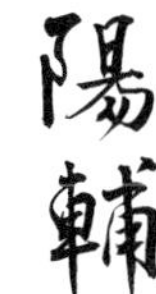

Jing-River and Fire point of the Gall Bladder channel

LOCATION

On the lateral aspect of the lower leg, 4 cun superior to the prominence of the lateral malleolus, at the anterior border of the fibula.

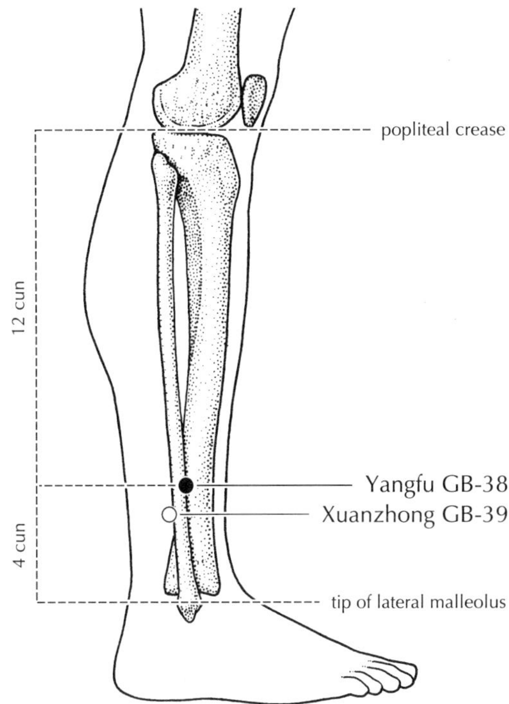

LOCATION NOTE

i. The distance between the tip of the lateral malleolus and the popliteal crease is 16 cun; locate Yangfu GB-38 at the junction of the upper three quarters and lower quarter of this line; ii. Above the region of Xuanzhong GB-39, the fibula is not easily palpable because it is covered by the peroneus brevis muscle; therefore feel for the anterior border of the fibula above the ankle joint where it is easily palpable and extend a line towards the head of the fibula.

NEEDLING

Perpendicular insertion 0.7 to 1 cun.

ACTIONS

Clears Gall Bladder channel heat
Harmonises shaoyang
Benefits the sinews and bones
Activates the channel and alleviates pain

INDICATIONS

- One-sided headache, pain of the outer canthus, throat painful obstruction.
- Bitter taste in the mouth, sighing, pain of the chest and lateral costal region, chills and fever, sweating with cold shivering, pain in the middle of the supraclavicular fossa, swelling and pain of the axilla, scrofula, malaria, blue-green (qing) complexion.
- Wind painful obstruction with numbness, wandering pain of the joints, hemiplegia, contracted sinews, pain of the hundred joints, pain and numbness of the lateral side of the lower limb, lower limb painful obstruction, oedema below the knee, leg qi, sensation in the lumbar region as if sitting in water, severe lumbar pain, lumbar pain like a small hammer in the middle of the back, pain of the lateral malleolus.

COMMENTARY

Yangfu GB-38 is the fire and jing-river point of the Gall Bladder channel. According to the *Great Compendium of Acupuncture and Moxibustion* "when the Gall Bladder is excess reduce Yangfu GB-38". The main actions of Yangfu GB-38 are to clear stagnation and heat from the entire course of the Gall Bladder channel, clear shaoyang heat, and benefit the sinews and bones of the whole body.

In the head, Yangfu GB-38 is an important point for one-sided headache, principally due to Liver qi stagnation or uprising of Liver fire or Liver yang which transmit along the Gall Bladder channel. In the upper part of the chest, the Gall Bladder channel passes anterior to the axilla. When qi and phlegm stagnate (and in some cases transform into heat), usually due to emotional causes, there may be swelling and pain of the axilla or scrofula. In the chest and lateral costal region, Yangfu GB-38 is indicated when qi stagnates and gives rise to pain accompanied by sighing. In the lower body, Yangfu GB-38 is indicated for pain extending along the Gall Bladder channel on the lateral side of the lower limb and the lateral malleolus. If pain in any of these regions is severe, a blue-green (qing) colour may be seen on the complexion. This colour, frequently observed around the mouth, eyes, nose or temples, has traditionally been linked with Liver disorders, severe pain or cold in the body.

According to both the *Spiritual Pivot*[16] and the *Essential Questions*[17] "Taiyang is the opening, yangming is the closing and shaoyang is the pivot". The shaoyang is the pivot between the interior and the exterior and Yangfu GB-38 is indicated for the classic symptoms seen when a pathogenic factor lodges in this 'half-interior, half-exterior' portion. These include distinct alternating phases of chills and fever, bitter taste in the mouth, pain of the chest and lateral costal region and sighing. Malaria, for which this point is indicated, is a classic example of shaoyang pattern.

According to the *Spiritual Pivot*[18] "When the disease is at the yin within yang (sinews and bones), needle the jing-river points of the yin channels". Although this passage emphasises the yin channels only, it is clear from an examination of the indications of Yangfu GB-38, the jing-river point of the yang Gall Bladder channel, that it is nevertheless an important point for wandering painful obstruction, contraction and pain of the sinews, and pain of the hundred joints (i.e. all the joints of the body). The Gall Bladder primary channel descends from Zhangmen LIV-13 to the sacral region, and Yangfu GB-38 is indicated for a sensation in the lumbar region as if one was sitting in water, severe lumbar pain, and lumbar pain like a small hammer in the middle of the back.

COMBINATIONS

- Swelling of the axilla: Yangfu GB-38, Zulinqi GB-41, Diwuhui GB-42, Weiyang BL-39, Shenmai BL-62 and Tianchi P-1 (*Thousand Ducat Formulas*).
- Swelling of the axilla: Yangfu GB-38, Qiuxu GB-40 and Zulinqi GB-41 (*Great Compendium*).
- Swelling and sabre lumps of the axilla: Yangfu GB-38, Xiaxi GB-43 and Taichong LIV-3 (*Thousand Ducat Formulas*).
- Scrofula: Yangfu GB-38, Shaohai HE-3, Tianchi P-1, Zhangmen LIV-13, Zulinqi GB-41, Zhigou SJ-6, Jianjing GB-21 and Shousanli L.I.-10 (*Great Compendium*).
- Wind painful obstruction: Yangfu GB-38 and Chize LU-5 (*Great Compendium*).
- Wind painful obstruction: Yangfu GB-38, Tianjing SJ-10, Chize LU-5, Shaohai HE-3 and Weizhong BL-40 (*Great Compendium*).
- Bone painful obstruction and numbness of the hip joint and knee: Yangfu GB-38, Yangjiao GB-35 and Yanglingquan GB-34 (*Thousand Ducat Formulas*).
- Paralysis of the lower extremity: Yangfu GB-38, Huantiao GB-30, Yinlingquan SP-9, Taixi KID-3 and Zhiyin BL-67 (*Great Compendium*).

XUANZHONG GB-39

Suspended Bell

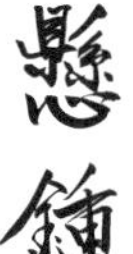

Hui-Meeting point for Marrow

LOCATION

Above the ankle joint, 3 cun superior to the prominence of the lateral malleolus, between the posterior border of the fibula and the tendons of peroneus longus and brevis.

LOCATION NOTE

Locate one handbreadth proximal to the prominence of the lateral malleolus.

NEEDLING

Perpendicular insertion 1 to 1.5 cun. The practitioner should use the index finger of one hand to separate the peroneal tendons from the fibula, to emphasise the groove. Needle into the groove, first slightly posteriorly for 0.5 cun and then perpendicularly, to avoid hitting the fibula. Movement of the patient's ankle after needling can result in a bent needle. For this reason, this point should be needled last and the patient instructed not to move the leg after needling.

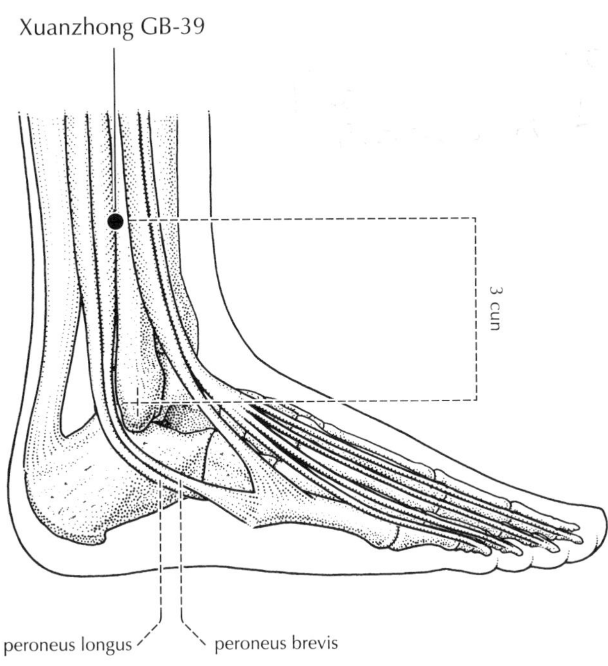

ACTIONS

Benefits the sinews and bones
Benefits the neck
Dispels wind-damp
Clears Gall Bladder fire
Activates the channel and alleviates pain

INDICATIONS

- Stiffness and pain of the neck, atrophy disorder, chronic painful obstruction, wind-taxation with heaviness of the body, injury by cold pathogen leading to taxation, deficiency-taxation, contracted sinews and pain of the bones, hip pain, numbness and pain of the knee and lower leg, sciatica, leg qi, sprain of the ankle joint, flaccidity of the foot.
- Hemiplegia, headache, dizziness, throat painful obstruction, nosebleed, dryness of the nose.
- Distention and fullness of the chest and abdomen, counterflow qi and cough, soreness and pain of the lateral costal region, swelling of the axilla.
- Fullness of the abdomen in children with inability to eat or drink, fullness and distention of the Heart and abdomen, heat in the Stomach, no pleasure in eating, watery diarrhoea.
- Injury by cold leading to heat with persistent fever, haemorrhoids, agitation and fullness, mania, anxiety, indignation and anger, the five types of painful urinary dysfunction.

COMMENTARY

Xuanzhong GB-39 is the hui-meeting point for the 'marrow' which is the source of both the 'sea of marrow' (the brain) and the bone marrow. There is little evidence in classical texts of the ability of Xuanzhong GB-39 to nourish the sea of marrow, in other words to treat diseases of the head and brain, and even headache and dizziness are modern rather than traditional indications.

Xuanzhong GB-39, however, has a strong action on benefiting the bone marrow, sinews and bones and is indicated for a wide range of disorders characterised by weakness, flaccidity, contraction and pain of the limbs. This latter action is complemented by its ability to dispel wind-damp. According to the *Essential Questions*[19] "In bone painful obstruction the pathogenic factor reaches the Kidneys; in sinew painful obstruction it reaches the Liver". In chronic painful obstruction, therefore, prolonged retention of wind-damp which injures the sinews and bones will eventually deplete the Liver and Kidneys and hence the marrow. Prolonged deficiency of the Liver and Kidneys and insufficiency of essence, resulting in malnourishment of the sinews, may also give rise to atrophy disorder. By its action of nourishing the marrow and benefiting the sinews and bones Xuanzhong GB-39 is therefore indicated for both chronic painful obstruction and atrophy disorder, hence the references to the use of Xuanzhong GB-39 in wind-taxation with heaviness of the body, injury by cold pathogen leading to taxation and deficiency-taxation. The term taxation here denotes the extreme deficiency that arises due to chronic retention of pathogenic factors. According to the *Ode to Elucidate Mysteries*, the great Han dynasty physician Hua Tuo needled Xuanzhong GB-39 and Huantiao GB-30 for lameness of the legs, and "immediately the patient was able to walk".

The Gall Bladder primary and sinew channels pass through different portions of the neck. By virtue of its actions of benefiting the sinews and bones and activating the channel and alleviating pain, Xuanzhong GB-39 is the main distal point on the Gall Bladder channel for disorders of the neck, both acute and chronic.

Xuanzhong GB-39 has a further action of promoting the smooth flow of Liver and Gall Bladder qi, and clearing Gall Bladder fire primarily arising from the transformation of stagnant qi. It is indicated for distention of the chest and abdomen, fullness and distention of the Heart and abdomen, soreness and pain of the lateral costal region, anxiety, indignation, anger and mania. Gall Bladder fire may easily transmit to the Stomach, resulting in Stomach heat, or obstruct the Stomach descending function leading to lack of appetite. The Gall Bladder sinew channel binds at the side of the nose and the primary channel connects with the Governing vessel at Changqiang DU-1. By clearing Gall Bladder fire, Xuanzhong GB-39 is also indicated for dryness of the nose, nosebleed and haemorrhoids.

COMBINATIONS

- Coldness and pain of the bone marrow: Xuanzhong GB-39, Dazhu BL-11, Fuliu KID-7, Shenmai BL-62, Lidui ST-45 and Shenshu BL-23 (*Compilation*).
- Curvature of the lumbar spine: reinforce Fengchi GB-20 and reduce Xuanzhong GB-39 (*Song of the Jade Dragon*).
- Windstroke with one-sided withering and incessant pain: Xuanzhong GB-39, Jianyu L.I.-15, Taixi KID-3, Quchi L.I.-11, Zusanli ST-36 and Kunlun BL-60 (*Great Compendium*).
- Flaccidity of the legs with difficulty in walking: first needle Xuanzhong GB-39 then needle Tiaokou ST-38 and Chongyang ST-42 (*Secrets of the Heavenly Star*).
- Leg qi: Xuanzhong GB-39, Zusanli ST-36 and Sanyinjiao SP-6 (*Ode of the Jade Dragon*).
- Pain of the ankle and heel: Xuanzhong GB-39, Kunlun BL-60 and Qiuxu GB-40 (*Song More Precious Than Jade*).
- Fullness and distention of the Heart and abdomen: Xuanzhong GB-39 and Neiting ST-44 (*Great Compendium*).
- Hot Stomach with no pleasure in eating: Xuanzhong GB-39 and Xialian L.I.-8 (*Supplementing Life*).
- Stiff neck: Xuanzhong GB-39, Tianzhu BL-10 and Houxi SI-3.

QIUXU GB-40

Mound of Ruins

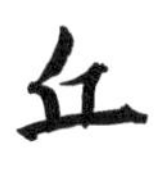
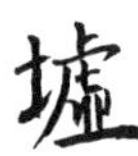

Yuan-Source point of the Gall Bladder channel

LOCATION

At the ankle joint, in the depression anterior and inferior to the lateral malleolus.

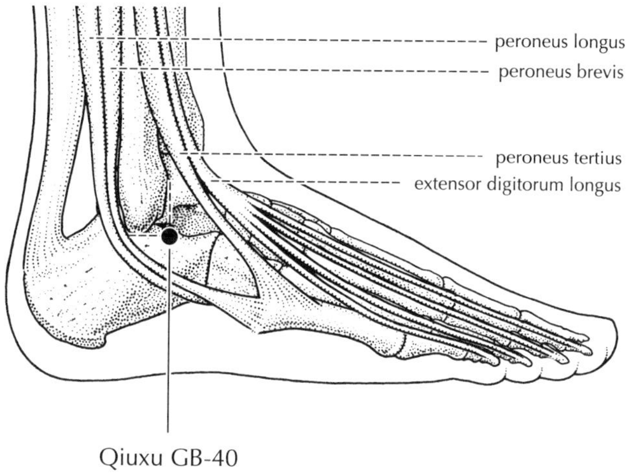

LOCATION NOTE

Locate at the junction of lines drawn along the anterior and inferior borders of the lateral malleolus.

NEEDLING

Perpendicular insertion 1 to 1.5 cun, directed towards Zhaohai KID 6.

ACTIONS

Spreads Liver qi and clears Gall Bladder heat and damp-heat
Activates the channel, alleviates pain and benefits the joints
Regulates shaoyang

INDICATIONS

- Distention and pain of the chest and lateral costal region with inability to catch the breath, sighing, swelling in the axilla, sudden shan disorder, hardness of the lower abdomen, herpes zoster.
- One-sided headache, redness, swelling and pain of the eyes, superficial visual obstruction, poor eyesight, throat painful obstruction.
- Vomiting, acid regurgitation, chronic malaria with cold shivering.

- Neck pain, chills and fever with swelling of the neck, windstroke, paralysis, pain of the lumbar spine, pain of the hip, atrophy disorder and painful obstruction of the lower limb, cramping and pain of the legs, sciatica, pain of the lower leg, drop foot, flaccidity of the ankle, swelling of the lateral ankle, pain of the wrist.

COMMENTARY

According to Chen Shi-dou "Only when the Liver acquires ming men is it able to plan strategies, only when the Gall Bladder acquires ming men are decisions made". The Liver and Gall Bladder are entrusted with the ministerial fire which corresponds to the energy of spring, growth, forcefulness and decision making. In disharmony, this indispensable fire is prone to flare up, principally when the Liver and Gall Bladder lose their free-flowing function and qi stagnates and transforms to fire. The fire is drawn into the Gall Bladder channel as a whole, and especially rises upwards to the head. Qiuxu GB-40, the yuan-source point of the Gall Bladder channel, is indicated when there is heat and stagnant qi in various portions of the Gall Bladder channel giving rise to distention, pain, redness or swelling of the head, eyes, neck, throat, axilla and abdomen, distention and pain of the chest and lateral costal region with sighing and inability to catch the breath, and shan disorder.

Qiuxu GB-40 is also indicated when heat and dampness combine, giving rise to such symptoms of damp-heat distressing the Gall Bladder fu or channel as cholecystitis and herpes zoster. If Liver and Gall Bladder heat or damp-heat transversely invade the Stomach, impairing its descending function, there may be vomiting and acid regurgitation.

Qiuxu GB-40 is able to treat disorders of the lower limb as a whole and is frequently employed in combination with points such as Juliao GB-29, Huantiao GB-30 and Yanglingquan GB-34 in the 'chain and lock' point association method. It is specifically indicated for hip pain, sciatica, cramping and pain of the legs, atrophy disorder, painful obstruction (especially of the ankle joint), drop foot and flaccidity or swelling of the ankle. In the cross-needling method of point selection, the wrist joint in the upper body corresponds to the ankle joint in the lower body, and Qiuxu GB-40 is indicated by a number of classical texts for contralateral wrist pain.

According to both the *Spiritual Pivot*[20] and the *Essential Questions*[21] "Taiyang is the opening, yangming is the closing and shaoyang is the pivot". In the differentiation of fevers expounded in the *Treatise on Injury by Cold* by Zhang Zhong-jing, shaoyang syndrome represents the 'half-exterior half-interior' stage. The pathogenic factor resides between the taiyang and yangming levels and in this sense shaoyang is the pivot or hinge between the exterior and interior. Qiuxu GB-40 has long been used for chronic malaria, a classic example of a disease where the pathogenic factor enters the body and lodges at the half-exterior half-interior level. The alternating fever and chills reflect the battle between the correct qi and the pathogenic qi. When the correct qi predominates and is able to struggle with the pathogen, there is fever, and when the pathogenic qi predominates there are chills. Qiuxu GB-40, the yuan-source point of the foot shaoyang channel, is chosen to regulate the shaoyang channel and expel the pathogen, especially when chills predominate.

COMBINATIONS

- Superficial visual obstruction: Qiuxu GB-40 and Tongziliao GB-1 (*Supplementing Life*).
- Pain of the lateral costal region: Qiuxu GB-40 and Zhongdu GB-32 (*Great Compendium*).
- Fullness of the chest and lateral costal region radiating to the abdomen: Qiuxu GB-40, Xiaxi GB-43, Xiajuxu ST-39 and Shenshu BL-23 (*Great Compendium*).
- Stabbing pain of the chest: Qiuxu GB-40 and Fenglong ST-40 (*Thousand Ducat Formulas*).
- Tension of the chest and back with a swollen sensation of the chest: Qiuxu GB-40 and Jingqu LU-8 (*Thousand Ducat Formulas*).
- Swelling of the axilla, chills and fever, swelling of the neck: Qiuxu GB-40 and Shenmai BL-62 (*Thousand Ducat Formulas*).
- Swelling of the axilla: Qiuxu GB-40, Yangfu GB-38 and Zulinqi GB-41 (*Great Compendium*).
- Manic raving: Qiuxu GB-40 and Xiajuxu ST-39 (*Thousand Ducat Formulas*).
- Cramping of the sinews: Qiuxu GB-40 and Jinmen BL-63 (*One Hundred Symptoms*).
- Hip pain: Qiuxu GB-40, Huantiao GB-30 and Yanglingquan GB-34 (*Great Compendium*).
- Flaccidity of the legs: Qiuxu GB-40, Yanglingquan GB-34, Chongyang ST-42 and Taichong LIV-3 (*Great Compendium*).
- Pain of the ankle and heel: Qiuxu GB-40, Xuanzhong GB-39 and Kunlun BL-60 (*Song More Precious Than Jade*).
- Chronic malaria: Qiuxu GB-40, Zhongzhu SJ-3 and Shangyang L.I.-1 (*Great Compendium*).

ZULINQI GB-41

Foot Governor of Tears

足臨泣

Shu-Stream and Wood point of the Gall Bladder channel
Confluent point of the Girdling vessel

LOCATION

In the depression distal to the junction of the 4th and 5th metatarsal bones, on the lateral side of the tendon of m. extensor digitorum longus (branch to little toe).

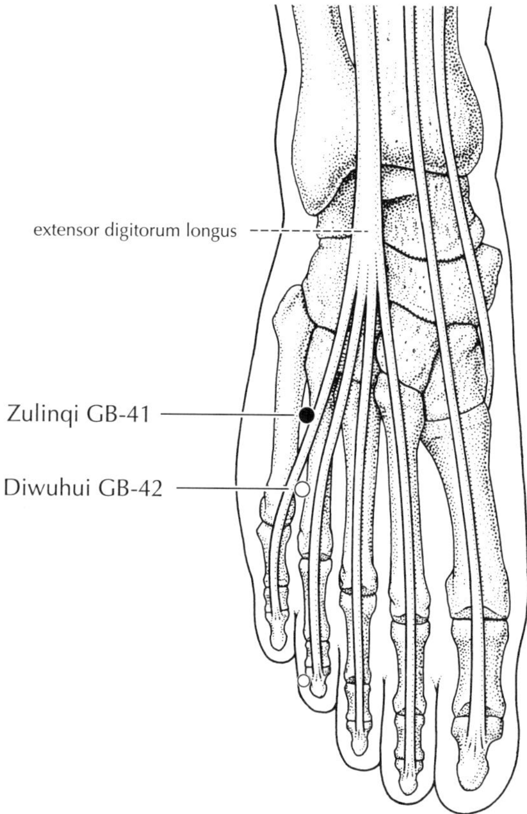

LOCATION NOTE

Ask the patient to abduct their little toe in order to make the branch of m. extensor digitorum longus more prominent. Run a finger from Xiaxi GB-43 towards the ankle, along the interspace between the fourth and fifth metatarsals until it passes over this branch into the significant depression immediately beyond the tendon.

NEEDLING

Perpendicular insertion 0.5 to 1 cun. Incorrect angle of insertion will not enable the needle to pass between the shafts of the fourth and fifth metatarsal bones.

ACTIONS

Spreads Liver qi
Benefits the chest, lateral costal region and breasts
Clears the head and benefits the eyes
Transforms phlegm and dissipates nodules

INDICATIONS

- Pain of the lateral costal region, fullness of the chest with inability to catch the breath, rebellious qi with dyspnoea, chest painful obstruction, pain of the supraclavicular fossa, inversion counterflow of the four limbs, scrofula, swelling of the axilla, enuresis, malaria.
- Headache, one-sided headache, head wind, dizziness, visual dizziness, pain of the occiput, pain of the vertex, pain of the outer canthus, redness, swelling and pain of the eyes, lacrimation, dry eyes, deafness and tinnitus, propensity to gnaw the tongue and cheek, swelling of the submandibular region and cheek, swelling of Tianyou SJ-16, toothache.
- Distention and pain of the breast, breast abscess, menstrual disorders, inhibited menstruation.
- Pain of the hip, pain of the lower leg, fixed painful obstruction, wandering pain, swelling and pain of the feet, pain and contraction of the toes, swelling and pain of the dorsum of the feet, all disorders of the feet.

COMMENTARY

Zulinqi GB-41 is an indispensable point to spread the Liver qi, especially when qi stagnation manifests along the course of the Gall Bladder channel, and this action underpins all the indications of this point. Although the primary cause of Liver qi stagnation is emotional, it may manifest both with physical symptoms and emotional changes. Zulinqi GB-41 predominantly treats the physical symptoms of Liver qi stagnation, namely distention, pressure and pain along the Gall Bladder channel in the chest, head, eyes, breast, lateral costal region and axilla.

The smooth flow of Liver qi assists the ascending and descending of the qi of all the zangfu. If Liver qi stagnates in the chest region, therefore, it may hinder the descent of Lung qi and prevent smooth respiration. As well as fullness of the chest, chest painful obstruction and dyspnoea, there may be inability to catch the breath. This symptom, which may be described by the patient as a kind of breathlessness, is more an abnormal awareness of breathing accompanied by a feeling that the Lungs cannot be filled adequately.

If Liver qi stagnation transforms to Liver fire, or if Liver fire subsequently consumes yin and leads to uprising of Liver yang, the fire or yang may ascend to the head along the Gall Bladder channel (occiput, temporal region and ears) or the Liver channel (vertex) and cause pain, dizziness, tinnitus or even deafness. Although Zulinqi GB-41 is much used in modern clinical practice for one-sided headache, particularly with Waiguan SJ-5 and especially for headaches associated with the menstrual cycle, it is interesting to note that all major classical references are to occipital pain and pain of the vertex.

In the *Ode of the Obstructed River* the use of Zulinqi GB-41 is referred to as one of 'the eight therapeutic methods'. In this description of the application of the eight confluent points of the extraordinary vessels to affect specific symptoms and areas of the body, Zulinqi GB-41 is indicated for disorders of the eyes. The Liver 'opens' into the eyes, and the Liver, Gall Bladder and Gall Bladder divergent channels all connect with the eye. When Liver fire or Liver yang rise to disturb the eyes, or exterior wind-heat enters the Liver channel, there may be lacrimation or dry eyes, redness, swelling and pain of the eyes, especially at the outer canthus, or visual dizziness. Zulinqi GB-41, as the name (Foot Governor of Tears) implies, is an important point to adjust the fluid in the eye and treat these conditions.

Zulinqi GB-41 is the confluent point of the Girdling vessel which encircles the waist and binds the Penetrating and Conception vessels and the Kidney, Liver and Spleen channels, all of which channels influence the menstrual cycle. Furthermore, the Gall Bladder primary channel descends through the chest region, the Gall Bladder sinew channel links with the breast, and the nipples are ascribed to the jueyin Liver channel. Zulinqi GB-41 is particularly used therefore in situations where Liver qi stagnation impairs the regularity of the menstrual cycle, and more especially for symptoms of stagnant qi such as distention and pain of the breast and headache which precede the menstrual period. Zulinqi GB-41 is also indicated for breast abscess and is combined in a modern prescription with Guangming GB-37 to stop lactation. After needling, moxibustion is applied to the points for ten minutes.

Liver qi stagnation may impair the smooth circulation of fluids resulting in their condensation into phlegm, or may transform into fire which scorches and condenses the body fluids leading to the formation of phlegm. Zulinqi GB-41 is indicated when phlegm and stagnant qi combine to form swelling and nodules in the neck, breast and axilla.

Finally, Zulinqi GB-41 is used for swelling and pain of the feet (especially the dorsum) and pain and contraction of the toes. According to *Investigation into Points Along the Channels* Zulinqi GB-41 is suitable for "all disorders of the feet".

COMBINATIONS

- Internal eye obstruction: Zulinqi GB-41, Jingming BL-1, Tongziliao GB-1 and Hegu L.I.-4 (*Great Compendium*).
- Cold lacrimation: Zulinqi GB-41, Jingming BL-1, Fengchi GB-20 and Wangu SI-4 (*Great Compendium*).
- Lacrimation: Zulinqi GB-41, Baihui DU-20, Yemen SJ-2, Houxi SI-3, Qiangu SI-2 and Ganshu BL-18 (*Great Compendium*).
- Deafness: Zulinqi GB-41, Jinmen BL-63 and Hegu L.I.-4 (*Song of Points*).
- Grinding of the teeth: Zulinqi GB-41 and Guangming GB-37 (*Thousand Ducat Formulas*).
- Swelling of the axilla: Zulinqi GB-41, Yangfu GB-38, Diwuhui GB-42, Weiyang BL-39, Shenmai BL-62 and Tianchi P-1 (*Thousand Ducat Formulas*).
- Swelling of the axilla: Zulinqi GB-41, Qiuxu GB-40 and Yangfu GB-38 (*Great Compendium*).
- Sabre lumps of the axilla: Zulinqi GB-41, Yuanye GB-22, Zhigou SJ-6 and Waiguan SJ-5 (*Illustrated Supplement*).
- Scrofula: Zulinqi GB-41, Shaohai HE-3, Tianchi P-1, Zhangmen LIV-13, Zhigou SJ-6, Yangfu GB-38, Jianjing GB-21 and Shousanli L.I.-10 (*Great Compendium*).
- Swelling of the supraclavicular fossa [Quepen ST-12]: Zulinqi GB-41, Shangyang L.I.-1 and Taixi KID-3 (*Great Compendium*).
- Heart pain: Zulinqi GB-41, Jueyinshu BL-14 and Shenmen HE-7 (*Supplementing Life*).
- Chest painful obstruction and Heart pain: Zulinqi GB-41 and Tianjing SJ-10 (*Supplementing Life*).
- Fullness of the chest: Zulinqi GB-41 and Yangjiao GB-35 (*Supplementing Life*).
- Fullness of the abdomen and lateral costal region: Zulinqi GB-41, Yanglingquan GB-34 and Shanglian L.I.-9 (*Great Compendium*).
- Swelling of the breasts in women: Zulinqi GB-41 and Shaoze SI-1 (*Divine Moxibustion*).
- Breast abscess: Zulinqi GB-41, Xiajuxu ST-39, Zusanli ST-36, Xiaxi GB-43, Yuji LU-10, Weizhong BL-40 and Shaoze SI-1 (*Great Compendium*).
- Inhibited menstruation: Zulinqi GB-41, Sanyinjiao SP-6 and Zhongji REN-3 (*Great Compendium*).
- Pain of the hip with difficulty in walking and pain of the skin of the lateral aspect of the leg: Zulinqi GB-41 and Sanyinjiao SP-6 (*Thousand Ducat Formulas*).
- To stop lactation: Zulinqi GB-41 and Guangming GB-37.

DIWUHUI GB-42

Earth Five Meetings

地五會

LOCATION

Between the 4th and 5th metatarsal bones, in the depression proximal to the metatarsal heads, on the medial side of the tendon of m. extensor digitorum longus (branch to little toe).

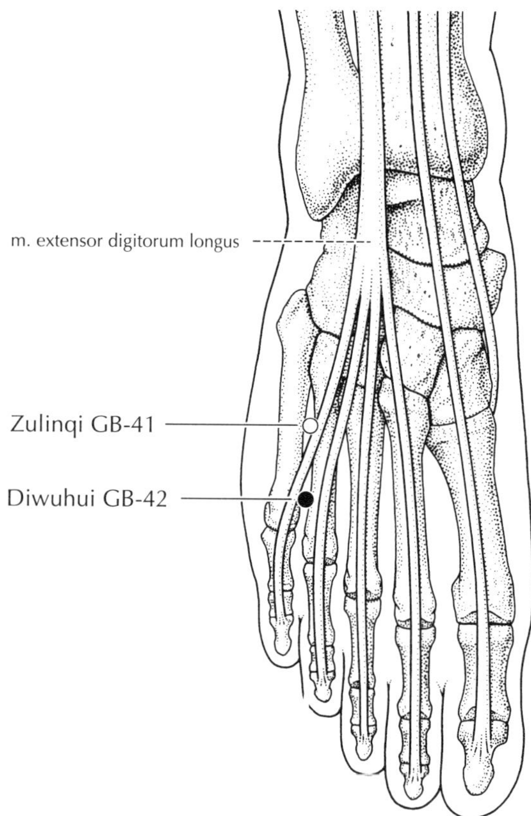

LOCATION NOTE

Ask the patient to abduct their little toe in order to make the branch of m. extensor digitorum longus more prominent. Run a finger from Xiaxi GB-43 towards the ankle, along the interspace between the fourth and fifth metatarsals, until it encounters the significant depression immediately before the tendon.

NEEDLING

Perpendicular insertion 0.5 to 0.8 cun. Incorrect angle of insertion will not enable the needle to pass between the shafts of the fourth and fifth metatarsal bones. **Note:** the *Systematic Classic of Acupuncture and Moxibustion*, *Great Compendium of Acupuncture and Moxibustion*, and *Illustrated Classic of Acupuncture Points on the Bronze Man* all say that this point should not be treated by moxibustion otherwise emaciation and death will follow within three years. Modern sources however agree that there are no contraindications to moxibustion.

ACTIONS

Spreads Liver qi
Clears Gall Bladder heat

INDICATIONS

- Headache, redness, itching and pain of the eyes, tinnitus, deafness.
- Fullness of the chest, pain of the lateral costal region, swelling and pain of the axilla, distention and pain of the breasts, breast abscess, spitting blood due to internal injury.
- Swelling, redness and pain of the dorsum of the foot, lumbar pain.

COMBINATIONS

- Pain and itching of the eyes: reduce Diwuhui GB-42 and Guangming GB-37 (*Ode to Elucidate Mysteries*).
- Swelling of the axilla: Diwuhui GB-42, Yangfu GB-38, Shenmai BL-62, Weiyang BL-39, Tianchi P-1 and Zulinqi GB-41 (*Thousand Ducat Formulas*).
- Breast abscess: Diwuhui GB-42 and Liangqiu ST-34 (*Supplementing Life*).

XIAXI GB-43

Clamped Stream

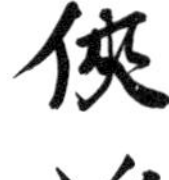

Ying-Spring and Water point of the Gall Bladder channel

LOCATION

Between the fourth toe and the little toe, 0.5 cun proximal to the margin of the web.

NEEDLING

i. Perpendicular insertion 0.3 to 0.5 cun; ii. Oblique insertion directed proximally, 0.5 to 1 cun.

ACTIONS

Clears heat and benefits the head, ears and eyes
Clears damp-heat from the channel and reduces swelling

INDICATIONS

- Headache, dizziness, visual dizziness, hypertension, redness and pain of the outer canthus, itching of the eyes, deafness, tinnitus, pain of the ears, pain and swelling of the cheek and submandibular region.

- Fullness and pain of the chest and lateral costal region, pain of the chest with inability to turn to the side, breast abscess, discharging breast abscess.
- Amenorrhoea, hardness and pain of the hypogastrium, swelling of the four limbs, pain of the whole body, febrile disease with absence of sweating, copious sweating, malaria, mania.
- Wandering pain, pain of the knee and thigh, swelling and pain of the lateral aspect of the knee, redness, swelling and pain of the dorsum of the foot, heat in the soles of the feet, damp erosion and cracks between the toes, contraction of the five toes.

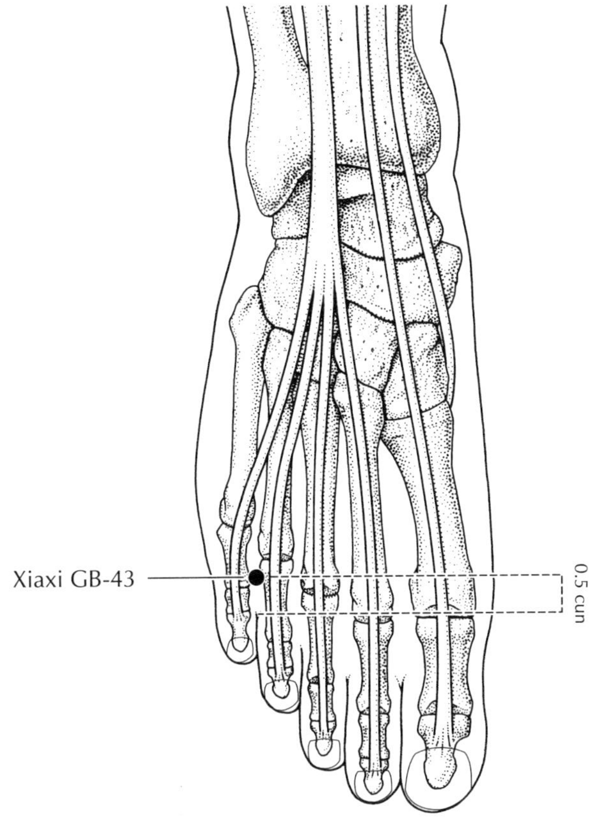

COMMENTARY

According to the *Classic of Difficulties*[22] ying-spring points are indicated for 'heat in the body'. The Gall Bladder channel traverses the sides of the head, enters the ear and connects with the eye. Xiaxi GB-43, the ying-spring point of the Gall Bladder channel, is indicated for Liver and Gall Bladder heat which ascends along the channel to the head and gives rise to such symptoms as headache, dizziness, deafness, tinnitus, ear pain, redness and pain of the outer canthus and itching of the eyes. It is interesting to note, however, that although much used for one-sided headache in modern-day clinical practice, headache is not mentioned as an indication for this point in any of the major classical texts, although Xiaxi GB-43 does appear in point combinations for head wind.

Both the Gall Bladder fu and the Gall Bladder channel are prone to suffer from damp-heat. It is a general principle of the channels, most clearly seen on the leg yang channels, that the points close to the knee (especially the he-sea points) treat the internal fu, and the more distal points (especially the jing-well and ying-spring points) treat disorders of the channel. Whilst not applicable for damp-heat distressing the Gall Bladder fu, therefore, Xiaxi GB-43 as befits its distal location is an important point for damp-heat (usually in combination with qi stagnation) which congests the channel giving rise to swelling in various regions of the body. In the upper body it is indicated for swelling of the cheek or submandibular region. In the chest it is able to treat pain of the chest and lateral costal region, breast abscess and discharging breast abscess (reflecting both the pathway of the Gall Bladder sinew channel to the breasts and the close relationship between the Gall Bladder's coupled Liver channel and the breasts). In the lower body it may be used for dampness and heat which sink downwards and give rise to swelling of the knee, toes or dorsum of the foot, and damp erosion and cracking between the toes.

COMBINATIONS

- Head wind: Xiaxi GB-43, Shangxing DU-23, Qianding DU-21, Baihui DU-20, Yanggu SI-5, Hegu L.I.-4, Guanchong SJ-1 and Kunlun BL-60 (*Great Compendium*).
- Impaired hearing and deafness: Xiaxi GB-43, Ermen SJ-21, Fengchi GB-20, Tinghui GB-2 and Tinggong SI-19 (*Great Compendium*).
- Pain of the submandibular region giving rise to tinnitus and difficult hearing: Xiaxi GB-43, Wangu SI-4, Yanggu SI-5, Jianzhen SI-9 and Zuqiaoyin GB-44 (*Thousand Ducat Formulas*).
- Swelling of the submandibular region with lockjaw: Xiaxi GB-43 and Yanggu SI-5 (*One Hundred Symptoms*).
- Swelling and sabre lumps of the axilla: Xiaxi GB-43, Yangfu GB-38 and Taichong LIV-3 (*Thousand Ducat Formulas*).
- Abscess, ulceration and swelling of the breast: Xiaxi GB-43 and Tianxi SP-18 (*Thousand Ducat Formulas*).
- Pain and hardness of the hypogastrium: Xiaxi GB-43 and Daimai GB-26 (*Supplementing Life*).
- Pain of the lateral aspect of the knee: Xiaxi GB-43 and Yanglingquan GB-34 (*Thousand Ducat Formulas*).
- The five types of haemorrhoids: Xiaxi GB-43, Weizhong BL-40, Chengshan BL-57, Feiyang BL-58, Yangfu GB-38, Fuliu KID-7, Taichong LIV-3, Qihai REN-6, Huiyin REN-1 and Changqiang DU-1 (*Great Compendium*).

ZUQIAOYIN GB-44

足竅陰

Yin Portals of the Foot

Jing-Well and Metal point of the Gall Bladder channel

LOCATION

On the dorsal aspect of the 4th toe, at the junction of lines drawn along the lateral border of the nail and the base of the nail, approximately 0.1 cun from the corner of the nail.

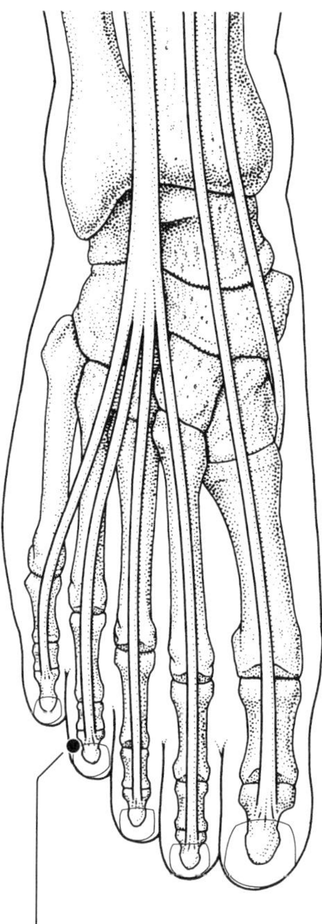

Zuqiaoyin GB-44

NEEDLING

Perpendicular or oblique insertion directed proximally 0.1 to 0.2 cun, or prick to bleed.

ACTIONS

Clears heat and benefits the head
Benefits the chest and lateral costal region
Calms the spirit

INDICATIONS

- Headache, headache with agitation, stabbing pain of the head, dizziness, sudden deafness, tinnitus, redness swelling and pain of the eyes, pain of the outer canthus, throat painful obstruction, stiffness of the tongue or curled tongue with dry mouth, stiffness of the tongue with inability to speak.
- Pain of the lateral costal region, pain of the lateral costal region with cough and inability to catch the breath.
- Nightmares, insomnia, somnolence, agitation and heat of the hands and feet.
- Irregular menstruation, febrile disease, absence of sweating.
- Contracted sinews, contraction of the sinews of the four limbs, inability to raise the elbow.

COMMENTARY

The name of Zuqiaoyin GB-44 (Yin Portals of the Foot) is said to refer to its ability to treat diseases of the sense organs associated with the five zang, namely the eyes (Liver), ears (Kidneys), tongue (Heart), mouth (Spleen) and nose (Lung). In fact, classical indications appear for all of these except the nose. In this respect, Zuqiaoyin GB-44 on the lower body mirrors Touqiaoyin GB-11 (Yin Portals of the Head) in the upper body.

Zuqiaoyin GB-44 is the jing-well, and therefore most distal, point of the Gall Bladder channel. According to the *Spiritual Pivot*[23] "for diseases of the head select [points from] the feet". Zuqiaoyin GB-44 has long been cited by numerous classical sources for disorders due to Gall Bladder fire rising to disturb the head, or exterior wind-heat attacking the head, giving rise to symptoms such as headache, headache with agitation, sudden deafness, tinnitus, dizziness, swollen red and painful eyes and throat painful obstruction. As the terminal, and therefore most dynamic point of the channel, Zuqiaoyin GB-44 is especially indicated when these conditions are severe and acute.

The *Classic of Difficulties*[24] states that jing-well points treat "fullness below the Heart". Whilst the region 'below the Heart' specifically refers to the apex of the epigastrium, like many of the jing-well points Zuqiaoyin GB-44 treats stagnation and fullness throughout the chest region. When Liver qi stagnates in the chest and lateral costal region there can be distention and pain. Zuqiaoyin GB-44 is the metal point of the Gall Bladder channel and its use was emphasised in classics such as the *Systematic Classic of Acupuncture and Moxibustion* and the *Great Compendium of Acupuncture and Moxibustion* for pain of the lateral costal region with cough and inability to catch the breath. These symptoms occur when Liver qi or Liver fire invade the Lung (wood insults metal).

The Gall Bladder divergent channel links with the Heart, and wood is the 'mother' of fire. Gall Bladder fire, therefore, may easily transmit to the Heart and disrupt the spirit (disease of the mother affecting the child). In common with many of the jing-well points, Zuqiaoyin GB-44 is effective to calm the spirit and like other jing-well points of the feet (e.g. Lidui ST-45 and Yinbai SP-1) to treat disorders of sleep such as insomnia and nightmares. In discussing Zuqiaoyin GB-44, the *Investigation into Points Along the Channels* said "[for] Gall Bladder heat somnolence reduce it, [for] Gall Bladder cold insomnia reinforce it".

Finally, unlike the majority of the jing-well points of the twelve channels, Zuqiaoyin GB-44 does not appear to be indicated in the major classics for restoring consciousness.

COMBINATIONS

- Stabbing pain of the head with inability to move: Zuqiaoyin GB-44 and Qiangjian DU-18 (*Thousand Ducat Formulas*).
- Deafness: Zuqiaoyin GB-44 and Guanchong SJ-1 (*Spiritual Pivot*).
- Throat painful obstruction, curled tongue and dry mouth: Zuqiaoyin GB-44, Guanchong SJ-1 and Shaoze SI-1 (*Thousand Ducat Formulas*).
- Absence of sweating: Zuqiaoyin GB-44, Fuliu KID-7, Quze P-3, Yuji LU-10, Shaoze SI-1, Shangxing DU-23, Ququan LIV-8, Kunlun BL-60 and Xiaxi GB-43 (*Great Compendium*).
- Contraction and inability to extend the arm and elbow: Zuqiaoyin GB-44 and Shousanli L.I.-10 (*Supplementing Life*).

NOTES

1 *Spiritual Pivot* Chapter 9 and *Essential Questions* Chapter 70.
2 *Spiritual Pivot* Chapter 9 and *Essential Questions* Chapter 70.
3 *Classic of Difficulties* 29th Difficulty.
4 *Essential Questions* Chapter 39.
5 *Fu Qing-zhu's Gynaecology*, Blue Poppy Press, page 164.
6 *Essential Questions* Chapter 8.
7 *Spiritual Pivot* Chapter 65.
8 *Extra Treatises Based on Investigation & Inquiry*, A Translation of Zhu Dan-xi's Ge Zhi Yu Lun by Yang Shou-zhong & Duan Wu-jin, Blue Poppy Press, 1994.
9 Ma Dan-yang was the originator of the *Song of the Eleven Heavenly Star Points*. They first appeared in print in the 12th century CE *Classic of the Jade Dragon*. Xu Feng included this text in his work *Complete Collection of Acupuncture and Moxibustion* and added a twelfth point, Taichong LIV-3.
10 *Essential Questions* Chapter 17.
11 *Spiritual Pivot* Chapter 4.
12 *Spiritual Pivot* Chapter 5.
13 *Essential Questions* Chapter 6.
14 *Spiritual Pivot* Chapter 44.
15 Quoted in *Chinese Acupuncture and Moxibustion*, Foreign Languages Press, Beijing.
16 *Spiritual Pivot* Chapter 5.
17 *Essential Questions* Chapter 6.
18 *Spiritual Pivot* Chapter 6.
19 *Essential Questions* Chapter 43.
20 *Spiritual Pivot* Chapter 5.
21 *Essential Questions* Chapter 6.
22 *Classic of Difficulties* 68th Difficulty.
23 *Spiritual Pivot* Chapter 9.
24 *Classic of Difficulties* 68th Difficulty.

足厥陰肝經

THE LIVER CHANNEL OF FOOT JUEYIN

THE LIVER CHANNEL OF FOOT JUEYIN

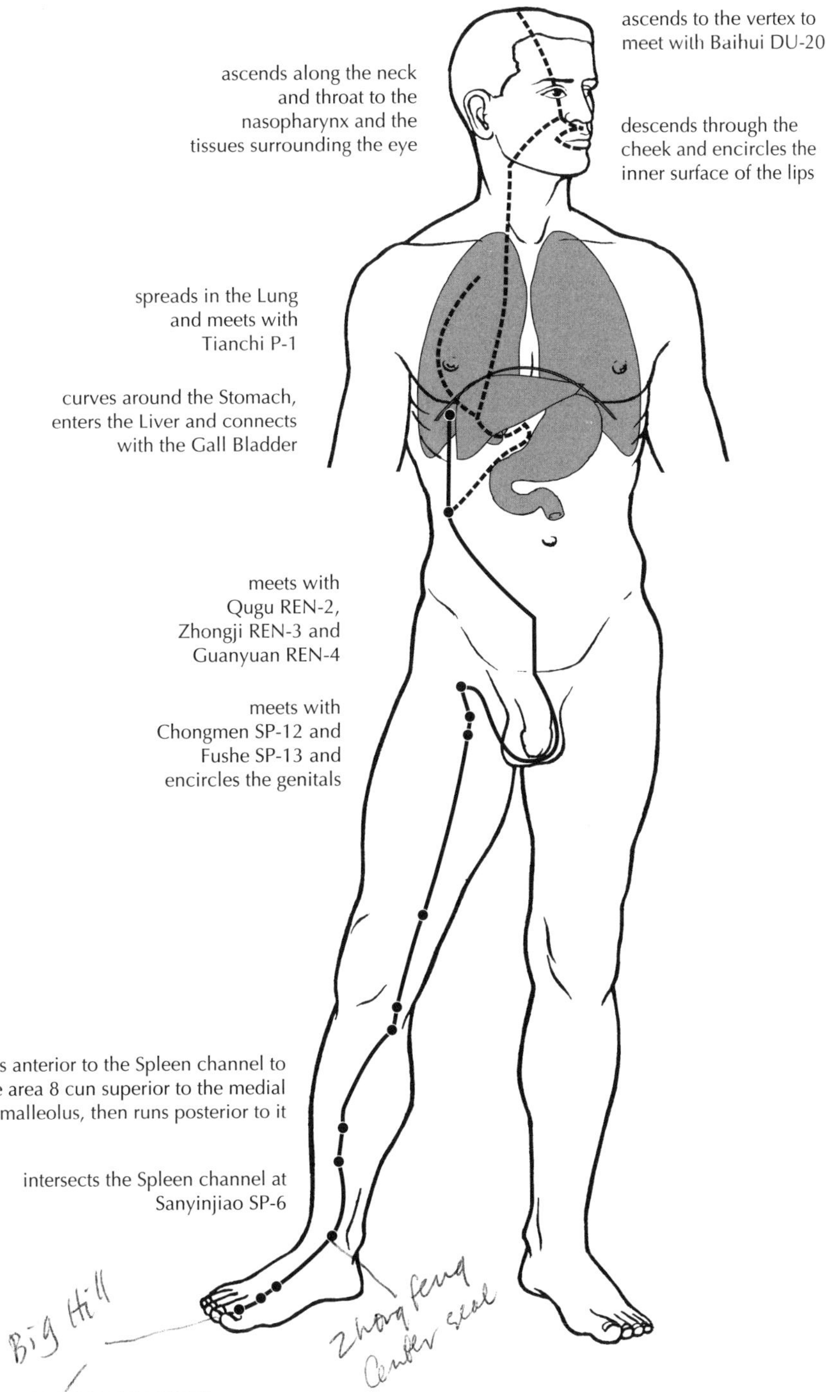

THE LIVER PRIMARY CHANNEL

- originates at the lateral aspect of the dorsum of the big toe at Dadun LIV-1, and runs along the foot to Zhongfeng LIV-4, 1 cun anterior to the medial malleolus,
- ascends along the medial aspect of the lower leg, intersecting the Spleen channel at Sanyinjiao SP-6, then continues to ascend anterior to the Spleen channel to an area 8 cun above the medial malleolus, where it crosses and continues posterior to the Spleen channel up to the knee and the medial aspect of the thigh,
- continues to the pubic region via Chingmen SP-12 and Fushe SP-13 where it encircles the genitals, then ascends to enter the lower abdomen where it intersects the Conception vessel at Qugu REN-2, Zhongji REN-3 and Guanyuan REN-4,

- continues upwards to curve round the Stomach before entering the Liver and connecting with the Gall Bladder,
- crosses the diaphragm and spreads in the costal and hypochondriac region,
- ascends along the neck and posterior aspect of the throat to the nasopharynx to link with the tissues surrounding the eye (the 'eye system'),
- ascends across the forehead to the vertex where it intersects with the Governing vessel at Baihui DU-20.

A branch
- descends from the eye system through the cheek and encircles the inner surface of the lips.

Another branch
- separates from the Liver, crosses the diaphragm and spreads in the Lung, meeting with Tianchi P-1.

The Liver primary channel connects with the following zangfu: Liver, Gall Bladder, Lung, Stomach.

The Liver primary channel meets with other channels at the following points: Sanyinjiao SP-6, Chongmen SP-12, Fushe SP-13, Qugu REN-2, Zhongji REN-3, Guanyuan REN-4, Tianchi P-1, Baihui DU-20.

THE LIVER LUO-CONNECTING CHANNEL
- separates from the primary channel at Ligou LIV-5 on the medial aspect of the lower leg,
- connects with the Gall Bladder channel,
- ascends to the genitals.

THE LIVER DIVERGENT CHANNEL
- separates from the primary channel on the dorsum of the foot,
- ascends to the pubic region where it converges with the Gall Bladder primary channel.

THE LIVER SINEW CHANNEL
- originates on the dorsum of the big toe, and ascends to bind at the anterior aspect of the medial malleolus,
- proceeds along the medial aspect of the tibia to bind at the medial condyle,
- continues upwards along the medial aspect of the thigh to the genitals where it connects with other sinew channels.

Pathological symptoms of the Liver sinew channel
Strain of the big toe, pain anterior to the medial malleolus, pain of the medial aspect of the knee, spasm and pain of the medial aspect of the thigh, dysfunction of the genitals (with internal injury there is inability to have an erection, with injury by cold there is retraction of the genitals, with injury by heat there is persistent erection).

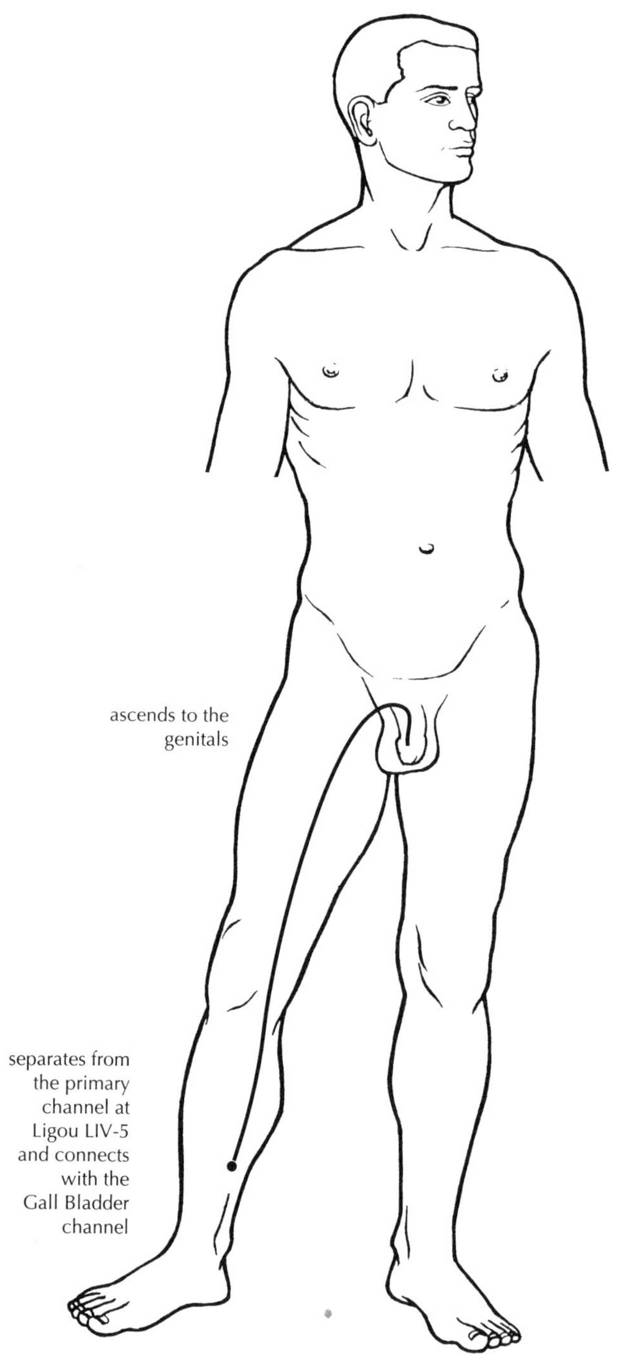

The Liver luo-connecting channel

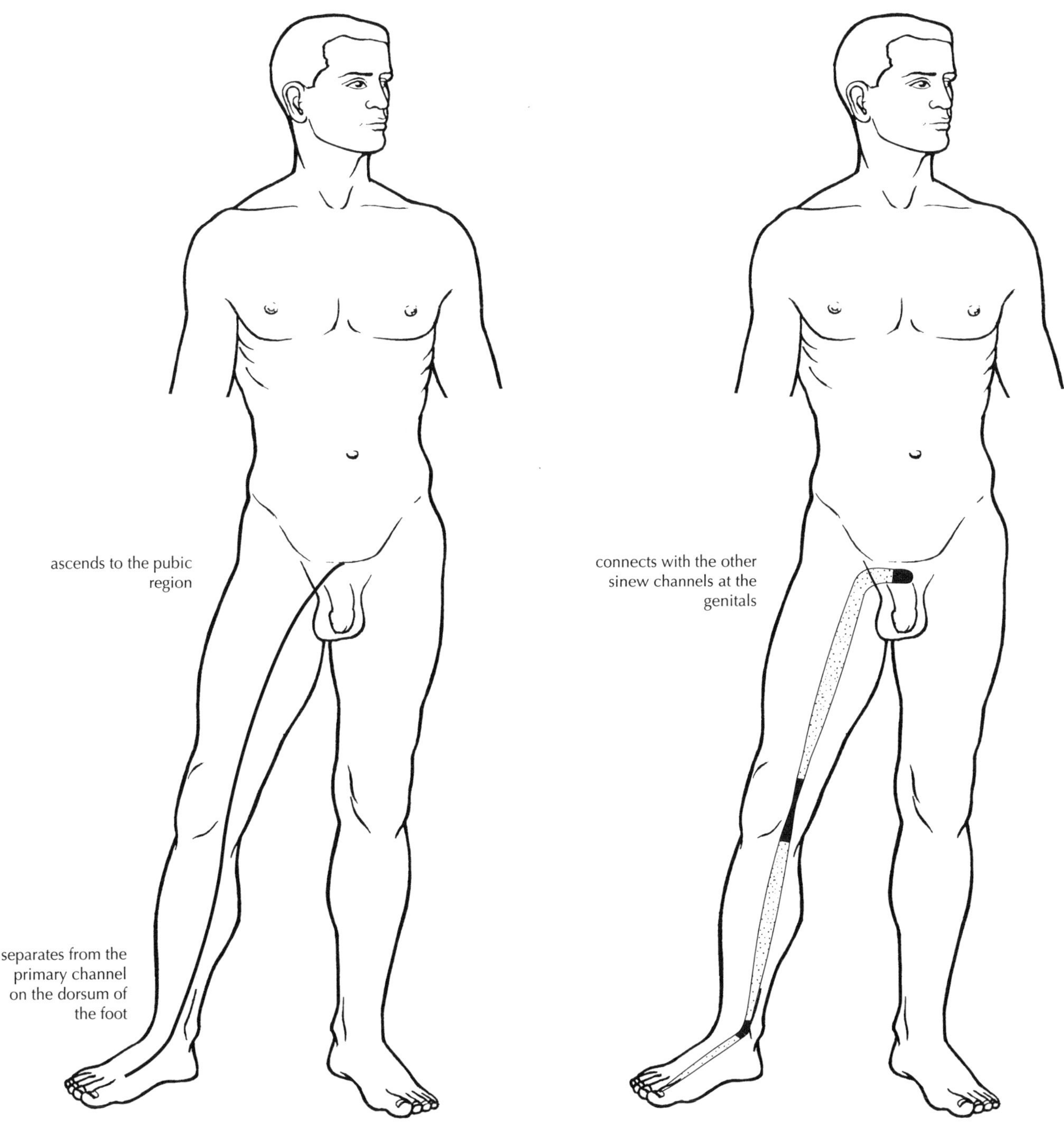

The Liver divergent channel

The Liver sinew channel

DISCUSSION

The Liver channel of foot jueyin is interiorly-exteriorly coupled with the Gall Bladder channel, and paired with the Pericardium channel of hand jueyin according to six channel theory. The Liver-Gall Bladder relationship is further strengthened by the fact that:

- the Liver primary channel connects with the Gall Bladder fu.
- the Liver luo-connecting and divergent channels connect with the Gall Bladder channel.

It is also interesting to note that:

- the Liver primary, luo-connecting and sinew channels go to the genitals, whilst the divergent channel ascends to the pubic region.
- the Liver primary channel enters the lower abdomen.
- the Liver primary channel curves around the Stomach.
- the Liver primary channel spreads in the Lung.
- the Liver primary channel ascends just posterior to the throat.
- the Liver primary channel passes through the nasopharynx.
- the Liver primary channel links with the eye system (the tissues surrounding the eye).
- the Liver primary channel ascends to the vertex to intersect the Governing vessel at Baihui DU-20, the highest point reached by any yin channel.

The Liver has five primary functions:

- storing the blood.
- spreading (maintaining the free flow of) the qi.
- dominating the sinews.
- opening into the eyes.
- manifesting in the nails.

In addition:

- the Liver zang belongs to the wood phase and corresponds to wind.
- the Liver governs uprising, and in disharmony its qi may therefore rise excessively.
- the Liver is entrusted with the ming men fire which in disharmony may easily flare upwards as pathological heat.
- the Liver free-flowing function assists the qi movement of the zangfu, especially the descending of Lung and Stomach qi and the ascending of Spleen qi.
- the Liver free-flowing function assists the qi transformation function of the Bladder.
- the Liver stores the ethereal soul (hun) and as the wood zang is the 'mother' of the Heart.
- the Liver stores the blood which flows into the Conception and Penetrating vessels to become menstrual blood, and its qi is responsible for the smooth flow of menstruatioin.
- the Liver is closely associated with such emotions as anger, irritability, fractiousness, frustration, resentment, depression weepiness and mood swings.

It is by virtue of these functions as well as the channel pathways discussed above, that many of the actions and indications of the points of the Liver channel can be explained. These can be summarised as:

- resolving distention and pain due to stagnation of Liver qi in the head, throat region, chest, Heart, Lung, Stomach, abdomen, lateral costal region, lower abdomen, intestines and genitals.
- assisting in the descent of Stomach and Lung qi and the ascent of Spleen qi
- pacifying interior wind and uprising of yang giving rise to headache, dizziness, epilepsy, spasm etc.
- cooling Liver fire affecting any region of the body.
- benefiting the eyes.
- treating disorders characterised by pain and swelling of the external genitals (especially in men) as well as seminal emission, ejaculatory disorders, priapism and impotence.
- regulating menstruation and the menstrual cycle.
- treating shan disorder (a broad category that includes hernia, genital swelling and pain, and severe pain of the lower abdomen).
- treating disorders of urination such as urinary retention, painful urinary dysfunction, incontinence, frequent urination etc.
- treating lumbar pain.
- treating psycho-emotional disorders deriving from Liver blood deficiency, Liver qi stagnation or Liver fire, all of which may disturb the ethereal soul and spirit.

DADUN LIV-1

Big Mound

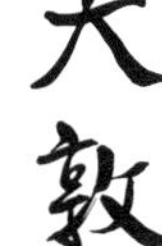

Jing-Well and Wood point of the Liver channel

LOCATION

On the dorsal aspect of the big toe, at the junction of lines drawn along the lateral border of the nail and the base of the nail, approximately 0.1 cun from the corner of the nail.

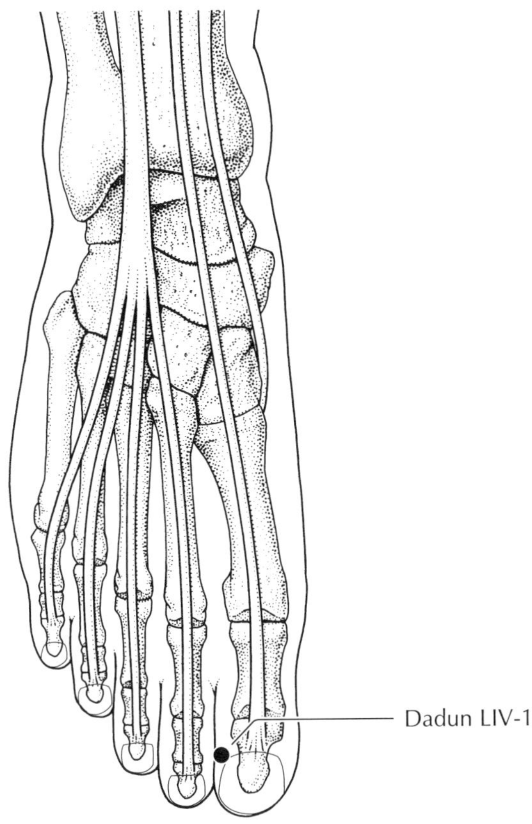

LOCATION NOTE

Some sources (including the *Spiritual Pivot*) locate this point on the dorsal aspect of the big toe, midway between the lateral corner of the nail (i.e. the location above) and the interphalangeal joint, 0.4 cun proximal to the corner of the nail.

NEEDLING

Perpendicular or oblique insertion directed proximally 0.1 to 0.2 cun, or prick to bleed.

ACTIONS

Regulates qi in the lower jiao, treats shan disorder and alleviates pain
Benefits the genitals and adjusts urination
Regulates Liver qi and stops menstrual bleeding
Revives consciousness and calms the spirit

INDICATIONS

- Shan disorder, sudden shan disorder, the seven kinds of shan disorder, hypogastric pain, pain of the umbilicus, abdominal distention and swelling, constipation, heat of the lower abdomen.
- Swelling and pain of the genitals, pain of the head of the penis, retraction of the genitals, swelling of the testicles.
- Painful retention of urine, blood in the urine, painful urinary dysfunction, the five types of painful urinary dysfunction, enuresis, frequent urination.
- Irregular menstruation, ceaseless uterine bleeding, menorrhagia, metrorrhagia, uterine prolapse.
- Epilepsy, loss of consciousness from windstroke, loss of consciousness, acute and chronic childhood fright wind, excessive fright and little strength, great fear as if seeing ghosts, mania-depression, worry and oppression, bitter taste in the mouth, sighing, somnolence, sudden Heart pain, tetany, ceaseless nosebleed, copious sweating.

COMMENTARY

According to the *Song of the Jade Dragon* "For the seven types of shan disorder, choose Dadun LIV-1", whilst the *Essential Questions*[1] says "when the pathogen resides in the foot jueyin luo, it will give rise to sudden pain of shan disorder; needle above the nail of the big toe". Shan disorder is a broad category that includes hernia, genital swelling and pain, and severe pain of the lower abdomen. The most common patterns for these disorders include stagnation of qi, accumulation of cold in the Liver channel, damp-heat, traumatic injury and deficiency. Dadun LIV-1 is the jing-well point of the Liver channel which encircles the genitals and enters the lower abdomen. It is an important point to regulate the qi in these areas and is the pre-eminent distal point in the treatment of any pattern of shan disorder, but as the jing-well point is especially suited to urgent conditions with acute and sudden pain. Both the *Yellow Emperor's Inner Classic* and later texts such as the *Great Compendium of Acupuncture and Moxibustion* recommend that cross-needling be applied at Dadun LIV-1, in other words left Dadun LIV-1 is needled for right shan disorder and vice-versa.

Through its action of regulating qi in the lower jiao Dadun LIV-1 is also indicated for a variety of disorders of both urination and menstruation. As far as urination is concerned, it is notable that all the distal points of the Liver channel are strongly indicated in classical texts for a wide range of urinary disorders. Some explanation may be offered by the fact that the Liver's free-flowing function is said to assist the qi transformation function of the Bladder, and therefore Liver qi stagnation, Liver damp-heat or Liver fire may all impair the smooth flow of urine giving rise to difficult and painful urination, painful urinary dysfunction (especially qi painful urinary dysfunction) etc. In modern clinical practice, points of the Liver channel are often selected in the treatment of such excess patterns, but it is clear from indications such as frequent urination, enuresis and urinary incontinence that Liver channel points were also considered effective in the treatment of deficiency patterns. This reflects the ability of points of the Liver channel to regulate any disorders of the genito-urinary region.

As far as menstrual disorders are concerned, the Liver stores the blood, and if Liver qi stagnation transforms to heat and enters the blood it will give rise to agitation and turbulence manifesting as irregular menstruation, ceaseless uterine bleeding, menorrhagia or metrorrhagia. The important action of Dadun LIV-1 on stopping excessive bleeding extends also to blood in the urine and, according to Sun Si-miao, to nosebleed, which is frequently due to upsurging heat of the Liver. It is useful to compare the application of Dadun LIV-1 with its neighbouring point Yinbai SP-1. Whilst Yinbai SP-1 has a wide application for haemorrhage due either to Spleen qi deficiency or blood heat, Dadun LIV-1 is primarily applicable for haemorrhage due to blood heat.

The focus of Dadun LIV-1 on shan disorder, disorders of the genitals, urinary diseases and uterine bleeding reflects its close affinity for the lower jiao. In this respect it is something of an exception among the jing-well points, which mostly treat disorders of the head and chest region.

Finally, in common with the majority of the jing-well points of the twelve channels, Dadun LIV-1 is indicated for restoring consciousness in cases of collapse and epilepsy, and calming the spirit, being indicated for fear and fright, mania-depression, worry and oppression and sighing.

COMBINATIONS

- Cold shan disorder: Dadun LIV-1 and Zhaohai KID-6 (*One Hundred Symptoms*).
- The seven kinds of shan disorder: Dadun LIV-1 and Taichong LIV-3 (*Song of Points*).
- Abdominal fullness that radiates to the back, one-sided swelling and sagging of the testicle: Dadun LIV-1 [7 moxa cones] and Guanyuan REN-4 [3 moxa cones] (*Great Compendium*).
- Sagging and swollen testicle without pain: Dadun LIV-1, Guilai ST-29 and Sanyinjiao SP-6 (*Great Compendium*).
- Involuntary erection with difficult urination: Dadun LIV-1, Weiyang BL-39, Yingu KID-10, Qimen LIV-14 and Weizhong BL-40 (*Supplementing Life*).
- Enuresis: Dadun LIV-1, Jimen SP-11, Tongli HE-5, Pangguangshu BL-28, Taichong LIV-3, Weizhong BL-40 and Shenmen HE-7 (*Supplementing Life*).
- The five types of painful urinary dysfunction: Dadun LIV-1 and Xuehai SP-10 (*Song of Points*).
- The five types of painful urinary dysfunction, with inability to urinate: Dadun LIV-1 and Qihai REN-6 (*Thousand Ducat Formulas*).
- Uterine prolapse: Dadun LIV-1, Ququan LIV-8 and Zhaohai KID-6 (*Great Compendium*).
- Hot constipation, qi constipation: first needle Changqiang DU-1 then Dadun LIV-1 and Yanglingquan GB-34 (*Song of Points*).
- Somnolence: Dadun LIV-1 and Lidui ST-45 (*Supplementing Life*).
- Loss of consciousness: Dadun LIV-1 and Yinbai SP-1 (*Systematic Classic*).

XÍNGJIĀN LIV-2

Moving Between

行間

Ying-Spring and Fire point of the Liver channel

LOCATION

On the dorsum of the foot, between the first and second toes, 0.5 cun proximal to the margin of the web.

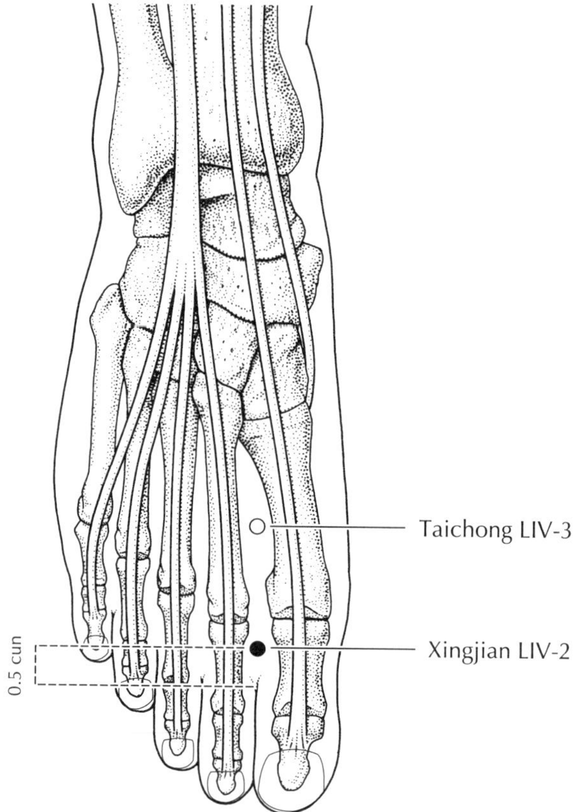

NEEDLING

0.5 to 1 cun obliquely towards the heel, or perpendicular insertion 0.5 cun to 0.8 cun.

ACTIONS

Clears Liver fire
Spreads Liver qi
Pacifies Liver wind
Clears heat and stops bleeding
Benefits the lower jiao

INDICATIONS

- Headache, dizziness, redness and pain of the eyes, lacrimation, eye diseases.
- Nosebleed, thirst, burning heat of the face, dark green complexion, death-like green colour.
- Throat painful obstruction, dry throat with agitation and thirst, clutching sensation in the throat, bitter taste in the mouth, heat in the body.
- Propensity to anger, sadness, propensity to fright, closes eyes and has no desire to look, excessive fright and little strength, propensity to fear as if seeing ghosts, madness, insomnia, palpitations, epilepsy, loss of consciousness, chronic and acute childhood fright wind.
- Contracted sinews, windstroke, fullness of the four limbs, deviation of the mouth, tetany, hypertension.
- Pain and itching of the genitals, pain of the penis, sudden involuntary erection, the seven kinds of shan disorder, cold shan disorder, painful urinary dysfunction, enuresis, retention of urine, difficult urination, white turbidity, red and white leucorrhoea, cold or damp (dong) diarrhoea, constipation, abdominal distention.
- Incessant uterine bleeding, menorrhagia, inhibited menstruation, early menstruation, lower abdominal fullness, abdominal (jia) masses in women, difficult lactation.
- Coughing blood, vomiting, pain of the Heart and the Liver, distention and pain of the chest and lateral costal region, pain of the chest and back, pain below the Heart, much sighing, inability to catch the breath all day long, difficulty in catching the breath, shortness of breath.
- Four limbs counterflow cold, wasting and thirsting disorder with desire to drink, malaria, lotus flower tongue in children.
- Lumbar pain with difficulty in flexing and extending the back, swelling of the knee, pain of the inner aspect of the leg, heat in the shin, leg qi with redness and swelling, pain and swelling of the instep.

COMMENTARY

The Liver, entrusted with the ministerial fire, is known as the 'indomitable zang' and corresponds to the energies of Spring, growth and forcefulness. Although the Liver free-flowing function assists the ascent and descent of the qi of all the zangfu, its own qi direction is upwards, hence the saying "The Liver governs uprising". Since its yang activity is by nature exuberant, fierce and strong, the Liver easily becomes overheated and the normal ascending of Liver qi readily flares up into excess. The *Great Compendium of Acupuncture and Moxibustion* says "When the Liver is excess, reduce Xingjian LIV-2" whilst according to the *Classic of Difficulties*[2] ying-spring points are indicated for 'heat in the body'. Xingjian LIV-2, the ying-spring and fire point of the Liver channel, is therefore the principal point on this channel, indeed in the whole body, to clear Liver fire and descend Liver yang. It has three principal spheres of activity: the head, the emotions and the lower jiao.

The Liver primary channel ascends along the neck and posterior aspect of the throat to the nasopharynx and the tissues surrounding the eye, and then ascends across the forehead to link with Baihui DU-20 at the vertex. Xingjian LIV-2 consequently is much used clinically to treat headache, dizziness, burning heat of the face, nosebleed, throat painful obstruction and dry throat, red and painful eyes, lacrimation and other eye diseases due to Liver fire ascending to the head, although it is interesting to note that headache, dizziness and nosebleed are modern indications and do not appear in any of the major classical acupuncture texts. When extreme, Liver fire or Liver yang may give rise to stirring of interior wind, and Xingjian LIV-2 is used to treat such consequences of this development as epilepsy, loss of consciousness, childhood fright wind, contracted sinews, windstroke and deviation of the mouth.

The *Spiritual Pivot*[3] says "The Liver stores blood and the blood is the residence of the ethereal soul [hun]; when Liver qi is deficient there is fear, when excess there is anger", whilst the *Essential Questions*[4] says "Anger easily injures the Liver". The free and unobstructed spreading of the Liver qi is closely related to the harmonious interplay of the seven emotions. Repression of any of the emotions will cause the Liver qi to stagnate, and after time to transform into fire. At the same time, stagnation of Liver qi, and even more so the blazing up of Liver fire, will render a person prone to experience feelings of irritability and anger. At the stage of qi stagnation, acknowledgement and expression of the appropriate emotion will help free the qi and dispel stagnation, thus Fei Bo-xiong said "Joy, anger, melancholy, anxiety, grief, fear and terror are common to everyone. Giving vent to joy, anger and melancholy as occasion requires is what is meant by venting emotions properly"[5]. When Liver fire is blazing, however, it is like a fire with an unlimited supply of fuel, and giving vent to rage and anger will not only fail to dispel the fire but will continually stoke and encourage it. At the same time, the anger itself will injure the body, and at this stage moderation of excessive emotion and not spontaneous expression must be practised. Thus Cao Tong of the Qing dynasty recommended in *Common Sayings on Gerontology* "When faced with something exasperating, one should calmly consider which is more important, anger or health. This comparison will enable one to gradually eliminate one's anger"[6]. Li Yi-ru of the Qing dynasty, however, said "Of the seven emotions, anger is the hardest to control". Acupuncture treatment seeks to quell and douse the fire, and Xingjian LIV-2 is the primary point to subdue blazing Liver fire giving rise to such manifestations as raging anger with a red face and clutching sensation in the throat. The *Spiritual Pivot*[7] says "with anger the qi rebels upwards and accumulates in the chest". If Liver fire and stagnant qi attack the chest and Lung they will give rise to distention and pain, shortness of breath, sighing and difficulty in catching the breath. If, as is commonly seen clinically, Liver fire and stagnant qi transmit to the Heart there will be pain of both the Liver and Heart, as well as severe disturbance of the spirit manifesting as mania disorder, insomnia, palpitations etc. If there is a deeply established pattern of repression of anger, usually deriving from early childhood experiences, then the stagnant qi and fire will have no appropriate outlet and a person may become sad and tearful. Anger, overt or hidden, is not the only emotion associated with the Liver however, as stressed by the statement in the *Spiritual Pivot* that "when Liver qi is deficient there is fear". The Liver and Gall Bladder are associated in Chinese culture with decisiveness and courage. If the Liver is deficient, especially Liver blood, or if a person is unable to acknowledge their anger and thus embrace their power and courage, there may be fear and fright with a feeling of lack of strength and a tendency to close the eyes and have "no desire to look".

The Liver stores the blood, and the Liver channel converges with the Conception vessel in the lower abdomen at Qugu REN-2, Zhongji REN-3 and Guanyuan REN-4. Liver fire can easily transmit to the uterine blood and induce wild and reckless flow, manifesting as ceaseless uterine bleeding, menorrhagia and early menstruation. If heat condenses the blood and causes stagnation, or if Liver qi stagnation is prolonged, uterine (jia) masses may form or there may be inhibited menstruation. Disturbance of the blood by Liver fire may also give rise to coughing of blood and nosebleed.

The Liver channel encircles the genitals and penetrates the lower abdomen, whilst the Liver assists the free movement of qi throughout the body. If there is qi stagnation or consequent fire or damp-heat in the lower jiao, especially the genital region or Bladder, there may be a variety of symptoms such as itching and pain of the genitals, sudden involuntary erection, painful urinary dysfunction, retention of urine, difficult and turbid urination, leucorrhoea and shan disorder. If qi stagnation binds the intestines there may be constipation. In all these cases Xingjian LIV-2 may be used.

One special condition for which Xingjian LIV-2 is indicated is the symptom of hands and feet counterflow cold, where only the hands and feet are cold but the body is warm. This may occur in the pattern known as 'true heat, false cold', where heat constrained in the interior prevents the yang qi from circulating to the limbs. Despite the apparent cold, the other symptoms, as well as the pulse and the tongue, are indicative of heat and constraint. In clinical practice, this symptom is often encountered in patients with Liver qi stagnation rather than heat, where the stagnant qi prevents adequate circulation of qi to the extremities.

According to the *Spiritual Pivot*[8] "The Liver governs the sinews", and Xingjian LIV-2 is indicated in many classical sources for pain of the lumbar region. Although more commonly ascribed to Kidney deficiency or painful obstruction, stagnation of Liver qi or Liver blood deficiency may also give rise to lumbar pain due to contraction and inflexibility of the sinews. However the frequency with which Xingjian LIV-2 appears in classical combinations for lumbar pain, points more towards an empirical application rather than a theoretical one.

Finally, Xingjian LIV-2 is indicated for swelling of the knee, pain of the inner aspect of the leg, heat in the shins and pain and swelling of the instep, and the *Song of Points for Miscellaneous Diseases* says "for leg and knee pain covet Xingjian LIV-2".

COMBINATIONS

- Lacrimation: Xingjian LIV-2 and Shenting DU-24 (*Supplementing Life*).
- Liver qi night blindness: Xingjian LIV-2 and Jingming BL-1 (*One Hundred Symptoms*).
- Dry throat with desire to drink: Xingjian LIV-2 and Taichong LIV-3 (*Thousand Ducat Formulas*).
- Pain of the Liver and Heart: Xingjian LIV-2 and Taichong LIV-3 (*Thousand Ducat Formulas*).
- Pain of the Heart with a green complexion like death, inability to catch the breath all day long, pain of the Liver and Heart: Xingjian LIV-2 and Taichong LIV-3 (*Systematic Classic*).
- Heart pain: Xingjian LIV-2 and Yinxi HE-6 (*Supplementing Life*).

- Fright epilepsy, mad walking and madness: Xingjian LIV-2, Jinsuo DU-8, Qugu REN-2 and Yingu KID-10 (*Thousand Ducat Formulas*).
- Retention of urine and pain of the penis: Xingjian LIV-2 and Ququan LIV-8 (*Supplementing Life*).
- Severe thirst of wasting and thirsting disorder: Xingjian LIV-2 and Yongquan KID-1 (*One Hundred Symptoms*).
- Lumbar pain with inability to stand for long or to move: Xingjian LIV-2 and Jingmen GB-25 (*Systematic Classic*).
- Lumbar pain that radiates down the leg: Xingjian LIV-2, Huantiao GB-30 and Fengshi GB-31 (*Song of Points*).
- Lumbar pain with inability to bend and extend: Xingjian LIV-2, Weiyang BL-39, Yinmen BL-37, Taibai SP-3 and Yinlingquan SP-9 (*Thousand Ducat Formulas*).
- Lumbar pain with difficulty in moving: Xingjian LIV-2, Fengshi GB-31 and Weizhong BL-40 (*Glorious Anthology*).
- Inability of the legs to support the body: Xingjian LIV-2 and Tianzhu BL-10 (*Thousand Ducat Formulas*).

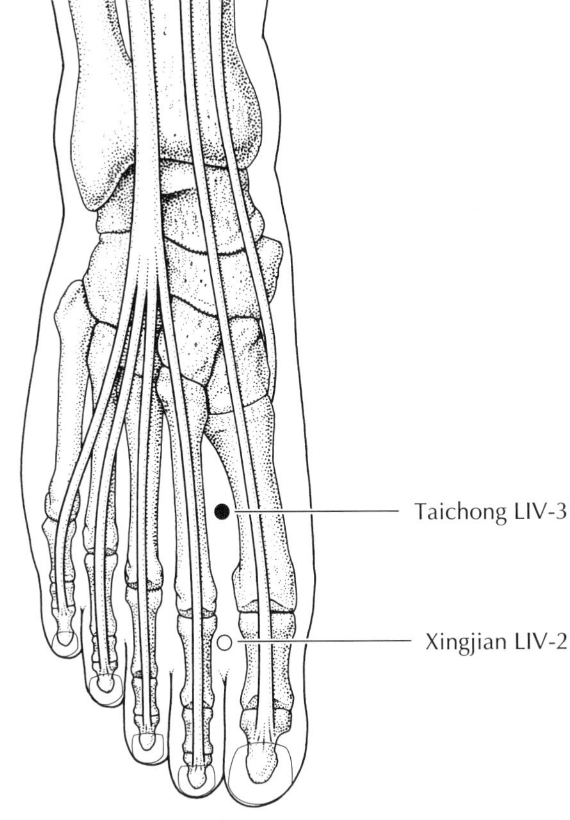

TÀICHŌNG LIV-3
Great Rushing

太冲

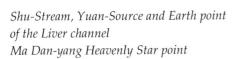

Shu-Stream, Yuan-Source and Earth point of the Liver channel
Ma Dan-yang Heavenly Star point

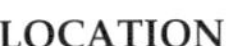

LOCATION
On the dorsum of the foot, in the hollow distal to the junction of the first and second metatarsal bones.

LOCATION NOTE
Run a finger from Xingjian LIV-2 along the interspace between the first and second metatarsal bones towards the ankle, into the pronounced depression before the junction of the bases of the first and second metatarsals.

NEEDLING
In the direction of Yongquan KID-1, 0.5 to 1.5 cun.

ACTIONS
Spreads Liver qi
Subdues Liver yang and extinguishes wind
Nourishes Liver blood and Liver yin
Clears the head and eyes
Regulates menstruation
Regulates the lower jiao

INDICATIONS
- Headache, dizziness, numbness of the head, opisthotonos, contraction of the sinews of the hands and feet, epilepsy, childhood fright wind, deviation of the mouth, tetany, hypertension.
- Distention and pain of the lateral costal region, inability to catch the breath all day long, sighing, swelling of the axilla, pain of the Liver and Heart, Heart pain with a wiry pulse, distention of the Heart, breast pain, epigastric or abdominal pain, periumbilical pain, pain and fullness of the hypogastrium, shan disorder, sudden shan disorder in children, swollen testicles, retracted testicles, unilateral sagging of the testicle, pain of the genitals.
- Insomnia, easily fearful.
- Blurred vision, cloudy vision, redness, swelling and pain of the eyes.
- Cracked lips, swelling of the lips, distention of the throat, pain of the throat, dry throat with desire to drink, internal heat with thirst, low grade fever, death-like green complexion.
- Amenorrhoea, irregular menstruation, incessant uterine bleeding, uterine prolapse, ceaseless and profuse sweating after childbirth, insufficient lactation.
- Enuresis, difficult urination, retention of urine, painful urinary dysfunction, the five types of painful urinary dysfunction, deficiency-taxation oedema.

- Jaundice, vomiting, vomiting blood, nausea, constipation, difficult defecation, borborygmus, diarrhoea containing undigested food, diarrhoea with thin stools, bloody diarrhoea and dysenteric disorder, blood in the stools.
- Emaciation, insufficiency of essence (semen) in men, seminal emission, insufficiency of qi.
- Lumbar pain radiating to the lower abdomen, lumbar pain, pain of the inner and outer knee, pain of the lower leg, flaccidity and weakness of the legs, inability to walk, cold sensation in the knees and feet, cold feet, pain of the inner malleolus, swelling of the elbow, contraction of the five fingers.

COMMENTARY

Taichong LIV-3 is the shu-stream and yuan-source point of the Liver channel. The *Spiritual Pivot* in Chapter 6 recommends the use of the shu-stream points in disorders of the zang, whilst in Chapter 1 it says "When the five zang are diseased, select [from] the twelve yuan-source [points]". Taichong LIV-3 is arguably the most important point of the Liver channel, with an extensive range of actions, and may be used with equal effect for both excess and deficiency patterns of the Liver zang and its channel. So important did the Ming dynasty physician Xu Feng consider Taichong LIV-3 to be, that he added it to Ma Danyang's 'eleven heavenly star points' when listing them in his work *Complete Collection of Acupuncture and Moxibustion*. Since this time, these points have become known as Ma Danyang's 'twelve heavenly star points'.

Master Zhu Dan-xi in the 14th century said "The Liver governs spreading and draining" and "When the qi and blood flow harmoniously, the ten thousand diseases will not arise. Once there is constraint, all diseases may arise". The Liver's function of spreading means that although the Liver is not considered responsible for the production of qi, it ensures that the flow of qi in the body remains free, easy, open, relaxed and unobstructed. This function may be impaired in three main ways. Firstly, and most commonly, it may develop when the spontaneous expression of any of the emotions is restricted, especially anger. Secondly, the spreading function of the Liver is an expression of its yang qi, and a saying of Chinese medicine stresses "The body of the Liver is yin whilst its function is yang". In other words, the Liver yang is dependent on Liver yin. Stagnation of Liver qi may therefore result from failure of yin or blood to moisten, nourish and soften the Liver. Thirdly, the ability of the Liver to spread qi may be obstructed by the presence of pathogenic damp-heat. A full understanding of Liver disharmony also stresses one further point which is that Liver qi stagnation may bring about the development of any other Liver pattern, for example by transformation into Liver fire, the consequent consumption of yin and hence the uprising of Liver yang, or by transformation of either Liver fire or Liver yang into wind. For this reason it is said that clinically any pattern of disharmony of the Liver may be accompanied by qi stagnation.

When Liver qi stagnates it gives rise to sensations of pressure, distention and pain, predominantly in those areas traversed by the Liver channel and its interiorly-exteriorly coupled Gall Bladder channel. Qi stagnation tends to move around and fluctuate, mainly according to emotional changes, and is relieved by emotional expressiveness and physical activity, both of which free the flow of qi. The name of Taichong LIV-3 'Great Rushing' refers to this point's function as the great passageway for the flow of qi in the channel. It is a primary point for promoting the free-flow of Liver qi, and can resolve Liver qi stagnation giving rise to distention and pain in any part of the body, whether the head, eyes, throat, chest, Heart, breasts, epigastrium, abdomen, lateral costal region, uterus or genitals.

According to the *Spiritual Pivot*[10] "The Liver stores blood, the blood is the residence of the ethereal soul (hun); when Liver qi is deficient there is fear". Although much used in modern clinical practice for emotional and psychological manifestations of qi stagnation such as depression, frustration, pent-up feelings, irritability, premenstrual tension, mood swings, weepiness etc., it is striking that with the exception of fearfulness, psycho-emotional indications are almost entirely absent from major classical sources.

Taichong LIV-3 is an essential point for subduing Liver yang and pacifying Liver wind. The Liver is the zang of wood and wind and is entrusted with the ministerial fire. Its qi is vigorous, forceful and active, and according to sayings of Chinese medicine "The Liver governs uprising" and "The Liver dominates physical movement". It is common, therefore, for the hot, aggressive, ascending, and moving nature of the Liver to exceed normal limits and manifest as upsurging of Liver yang, or progress to the stirring up of Liver wind. Alternatively wind may stir due to deficient blood and consequent emptiness of the blood vessels. Typical manifestations of wind for which Taichong LIV-3 is indicated include headache, dizziness, numbness of the head, childhood fright wind, tetany, epilepsy, opisthotonos and deviation of the mouth.

Taichong LIV-3 is equally important for all deficiency patterns of the Liver. It promotes the generation of both Liver blood and Liver yin and hence nourishes those areas of the body dominated by the Liver, namely the eyes, sinews and uterus. Liver yin deficiency is the root of hyperactivity of Liver yang, whilst Liver blood or yin deficiency frequently lie at the root of Liver wind. Taichong LIV-3, therefore, is able both to subdue excess and nourish deficiency, and thus treat both the root and manifestation of these patterns.

The *Spiritual Pivot*[11] says "Liver qi opens into the eyes, when the Liver is in harmony the eyes are able to distinguish the five colours" whilst the *Essential Questions*[12] states "When the Liver receives blood it gives rise to vision". Taichong LIV-3 is indicated for failure of the Liver blood or yin to nourish the eyes resulting in blurred or failing vision, as well as for excess disharmonies where Liver fire, Liver yang, or Liver channel wind-heat result in red, swollen, and painful eyes, or where Liver wind leads to unusual movement of the eyes or eyelids.

The Liver channel connects with the brain at Baihui DU-20, the topmost point of the body, and is the only yin channel to ascend directly to the upper part of the head. Taichong LIV-3, therefore, is used to treat many disorders of the head, especially headache and dizziness, due to both excess and deficiency patterns of the Liver. It is specifically indicated for vertex headaches, although it is worth noting that neither headache nor dizziness are found as indications for this point in any major classic.

The Liver is closely related to the menstrual cycle. The Liver stores the blood and its channel enters the lower abdomen and connects with the Conception vessel at Qugu REN-2, Zhongji REN-3 and Guanyuan REN-4, whilst it is the free movement of Liver qi prior to menstruation which ensures the smooth flow of blood. So important is the Liver to menstruation that Ye Tian-shi stated "the Liver is the pre-heaven qi of women". Liver qi stagnation, Liver fire or deficiency of Liver blood may therefore give rise to such disorders as amenorrhoea, irregular menstruation and incessant uterine bleeding. Taichong LIV-3 is an important point in the treatment of any of these disorders.

The Liver channel passes through the genitals and lower abdomen, and is closely related to the genito-urinary organs. Normal excretion of urine depends mainly on the Kidneys and Bladder but is also assisted by the Liver's spreading function. Taichong LIV-3 is indicated for retention of urine, painful urinary dysfunction or difficult urination characterised by qi stagnation, as well as for shan disorder, pain of the genitals and swelling or retraction of the testicles. Due to its general affinity for this area, however, Taichong LIV-3 is also indicated for deficiency urinary patterns such as enuresis, incontinence and deficiency-taxation oedema. In fact there are other indications of the ability of Taichong LIV-3 to tonify deficiency in this region, for example insufficiency of essence (semen) in men and seminal emission.

In the intestinal region, failure of the qi to flow freely may lead to binding of the stools, and Taichong LIV-3 may be used for constipation or difficult defecation due to qi stagnation or stagnant heat. When Liver qi stagnation co-exists with Spleen deficiency, the commonly-seen clinical pattern of abdominal pain and diarrhoea with thin stools, alternating with difficult defecation or constipation, may be encountered. Taichong LIV-3 is an important point for the treatment of this pattern, and may be combined for example with Zhangmen LIV-13, the front-mu point of the Spleen. In the middle jiao, Taichong LIV-3 is indicated for vomiting due to Liver-Stomach disharmony and jaundice due to Liver and Gall Bladder damp-heat.

Bilateral Taichong LIV-3 and Hegu L.I.-4 are known as 'the four gates'. This combination first appeared in the *Ode to Elucidate Mysteries* which said "for cold and heat with painful obstruction, open the four gates". The text goes on to imply that the yuan-source points of the six yang channels emerge at the four gates. Since a fundamental principle for treating painful obstruction is to select points from yang channels, this helps to explain why these two points are considered so effective in treating painful obstruction. Subsequently, the use of these points has been extended to treat a variety of disorders involving pain and spasm. This is an elegant combination. Hegu L.I.-4 on the upper extremity lies in the wide valley between the first and second metacarpals, whilst Taichong LIV-3 on the lower extremity lies in the wide valley between the first and second metatarsals. Hegu L.I.-4, the yuan-source point, belongs to yangming channel which is 'abundant in qi and blood' whilst Taichong LIV-3, the shu-stream and yuan-source point of the Liver channel, has the function of spreading the qi. Together they are able to vigorously activate the qi and blood and ensure their free and smooth passage throughout the body.

Finally Taichong LIV-3 is indicated for a variety of channel disorders such as lumbar pain, pain or weakness of the knee and leg, coldness of the knees and feet and contraction of the five fingers.

COMBINATIONS

- Red eyes and bleeding from Yingxiang L.I.-20 (i.e. nosebleed): Taichong LIV-3, Toulinqi GB-15 and Hegu L.I.-4 (*Song of Points*).
- Nasal congestion, nasal polyp and nasal congestion and discharge: Taichong LIV-3 and Hegu L.I.-4 (*Song of Points*).
- Swelling of the lips: Taichong LIV-3 and Yingchuang ST-16 (*Supplementing Life*).
- Cracked and bleeding tongue: Taichong LIV-3, Neiguan P-6 and Yinjiao REN-7 (*Miscellaneous Diseases*).
- Erosion, heat and dryness of the mouth: Taichong LIV-3, Laogong P-8, Shaoze SI-1 and Sanjian L.I.-3 (*Thousand Ducat Formulas*).

- For most types of acute throat pain: first needle Baihui DU-20 then Taichong LIV-3, Zhaohai KID-6 and Sanyinjiao SP-6 (*Ode of Xi-hong*).
- Dry throat with desire to drink: Taichong LIV-3 and Xingjian LIV-2 (*Thousand Ducat Formulas*).
- Pain of the Liver and Heart: Taichong LIV-3 and Xingjian LIV-2 (*Thousand Ducat Formulas*).
- Pain of the Heart with a green complexion like death, inability to catch the breath all day long, pain of the Liver and Heart: Taichong LIV-3 and Xingjian LIV-2 (*Systematic Classic*).
- Breast pain: Taichong LIV-3 and Fuliu KID-7 (*Systematic Classic*).
- Swelling and sabre lumps of the axilla: Taichong LIV-3, Xiaxi GB-43 and Yangfu GB-38 (*Thousand Ducat Formulas*).
- Abdominal distention leading to back pain: Taichong LIV-3 and Taibai SP-3 (*Great Compendium*).
- Pain of the genitals: Taichong LIV-3, Shenshu BL-23, Zhishi BL-52 and Jinggu BL-64 (*Supplementing Life*).
- The seven kinds of shan disorder: Taichong LIV-3 and Dadun LIV-1 (*Song of Points*).
- Profuse and ceaseless uterine bleeding: Taichong LIV-3, Jiaoxin KID-8, Yingu KID-10 and Sanyinjiao SP-6 (*Supplementing Life*).
- Profuse and ceaseless uterine bleeding: Taichong LIV-3 and Sanyinjiao SP-6 (*Great Compendium*).
- Uterine prolapse: Taichong LIV-3, Shaofu HE-8, Zhaohai KID-6 and Ququan LIV-8 (*Great Compendium*).
- Difficult delivery: reduce Taichong LIV-3 and Sanyinjiao SP-6, reinforce Hegu L.I.-4 (*Great Compendium*).
- Red and white leucorrhoea: Qugu REN-2 [7 cones of moxa], Taichong LIV-3, Guanyuan REN-4, Fuliu KID-7, Sanyinjiao SP-6 and Tianshu ST-25 [one hundred cones of moxa] (*Compilation*).
- Difficulty in defecation: Taichong LIV-3, Zhongliao BL-33, Shimen REN-5, Chengshan BL-57, Zhongwan REN-12, Taixi KID-3, Dazhong KID-4 and Chengjin BL-56 (*Supplementing Life*).
- Diarrhoea with thin stools, dysenteric disorder with blood in the stools: Taichong LIV-3 and Ququan LIV-8 (*Thousand Ducat Formulas*).
- Diarrhoea with thin stools: Taichong LIV-3, Shenque REN-8 and Sanyinjiao SP-6 (*Great Compendium*).
- The five types of haemorrhoids: Taichong LIV-3, Weizhong BL-40, Chengshan BL-57, Feiyang BL-58, Yangfu GB-38, Fuliu KID-7, Xiaxi GB-43, Qihai REN-6, Huiyin REN-1 and Changqiang DU-1 (*Great Compendium*).
- Blood in the stool: Taichong LIV-3, Chengshan BL-57, Fuliu KID-7 and Taibai SP-3 (*Great Compendium*).
- Deficiency-taxation oedema: moxa Taichong LIV-3 one hundred times, also moxa Shenshu BL-23 (*Thousand Ducat Formulas*).
- Enuresis: Taichong LIV-3, Jimen SP-11, Tongli HE-5, Dadun LIV-1, Pangguangshu BL-28, Weizhong BL-40 and Shenmen HE-7 (*Supplementing Life*).
- Wasting and thirsting disorder: Taichong LIV-3, Xingjian LIV-2, Chengjiang REN-24, Jinjin (M-HN-20), Yuye (M-HN-20), Renzhong DU-26, Lianquan REN-23, Quchi L.I-11, Laogong P-8, Shangqiu SP-5, Ranggu KID-2 and Yinbai SP-1 (*Great Compendium*).
- "For cold and heat with painful obstruction, open the Four Gates" [Taichong LIV-3 and Hegu L.I.-4] (*Ode to Elucidate Mysteries*).
- Unendurable pain of the arm that radiates to the shoulder and spine: Taichong LIV-3 and Hegu L.I.-4 (*Ode of Xi-hong*).
- Flaccidity of the legs: Taichong LIV-3, Yanglingquan GB-34, Chongyang ST-42 and Qiuxu GB-40 (*Great Compendium*).
- Weakness of the legs: moxa Taichong LIV-3, Lidui ST-45 and Fengshi GB-31 (*Outline of Medicine*).
- Inability to walk: Taichong LIV-3, Zusanli ST-36 and Zhongfeng LIV-4 (*Ode of the Jade Dragon*).
- Difficulty in walking: Taichong LIV-3 and Zhongfeng LIV-4 (*Song More Precious Than Jade*).

ZHONGFENG LIV-4

Middle Seal

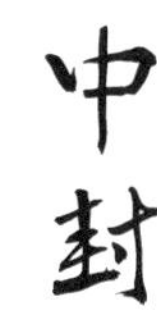

Jing-River and Metal point of the Liver channel

LOCATION

On the ankle, anterior to the prominence of the medial malleolus, in the significant depression just medial to the tendon of tibialis anterior when the ankle is extended (dorsiflexed).

LOCATION NOTE

i. It is important to extend (dorsiflex) the ankle (by drawing the toes upwards towards the shin) before locating this point; ii. This point is also described as midway between Shangqiu SP-5 and Jiexi ST-41; iii. The distance of this point from the prominence of the medial malleolus is given variously in classical sources as either 1 or 1.5 cun.

NEEDLING

Perpendicular insertion 0.3 to 0.5 cun, or oblique insertion medially towards Shangqiu SP-5 or laterally towards Jiexi ST-41.

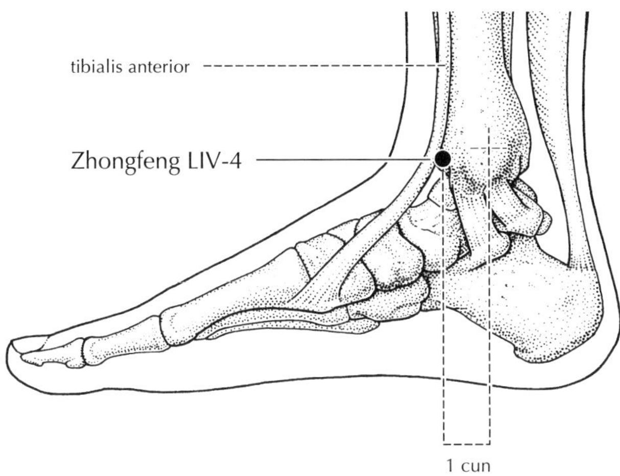

ACTIONS

Spreads Liver qi and regulates the lower jiao
Clears Liver channel stagnant heat

INDICATIONS

- Pain and retraction of the genitals, hypogastric pain, shan disorder, cold shan disorder, seminal emission, seminal emission due to deficiency-taxation, seminal emission with dreams, difficult urination, the five types of painful urinary dysfunction, retention of urine.
- Pain and swelling of the lower abdomen, abdominal discomfort after eating, periumbilical pain, difficult defecation, no pleasure in eating.
- Green complexion, sighing, jaundice, yellow body with low grade fever, low grade fever, malaria, goitre, dry throat.
- Lumbar pain, contracted sinews, numbness of the body, diminished qi, heaviness of the body, pain of the medial aspect of the knee, cold inversion of the feet, pain and swelling of the medial malleolus.

COMMENTARY

Zhongfeng LIV-4 is the jing-river point of the Liver channel. Like Dadun LIV-1, its main action is to regulate qi in the lower jiao portion of the Liver channel, specifically the genitals, the urinary system and the region around and below the umbilicus.

In the genital region Zhongfeng LIV-4 is indicated for hypogastric pain, pain and retraction of the genitals and shan disorder due to stagnation of Liver qi, traumatic injury or penetration of cold into the Liver channel. It is also indicated for various kinds of seminal emission. The Liver is entrusted with the ministerial fire, and the Liver channel dominates the genitals. Sexual desire, therefore, is a manifestation of the fire of both the Kidneys and the Liver. The ejaculatory function in men is dominated by the free flow of Liver qi, in the same way that it dominates the regularity of the menstrual cycle in women. Heat due to Liver fire, damp-heat in the Liver channel, or Liver and Kidney yin deficiency may agitate and disturb the 'gate of essence' leading to seminal emission. Zhongfeng LIV-4 is primarily indicated for seminal emission due to heat, but owing to its regulatory action on the genital region may be used in all patterns. Thus the *Classic of Supplementing Life* recommended it for seminal emission with dreams (indicative of heat), whilst Sun Si-miao in the *Thousand Ducat Formulas* recommended it for seminal emission due to deficiency-taxation.

Normal excretion of urine depends mainly on the Kidneys and Bladder but is also assisted by the Liver's spreading function. Like all the more distal points of the channel, Zhongfeng LIV-4 is indicated for disorders such as difficult urination, painful urinary dysfunction and retention of urine, especially those characterised either by stagnation of qi, stagnant heat, or damp-heat in the Liver channel.

Liver qi stagnation can affect many different regions of the body. Zhongfeng LIV-4 focuses primarily on stagnation of qi in the lower abdominal region and is indicated for pain and swelling (especially in the umbilical region), discomfort after eating and difficulty in defecating. Its ability to treat Liver qi stagnation is not confined to the abdomen, however, and it has long been indicated for stagnation of qi in the chest region giving rise to excessive sighing. The *Systematic Classic of Acupuncture and Moxibustion*, for example, states that Zhongfeng LIV-4 is indicated for "sighing as if [the patient is] about to die".

Zhongfeng LIV-4 is also classically indicated for jaundice and malaria, especially when accompanied by low-grade fever, a clear reflection of the presence of damp-heat.

Finally Zhongfeng LIV-4 is indicated for inversion counterflow of the feet, a term identical in meaning to counterflow cold (see Xingjian LIV-2). This kind of cold may be seen when heat is constrained on the interior, or when qi stagnation prevents the smooth flow of warming qi from reaching the extremities.

COMBINATIONS

- Periumbilical pain: Zhongfeng LIV-4, Shuifen REN-9 and Shenque REN-8 (*Supplementing Life*).
- Pain of the umbilical region: Zhongfeng LIV-4, Ququan LIV-8 and Shuifen REN-9 (*Great Compendium*).
- Drum distention: Zhongfeng LIV-4, Fuliu KID-7, Gongsun SP-4, Taibai SP-3 and Shuifen REN-9 (*Bronze Man*).
- Swelling of the throat with inability to swallow: Zhongfeng LIV-4, Qiangu SI-2 and Zhaohai KID-6 (*Thousand Ducat Formulas*).

- Oesophageal constriction: Zhongfeng LIV-4 and Shentang BL-44 (*Supplementing Life*).
- Jaundice with periodic low grade fever: Zhongfeng LIV-4 and Zuwuli LIV-10 (*Thousand Ducat Formulas*).
- Difficulty in walking: apply moxa to Zhongfeng LIV-4 and Zusanli ST-36 (*Golden Mirror*).
- Difficulty in walking: Zhongfeng LIV-4 and Taichong LIV-3 (*Song More Precious Than Jade*).
- Inability to walk: Zhongfeng LIV-4, Taichong LIV-3 and Zusanli ST-36 (*Ode of the Jade Dragon*).

LIGOU LIV-5

Woodworm Canal

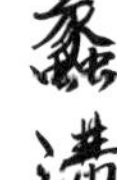

Luo-Connecting point of the Liver channel.

LOCATION

5 cun above the prominence of the medial malleolus, immediately posterior to the medial crest of the tibia, in the depression between the medial crest of the tibia and the gastrocnemius muscle.

LOCATION NOTE

Divide the distance between the tip of the medial malleolus and the popliteal crease into thirds; Ligou LIV-5 is located at the junction of the distal third and proximal two thirds.

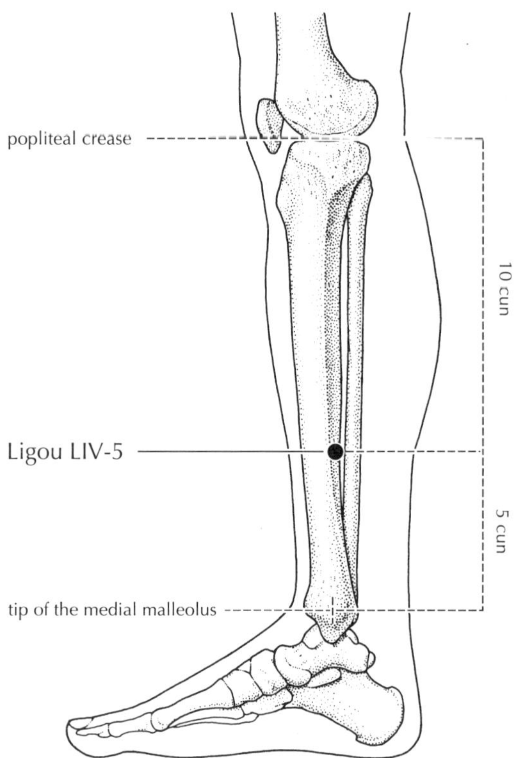

NEEDLING

i. Perpendicular insertion 0.5 to 1 cun; ii. Oblique insertion directed proximally towards the abdomen, 1 to 2 cun.

ACTIONS

Spreads the Liver, regulates qi and benefits the genitals
Clears dampness and heat from the lower jiao
Regulates menstruation
Treats plumstone qi

INDICATIONS

- Itching, swelling and pain of the genitals, sudden itching of the genitals, sudden swelling and pain of the testicles, incessant erection, shan disorder, cold shan disorder, distention and fullness of the lower abdomen, qi accumulation below the umbilicus like a stone.
- Difficult urination, retention of urine.
- Dysmenorrhoea, irregular menstruation, red and white leucorrhoea, prolapse of the uterus.
- Plumstone qi (globus hystericus), depression, much belching, fright palpitations, fear and fright, worry and oppression.
- Inflexibility of the back with inability to turn, lumbar pain, cold and pain of the feet and lower leg.

COMMENTARY

According to the *Spiritual Pivot*[13] "The Liver governs the sinews", whilst the *Essential Questions*[14] says "The genitals are the gathering place of the sinews". The Liver primary channel encircles the genitals, and the Liver sinew channel and the Liver luo-connecting channel from Ligou LIV-5 ascend to the genitals.

Ligou LIV-5, the luo-connecting point of the Liver channel, is a major point for treating diseases of this area and is indicated for itching, swelling and pain of the genitals and sudden pain and swelling of the testicles due to both Liver qi stagnation and damp-heat in the Liver channel. Ligou LIV-5 is also indicated for incessant erection (priapism). The Liver belongs to wood and spring, which manifest the energy of growth, spreading and ascending, and is entrusted with ministerial (ming men) fire which has its source in the Kidneys. Normal erection is dependent both on the flourishing of the Kidneys and harmony of the Liver. Incessant erection may arise either in the springtime of adolescence, when the Kidney essence becomes abundant and the Liver is exuberant, in which case it may be embarrassing but is not considered abnormal, or when pathological flaring of Liver fire agitates and inflames the penis, in which case it is a pathological and distressing condition. Ligou LIV-5 is one of the few points especially indicated for this disorder.

The ability of Ligou LIV-5 to clear Liver qi stagnation and damp-heat extends to the lower jiao as a whole, and it is indicated for red and white leucorrhoea, shan disorder, distention of the lower abdomen, qi accumulation below the umbilicus like a stone, prolapse of the uterus, difficult urination and retention of urine.

In common with many of the luo-connecting points, especially of the yin channels, Ligou LIV-5 treats a variety of psycho-emotional disorders. The Liver channel ascends to the throat and according to a number of classics, including the *Great Compendium of Acupuncture and Moxibustion* Ligou LIV-5 is indicated for " ... worry and oppression, stuffiness in the throat as if [obstructed by] a polyp". This refers to what is more commonly known in Chinese medicine as plumstone qi (globus hystericus), a sensation of physical obstruction that fluctuates according to a person's mood. Plumstone qi is most commonly due to stagnation of Liver qi and accumulation of phlegm. Ligou LIV-5 is further indicated for depression, fright palpitations and fear and fright, these latter indications reflecting the statement in the *Spiritual Pivot*[15] "when Liver qi is deficient there is fear".

The Liver stores the blood, and the smooth flow of blood depends on the free-flowing of Liver qi. The Liver therefore has a close relationship to the menstrual cycle and Ligou LIV-5 is able to treat menstrual disorders such as dysmenorrhoea and irregular menstruation due to qi stagnation or blood stasis. Due to its ability to treat depression, it is especially indicated when this symptom accompanies menstrual disorders.

The Liver has the functions of both spreading the qi and nourishing the sinews. It is interesting to note that in common with several other points of the Liver channel, Ligou LIV-5 is indicated for inflexibility and pain of the lumbar region, reflecting the clinical importance of Liver pathology (see Xingjian LIV-2) in some disorders of this area.

Finally the *Great Compendium of Acupuncture and Moxibustion* gives specific indications for excess and deficiency of the luo-connecting points. In the case of Ligou LIV-5, these are persistent erection (excess); sudden itching of the genitals (deficiency).

COMBINATIONS

- Difficult urination and seminal emission: Ligou LIV-5, Lougu SP-7, Zhongji REN-3, Chengfu BL-36 and Zhiyin BL-67 (*Supplementing Life*).
- Irregular menstruation: Ligou LIV-5 and Yinbao LIV-9 (*Supplementing Life*).
- Qi [stagnation] in the throat as if [obstructed by] a polyp: Ligou LIV-5 and Shaofu HE-8 (*Thousand Ducat Formulas*).
- Fright palpitations with diminished qi: Ligou LIV-5, Shenmen HE-7 and Juque REN-14 (*Supplementing Life*).
- Swelling of the lower abdomen: Ligou LIV-5, Jingmen GB-25 and Zhongfeng LIV-4 (*Supplementing Life*).

ZHONGDU LIV-6

Central Capital

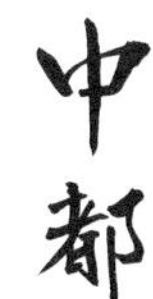

Xi-Cleft point of the Liver channel

LOCATION

7 cun above the prominence of the medial malleolus, immediately posterior to the medial border of the tibia, in the depression between the medial border of the tibia and the gastrocnemius muscle.

LOCATION NOTE

Divide the distance between the tip of the medial malleolus and the popliteal crease into half and locate Zhongdu LIV-6 at 0.5 cun distal to the midpoint.

NEEDLING

i. Perpendicular insertion 0.5 to 1 cun; ii. Oblique insertion directed proximally towards the abdomen, 1 to 2 cun.

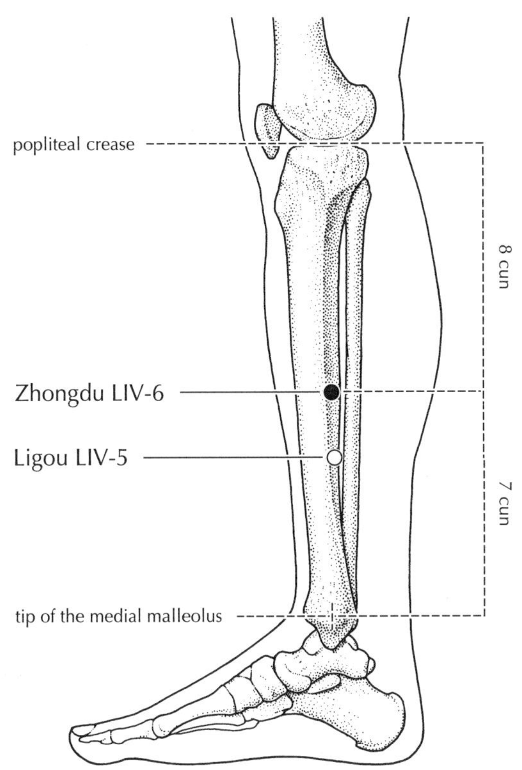

ACTIONS:

Spreads Liver qi and regulates the lower jiao
Regulates blood
Drains damp

INDICATIONS

- Shan disorder, lower abdominal pain, hypogastric pain, diarrhoea, persistent flow of lochia, uterine bleeding.
- Damp painful obstruction with inability to walk, flaccidity and emaciation of the legs, numbness of the body, numbness of the hands and feet, cold sensation of the lower legs with inability to stand for long, hot sensation of the soles of the feet.

COMMENTARY

Zhongdu LIV-6 is the xi-cleft point of the Liver channel. The xi-cleft points are where the qi and blood, which flow relatively superficially along the channels from the jing-well points, gather and plunge more deeply. The xi-cleft points in general are indicated in the treatment of acute conditions and pain, whilst the xi-cleft points of the yin channels have an additional action of treating disorders of blood. Despite the status of Zhongdu LIV-6 as a xi-cleft point, however, other than treating persistent flow of lochia and uterine bleeding it has relatively few indications of this kind.

The *Classic of the Jade Dragon* recommends Zhongdu LIV-6 for numbness of the body and numbness of the hands and feet, the *Investigation into Points Along the Channels* for flaccidity and emaciation of the legs, and the *Thousand Ducat Formulas* for heat in the soles, which together reflect a clinical picture of atrophy disorder due to damp-heat. In modern clinical practice, however, Zhongdu LIV-6 is rarely used, and from the paucity of classical combinations for this point it seems that this has always been the case.

COMBINATIONS

- Oedema of the four limbs: Zhongdu LIV-6, Hegu L.I.-4, Quchi L.I.-11, Zhongzhu SJ-3, Yemen SJ-2, Xingjian LIV-2, Neiting ST-44, Sanyinjiao SP-6 and Yinlingquan SP-9 (*Great Compendium*).
- Cold-damp shan disorder: Zhongdu LIV-6, Daju ST-27 and Diji SP-8 (*Systematic Classic*).

XIGUAN LIV-7

Knee Joint

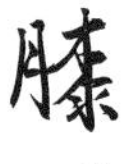
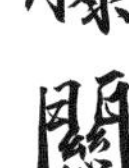

LOCATION

Posterior and inferior to the medial condyle of the tibia, 1 cun posterior to Yinlingquan SP-9.

LOCATION NOTE

Locate Yinlingquan SP-9 in the depression in the angle formed by the medial condyle of the tibia and the posterior border of the tibia, and then locate Xiguan LIV-7 one cun posterior to it.

NEEDLING

Perpendicular insertion 1 to 2 cun.

ACTIONS

Dispels wind-damp
Benefits the knee and relaxes the sinews

INDICATIONS

- Swelling and pain of the knee, pain of the inner aspect of the knee radiating to the patella, crane's knee wind, wind painful obstruction, white tiger joint wind pain, difficulty in flexing and extending the knee, cold damp pouring downwards.
- Abdominal pain, pain of the throat.

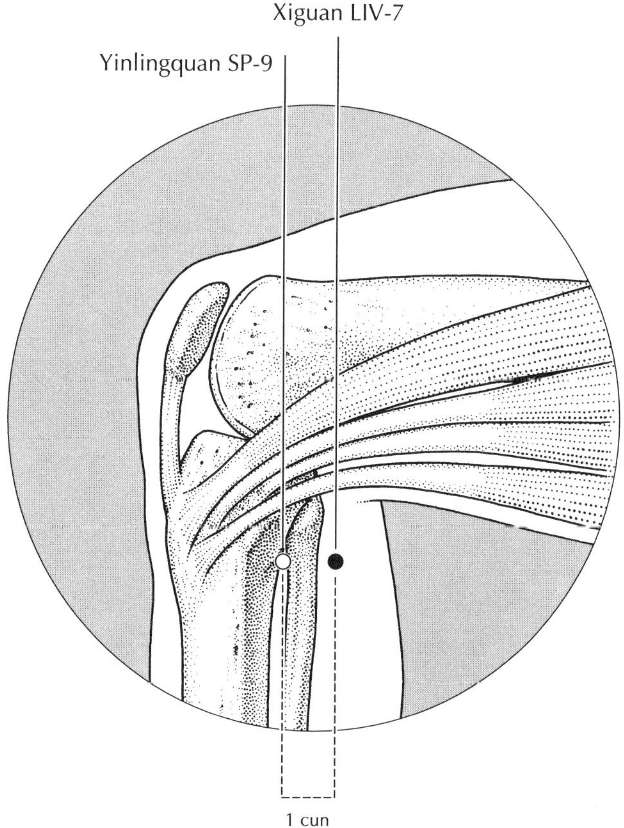

COMBINATIONS

- Disorders of the knee and below the knee: moxa Xiguan LIV-7, Dubi ST-35, Zusanli ST-36 and Yanglingquan GB-34 (*Supplementing Life*).

- Redness, swelling and pain of the knees: Xiguan LIV-7, Weizhong BL-40, Zusanli ST-36 and Yinshi ST-33 (*Great Compendium*).
- Redness, swelling and pain of the knees with inability to walk: Xiguan LIV-7 and Xiyan (MN-LE-16) (*Song of the Jade Dragon*).
- Pain of the medial aspect of the knee: Xiguan LIV-7 and Ququan LIV-8 (*Supplementing Life*).

QUQUAN LIV-8

Spring at the Crook

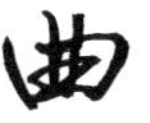

He-Sea and Water point of the Liver channel

LOCATION

Just superior to the medial end of the popliteal crease, in the depression anterior to the tendons of m. semitendinosus and m. semimembranosus, about 1 cun anterior to Yingu KID-10.

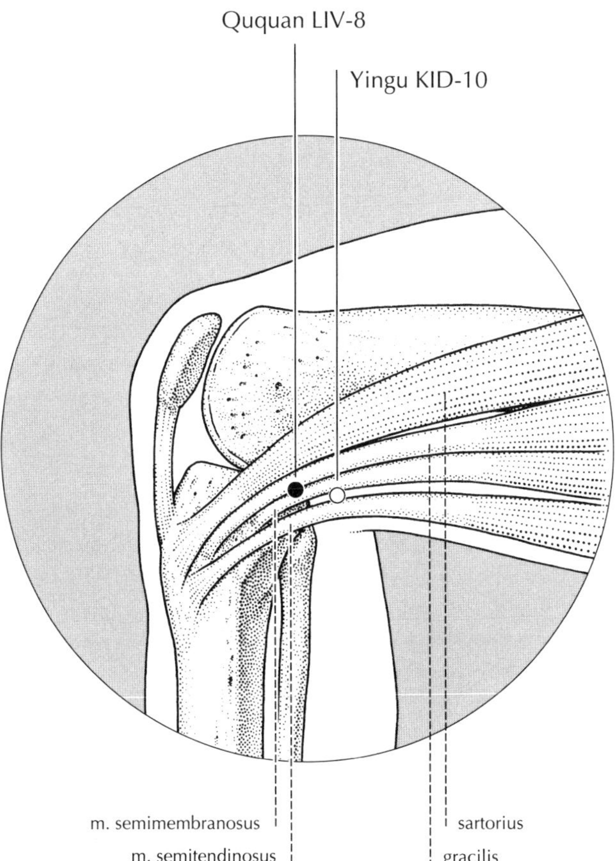

LOCATION NOTE

i. It is helpful to flex the knee to locate the popliteal crease and identify the tendons of m. semitendinosus and m. semimembranosus, although the point may subsequently be needled with a pillow under the leg to semi-flex it; ii. The tendon of semitendinosus, which lies posteriorly to semimembranosus, is the most prominent of the two tendons.

NEEDLING

Perpendicular or slightly posterior insertion 1 to 1.5 cun.

ACTIONS

Clears damp-heat from the lower jiao
Benefits the genitals
Invigorates blood and benefits the uterus
Nourishes blood and yin

INDICATIONS

- Swelling and itching of the genitals, pain of the genitals, pain of the penis, impotence, seminal emission, seminal emission associated with sexual taxation.
- Difficult urination, retention of urine, enuresis.
- Diarrhoea containing undigested food, diarrhoea containing blood and pus, no pleasure in eating.
- Uterine prolapse, abdominal masses in women due to blood stasis, masses (zheng jia) of the hypogastrium, infertility due to blood stasis, amenorrhoea, swelling of the hypogastrium, shan disorder, pain of the abdomen and lateral costal region, umbilical pain.
- Mania disorder, headache, visual dizziness, nosebleed, redness, heat, swelling and pain of the eyes, dyspnoea.
- Knee pain, swelling and pain of the patella, coldness and pain of the knee and lower leg, pain of the inner thigh, extreme pain of the body.

COMMENTARY

Ququan LIV-8 is the he-sea and water point of the Liver channel. The he-sea points of the three leg yin channels, all water points, share the common property of draining dampness and damp-heat from the lower jiao. Yingu KID-10 predominantly clears damp-heat from the urogenital system (dominated by the Kidneys) whilst Yinlingquan SP-9, by virtue of the intimate relationship between the Spleen and dampness, is able to treat all dampness disorders of the lower jiao. Because of the close relationship between the Liver channel and the genitals, Ququan LIV-8 primarily drains Liver damp-heat sinking down to this region.

Liver damp-heat may be due to i. the combination of Liver stagnant heat and Spleen dampness, ii. invasion of exterior damp-heat, or iii. excessive consumption of greasy food and alcohol. When damp-heat pours into the Liver channel it may give rise to genital itching, swelling and pain. If damp-heat agitates the 'gate of essence' there may be seminal emission. The Liver dominates the sinews, and according to the *Essential Questions*[16] "The genitals are the gathering place of the sinews". If damp-heat sinks to the genital region it can cause impotence due to flaccidity, in much the same way that damp-heat may cause atrophy disorder. Ququan LIV-8 is primarily indicated for these excess kinds of seminal emission and impotence, but in view of its secondary action of nourishing the Liver (see below), may be used in cases of deficiency, for example the *Great Compendium of Acupuncture and Moxibustion recommends* Ququan LIV-8 for seminal emission associated with sexual taxation.

The damp-heat draining action of Ququan LIV-8 extends to the Bladder (difficult urination or retention of urine), and the intestines (diarrhoea containing undigested food as well as diarrhoea containing blood and pus).

The Liver stores the blood which flows into the Conception and Penetrating vessels and thence the uterus to become menstrual blood, and its qi is responsible for the smooth flow of menstruation. When Liver qi stagnates, therefore, menstrual blood may also stagnate. Ququan LIV-8 is indicated in various classical sources for blood stasis in the uterus giving rise to infertility, abdominal masses and amenorrhoea. Clinically the combination of damp-heat and blood stasis is frequently encountered in gynaecological disorders, since stagnant blood may generate heat whilst the presence of damp-heat may obstruct blood. The action of Ququan LIV-8 on both these pathogenic factors renders it particularly suited to treating such dual disharmony. Uterine prolapse predominantly results from qi deficiency or damp-heat, and Ququan LIV-8 is particularly indicated for the latter.

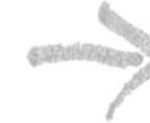

As the water point of the Liver channel, Ququan LIV-8 links the Liver with its 'mother' the Kidneys. It therefore has a secondary function of both 'generating water to submerge wood' and nourishing the Liver yin and blood. It can be used to help subdue Liver yang in cases of headache and visual dizziness, and to nourish yin and blood in menstrual disorders. It should be said that the degree to which Ququan LIV-8 is considered an important point for nourishing the Liver varies considerably among different practitioners. An examination of its traditional indications and combinations, however, reveals that historically it has primarily been used for excess patterns. Finally Ququan LIV-8 is used for local disorders and is indicated for swelling, pain and coldness of the knee joint and surrounding area.

COMBINATIONS

- Itching of the genitals: Ququan LIV-8 and Yinjiao REN-7 (*Supplementing Life*).
- Retention of urine and pain of the penis: Ququan LIV-8 and Xingjian LIV-2 (*Supplementing Life*).
- Seminal emission: Ququan LIV-8, Zhiyin BL-67 and Zhongji REN-3 (*Supplementing Life*).
- Seminal emission with dreams: Ququan LIV-8 [one hundred cones of moxa], Zhongfeng LIV-4, Taichong LIV-3, Zhiyin BL-67, Geshu BL-17, Pishu BL-20, Sanyinjiao SP-6, Shenshu BL-23, Guanyuan REN-4 and Sanjiaoshu BL-22 (*Great Compendium*).
- Uterine prolapse: Ququan LIV-8, Shuiquan KID-5, Zhaohai KID-6 and Shenmai BL-62 (*Supplementing Life*).
- Uterine prolapse: Ququan LIV-8, Zhaohai KID-6 and Dadun LIV-1 (*Great Compendium*).
- Uterine prolapse: Ququan LIV-8, Taichong LIV-3, Zhaohai KID-6 and Shaofu HE-8 (*Great Compendium*).
- Lower abdominal pain from the seven kinds of shan disorder: Ququan LIV-8, Zhaohai KID-6 and Sanyinjiao SP-6 (*Ode of Xi-hong*).
- Pain of the umbilical region: Ququan LIV-8, Zhongfeng LIV-4 and Shuifen REN-9 (*Great Compendium*).
- Diarrhoea with thin stools, dysenteric disorder with blood in the stools: Ququan LIV-8 and Taichong LIV-3 (*Thousand Ducat Formulas*).
- Headache and dizziness: Ququan LIV-8, Kunlun BL-60, Feiyang BL-58, Qiangu SI-2, Shaoze SI-1 and Tongli HE-5 (*Thousand Ducat Formulas*).
- All wind, painful obstruction, atrophy and inversion diseases: Ququan LIV-8 and Dazhu BL-11 (*Song to Keep Up Your Sleeve*).
- Pain of the medial aspect of the knee: Ququan LIV-8 and Xiguan LIV-7 (*Supplementing Life*).
- Contraction of the sinews and difficulty in flexing and extending the knee, with inability to walk: Ququan LIV-8, Liangqiu ST-34 and Xiyangguan GB-33 (*Thousand Ducat Formulas*).

YINBAO LIV-9

Yin Wrapping

陰包

LOCATION

Directly superior to the medial epicondyle of the femur, 4 cun superior to Ququan LIV-8, in the cleft between m. vastus medialis and m. sartorius.

LOCATION NOTE

Locate one patella's height (2 cun) above the superior border of the patella, in the tender depression between m. vastus medialis and m. sartorius, directly above Ququan LIV-8.

NEEDLING

Perpendicular or oblique insertion 1-2 cun.

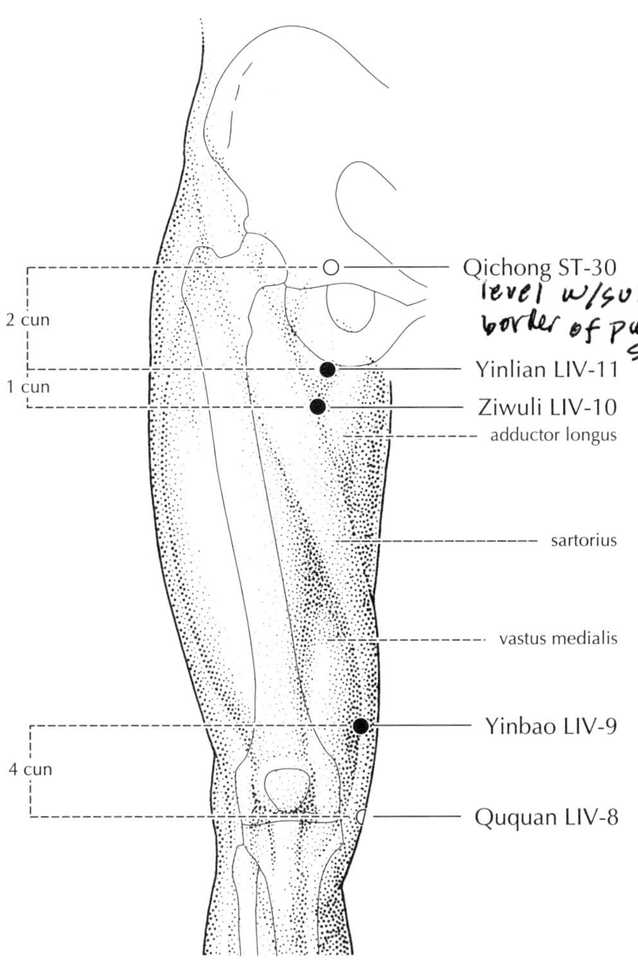

ACTIONS

Adjusts menstruation and regulates the lower jiao

INDICATIONS

- Irregular menstruation, disorders of menstruation, difficult urination, retention of urine, enuresis.
- Lumbo-sacral pain extending to the lower abdomen.

COMBINATIONS

- Irregular menstruation: Yinbao LIV-9 and Ligou LIV-5 (*Supplementing Life*).

ZUWULI LIV-10

Leg Five Miles

足五里

LOCATION

3 cun inferior to Qichong ST-30 on the anterior border of m. adductor longus.

LOCATION NOTE

i. Qichong ST-30 is located on the lower abdomen, 2 cun lateral to the midline, level with the superior border of the pubic symphysis (Qugu REN-2); ii. Measure the 3 cun as one handbreadth inferior to Qichong ST-30; iii. The tendon of origin of adductor longus arises from the pubic bone and is identified as the most prominent tendon in the groin.

NEEDLING

Perpendicular or oblique insertion 0.5 to 1.5 cun.

ACTIONS

Clears damp-heat and benefits the lower jiao

INDICATIONS

- Difficult urination, retention of urine, enuresis, itching of the genitals, swelling and pain of the testicles, fullness of the abdomen, fullness of the lower abdomen.
- Wind-taxation somnolence, difficult respiration, cough.

COMBINATIONS

- Somnolence with no desire to move the four limbs: Zuwuli LIV-10, Sanyangluo SJ-8, Tianjing SJ-10, Lidui ST-45 and Sanjian L.I.-3 (*Thousand Ducat Formulas*).
- Jaundice with periodic low grade fever: Zuwuli LIV-10 and Zhongfeng LIV-4 (*Thousand Ducat Formulas*).

YINLIAN LIV-11

Yin Corner

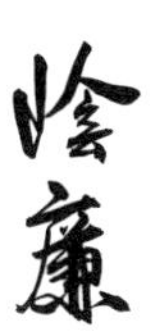

LOCATION

2 cun inferior to Qichong ST-30 on the anterior border of m. adductor longus.

LOCATION NOTE

i. Qichong ST-30 is located on the lower abdomen, 2 cun lateral to the midline, level with the superior border of the pubic symphysis (Qugu REN-2); ii. The tendon of origin of adductor longus arises from the pubic bone and is identified as the most prominent tendon in the groin.

NEEDLING

Perpendicular or oblique insertion 0.5 to 1.5 cun.

ACTIONS

Benefits the uterus

INDICATIONS

- Infertility, irregular menstruation, pain in the inner thigh and knee.

COMMENTARY

Many classical texts recommend moxibustion at this point for the treatment of infertility.

JIMAI LIV-12

Urgent Pulse

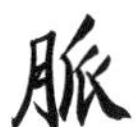

LOCATION

1 cun inferior and 2.5 cun lateral to Qugu REN-2, in the crease of the groin, medial to the femoral vein.

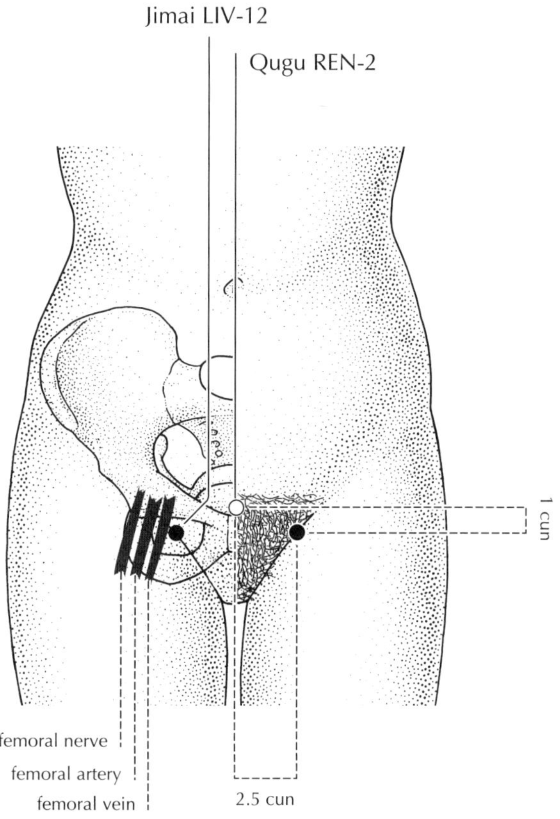

LOCATION NOTE

Locate the pulsation of the femoral artery in the groin, approximately midway between the pubic symphysis and the anterior superior iliac spine. The femoral vein runs along the medial side of the artery and is approximately one fingerbreadth in diameter. Jimai LIV-12 is then located just medial to the vein on the groin crease.

NEEDLING

Medial, slightly oblique insertion 0.5 to 0.8 cun.
Caution: care should be taken to avoid penetrating the femoral vein. The *Essential Questions* advises that this point should be treated by moxibustion rather than needling. Modern texts, however, say that moxibustion is contraindicated due to the proximity of this point both to the femoral vessels and to the pubic hair, and that the point should rather be treated by needling.

ACTIONS

Eliminates cold from the Liver channel and benefits the lower jiao

INDICATIONS

- Pain of the genitals, pain of the penis, swelling of the testicles, uterine prolapse.
- Pain of the hypogastrium, shan disorder, pain of the inner thigh.

COMMENTARY

Jimai LIV-12 was first mentioned in the *Essential Questions*. It was not discussed however in either the *Systematic Classic of Acupuncture and Moxibustion* nor the *Great Compendium of Acupuncture and* Moxibustion which refer to the "thirteen points of the Liver channel".

ZHANGMEN LIV-13

Completion Gate

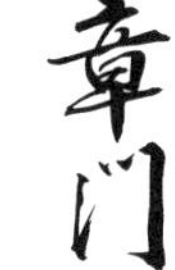

Front-Mu point of the Spleen
Hui-Meeting point of the zang
Meeting point of the Liver and Gall Bladder channels

LOCATION

Directly anterior and inferior to the free end of the eleventh rib.

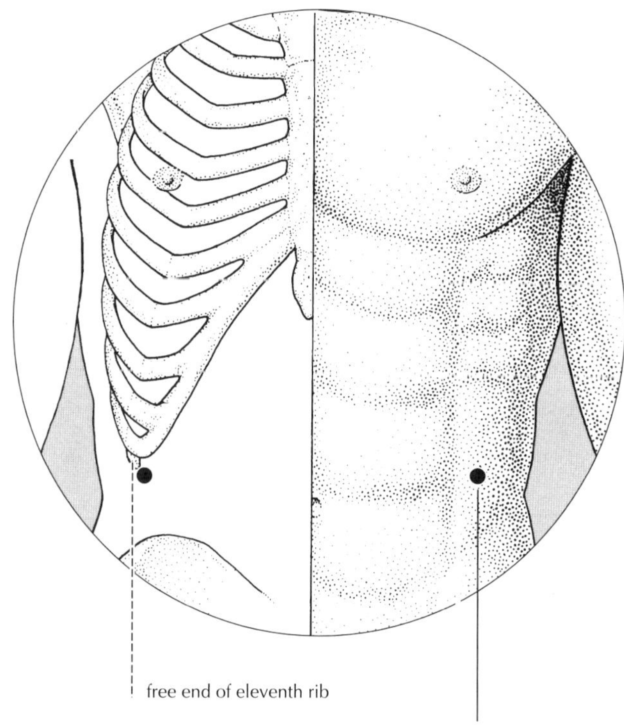

LOCATION NOTE

i. To locate the free end of the eleventh rib, first place the entire hand on the upper abdomen and with gentle finger pressure palpate downwards along the costal margin, until the end of the eleventh rib is located just above the level of the umbilicus; ii. This point usually lies on or near the mid-axillary line which is drawn vertically down from the apex of the axilla (Jiquan HE-1).

NEEDLING

Transverse or oblique insertion medially or laterally (along the line of the rib) 0.5 to 1 cun. **Caution:** deep perpendicular needling may damage an enlarged liver or spleen.

ACTIONS

Harmonises the Liver and Spleen
Regulates the middle and lower jiao
Fortifies the Spleen
Spreads the Liver and regulates qi

INDICATIONS

- Injury to the Stomach and Spleen from overindulgence in eating, focal distention, distention and pain of the abdomen, drum distention, abdominal (ji ju) masses, oesophageal constriction, vomiting, pain of the Heart with vomiting, no pleasure in eating, undigested food (in the stool), borborygmus, diarrhoea, constipation, emaciation and jaundice, frequent urination with turbid white discharge.
- Fullness of the chest and lateral costal region, pain of the ribs, sudden difficulty in breathing, inability to catch the breath, dyspnoea, cough, stone oedema.
- Weariness of the four limbs, running piglet qi with distention of the abdomen, diminished qi with inversion counterflow.
- Agitation and heat with dry mouth, propensity to anger, propensity to fear, mad walking, epilepsy.
- Cold and pain of the lumbar spine, rigidity of the spine, lumbar pain with inability to turn and bend the waist, inability to raise the arm and shoulder.

COMMENTARY

Zhangmen LIV-13, located midway between the middle and lower jiao, is both a point of the Liver channel and the front-mu point of the Spleen. The term 'mu' means to gather or to collect, and the front-mu points are where the qi of the zangfu gathers and concentrates on the anterior surface of the body. Zhangmen LIV-13 is therefore an important point to harmonise the relationship both between the Liver and Spleen, and between the middle and lower jiao, with the emphasis on disorders of the abdomen and intestines.

According to *Standards of Patterns and Treatments* "The essence of the five zang is all transported from the Spleen". As the origin of the post-natal qi, the Spleen and Stomach are considered to play a central role among the zangfu, transforming and distributing the essence of food and drink throughout the body. For this reason, the Spleen may be said to dominate the zang and the Stomach the fu. The close relationship of Zhangmen LIV-13 to the Spleen, therefore, is further reflected in its status as the hui-meeting point of the zang, in the same way that Zhongwan REN-12, the front-mu point of the Stomach, is also the hui-meeting point of the fu.

The Liver tends to excess patterns and the Spleen to deficiency. Liver-Spleen disharmony may originate either from the Liver, when qi stagnation aggressively invades, obstructs and suppresses the transportation and transformation function of the Spleen, or from the Spleen, when Spleen qi deficiency is unable to resist the encroachment of exuberant Liver qi. This process is reflected in the saying "Anger is hard and the zangfu are soft; what is hard easily injures what is soft" and by Zhang Jing-yue's observation "If anger occurs during or after eating it injures the Stomach and Spleen"[17]. The origin of Liver-Spleen disharmony, therefore, may be either an excess condition of the Liver or a deficient condition of the Spleen, or a combination of the two. One characteristic of this disharmony is the fluctuation in severity of symptoms with changes in the emotional state, and the tendency for either Liver qi stagnation or Spleen deficiency to predominate at different times. Zhangmen LIV-13, which is able both to regulate the Liver qi and to tonify the Spleen, is the main point on the abdomen to treat all gradations of Liver-Spleen disharmony giving rise to symptoms such as propensity to anger, distention and pain of the abdomen, borborygmus, diarrhoea and loss of appetite. Diarrhoea due to Liver-Spleen disharmony is distinguished by two main characteristics. The first is that the diarrhoea is often preceded by distention and pain, both of which are relieved after passing stools. The second is that the diarrhoea frequently alternates with constipation, for which this point is also indicated. This pattern is frequently encountered in irritable bowel syndrome and premenstrual bowel disorders.

Zhangmen LIV-13 may also be used for Spleen disharmony without Liver complications, or Liver disharmony without Spleen complications. Through its action of fortifying the Spleen, it is indicated for weariness of the limbs, emaciation, injury to the Stomach and Spleen from overindulgence in eating, and diarrhoea containing undigested food. By resolving Liver qi stagnation it is able to treat oesophageal constriction, fullness of the chest, focal distention, pain of the lateral costal region and constipation.

If Liver qi stagnation leads to stasis of blood, there may be abdominal masses and (in terms of western medicine) enlargement of the liver and/or spleen. If Liver qi stagnation transforms to fire, there may be agitation and heat with a dry mouth, mad walking and propensity to anger. If the Liver is deficient, there will be propensity to fear. If Liver qi invades the Stomach or Lung, and impairs their descending function, there will be vomiting, cough or dyspnoea. Through its dual action on the Liver and Spleen, Zhangmen LIV-13 is also able to drain dampness or damp-heat from the middle and lower jiao with such symptoms as jaundice and frequent urination with turbid white discharge.

The Liver channel is interiorly-exteriorly coupled with the Gall Bladder channel which controls the sides of the body and facilitates turning and bending. Zhangmen LIV-13, a meeting point of the Liver and Gall Bladder channels, is located close to the waist and lumbar region and is indicated for rigidity of the spine, lumbar pain and inability to turn and bend the waist. The *Great Compendium of Acupuncture and Moxibustion* recommends Zhangmen LIV-13 for cold and pain of the lumbar spine, whilst Sun Si-miao in the *Thousand Ducat Formulas* is more specific and recommends it for cold and painful lumbar spine in men.

Finally, Zhangmen LIV-13 is indicated for the pattern of running piglet qi arising from severe stagnation of qi. According to the *Essentials From the Golden Cabinet* "Running piglet disorder arises from the lower abdomen; it rushes up to the throat with such ferocity that the patient feels he is close to death. It attacks and then remits. It is brought about by fear and fright". Running piglet qi primarily arises when stagnant Liver qi transforms to heat, or when Kidney yang deficiency leads to accumulation of cold in the lower jiao. In both cases, qi is violently discharged and rushes upwards along the Penetrating vessel. In clinical practice, running piglet qi may be encountered in a number of variants, all involving a rushing sensation, usually upwards, along the trunk, back or limbs. It is usually accompanied by feelings of intense anxiety.

COMBINATIONS

- Invasion by cold or damp (dong) diarrhoea containing undigested food: Zhangmen LIV-13 and Shenshu BL-23 (*Thousand Ducat Formulas*).
- Borborygmus, abdominal distention and watery diarrhoea: Zhangmen LIV-13, Sanjiaoshu BL-22, Xiaochangshu BL-27, Xialiao BL-34 and Yishe BL-49 (*Thousand Ducat Formulas*).
- Vomiting: Zhangmen LIV-13, Zhongwan REN-12 and Geshu BL-17 (*Thousand Ducat Formulas*).
- Constipation: Zhangmen LIV-13, Taibai SP-3 and Zhaohai KID-6 (*Great Compendium*).
- Constipation: Zhangmen LIV-13, Taibai SP-3, Zhaohai KID-6 and Zhigou SJ-6 (*Great Compendium*).
- Pain of the lateral costal region: Zhangmen LIV-13 and Danshu BL-19 (*Thousand Ducat Formulas*).
- Pain of the lateral costal region: Zhangmen LIV-13, Gongsun SP-4, Zhigou SJ-6 and Yanglingquan GB-34 (*Complete Collection*).
- Pain of the lateral costal region: Zhangmen LIV-13, Zhigou SJ-6 and Waiguan SJ-5 (*Great Compendium*).
- Stone oedema of the upper abdomen: moxa Zhangmen LIV-13, Qichong ST-30, Rangu KID-2 and Siman KID-14 (*Thousand Ducat Formulas*).
- Running piglet qi: Zhangmen LIV-13, Shimen REN-5 and Sanyinjiao SP-6 (*Thousand Ducat Formulas*).
- Insomnia: Zhangmen LIV-13 and Qichong ST-30 (*Supplementing Life*).
- Rigidity of the lumbar spine with inability to turn: Zhangmen LIV-13 and Ciliao BL-32 (*Supplementing Life*).

QIMEN LIV-14

Cycle Gate

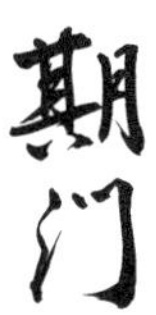

Front-Mu point of the Liver
Meeting point of the Liver and Spleen channels with the Yin Linking vessel

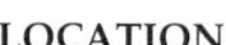

LOCATION

On the mamillary line, in the sixth intercostal space, 4 cun lateral to the midline.

LOCATION NOTE

i. First locate the costal cartilage of the second rib which is level with the sternal angle, then locate the second inter costal space below it and count down to the sixth space; ii. Note that there is another point known as 'lower Qimen' located on the mamillary line, 4 cun lateral to the midline, on the lower border of the tenth rib.

NEEDLING

Oblique medial or lateral insertion 0.5 to 1 cun.
Caution: deep perpendicular or oblique insertion carries a substantial risk of causing a pneumothorax.

ACTIONS

Spreads the Liver and regulates qi
Invigorates blood and disperses masses
Harmonises the Liver and Stomach

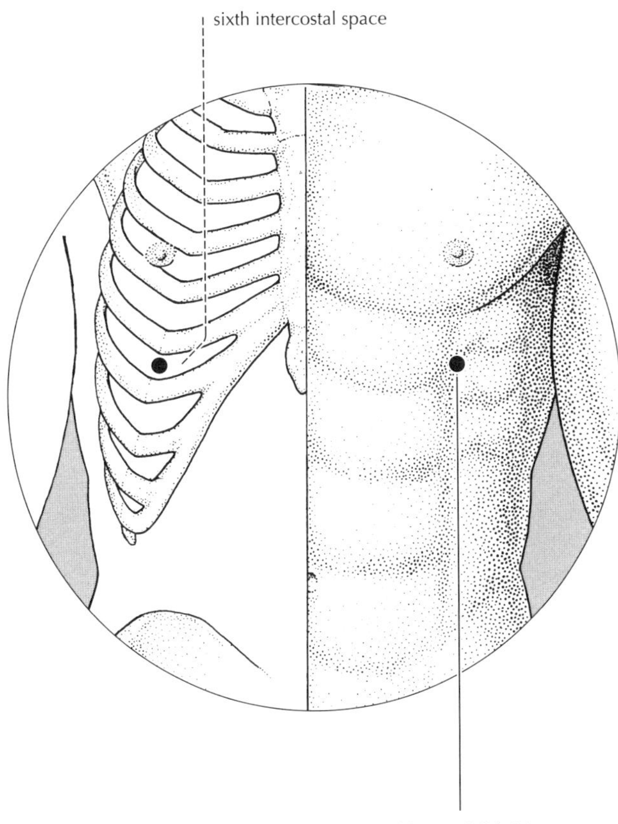

INDICATIONS

- Pain, distention and fullness of the chest, (ji ju) masses in the lateral costal region, pain of the lateral costal region, much sighing, cutting pain of the Heart, distention and pain of the breast, agitation and heat of the chest, cough, dyspnoea, enlarged and hard abdomen with difficulty in breathing.
- Epigastric distention and pain, acid regurgitation, vomiting and hiccup, vomiting fluid after eating, sudden turmoil disorder, desire to eat despite difficult ingestion, abdominal distention and watery diarrhoea, hardness of the epigastrium, hypogastrium and abdomen.
- Injury by cold leading to heat which enters the blood chamber, manic raving, alternating chills and fever, uterine bleeding, post-partum disorders, red face, tetany, dry mouth.
- Malaria, jaundice, gallstones, wasting and thirsting disorder, running piglet qi, stiffness and pain of the head and neck, visual dizziness.

COMMENTARY

Qimen LIV-14 is the last point on the Liver channel and indeed the last point in the great circulation of qi which begins at Zhongfu LU-1 and passes through all the twelve channels, ending one complete cycle at this point. This is reflected in its name 'Cycle Gate'.

Qimen LIV-14 is the front-mu point of the Liver. The term 'mu' means to gather or to collect, and the front-mu points are where the qi of the zangfu gathers and concentrates on the anterior surface of the body. It is in the region of this point that the Liver channel spreads through the lateral costal region, diaphragm and chest. Its main sphere of action therefore is on regulating the free flow of qi in these areas, and in contrast to Zhangmen LIV-13 which focuses on the middle and lower jiao, Qimen LIV-14 acts primarily on the middle and upper jiao.

The *Spiritual Pivot*[18] states "With anger the qi rebels upwards and accumulates in the chest". If Liver qi is obstructed in the chest or lateral costal region, there will be pain, distention or fullness, whilst if Liver qi invades the Lung and obstructs its descending function, it will give rise to cough, sighing and dyspnoea. The Liver sinew channel links with the breast, and the entire breast region is strongly influenced by the Liver. If Liver qi is obstructed in the breast region, therefore, there will be pain, distention and even masses, all of which may fluctuate with the menstrual cycle, being most pronounced in the days immediately prior to menstruation. Qimen LIV-14 is an important adjacent point in the treatment of this common condition.

The intimate relationship between qi and blood is clearly expressed in the saying "Qi is the commander of blood ... when qi moves, blood moves". Severe or prolonged qi stagnation, therefore, will lead to blood stasis manifesting as hardness or masses with cutting pain in the chest, lateral costal region, abdomen or hypogastrium. Qimen LIV-14, by virtue of its ability to circulate both qi and blood, is indicated in all these situations. Qimen LIV-14 is also specifically indicated for cutting or stabbing pain of the Heart, reflecting its status as a meeting point of the Liver channel with the Yin Linking vessel. According to the *Classic of Difficulties*[19] "When the Yin Linking vessel is diseased, Heart pain will result".

According to Zhang Jing-yue "If anger occurs during or after eating it injures the Stomach and Spleen"[17]. This vital observation emphasises the great importance ascribed to a peaceful and harmonious state of mind during mealtimes. If instead there is disturbance, conflict, frustration, resentment or outright anger they may wreak turmoil in the digestive system. If Liver qi transversely invades the Stomach in this way and impairs its descending function, the Stomach qi will stagnate or rebel upwards leading to epigastric distention and pain, acid regurgitation, vomiting and hiccup. Qimen LIV-14 is an essential local point in the treatment of this pattern of Liver-Stomach disharmony. If Liver qi transversely invades the Spleen and impairs the Spleen transportation and transformation function, there will be abdominal distention and diarrhoea, although Qimen LIV-14 is less used clinically in this situation than Zhangmen LIV-13.

A specific indication for Qimen LIV-14 is 'injury by cold leading to heat which enters the blood chamber'. This refers to attack and penetration of cold during menstruation or after childbirth. The cold transforms to heat and gives rise to alternating fever and chills, hardness and fullness in the lower abdomen, chest and lateral costal region, and clear consciousness during the day with disordered speech at night. This pattern was first described in the *Treatise on Injury by Cold* by Zhang Zhong-jing who recommended the administration of *Xiao Chai Hu Tang* (Minor Bupleurum Decoction) and needling Qimen LIV-14, especially in the case of manic raving. The Tang dynasty author Xu Xue-shi, a scholar of the works of Zhang Zhong-jing, in his discussion of the *Treatise on Injury by Cold* said "Concerning heat entering the blood chamber in women, when *Xiao Chai Hu Tang* is too slow, needle Qimen LIV-14". Qimen LIV-14 is also indicated for uterine bleeding.

Finally, like Zhangmen LIV-13, Qimen LIV-14 is an important point in the treatment of running piglet qi (see Zhangmen LIV-13 for a fuller discussion).

COMBINATIONS

- Pain of the Heart with shortness of breath: Qimen LIV-14, Changqiang DU-1, Tiantu REN-22, Xiabai LU-4 and Zhongchong P-9 (*Thousand Ducat Formulas*).
- Stabbing pain of the Heart: Qimen LIV-14 and Burong ST-19 (*Thousand Ducat Formulas*).
- Chest pain: Qimen LIV-14, Feishu BL-13, Yunmen LU-2, Zhongfu LU-1, Yinbai SP-1, Hunmen BL-47 and Daling P-7 (*Thousand Ducat Formulas*).
- Heat in the chest: Qimen LIV-14 and Quepen ST-12 (*Thousand Ducat Formulas*).
- Chest pain due to injury by cold: Qimen LIV-14 and Daling P-7 (*Great Compendium*).
- Dyspnoea with inability to walk: Qimen LIV-14, Zhongwan REN-12 and Shanglian L.I.-9 (*Great Compendium*).
- Rebellion of qi with cough, fullness of the chest, shortness of breath with pain that radiates to the back: 50 moxa cones each on Qimen LIV-14 and Juque REN-14 (*Thousand Ducat Formulas*).
- Distention of the lateral costal region: Qimen LIV-14, Guanyuan REN-4 and Shaoshang LU-11 (*Thousand Ducat Formulas*).
- Difficult ingestion: Qimen LIV-14, Yanggang BL-48, Shaoshang LU-11 and Laogong P-8 (*Thousand Ducat Formulas*).
- Post-partum belching: Qimen LIV-14 and Xiangu ST-43 (*Supplementing Life*).
- Running piglet qi in women: Qimen LIV-14, Guanyuan REN-4, Zhongji REN-3, Sanyinjiao SP-6, Shimen REN-5 and Xuehai SP-10 (*Supplementing Life*).
- Stiffness of the nape of the neck due to injury by cold: Qimen LIV-14 and Wenliu L.I.-7 (*One Hundred Symptoms*).
- Involuntary erection with difficult urination: Dadun LIV-1, Qimen LIV-14, Yingu KID-10, Weizhong BL-40 and Weiyang BL-39 (*Supplementing Life*).

NOTES

1 *Essential Questions* Chapter 68.
2 *Classic of Difficulties* 68th Difficulty.
3 *Spiritual Pivot* Chapter 8.
4 *Essential Questions* Chapter 5.
5 Fei Bo Xiong in *Surplus Parts of Pure Medicine* quoted in *Health Preservation and Rehabilitation*, Publishing House of Shanghai College of Traditional Chinese Medicine, p. 72.
6 *Common Sayings on Gerontology* by Cao Tong, quoted in *Health Preservation and Rehabilitation*, Publishing House of Shanghai College of Traditional Chinese Medicine, p. 66.
7 *Spiritual Pivot* Chapter 46.
8 *Spiritual Pivot* Chapter 78.
9 Ma Dan-yang was the originator of the *Song of the Eleven Heavenly Star Points*. They first appeared in print in the 12th century CE *Classic of the Jade Dragon*. Xu Feng included this text in his work *Complete Collection of Acupuncture and Moxibustion* and added a twelfth point, Taichong LIV-3 and gave the following indications: fright epilepsy wind, distention of the throat and Heart, both legs unable to walk, the seven shan, unilateral sagging and swelling of the testicle, cloudy vision and lumbar pain.
10 *Spiritual Pivot* Chapter 8.
11 *Spiritual Pivot* Chapter 17.
12 *Essential Questions* Chapter 10.
13 *Spiritual Pivot* Chapter 78.
14 *Essential Questions* Chapter 45.
15 *Spiritual Pivot* Chapter 8.
16 *Essential Questions* Chapter 45.
17 Zhang Jing-yue 1986 *Complete Book of Jing-yue* (Jing Yue Quan Shu), Shanghai Scientific Publishing House, Shanghai p.415. First published in 1624. Quoted in *The Practice of Chinese Medicine*, Maciocia, G., Churchill Livingstone.
18 *Spiritual Pivot* Chapter 46.
19 *Classic of Difficulties* 29th Difficulty.

任脈經穴

THE CONCEPTION VESSEL

THE CONCEPTION VESSEL

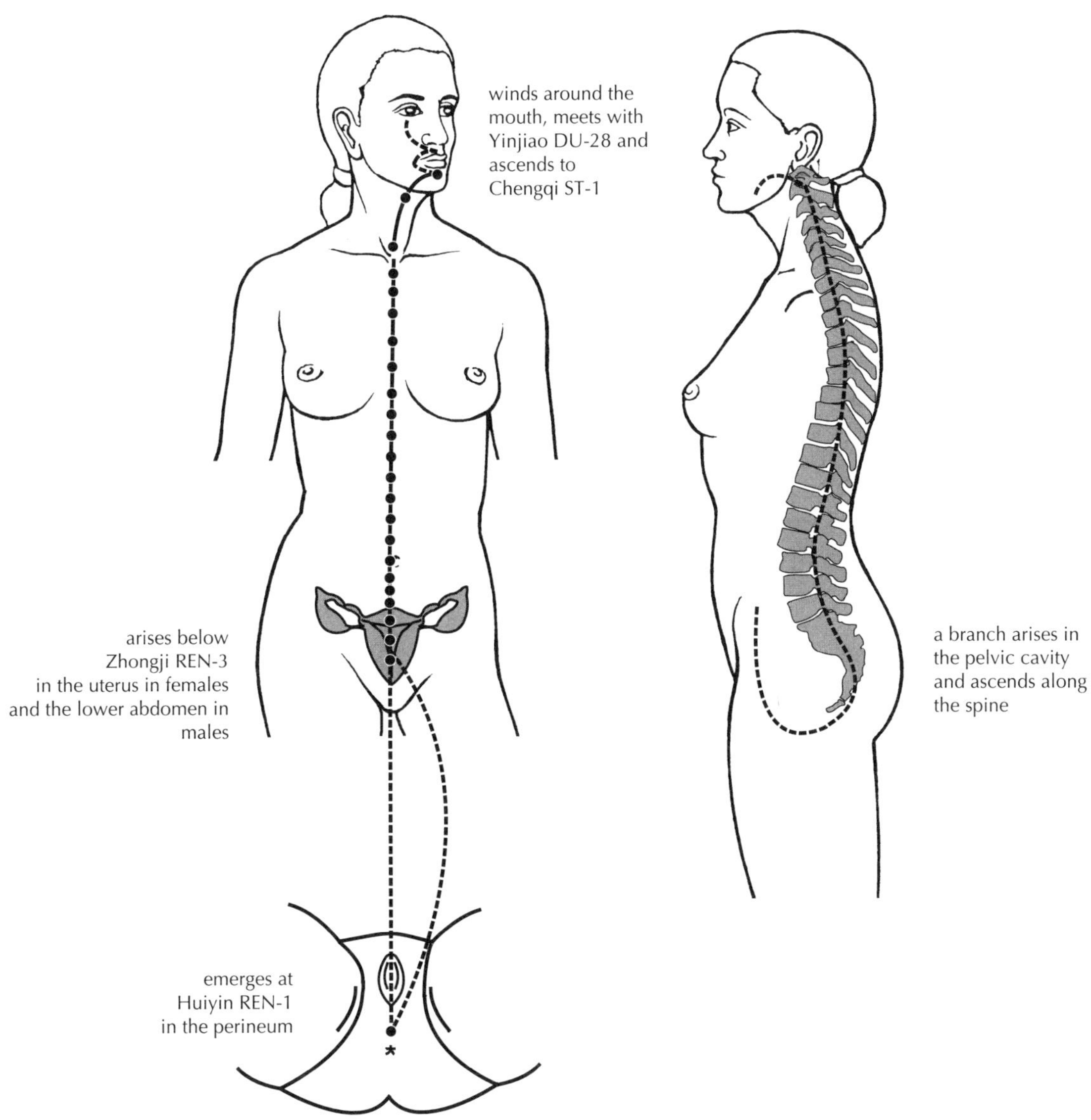

The Conception vessel primary pathway

THE CONCEPTION VESSEL PRIMARY PATHWAY

- arises (below Zhongji REN-3) in the uterus in females and the lower abdomen in males and emerges at Huiyin REN-1 in the perineum,
- ascends along the midline of the abdomen, chest, throat and jaw, terminating at Chengjiang REN-24,
- the interior portion of the channel winds around the mouth, connects with the Governing vessel at Yinjiao DU-28 and terminates below the eye at Chengqi ST-1.

A branch

- arises in the pelvic cavity, enters the spine and ascends along the back.

Note

- Changqiang DU-1 is classified as a meeting point of the Conception and Governing vessels, although it is not normally shown as such on illustrations of the Conception vessel primary pathway.

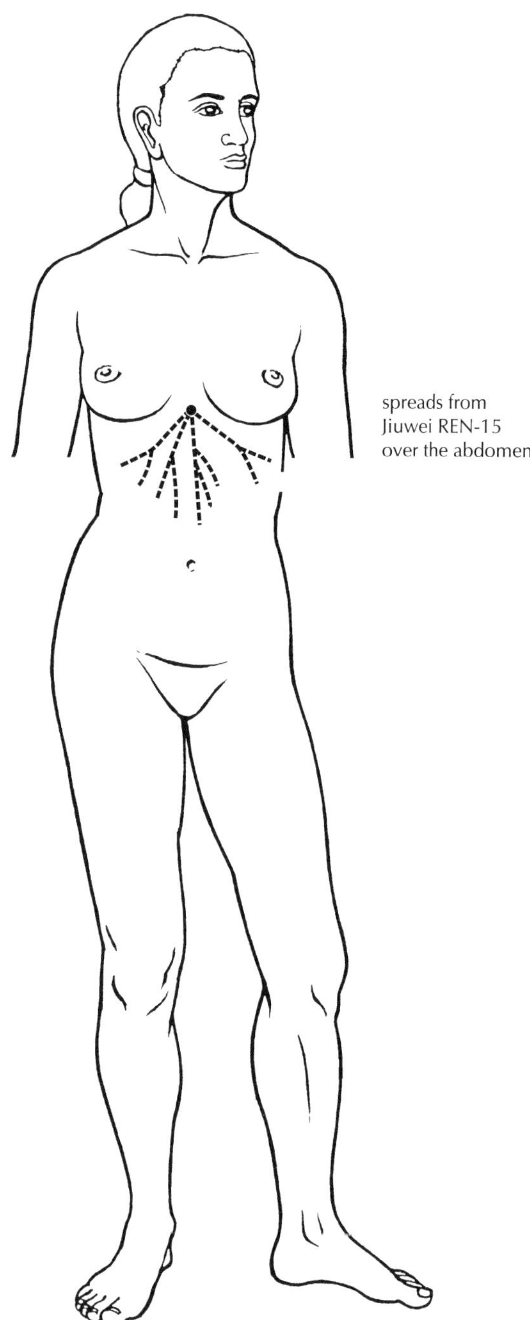

The Conception luo-connecting vessel

THE CONCEPTION LUO-CONNECTING VESSEL

- descends from Jiuwei REN-15 and disperses over the abdomen.

DISCUSSION

The Conception vessel is one of the eight extraordinary vessels, but along with the Governing vessel is exceptional among these eight in that it has its own acupuncture points. For this reason the Conception and Governing vessels are often included with the twelve primary channels (and together known as the fourteen channels). The other six extraordinary vessels have no points of their own, passing instead through points of the fourteen channels.

The Conception vessel is principally understood to be the channel that ascends along the midline of the anterior of the body. As the above description shows however, a branch enters the spine and ascends along the back, whilst a branch of the Governing vessel also ascends along the midline of the anterior of the body. Li Shi-zhen therefore said "The Conception and Governing vessels are like midnight and midday, they are the polar axis of the body ... there is one source and two branches, one goes to the front and the other to the back of the body ... When we try to divide these, we see that yin and yang are inseparable. When we try to see them as one, we see that it is an indivisible whole"[1].

As far as the pathway of the Conception vessel is concerned, it is important to note that:

- according to the *Spiritual Pivot*[2] the Conception vessel originates in the uterus in females.
- the primary channel winds around the mouth and terminates below the eye.

The actions of the points of the Conception vessel can be summarised as follows:

- Treating disorders of their local area. All the Conception vessel points below the umbilicus treat disorders of urination and defecation, genital diseases, stagnation in the lower abdomen and uterine and menstrual diseases. Shenque REN-8 and Shuifen REN-9 treat disorders of the intestines and abdomen. From Xiawan REN-10 up to Xuanji REN-21 all the Conception vessel points treat stagnation and rebellion of Stomach qi, even when their location is high up on the chest. From Shangwan REN-13 upwards, most points treat disorders of the Heart, and from Juque REN-14 upwards, of the Lung and chest.
- Located on the soft, yielding and yin anterior surface of the body, the Conception vessel points allow direct access to the zangfu. Six of the front-mu points therefore are located on this channel (Zhongji REN-3: the Bladder, Guanyuan REN-4: the Small Intestine; Shimen REN-5: the Sanjiao; Zhongwan REN-12: the Stomach; Juque REN-14: the Heart; Shanzhong

REN-17: the Pericardium). In most cases these are fundamentally important points to regulate their respective zangfu.

- The lower abdomen is the location of the dantian (cinnabar field), the residence of the deepest energies of the body. Guanyuan REN-4 and Qihai REN-6 are therefore among the most important tonifying and nourishing points of the body. Along with Shenque REN-8, they are also able to rescue yang and restore consciousness in cases of yang collapse.

HUIYIN REN-1

Meeting of Yin

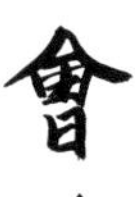

Meeting point of the Conception, Penetrating and Governing vessels
Sun Si-miao Ghost point

LOCATION

At the perineum, midway between the anus and the scrotum in men, and the anus and the posterior labial commissure in women.

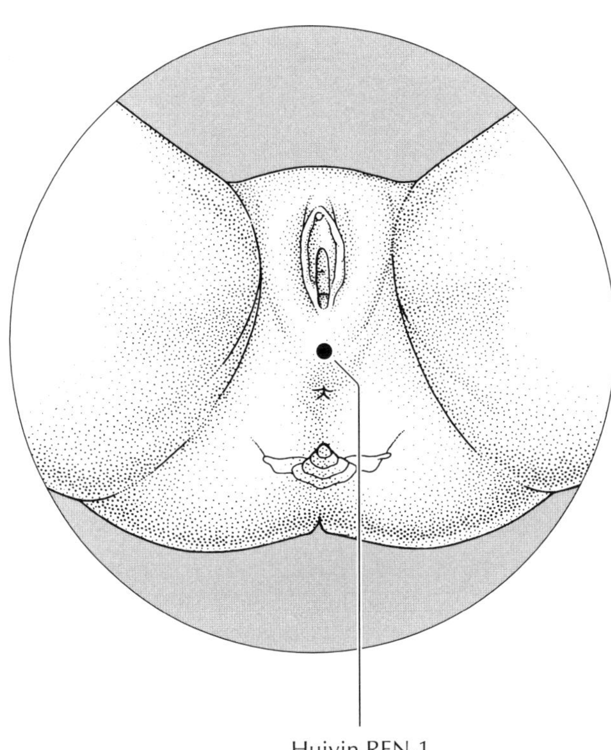

LOCATION NOTE

In males the scrotum may need to be lifted away from the point.

NEEDLING

Perpendicular insertion 0.5 to 1 cun. **Note:** according to the *Great Compendium of Acupuncture and Moxibustion*, this point is contraindicated to needling.
Caution: contraindicated in pregnancy.

ACTIONS

Regulates the anterior and posterior yin
Drains damp heat
Calms the spirit
Promotes resuscitation and revives from drowning

INDICATIONS

- Difficult urination and defecation, enuresis, seminal emission, impotence, genital diseases, sweating of the genitals, pain of the head of the penis, cold sensation of the head of the penis, swelling of the testicles, swelling and pain of the vagina, prolapse of the rectum, haemorrhoids, pain of the anus and urethra, sensation of heat in the urethra, itching and pain of the perineum, shan disorder.
- Amenorrhoea, irregular menstruation, uterine prolapse.
- Coma, suffocation by water (drowning), mania-depression.
- Pain of the skin of the abdomen, itching of the skin of the abdomen.

COMMENTARY

Huiyin REN-1 (Meeting of Yin) derives its name from its location in the area between the anus and the external genitalia (the two lower yin) and the fact that the perineum is where the Conception and Penetrating vessels meet (with the Governing vessel). It is also directly beneath and opposite to Baihui DU-20 (the point at which all the yang gathers) and hence the deep, dark, hidden and protected place where yin meets. This is reflected in the importance of Huiyin REN-1 in qigong practice. In the practice of small heavenly circuit rotation, qi is focused in the lower dantian (cinnabar field), directed to Huiyin REN-1 and then to Changqiang DU-1 before being directed up the Governing vessel to Baihui DU-20 and then down the Conception vessel to return to the lower dantian.

Historically there has been some discussion as to whether Huiyin REN-1 rather than Jiuwei REN-15 is the luo-connecting point of the Conception vessel. The *Spiritual Pivot*[3] refers to the luo-connecting point of the Conception vessel as Weiyi (Tail Screen), an alternative name for Jiuwei REN-15, and gives symptoms of excess (pain of the skin of the abdomen) and deficiency (itching of the skin of the abdomen). Later classics, including both the *Systematic Classic of Acupuncture and Moxibustion* and the *Great Compendium of Acupuncture and Moxibustion* refer to the luo-connecting point of the Conception vessel as Pingyi (Flat Screen), an alternative name for Huiyin REN-1, and ascribe these symptoms of excess and deficiency to this point. Huiyin REN-1 as the luo-connecting point of the Conception vessel would reflect a neat symmetry with Chengqiang DU-1 as the luo-connecting point of the Governing vessel.

Huiyin REN-1 has a strong action on the genito-urinary and anal regions, especially in disorders due to damp-heat, and is indicated for genital pain and swelling, as well as recalcitrant urinary disorders. It is unfortunate that due to its location it is clinically less used than it otherwise might be.

Huiyin REN-1, under its alternative name of Guicang (Ghost Store) is one of the 'thirteen ghost points' of Sun Simiao, used in the treatment of epilepsy and mania disorder. The *Supplement to the Thousand Ducat Formulas* in fact specified that in men Yinxiafeng (Extra) should be needled, whilst in women Yumentou (Extra), located at the posterior labial commissure, should be needled. Both points more or less correspond to Huiyin REN-1.

Finally, Huiyin REN-1 is indicated (for example in the *Great Compendium of Acupuncture and Moxibustion*) for reviving from drowning and is said to have the ability to promote the expulsion of water from the lungs.

COMBINATIONS

- Sudden swelling, redness and pain of the vagina: Huiyin REN-1, Zhongji REN-3 and Sanyinjiao SP-6 (*Great Compendium*).
- The five types of haemorrhoids: Huiyin REN-1, Weizhong BL-40, Chengshan BL-57, Feiyang BL-58, Yangfu GB-38, Fuliu KID-7, Taichong LIV-3, Xiaxi GB-43, Qihai REN-6 and Changqiang DU-1 (*Great Compendium*).

QUGU REN-2

Curved Bone

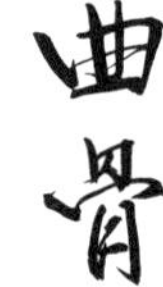

Meeting point of the Conception vessel with the Liver channel

LOCATION

On the midline of the lower abdomen, at the superior border of the pubic symphysis, 5 cun below the umbilicus.

NEEDLING

Perpendicular insertion 0.5 to 1 cun.

Caution: deep insertion will penetrate a full bladder which should therefore be emptied before treatment.

ACTIONS

Benefits urination

Regulates the lower jiao

Warms and invigorates the Kidneys

INDICATIONS

- Dribbling and hesitant flow of urine, difficult urination, retention of urine due to foetal pressure, enuresis, the five types of painful urinary dysfunction.
- Fullness, distention and pain of the lower abdomen, acute lower abdominal pain, painful shan disorder.

- Impotence, seminal emission, dampness and itching of the scrotum, contraction of the penis, dryness and pain of the genitals.
- Red and white leucorrhoea, irregular menstruation, dysmenorrhoea.
- Deficiency and exhaustion of the five zang, deficiency and weariness with extreme cold.

COMMENTARY

Qugu REN-2 acts primarily on the genito-urinary regions, being able to treat a variety of urinary, lower abdominal, sexual, genital and gynaecological diseases. Its importance in the treatment of these disorders however, is overshadowed by neighbouring points such as Qichong ST-30 and Zhongji REN-3.

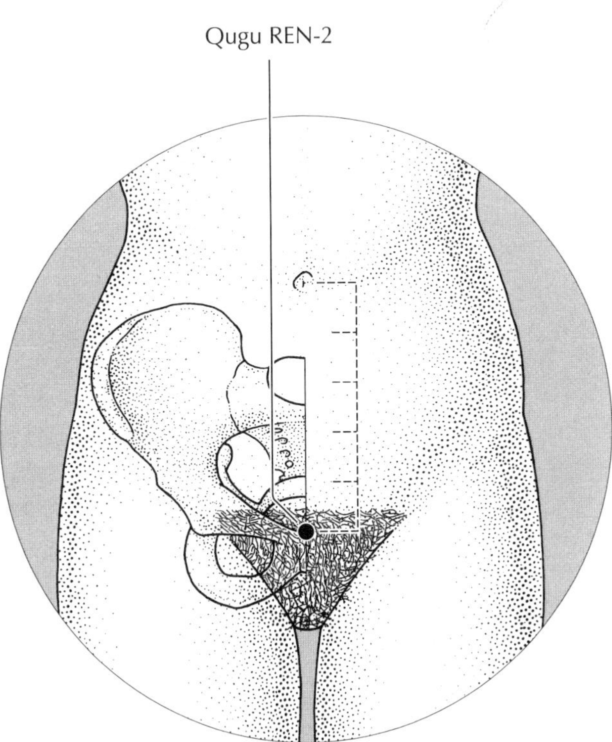

COMBINATIONS

- Inability to urinate: Qugu REN-2, Shimen REN-5, Guanyuan REN-4, Zhongji REN-3 and Sanyinjiao SP-6 (*Supplementing Life*).
- Red and white leucorrhoea: Qugu REN-2 [7 cones of moxa], Taichong LIV-3, Guanyuan REN-4, Fuliu KID-7, Sanyinjiao SP-6, Tianshu ST-25 [one hundred cones of moxa] (*Compilation*).
- Fright epilepsy, mad walking and madness: Qugu REN-2, Xingjian LIV-2, Jinsuo DU-8 and Yingu KID-10 (*Thousand Ducat Formulas*).

ZHONGJI REN-3

Middle Pole

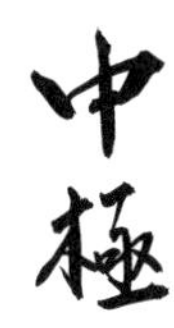

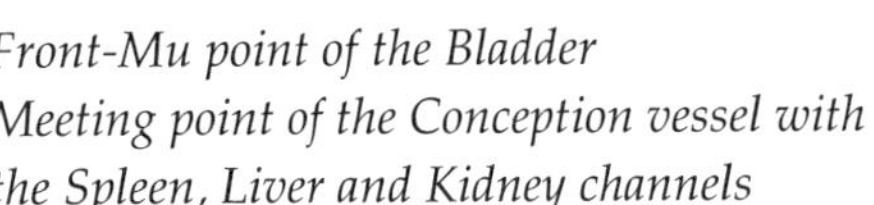
Front-Mu point of the Bladder
Meeting point of the Conception vessel with the Spleen, Liver and Kidney channels

LOCATION

On the midline of the lower abdomen, 4 cun inferior to the umbilicus and 1 cun superior to the pubic symphysis.

NEEDLING

Perpendicular insertion 0.5 to 1 cun.
Caution: deep insertion will penetrate a full bladder which should therefore be emptied before treatment.

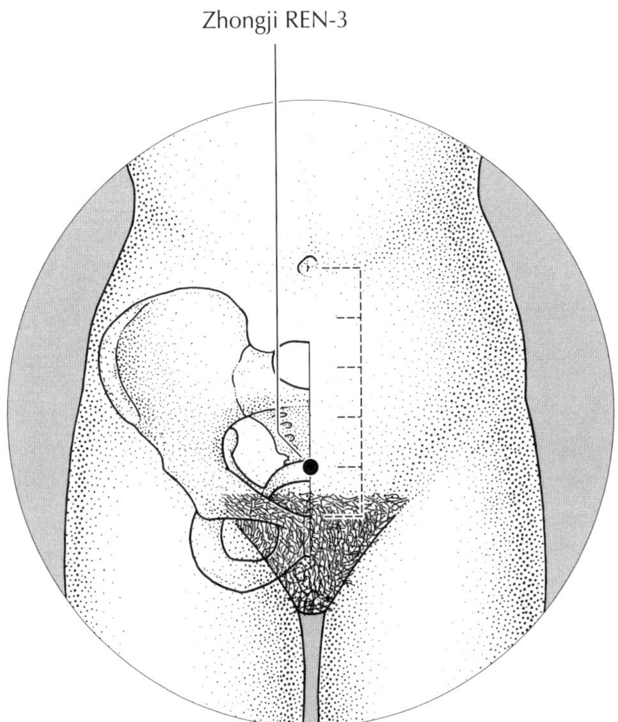

ACTIONS

Benefits the Bladder, regulates qi transformation and drains damp-heat
Drains dampness and treats leucorrhoea
Benefits the uterus and regulates menstruation
Dispels stagnation and benefits the lower jiao
Fortifies the Kidneys

INDICATIONS

- Severe pain of the lower abdomen with retention of urine (in pregnancy), frequent urination, dark urination, urethral pain, the five types of painful urinary dysfunction, oedema.

- Genital itching with heat sensation, pain of the genitals, red and white leucorrhoea, seminal emission, seminal emission with dreams.
- Pain and swelling of the child gate (cervix), infertility, irregular menstruation, amenorrhoea, menorrhagia, uterine prolapse, abdominal (zheng jia) masses, retention of the placenta, retention of lochia, persistent flow of lochia.
- Masses below the umbilicus, severe twisting pain below the umbilicus, the seven kinds of shan disorder, cold sensation of the lower abdomen, heat sensation of the abdomen, sudden severe pain of the lower abdomen and back.
- Accumulation of cold qi rising to invade the Heart, running piglet qi rising to the Heart causing inability to breathe.
- Lumbar pain, deficiency of yang qi, lower origin (yuan) deficient, loss of consciousness, hunger with inability to eat.

COMMENTARY

Zhongji REN-3 is the front-mu point of the Bladder and a meeting point of the Conception vessel with the Spleen, Liver and Kidney channels. The term 'mu' means to gather or to collect, and the front-mu points are where the qi of the zangfu gathers and concentrates on the anterior surface of the body. Zhongji REN-3 therefore has a direct action on the Bladder fu. Urinary disorders characterised by retention, pain, frequency and urgency of urination may be excess or deficient in nature. Excess patterns include accumulation of dampness or damp-heat and stagnation of qi, and may be complicated by the presence of stones or bleeding. Deficiency patterns primarily involve deficiency of qi and yang. Due to its ability to regulate the qi transformation function of the Bladder, drain dampness and heat, and strengthen the Kidneys, Zhongji REN-3 is a primary point in the treatment of a variety of urinary disorders involving any of these disharmonies. In clinical practice however, Zhongji REN-3 is favoured for excess patterns, whilst Guanyuan REN-4 is favoured for deficiency patterns. By virtue of its ability to promote smooth urination, Zhongji REN-3 is also indicated for oedema.

The ability of Zhongji REN-3 to drain dampness and heat extends to the genital region where it is an important point for itching, swelling and pain as well as leucorrhoea and seminal emission. The *Great Compendium of Acupuncture and Moxibustion* specifically recommends Zhongji REN-3 for pain and swelling of the cervix.

The Spleen controls blood, the Liver stores blood, and the Kidneys and the Conception vessel dominate the uterus and conception. Zhongji REN-3, as a meeting point of all these channels, is able to regulate the uterus and menstruation and is primarily indicated for excess patterns giving rise to abdominal (zheng jia) masses, irregular or absent menstruation, infertility, and especially retention of the placenta or lochia.

The three leg yin channels of Spleen, Liver and Kidney all pass through and dominate the lower abdomen. As a meeting point of the Conception vessel with these three channels, Zhongji REN-3 therefore has a strong action on the lower abdomen as a whole, predominantly in excess patterns involving stagnation and accumulation of cold or heat. It is indicated for masses, shan disorder and severe twisting pain, and both hot and cold sensations in the abdomen.

Zhongji REN-3 is also used for the condition known as running piglet qi, particularly when due to Kidney yang deficiency with invasion of cold. According to the *Essentials From the Golden Cabinet* "Running piglet disorder arises from the lower abdomen; it rushes up to the throat with such ferocity that the patient feels he is close to death. It attacks and then remits. It is brought about by fear and fright".

Finally, Zhongji REN-3 is indicated for deficiency of yang qi and lower origin (yuan) deficiency. However, so great are the tonifying properties of Guanyuan REN-4 that in clinical practice this latter point is almost invariably used for this purpose. Like Guanyuan REN-4 also, Zhongji REN-3 is indicated for lumbar pain, reflecting the principle of selecting points from the front of the body to treat the back.

COMBINATIONS

- Inability to urinate: Zhongji REN-3, Qugu REN-2, Shimen REN-5, Guanyuan REN-4 and Sanyinjiao SP-6 (*Supplementing Life*).
- Difficult urination and seminal emission: Zhongji REN-3, Ligou LIV-5, Lougu SP-7, Chengfu BL-36 and Zhiyin BL-67 (*Supplementing Life*).
- Seminal emission: Zhongji REN-3, Zhiyin BL-67 and Ququan LIV-8 (*Supplementing Life*).
- Pain of the penis: Zhongji REN-3, Taixi KID-3, Yuji LU-10 and Sanyinjiao SP-6 (*Great Compendium*).
- Sudden swelling, redness and pain of the vagina: Zhongji REN-3, Huiyin REN-1 and Sanyinjiao SP-6 (*Great Compendium*).
- Infertility: Zhongji REN-3 and Zigong (M-CA-18) (*Great Compendium*).
- Uterine bleeding: Zhongji REN-3 and Zigong (M-CA-18) (*Great Compendium*).
- Ceaseless uterine bleeding: Zhongji REN-3, Shimen REN-5, Zigong (M-CA-18) and Shenshu BL-23 (*Great Compendium*).

- Irregular menstruation: Zhongji REN-3, Sanyinjiao SP-6, Daimai GB-26, Qihai REN-6 and Shenshu BL-23 (*Great Compendium*).
- Inhibited menstruation: Zhongji REN-3, Sanyinjiao SP-6 and Zulinqi GB-41 (*Great Compendium*).
- Infertility: Zhongji REN-3 and Shangqiu SP-5 (*Great Compendium*).
- Retention of the placenta: reduce Zhongji REN-3 and Sanyinjiao SP-6 (*Great Compendium*).
- Retention of the placenta: Zhongji REN-3 and Jianjing GB-21 *Great Compendium*).
- Retention of the placenta: Zhongji REN-3, Jianjing GB-21 and Sanyinjiao SP-6 (*Meeting the Source*).
- Ceaseless diarrhoea: Zhongji REN-3, Tianshu ST-25 and Zhongwan REN-12 (*Great Compendium*).

GUANYUAN REN-4

Gate of Origin

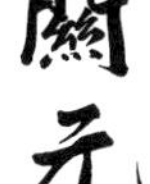

Front-Mu point of the Small Intestine
Meeting point of the Conception vessel with the Spleen, Liver and Kidney channels

LOCATION

On the midline of the lower abdomen, 3 cun inferior to the umbilicus and 2 cun superior to the pubic symphysis.

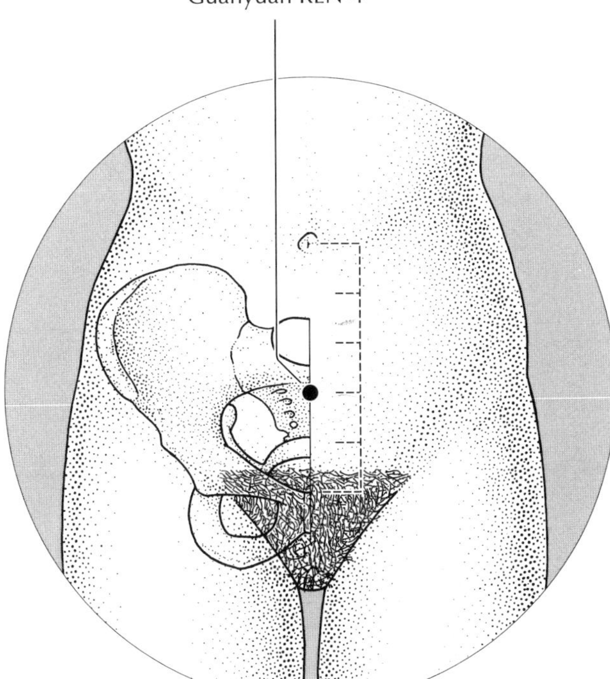

NEEDLING

Perpendicular insertion 0.5 to 1 cun, or oblique insertion directed inferiorly, 1 to 1.5 cun.
Caution: deep insertion may penetrate a full bladder which should therefore be emptied before treatment.

ACTIONS

Fortifies the original qi and benefits essence
Tonifies and nourishes the Kidneys
Warms and fortifies the Spleen
Benefits the uterus and assists conception
Regulates the lower jiao and benefits the Bladder
Regulates Small Intestine qi
Restores collapse

INDICATIONS

- Kidney deficiency, Kidney taxation, weakness of the lumbar region and legs, pain of the lumbar region and the bones and joints of the legs in the middle-aged and elderly, aversion to cold in the back, withered ears, gradual darkening of the face, fear, fright, fear leading to deficiency consumption, deep-rooted bone ulcers due to fear, frequent urination, enuresis, seminal emission, white turbidity, impotence.
- Infertility, infertility with cold sensation in the vagina, amenorrhoea, bleeding during pregnancy, persistent flow of lochia, post-partum abdominal pain, red and white leucorrhoea.
- Taxation heat, deficiency consumption with cough, tidal fever with coughing of blood, dyspnoea with inability to lie down, Kidney deficiency dyspnoea, insomnia, dizziness, wind dizziness, headache, wasting and thirsting disorder.
- Lethargy and lack of strength, emaciation of the four limbs despite much eating, weariness of the four limbs, weakness of Spleen qi, undigested food (in the stool), diarrhoea, dysenteric disorder, incontinence of the stool in the elderly, belching, vomiting of phlegm.
- Retention of urine due to foetal pressure, retention of urine, dark urine, stone painful urinary dysfunction, the five types of painful urinary dysfunction, blood in the urine, burning pain on urination, oedema that leads to pain of the lateral costal region.
- Cold qi entering the lower abdomen giving rise to pain, cold accumulation with deficiency, running piglet qi rising to the Heart, fullness of the lower abdomen, back pain and twisting pain below the umbilicus that gradually radiates to the genitals, sudden painful shan disorder, intense heat in the hypogastrium.
- Sudden turmoil disorder, windstroke, heaviness of the body like a mountain, tremor of the hands.

COMMENTARY

Guanyuan REN-4 is one of the principle acupuncture points to promote and foster the original qi, benefit essence, fortify Kidney yang and nourish Kidney yin. As well as Guanyuan (Gate of Origin) several of the numerous different names given to this point reflect its deeply tonifying properties, for example Mingmen (Gate of Life), Huangzhiyuan (Origin of Huang), Xuehai (Sea of Blood), Qihai (Sea of Qi), Dahai (Great Sea) and of course Dantian (Cinnabar Field). According to classical Chinese thought, the lower dantian, located in the lower abdomen and extending from Yinjiao REN-7 to Guanyuan REN-4, is the residence of the deepest energies of the body and the source of all movement. According to the *Classic of Difficulties*[4] "The dynamic qi that moves between the Kidneys is [the basis] of human life, the source of the five zang and six fu, the root of the twelve channels, the door of respiration and the origin of the sanjiao". According to the *Discourse into the Origin and Development of Medicine*[5] "Original qi is distributed to the five zang and forms the essence of the five zang. Where is the place of origin of the original qi? The Daoists believe it is dantian".

Due to its location at the heart of the lower dantian (cinnabar field) and its close relationship with the original qi and hence essence, Guanyuan REN-4 is an indispensable point to tonify and nourish the Kidneys. This action is made abundantly clear by the long list of classical indications which reads like a textbook description of Kidney deficiency. The Kidneys dominate the bones and lumbar region, and Guanyuan REN-4 is indicated for weakness, pain and cold sensations of the lumbar region and legs, especially in the middle-aged and elderly. In severe cases Kidney deficiency may give rise to withered ears, darkness of the complexion and Kidney taxation. According to the *Essential Questions*[6] "fear depletes the essence". Fear is closely linked to the Kidneys, and prolonged fear may injure and weaken the Kidneys and the essence, whilst Kidney deficiency may render a person prone to deep-seated fear. The powerful effect that fear may have on the body is reflected in classical sources which ascribe even deep-rooted bone ulcers and deficiency consumption to this aetiology. When the Kidneys are deficient and fail to dominate the Bladder there may be urinary frequency or enuresis. In all such cases Guanyuan REN-4 is of fundamental importance. Guanyuan REN-4 is also used for the condition known as running piglet qi, especially when due to Kidney yang deficiency with invasion of cold. According to the *Essentials From the Golden Cabinet* "Running piglet disorder arises from the lower abdomen; it rushes up to the throat with such ferocity that the patient feels he is close to death. It attacks and then remits. It is brought about by fear and fright". Not only may this pattern be induced by fear, but when the qi rushes upwards in this way it can induce uncontrollable anxiety and panic.

The Spleen controls blood, the Liver stores blood, and the Kidneys and the Conception vessel dominate the uterus and conception. Guanyuan REN-4, also known as Sanjiejiao (Triple Intersection), is a meeting point of the Conception vessel with these three channels and is an essential point to regulate the uterus and promote fertility. When Kidney deficiency leads to deficiency and coldness of what is known as the 'palace of the child' (i.e. the uterus) in women there may be infertility, amenorrhoea and cold leucorrhoea. The importance of this point in assisting conception is reflected in further alternative names, for example Zihu (Infant's Door) and Zigong (Infant's Palace). If deficiency of Kidney fire leads to coldness and weakness of the 'essence gate' in men, there may be seminal emission and impotence.

According to the *True Lineage of Medicine*[7] "When Kidney origin (yuan) is abundant, then life is long, when Kidney origin (yuan) is in decline, life is short". For this reason, traditional health preservation practitioners in China recommend the regular application of moxibustion to Guanyuan REN-4 in later life.

The strong tonifying and nourishing action of Guanyuan REN-4 is not limited to the Kidneys alone. Since the Kidneys are the root of both the yin and yang of the body, and "the original qi is distributed to the five zang and forms the essence of the five zang", Guanyuan REN-4 may be used in the treatment of any profound deficiency of the zangfu, whether of qi, blood, yin or yang. Thus, for example, when the yin of the Kidneys and Lung is deficient, Guanyuan REN-4 may be used to treat taxation heat, deficiency consumption with cough, tidal fever with coughing of blood, Kidney deficiency dyspnoea, dyspnoea with inability to lie down, and wasting and thirsting disorder. When the Kidney fire fails to provide sufficient heat for the Spleen's transportation and transformation function there may be chronic diarrhoea, incontinence of the stool in the elderly, lethargy, weakness of the four limbs and undigested food (in the stool).

The action of Guanyuan REN-4 is not limited to tonifying deficiency, however. If exterior cold attacks the lower abdomen, and particularly the Liver channel, especially when there is underlying yang deficiency, there may be severe twisting lower abdominal pain radiating to the genitals and sudden painful shan disorder. These symptoms are commonly ascribed to disharmony of the Small Intestine (Small Intestine qi pain), and this is the principal significance of the status of Guanyuan REN-4 as the front-mu point of the Small Intestine.

When damp-heat knots the Bladder there may be various kinds of urinary disorders characterised by frequency, urgency, pain and dark or bloody urination as well as an intense sensation of heat in the hypogastrium. Guanyuan REN-4 may be used to drain these excess pathogenic factors. According to Zhu Dan-xi "When the Kidneys are deficient the Bladder will generate heat", whilst the *General Treatise on the Aetiology and Symptomatology of Diseases*[8] says "Where painful urinary dysfunction is concerned there is Kidney deficiency and Bladder heat". Guanyuan REN-4 is especially indicated when, as is commonly the case, deficiency and excess co-exist and there is underlying Kidney deficiency. Guanyuan REN-4 is also an important point in the treatment of post-partum disorders such as pain and persistent flow of lochia, which are also frequently due to a combination of deficiency and excess.

Finally, due to its powerful ability to restore the yang, Guanyuan REN-4 is used to treat collapse of yang characterised by chills, breathlessness, minute pulse, profuse sweating and unconsciousness. In such cases, Guanyuan REN-4, in combination with Qihai REN-6 and Shenque REN-8, is treated by continuous indirect moxibustion.

COMBINATIONS

- Wind dizziness and headache: Guanyuan REN-4, Fengmen BL-12, Kunlun BL-60, Tianyou SJ-16 and Guanchong SJ-1 (*Thousand Ducat Formulas*).
- Heat in the body with headache that comes and goes: Guanyuan REN-4 and Shendao DU-11 (*Thousand Ducat Formulas*).
- Distention of the lateral costal region: Guanyuan REN-4, Qimen LIV-14 and Shaoshang LU-11 (*Thousand Ducat Formulas*).
- Heat sensation and pain of the hypogastrium: Guanyuan REN-4, Weizhong BL-40, Zhaohai KID-6 and Taixi KID-3 (*Thousand Ducat Formulas*).
- Abdominal fullness that radiates to the back, one-sided swelling and sagging of the testicle: Guanyuan REN-4 [3 moxa cones] and Dadun LIV-1 [7 moxa cones] (*Great Compendium*).
- Running piglet qi in women: Guanyuan REN-4, Zhongji REN-3, Sanyinjiao SP-6, Shimen REN-5, Xuehai SP-10 and Qimen LIV-14 (*Supplementing Life*).
- Red and hesitant urinary flow: Guanyuan REN-4, Zhibian BL-54, Qihai REN-6 and Yanggang BL-48 (*Supplementing Life*).
- Inability to urinate: Guanyuan REN-4, Shimen REN-5, Zhongji REN-3, Qugu REN-2 and Sanyinjiao SP-6 (*Supplementing Life*).
- Dark urine: Guanyuan REN-4, Qihai REN-6, Taixi KID-3, Yingu KID-10, Shenshu BL-23 and Pangguangshu BL-28 (*Great Compendium*).
- Incontinence of faeces: Guanyuan REN-4 and Dachangshu BL-25 (*Great Compendium*).
- Difficulty in defecation: Guanyuan REN-4, Dazhong KID-4, Zhongliao BL-33, Chengjin BL-56, Taichong LIV-3, Chengshan BL-57, Taixi KID-3 and Zhongwan REN-12 (*Supplementing Life*).
- Ceaseless diarrhoea and dysenteric disorder: Guanyuan REN-4 and Taixi KID-3 (*Thousand Ducat Formulas*).

SHIMEN REN-5

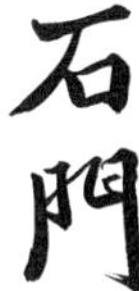

Stone Gate

Front-Mu point of the Sanjiao

LOCATION

On the midline of the lower abdomen, 2 cun inferior to the umbilicus and 3 cun superior to the pubic symphysis.

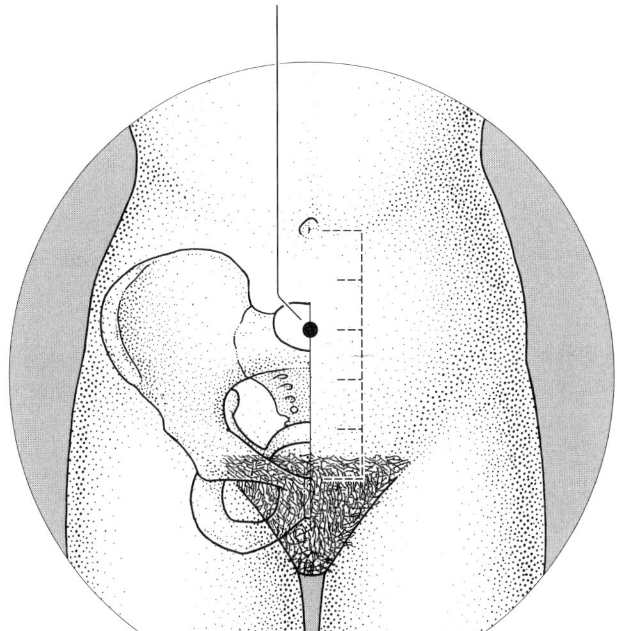

NEEDLING

Perpendicular insertion 0.8 to 1.5 cun. **Note**: according to several classical texts, this point is contraindicated to needling and moxibustion during pregnancy.

Caution: deep needling may penetrate the peritoneal cavity.

ACTIONS

Moves and benefits the water passages
Regulates qi and alleviates pain
Regulates the uterus

INDICATIONS

- Difficult urination, difficult urination due to injury by cold, retention of urine, qi painful urinary dysfunction, blood painful urinary dysfunction, dark urine, oedema.
- Diarrhoea, undigested food (in the stool), dysenteric disorder, vomiting blood with inability to eat.
- Twisting pain of the lower abdomen, shan disorder with severe periumbilical pain, lower abdominal distention, retraction of the testicles, genital itching, swelling of the penis giving rise to pain of the lower abdomen and lumbar region, running piglet qi attacking the Heart.
- Persistent flow of lochia, abdominal masses, uterine bleeding, stone-like hardness of the lower abdomen, diseases of the breast, leucorrhoea.
- Deficiency-taxation, lower origin (yuan) deficient and cold.

COMMENTARY

Shimen REN-5 is the front-mu point of the Sanjiao. The term 'mu' means to gather or to collect, and the front-mu points are where the qi of the zangfu gathers and concentrates on the anterior surface of the body. The *Essential Questions* says "the Sanjiao is the official in charge of drainage and controls the water passages"[9], the *Classic of Difficulties* says "the Sanjiao is the pathway of water and grain"[10] and the *Classic of Categories* states "when the lower jiao is not treated there is water disorder in the bowels and Bladder". Shimen REN-5 is indicated for stagnation of fluids characterised by difficult urination or retention of urine, painful urinary dysfunction and oedema, as well as for diarrhoea, undigested food in the stool and dysenteric disorder.

Shimen REN-5 is also able to regulate qi stagnation and alleviate pain in the lower abdomen and genital region and is strongly indicated in the treatment of conditions such as twisting pain of the lower abdomen, shan disorder with severe periumbilical pain, abdominal distention, and retraction, swelling and pain of the genitals.

In colloquial Chinese a woman who is infertile is known as a 'stone woman', whilst the name Shimen means 'Stone Gate' or 'Stone Door'. An alternative name for this point is Jueyun (Infertility). These names refer to the unique quality classically attributed to this point of inducing infertility. Texts such as the *Great Compendium of Acupuncture and Moxibustion*, the *Systematic Classic of Acupuncture and Moxibustion*, the *Illustrated Classic of Acupuncture Points on the Bronze Man* and the *Illustrated Supplement to the Classic of Categories* all warn that needling this point can make a woman infertile for life. Modern acupuncture texts, however, make no mention of this warning. The effect of Shimen REN-5 on regulating the function of the uterus and adjusting menstruation is further illustrated by its indications for persistent flow of lochia, abdominal masses, uterine bleeding and leucorrhoea.

Finally, although indicated for deficiency-taxation and lower origin (yuan) deficient and cold, compared with its neighbouring points Guanyuan REN-4 and Qihai REN-6, Shimen REN-5 is notable for the absence of indications of deficiency, and is principally indicated for excess patterns.

COMBINATIONS

- Inability to urinate: Shimen REN-5, Guanyuan REN-4, Sanyinjiao SP-6, Zhongji REN-3 and Qugu REN-2 (*Supplementing Life*).
- Hardness and pain in the lower abdomen that radiates to the genitals with inability to urinate: Shimen REN-5, Weiyang BL-39 and Yinjiao REN-7 (*Supplementing Life*).
- Hypogastric pain radiating to the genitals: Shimen REN-5 and Shangqiu SP-5 (*Thousand Ducat Formulas*).
- Spasmodic pain of the hypogastrium: Shimen REN-5 and Shuifen REN-9 (*Thousand Ducat Formulas*).
- Hypogastric shan disorder: Shimen REN-5, Tianshu ST-25, Shenque REN-8 and Qihai REN-6 (*Thousand Ducat Formulas*).
- Umbilical shan disorder: Shimen REN-5, Shenque REN-8 and Tianshu ST-25 (*Supplementing Life*).
- Women who have had too many children: Shimen REN-5 and Sanyinjiao SP-6 (*Great Compendium*).
- Profuse uterine bleeding: Shimen REN-5 and Yinjiao REN-7 (*Supplementing Life*).
- Ceaseless uterine bleeding: Shimen REN-5, Zhongji REN-3, Zigong (M-CA-18) and Shenshu BL-23 (*Great Compendium*).
- Running piglet qi: Shimen REN-5, Zhangmen LIV-13 and Sanyinjiao SP-6 (*Thousand Ducat Formulas*).
- Running piglet qi in women: Shimen REN-5, Zhongji REN-3, Guanyuan REN-4, Qimen LIV-14, Sanyinjiao SP-6 and Xuehai SP-10 (*Supplementing Life*).

QIHAI REN-6

Sea of Qi

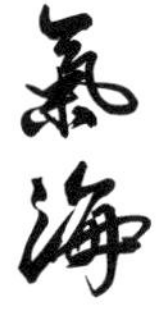

LOCATION

On the midline of the lower abdomen, 1.5 cun inferior to the umbilicus and 3.5 cun superior to the pubic symphysis.

NEEDLING

Perpendicular insertion 0.8 to 1.5 cun.

Caution: deep needling may penetrate the peritoneal cavity.

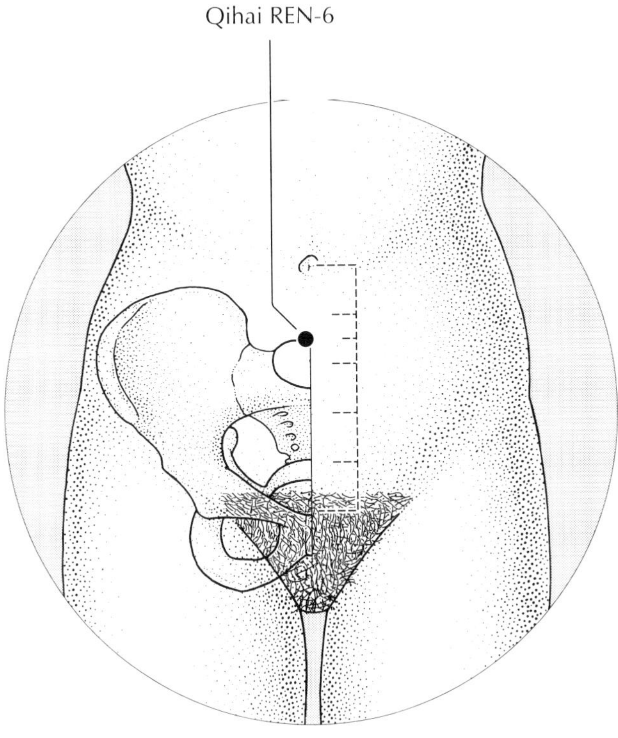

ACTIONS

Fosters original qi
Tonifies qi
Tonifies the Kidneys and fortifies yang
Rescues collapse of yang
Regulates qi and harmonises blood

INDICATIONS

- Zang deficiency with qi exhaustion, original qi deficiency, sudden collapse of yang, slow and minute pulse, yin deficiency with sudden collapse of yang, loss of consciousness from windstroke, all kinds of chronic qi disease that do not respond to treatment, emaciation of the muscles and body, feebleness and weakness of the muscles, failure of the fontanelle to close in babies, upward attack of the qi of the five zang.
- Impotence, seminal emission, prolapse of the uterus, prolapse of the rectum.
- Deficiency and cold of the lower jiao, inversion counterflow of the four limbs, cold illness with dark face, diarrhoea, dysenteric disorder, white and turbid urine, dark urine, hesitant urination, childhood enuresis.
- Uterine bleeding, persistent flow of lochia, postpartum bleeding, irregular menstruation, dysmenorrhoea, red and white leucorrhoea, infertility.
- The seven kinds of shan disorder, twisting pain of the umbilicus, abdominal (zheng jia) masses, abdominal distention, pain and cold sensation below the umbilicus, retraction of the testicles.
- Upward staring eyes, constipation, sudden pain of the Heart, dyspnoea, lumbar sprain.

COMMENTARY

Qihai REN-6, like Guanyuan REN-4, is also known by the name of 'Dantian' (Cinnabar Field). This reflects its location in the vital centre of the body where the deepest energies are stored and generated, and which plays a pivotal role in the treatment of disease and in Chinese martial arts and qigong practices. (For a fuller discussion of the dantian see the commentary on Guanyuan REN-4).

The name Qihai (Sea of Qi) emphasises the principal difference between Qihai REN-6 and Guanyuan REN-4. Whilst both have a powerful action on tonifying the Kidneys, the forte of Qihai REN-6 is generating qi and yang and it does not share the yin and blood nourishing qualities of Guanyuan REN-4.

According to the *Great Compendium of Acupuncture and Moxibustion* Qihai REN-6 is indicated for deficiency of the original qi and for qi deficiency of all the five zang. In fact the original qi is considered to be the basis for the formation and activity of all the zangfu. This concept is explained in the *Classic of Difficulties*[11] which states "The dynamic qi that moves between the Kidneys is [the basis] of human life, the source of the five zang and six fu, the root of the twelve channels, the door of respiration and the origin of the sanjiao", and in the *Discourse into the Origin and Development of Medicine*[12] which says "Original qi is distributed to the five zang and forms the essence of the five zang". Original qi is formed from the combination of pre- and post- heaven qi. In comparison with Zusanli ST-36 which tonifies the source of post-heaven qi in the Stomach and Spleen, Qihai REN-6 activates and mobilises the pre-heaven qi stored in the Kidneys. It is thus indicated in the widest possible range of disorders involving qi deficiency and exhaustion. By promoting the pre-heaven qi, Qihai REN-6 is able to foster the post-heaven qi of the Stomach and Spleen and is thus indicated for emaciation and feebleness of the muscles and diarrhoea. By warming and firming the Kidney yang, Qihai REN-6 is able to treat impotence, seminal emission, cold illness and dark face. By promoting the central qi, Qihai REN-6 is able to treat prolapse of the rectum and uterus. So strong are its qi and yang restoring properties that it is a vital point for rescuing yang in cases of collapse with a slow and minute pulse. For this purpose strong moxibustion either by moxa stick or by large moxa cones mediated by sliced fresh ginger or aconite cake is administered. Zhu Dan-xi of the Jin-Yuan dynasty describes a case of "yin depletion followed by sudden expiry of yang" with pouring sweat, faint respiration, urinary incontinence and a large irregular and arrhythmic pulse. He applied moxa to Qihai REN-6 "with the moxa cones as big as the small finger. When the eighteenth cone was burned up, his right hand was able to move. Another three cones and his lips began to move a little". He also describes a case of violent diarrhoea resulting in loss of consciousness and extremely faint breathing as if on the verge of death. Moxa was performed at Qihai REN-6 without delay[13]. The ability of Qihai REN-6 to treat disorders of profound deficiency is further reflected in its designation in the *Spiritual Pivot*[14] as the shu point of the 'huang'. The huang, which refers to the area just above the diaphragm and which also appears in the name of Gaohuangshu BL-43, implies one of the deepest and most vital regions of the body.

It is important to emphasise that due to its intimate relationship with the qi, Qihai REN-6 is equally important in the treatment of diseases due to qi stagnation affecting the lower jiao. It is indicated for distention and pain of the abdomen, constipation, qi stagnation due to pathogenic cold giving rise to retraction of the testicles, and cold pain of the abdomen. Since "qi is the master of blood" Qihai REN-6 is also indicated for abdominal masses whether due to stagnation of qi or stasis of blood.

By virtue of its dual actions of tonifying and regulating qi, Qihai REN-6 is able to treat a variety of gynaecological disorders. Uterine bleeding, persistent flow of lochia and post-partum bleeding may be due to failure of the qi to hold the blood, and along with irregular menstruation and dysmenorrhoea may also involve blood stasis, either as a sequela of haemorrhage or as a consequence of qi stagnation.

COMBINATIONS

- Distressed rapid dyspnoea: Qihai REN-6 and Xuanji REN-21 (*Ode of the Jade Dragon*).
- Impotence: Qihai REN-6, Mingmen DU-4, Shenshu BL-23 and Rangu KID-2 (*Illustrated Supplement*).
- White turbidity and chronic seminal emission: Qihai REN-6 and Sanyinjiao SP-6 (*One Hundred Symptoms*).
- Palpitations and insomnia: Qihai REN-6, Sanyinjiao SP-6 and Daju ST-27 (*Supplementing Life*).
- Irregular menstruation: Qihai REN-6, Zhongji REN-3, Daimai GB-26, Shenshu BL-23 and Sanyinjiao SP-6 (*Great Compendium*).
- Post-partum blood clot pain: Qihai REN-6 and Sanyinjiao SP-6 (*Great Compendium*).
- Dysmenorrhoea: Qihai REN-6 and Xiaochangshu BL-27 (*Supplementing Life*).
- Red and white leucorrhoea: Qihai REN-6, Guanyuan REN-4, Jianshi P-5, Baihuanshu BL-30, Daimai GB-26 and Sanyinjiao SP-6 (*Great Compendium*).
- Red (bloody) dysenteric disorder: Qihai REN-6, Neiguan P-6, Tianshu ST-25, Neiting ST-44, Yinbai SP-1 and Zhaohai KID-6 (*Great Compendium*).
- Blood in the stool: Qihai REN-6, Zhongwan REN-12 and Zusanli ST-36 (*Glorious Anthology*).
- Red and hesitant urinary flow: Qihai REN-6, Guanyuan REN-4, Zhibian BL-54 and Yanggang BL-48 (*Supplementing Life*).
- Dark urine: Qihai REN-6, Guanyuan REN-4, Taixi KID-3, Yingu KID-10, Shenshu BL-23 and Pangguangshu BL-28 (*Great Compendium*).
- Obstructed urination: Qihai REN-6, Sanyinjiao SP-6 and Yinlingquan SP-9, followed by Yingu KID-10 and Daling P-7 (*Great Compendium*).
- The five types of painful urinary dysfunction, with inability to urinate: Qihai REN-6 and Dadun LIV-1 (*Thousand Ducat Formulas*).
- The five types of painful urinary dysfunction: Qihai REN-6 and Xuehai SP-10 (*Great Compendium*).
- Periumbilical pain: Qihai REN-6, Shuifen REN-9 and Shenque REN-8 (*Great Compendium*).

YINJIAO REN-7

陰交

Yin Intersection

Meeting point of the Conception and Penetrating vessels and the Kidney channel

LOCATION

On the midline of the lower abdomen, 1 cun inferior to the umbilicus and 4 cun superior to the pubic symphysis.

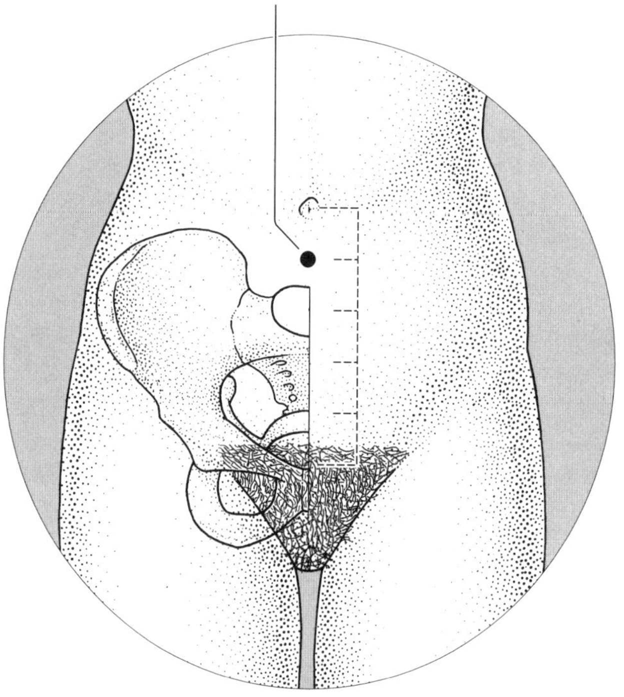

NEEDLING

Perpendicular insertion 0.8 to 1.5 cun.

Caution: deep needling may penetrate the peritoneal cavity.

ACTIONS

Regulates menstruation

Benefits the lower abdomen and genital region

INDICATIONS

- Uterine bleeding, irregular menstruation, amenorrhoea, infertility, leucorrhoea, persistent flow of lochia, diseases of the breast.
- Hardness and pain of the abdomen radiating to the genitals, retraction of the testicles, painful shan disorder, cold shan disorder, sweating of the genitals, damp itching of the genitals, pain of the hypogastrium, heat sensation below the umbilicus, pain and cold around the umbilicus.
- Retention of urine and faeces, inability to urinate, dark urine, oedema, sudden turmoil disorder, borborygmus.
- Pain of the lumbar spine, contraction of the lumbar spine and knees, failure of the fontanelle to close.
- Nosebleed, running piglet qi, vomiting blood, pain of the chest and lateral costal region.

COMMENTARY

Yinjiao REN-7 (Yin Intersection) is a meeting point of the Conception and Penetrating vessels with the Kidney channel, all of which have an intimate relationship with the uterus. The Conception vessel, known as the 'sea of the yin channels' and the Penetrating vessel, known as the 'sea of blood', both originate in the uterus in women and their maturation depends on the flourishing of the Kidneys. The *Essential Questions*[15] states "At the age of fourteen, the tian gui[16] matures, the Conception vessel flows and the Penetrating vessel fills, the menses come according to their times, thus conception is possible". Disorders of menstruation may be of excess or deficiency type, due to cold or heat, exterior pathogens or interior disharmony. Due to the close relationship of Yinjiao REN-7 to the uterus however, it may be used to treat such disorders as irregular menstruation, amenorrhoea, uterine bleeding, persistent flow of lochia or infertility due to any aetiology.

The Conception vessel emerges at the perineum and ascends through the genital region, whilst the Penetrating vessel emerges at Qichong ST-30 and ascends the lower abdomen. Both channels therefore have a strong influence on the lower abdomen and genitals, and Yinjiao REN-7 is indicated for such disorders as pain, retraction, itching and sweating of the genitals, shan disorder and abdominal and umbilical pain.

Finally, like several points which affect the Penetrating vessel, Yinjiao REN-7 is indicated for running piglet qi (see Qichong ST-30).

COMBINATIONS

- Profuse uterine bleeding: Yinjiao REN-7 and Shimen REN-5 (*Supplementing Life*).
- Infertility: Yinjiao REN-7 and Shimen REN-5 (*One Hundred Symptoms*).
- Itching of the genitals: Yinjiao REN-7 and Ququan LIV-8 (*Supplementing Life*).
- Hardness and pain in the lower abdomen that radiates to the genitals with inability to urinate: Yinjiao REN-7, Shimen REN-5 and Weiyang BL-39 (*Supplementing Life*).
- Cracked and bleeding tongue: Yinjiao REN-7, Neiguan P-6 and Taichong LIV-3 (*Miscellaneous Diseases*).

SHENQUE REN-8

Spirit Gateway

神闕

LOCATION

In the centre of the umbilicus.

NEEDLING

Needling is contraindicated at this point, which is normally treated by moxibustion or massage. Moxibustion may be indirect (moxa stick) or mediated by substances such as salt, sliced ginger, crushed garlic or aconite cake.

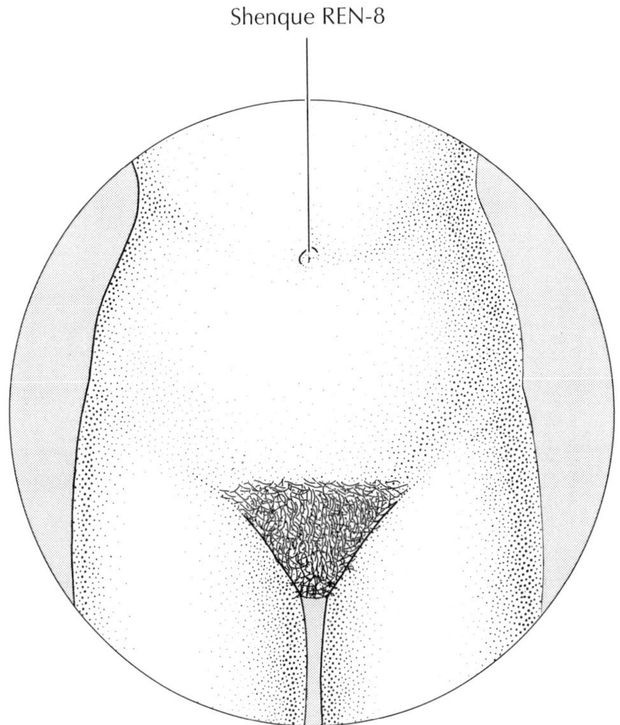

ACTIONS
Warms the yang and rescues collapse
Warms and harmonises the intestines

INDICATIONS
- Loss of consciousness from windstroke, collapse of yang qi, loss of consciousness.
- Deficiency cold of the abdomen, incessant diarrhoea, borborygmus, diarrhoea in the elderly or in deficient people, infantile diarrhoea following breast-feeding, prolapse of the rectum, sudden turmoil disorder, pain around the umbilicus, oedema and drum distention.
- Abdominal distention and retention of urine in post-partum women, infertility from cold in the blood.
- Qi painful urinary dysfunction, wind epilepsy, opisthotonos.

COMMENTARY
Shenque REN-8 is located in the centre of the umbilicus. Shen is translated as spirit, whilst Que literally refers to the watchtower above the gates which protect a city. This point is also known as Qishe (Abode of Qi) or Qihe (Joining of Qi). These various names reflect the importance of the umbilicus as i. the entry and exit point of the spirit, ii. the source of foetal nourishment, and iii. in later life an important point to rescue the qi or yang.

Shenque REN-8 is one of only two points (with Ruzhong ST-17) considered forbidden to needle in current clinical practice, and is exclusively treated by strong moxibustion or massage. When moxibustion is applied, it may be in the form of indirect moxibustion with a moxa stick, or by large moxa cones placed over a mound of salt, sliced ginger, aconite cake etc.

Shenque REN-8 has two principal actions. Firstly it is an important point to warm and rescue yang in cases of collapse due to extreme cold or sudden and severe exhaustion of yang, for example deficiency type windstroke or shock. Secondly it is able to warm a "deficient cold abdomen", and is indicated for ceaseless diarrhoea, diarrhoea in breast feeding infants, diarrhoea in the elderly and deficient, borborygmus, umbilical pain and prolapse of the rectum due to yang deficiency of the Spleen.

COMBINATIONS
- Borborygmus and diarrhoea: Shenque REN-8, Shuifen REN-9 and Sanjian L.I.-3 (*Great Compendium*).
- Diarrhoea with thin stools: Shenque REN-8, Taichong LIV-3 and Sanyinjiao SP-6 (*Great Compendium*).
- Prolapse of the rectum: Shenque REN-8, Baihui DU-20 and Pangguangshu BL-28 (*Compilation*).
- Umbilical shan disorder: Shenque REN-8, Tianshu ST-25 and Shimen REN-5 (*Supplementing Life*).
- Periumbilical pain: Shenque REN-8, Shuifen REN-9 and Zhongfeng LIV-4 (*Supplementing Life*).
- Periumbilical pain: Shenque REN-8, Shuifen REN-9 and Qihai REN-6 (*Great Compendium*).
- Hypogastric shan disorder: Shenque REN-8, Shimen REN-5, Tianshu ST-25 and Qihai REN-6 (*Thousand Ducat Formulas*).
- Oedema with qi distention and fullness: Shenque REN-8 and Fuliu KID-7 (*Great Compendium*).

SHUIFEN REN-9
Water Separation

水分

LOCATION
On the midline of the abdomen, 1 cun above the umbilicus and 7 cun below the sternocostal angle.

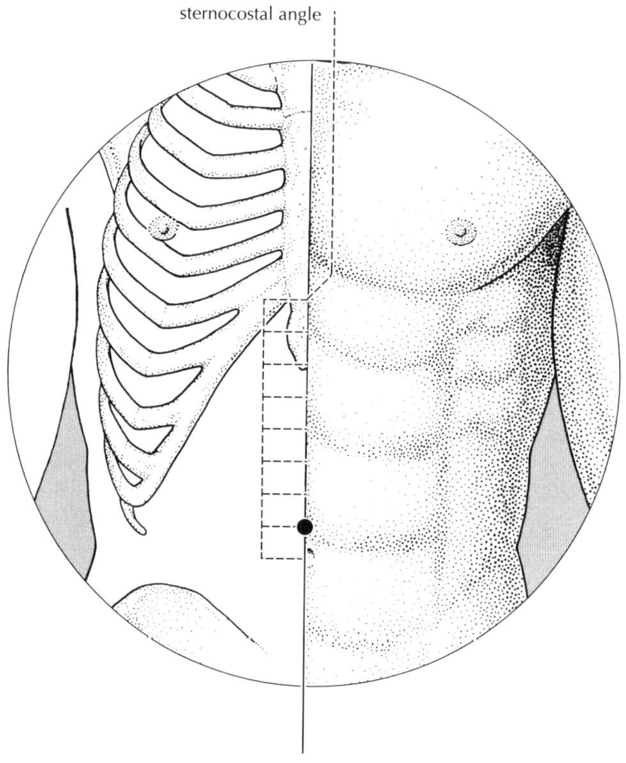

LOCATION NOTE
To locate the sternocostal angle see page 69.

NEEDLING
Perpendicular insertion 0.8 to 1.5 cun. **Note**: according to the *Illustrated Classic of Acupuncture Points on the Bronze Man* and the *Illustrated Supplement to the Classic of Categories*, this point is contraindicated to needling in cases of 'water illness', and plentiful moxibustion should rather

be used. Moxibustion is contraindicated in pregnancy. **Caution:** in thin patients deep needling may penetrate the peritoneal cavity.

ACTIONS

Regulates the water passages and treats oedema
Harmonises the intestines and dispels accumulation

INDICATIONS

- Water diseases, oedema.
- Deficiency and distention of the intestines and Stomach, borborygmus, no pleasure in eating, acid regurgitation, vomiting after eating, sudden turmoil disorder with cramps, abdomen swollen and hard like a drum, periumbilical pain rushing up to the chest and Heart causing difficulty in breathing.
- Nosebleed, failure of the fontanelle to close, tetany, contracted sinews, rigidity of the lumbar spine.

COMMENTARY

As its name implies, Shuifen REN-9 (Water Separation) has a strong action on fluid transformation and distribution and is particularly indicated for oedema. According to the *Great Compendium of Acupuncture and Moxibustion* Shuifen REN-9 is located over the Small Intestine which has the function of 'separating the clear from the turbid' and sending fluids to the Bladder and solid dregs to the Large Intestine for excretion. This Small Intestine function is dominated by the Spleen and Kidneys, and Shuifen REN-9 is particularly indicated for yin oedema due to deficiency of the Spleen and/or Kidneys, especially oedema of the abdominal region. Many early texts specify that in the treatment of oedema this point should be treated by moxibustion rather than needling.

Impairment of the function of the intestines may give rise to severe stagnation and, by blocking its descent, cause rebellion of Stomach qi. Shuifen REN-9 is indicated for distention and pain of the abdomen, drum-like swelling and hardness of the abdomen, periumbilical pain rushing up to the chest and Heart causing difficulty in breathing, loss of appetite, acid regurgitation and vomiting.

The action of Shuifen REN-9 in treating these kinds of accumulation of water, qi and food reflects its ability to harmonise the intestinal region and promote smooth circulation rather than to directly tonify the Spleen or Kidneys.

COMBINATIONS

- Oedema: Shuifen REN-9 and Fuliu KID-7 (*Song of Points*).
- Oedema around the umbilical region: Shuifen REN-9 and Yinlingquan SP-9 (*One Hundred Symptoms*).
- Oedema of the abdomen with drum-like distention: Shuifen REN-9 and Jianli REN-11 [reduce] (*Secrets of the Celestial Star*).
- Spasmodic pain of the hypogastrium: Shuifen REN-9 and Shimen REN-5 (*Thousand Ducat Formulas*).
- Periumbilical pain: Shuifen REN-9, Shenque REN-8 and Qihai REN-6 (*Great Compendium*).
- Periumbilical pain: Shuifen REN-9, Shenque REN-8 and Zhongfeng LIV-4 (*Supplementing Life*).
- Pain of the umbilical region: Shuifen REN-9, Zhongfeng LIV-4 and Ququan LIV-8 (*Great Compendium*).
- No pleasure in eating: Shuifen REN-9, Diji SP-8, Yinlingquan SP-9, Youmen KID-21 and Xiaochangshu BL-27 (*Supplementing Life*).

XIAWAN REN-10

Lower Cavity

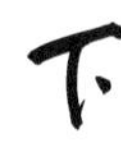
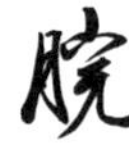

Meeting point of the Conception vessel with the Spleen channel

LOCATION

On the midline of the abdomen, 2 cun above the umbilicus and 6 cun below the sternocostal angle.

LOCATION NOTE

To locate the sternocostal angle see page 69.

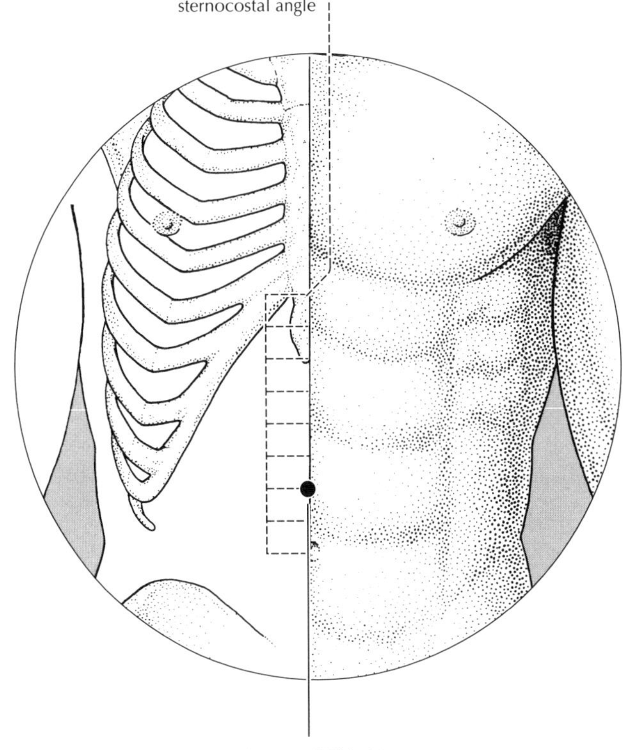

Xiawan REN-10

NEEDLING

Perpendicular insertion 0.8 to 1.5 cun. **Caution:** in thin patients deep needling may penetrate the peritoneal cavity. According to the *Illustrated Supplement to the Classic of Categories*, moxibustion is contraindicated in pregnancy.

ACTIONS

Harmonises the Stomach and regulates qi
Dispels food stagnation

INDICATIONS

- Abdominal fullness, abdominal hardness, epigastric pain, nausea and vomiting after eating, focal distention, undigested food (in the stool), no pleasure in eating, cold qi of the six fu.
- Thready pulse lacking in force, emaciation, dark urine.

COMMENTARY

Xiawan REN-10 (Lower Cavity) is also known as Xiaguan (Lower Controller). This point was traditionally considered to affect the lower portion of the Stomach, whilst Shangwan REN-13 (Upper Cavity) was considered to affect its upper portion. Between these two points lies Zhongwan REN-12 (Middle Cavity). The *Spiritual Pivot*[17] states "When there is difficult ingestion and obstruction in the diaphragm, this indicates the pathogen is in the Stomach. When the disorder is in the upper cavity, then needle Shangwan REN-13 to restrain the rebellion and descend it. When the disorder is in the lower cavity, then needle Xiawan REN-10 to scatter and move it". The *Song More Precious Than Jade* says "when the Stomach is cold, Xiawan REN-10 is excellent" whilst the *Systematic Classic of Acupuncture and Moxibustion* states "Xiawan REN-10 is the main point to use when food and drink are not digested and regurgitated after ingestion".

The principal use of this point is in cases of food stagnation with such symptoms as abdominal fullness, epigastric pain, nausea and vomiting after eating, lack of appetite, and undigested food in the stools.

COMBINATIONS

- Undigested food (in the stool), vomiting immediately after ingestion: first needle Xiawan REN-10 and then reduce Zusanli ST-36 (*Thousand Ducat Formulas*).
- Undigested food (in the stool): Xiawan REN-10, Zusanli ST-36, Liangmen ST-21, Sanyinjiao SP-6, Dachangshu BL-25, Sanjiaoshu BL-22 and Xuanshu DU-5 (*Supplementing Life*).
- Borborygmus: Xiawan REN-10 and Xiangu ST-43 (*One Hundred Symptoms*).
- Hardness of the abdomen: Xiawan REN-10 and Zhongwan REN-12 (*Ode of Spiritual Brightness*).

JIANLI REN-11

Strengthen the Interior

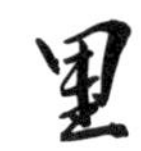

LOCATION

On the midline of the abdomen, 3 cun above the umbilicus and 5 cun below the sternocostal angle.

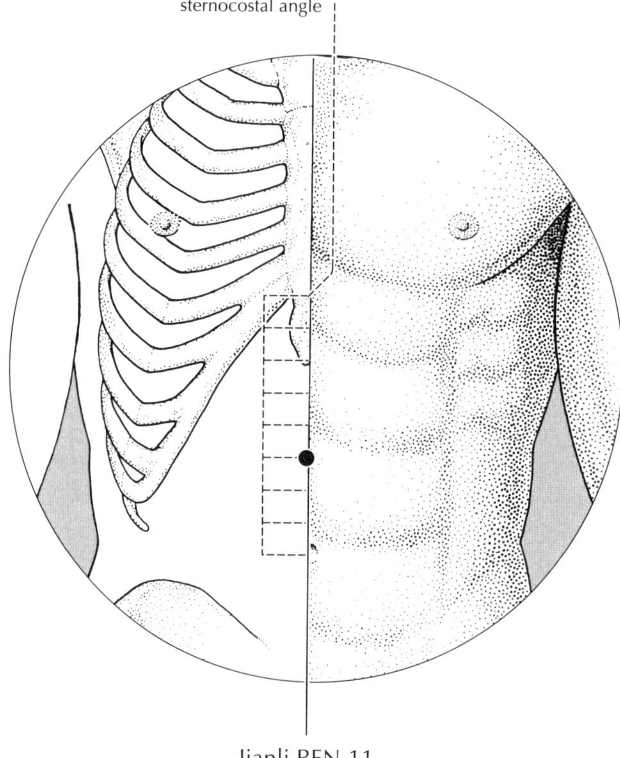

LOCATION NOTE

To locate the sternocostal angle see page 69.

NEEDLING

Perpendicular insertion 0.8 to 1.5 cun.
Caution: in thin patients deep needling may penetrate the peritoneal cavity.

ACTIONS

Harmonises the middle jiao and regulates qi

INDICATIONS

- Abdominal distention, pain of the intestines, vomiting, no pleasure in eating, sudden turmoil disorder, Heart pain, oedema of the body.

COMBINATIONS

- Oppression of the chest: Jianli REN-11 and Neiguan P-6 (*One Hundred Symptoms*).
- Oedema of the abdomen with drum-like distention: Jianli REN-11 (reduce) and Shuifen REN-9 (*Secrets of the Celestial Star*).

ZHONGWAN REN-12

Middle Cavity

中脘

Front-Mu point of the Stomach
Hui-Meeting point of the Fu
Meeting point of the Conception vessel with the Small Intestine, Sanjiao and Stomach channels

LOCATION

On the midline of the abdomen, 4 cun above the umbilicus and midway between the umbilicus and the sternocostal angle.

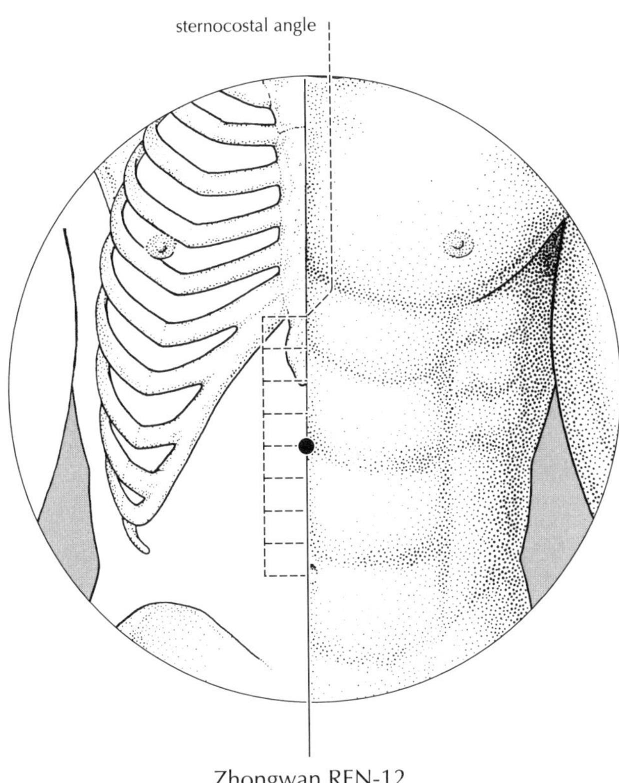

LOCATION NOTE

To locate the sternocostal angle see page 69.

NEEDLING

Perpendicular insertion 0.8 to 1.5 cun.
Caution: in thin patients deep needling may penetrate the peritoneal cavity.

ACTIONS

Harmonises the middle jiao and descends rebellion
Tonifies the Stomach and fortifies the Spleen
Regulates qi and alleviates pain

INDICATIONS

- All diseases of the Stomach and Spleen, interior injury to the Stomach and Spleen, epigastric pain and fullness, difficult ingestion, eats little but is easily full, nausea, Stomach reflux, vomiting, vomiting blood, abdominal distention, severe pain of the abdomen, sudden abdominal fullness, focal distention and fullness, pain of the Spleen, hardness and pain of the lateral costal region.
- Injury by worry, anxiety and overthinking, injury by the seven emotions leading to epigastric pain.
- Diarrhoea, undigested food (in the stool), red and white dysenteric disorder, difficulty in defecation, heat in the Small Intestine, dark urine, sudden turmoil disorder.
- Deficiency-taxation, sallow complexion, post-partum blood dizziness.
- Heart pain, chronic and acute childhood fright wind, loss of consciousness, mania-depression, epilepsy, tongue thrusting.
- Cold body, scorched foul odour in the nose, running piglet qi, warm malaria, dyspnoea.

COMMENTARY

Zhongwan REN-12 (Middle Cavity), also known as Zhongguan (Middle Controller), is the front-mu point of the Stomach and the hui-meeting point of the fu. The term 'mu' means to gather or to collect, and the front-mu points are where the qi of the zangfu gathers on the anterior surface of the body. As the origin of the post-heaven qi, the Stomach and Spleen are considered to play a central role among the zangfu, transforming and distributing the essence of food and drink throughout the body. For this reason, the Stomach may be said to dominate the fu and the Spleen the zang. The close relationship of Zhongwan REN-12 to the Stomach, therefore, is further reflected in its status as the hui-meeting point of the fu, in the same way that Zhangmen LIV-13, the front-mu point of the Spleen, is also the hui-meeting point of the zang.

Zhongwan REN-12 is the principal point on the abdomen to regulate the function of the Stomach. The *Investigation into Points Along the Channels* simply states that Zhongwan REN-12 can treat "all diseases of the Stomach and Spleen". In comparison with neighbouring points such as Liangmen ST-21, Shangwan REN-13 and Xiawan REN-10 which are predominantly indicated in excess patterns, Zhongwan REN-12 is equally applicable in disorders characterised by either excess or deficiency.

The Stomach is the 'sea of water and grain' and its principal functions are to receive food and drink, 'rot and ripen' them and then descend these transformed products. Disorders of the Stomach may be deficient or excess in nature, due to cold or heat, exterior pathogens or interior disharmony. Whatever the aetiology, disharmony of the Stomach will always manifest in disturbance of one or more of these functions. If the Stomach fails to receive food and drink, there will be inability to eat and difficult ingestion; if the Stomach fails to 'rot and ripen' and to descend there will be fullness, distention and pain; if the Stomach qi rebels upwards there will be nausea, vomiting, Stomach reflux and hiccup.

Traditional Chinese methods of health preservation have long recognised the importance of emotional harmony in the smooth functioning of the Stomach. The constant dissipation of qi resulting from worry, anxiety and overthinking may deplete the Stomach and Spleen and impair the function of the Stomach. Excess of any of the seven emotions may result in stagnation of qi which then injures the Stomach leading to epigastric pain. Most injurious of all the emotions are anger, frustration or resentment, particularly if experienced whilst eating. At this time the qi is focused on the Stomach, rendering it particularly susceptible to qi stagnation. In all these cases Zhongwan REN-12 is a primary point. In practice, epigastric pain or distention deriving from Liver qi stagnation may be accompanied by pain or distention of the lateral costal region. Not only is Zhongwan REN-12 indicated for this symptom, but the needling sensation from Zhongwan REN-12 commonly transmits to this area.

The Stomach and Spleen are intimately related. According to the *Treatise on the Spleen and Stomach* by Li Dong-yuan "when Stomach deficiency gives rise to failure of the taiyin to receive [what is naturally due it], the foot yangming mu point [Zhongwan REN-12] will lead it through". This highlights the important secondary action of Zhongwan REN-12 in strengthening the Spleen in cases of deficiency. It is indicated for diarrhoea, undigested food (in the stool), deficiency-taxation, post-partum dizziness and sallow complexion.

Finally Zhongwan REN-12 is cited in the *Song of the Nine Needles for Returning the Yang* for the treatment of collapse of yang characterised by loss of consciousness, aversion to cold, cold counterflow of the limbs, purple lips etc.

COMBINATIONS

- Vomiting: Zhongwan REN-12, Geshu BL-17 and Zhangmen LIV-13 (*Thousand Ducat Formulas*).
- Vomiting clear (watery) saliva: Zhongwan REN-12, Shanzhong REN-17, Daling P-7 and Laogong P-8 (*Great Compendium*).
- Stagnation of food in the mid-abdomen, stabbing pain that does not cease: Zhongwan REN-12, Gongsun SP-4, Jiexi ST-41 and Zusanli ST-36 (*Complete Collection*).
- Abdominal pain: Zhongwan REN-12, Neiguan P-6 and Zusanli ST-36 (*Great Compendium*).
- Hardness of the abdomen: Zhongwan REN-12 and Xiawan REN-10 (*Ode of Spiritual Brightness*).
- Hardness and pain of the lateral costal region: Zhongwan REN-12 and Chengman ST-20 (*Thousand Ducat Formulas*).
- Abdominal masses in the hypogastrium due to qi stagnation and blood stasis that are hard and big like a plate, with epigastric distention and undigested food (in the stool): Zhongwan REN-12 and Sanjiaoshu BL-22 (*Thousand Ducat Formulas*).
- Undigested food (in the stool): Zhongwan REN-12 and Sanyinjiao SP-6 (*Supplementing Life*).
- Ceaseless diarrhoea: Zhongwan REN-12, Tianshu ST-25 and Zhongji REN-3 (*Great Compendium*).
- Blood in the stool: Zhongwan REN-12, Zusanli ST-36 and Qihai REN-6 (*Glorious Anthology*).
- Difficulty in defecation: Zhongwan REN-12, Dazhong KID-4, Zhongliao BL-33, Guanyuan REN-4, Chengjin BL-56, Taichong LIV-3, Chengshan BL-57 and Taixi KID-3 (*Supplementing Life*).
- All phlegm disease, head wind, dyspnoea and cough, all types of tanyin (phlegm-fluid): Zhongwan REN-12 and Fenglong ST-40 (*Outline of Medicine*).
- Dyspnoea with inability to walk: Zhongwan REN-12, Qimen LIV-14 and Shanglian L.I.-9 (*Great Compendium*).
- Jaundice with weakness of the four limbs: Zhongwan REN-12 and Zusanli ST-36 (*Classic of the Jade Dragon*).
- Spleen deficiency jaundice: Zhongwan REN-12 and Wangu SI-4 (*Ode of the Jade Dragon*).

SHANGWAN REN-13

Upper Cavity

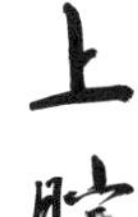

Meeting point of the Conception vessel with the Stomach and Small Intestine channels

LOCATION

On the midline of the abdomen, 5 cun above the umbilicus and 3 cun below the sternocostal angle.

LOCATION NOTE

To locate the sternocostal angle see page 69.

NEEDLING

Perpendicular insertion 0.8 to 1.5 cun.

Caution: in thin patients deep needling may penetrate the peritoneal cavity.

ACTIONS

Harmonises the Stomach and regulates qi
Descends rebellion and alleviates vomiting
Regulates the Heart

INDICATIONS

- Nausea, vomiting, deficiency-taxation vomiting of blood, difficult ingestion, Stomach reflux, sudden turmoil disorder, abdominal pain, abdominal distention and fullness, abdominal (ji ju) masses, pain of the Spleen, undigested food (in the stool), borborygmus.
- Sudden Heart pain, sensation of heat and agitation in the Heart, fright palpitations.
- Heat in the body with absence of sweating, febrile disease, jaundice.
- Wind epilepsy, much phlegm, running piglet qi, visual dizziness.

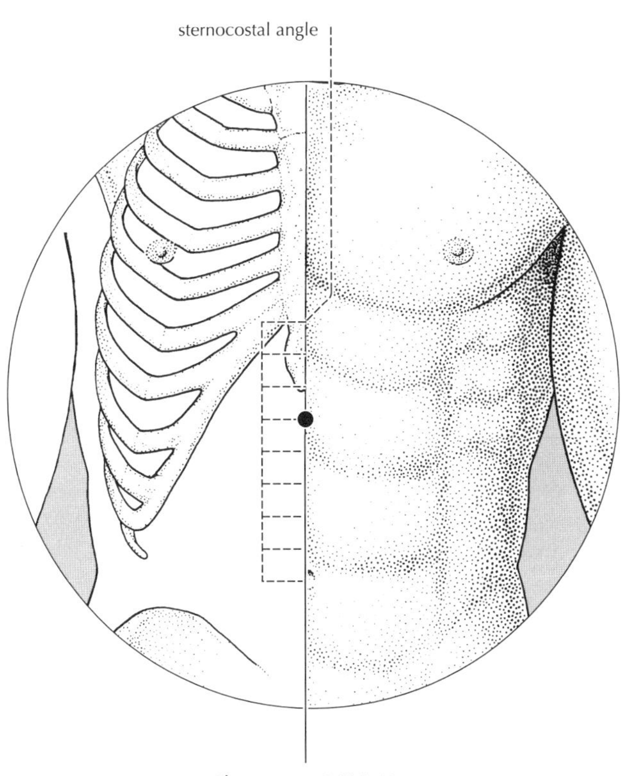

COMMENTARY

Shangwan REN-13 (Upper Cavity) is also known as Shangguan (Upper Controller). This point was traditionally considered to affect the upper portion of the Stomach whilst Xiawan REN-10 (Lower Cavity) was considered to affect its lower portion. Between these two points lies Zhongwan REN-12 (Middle Cavity). The *Spiritual Pivot*[18] states "When there is difficult ingestion and obstruction in the diaphragm, this indicates the pathogen is in the Stomach. When the disorder is in the upper cavity, then needle Shangwan REN-13 to restrain the rebellion and descend it. When the disorder is in the lower cavity, then needle Xiawan REN-10 to scatter and move it". Shangwan REN-13 is indicated for rebellion of Stomach qi manifesting as nausea, vomiting, vomiting of blood and Stomach reflux and for stagnation in the epigastrium and abdomen manifesting as pain, distention, fullness and masses.

The Conception vessel ascends through the middle of the chest, whilst Shangwan REN-13 is a meeting point of the Conception vessel with the Stomach and Small Intestine channels, both of which connect with the Heart via their primary or secondary pathways. Shangwan REN-13 is indicated (and included in classical combinations) for heat, agitation and pain of the Heart and palpitations. In clinical practice however, Juque REN-14, the next point along the channel and the front-mu point of the Heart, is more commonly used for such Heart disorders.

COMBINATIONS

- Vomiting blood and spontaneous external bleeding: Shangwan REN-13, Pishu BL-20, Ganshu BL-18 and Yinbai SP-1 (*Great Compendium*).
- Vomiting blood: Shangwan REN-13, Burong ST-19 and Daling P-7 (*Thousand Ducat Formulas*).
- Vomiting: Shangwan REN-13, Burong ST-19 and Daling P-7 (*Supplementing Life*).
- The nine types of Heart pain: Shangwan REN-13 and Zhongwan REN-12 (*Ode of the Jade Dragon*).
- Unbearable Heart pain: Shangwan REN-13 and Daling P-7 (*Thousand Ducat Formulas*).
- Distention and fullness of the Heart and abdomen: Shangwan REN-13 and Juque REN-14 (*Supplementing Life*).
- Manic rushing around: Shangwan REN-13 and Shenmen HE-7 (*One Hundred Symptoms*).

JUQUE REN-14

Great Gateway

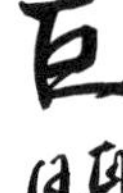
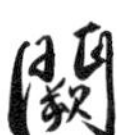

Front-Mu point of the Heart

LOCATION

On the midline of the abdomen, 6 cun above the umbilicus and 2 cun below the sternocostal angle.

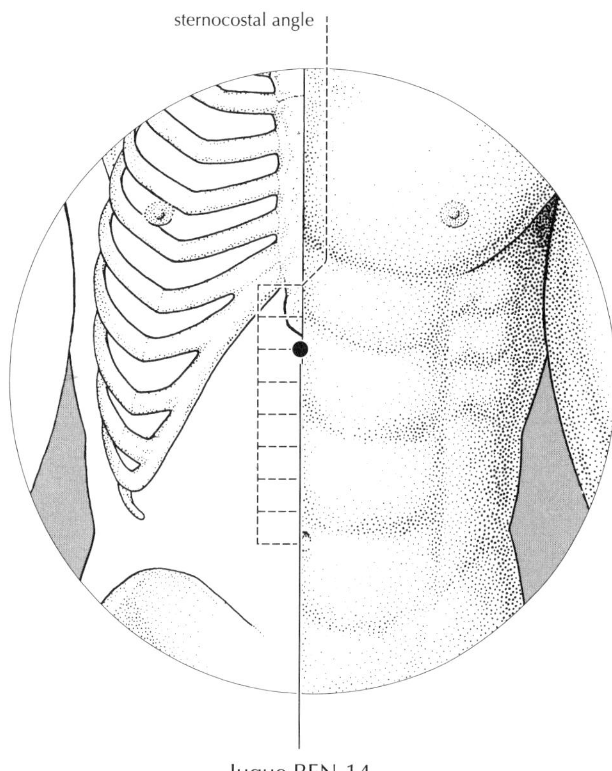

LOCATION NOTE

i. In some patients the xiphoid process may extend to this point; ii. To locate the sternocostal angle see page 69.

NEEDLING

Perpendicular insertion 0.5 to 1 cun, or oblique insertion directed inferiorly 1 to 1.5 cun.

Caution: i. deep insertion, especially in thin subjects, may damage the left lobe of the liver or the heart if either is enlarged, ii. oblique superior insertion towards the heart is contraindicated in all cases.

ACTIONS

Regulates the Heart and alleviates pain
Descends Lung qi and unbinds the chest
Transforms phlegm and calms the spirit
Harmonises the Stomach and descends rebellion

INDICATIONS

- Heart pain, sudden Heart pain, Heart pain due to cold, injury by cold leading to agitation of the Heart, pain of the chest radiating to the back, chest pain radiating to the lateral costal region, accumulation of phlegm in the chest, rebellious qi, cough, fullness of the chest with shortness of breath, spitting blood.
- Mania-disorder, mania-depression, aversion to fire, tendency to curse and scold others, ranting and raving, anger, disorientation, loss of consciousness, epilepsy with vomiting of foam, fright palpitations, poor memory, agitation and heat.
- Sudden turmoil disorder, abdominal distention, sudden abdominal pain, focal distention, oesophageal constriction, nausea, vomiting, Stomach reflux, acid regurgitation, obstruction of the diaphragm, jaundice, acute jaundice, shan disorder, distention and fullness of the lower abdomen, pain due to roundworms.
- Mutual overacting of the five phases, diminished qi, febrile disease, clonic spasm.

COMMENTARY

According to the *Essential Questions* the front-mu points are where the qi of the zangfu gathers and concentrates, and Juque REN-14, the front-mu point of the Heart, is indicated for disorders both of the Heart zang and of the spirit. The *Introduction to Medicine* by Li Ting of the Ming dynasty states that Juque REN-14 treats the "nine types of Heart pain". According to the principles "without movement there is pain" and "where there is malnourishment there is pain", Heart pain always involves either stagnation of qi and blood or deficiency of qi, blood, yin or yang. In clinical practice such excess and deficiency patterns often combine, and even when the manifestation is excess (for example blood stasis or obstruction of blood by phlegm), the root may involve deficiency. Whatever the aetiology or pattern, as the front-mu point of the Heart Juque REN-14 is the principal local point for these disorders, particularly, according to many classical sources, when cold attacks the Heart. It is also indicated for chest pain, especially when it radiates to the back, a symptom of what is known as chest painful obstruction. This disorder, characterised by stasis of phlegm and blood and impaired circulation of yang qi, may also disrupt the function of the Lung resulting in cough and shortness of breath.

Any disharmony of the Heart may give rise to disturbance of the spirit, but the most serious occurs when phlegm obscures the portals of the Heart. In the context of the traditional indications for Juque REN-14, when phlegm alone predominates there may be poor memory, disorientation, loss of consciousness or epilepsy with vomiting of foam, whilst if phlegm combines with heat there will be various manifestations of mania disorder such as ranting and raving, great anger and fury, a tendency to curse and scold others etc. Alternatively, if i. Heart blood is deficient, ii. blood stasis hinders the proper nourishment of the Heart by fresh blood, or iii. either Heart yin deficiency or the transformation of blood stasis generate heat which agitates the spirit, there may be anxiety, palpitations and a nervous, agitated sensation in the pit of the epigastrium (below the Heart). Juque REN-14 is the principal local point for the treatment of these disorders.

The main pathway of the Conception vessel ascends from the perineum to the region of the mouth. Notwithstanding this upward movement of the channel, the points of the Conception vessel on the chest and abdomen have a strong action on descending qi, especially of the Lung and Stomach. This downward movement is reflected in the qigong 'small heavenly circuit' practice which ascends the qi through the Governing vessel and descends it through the Conception vessel. Located in the region between the Lung and Stomach, Juque REN-14 has a strong action on subduing rebellious qi in these two zangfu.

As far as the Lung is concerned, Juque REN-14 is indicated for rebellious qi manifesting as cough and fullness of the chest with shortness of breath. As for the Stomach, Juque REN-14 is able to regulate rebellion of qi manifesting as nausea, Stomach reflux, vomiting and acid regurgitation, and stagnation of qi giving rise to abdominal distention, oesophageal constriction, focal distention and obstruction of the diaphragm.

Finally the *Great Compendium of Acupuncture and Moxibustion recommends* Juque REN-14 for mutual overacting of the five phases. This extremely broad indication is usually interpreted as a reflection of the status of the Heart, of which Juque REN-14 is the front-mu point, as the sovereign ruler of all the zangfu.

COMBINATIONS

- Agitation of the Heart: Juque REN-14 and Xinshu BL-15 (*Supplementing Life*).
- Agitation and fullness of the Heart: Juque REN-14 and Yindu KID-19 (*Supplementing Life*).
- Distention and fullness of the Heart and abdomen: Juque REN-14 and Shangwan REN-13 (*Supplementing Life*).
- Fright palpitations with diminished qi: Juque REN-14, Shenmen HE-7 and Ligou LIV-5 (*Supplementing Life*).
- Heart disorientation: Juque REN-14, Tianjing SJ-10 and Xinshu BL-15 (*Great Compendium*).
- Mania disorder, raving, fury and cursing: Juque REN-14 and Zhubin KID-9 (*Thousand Ducat Formulas*).
- Rebellion of qi with cough, fullness of the chest and shortness of breath with pain that radiates to the back: 50 moxa cones each on Juque REN-14 and Qimen LIV-14 (*Thousand Ducat Formulas*).
- Cough: Juque REN-14, Shanzhong REN-17 and Quepen ST-12 (*Thousand Ducat Formulas*).
- Vomiting with fullness of the chest: Juque REN-14, Shufu KID-27, Shencang KID-25 and Lingxu KID-24 (*Thousand Ducat Formulas*).
- Sudden turmoil disorder: Juque REN-14, Guanchong SJ-1, Zhigou SJ-6, Gongsun SP-4 and Jiexi ST-41 (*Systematic Classic*).
- Pain of the diaphragm from accumulation of fluid that is difficult to endure: Juque REN-14 and Shanzhong REN-17 (*One Hundred Symptoms*).

JIUWEI REN-15

Turtledove Tail

鳩尾

Luo-Connecting point of the Conception vessel

LOCATION

On the midline of the abdomen, 7 cun above the umbilicus and 1 cun below the sternocostal angle.

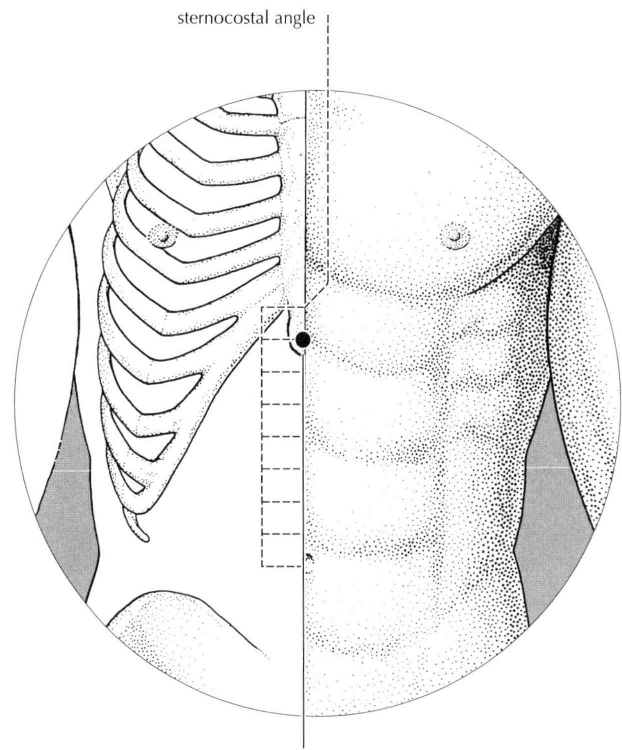

LOCATION NOTE

i. Many sources locate this point below the xiphoid process. In practice however, the xiphoid process varies considerably in length, and this point may lie on the xiphoid process itself; ii. To locate the sternocostal angle see page 69.

NEEDLING

Oblique insertion directed inferiorly 0.5 to 1 cun. **Note:** according to several classical texts, this point is contraindicated to moxibustion.

Caution: i. deep insertion, especially in thin subjects, may damage the left lobe of the liver or the heart if either is enlarged, ii. oblique superior insertion towards the heart is contraindicated in all cases.

ACTIONS

Regulates the Heart and calms the spirit
Descends Lung qi and unbinds the chest

INDICATIONS

- The five types of epilepsy, mania, mad walking, mad singing, aversion to the sound of people talking, fright palpitations.
- Oppressive sensation in the Heart, chest pain, excessive sighing, pain radiating from the Heart to the back.
- Pain of the skin of the abdomen, itching of the skin of the abdomen.
- Wheezing, dyspnoea, fullness of the chest, cough, coughing blood, diminished qi, rattling sound in the throat, throat painful obstruction, swelling of the throat.
- Difficult ingestion, Stomach reflux, prolapse of the rectum, febrile disease, one-sided headache extending to the outer canthus, excessive sexual activity leading to exhaustion in youths.

COMMENTARY

Jiuwei REN-15 is the luo-connecting point of the Conception vessel, from where the qi of this channel disperses and spreads down over the abdomen. The name of Jiuwei REN-15 (Turtledove Tail) reflects the shape of the xiphoid process, likened to the tail of a dove, with the ribs forming the wings. In fact, historically there has been some discussion as to whether Huiyin REN-1, rather than Jiuwei REN-15, is the luo-connecting point of the Conception vessel. The *Spiritual Pivot*[19] refers to the luo-connecting point of the Conception vessel as Weiyi (Tail Screen), an alternative name for Jiuwei REN-15, and gives symptoms of excess (pain of the skin of the abdomen) and deficiency (itching of the skin of the abdomen). Later classics, however, including both the *Systematic Classic of Acupuncture and Moxibustion* and the *Great Compendium of Acupuncture and Moxibustion* refer to the luo-connecting point of the Conception vessel as Pingyi (Flat Screen), an alternative name for Huiyin REN-1, and ascribe these symptoms of excess and deficiency to that point. Huiyin REN-1 rather than Jiuwei REN-15 as the luo-connecting point of the Conception vessel would reflect a neat symmetry with Chengqiang DU-1 as the luo-connecting point of the Governing vessel.

Like Juque REN-14, the front-mu point of the Heart, Jiuwei REN-15 has a powerful action on calming the spirit in cases of phlegm obscuring the Heart (epilepsy, mania disorder, mad singing and walking and aversion to the sound of people talking), as well as regulating stagnation of qi and blood in the Heart region giving rise to oppression and pain. Also like Juque REN-14, Jiuwei REN-15 is able to regulate and descend Lung qi in cases of wheezing, cough, dyspnoea etc.

In the *Spiritual Pivot*[20] Jiuwei REN-15 is listed as the yuan point of the 'gao'. This term, the same gao as in Gaohuangshu BL-43, refers to the area below the Heart, whilst 'huang' refers to the area above the diaphragm. It is said that when a disease enters the gaohuang it is difficult to cure. *Master Zuo-jiu's Tradition of the Spring and Autumn Annals*[21], one of the earliest textual references to acupuncture, describes how when the Prince of Jin was gravely ill, he sent for the famous Doctor Yi Huan. After examining the patient, Doctor Huan declared that the disease had settled in the gaohuang region (between the Heart and the diaphragm) and hence "it cannot be purged, it cannot be reached [by needling], herbs will not penetrate it, there is nothing to be done". Despite the statement by the *Spiritual Pivot* which implies that the gao originates at Jiuwei REN-15, this point is not normally understood to treat deep and chronic deficiency diseases, the only relevant indications being 'diminished qi' and 'excessive sexual activity leading to exhaustion in youths'.

COMBINATIONS

- The five types of epilepsy: Jiuwei REN-15, Houxi SI-3 and Shenmen HE-7 (*Song More Precious Than Jade*).
- Coughing and spitting blood: Jiuwei REN-15, Ganshu BL-18, Quepen ST-12, Xinshu BL-15 and Juque REN-14 (*Supplementing Life*).
- Prolapse of the rectum in children: moxa Jiuwei REN-15 and Baihui DU-20 (*Ode of Xi-hong*).
- Prolapse of the rectum: Jiuwei REN-15 and Baihui DU-20 (*One Hundred Symptoms*).
- Dysenteric disorder: Jiuwei REN-15 and Baihui DU-20 (*Ode of Spiritual Brightness*).
- Febrile disease with one-sided headache: Jiuwei REN-15 and Xuanli GB-6 (*Thousand Ducat Formulas*).

ZHONGTING REN-16

中庭

Central Courtyard

LOCATION

On the midline of the sternum at the sternocostal angle.

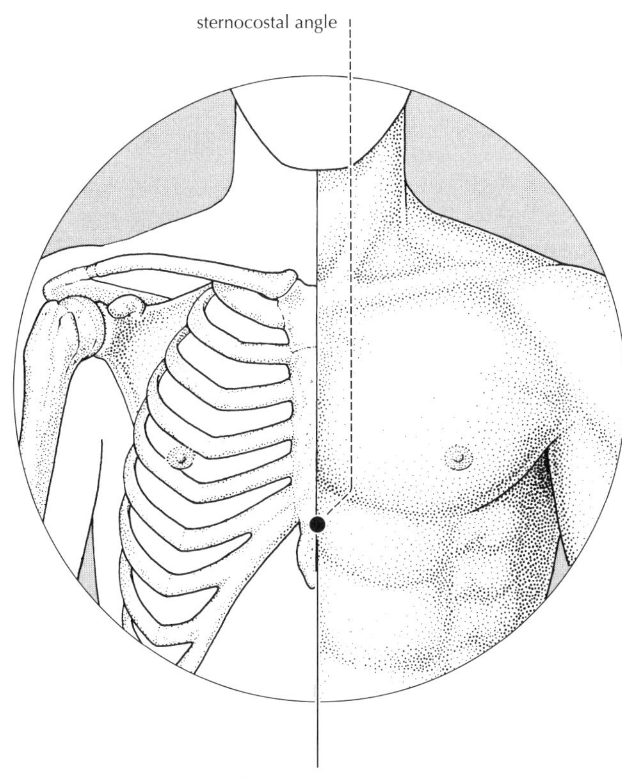

Zhongting REN-16

LOCATION NOTE

i. To locate the sternocostal angle see page 69; ii. This point is level with the fifth intercostal space at the mamillary line.

NEEDLING

Transverse insertion, directed superiorly or inferiorly along the midline, 0.5 cun.

ACTIONS

Unbinds the chest

Regulates the Stomach and descends rebellion

INDICATIONS

- Fullness of the chest and lateral costal region, oesophageal constriction, difficult ingestion, vomiting after eating, vomiting of breast milk in infants, cold and pain of the umbilicus.

COMBINATIONS

- Vomiting: Zhongting REN-16, Shufu KID-27 and Yishe BL-49 (*Supplementing Life*).
- Oesophageal constriction, with difficult ingestion and vomiting: Zhongting REN-16 and Zhongfu LU-1 (*Thousand Ducat Formulas*).
- Difficult ingestion: Zhongting REN-16, Zigong REN-19 and Danshu BL-19 (*Thousand Ducat Formulas*).

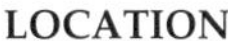

SHANZHONG REN-17

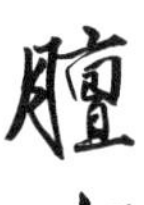
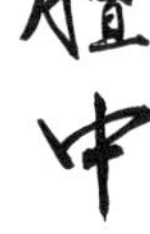

Chest Centre

Front-Mu point of the Pericardium
Hui-Meeting point of the Qi
Point of the Sea of Qi
Meeting point of the Conception vessel with the Spleen, Kidney, Small Intestine and Sanjiao channels

LOCATION

On the midline of the sternum, in a depression level with the junction of the fourth intercostal space and the sternum.

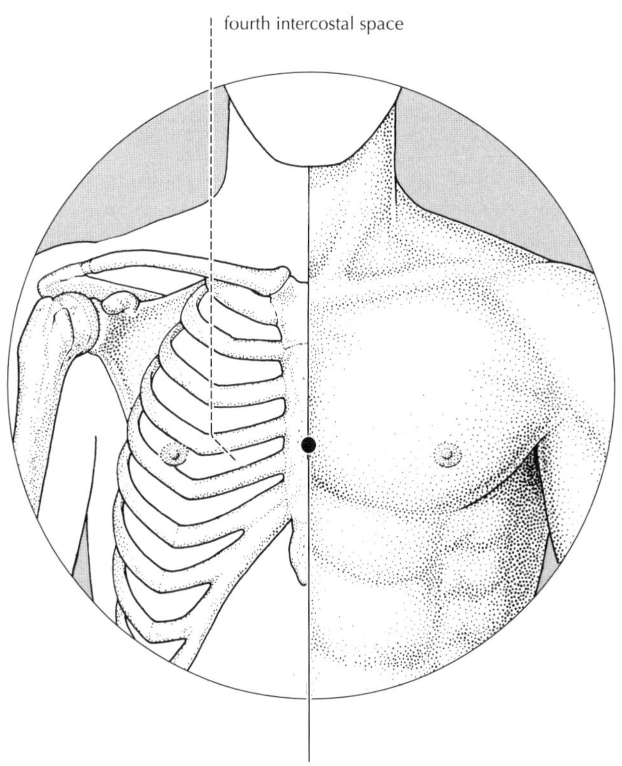

Shanzhong REN-17

LOCATION NOTE

i. First locate the costal cartilage of the second rib which is level with the sternal angle, then locate the second intercostal space below it and count down to the fourth space; ii. This point can be located directly between the nipples in men.

NEEDLING

i. Transverse insertion directed superiorly or inferiorly along the channel 0.5 to 1 cun; ii. Transverse insertion directed laterally towards the breasts, 1 to 1.5 cun, for breast disorders. **Note**: according to several classical texts, this point is contraindicated to needling.

ACTIONS

Regulates qi and unbinds the chest
Descends rebellion of the Lung and Stomach
Benefits gathering qi
Benefits the breasts and promotes lactation

INDICATIONS

- Shortness of breath with rebellious qi, inability to speak, dyspnoea, wheezing, rattling sound in the throat, cough, asthma, fullness and oppression of the chest and diaphragm, obstruction of the chest, pain of the chest and Heart, coughing blood, chest painful obstruction, Lung abscess with purulent coughing.
- Difficult ingestion, acid regurgitation, oesophageal constriction, vomiting of foamy (watery) saliva.
- Insufficient lactation, breast abscess, distention and pain of the breast.
- Goitre, wind painful obstruction, loss of consciousness.

COMMENTARY

Shanzhong REN-17 is also known as Shangqihai (Upper Sea of Qi) and Danzhong (another name for the Pericardium). These alternative names reflect the status of Shanzhong REN-17 as both the hui-meeting point of qi and the front-mu point of the Pericardium. The term 'mu' means to gather or to collect, and the front-mu points are where the qi of the zangfu gathers and concentrates on the anterior surface of the body.

According to the *Spiritual Pivot*[22] Shanzhong REN-17 is the 'sea of qi' (linking with Dazhui DU-14, Yamen DU-15 and Renying ST-9). This passage states "When the sea of qi is in excess there is fullness in the chest, urgent breathing and a red complexion. When the sea of qi is deficient, there is scanty energy insufficient for speech". These indications reflect the ability of Shanzhong REN-17 to regulate qi in the chest, as well as to treat breathlessness with inability to speak.

The *Spiritual Pivot*[23] says that the gathering qi accumulates in the 'upper sea', with its lower pathway flowing down to Qichong ST-30 and its upper pathway entering the respiratory passages. Located in the centre of the chest, Shanzhong REN-17 has a strong effect on the gathering qi which in turn oversees both the Lung functions of dominating qi and controlling respiration and speech, and the Heart function of governing the blood and blood vessels. According to the *Illustrated Supplement to The Classic of Categories*[24] Shanzhong REN-17 can treat "all types of uprising qi and dyspnoea". When the Lung fails to descend qi and control respiration, whether due to attack by exterior pathogens or to interior disharmony, there will be various manifestations of accumulation or rebellion of qi such as cough, dyspnoea, wheezing, asthma and fullness and oppression of the chest. Shanzhong REN-17 is an important local point to relieve such accumulation of qi in the chest and to descend rebellion of Lung qi. When the gathering qi is deficient, then both Lung and Heart qi will be deficient. In the Lung there will be shortness of breath, whilst if the Heart qi fails to move the blood and the blood vessels in the chest, there will be chest painful obstruction and pain of the Heart and chest with fullness and oppression. Shanzhong REN-17 is one of the primary points to regulate the gathering qi.

The action of Shanzhong REN-17 on descending rebellion of qi extends to the middle jiao, and it is able to restore harmony to the Stomach in cases of difficult ingestion, acid regurgitation, oesophageal constriction and vomiting.

Located midway between the breasts, Shanzhong REN-17 is a principal point in the treatment of insufficient lactation. According to *Observations of Women* by Zhang Jing-yue "Qi and blood in the Conception and Penetrating vessels in women transforms into menstrual blood when it descends, and into milk when it ascends; delayed or insufficient production of milk after delivery is due to deficiency of qi and blood", whilst the book *Literati's Care of Parents* states "Sobbing, crying, grief, anger or depression lead to obstruction of the milk passage". These two quotations illustrate the two main patterns underlying insufficient lactation, namely i. deficiency of qi, and ii. blood and qi stagnation. In either case, Shanzhong REN-17 may be used in combination with other suitable points, and is frequently found in combination with Shaoze SI-1 in classical combinations. Similarly, Shanzhong REN-17 is often used clinically in the treatment of distention and pain of the breast and breast abscess. Where any of these breast disorders is unilateral, the needle at Shanzhong REN-17 may be directed towards the affected side to induce qi sensation into the breast, whilst if the disorder is bilateral, the needle may be directed first to one side and then to the other.

COMBINATIONS

- Dyspnoea and cough: Shanzhong REN-17 and Tiantu REN-22 (*Ode of the Jade Dragon*).
- Cough: Shanzhong REN-17, Quepen ST-12 and Juque REN-14 (*Thousand Ducat Formulas*).
- Rebellious qi cough: Shanzhong REN-17, Tianchi P-1, Tiantu REN-22, Jiexi ST-41 and Jianzhongshu SI-15 (*Supplementing Life*).
- Asthma, inability to sleep at night and agitated mind: Shanzhong REN-17 and Tiantu REN-22 (*Song of the Jade Dragon*).
- Shortness of breath and difficulty catching the breath with inability to speak: Shanzhong REN-17 and Huagai REN-20 (*Thousand Ducat Formulas*).
- Abdominal fullness, shortness of breath with a rattling sound: moxa Shanzhong REN-17, Zhongfu LU-1 and Shenque REN-8 (*Thousand Ducat Formulas*).
- Chest painful obstruction, Heart pain and fullness of the Heart and abdomen: Shanzhong REN-17 and Tianjing SJ-10 (*Supplementing Life*).
- Pain of the diaphragm from accumulation of fluid that is difficult to endure: Shanzhong REN-17 and Juque REN-14 (*One Hundred Symptoms*).
- Vomiting phlegm and watery saliva, dizziness that does not cease: Shanzhong REN-17, Yangxi L.I.-5, Gongsun SP-4 and Fenglong ST-40 (*Complete Collection*).
- Vomiting clear (watery) saliva: Shanzhong REN-17, Zhongwan REN-12, Daling P-7 and Laogong P-8 (*Great Compendium*).
- Absence of lactation: moxa Shanzhong REN-17 and reinforce Shaoze SI-1 (*Great Compendium*).
- Absence of lactation: Shanzhong REN-17, Shaoze SI-1 and Hegu L.I.-4 (*Great Compendium*).

YUTANG REN-18

Jade Hall

玉堂

LOCATION

On the midline of the sternum, level with the junction of the third intercostal space and the sternum.

LOCATION NOTE

First locate the costal cartilage of the second rib which is level with the sternal angle, then locate the second intercostal space below it and count down to the third space.

NEEDLING

Transverse insertion directed superiorly or inferiorly along the channel, 0.5 to 1 cun.

ACTIONS

Unbinds the chest

Regulates and descends qi

INDICATIONS

- Pain of the chest and sternum, agitation with cough, uprising qi, fullness of the chest with difficulty in breathing, wheezing and dyspnoea, cold phlegm.
- Vomiting, difficult ingestion.
- Throat painful obstruction, swelling of the throat, swelling and pain of the breasts, pain of the lateral costal region.

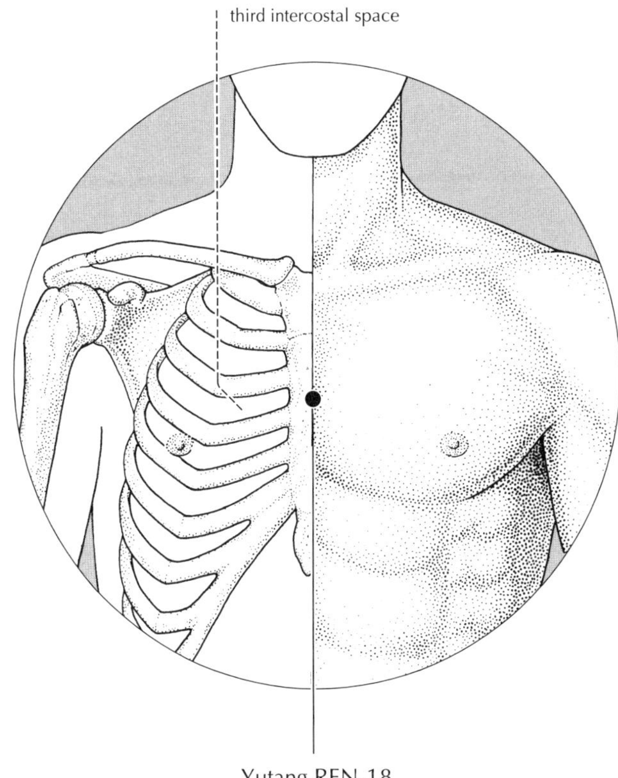

COMBINATIONS

- Cough with rebellious qi and agitation: Yutang REN-18, Zigong REN-19 and Taixi KID-3 (*Thousand Ducat Formulas*).
- Agitation of the Heart and vomiting: Yutang REN-18 and Youmen KID-21 (*One Hundred Symptoms*).
- Bone pain: Yutang REN-18, Zigong REN-19 and Geshu BL-17 (*Supplementing Life*).

ZIGONG REN-19

紫宮

Purple Palace

LOCATION

On the midline of the sternum, level with the junction of the second intercostal space and the sternum.

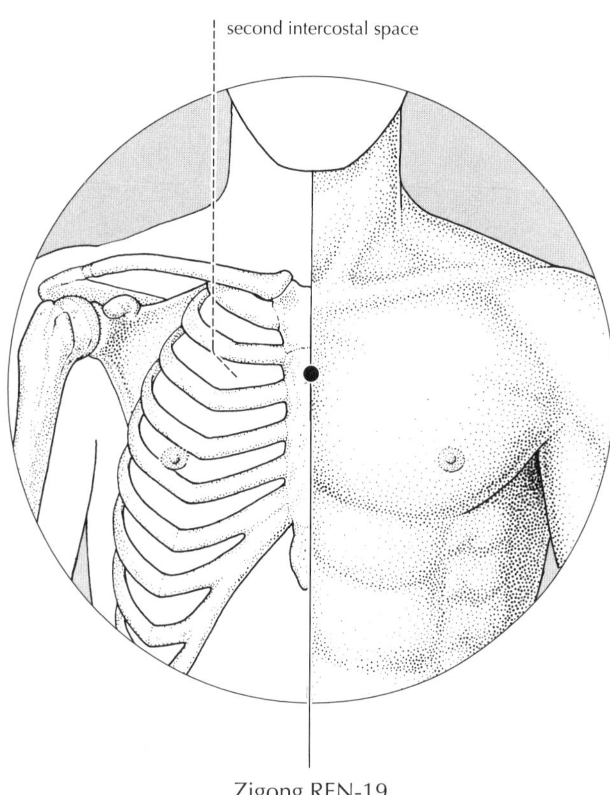

LOCATION NOTE

Locate the costal cartilage of the second rib which is level with the sternal angle, then locate the second intercostal space below it.

NEEDLING

Transverse insertion directed superiorly or inferiorly along the channel, 0.5 to 1 cun.

ACTIONS

Unbinds the chest
Regulates and descends qi

INDICATIONS

- Pain of the chest, pain of the sternum, cough, coughing blood, saliva like white glue.
- Vomiting with uprising qi, difficult ingestion, agitation, painful obstruction, bone pain.

COMBINATIONS

- Cough with rebellious qi and agitation: Zigong REN-19, Yutang REN-18 and Taixi KID-3 (*Thousand Ducat Formulas*).
- Difficult ingestion: Zigong REN-19, Zhongting REN-16 and Danshu BL-19 (*Thousand Ducat Formulas*).
- Bone pain: Zigong REN-19, Yutang REN-18 and Geshu BL-17 (*Supplementing Life*).

HUAGAI REN-20

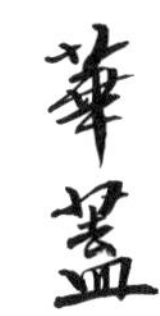

Magnificent Canopy

LOCATION

On the midline of the sternum, level with the junction of the first intercostal space and the sternum.

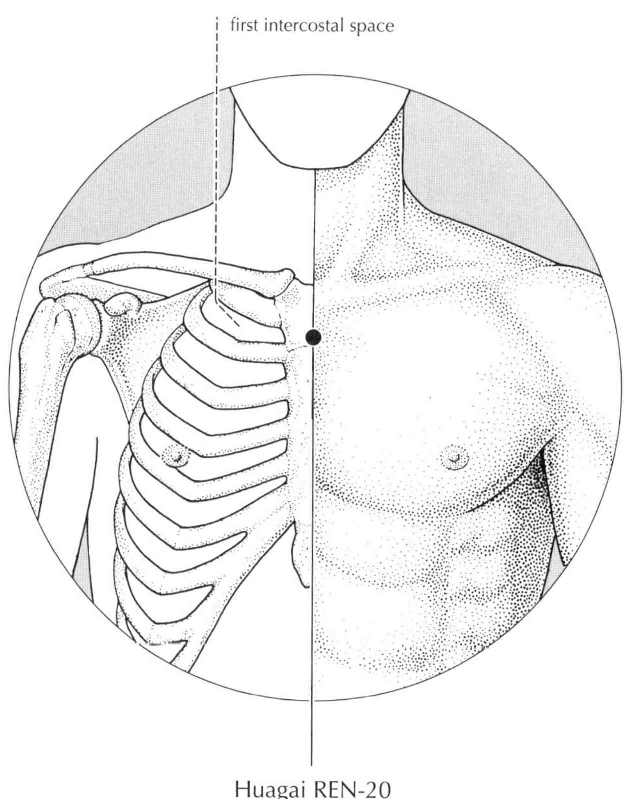

LOCATION NOTE

First locate the costal cartilage of the second rib which is level with the sternal angle, then locate the first intercostal space above it.

NEEDLING

Transverse insertion directed superiorly or inferiorly along the channel, 0.5 to 1 cun.

ACTIONS

Unbinds the chest
Regulates and descends qi

INDICATIONS

- Dyspnoea, wheezing, asthma, cough, rebellious qi, dyspnoea with inability to speak, pain and fullness of the chest and lateral costal region.
- Difficult ingestion.

COMBINATIONS

- Shortness of breath and difficulty catching the breath with inability to speak: Huagai REN-20 and Shanzhong REN-17 (*Thousand Ducat Formulas*).
- Chronic pain of the lateral costal region: Huagai REN-20 and Qihu ST-13 (*One Hundred Symptoms*).

XUANJI REN-21

Jade Pivot

璇璣

LOCATION

On the midline of the manubrium of the sternum, midway between Huagai REN-20 and Tiantu REN-22.

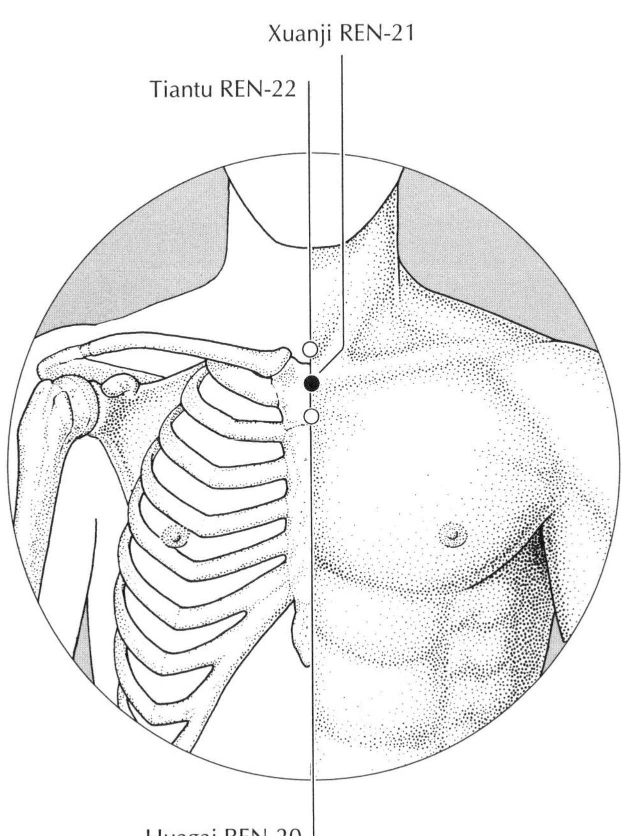

NEEDLING

Transverse insertion directed inferiorly, 0.5 to 1 cun.

ACTIONS

Descends Stomach qi and dispels food accumulation
Unbinds the chest and descends Lung qi
Benefits the throat

INDICATIONS

- Accumulation in the Stomach, difficult ingestion.
- Pain and fullness of the chest and lateral costal region, cough, rebellious qi, wheezing, dyspnoea with inability to speak.
- Rattling sound in the throat, throat painful obstruction.

COMMENTARY

The combination of Xuanji REN-21 and Zusanli ST-36 has long been considered pre-eminent for treating accumulation of food in the Stomach. Whilst Xuanji REN-21 shares with many points of the Conception vessel the ability to regulate the Stomach, it is interesting to note the statement in the *Ode to Elucidate Mysteries*, "Heaven, earth and man are the three powers. Baihui DU-20 ... echoes heaven, Xuanji REN-21 ... echoes man and Yongquan KID-1 ... echoes the earth". When this threefold division is applied to the body, heaven corresponds to the upper jiao which absorbs the heavenly qi, earth corresponds to the lower jiao and especially the Kidneys, whilst 'man', lying in-between heaven and earth, corresponds to the middle jiao and hence the Stomach.

The strong descending action of this point extends also to the Lung and it is indicated for rebellion of Lung qi giving rise to cough, wheezing and dyspnoea.

COMBINATIONS

- Internal injury by accumulation of food in the Stomach: Xuanji REN-21 and Zusanli ST-36 (*Miscellaneous Diseases*).
- Accumulation in the Stomach: Xuanji REN-21 and Zusanli ST-36 (*Ode of Xi-hong*).
- Obstruction of food in the Stomach: Xuanji REN-21 and Zusanli ST-36 (*Heavenly Star Points*).
- Distressed, rapid dyspnoea: Xuanji REN-21 and Qihai REN-6 (*Ode of the Jade Dragon*).
- Fullness of the chest with stiffness of the neck: Xuanji REN-21 and Shencang KID-25 (*One Hundred Symptoms*).

TIANTU REN-22
Heavenly Prominence

天突

Meeting point of the Conception and Yin Linking vessels
Point of the Window of Heaven

LOCATION

On the midline, in the centre of the suprasternal fossa, 0.5 cun superior to the suprasternal notch.

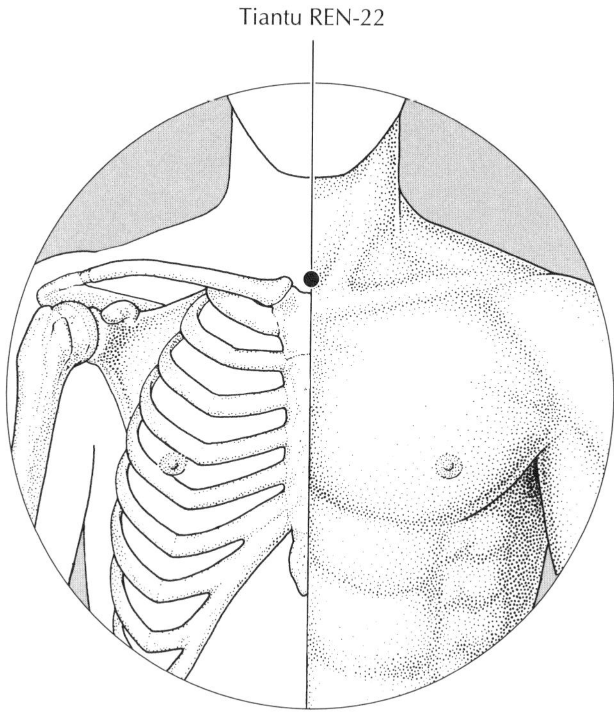

NEEDLING

i. Perpendicular insertion 0.3 cun; ii. With the neck extended (remove head pillow), needle first perpendicularly 0.2 to 0.3 cun, then direct the needle inferiorly along the posterior border of the manubrium of the sternum 0.5 to 1 cun.
Caution: this second method should not be attempted by practitioners without clinical experience under supervision.

ACTIONS

Descends rebellious qi and alleviates cough and wheezing
Benefits the throat and voice

INDICATIONS

- Obstruction in the chest, fullness of the chest, obstruction of qi with Heart pain, pain of the Heart and back, rebellious qi with cough, asthma, sudden dyspnoea, inability to breathe, abscess of the Lung with purulent bloody coughing.
- Rattling sound in the throat, accumulation of phlegm in the throat, plumstone qi, ulceration of the throat which prevents eating, swelling of the throat, cold sensation of the throat, dry throat, much spittle, throat painful obstruction, cracked voice, sudden loss of voice, inability to speak, swelling of the neck, goitre.
- Oesophageal constriction, vomiting, jaundice.
- Purple-green veins beneath the tongue, nosebleed, heat sensation of the skin of the face, red face, swelling of the back of the neck and shoulder, chills and fever, heat sensation of the skin of the abdomen, urticaria, numbness of the flesh of the body.

COMMENTARY

In common with many points of the Conception vessel, Tiantu REN-22 has a strong action on descending qi. Located in-between the lungs and below the throat, its principal application is in the treatment of a wide variety of disorders affecting these two areas.

Tiantu REN-22 has long been recognised as an important point to treat Lung disorders, for example the *Essential Questions*[25] recommended it for rebellious qi, inability to breathe and shortness of breath. Like other points situated in the uppermost portion of the chest (for example Zhongfu LU-1), Tiantu REN-22 is principally used to treat excess patterns characterised by upward rebellion of Lung qi, including cough, asthma, sudden dyspnoea, inability to breathe and Lung abscess with purulent bloody coughing.

As far as throat disorders are concerned, Tiantu REN-22 may be used in virtually any clinical situation, ranging from dryness, cold sensation, swelling and pain, to plumstone qi and severe ulceration which prevents eating. It is also an important point for disorders of the voice including cracked voice, loss of voice and inability to speak. In modern clinical practice, the most common application of this point is in the treatment of wheezing and asthma, especially when accompanied by accumulation of phlegm in the throat.

Tiantu REN-22 is a meeting point of the Conception vessel with the Yin Linking vessel. The Yin Linking vessel ascends through the chest region and according to the *Classic of Difficulties*[26] "when the Yin Linking vessel alone is diseased it will cause Heart pain". Tiantu REN-22 is specifically indicated for obstruction of qi with Heart pain and pain of the Heart and the back.

Finally, Tiantu REN-22 is one of ten points listed in Chapter 2 of the *Spiritual Pivot* that have come to be known as Window of Heaven points (for a fuller discussion see page 48). It illustrates many of the characteristic actions of these points in its ability to treat goitre, rebellious qi of the Lung and Stomach and sudden onset of disorders (sudden loss of voice).

COMBINATIONS
- Rebellious qi cough: Tiantu REN-22, Shanzhong REN-17, Tianchi P-1, Jiexi ST-41 and Jianzhongshu SI-15 (*Supplementing Life*).
- Asthma, inability to sleep at night and agitated mind: Tiantu REN-22 and Shanzhong REN-17 (*Song of the Jade Dragon*).
- Dyspnoea and cough: Shanzhong REN-17 and Tiantu REN-22 (*Ode of the Jade Dragon*).
- Cough that reaches the voice (hoarse voice): Tiantu REN-22 and Feishu BL-13 (*One Hundred Symptoms*).
- Loss of voice: Tiantu REN-22, Lingdao HE-4, Yingu KID-10, Fuliu KID-7, Fenglong ST-40 and Rangu KID-2 (*Illustrated Supplement*).
- Sudden loss of voice with lockjaw: Tiantu REN-22, Lingdao HE-4 and Tianchuang SI-16 (*Supplementing Life*).
- Swollen painful throat: Tiantu REN-22, Shaoshang LU-11 and Hegu L.I.-4 (*Great Compendium*).
- Pain of the Heart with shortness of breath: Tiantu REN-22, Qimen LIV-14, Changqiang DU-1, Xiabai LU-4 and Zhongchong P-9 (*Thousand Ducat Formulas*).
- Heat sensation of the skin of the face: Tiantu REN-22 and Tianchuang SI-16 (*Supplementing Life*).

LIANQUAN REN-23
Corner Spring

廉泉

Meeting point of the Conception and Yin Linking vessels

LOCATION
On the anterior midline of the neck, in the depression above the hyoid bone.

LOCATION NOTE
i. Run a finger gently along the underside of the chin towards the throat until it falls into the deep depression just in front of the hyoid bone; ii. the hyoid bone is readily located as the most superior palpable bony structure at the midline of the throat and runs transversely above the laryngeal prominence; this point is located at its superior border.

NEEDLING
Oblique insertion in the direction of Baihui DU-20, 0.5 to 1.2 cun. **Note**: according to several modern texts, this point is contraindicated to moxibustion.

ACTIONS
Benefits the tongue
Descends qi and alleviates cough

INDICATIONS
- Swelling below the tongue with difficulty speaking, sudden loss of voice, loss of voice following windstroke, contraction of the root of the tongue with difficulty in eating, protrusion of the tongue, much spittle, dryness of the mouth, thirst, mouth ulcers, lockjaw.
- Cough, rebellious qi, dyspnoea, chest pain, vomiting of foam.

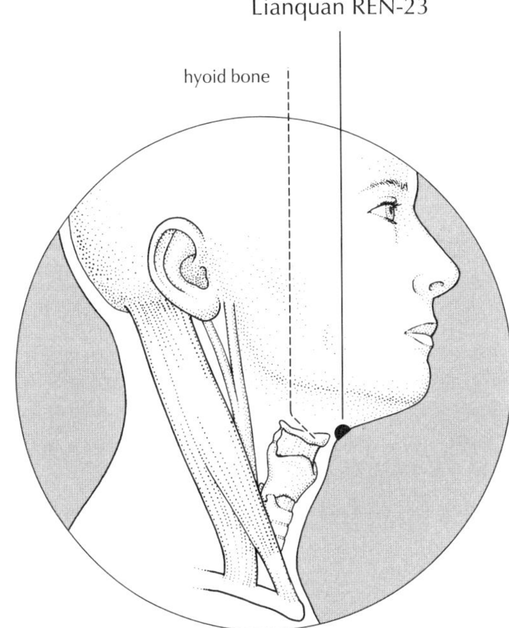

COMMENTARY
Lianquan REN-23, a meeting point of the Conception vessel with the Yin Linking vessel and located at the root of the tongue, is much used clinically in the treatment of loss of voice and stiffness of the tongue following windstroke. Lianquan REN-23 may also be used to regulate the production of fluids in the mouth, either in the case of excess spittle or for dryness of the mouth and thirst. For this purpose the needle is directed alternately towards the extraordinary points Jinjin (M-HN-20) and Yuye (M-HN-20) located below the tongue.

COMBINATIONS
- Swelling below the tongue with difficulty speaking, protrusion of the tongue with drooling: Lianquan REN-23, Rangu KID-2 and Yingu KID-10 (*Thousand Ducat Formulas*).
- Swelling and pain below the tongue: Lianquan REN-23 and Zhongchong P-9 (*One Hundred Symptoms*).

- Swelling of the tongue with difficulty speaking: Lianquan REN-23, Jinjin (M-HN-20) and Yuye (M-HN-20) (*Great Compendium*).
- Cough with rebellious qi, dyspnoea, vomiting of foam, and lockjaw: Lianquan REN-23, Futu L.I.-18, Tianrong SI-17, Pohu BL-42, Qishe ST-11 and Yixi BL-45 (*Thousand Ducat Formulas*).

CHENGJIANG REN-24

Container of Fluids

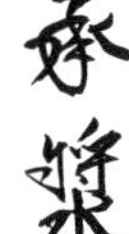

Meeting point of the Conception vessel with the Governing vessel and the Large Intestine and Stomach channels
Sun Si-miao Ghost point

LOCATION

Above the chin, in the depression in the centre of the mentolabial groove.

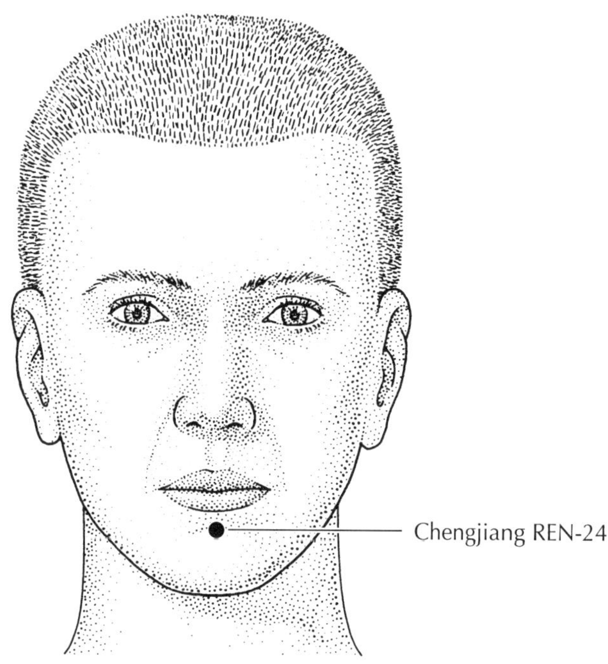

LOCATION NOTE

The mentolabial groove runs horizontally, approximately midway between the chin and the lower lip.

NEEDLING

i. Transverse-oblique insertion directed superiorly 0.2 to 0.3 cun; ii. Transverse insertion along the lower lip to join with Dicang ST-4.

ACTIONS

Extinguishes wind and benefits the face
Regulates the Conception vessel

INDICATIONS

- Hemiplegia, deviation of the mouth and eye, lockjaw, wind epilepsy, stiffness of the head and nape, tetany, mania-depression.
- Pain and numbness of the face, swelling of the face, pain of the teeth and gums, sudden loss of voice, purple lips, excessive production of watery saliva, dry mouth, wasting and thirsting disorder with great desire to drink, nosebleed.
- Dark urine, sweating, shan disorder in men, abdominal (zheng jia) masses in women.

COMMENTARY

Chengjiang REN-24 is a meeting point of the Conception vessel with the hand and foot yangming channels (Large Intestine and Stomach). Yangming channel dominates the facial region whilst Chengjiang REN-24 is located just inferior to the mouth. Its principal clinical application, therefore, is in the treatment of facial disorders, especially pain and numbness of the face and deviation of the mouth and eye (i.e. facial paralysis). Facial paralysis may be due either to exterior wind, which attacks and obstructs the channels of the face, or to interior wind which stirs upwards and leads to malnourishment of the channels. These two patterns correspond more or less exactly to peripheral and central nervous system facial paralysis in modern medicine. In the treatment of this disorder, Chengjiang REN-24 is usually joined by through-needling to points such as Dicang ST-4 or Jiache ST-6. The ability of Chengjiang REN-24 to extinguish wind, especially in the region of the face and jaw, extends to the treatment of hemiplegia, lockjaw and epilepsy.

As its name 'Contain Fluid' implies, Chengjiang REN-24 is able to affect the production of fluids in the mouth and is indicated for excessive production of watery saliva, dry mouth and wasting and thirsting disorder with great desire to drink.

Chengjiang REN-24 is a meeting point of the Conception and Governing vessels and lies directly opposite the neck which is traversed by the Governing vessel. A number of classics, for example the *Ode of the Essentials of Understanding*, recommend it for stiffness and pain of the nape of the neck.

As the terminal point of the Conception vessel, Chengjiang REN-24 is indicated for disorders of the lower portion of the channel such as dark urination, shan disorder in men and abdominal masses in women. Finally, Chengjiang REN-24 was included under its alternative name Guishi (Ghost Market) by Sun Si-miao among his 'thirteen ghost points' for the treatment of epilepsy and mania-depression.

COMBINATIONS

- Deviation of the mouth and eye: Chengjiang REN-24, Hegu L.I.-4, Jiache ST-6, Dicang ST-4, Renzhong DU-26 and Tinghui GB-2 (*Illustrated Supplement*).
- Lockjaw following windstroke: reduce Chengjiang REN-24, Hegu L.I.-4, Jiache ST-6, Renzhong DU-26 and Baihui DU-20 (*Great Compendium*).
- Loss of voice: Chengjiang REN-24 and Fengfu DU-16 (*Supplementing Life*).
- Ceaseless nosebleed: Chengjiang REN-24 and Weizhong BL-40 (*Systematic Classic*).
- Wasting and thirsting disorder with great desire to drink: Chengjiang REN-24, Yishe BL-49, Rangu KID-2 and Guanchong SJ-1 (*Thousand Ducat Formulas*).
- Wasting and thirsting disorder: Chengjiang REN-24, Jinjin (M-HN-20), Yuye (M-HN-20), Renzhong DU-26, Lianquan REN-23, Quchi L.I-11, Laogong P-8, Taichong LIV-3, Xingjian LIV-2, Shangqiu SP-5, Ranggu KID-2 and Yinbai SP-1 (*Great Compendium*).
- Mouth ulcers: Chengjiang REN-24 and Laogong P-8 (*Compilation*).
- Stiffness and pain of the head and nape with difficult rotation: Chengjiang REN-24 and Fengfu DU-16 (*Song of the Jade Dragon*).

NOTES

1 Translated by Giovanni Maciocia.

2 *Spiritual Pivot* Chapter 65.

3 *Essential Questions* Chapter 10.

4 *Classic of Difficulties* 8th Difficulty.

5 *Discourse into the Origin and Development of Medicine* by Xu Da-cun, 1704.

6 *Essential Questions* Chapter 39.

7 *True Lineage of Medicine* by Yu Tian-min, Ming dynasty.

8 *General Treatise on the Aetiology and Symptomatology of Diseases* by Chao Yuan-fang.

9 *Essential Questions* Chapter 8.

10 *Classic of Difficulties* 31st Difficulty.

11 *Classic of Difficulties* 8th Difficulty.

12 *Discourse into the Origin and Development of Medicine* by Xu Da-cun, 1704.

13 *The Heart & Essence of Dan-xi's Methods of Treatment*, A Translation of Zhu Dan-xi's Dan Xi Zhi Fa Xin Yao, Blue Poppy Press, pp. 9 and 102.

14 *Spiritual Pivot* Chapter 1.

15 *Essential Questions* Chapter 1.

16 Tian Gui: see glossary.

17 *Spiritual Pivot* Chapter 19.

18 Ibid.

19 *Spiritual Pivot* Chapter 10.

20 *Spiritual Pivot* Chapter 1.

21 Cited in *Celestial Lancets* by Lu Gwei-Djen & Joseph Needham, p. 78, Cambridge University Press.

22 *Spiritual Pivot* Chapter 33.

23 *Spiritual Pivot* Chapter 75.

24 *Illustrated Supplement to The Classic of Categories* by Zhang Jie-bin.

25 *Essential Questions* Chapter 58.

26 *Classic of Difficulties* 29th Difficulty.

督脈經穴

THE GOVERNING VESSEL

THE GOVERNING VESSEL

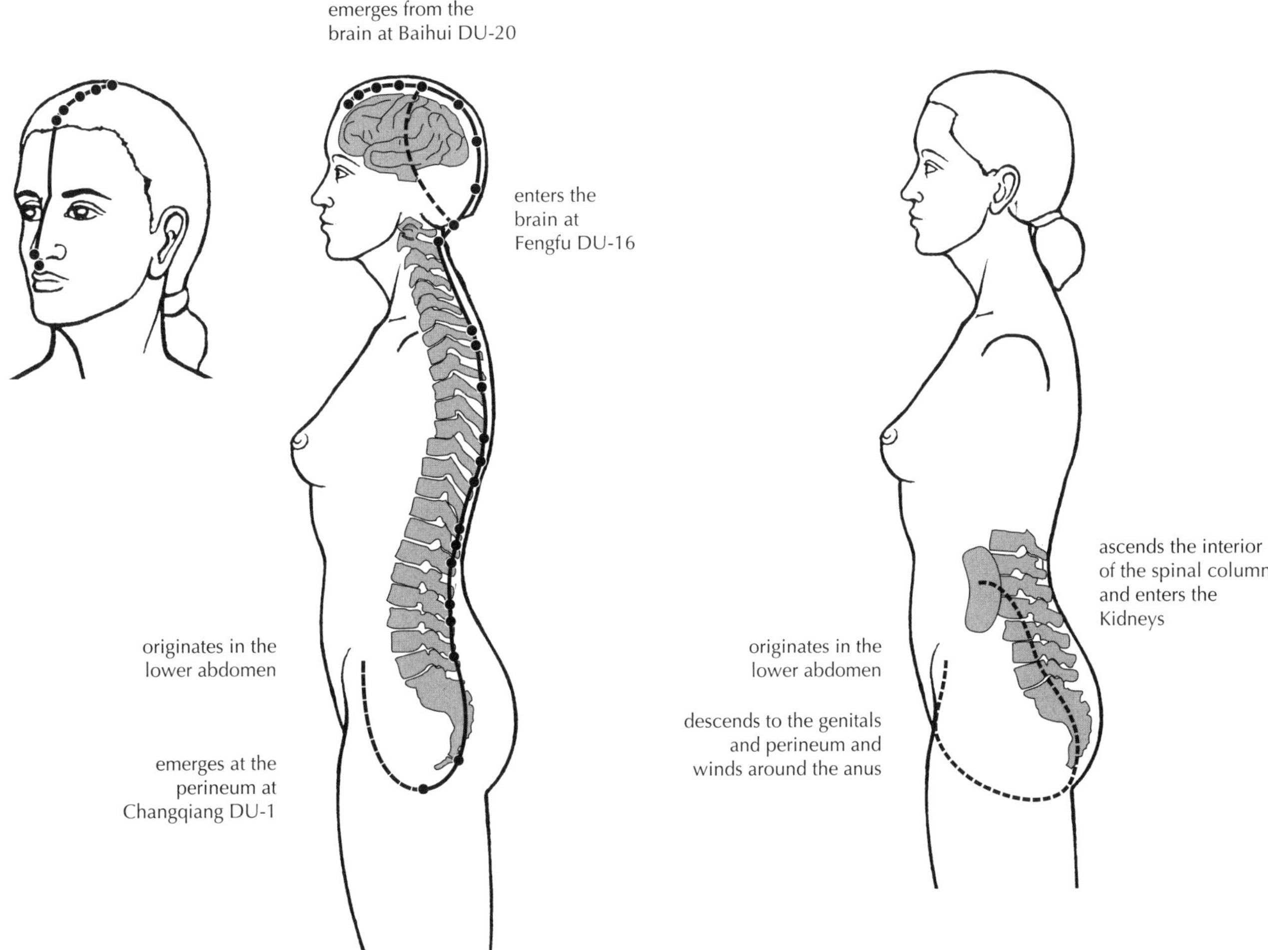

The Governing vessel primary pathway

The Governing vessel first branch

GOVERNING VESSEL PRIMARY PATHWAY

- originates in the lower abdomen,
- emerges at the perineum at Changqiang DU-1,
- runs posteriorly along the midline of the sacrum and the interior of the spinal column to Fengfu DU-16 at the nape of the neck,
- enters the brain,
- ascends to the vertex at Baihui DU-20,
- descends along the midline of the head to the bridge of the nose and the philtrum at Renzhong DU-26
- terminates at the junction of the upper lip and the gum.

Note

- Huiyin REN-1 and Chengjiang REN-24 are classified as meeting points of the Governing vessel with the Conception vessel.

The Governing vessel first branch

- originates in the lower abdomen,
- descends to the genitals and perineum,
- winds around the anus,
- ascends the interior of the spinal column,
- enters the Kidneys.

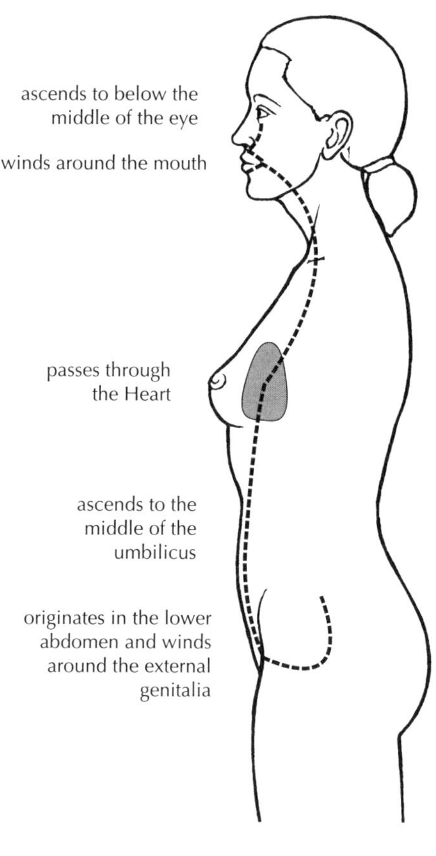

The Governing vessel second branch

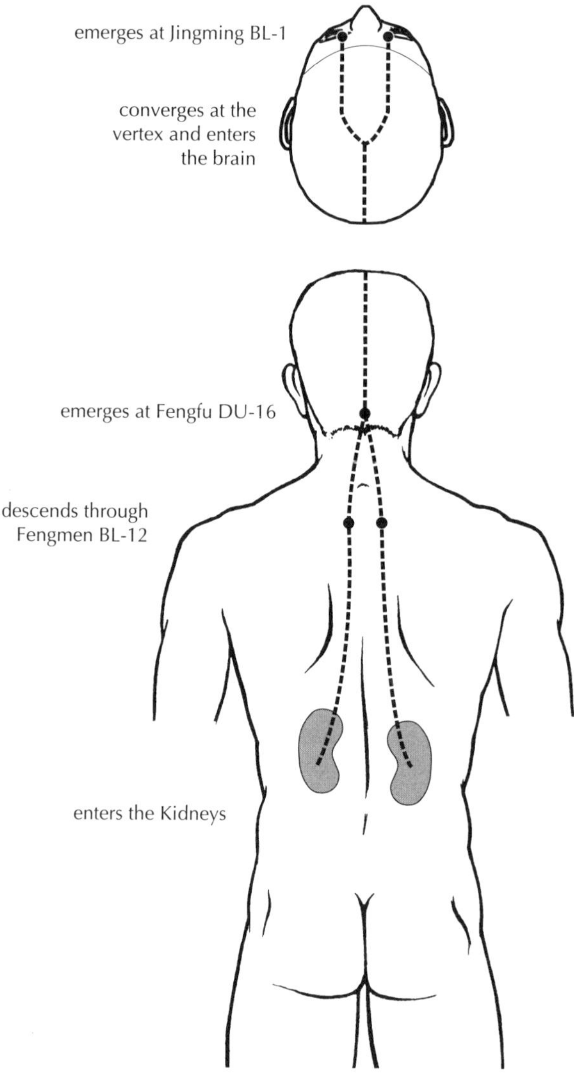

The Governing vessel third branch

The Governing vessel second branch
- originates in the lower abdomen,
- winds around the external genitalia,
- ascends to the middle of the umbilicus,
- passes through the Heart,
- ascends to the throat,
- winds around the mouth,
- ascends to below the middle of the eyes.

The Governing vessel third branch
- emerges at Jingming BL-1,
- follows the Bladder channel bilaterally along the forehead,
- the bilateral branches converge at the vertex and enter the brain,
- the single channel emerges at Fengfu DU-16,
- then divides again, descending through Fengmen BL-12 along either side of the spine to the Kidneys.

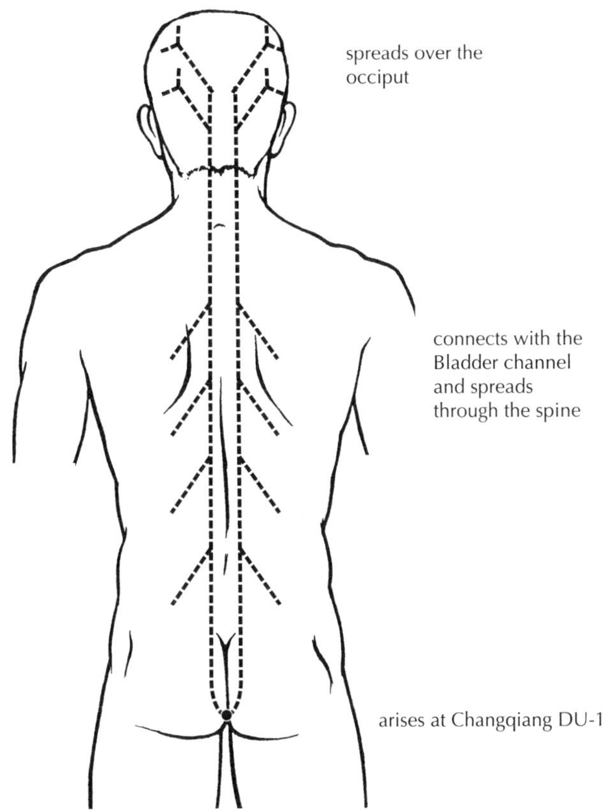

The Governing luo-connecting vessel

THE GOVERNING LUO-CONNECTING VESSEL

- arises at Changqiang DU-1 and ascends bilaterally along the sides of the spine to the nape of the neck and spreads over the occiput.
- at the scapular region it connects with the Bladder channel and threads through the spine.

DISCUSSION

The Governing vessel is one of the eight extraordinary vessels, but along with the Conception vessel is exceptional among these eight in that it has its own acupuncture points. For this reason the Governing and Conception vessels are often included with the twelve primary channels (and together known as the fourteen channels). The other six extraordinary vessels have no points of their own, passing instead through points of the fourteen channels.

The Governing vessel is principally understood to be the channel that ascends through the spine to the brain. As the above description shows, however, its third pathway ascends the front of the body, whilst a branch of the Conception vessel arises in the pelvic cavity, enters the spine and ascends along the back. Li Shi-zhen, therefore, said "The Conception and Governing vessels are like midnight and midday, they are the polar axis of the body ... there is one source and two branches, one goes to the front and the other to the back of the body ... When we try to divide these, we see that yin and yang are inseparable. When we try to see them as one, we see that it is an indivisible whole"[1].

As far as the pathway of the Governing vessel is concerned, it is important to note that:

- the primary channel ascends both inside the spine and alongside the spine.
- the primary channel enters the brain at Fengfu DU-16 and at the vertex (Baihui DU-20).
- the primary channel enters the Kidneys.
- the primary channel passes through the Heart.
- the primary channel winds around the anus.
- the primary channel winds around the external genitals.
- the luo-connecting channel spreads through the occiput.

As a consequence of the various pathways of the Governing vessel and its relationship with the Kidneys, Heart and brain, we can summarise the actions of the points of the Governing vessel as follows:

- Treating diseases of the anus, rectum, and intestines. The Governing vessel winds around the anal region and the lower points of this channel (Changqiang DU-1 to Xuanshu DU-5) as well as Renzhong DU-26 above, treat diseases such as haemorrhoids, prolapse of the rectum and intestinal disorders.
- Treating diseases of the genitals, urinary system and uterus. The anterior pathway of the Governing vessel winds around the genitals, and points Changqiang DU-1 to Mingmen DU-4 treat diseases such as

painful urinary dysfunction, urinary retention or difficulty, seminal emission, leucorrhoea and menstrual disturbance.

- Treating disorders of the spine. The Governing vessel ascends through the spinal column, and its points treat disorders of the spine, predominantly at their corresponding level.
- Treating febrile diseases and reducing heat in the body. The Governing vessel is the 'sea of the yang channels' and its points are effective to reduce yang heat manifesting as heat of the body, fever and especially malaria.
- Treating diseases of the zangfu. As the Governing vessel ascends along the spine, its points have the ability to treat diseases of the zangfu roughly corresponding to their location. This correspondence does not exactly mirror the back-shu points. For example Jinsuo DU-8 (which lies level with Ganshu BL-18, the back-shu point of the Liver) treats disharmony of the Liver, and points Shendao DU-11 (level with Xinshu BL-15 the back-shu point of the Heart) and Shenzhu DU-12 (level with Feishu BL-13 the back-shu point of the Lung) treat diseases of the Heart and Lung respectively. Zhiyang DU-9, however which lies beneath the seventh thoracic vertebra level with Geshu BL-17, treats diseases of the Stomach and Spleen. There is also a system of correspondence mentioned in the *Essential Questions*[2] which was discontinued in later texts, whereby for example Zhiyang DU-9 was said to treat heat in the Kidney, Lingtai DU-10 heat in the Spleen, Shendao DU-11 heat in the Liver etc.
- Treating disorders of exterior or interior wind. Wind is a yang pathogen, and the Governing vessel is the 'sea of the yang channels'. Many of its points are of vital importance in the treatment of exterior wind (especially Dazhui DU-14 and Fengfu DU-16), whilst from Jinsuo DU-8 upwards most points have a strong action on pacifying interior wind giving rise to such disorders as upward staring eyes, opisthotonos, lockjaw, dizziness, head wind, windstroke, spasm and especially epilepsy.
- Treating disorders of the sense organs. From Yamen DU-15 upwards, the points of the Governing vessel treat disorders of the tongue, eyes, face and especially the nose, through which the central portion of the channel descends.
- Treating disorders of the Heart zang, primarily pain and palpitations. This may be explained by the passage of the anterior portion of the Governing vessel through the Heart.
- Treating disorders of the brain and spirit. It is striking how many points of the Governing vessel are indicated for the kind of disharmony usually associated with the Heart and spirit, for example mania-depression, manic behaviour, agitation, poor memory, disorientation, palpitations, insomnia, loss of consciousness and epilepsy. (see especially Baihui DU-20 and Shenting DU-24). There is indeed an apparent contradiction here within Chinese medicine theory. The concept that the spirit is stored in the Heart is of course an axiom of Chinese medicine and is attested to in various classics. The *Spiritual Pivot* says "The Heart controls the vessels; the vessels are the residence of the spirit"[3], "When the blood and qi are already in harmony, the nutritive qi and defensive qi already communicating, the five zang already formed, the spirit will reside in the Heart"[4], and "The Heart is the great master of the five zang and six fu and the residence of the essence spirit"[5], whilst the *Essential Questions* says "The Heart stores the spirit"[6]. At the same time, there are many classical references to the idea that the spirit concentrates in the head and brain, for example the *Essential Questions* says "the head is the residence of the intelligence"[7], the *Ten Works on Practice Toward the Attainment of Truth* says "The brain is the ancestor of the body's form and the meeting place of the hundred spirits"[8], the *Daoist Internal Mirror* says "The brain is the ancestral portal of the body, the capital where the ten thousand spirits meet"[9], Sun Si-miao, in the *Thousand Ducat Formulas* says "The head is the supreme leader, the place where man's spirit concentrates", Li Shi-zhen says "The brain is the residence of the original spirit", and the *Essentials of Materia Medica* says "All of a person's memory resides in the brain"[10].

Three main factors may help to illuminate this theoretical difficulty: i. different traditions within Chinese medicine, ii. the influence of modern medicine, and iii. the interrelationship of the Heart, blood, essence, brain and spirit.

Different traditions within Chinese Medicine

Both before and after the appearance of the *Yellow Emperor's Inner Classic*, different traditions are apparent within the broad fields of Chinese medicine, spiritual practice and health preservation. In pre-*Inner Classic* times, a more structural perception of the human body placed the brain as the main organ in charge of mental activity[11]. After the *Inner Classic*, when the study of medicine diverged and grew more independent of its Daoist roots, a more functional view of the body developed, based on the predominance of the five zang and six fu and their correspondences (especially five phase correspondences), the brain being 'relegated' to the status of an extra fu, and the Heart becoming the sovereign of the body and the residence of the spirit. This divergence is reflected in the *Essential Questions* which says "I understand that there are some Daoists who have a completely different understanding of the nature of a zang and a fu. Some say the brain and the marrow are zang ... whereas others think of them as fu. If presented with a view other than their own, they insist that only their own interpretation is right"[12]. Later esoteric Daoist texts strongly influenced certain great doctors of the Tang, Yuan and Ming dynasties such as Sun Si-miao, Zhang Jing-yue and Li Shi-zhen[13]. Their understanding of the role of the brain, and the principal acupuncture channel which influences it, the Governing vessel, again entered the corpus of Chinese medicine theory. At the same time, none of these doctors challenged the theory of the Heart and spirit as being essentially contradictory to the brain spirit theory.

The influence of modern medicine

During the Qing dynasty and the Republican era, knowledge of Western anatomy began to infiltrate China. One author who is considered to have been influenced by these developments was Wang Qing-ren who in the chapter 'On the Brain' (in *Correcting the Errors of Medicine* 1830) stated "intelligence and memory rely on the brain"[14]. Wang's book was published and distributed along with *A New Treatise on Anatomy*, a translation of basic Western medicine texts by an English medical missionary Benjamin Hobson and his assistant Chen Xiu-tang.

The inter-relationship of the Heart, Kidneys, essence, brain and spirit.

The *Spiritual Pivot*[15] states "The brain is the sea of marrow", and it is a basic tenet of Chinese medicine that the Kidneys produce marrow to fill up the brain. The Kidneys' relationship to marrow is intimately tied up with the Kidney function of storing essence, which nourishes the brain and spinal cord. All aspects of the human organism derive from the coming together of the essence of the parents. The *Spiritual Pivot*[16] says "Essence is the source of life, when the two essences unite [literally: struggle against each other] the spirit is formed", and the *Classic of Categories* says "The two essences, one yin and one yang, unite ... to form life; the essence of mother and father unite to form the spirit"[17]. In other words the pre-natal essence, derived from the parents, is intimately related to the Kidneys and brain and is the origin of the existence of the human being and the original source of the spirit. This is the meaning of the statements by Li Shi-zhen "The brain is the residence of the original spirit", and found in *A Record of Nourishing Xing and Extending Ming* "Spirit, that is essence. If we can preserve essence, then the spirit will be bright; if spirit is bright, there will be long life"[18]. At the same time, various authors have stressed the relationship between the brain and the Heart, which is a reflection of the vital relationship between the Kidneys and Heart, water and fire. The *Differentiation and Treatment of Disease* stated "The spirit of the human being resides in the Heart, and the Heart's essence relies entirely on the Kidneys. Thus, the brain is the store house of the original spirit, the sea of essence marrow, and this is where memory comes from"[19], and the Daoist classic *Collected Wisdom by Master Magic Sword* states "The qi of the Heart is connected with the Niwan Palace above"[20]. Niwan ('Sticky Pellet' or 'Mud Ball Palace') in the Daoist tradition is the central one of the nine palaces of the brain where all the various spirits meet, and is considered to be the location of the material basis of the spirit. Niwan is discussed in various Daoist classics, for example "The origin of essence-spirit in the brain is also called Niwan" and "The entire spirit that expresses in the face has its origin in Niwan"[21], and "At the top of the human body, there is Tiangu Niwan, this is where the spirit is stored ... Tiangu, that is the Original Palace, the residence of the original spirit, where mental and spiritual brightness exists, the most important aspect of spirit"[22].

The Governing vessel in its anterior pathway passes through the Heart, and in its posterior pathway penetrates the brain. This linkage between the brain and Heart was discussed by Cheng Xing-gan who said "When marrow is full, thinking is clear. Too much thinking leads to Heart fire which burns the brain ... the marrow is rooted in the essence and connects downwards with the Governing vessel; when the ming men warms and nourishes, the marrow is full"[23].

In conclusion, the Governing vessel is the channel that mediates between the brain and the Heart. Clinically many of its points may be used to treat a variety of psycho-emotional disorders, in much the same way that points of the twelve principal channels may be used, especially those of the Heart and Pericardium. If we try to be more precise about the use of the Governing vessel points, we can suggest that i. their indications generally reflect excess patterns of spirit disharmony such as mania-depression, and ii. they are especially indicated when psycho-emotional disorders are accompanied by fullness and discomfort of the head, dizziness, disturbance of consciousness and epilepsy.

CHANGQIANG DU-1

Long Strong

長強

Luo-Connecting point of the Governing vessel
Meeting point of the Governing vessel with the Conception vessel and the Gall Bladder and Kidney channels

LOCATION

On the midline, midway between the tip of the coccyx and the anus.

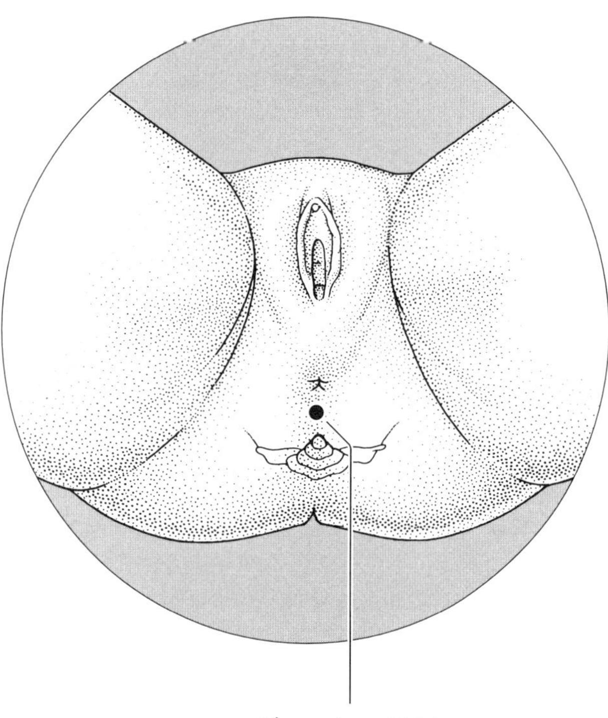

LOCATION NOTE

This point may be located and needled with the patient either: i. lying on the front, ii. lying on the side with knees drawn up, or iii. first sitting on the heels and then leaning forwards and resting the upper body weight on the elbows with the head on the hands.

NEEDLING

Perpendicular insertion 0.5 to 1 cun.

ACTIONS

Treats haemorrhoids
Benefits the two lower yin
Activates the channel and alleviates pain
Calms the spirit

INDICATIONS

- Haemorrhoids, the five types of haemorrhoids, chronic haemorrhoids, difficult defecation, cold or damp (dong) diarrhoea, blood in the stool, prolapse of the rectum.
- The five types of painful urinary dysfunction, difficult urination, retention of urine, dark urine, sexual taxation, seminal emission due to fear and fright.
- Pain of the lumbar region, heavy sensation of the sacrum, heaviness of the head, shaking of the head, stiffness of the spine, pain of the Heart.
- Mania, fright epilepsy, upward staring eyes, mad walking, tetany, clonic spasm, vomiting blood.

COMMENTARY

Changqiang DU-1 is the first point and the luo-connecting point of the Governing vessel, and all its indications reflect the pathways and functions of the Governing vessel principal and luo-connecting pathways.

The Governing vessel winds around the anus, and Changqiang DU-1 is an important local point in the treatment of haemorrhoids, prolapse of the rectum and disorders of defecation. The Governing vessel enters the Kidneys and its anterior pathway winds around the genitals. Changqiang DU-1 is therefore also indicated for various disorders of urination such as painful urinary dysfunction, difficult urination and retention of urine, as well as sexual taxation and the unusual symptom of seminal emission induced by fear and fright, emotions which are classically considered to injure the Kidneys and Heart.

The Governing vessel ascends along the entire length of the spinal column and enters the brain, whilst its luo-connecting channel spreads in the occiput. As well as lumbar and sacral pain and stiffness of the spine, Changqiang DU-1 is indicated for heaviness of the head. The *Spiritual Pivot*[24] gives specific indications for disorders of the Governing luo-connecting channel. If it is excess there is stiffness of the spine, and if deficient there is heaviness of the head and shaking of the head.

Although the Heart is most frequently cited as the residence of the spirit, since its early beginnings Chinese medicine has been able to hold the concurrent belief that the head and brain also influence the spirit (see introductory discussion above). Thus the *Essential Questions*[25] stated "the head is the residence of the intelligence" and Sun Simiao, in the *Thousand Ducat Formulas* said "The head is the supreme leader, the place where man's spirit concentrates". Since the Governing vessel enters the brain and its anterior pathway ascends through the Heart, Changqiang DU-1 is indicated for such manifestations of disordered spirit as mania, mad walking and fright epilepsy, as well as for pain of the Heart.

According to qigong theory, there are three important gates or passes (sanguan) in the practice of qi circulation through the Governing vessel. These gates, through which it is more difficult to circulate the qi are the Coccyx Pass (Weiluguan) in the region of Changqiang DU-1, the Lumbar Pass (Jiajiguan) in the region of Mingmen DU-4, and the Occipital Pass (Yuzhenwan) in the region of Yuzhen BL-9.

Changqiang DU-1 has been accorded a great variety of different names. Its best known, Changqiang (Long Strong), is said to refer either to the Governing vessel (of which this is the first point) which is long and strong, or to this point's ability to make the penis long and strong. Alternative names include Longhuxue (Dragon and Tiger Point), Chaotiandian (Heavenward-Looking Summit) and Shangtianti (Stairway to Heaven).

COMBINATIONS

- The five types of haemorrhoids: Changqiang DU-1, Weizhong BL-40, Chengshan BL-57, Feiyang BL-58, Yangfu GB-38, Fuliu KID-7, Taichong LIV-3, Xiaxi GB-43, Qihai REN-6 and Huiyin REN-1 (*Great Compendium*).
- The nine types of haemorrhoids (with bleeding): Changqiang DU-1 and Chengshan BL-57 (*Song of the Jade Dragon*).
- Chronic haemorrhoids: Changqiang DU-1, Erbai (M-UE-29) and Chengshan BL-57 (*Great Compendium*).
- Prolapse of the rectum and haemorrhoids: Changqiang DU-1, Erbai (M-UE-29), Baihui DU-20 and Zhishi BL-52 (*Great Compendium*).
- Prolapse of the rectum: Changqiang DU-1, Dachangshu BL-25, Baihui DU-20, Jianjing GB-21, Hegu L.I.-4 and Qichong ST-30 (*Compilation*).
- Prolapse of the rectum in children: Changqiang DU-1, Baihui DU-20 and Dachangshu BL-25 (*Great Compendium*).
- Difficult urination and defecation, dribbling and retention of urine: Changqiang DU-1 and Xiaochangshu BL-27 (*Thousand Ducat Formulas*).
- Hot constipation, qi constipation: first needle Changqiang DU-1 then Dadun LIV-1 and Yanglingquan GB-34 (*Song of Points*).
- Intestinal wind (blood in the stools): Changqiang DU-1 and Chengshan BL-57 (*One Hundred Symptoms*).
- Childhood fright epilepsy: Changqiang DU-1 and Shenzhu DU-12 (*Supplementing Life*).
- Childhood epileptic convulsions, vomiting and diarrhoea, fright and fear: Changqiang DU-1 and Qimai SJ-18 (*Systematic Classic*).
- Pain of the Heart with shortness of breath: Changqiang DU-1, Qimen LIV-14, Tiantu REN-22, Xiabai LU-4 and Zhongchong P-9 (*Thousand Ducat Formulas*).

YAOSHU DU-2

Lumbar Shu

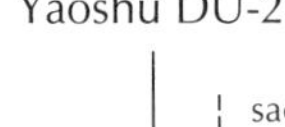

LOCATION

On the midline, in the sacro-coccygeal hiatus.

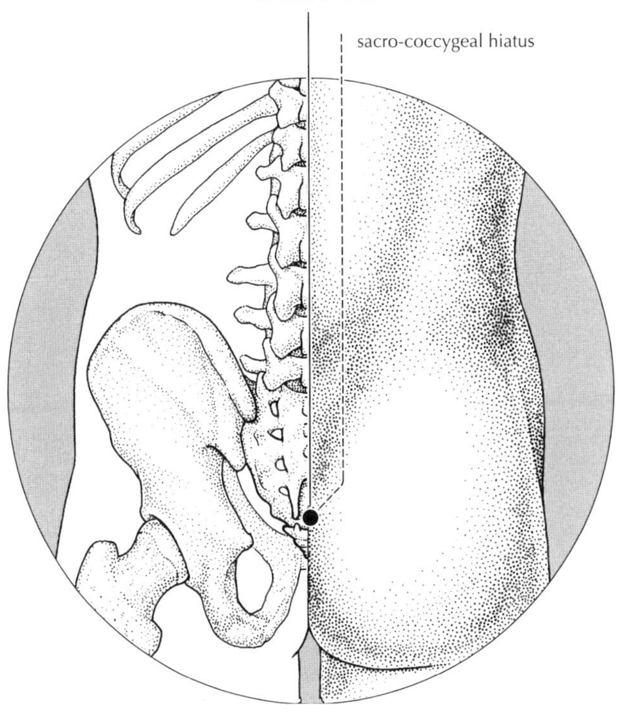

LOCATION NOTE

The sacro-coccygeal hiatus is located in-between the cornua of the sacrum and coccyx, in the depression inferior to the fourth sacral spinous process if this is palpable. Note, however, that the sacro-coccygeal hiatus may sometimes extend as high as the level of the third sacral foramina.

NEEDLING

Oblique superior insertion 0.5 to 1 cun.

ACTIONS

Benefits the lumbar region and legs
Dispels wind-damp

INDICATIONS

- Pain of the sacrum, pain of the lumbar region and hips with inability to flex and extend, lumbar pain radiating to the foot, cold painful obstruction with numbness of the leg.
- Irregular menstruation, red and white leucorrhoea, dark urine, haemorrhoids.
- Warm malaria with absence of sweating, epilepsy, injury by cold with ceaseless heat in the four limbs.

COMMENTARY

The primary clinical use of Yaoshu DU-2 is to treat pain of the sacrum and lumbar region, especially when it radiates to the hips and down the legs.

According to the *Essential Questions*[26] Yaoshu DU-2 is one of the 'eight points for draining heat from the extremities' (although in fact only seven are listed) namely Yunmen LU-2, Jianyu L.I.-15, Weizhong BL-40 and Yaoshu DU-2, and is indicated for 'injury by cold with ceaseless heat in the four limbs'.

COMBINATIONS

- Stiffness and pain of the lumbar region: Yaoshu DU-2, Weizhong BL-40, Yongquan KID-1, Xiaochangshu BL-27 and Pangguangshu BL-28 (*Great Compendium*).
- Stiffness of the lumbar region and back with inability to bend to the side: Yaoshu DU-2 and Feishu BL-13 (*Great Compendium*).
- Cold wind painful obstruction that is difficult to cure: Yaoshu DU-2 and Huantiao GB-30 (*Ode of Xi-hong*).
- Numbness of the legs: Yaoshu DU-2 and Fengfu DU-16 (*Thousand Ducat Formulas*).
- Malaria: Yaoshu DU-2 and Dazhui DU-14 (*Supplementing Life*).

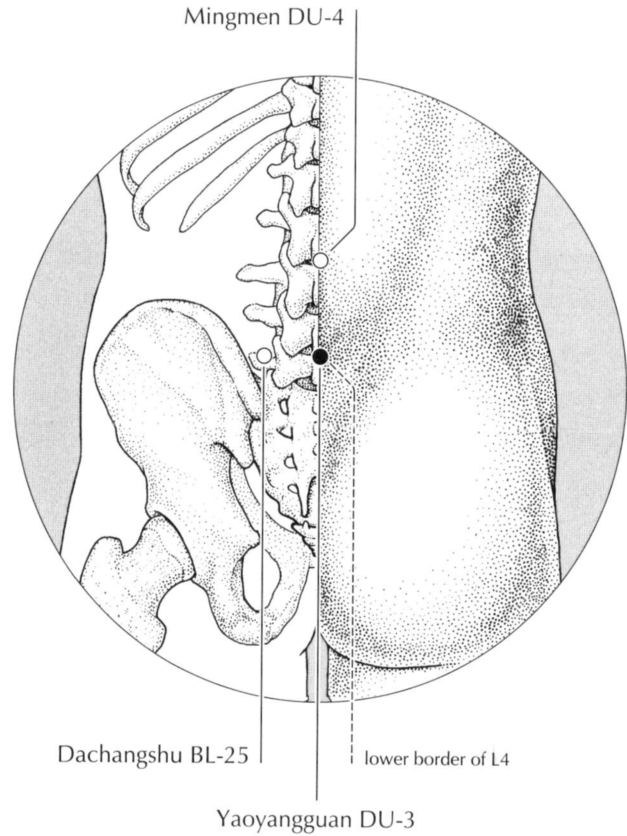

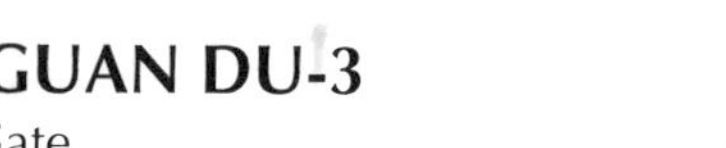

YAOYANGGUAN DU-3

Lumbar Yang Gate

腰陽關

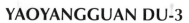

LOCATION

On the midline of the lower back, in the depression below the spinous process of the fourth lumbar vertebra.

LOCATION NOTE

This point is located one intervertebral space below the line connecting the highest points of the two iliac crests (level with the lower border of L3).

NEEDLING

Perpendicular insertion 0.5 to 1 cun.

Caution: the spinal canal lies between 1.25 and 1.75 cun deep to the skin surface, varying according to body build.

ACTIONS

Dispels wind-damp
Benefits the lumbar region and legs
Regulates the lower jiao

INDICATIONS

- Inability to flex and extend the knee, pain of the outer aspect of the knee, wind painful obstruction with numbness, contraction of the sinews, inability to walk, pain of the crotch and lumbar region due to taxation injury.
- Seminal emission, impotence, white turbidity, disorders of menstruation, leucorrhoea.

COMMENTARY

The principal clinical use of Yaoyangguan DU-3 is in the treatment of dual disorders of the lumbar region and legs, and it is one of the main points on the back itself which treats disorders of the lower limb.

MINGMEN DU-4

Gate of Life

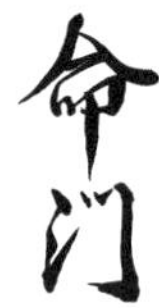

LOCATION

On the midline of the lower back, in the depression below the spinous process of the second lumbar vertebra.

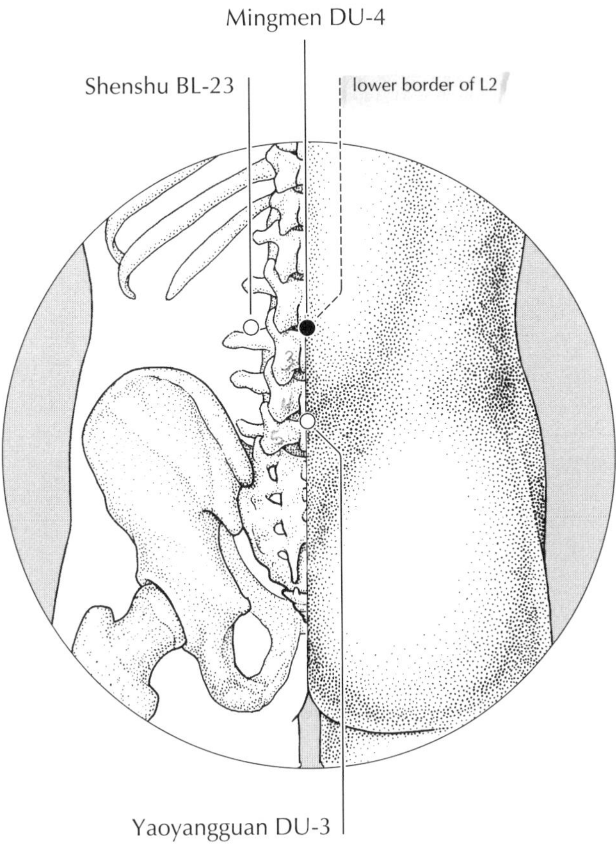

LOCATION NOTE

This point is located one intervertebral space above the line connecting the highest points of the two iliac crests (level with the lower border of L3).

NEEDLING

Perpendicular insertion 0.5 to 1 cun.

Caution: the spinal canal lies between 1.25 and 1.75 cun deep to the skin surface, varying according to body build.

Note: according to a number of classical texts, this point is contraindicated to moxibustion in those who are under 20 years of age.

ACTIONS

Clears heat
Regulates the Governing vessel
Tonifies the Kidneys
Benefits the lumbar spine

INDICATIONS

- Heat in the body like fire, absence of sweating, steaming bones, heat of the five zang, malaria with alternating chills and fever.
- Shaking of the head with open mouth, tinnitus, dizziness, opisthotonos, splitting headache, childhood epilepsy, fear and fright.
- Seminal emission, white turbidity, red and white leucorrhoea, shan disorder.
- Prolapse of the rectum, haemorrhoids, blood in the stool.
- Stiffness of the lumbar spine, pain of the lumbar spine radiating to the abdomen, Kidney deficiency lumbar pain, all types of lumbar pain due to deficiency, spinal rigidity with inability to flex and extend the back, cold painful obstruction of the hands and feet.

COMMENTARY

The *Classic of Difficulties*[27] said "On the left is the Kidney, on the right is ming men" whilst according to Zhang Jing-yue "Ming men resides between the Kidneys". The exact location of ming men (Gate of Life) has been described differently at different times, but as its name makes clear, Mingmen DU-4, located between the Kidney back-shu points, is an important point to influence the ming men and the ministerial fire to which it is closely related. As well as influencing the ming men fire, Mingmen DU-4 is a point of the Governing vessel, which is known as the 'sea of the yang channels', and therefore has a strong regulatory effect on the yang qi and the exterior portion of the body. These two considerations help explain the fact that the indications given for Mingmen DU-4 in classical texts emphasise the treatment of heat disorders, whether interior or exterior, excess or deficient. Mingmen DU-4 is able to drain heat manifesting as 'heat in the body like fire', steaming bone disorder and malaria. According to the *Classic of Difficulties*, the ministerial fire is the "root of the five zang". Mingmen DU-4 is specifically indicated for heat of the five zang and shares this special indication with Xinshu BL-15, the back-shu point of the Heart which dominates sovereign fire.

An alternative name for this point is Jinggong (Palace of Essence). The Governing vessel ascends through the spinal cord and enters the brain (the sea of marrow) as well as entering the Kidneys. Mingmen DU-4 is indicated for such manifestations of Kidney essence deficiency as shaking of the head, tinnitus and dizziness, and this reflects the ability of Mingmen DU-4 both to strengthen the Kidneys, and to open the Governing vessel and assist the ascent of essence. According to the *Classic of Difficulties*[28] "When the Governing vessel is diseased, symptoms such as opisthotonos and fainting may occur". Mingmen DU-4 is able to pacify wind in the Governing vessel, reflected in indications such as opisthotonos, splitting headache and epilepsy.

The Governing vessel dominates the spinal column, the pillar of the body, and as reflects its location Mingmen DU-4 has its strongest action on the lumbar region. It may be used for rigidity and stiffness of the lumbar spine and is strongly indicated in classical sources for lumbar pain due to any kind of deficiency, especially of the Kidneys.

According to the *Classic of Difficulties*[29] "The ming men is the residence of essence ... and stores semen in the male and connects with the uterus in the female". The anterior pathway of the Governing vessel encircles the genitals, and Mingmen DU-4 is indicated for such disorders as seminal emission, white turbidity and leucorrhoea.

The Governing vessel winds around the anus, and like several of the lower points of this channel, Mingmen DU-4 is indicated for prolapse of the rectum, haemorrhoids and blood in the stool.

Despite the common perception of Mingmen DU-4 as a major point to tonify and warm the ming men fire, it is remarkable that there are no clear classical indications for Kidney yang deficiency (compared for example with Shenshu BL-23, Guanyuan REN-4 and Qihai REN-6). Interestingly, however, the classical combinations for this point much more strongly emphasise its yang tonifying properties (see below).

Finally, according to qigong theory, there are three important gates or passes (sanguan) in the practice of qi circulation through the Governing vessel. These gates, through which it is more difficult to circulate the qi are the Coccyx Pass (Weiluguan) in the region of Changqiang DU-1, the Lumbar Pass (Jiajiguan) in the region of Mingmen DU-4, and the Occipital Pass (Yuzhenwan) in the region of Yuzhen BL-9.

COMBINATIONS

- Heat in the body like fire and splitting headache: Mingmen DU-4 and Zhongchong P-9 (*Supplementing Life*).
- Lumbar pain in the elderly: Mingmen DU-4 and Shenshu BL-23 (*Compilation*).
- Incontinence of urine and faeces in the elderly: moxa Mingmen DU-4 and Shenshu BL-23 (*Ode of the Jade Dragon*).
- Impotence: Mingmen DU-4, Shenshu BL-23, Qihai REN-6 and Rangu KID-2 (*Illustrated Supplement*).

XUANSHU DU-5

Suspended Pivot

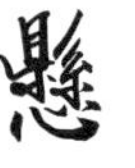
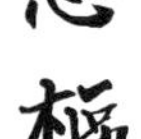

LOCATION

On the midline of the lower back, in the depression below the spinous process of the first lumbar vertebra.

LOCATION NOTE

This point is located two intervertebral spaces above the line connecting the highest points of the two iliac crests (level with the lower border of L3).

NEEDLING

Perpendicular insertion 0.5 to 1 cun.

Caution: the spinal canal lies between 1.25 and 1.75 cun deep to the skin surface, varying according to body build.

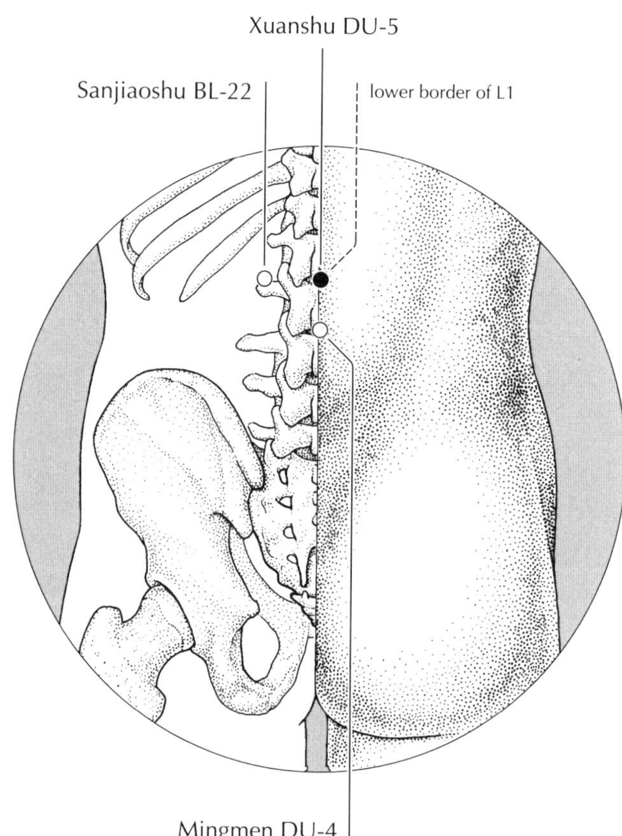

ACTIONS

Benefits the lumbar spine
Benefits the lower jiao

INDICATIONS

- Stiffness of the lumbar spine with inability to flex and extend.
- Undigested food (in the stool), diarrhoea, running piglet qi, shan disorder, retraction of the testicles.

COMBINATIONS

- Undigested food (in the stool): Xuanshu DU-5, Zusanli ST-36, Dachangshu BL-25, Sanyinjiao SP-6, Xiawan REN-10, Sanjiaoshu BL-22 and Liangmen ST-21 (*Supplementing Life*).

JIZHONG DU-6

Centre of the Spine

脊中

LOCATION

On the midline of the back, in the depression below the spinous process of the eleventh thoracic vertebra.

LOCATION NOTE

This point is located four intervertebral spaces above the line connecting the highest points of the two iliac crests (level with the lower border of L3).

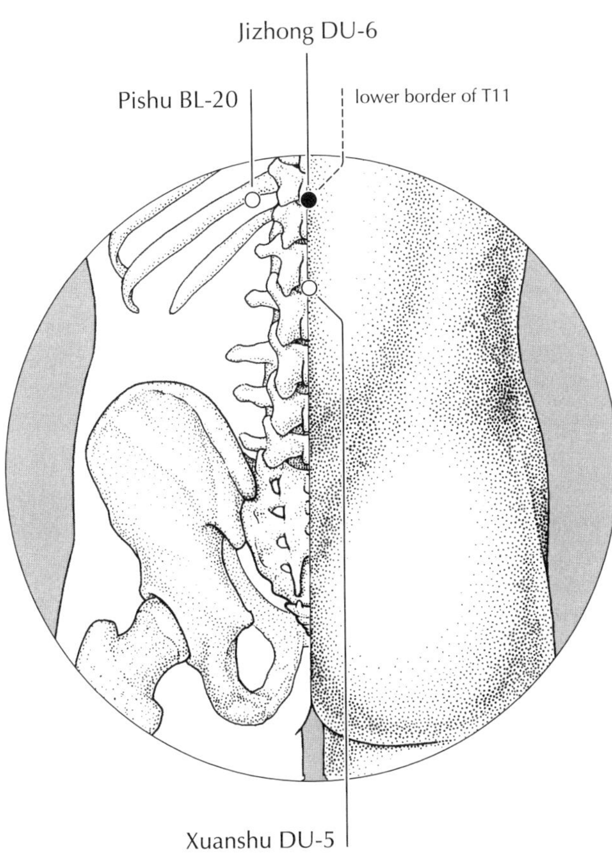

NEEDLING

Perpendicular-oblique superior insertion 0.5 to 1 cun. **Caution:** the spinal canal lies between 1.25 and 1.75 cun deep to the skin surface, varying according to body build. **Note**: according to a number of classical texts, this point is contraindicated to moxibustion.

ACTIONS

Fortifies the Spleen and drains damp

Benefits the spine

INDICATIONS

- Abdominal fullness with no pleasure in eating, abdominal (ji ju) masses, jaundice, diarrhoea, diarrhoea with inability to eat, blood in the stool, the five types of haemorrhoids, prolapse of the rectum in children.
- Stiffness of the lumbar spine, wind epilepsy, warm febrile disease.

COMBINATIONS

- Wind epilepsy: Jizhong DU-6 and Yongquan KID-1 (*Supplementing Life*).

ZHONGSHU DU-7

Central Pivot

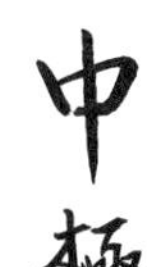

LOCATION

On the midline of the back, in the depression below the spinous process of the tenth thoracic vertebra.

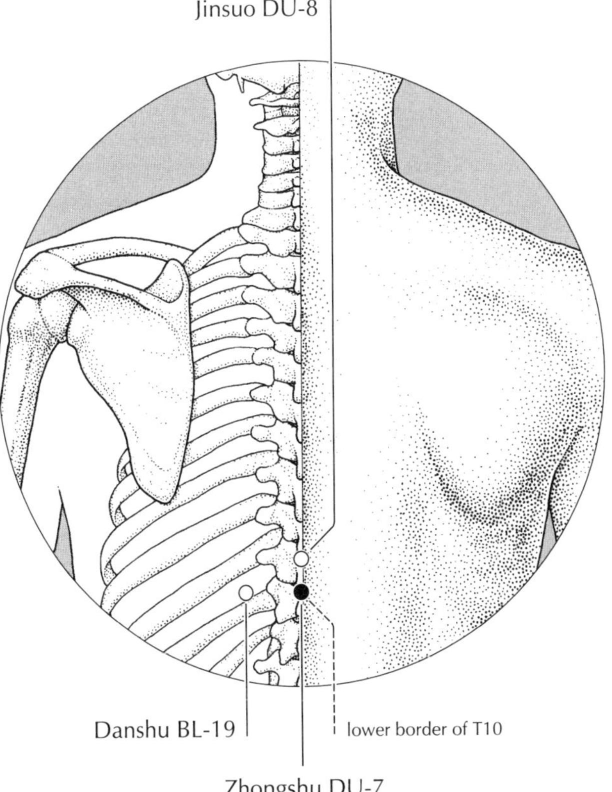

LOCATION NOTE

This point is located five intervertebral spaces above the line connecting the highest points of the two iliac crests (level with the lower border of L3). **Note**: according to the *Illustrated Supplement to the Classic of Categories* this point is contraindicated to moxibustion.

NEEDLING

Perpendicular-oblique superior insertion 0.5 to 1 cun.
Caution: the spinal canal lies between 1.25 and 1.75 cun deep to the skin surface, varying according to body build.

ACTIONS

Benefits the spine
Benefits the middle jiao

INDICATIONS

- Pain of the lumbar region and back.
- Abdominal fullness, no desire to eat, jaundice, amenorrhoea.

JINSUO DU-8

Sinew Contraction

筋縮

LOCATION

On the midline of the back, in the depression below the spinous process of the ninth thoracic vertebra.

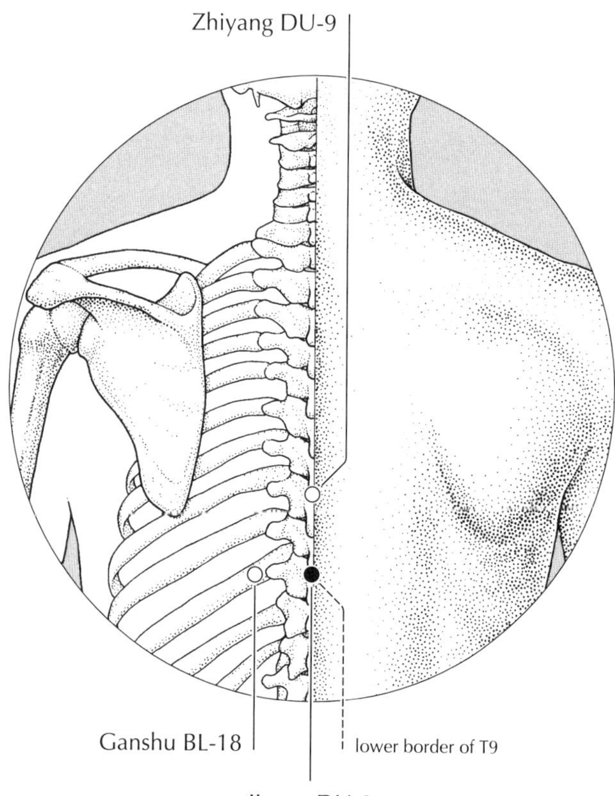

LOCATION NOTE

This point is located six intervertebral spaces above the line connecting the highest points of the two iliac crests (level with the lower border of L3).

NEEDLING

Oblique superior insertion 0.5 to 1 cun.
Caution: the spinal canal lies between 1.25 and 1.75 cun deep to the skin surface, varying according to body build.

ACTIONS

Soothes the Liver, pacifies wind and relieves spasm
Calms the spirit

INDICATIONS

- Upward staring eyes, clonic spasm, epilepsy, childhood fright epilepsy, stiffness and contraction of the spine, pain of the Heart.
- Mania, mad walking, incessant talking, jaundice, anger injuring the Liver.

COMMENTARY

The name of this point (Sinew Contraction) and its location at the level of Ganshu BL-18 the back-shu point of the Liver, illuminate its function. Firstly, it is indicated for a wide variety of disorders resulting from the stirring upwards of Liver wind and characterised by abnormal movement, stiffness, contraction and spasm of the sinews (upward staring eyes, clonic spasm, epilepsy etc.).

Secondly, according to *Investigation into Points Along the Channels*, Jinsuo DU-8 may be selected for 'anger injuring the Liver', and its classical indications also include mania, mad walking and incessant talking, signs of Liver qi stagnation transforming to fire and disrupting the Heart and spirit.

COMBINATIONS

- Fright epilepsy, mad walking and madness: Jinsuo DU-8, Qugu REN-2, Yingu KID-10 and Xingjian LIV-2 (*Thousand Ducat Formulas*).
- Stiffness of the spine: Jinsuo DU-8 and Shuidao ST-28 (*One Hundred Symptoms*).

ZHIYANG DU-9

Reaching Yang

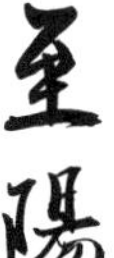

LOCATION

On the midline of the back, in the depression below the spinous process of the seventh thoracic vertebra.

LOCATION NOTE

This point is located seven intervertebral spaces below C7. To locate C7 see page 68.

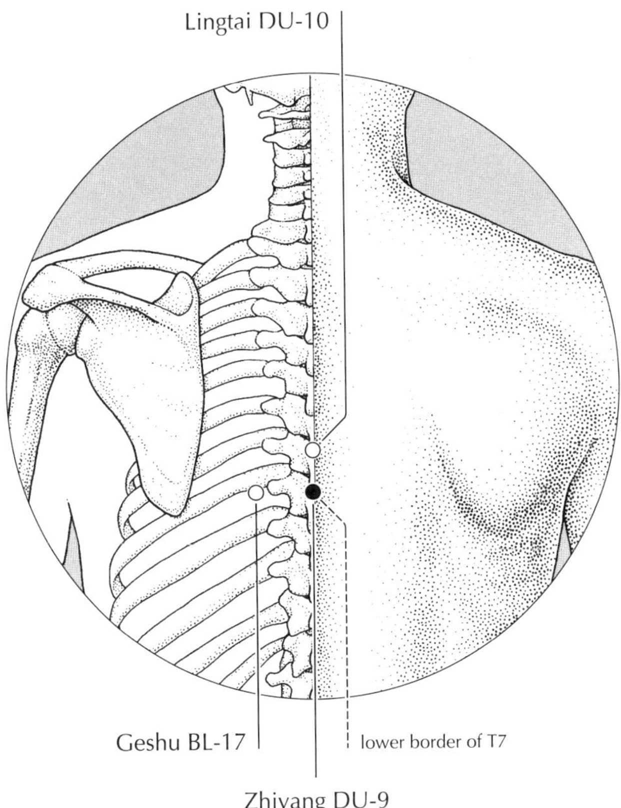

NEEDLING

Oblique superior insertion 0.5 to 1 cun.

Caution: the spinal canal lies between 1.25 and 1.75 cun deep to the skin surface, varying according to body build.

ACTIONS

Fortifies the Spleen, drains dampness and regulates the middle jiao

Treats jaundice

Unbinds the chest

INDICATIONS

- Cold in the Stomach, inability to eat, emaciation, borborygmus, heaviness and pain of the four limbs, weakness of the four limbs with malaise of the whole body due to exterior heat or cold pathogen, diminished qi difficulty in speaking.
- The five types of jaundice, fullness of the chest and lateral costal region, cough, dyspnoea, heat in the Kidneys.
- Pain of the lumbar spine, stiffness of the spine.

COMMENTARY

Zhiyang DU-9 is located at the level of Geshu BL-17 (Diaphragm Shu). The diaphragm separates the middle and upper jiao, and Zhiyang DU-9 acts on both these areas. In fact an alternative name for this point is Feidi (Bottom of the Lung), again reflecting its location at the intersection of these two jiao.

In the middle jiao it is able to tonify and warm the Stomach and Spleen (cold in the Stomach, inability to eat, emaciation), as well as to drain dampness or damp-heat, especially of exterior origin (heaviness of the four limbs, and general malaise of the body). In modern clinical practice this point is much emphasised in the treatment of jaundice and was classically indicated for the five types of jaundice.

In the upper jiao it is able to unbind the chest (fullness of the chest and lateral costal region, cough and dyspnoea), and in common with many of the points of the Governing vessel is indicated for stiffness of the spine and lumbar pain.

Finally in the *Essential Questions*[30] Zhiyang DU-9 is indicated for heat in the Kidneys. This indication clearly fell out of favour and was not mentioned in subsequent texts.

COMBINATIONS

- Jaundice: Zhiyang DU-9, Yinlingquan SP-9, Zusanli ST-36, Riyue GB-24, Danshu BL-19 and Yanggang BL-48.

LINGTAI DU-10

Spirit Tower

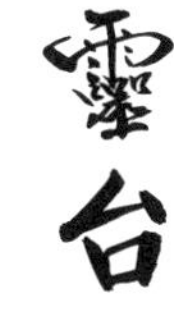

LOCATION

On the midline of the back, in the depression below the spinous process of the sixth thoracic vertebra.

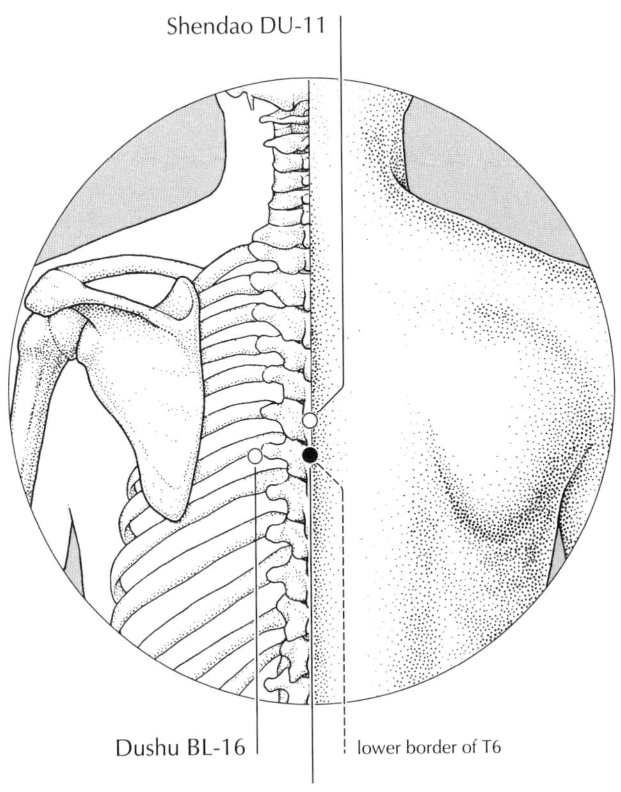

LOCATION NOTE

This point is located six intervertebral spaces below C7. To locate C7 see page 68.

NEEDLING

Oblique superior insertion 0.5 to 1 cun. **Note**: according to several classical texts, this point is contraindicated to needling.

Caution: the spinal canal lies between 1.25 and 1.75 cun deep to the skin surface, varying according to body build.

ACTIONS

Alleviates cough and wheezing

Clears heat and detoxifies poison

INDICATIONS

- Dyspnoea, asthma, chronic cough, wind cold chronic cough.
- Heat in the Spleen, steaming bone taxation consumption, carbuncles and furuncles, clove sores.
- Back pain, stiffness of the neck.

COMMENTARY

The name Lingtai (Spirit Tower) is a traditional term for the Heart and has come to denote the reasoning faculty. It originated with the Spirit Tower built by the emperor Wen Wang as a vantage point to survey all that lay beneath him. Despite this name and the fact that Lingtai DU-10 is located one vertebra below Xinshu BL-15, the back-shu point of the Heart, there are no indications or combinations reflecting this association in any major classic.

Lingtai DU-10 is an empirical point in the treatment of furuncle and red-thread furuncle (lymphangitis) as well as for clove sores (small, hard, deep-rooted, clove-shaped purulent lesions), and is used for this purpose in modern clinical practice. It is also indicated in the *Essential Questions*[31] for heat in the Spleen. This indication clearly fell out of favour and was not mentioned in subsequent texts.

COMBINATIONS

- Furuncle: Lingtai DU-10, Shenzhu DU-12, Ximen P-4, Hegu L.I.-4 and Weizhong BL-40.

SHENDAO DU-11

Spirit Pathway

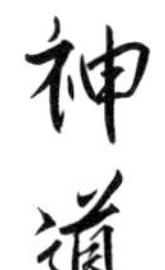

LOCATION

On the midline of the upper back, in the depression below the spinous process of the fifth thoracic vertebra.

LOCATION NOTE

This point is located five intervertebral spaces below C7. To locate C7 see page 68.

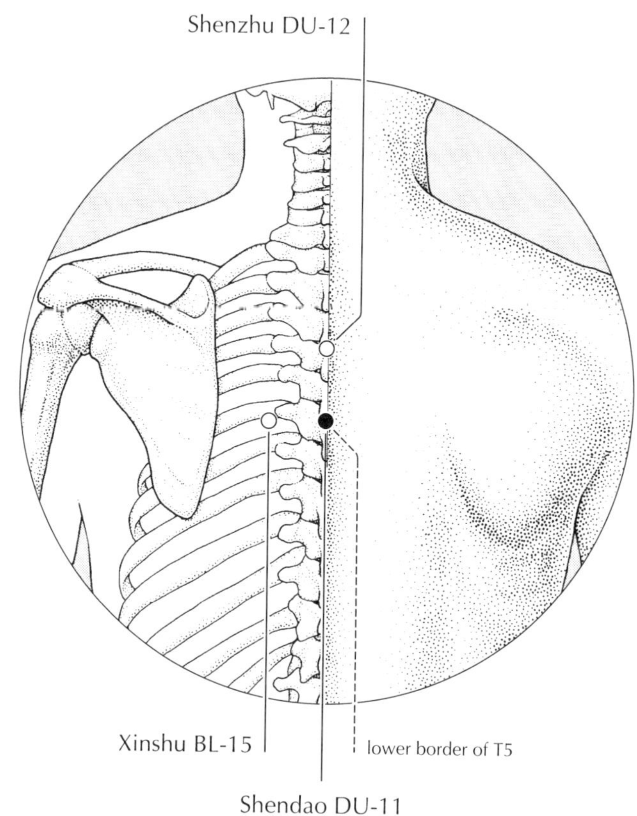

NEEDLING

Oblique superior insertion 0.5 to 1 cun. **Note**: according to several classical texts, this point is contraindicated to needling.

Caution: the spinal canal lies between 1.25 and 1.75 cun deep to the skin surface, varying according to body build.

ACTIONS

Tonifies the Heart and Lung and calms the spirit

Clears heat and pacifies wind

INDICATIONS

- Sadness and anxiety, poor memory, fright palpitations, disorientation, timidity with shortness of breath, lack of qi, taxation consumption.
- Childhood wind epilepsy, clonic spasm, childhood fright wind, lockjaw.
- Fever due to injury by cold with headache that comes and goes, heat in the body, cough and hot dyspnoea, malaria, dizziness, heat in the Liver.
- Pain and cold sensation of the upper back.

COMMENTARY

Shendao DU-11 (Spirit Pathway) is located on the upper back in the region of the Lung, at the level of Xinshu BL-15 the back-shu point of the Heart. The Lung dominates qi and the Heart stores the spirit, and together they are activated by the gathering qi. Shendao DU-11 is indicated for deficiency of the gathering qi and malnourishment of the Heart and spirit giving rise to such indications as lack of qi, timidity with shortness of breath, palpitations, disorientation, poor memory and sadness and anxiety.

In common with many points of this channel, Shendao DU-11 is also able to pacify internally generated wind which ascends along the Governing vessel and gives rise to such disorders as epilepsy, clonic spasm, childhood fright wind and lockjaw.

Finally Shendao DU-11 is indicated for a variety of heat symptoms including fever, heat in the body, hot dyspnoea and, according to the *Essential Questions*[32], heat in the Liver. This last indication clearly fell out of favour and was not mentioned in subsequent texts.

COMBINATIONS

- Poor memory: Shendao DU-11, Youmen KID-21, Lieque LU-7 and Gaohuangshu BL-43 (*Supplementing Life*).
- Sadness, anxiety and disorientation: Shendao DU-11, Xinshu BL-15 and Tianjing SJ-10 (*Supplementing Life*).
- Fright palpitations: Shendao DU-11, Yemen SJ-2, Tianjing SJ-10 and Baihui DU-20 (*Supplementing Life*).
- Frequent attacks of wind epilepsy: Shendao DU-11 and Xinshu BL-15 (*One Hundred Symptoms*).
- Heat in the body with headache that comes and goes: Shendao DU-11 and Guanyuan REN-4 (*Thousand Ducat Formulas*).

SHENZHU DU-12

Body Pillar

身柱

LOCATION

On the midline of the upper back, in the depression below the spinous process of the third thoracic vertebra.

LOCATION NOTE

This point is located three intervertebral spaces below C7. To locate C7 see page 68.

NEEDLING

Perpendicular-oblique superior insertion 0.5 to 1 cun.

Caution: the spinal canal lies between 1.25 and 1.75 cun deep to the skin surface, varying according to body build.

ACTIONS

Clears heat from the Lung and Heart
Calms the spirit
Pacifies wind

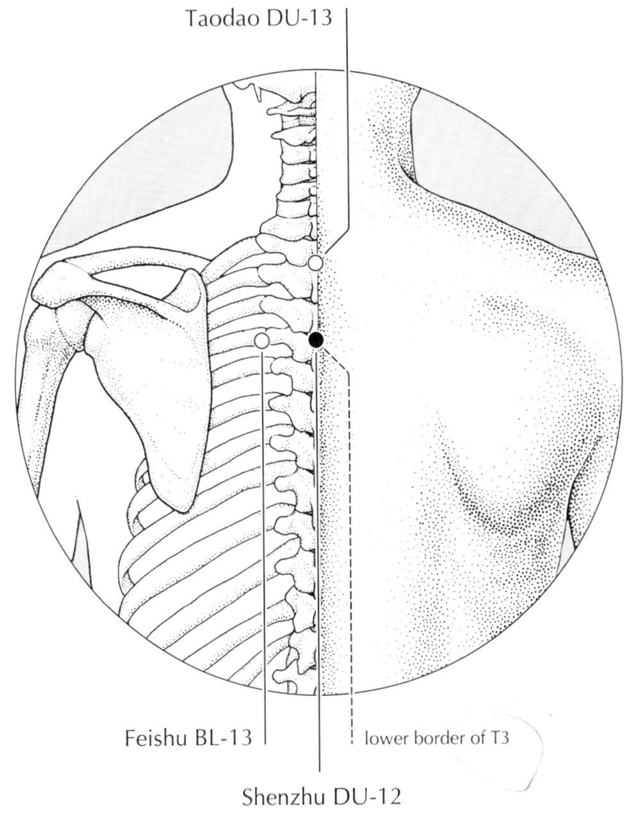

INDICATIONS

- Heat in the chest, dyspnoea, sudden cough with lumbar pain, heat in the body, dry mouth, agitation with thirst, headache and sweating.
- Mad walking, delirious raving, seeing ghosts, rage with desire to kill people.
- Childhood fright epilepsy, clonic spasm, opisthotonos, clove sores.

COMMENTARY

As early as the *Essential Questions*[33] Shenzhu DU-12 was said to clear heat from the chest, and this is reinforced by many indications found in subsequent classical texts. Shenzhu DU-12, located below the third thoracic vertebra at the level of Feishu BL-13 the back-shu point of the Lung, is able to clear heat from the Lung, giving rise to cough, dyspnoea and fever. According to the *Warp and Woof of Warm Febrile Diseases* "The Lung and Heart are mutually connected; when there is Lung heat it most easily enters the Heart". This passage helps explain why Shenzhu DU-12 is also indicated for heat in the Heart which gives rise to such excess pattern manifestations of spirit disturbance as mad walking, ranting and raving, 'seeing ghosts' and rage with desire to kill. This ability to clear heat from the Lung and calm the spirit in excess patterns can be contrasted to the action of the previous point, Shendao DU-11, which is primarily used for deficiency patterns of the Heart and Lung.

Like many other points of this channel, Shenzhu DU-12 is also able to pacify wind in the Governing vessel and is indicated for epilepsy and clonic spasm.

COMBINATIONS

- Madness: Shenzhu DU-12 and Benshen GB-13 (*One Hundred Symptoms*).
- Childhood fright epilepsy: Shenzhu DU-12 and Changqiang DU-1 (*Supplementing Life*).
- Opisthotonos, clonic spasm, epilepsy and headache: Shenzhu DU-12, Wuchu BL-5, Weizhong BL-40, Weiyang BL-39 and Kunlun BL-60 (*Thousand Ducat Formulas*).

TAODAO DU-13

Way of Happiness

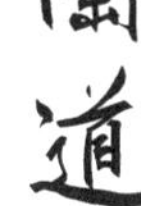

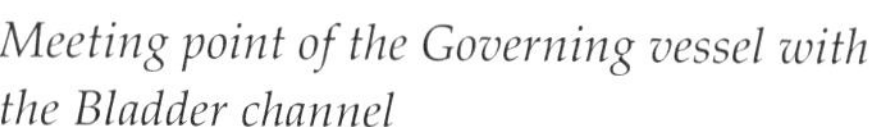

Meeting point of the Governing vessel with the Bladder channel

LOCATION

On the midline of the upper back, in the depression below the spinous process of the first thoracic vertebra.

LOCATION NOTE

This point is located one intervertebral space below C7. To locate C7 see page 68.

NEEDLING

Perpendicular-oblique superior insertion 0.5 to 1 cun.
Caution: the spinal canal lies between 1.25 and 1.75 cun deep to the skin surface, varying according to body build.

ACTIONS

Clears heat and treats malaria
Regulates the Governing vessel

INDICATIONS

- Malaria, chronic malaria, chills and fever, absence of sweating, steaming bone disorder.
- Stiffness of the spine, heaviness of the head, visual dizziness, clonic spasm, agitation and fullness, unhappiness and disorientation.

COMMENTARY

The Governing vessel is the 'sea of the yang channels' and many of its points are effective to reduce yang heat in the body, including febrile diseases and most especially malaria. In both traditional and modern clinical practice Taodao DU-13 has been an important point in the treatment of malaria, whether acute or chronic. This is primarily due to its ability to clear heat from the Governing vessel, and this action is reflected also in the indications for chills and fever and steaming bone disorder.

Like many points of the Governing vessel, Taodao DU-13 is also able to regulate the channel and to clear wind and is indicated for stiffness of the spine, heaviness of the head and clonic spasm.

Finally, as its name 'Way of Happiness' suggests, Taodao DU-13 is indicated for unhappiness and disorientation.

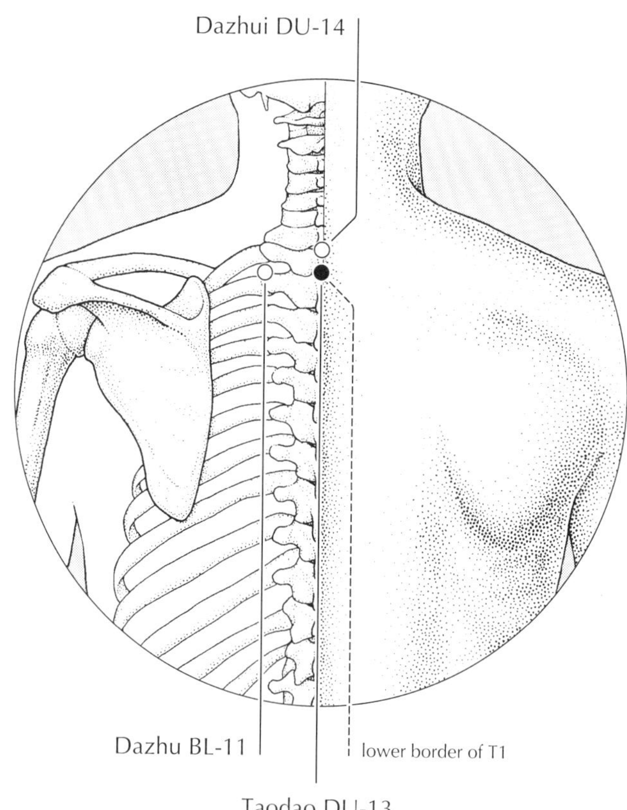

COMBINATIONS

- Seasonal fever: Taodao DU-13 and Feishu BL-13 (*Glorious Anthology*).
- Headache: Taodao DU-13, Houxi SI-3, Tianzhu BL-10, Dazhu BL-11 and Kongzui LU-6 (*Thousand Ducat Formulas*).
- Visual dizziness, dimness of vision with bursting eye pain: Taodao DU-13, Tianzhu BL-10 and Kunlun BL-60 (*Supplementing Life*).

DAZHUI DU-14

Great Vertebra

大椎

Meeting point of the Governing vessel with the six yang channels of the hand and foot
Point of the Sea of Qi

LOCATION

On the midline at the base of the neck, in the depression below the spinous process of the seventh cervical vertebra.

LOCATION NOTE

To locate C7 see page 69.

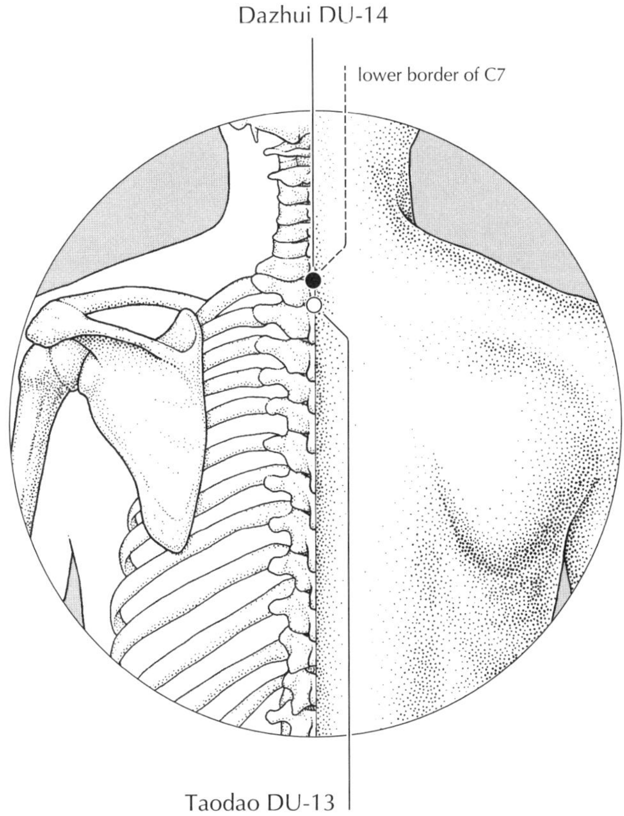

NEEDLING

Perpendicular-oblique superior insertion 0.5 to 1 cun. **Caution:** the spinal canal lies between 1.25 and 1.75 cun deep to the skin surface, varying according to body build.

ACTIONS

Expels wind and firms the exterior
Clears heat
Treats malaria
Tonifies deficiency
Pacifies wind

INDICATIONS

- Injury by cold leading to high fever with agitation and vomiting, aversion to wind with shivering, chills and fever, warm malaria, chronic malaria, throat painful obstruction, fullness of the chest and lateral costal region with dyspnoea.
- Deficiency sweating, night sweating, steaming bone disorder, heat in the bones, lack of strength, shortness of breath with inability to speak, the five taxations and the seven injuries, wind-taxation, pain of the hundred joints.
- Epilepsy, chronic and acute childhood fright wind, hypertension, insomnia, vomiting blood, nosebleed that does not stop.
- Stiffness of the spine, stiffness of the nape and neck with inability to turn the head.

COMMENTARY

The Governing vessel is known as the 'sea of the yang channels' and Dazhui DU-14 is the meeting point of the Governing vessel with the six yang channels of the hand and foot. As a consequence, Dazhui DU-14 has a strong action on i. clearing pathogenic factors from and firming the exterior yang portion of the body, ii. clearing yang heat, and iii. tonifying qi and yang.

When exterior pathogenic factors attack the body they most commonly first lodge in the exterior portion, known in the six channel and four level theories of febrile diseases as the taiyang stage and defensive level respectively. Typical symptoms of this pattern are chills and fever, aversion to wind, shivering, and throat painful obstruction. If the pathogen penetrates to the interior (yangming stage or qi level) there will be high fever with agitation. If the pathogen resides between the exterior and interior (shaoyang stage) there will be alternating chills and fever, epitomised by malaria. Dazhui DU-14 is unique in its ability to clear pathogens from all these three stages. Zhang Zhong-jing, in the *Treatise on Injury by Cold* which otherwise discusses few acupuncture points, recommends needling Dazhui DU-14 in combination with Feishu BL-13 and Ganshu BL-18 for the treatment of overlapping taiyang and shaoyang patterns.

According to the Ming dynasty author Zhang Jing-yue "Malaria is an exogenous disease .... only in the condition of delicate health or overstrain or stress, is one apt to be attacked by the malarial pathogenic factor". By virtue of its ability to clear pathogenic factors from shaoyang and to tonify qi and yang, Dazhui DU-14 is ideally suited to treat both the root and manifestation of malaria.

Dazhui DU-14 is one of the principal acupuncture points to treat disorders of sweating. Deficiency sweating arises either when pathogenic wind attacks the exterior and leads to disharmony of the nutritive qi and defensive qi, or when the defensive qi is deficient and unable to firm and control the pores. By virtue of its ability both to tonify the qi and to regulate the exterior, Dazhui DU-14 is able to treat both these forms of deficiency sweating. Night sweating and steaming bone disorder are most commonly seen in patterns of yin deficiency with heat, and here the action of Dazhui DU-14 is both to control the pores and clear the heat, and to tonify the deficiency.

Bailao (Hundred Taxations) is an alternative name for this point found in the *Glorious Anthology of Acupuncture and Moxibustion* and other classics. This name vividly illustrates the ability of Dazhui DU-14 to treat deficiency and exhaustion of the whole body manifesting as lack of strength, the five taxations and the seven injuries. Another indication that reflects the ability of Dazhui DU-14 to tonify and strengthen the body is shortness of breath with inability to speak. This is explained in the *Spiritual Pivot*[34] which classifies Dazhui DU-14 (along with Renying ST-9, Shanzhong REN-17 and Yamen DU-15) as a point of the 'sea of qi'. This passage states "When the sea of qi is deficient, there is scanty energy insufficient for speech".

According to the *Treatment Strategies for Assorted Syndromes*[35] "Painful obstruction syndrome ... is due to deficiency of nutritive and defensive qi and to the space between skin and muscles being open, thus allowing wind-cold-dampness to ride the deficiency". Not only can underlying deficiency render a person prone to painful obstruction in this way, but if pathogenic wind-damp penetrates the bones and joints, over time it may lead to exhaustion. Dazhui DU-14, which is able to expel wind, regulate the pores and tonify qi, is specifically indicated for pain of the hundred joints (i.e. all the joints) and for wind-taxation (chronic painful obstruction leading to exhaustion of qi and blood).

Like many points of the Governing vessel, Dazhui DU-14 is able to pacify interior wind (epilepsy and acute childhood fright wind), and to benefit the entire spine, particularly in the neck region. In clinical practice, Dazhui DU-14 is often needled towards one or other shoulder when neck pain radiates laterally.

After ascending to the vertex, the Governing vessel descends through the midline of the nose. Dazhui DU-14 is indicated for nosebleed which does not stop, an indication that mirrors the folk practice of placing a key or other piece of cold metal, or a cold sponge, at the back of the neck to stop nosebleed.

COMBINATIONS

- Malaria with much heat and little cold: Dazhui DU-14, Houxi SI-3, Jianshi P-5 and Quchi L.I.-11 (*Great Compendium*).
- Malaria with much cold and little heat: Dazhui DU-14, Houxi SI-3 and Quchi L.I.-11 (*Great Compendium*).
- Malaria: Dazhui DU-14 and Yaoshu DU-2 (*Supplementing Life*).
- Injury by cold with great heat that does not recede: reduce Dazhui DU-14, Quchi L.I.-11, Xuanzhong GB-39, Zusanli ST-36, Yongquan KID-1 and Hegu L.I.-4 (*Great Compendium*).
- Spleen cold malaria: Dazhui DU-14, Jianshi P-5 and Rugen ST-18 (*Great Compendium*).
- Spontaneous sweating: Dazhui DU-14, Fuliu KID-7 and moxa Gaohuangshu BL-43 (*Divine Moxibustion*).
- Nosebleed: moxa Dazhui DU-14 and Yamen DU-15 (*Secrets of the Master of Cinnabar Creek*).

YAMEN DU-15

Gate of Muteness

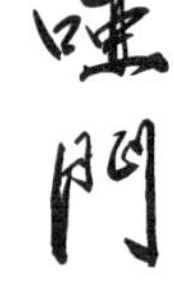

Meeting point of the Governing and Yang Linking vessels
Point of the Sea of Qi

LOCATION

On the midline at the nape of the neck, in the depression 0.5 cun inferior to Fengfu DU-16, below the spinous process of the first cervical vertebra (impalpable).

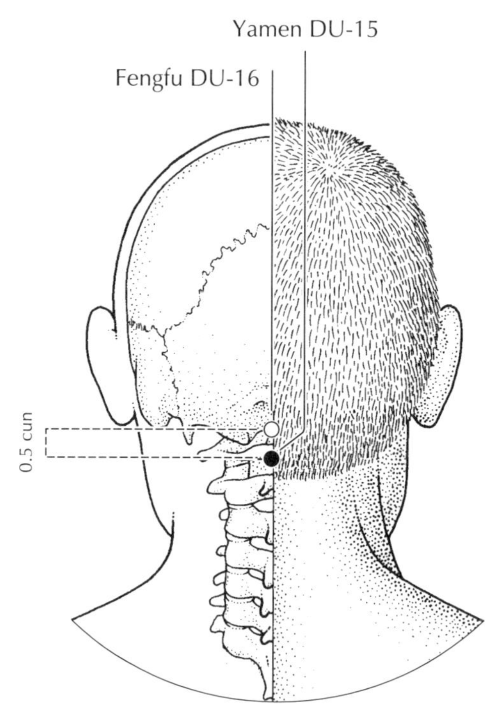

LOCATION NOTE

The posterior hairline is measured as 1 cun inferior to Fengfu DU-16. Locate Yamen DU-15 at the midpoint, i.e. 0.5 cun above the posterior hairline.

NEEDLING

Perpendicular insertion slightly inferiorly, 0.5 to 1 cun. **Note**: according to several classical texts, this point is contraindicated to moxibustion.

Caution: the spinal canal lies between 1.5 and 2 cun deep to the skin surface, varying according to body build. Deep perpendicular insertion is therefore strictly contraindicated, as is superior oblique insertion towards the brain.

ACTIONS

Benefits the tongue and treats muteness
Eliminates wind
Benefits the neck and spine

INDICATIONS

- Stiffness of the tongue with inability to speak, loss of voice, lotus flower tongue, flaccidity of the tongue.
- Heaviness of the head, head wind, loss of consciousness from windstroke, epilepsy, clonic spasm, mania-depression, loss of consciousness, all kinds of yang heat and qi exuberance.
- Absence of sweating, chills and fever, nosebleed that does not stop.
- Stiffness of the neck, stiffness of the spine, sprain of the spine.

COMMENTARY

Yamen DU-15, on the back of the neck just above the hairline, lies directly opposite the root of the tongue, and according the *Great Compendium of Acupuncture and Moxibustion* a channel from Yamen DU-15 (Gate of Muteness) binds at the root of the tongue. The *Spiritual Pivot*[36] lists Yamen DU-15 as a point of the 'sea of qi' and states "When the sea of qi is deficient, there is scanty energy insufficient for speech". As early as the *Systematic Classic of Acupuncture and Moxibustion*, and reasserted in later texts, it was said that moxibustion at this point could cause a person to become mute, whilst needling it could cure muteness. These classical references provided the basis for the claims made during the turbulent years of the Cultural Revolution that deep needling of Yamen DU-15 could have almost miraculous effects in the treatment of deaf-mute children. Photographs were published of whole classrooms of previously deaf-mute children singing 'The East is Red'. Like many of the extreme claims made during this period, this was later discredited, indeed it was confirmed that many patients suffered injury to the spinal cord from excessively deep needling. Notwithstanding this reservation, Yamen DU-15 is one of the few acupuncture points classically indicated for loss of voice and muteness, as well as for stiffness and flaccidity of the tongue, and the condition known as lotus flower tongue (distention and prominence of the blood vessels beneath the tongue), all of which may prevent normal speech. The *Great Compendium of Acupuncture and Moxibustion* advises the use of Yamen DU-15 for "all kinds of yang heat and qi exuberance", whilst the *Secrets of A Border Official* says that it "drains all yang qi and heat". In this context, it is interesting to note that many of the tongue disorders referred to arise due to excess heat and yang exuberance.

The second principal action of Yamen DU-15 is to eliminate either exterior or interior wind giving rise to such symptoms as head wind, stiff neck, loss of consciousness, epilepsy, clonic spasm and chills and fever with absence of sweating. Moreover the location of this point on the neck, and the pathway of the Governing vessel through the spine, renders it suitable for the treatment of stiff neck and spine due to any aetiology.

Like Dazhui DU-14, Yamen DU-15 is also indicated for nosebleed that does not stop.

Finally Yamen DU-15 is cited in the *Song of the Nine Needles for Returning the Yang* for the treatment of collapse of yang characterised by loss of consciousness, aversion to cold, cold counterflow of the limbs, purple lips etc.

COMBINATIONS

- Loss of voice: Yamen DU-15 and Kongzui LU-6 (*Supplementing Life*).
- Sudden loss of voice: Yamen DU-15 and Sanyangluo SJ-8 (*Supplementing Life*).
- Flaccidity of the tongue with inability to speak: Yamen DU-15 and Guanchong SJ-1 (*One Hundred Patterns*).
- Windstroke, flaccidity of the tongue and sudden loss of voice: Yamen DU-15 and Fengfu DU-16 (*Golden Mirror*).
- Stiffness of the tongue: Yamen DU-15, Shaoshang LU-11, Yuji LU-10, Erjian L.I.-2, Zhongchong P-9, Yingu KID-10 and Rangu KID-2 (*Great Compendium*).
- Heaviness of the head: Yamen DU-15, Tongtian BL-7 and Fuyang BL-59 (*Supplementing Life*).
- Nosebleed: moxa Yamen DU-15 and Dazhui DU-14 (*Secrets of the Master of Cinnabar Creek*).

FENGFU DU-16

Palace of Wind

風府

Meeting point of the Governing and Yang Linking vessels
Point of the Sea of Marrow
Point of the Window of Heaven
Sun Si-miao Ghost point

LOCATION

On the midline at the nape of the neck, in the depression immediately below the external occipital protuberance.

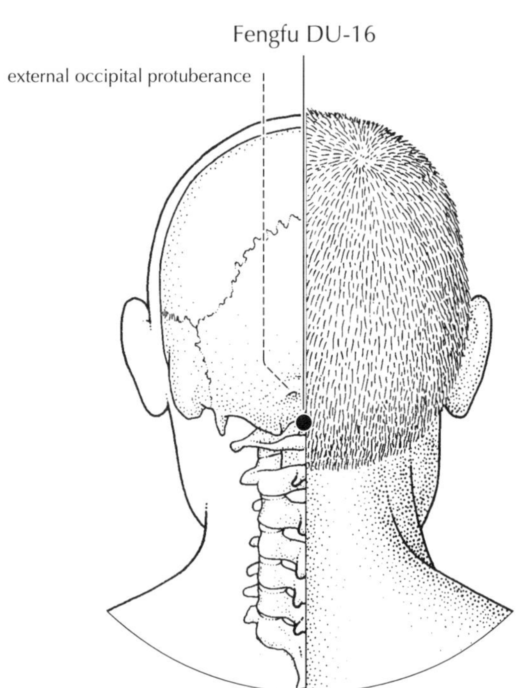

LOCATION NOTE

i. The external occipital protuberance is found as the bony prominence at the base of the skull on the midline, though in some individuals it may be difficult to feel; ii. This point lies approximately 1 cun above the posterior hairline.

NEEDLING

Perpendicular insertion slightly inferiorly, 0.5 to 1 cun. **Note**: according to several classical texts, this point is contraindicated to moxibustion.

Caution: the spinal canal lies between 1.5 and 2 cun deep to the skin surface, varying according to body build. Deep perpendicular or superior oblique insertion is therefore strictly contraindicated.

ACTIONS

Eliminates wind
Nourishes the sea of marrow and benefits the head and neck
Calms the spirit

INDICATIONS

- Heaviness of the body with aversion to cold, cold shivering with sweating, swelling and pain of the throat, wind painful obstruction, all types of wind disease, injury by wind.
- Headache, head wind, the hundred diseases of the head, visual dizziness, dizziness, blurred vision, nosebleed, upward staring eyes, sudden loss of voice, sudden inability to speak following windstroke, flaccid tongue with inability to speak, windstroke, numbness of the legs, hemiplegia, hypertension.
- Mania, incessant talking, mad walking and desire to commit suicide, sadness and fear with fright palpitations.
- Difficulty in breathing, heat in the chest, ceaseless vomiting, jaundice.
- Pain of the neck with inability to turn the head, stiff neck.

COMMENTARY

In the *Essential Questions*[37] the Yellow Emperor says "I have heard that wind is the beginning of the hundred diseases; what is the method of treating it by acupuncture"? His adviser Qi Bo replies "Wind enters from the exterior giving rise to shivering, sweating, headache, heaviness of the body and aversion to cold. Treat it by needling Fengfu DU-16".

Wind, which may be of exterior or interior origin, is a yang pathogenic factor that therefore tends to affect the outer and upper (yang) portions of the body. Exterior wind predominantly injures the head and the superficial portion of the body, whilst interior wind stirs upwards and harasses the top of the body. The Governing vessel is known as the 'sea of the yang channels', and whilst many of its points are effective to eliminate both exterior and interior wind, Fengfu DU-16 (Palace of Wind) is pre-eminent for this purpose. Its importance in the treatment of both kinds of wind disorder is emphasised in *Investigation into Points Along the Channels* by the Ming dynasty author Yan Zhen-shi, who said that Fengfu DU-16 is indicated for "all types of wind disease".

When pathogenic wind invades the exterior portion of the body and impairs the ability of defensive qi to warm the skin, there will aversion to cold and shivering. If defensive qi is deficient and pathogenic wind attacks, the pattern known as disharmony of the nutritive qi and defensive qi may ensue, characterised by chills and shivering accompanied by sweating. The application of Fengfu

DU-16 in the treatment of this particular pattern of taiyang wind disorder is emphasised in the *Treatise on Injury by Cold* which says "In taiyang disorder, initially prescribe *Gui Zhi Tang* (Cinnamon Twig Decoction). If this causes agitation, needle Fengchi GB-20 and Fengfu DU-16 then (once again) represcribe *Gui Zhi Tang*. Recovery will follow". If pathogenic wind enters the channels and collaterals and penetrates the joints, there may be migratory aching and pain, known as 'wind painful obstruction'. In all such cases Fengfu DU-16 is indicated.

Fengfu DU-16 is of equal importance in the treatment of interior wind which derives from disharmony of the zangfu, particularly the Liver, and rushes upwards to the neck, head and brain. It is therefore indicated for headache, head wind, dizziness, blurred vision, upward staring eyes and windstroke. Not only is Fengfu DU-16 able to descend pathogenic wind from the head in such cases, but it is also an important point to nourish the brain. According to the *Spiritual Pivot*[38] Fengfu DU-16 is a point of the sea of marrow, "Its point above is the top of the head; below it is Fengfu" and "When the sea of marrow is in excess then there is lightness of the body and much strength and a person's self exceeds the normal level; when the sea of marrow is insufficient there is a whirling sensation of the brain, dizziness, tinnitus, pain of the lower legs, impairment of vision, indolence and desire to sleep". The wide-ranging effect of Fengfu DU-16 on the head region is further emphasised both by the statement by Sun Si-miao in the *Thousand Ducat Formulas* that Fengfu DU-16 treats 'the hundred diseases of the head', and by the alternative name Xingxing (Clear Headedness) given to this point in the classic *Song to Keep Up Your Sleeve*.

Due to the location of Fengfu DU-16 in the neck region, the pivot of the head, as well as to its ability to eliminate wind and nourish the sea of marrow, Fengfu DU-16 is an important point in the treatment of headache, head wind and neck disorders. The traditional term head wind has two principal meanings. Firstly it is used to refer to severe, long-standing and recurring headaches (for example migraine) that are recalcitrant to treatment, in contrast to a single incident of headache. Secondly, it describes a condition deriving from attack by exterior wind which invades the channels of the head and gives rise to headache, dizziness and deviation of the mouth and eye. Although primarily indicated for occipital (taiyang region) headache, as would be expected from its location, Fengfu DU-16 is a meeting point of the Governing vessel with the Yang Linking vessel. This extraordinary vessel also links all the yang channels, and specifically connects with such important points for headache as Benshen GB-13 through to Fengchi GB-20 on the lateral side of the head, and Touwei ST-8 on the forehead. Fengfu DU-16 may therefore be needled in shaoyang (temporal) or yangming (frontal) region headaches when the primary pathogen is wind. As far as the neck is concerned, the ability of Fengfu DU-16 to benefit this region is emphasised in the *Great Compendium of Acupuncture and Moxibustion* which recounts how the great 2nd century physician Hua Tuo treated the Emperor Wu of the Three Kingdoms era for stiff neck. It is related that as soon as Hua Tuo needled Fengfu DU-16, the Emperor was cured.

It is a reflection of yin-yang theory that when excess accumulates at the top of the body there is often a corresponding deficiency below, and this is borne out in the statement in the classic *Song to Keep Up Your Sleeve* "when the legs and feet are diseased choose Fengfu DU-16". The ability of Fengfu DU-16 to treat numbness of the legs reflects the principle stated in the *Yellow Emperor's Inner Classic*[39] "When the disease is below select [points] from above".

Although the Heart is most frequently cited as the residence of the spirit, since its early beginnings Chinese medicine (particularly in the Daoist tradition) has been able to hold the concurrent belief that the head and brain also influence the spirit. Thus the *Essential Questions*[40] said "the head is the residence of the intelligence", Sun Si-miao in the *Thousand Ducat Formulas* said "The head is the supreme leader, the place where man's spirit concentrates" and Li Shi-zhen said "The brain is the residence of the original spirit". The Governing vessel enters the brain at Fengfu DU-16, which is also said to mark its lower border, whilst another branch of the vessel passes through the Heart. Fengfu DU-16 is therefore indicated for various mental disorders such as mania, incessant talking with inability to rest, mad walking and desire to commit suicide, as well as sadness and fear with fright palpitations. It was included under its alternative name of Guizhen (Ghost Pillow) by Sun Si-miao in his 'thirteen ghost points' for the treatment of mania disorder and epilepsy.

Finally, Fengfu DU-16 is one of ten points listed in Chapter 2 of the *Spiritual Pivot* that have come to be known as Window of Heaven points (for a fuller discussion see page 48). It shares with the other points of this group the ability to i. treat headache and dizziness, ii. descend rebellious qi (vomiting), iii. treat throat disorders, iv. benefit the sense organs (eyes, nose and tongue), and v. treat sudden onset of disorders (sudden inability to speak following windstroke, sudden loss of voice).

COMBINATIONS

- "In taiyang disorder, initially prescribe *Gui Zhi Tang* (Cinnamon Twig Decoction). If this causes agitation, needle Fengchi GB-20 and Fengfu DU-16, then represcribe *Gui Zhi Tang*. Recovery will follow" (*Treatise on Injury by Cold*).

- The hundred disorders due to injury by cold: Fengfu DU-16 and Fengchi GB-20 (*Ode of Xi-hong*).
- Throat pain: Fengfu DU-16, Tianchuang SI-16 and Laogong P-8 (*Thousand Ducat Formulas*).
- Loss of voice: Fengfu DU-16 and Chengjiang REN-24 (*Supplementing Life*).
- Windstroke, flaccidity of the tongue and sudden loss of voice: Fengfu DU-16 and Yamen DU-15 (*Golden Mirror*).
- Pain of the eyes with inability to see: Fengfu DU-16, Fengchi GB-20, Naohu DU-17, Yuzhen BL-9 and Shangxing DU-23 (*Thousand Ducat Formulas*).
- Rhinitis with nose bleed: Fengfu DU-16, Erjian L.I.-2 and Yingxiang L.I.-20 (*Great Compendium*).
- Stiffness and pain of the neck with inability to turn the head: Fengfu DU-16 and Yinjiao DU-28 (*Supplementing Life*).
- Stiffness and pain of the head and nape with difficult rotation: Fengfu DU-16 and Chengjiang REN-24 (*Song of the Jade Dragon*).
- Mania, incessant talking without rest: Fengfu DU-16, Kunlun BL-60 and Shugu BL-65 (*Thousand Ducat Formulas*).
- Mad walking with desire to commit suicide: Fengfu DU-16 and Feishu BL-13 (*Thousand Ducat Formulas*).
- Mad walking: Fengfu DU-16 and Yanggu SI.-5 (*Great Compendium*).
- Numbness of the legs: Fengfu DU-16 and Yaoshu DU-2 (*Thousand Ducat Formulas*).

NAOHU DU-17

Brain's Door

腦戶

Meeting point of the Governing vessel with the Bladder channel

LOCATION

At the back of the head on the midline, 1.5 cun directly above Fengfu DU-16, in the depression directly superior to the external occipital protuberance.

LOCATION NOTE

This point may be located at the junction of the lower quarter and the upper three quarters of the line connecting Fengfu DU-16 and Baihui DU-20.

NEEDLING

Transverse insertion superiorly or inferiorly 0.5 to 1 cun. **Note**: according to several classical texts, this point is contraindicated to both needling and moxibustion.

ACTIONS

Eliminates wind and alleviates pain
Benefits the eyes
Calms the spirit

INDICATIONS

- Heaviness of the head, head wind, aversion to wind in the head, wind dizziness, swelling and pain of the head, pain of the face, red face, stiffness and pain of the neck.
- Dimness of vision, short sightedness, eye pain, excessive lacrimation, yellow eyes, jaundice.
- Mania, epilepsy, clonic spasm, lockjaw, loss of voice, bleeding from the root of the tongue, goitre, chills and fever, sweating, pain of the bones.

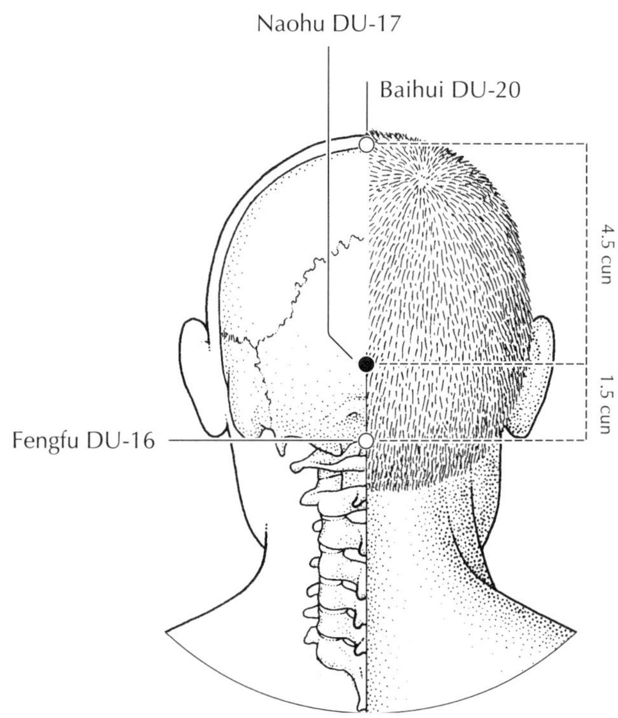

COMBINATIONS

- Pain and heaviness of the head: Naohu DU-17, Tongtian BL-7 and Naokong GB-19 (*Thousand Ducat Formulas*).
- Yellow eyes: Naohu DU-17, Danshu BL-19, Yishe BL-49 and Yanggang BL-48 (*Supplementing Life*).
- Pain of the eyes with inability to see: Naohu DU-17, Fengchi GB-20, Yuzhen BL-9, Fengfu DU-16 and Shangxing DU-23 (*Thousand Ducat Formulas*).
- Madness with vomiting: Naohu DU-17, Luoque BL-8, Zhubin KID-9, Yanggu SI-5, Houding DU-19, Qiangjian DU-18 and Yuzhen BL-9 (*Thousand Ducat Formulas*).

QIANGJIAN DU-18

Unyielding Space

強間

LOCATION

At the back of the head on the midline, 1.5 cun directly superior to Naohu DU-17, midway between Fengfu DU-16 and Baihui DU-20.

LOCATION NOTE

This point may be located at the midpoint of the line connecting Fengfu DU-16 and Baihui DU-20.

NEEDLING

Transverse insertion 0.5 to 1 cun.

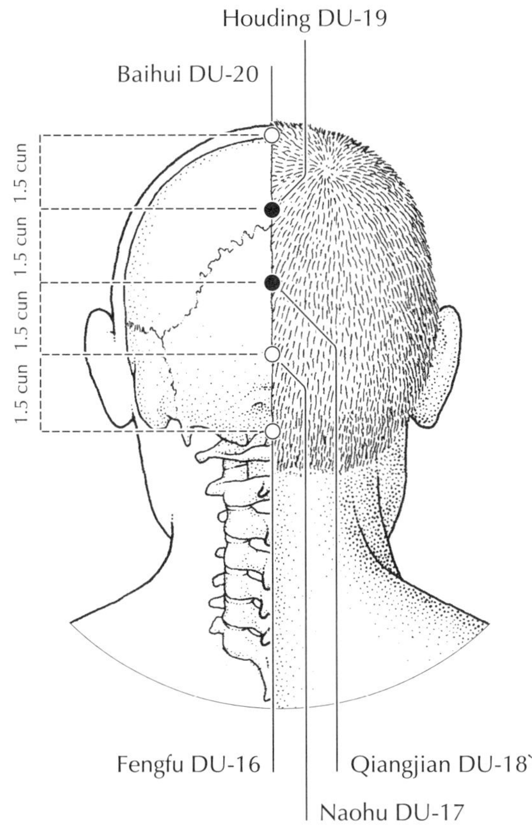

ACTIONS

Pacifies wind and alleviates pain
Calms the spirit

INDICATIONS

- Headache, dizziness with agitation, nausea and vomiting of foamy (watery) saliva, stiffness of the neck with inability to turn the head.
- Epilepsy, shaking of the head, mad walking, insomnia, mania-depression, clonic spasm.

COMMENTARY

As is often the case, a point such as Qiangjian DU-18 which is considered of minimal importance in modern clinical practice, was clearly ascribed greater significance in classical texts, witnessed by numerous traditional combinations. It shares with many points of the head region, particularly its neighbouring points of the Governing vessel (Naohu DU-17 and Houding DU-19) the ability to pacify interior wind and calm the spirit. It was primarily applied, however, for unendurable stabbing pain in the head.

COMBINATIONS

- Headache that is difficult to endure: Qiangjian DU-18 and Fenglong ST-40 (*One Hundred Symptoms*).
- Stabbing pain of the head with inability to move: Qiangjian DU-18 and Touqiaoyin GB-11 (*Supplementing Life*).
- Stabbing pain of the head with inability to move: Qiangjian DU-18 and Zuqiaoyin GB-44 (*Thousand Ducat Formulas*).
- Deviation of the mouth with inability to speak: Qiangjian DU-18, Chengqi ST-1, Sibai ST-2, Juliao ST-3, Kouheliao L.I.-19, Shangguan GB-3, Daying ST-5, Quanliao SI-18, Fengchi GB-20, Yingxiang L.I.-20 and Renzhong DU-26 (*Supplementing Life*).
- Agitation of the Heart: Qiangjian DU-18, Baihui DU-20 and Chengguang BL-6 (*Supplementing Life*).
- Epileptic convulsions, mad walking, inability to sleep, agitation of the Heart: Qiangjian DU-18, Zanzhu BL-2, Xiaohai SI-8 and Houxi SI-3 (*Thousand Ducat Formulas*).

HOUDING DU-19

Behind the Crown

後頂

LOCATION

At the back of the head on the midline, 1.5 cun directly superior to Qiangjian DU-18 and 1.5 cun posterior to Baihui DU-20.

LOCATION NOTE

This point may be located at the junction of the lower three quarters and the upper quarter of the line connecting Fengfu DU-16 and Baihui DU-20.

NEEDLING

Transverse insertion 0.5 to 1 cun.

ACTIONS

Eliminates wind and alleviates pain
Calms the spirit

INDICATIONS

- Stiffness and pain of the head and neck, one-sided headache, pain of the vertex, wind dizziness, aversion to wind and cold, painful obstruction with sweating.
- Mad walking, insomnia, epileptic convulsions.

COMBINATIONS

- Wind dizziness: Houding DU-19, Yuzhen BL-9 and Hanyan GB-4 (*Supplementing Life*).
- Wind dizziness and one-sided headache: Houding DU-19, Hanyan GB-4 and Qianding DU-21 (*Thousand Ducat Formulas*).
- Pain of the neck with aversion to wind-cold: Houding DU-19 and Waiqiu GB-36 (*Supplementing Life*).
- Pain of the head and nape: Houding DU-19, Baihui DU-20 and Hegu L.I.-4 (*Great Compendium*).
- Pain of the head and eyes: Houding DU-19, Tongli HE-5 and Baihui DU-20 (*Supplementing Life*).

BAIHUI DU-20

Hundred Meetings

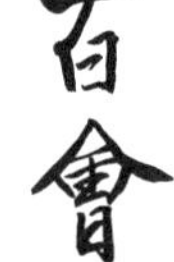

Meeting point of the Governing vessel with the Bladder, Gall Bladder, Sanjiao and Liver channels
Point of the Sea of Marrow

LOCATION

At the vertex on the midline, in the depression 5 cun posterior to the anterior hairline and 7 cun superior to the posterior hairline. This point may also be measured as 8 cun posterior to the glabella and 6 cun superior to the external occipital protuberance.

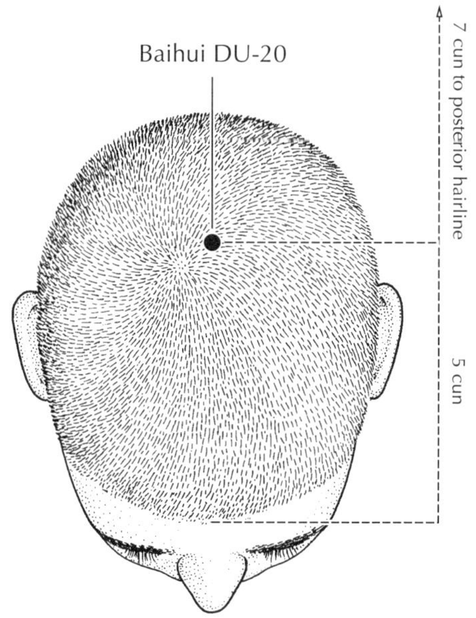

LOCATION NOTE

i. Place the heels of the hands on the anterior and posterior hairlines and extend the middle fingers towards each other; Baihui DU-20 is located 1 cun anterior to where the middle fingers meet; ii. If the anterior hairline is indistinct, place the heels of the hands on the glabella and external occipital protuberance and extend the middle fingers towards each other; Baihui DU-20 is located 1 cun posterior to where the middle fingers meet; iii. Extend a line along the long axis of the ear (from the midpoint of the lobe to the midpoint of the apex) in its slightly posterior direction to the top of the head where Baihui DU-20 may be found.

NEEDLING

Transverse insertion 0.5 to 1 cun.

ACTIONS

Pacifies wind and subdues yang
Raises yang and counters prolapse
Benefits the head and sense organs
Nourishes the sea of marrow
Benefits the brain and calms the spirit

INDICATIONS

- Head wind, one-sided headache, pain of the vertex, heaviness of the head, dizziness, wind dizziness, visual dizziness, tinnitus, protruding eyes, blindness, hypertension, hypotension.
- Windstroke, hemiplegia, opisthotonos, tetany, loss of consciousness, vomiting of foam, wind epilepsy, lockjaw.
- Prolapse of the rectum, prolapse of the uterus.
- Agitation and oppression, sensation of heat and oppression of the Heart, fright palpitations, poor memory, lack of mental vigour, disorientation, much crying, sadness and crying with desire to die, mania.
- Obstruction of the nose, nasal discharge, nosebleed, inability to taste food or drink.
- Redness of the face after consumption of alcohol, heat in the body, malaria.

COMMENTARY

The name Baihui DU-20 (Hundred Meetings) reflects the location of this point at the crown of the head which is the meeting of all the yang qi of the body, and its ability, according to the *Classic of Supplementing Life with Acupuncture and Moxibustion* to treat the 'one hundred diseases'. Like many acupuncture points, Baihui DU-20 has also been given a variety of alternative names in classical texts, reflecting different aspects of its nature. The name Sanyangwuhui (Three Yang Five Meetings) emphasises that Baihui DU-20 is the meeting point of the Governing vessel with the three yang channels of the Bladder, Gall Bladder and Sanjiao, as well as the Liver channel. Another name, Niwangong (Mud Ball Palace), is used in qigong theory. Niwan (Mud Ball) refers to the material aspect of the spirit which is located in the brain (see also Shenting DU-24), and accordingly Baihui DU-20 is sometimes considered to be the location of the upper dantian (cinnabar field). Further names include Tianshan (Mountain of Heaven) reflecting its location at the highest point of the body, and Guimen (Ghost Gate) reflecting its influence on psycho-emotional disorders.

Baihui DU-20 is located at the apex of the head, the highest and hence most yang point of the body. It therefore has a profound effect on regulating yang, both to descend excess yang and to raise deficient yang. Interior wind is a yang pathogen characterised by vigorous upward movement and is most commonly generated when the Liver's spreading and rising movement exceeds its normal bounds. Baihui DU-20, the meeting of the Governing and Liver channels, is able to descend such manifestations of interior wind and uprising of yang as windstroke, dizziness, tinnitus, headache, head wind, pain of the vertex, opisthotonos, lockjaw and loss of consciousness. A number of different classics state that Baihui DU-20 should be bled in such excess patterns. The pronounced ability of this point to descend excess from the head should not obscure its importance in nourishing the brain. According to the *Spiritual* Pivot[41] Baihui DU-20 is a point of the sea of marrow "Its point above is the top of the head; below it is Fengfu" and "When the sea of marrow is in excess then there is lightness of the body and much strength and a person's self exceeds the normal level; when the sea of marrow is insufficient there is a whirling sensation of the brain, tinnitus, pain of the lower legs, dizziness, impairment of vision, indolence and desire to sleep".

As well as treating disorders at the top of the body, Baihui DU-20 is able to raise sinking of yang at the lower end of the Governing vessel leading to prolapse of the rectum. This action of raising yang has been extended in modern clinical practice to the treatment of prolapse of the uterus and vagina. For this purpose Baihui DU-20 is often treated by moxibustion. Zhu Dan-xi recommends the application of three cones of moxa to Baihui DU-20 for chronic disease with qi deficiency and incessant diarrhoea[42]. All these indications reflect the principle stated in the *Yellow Emperor's Inner Classic*[43] "When the disease is below select [points] from above".

This effect of raising yang is emphasised in qigong practice. Attention is focused on the upper dantian [either Baihui DU-20 or Yintang (M-HN-3)] in cases of sinking of qi, aversion to wind and cold in the head, hypotension etc., but contraindicated in cases of excessive yang, fire or wind. According to the *Ode to Elucidate Mysteries* "Heaven, earth and man are the three powers. Baihui DU-20 ... echoes Heaven, Xuanji REN-21 ... echoes man and Yongquan KID-1 ... echoes the earth". It is by opening Baihui DU-20 that we can better absorb the energy of heaven, and through focusing on Yongquan KID-1 that we can root to the energy of the earth. It is strongly emphasised, however, that since yang has a natural tendency to rise to the head, most people should first master sinking the qi to the lower dantian, in the lower abdomen, or to Yongquan KID-1, and circulating the qi through the small heavenly circuit (the Governing and Conception vessels) before focusing unduly on the upper dantian.

One of the most striking groups of indications found in classical texts for Baihui DU-20 is disorders of the spirit and Heart, for example heat and oppression of the Heart, fright palpitations, poor memory, disorientation, sadness and crying with desire to die etc. As considered at length in the introductory discussion to the Governing vessel (above), this reflects the overlap between different theories in Chinese medicine concerning the residence of the spirit, some schools emphasising the Heart and others the brain. The *Essential Questions* for example states "The Heart stores the spirit"[44] and "The head is the residence of the intelligence"[45]. As stated above, the Governing vessel, and Baihui DU-20 in particular, has an especially close relationship with the brain. At the same time, the anterior pathway of the Governing vessel ascends through the Heart. The Governing vessel, therefore, can be seen as the channel which integrates these two theories, and Baihui DU-20 may be selected especially when psycho-emotional disturbance manifests with indications of disharmony both of the Heart (palpitations, oppression etc.) and the head and brain (heaviness of the head, epilepsy, dizziness etc.).

From Baihui DU-20, the Governing vessel starts to descend down the midline of the front of the head, traversing the nose. This point is therefore indicated for a variety of nasal disorders including discharge, obstruction and bleeding.

Finally, according to the *Spiritual Pivot*[46] Baihui DU-20 is listed as one of a group of twenty-five points for treating headache caused by inversion qi (disordered and contrary flow of qi): Qiangjian DU-18, Houding DU-19, Baihui DU-20, Qianding DU-21, Xinhui DU-22, Wuchu BL-5, Chengguang BL-6, Tongtian BL-7, Luoque BL-8, Yuzhen BL-9, Toulinqi GB-15, Muchuang GB-16, Zhengying GB-17, Chengling GB-18 and Naokong GB-19.

COMBINATIONS

- Somnolence: Baihui DU-20 and Xinhui DU-22 (*Supplementing Life*).
- Somnolence: Baihui DU-20, Tianjing GB-21, Erjian L.I.-2, Sanjian L.I.-3, Taixi KID-3, Zhaohai KID-6, Lidui ST-45 and Ganshu BL-18 (*Great Compendium*).
- Fright palpitations: Baihui DU-20, Shendao DU-11, Tianjing SJ-10 and Yemen SJ-2 (*Supplementing Life*).
- Agitation of the Heart: Baihui DU-20, Qiangjian DU-18 and Chengguang BL-6 (*Supplementing Life*).
- Mania: Baihui DU-20, Jianshi P-5, Fuliu KID-7, Yingu KID-10 and Zusanli ST-36 (*Illustrated Supplement*).
- Tendency to excessive crying: Baihui DU-20 and Renzhong DU-26 (*Great Compendium*).
- Wind epilepsy with upward staring eyes: Baihui DU-20, Kunlun BL-60 and Sizhukong SJ-23 (*Great Compendium*).
- Head wind: Baihui DU-20, Naokong GB-19 and Tianzhu BL-10 (*Supplementing Life*).
- Head wind: Baihui DU-20, Xiaxi GB-43, Shangxing DU-23, Qianding DU-21, Yanggu SI-5, Hegu L.I.-4, Guanchong SJ-1 and Kunlun BL-60 (*Great Compendium*).
- One-sided or generalised head wind: Baihui DU-20, Qianding DU-21, Shenting DU-24, Shangxing DU-23, Sizhukong SJ-23, Fengchi GB-20, Hegu L.I.-4, Zanzhu BL-2 and Touwei ST-8 (*Great Compendium*).
- Pain of the head and eyes: Baihui DU-20, Tongli HE-5 and Houding DU-19 (*Supplementing Life*).
- Pain of the head and nape: Baihui DU-20, Houding DU-19 and Hegu L.I.-4 (*Great Compendium*).
- Lockjaw following windstroke: Baihui DU-20, Renzhong DU-26, Jiache ST-6, Chengjiang REN-24 and Hegu L.I.-4 (*Great Compendium*).
- For most types of acute throat pain: first needle Baihui DU-20 then Taichong LIV-3, Zhaohai KID-6 and Sanyinjiao SP-6 (*Ode of Xi-hong*).
- Tinnitus: Baihui DU-20, Tinggong SI-19, Tinghui GB-2, Ermen SJ-21, Luoque BL-8, Yangxi L.I.-5, Qiangu SI-2, Houxi SI-3, Wangu SI-4, Zhongzhu SJ-3, Yemen SJ-2, Shangyang L.I.-1 and Shenshu BL-23 (*Great Compendium*).
- Obstruction of the nose with inability to distinguish the fragrant from the foul: Baihui DU-20, Shangxing DU-23, Xinhui DU-22 and Chengguang BL-6 (*Supplementing Life*).
- Nasal congestion: Baihui DU-20, Yuzhen BL-9, Toulinqi GB-15, Shangxing DU-23 and Danyang (Extra)[47] (*Supplementing Life*).
- Dysenteric disorder: Baihui DU-20 and Jiuwei REN-15 (*Ode of Spiritual Brightness*).
- Prolapse of the rectum in children: Baihui DU-20, Changqiang DU-1 and Dachangshu BL-25 (*Great Compendium*).
- Prolapse of the rectum in children: first moxa Baihui DU-20 then Jiuwei REN-15 (*Ode of Xi-hong*).
- Prolapse of the rectum: Baihui DU-20, Dachangshu BL-25, Changqiang DU-1, Jianjing GB-21, Hegu L.I.-4 and Qichong ST-30 (*Compilation*).
- Prolapse of the rectum: Baihui DU-20, Shenque REN-8 and Pangguangshu BL-28 (*Compilation*).
- Prolapse of the rectum and haemorrhoids: Baihui DU-20, Erbai (M-UE-29), Zhishi BL-52 and Changqiang DU-1 (*The Great Compendium of Acupuncture and Moxibustion*).

QIANDING DU-21

In Front of the Crown

前頂

LOCATION

At the top of the head on the midline, 1.5 cun directly anterior to Baihui DU-20 and 3.5 cun posterior to the anterior hairline.

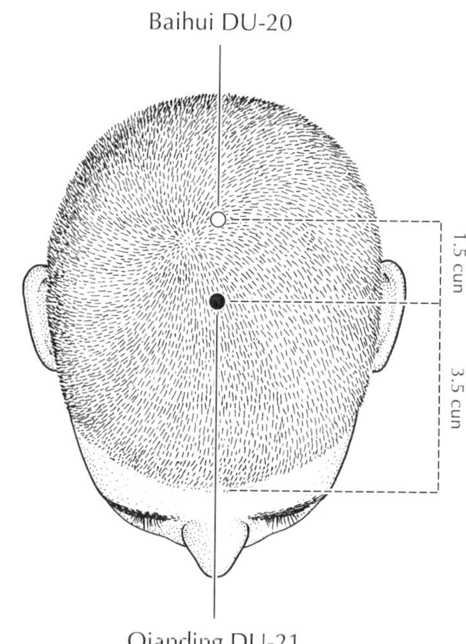

LOCATION NOTE

i. Divide the distance between Baihui DU-20 and the anterior hairline into thirds. Qianding DU-21 lies slightly posterior to the junction of the first and middle thirds; ii. If the anterior hairline is indistinct, locate it 3 cun superior to the glabella and 5 cun anterior to Baihui DU-20.

NEEDLING

Transverse insertion 0.5 to 1 cun.

Caution: this point should not be needled in infants whose fontanelle has not yet closed.

ACTIONS

Eliminates wind and treats convulsions

Benefits the head

INDICATIONS

- Head wind, visual dizziness, wind epilepsy, childhood fright epilepsy, acute and chronic childhood fright wind, clonic spasm.
- Pain and swelling of the vertex, swelling and redness of the face, oedema, aversion to wind-cold, copious clear nasal discharge.

COMBINATIONS

- Childhood fright epilepsy: Qianding DU-21, Xinhui DU-22, Benshen GB-13 and Tianzhu BL-10 (*Supplementing Life*).
- Wind dizziness and one-sided headache: Qianding DU-21, Houding DU-19 and Hanyan GB-4 (*Thousand Ducat Formulas*).
- One-sided or generalised head wind: Qianding DU-21, Baihui DU-20, Shenting DU-24, Shangxing DU-23, Sizhukong SJ-23, Fengchi GB-20, Hegu L.I.-4, Zanzhu BL-2 and Touwei ST-8 (*Great Compendium*).
- Inability to speak following windstroke: Qianding DU- 21 and Shenting DU-24 (*Song of the Jade Dragon*).
- Sudden swelling of the face: Qianding DU-21, Xinhui DU-22, Shangxing DU-23, Xiangu ST-43 and Gongsun SP-4 (*Supplementing Life*).
- Redness and swelling of the face: Qianding DU-21, Xinhui DU-22, Shangxing DU-23, Naohu DU-17 and Fengchi GB-20 (*Thousand Ducat Formulas*).
- Deficiency swelling of the face: Qianding DU-21 and Renzhong DU-26 (*One Hundred Symptoms*).

XINHUI DU-22

Fontanelle Meeting

顖會

LOCATION

At the top of the head on the midline, 2 cun posterior to the anterior hairline.

LOCATION NOTE

i. Divide the distance between Baihui DU-20 and the anterior hairline in half and locate Xinhui DU-22 at 0.5 cun anterior to this midpoint; ii. Locate 1 cun posterior to Shangxing DU-23; iii. If the anterior hairline is indistinct, locate it 3 cun superior to the glabella and 5 cun anterior to Baihui DU-20.

NEEDLING

Transverse insertion 0.5 to 1 cun.

Caution: this point should not be needled in infants whose fontanelle has not yet closed.

ACTIONS

Benefits the nose

Eliminates wind and benefits the head

INDICATIONS

- Nosebleed, nasal congestion, inability to distinguish the fragrant from the foul, excessive nasal discharge in children, pain of the nose, nasal polyps.
- Head wind, chronic headache, deficiency and cold of the brain, bursting headache due to excessive consumption of alcohol, dizziness, visual dizziness, chronic and acute childhood fright wind.
- Blue-green (qing) complexion, red and swollen face, swelling of the skin of the head, dandruff.
- Somnolence, fright palpitations.

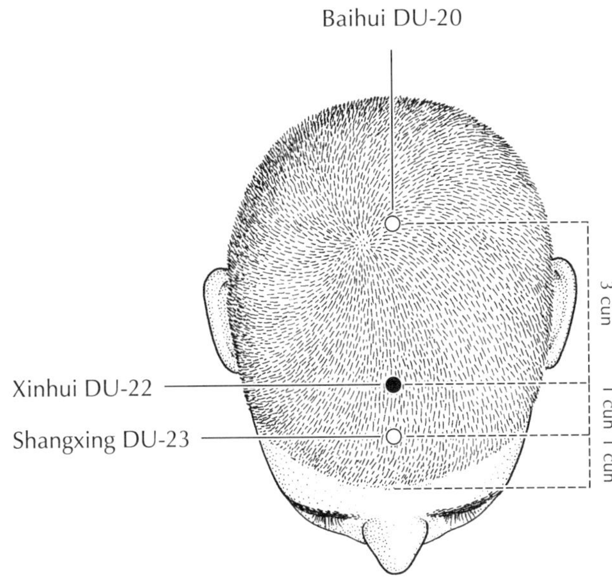

COMMENTARY

As is often the case, a point such as Xinhui DU-22 which is considered of minimal importance in modern clinical practice, was clearly ascribed greater significance in classical texts, witnessed by the many traditional indications and combinations. It shares with many points of the head region the ability to pacify interior wind and treat various disorders of the head. Its application in nose disorders, however, is overshadowed by Shangxing DU-23, and in head wind, headache and dizziness, by Baihui DU-20.

COMBINATIONS

- Somnolence: Xinhui DU-22 and Baihui DU-20 (*Supplementing Life*).

- Childhood fright epilepsy: Xinhui DU-22, Qianding DU-21, Benshen GB-13 and Tianzhu BL-10 (*Supplementing Life*).
- Head wind: Xinhui DU-22 and Yuzhen BL-9 (*One Hundred Symptoms*).
- Head wind and dizziness: Xinhui DU-22, Shenting DU-24 and Shangxing DU-23 (*Supplementing Life*).
- Obstruction of the nose with inability to distinguish the fragrant from the foul: Xinhui DU-22, Shangxing DU-23, Baihui DU-20 and Chengguang BL-6 (*Supplementing Life*).

SHANGXING DU-23

Upper Star

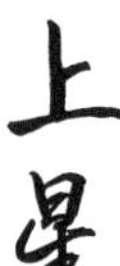

Sun Si-miao Ghost point

LOCATION

At the top of the head on the midline, 1 cun posterior to the anterior hairline and 0.5 cun posterior to Shenting DU-24.

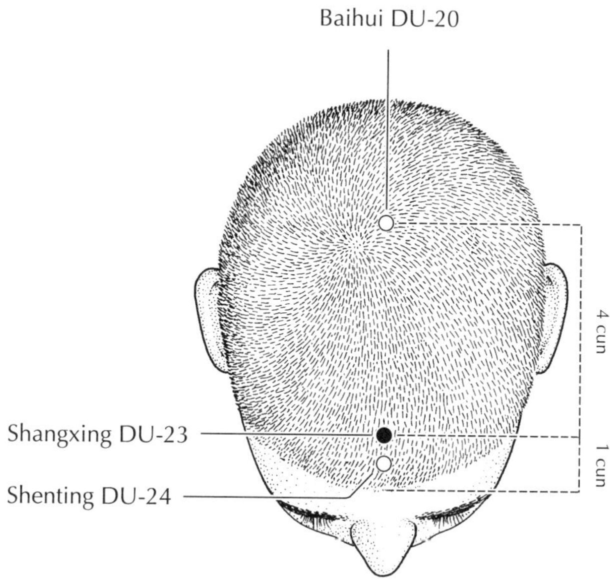

LOCATION NOTE

If the anterior hairline is indistinct, locate it 3 cun superior to the glabella and 5 cun anterior to Baihui DU-20.

NEEDLING

Transverse insertion 0.5 to 1 cun.

ACTIONS

Benefits the nose and eyes
Eliminates wind, benefits the head and face and dispels swelling
Calms the spirit

INDICATIONS

- Nasal obstruction and discharge, nasal obstruction accompanied by headache, inability to distinguish the fragrant from the foul, nasal polyps, clear nasal discharge, rhinitis, ceaseless bleeding from the nose and mouth.
- Visual dizziness, pain of the eyes, short sightedness, redness and swelling of the face, deficiency swelling of the face, swelling of the skin of the head, head wind.
- Malaria, febrile disease with absence of sweating, mania-depression.

COMMENTARY

After passing over the vertex of the head, the Governing vessel descends through the nose. Shangxing DU-23, located directly above the nose, is in a commanding position to regulate the widest range of nasal disorders and is an important point clinically in the treatment of nasal obstruction and discharge, pain of sinusitis, rhinitis, inability to smell, nosebleed and nasal polyps.

An alternative name for this point is Mingtang (Hall of Brightness) reflecting the fact that from the earliest times Shangxing DU-23 has also been considered valuable in treating eye diseases including short sightedness, eye pain, visual impairment and visual dizziness. This may be explained both by the proximity of this point to the eye region and by the fact that the anterior pathway of the Governing vessel ascends to below the middle of the eye. Interestingly, several classical texts warn that if this point is treated by excessive moxibustion it will raise the yang and lead to lack of clarity of vision.

A number of further alternative names for this point reflect its status as one of the 'thirteen ghost points' listed in the *Supplement to the Thousand Ducat Formulas* of Sun Si-miao for the treatment of mania disorder and epilepsy. These include Guitang (Ghost Hall), Guigong (Ghost Palace) and Shentang (Hall of the Spirit).

Finally Shangxing DU-23 is indicated for various kinds of swelling in the upper region, including redness and swelling of the face, deficiency swelling of the face, and swelling of the skin of the head.

COMBINATIONS

- Obstruction of the nose with inability to distinguish the fragrant from the foul: Shangxing DU-23, Baihui DU-20, Xinhui DU-22 and Chengguang BL-6 (*Supplementing Life*).
- Nasal congestion with inability to distinguish the fragrant from the foul: Shangxing DU-23, Yingxiang L.I.-20, Wuchu BL-5 and Kouheliao L.I.-19 (*Great Compendium*).

- Nasal congestion: Shangxing DU-23, Yuzhen BL-9, Baihui DU-20, Toulinqi GB-15 and Danyang (Extra)[47] (*Supplementing Life*).
- Nasal obstruction and discharge: Shangxing DU-23 and Tongtian BL-7 (*Primary Points of the Fourteen Channels*).
- Nosebleed: Shangxing DU-23 and Kouheliao L.I.-19 (*Song of Points*).
- Eye pain: Shangxing DU-23, Yangxi L.I.-5, Erjian L.I.-2, Daling P-7, Sanjian L.I.-3 and Qiangu SI-2 (*Great Compendium*).
- Pain of the eyeball: Shangxing DU-23 and Neiting ST-44 (*Great Compendium*).
- Pain of the eyes with inability to see: Shangxing DU-23, Fengchi GB-20, Naohu DU-17, Yuzhen BL-9 and Fengfu DU-16 (*Thousand Ducat Formulas*).
- Visual dizziness: Shangxing DU-23, Shenting DU-24, Yongquan KID-1, Yixi BL-45, Yuji LU-10 and Dadu SP-2 (*Supplementing Life*).
- Dizziness: Shangxing DU-23, Fengchi GB-20 and Tianzhu BL-10 (*Glorious Anthology*).
- Head wind and dizziness: Shangxing DU-23, Shenting DU-24 and Xinhui DU-22 (*Supplementing Life*).
- Head wind: Shangxing DU-23, Baihui DU-20, Xiaxi GB-43, Qianding DU-21, Yanggu SI-5, Hegu L.I.-4, Guanchong SJ-1 and Kunlun BL-60 (*Great Compendium*).
- Sudden swelling of the face: Shangxing DU-23, Xinhui DU-22, Qianding DU-21, Xiangu ST-43 and Gongsun SP-4 (*Supplementing Life*).
- Redness and swelling of the face: Shangxing DU-23, Xinhui DU-22, Qianding DU-21, Naohu DU-17 and Fengchi GB-20 (*Thousand Ducat Formulas*).

SHENTING DU-24

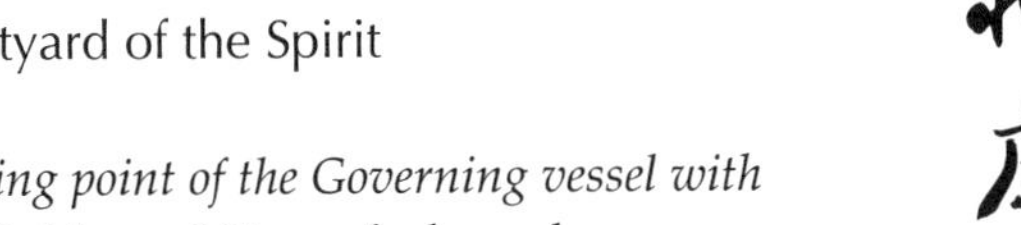

Courtyard of the Spirit

神庭

Meeting point of the Governing vessel with the Bladder and Stomach channels

LOCATION
At the top of the head on the midline, 0.5 cun posterior to the anterior hairline and 0.5 cun anterior to Shangxing DU-23.

LOCATION NOTE
If the anterior hairline is indistinct, locate it 3 cun superior to the glabella and 5 cun anterior to Baihui DU-20.

NEEDLING
Transverse insertion 0.5 to 1 cun. **Note**: according to several classical texts, this point is contraindicated to needling.

ACTIONS
Benefits the brain and calms the spirit
Eliminates wind and benefits the head
Benefits the nose and eyes

INDICATIONS
- Mania-depression, ascends to high places and sings, discards clothing and runs around, mimics other people's speech, fright palpitations, insomnia, loss of consciousness, tongue thrusting.
- Upward staring eyes, opisthotonos, wind epilepsy, wind dizziness accompanied by vomiting, vomiting with agitation and fullness, dizziness, head wind, headache with chills and fever, cold sensation of the head.
- Clear and ceaseless nasal discharge, nasal congestion and discharge, nosebleed, lacrimation, lack of visual clarity, dyspnoea.

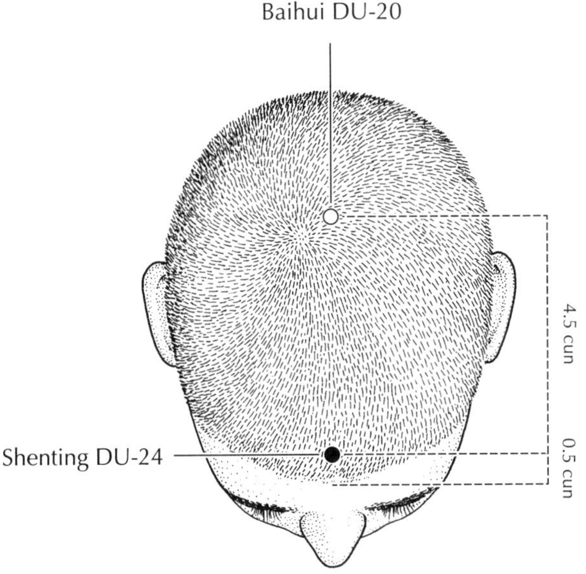

COMMENTARY
Shenting DU-24 (Courtyard of the Spirit) is also known as Tianting (Courtyard of Heaven). Like several of the points of the Governing vessel, it has a strong action on calming the spirit and treating epilepsy and mania disorder. It is dramatically and graphically indicated for the treatment of those who undress, climb to high places, sing and mimic other people's speech. The action of the Governing vessel points on the spirit can be explained in three ways. Firstly, of all the channels, the Governing vessel has the closest relationship with the brain. As explained in the introductory discussion to the Governing vessel (see above) the head and brain were considered among pre-*Inner Classic* and later Daoist traditions to be the seat of the

spirit, and one cause of mental disorders was traditionally perceived to be wind entering the brain through the Governing vessel. Secondly, the Governing vessel anterior pathway enters the Heart, and thus strongly links the brain and Heart which is more commonly understood to be the residence of the spirit. Thirdly, mania disorder is characterised by heat, and points of the Governing vessel, the 'sea of the yang channels', are important to clear pathogenic heat from the whole body. As far as Shenting DU-24 in particular is concerned, it is said to directly access Niwan (Mud Ball), also known as Huangting (The Yellow Courtyard). The Niwan in the Daoist tradition is the central one of the nine palaces of the brain and is considered to be the location of the material basis of the spirit. The *Classic on the Central Void in the Inner Sphere* said "The origin of essence-spirit in the brain is also called Niwan" and "The entire spirit that expresses in the face has its origin in Niwan"[48], whilst the Daoist Classic *Collected Wisdom by Master Magic Sword* stated "The qi of the Heart is connected with the Niwan Palace above"[49].

The second principal action of Shenting DU-24 is to pacify pathologically ascending interior wind (upward staring eyes, dizziness and epilepsy), and to dispel exterior pathogenic wind (head wind, headache with chills and fever and cold sensation of the head). Since Shenting DU-24 is a meeting point of the Governing vessel with the Stomach channel, it is specifically indicated for wind dizziness accompanied by vomiting, and vomiting with agitation and fullness.

Finally, like Shangxing DU-23, Shenting DU-24 is indicated for a variety of nasal and eye disorders including clear and ceaseless nasal discharge, nasal congestion and discharge, nosebleed, lacrimation and lack of visual clarity. It is interesting to note, however, that a number of classics including the *Systematic Classic of Acupuncture and Moxibustion* and the *Illustrated Classic of Acupuncture Points on the Bronze Man* warn that this point is contraindicated for needling as it may give rise to adverse effects such as damage to the eyesight or mania.

COMBINATIONS

- Madness with vomiting of foam: Shenting DU-24, Duiduan DU-27 and Chengjiang REN-24 (*Systematic Classic*).
- Wind epilepsy: Shenting DU-24, Suliao DU-25 and Yongquan KID-1 (*Great Compendium*).
- Inability to speak following windstroke: Shenting DU-24 and Qianding DU-21 (*Song of the Jade Dragon*).
- One-sided or generalised head wind: Shenting DU-24, Baihui DU-20, Qianding DU-21, Shangxing DU-23, Sizhukong SJ-23, Fengchi GB-20, Hegu L.I.-4, Zanzhu BL-2 and Touwei ST-8 (*Great Compendium*).
- Head wind and dizziness: Shenting DU-24, Shangxing DU-23 and Xinhui DU-22 (*Supplementing Life*).
- Visual dizziness: Shenting DU-24, Shangxing DU-23, Yongquan KID-1, Yixi BL-45, Yuji LU-10 and Dadu SP-2 (*Supplementing Life*).
- Rhinitis with clear nasal discharge: Shenting DU-24, Fengmen BL-12, Hegu L.I.-4, Zanzhu BL-2, Yingxiang L.I.-20, Zhiyin BL-67 and Futonggu KID-20 (*Thousand Ducat Formulas*).
- Lacrimation: Shenting DU-24 and Xingjian LIV-2 (*Supplementing Life*).

SULIAO DU-25

White Crevice

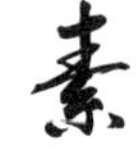

LOCATION

On the midline at the tip of the nose.

NEEDLING

i. Perpendicular insertion 0.2 to 0.3 cun; ii. Transverse insertion directed superiorly 0.5 to 1 cun; iii. Prick to bleed. **Note**: according to several classical texts, this point is contraindicated to moxibustion.

ACTIONS

Benefits the nose

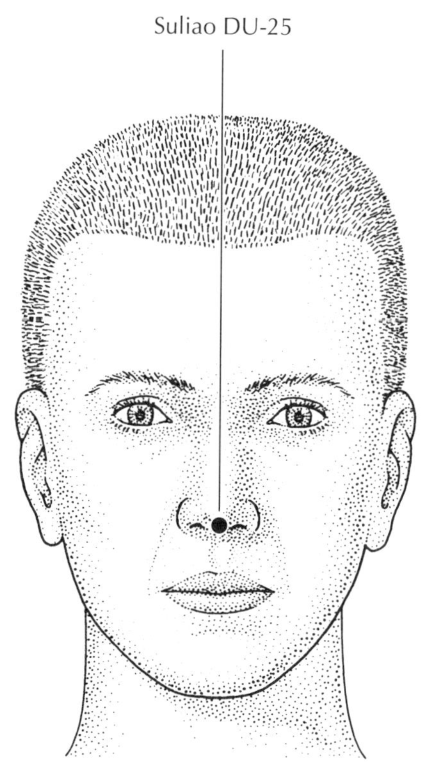

INDICATIONS

- Copious nasal discharge, rhinitis, inability to distinguish the fragrant from the foul, nasal obstruction, nasal sores, nosebleed, drinker's nose, nasal polyps, dyspnoea, hypotension.

COMMENTARY

In recent times this point has been found to be effective in reducing alcohol intoxication by redirecting the route of elimination from the liver to the lung and thereby increasing the volume of alcohol present in the expired air. Other recent research has shown this point to be more effective than Renzhong DU-26 in restoring loss of consciousness.

COMBINATIONS

- Wind epilepsy: Suliao DU-25, Shenting DU-24 and Yongquan KID-1 (*Great Compendium*).

RENZHONG DU-26

Man's Middle

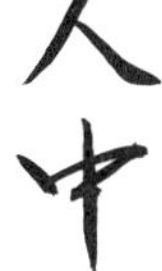

Meeting point of the Governing vessel with the Large Intestine and Stomach channels
Sun Si-miao Ghost point

LOCATION

Above the upper lip on the midline, at the junction of the upper third and lower two thirds of the philtrum.

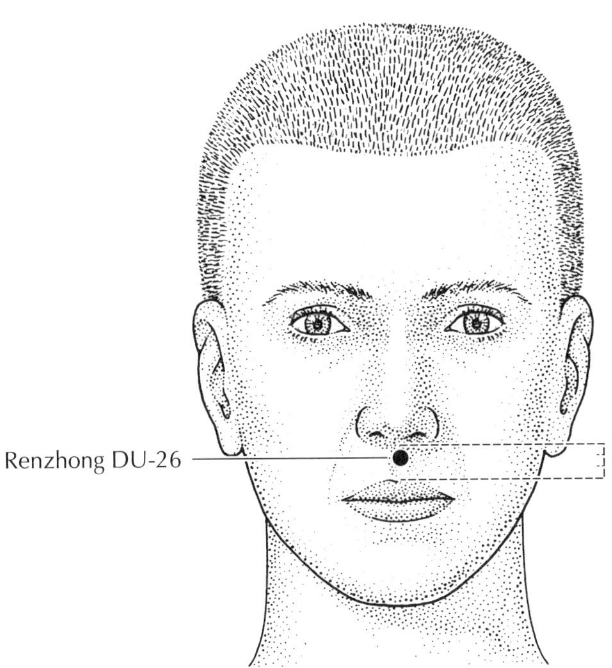

LOCATION NOTE

The philtrum is the marked indentation found on the midline between the root of the nose and the margin of the upper lip.

NEEDLING

Oblique insertion directed superiorly 0.3 to 0.5 cun.

ACTIONS

Restores consciousness and calms the spirit
Benefits the face and nose and expels wind
Benefits the spine and treats acute lumbar sprain

INDICATIONS

- Sudden loss of consciousness, coma, acute and chronic childhood fright wind, loss of consciousness from windstroke, lockjaw, deviation of the face and mouth, headache with chills and fever, hypertension.
- Mania-depression, epilepsy, inappropriate laughter, unexpected laughter and crying.
- Ceaseless nosebleed, clear nasal discharge, constant nasal discharge with difficulty in breathing, inability to distinguish the fragrant from the foul.
- Wasting and thirsting disorder, drinking water without limit, oedema of the body, swelling of the face with trembling lips, jaundice.
- Stiffness and pain of the spine, sprain and pain of the lumbar spine.

COMMENTARY

The name of this point (Man's Middle) reflects the location of this point close to the junction of the Governing and Conception vessels, and between the nose and mouth. The Governing vessel which governs all the yang channels, and the nose which receives heavenly qi, both correspond to heaven (yang). The Conception vessel which governs all the yin channels, and the mouth which receives earthly sustenance, both correspond to earth (yin). According to Chinese cosmology 'man' lies between heaven and earth, and Renzhong DU-26 is considered to establish connection between the two.

When the harmonious interaction of yin and yang is lost and they begin to separate, there is loss of consciousness (death being the ultimate manifestation of this separation). Renzhong DU-26 (along with Neiguan P-6) was one of two points added by later commentators to Gao Wu's 'four command points' to make the 'six command points'. In this grouping of the most essential acupuncture points, Renzhong DU-26 was indicated for resuscitation, and it is the single most important acupuncture point to revive consciousness and re-establish yin-yang harmony. In any kind of fainting or loss of consciousness, including needle shock, Renzhong DU-26 may be needled or strongly pressed (obliquely upwards towards the root of the nose). The *Ode of the Golden Needle* specifically recommends needling Renzhong DU-26 and Zusanli ST-36 for dizziness following needling (needle shock).

The powerful effect of Renzhong DU-26 on restoring consciousness is mirrored in its equally strong effect on calming the mind. The Governing vessel both enters the brain and connects (via its anterior pathway) with the Heart. Renzhong DU-26 is an important point in the treatment of severe psycho-emotional disorders, and is indicated in classical texts for unexpected and inappropriate laughter and crying. The importance of Renzhong DU-26 in the treatment of mania disorder and epilepsy is reflected in its inclusion under its alternative name of Guigong (Ghost Palace) among the 'thirteen ghost points' of Sun Si-miao for the treatment of mania disorder and epilepsy. According to the *Ode of Xi-hong* "the ability of Renzhong DU-26 to treat mania disorder is supreme; the thirteen ghost points must not be overlooked".

Renzhong DU-26 is a meeting point of the Governing vessel with the hand and foot yangming (Large Intestine and Stomach) channels which dominate the face and nose. It is therefore indicated for various disorders of the nose, including blockage, discharge, bleeding and loss of sense of smell, as well as swelling of the face and wind disorders such as deviation of the face and mouth and lockjaw.

According to the *Yellow Emperor's Inner Classic*[50] "When the disease is below select [points] from above". Renzhong DU-26, located close to the termination of the Governing vessel, is therefore an important point clinically in the treatment of sprain of the lumbar spine, traversed by the lower portion of the Governing vessel and close to its origin. It is normally selected when the pain is acute and on the midline, and needled whilst the patient stands and rotates and bends the waist.

COMBINATIONS

- Loss of consciousness from windstroke: Renzhong DU-26, Zhongchong P-9 and Hegu L.I.-4; if this is ineffective, needle Yamen DU-15 and Dadun LIV-1 (*Great Compendium*).
- Loss of consciousness from summerheat stroke: Renzhong DU-26, Hegu L.I-4, Neiting ST-44, Baihui DU-20, Zhongji REN-3 and Qihai REN-6 (*Great Compendium*).
- Tendency to excessive crying: Renzhong DU-26 and Baihui DU-20 (*Great Compendium*).
- Frequent laughter: Renzhong DU-26, Lieque LU-7, Yangxi L.I.-5 and Daling P-7 (*Great Compendium*).
- Madness: Renzhong DU-26 and Yinjiao DU-28 (*Systematic Classic*)
- Epilepsy: Renzhong DU-26 and Jianshi P-5 (*Ode of Spiritual Brightness*).
- Nasal discharge with inability to distinguish the fragrant from the foul: Renzhong DU-26 and Tianyou SJ-16 (*Thousand Ducat Formulas*).
- Deficiency swelling of the face: Renzhong DU-26 and Qianding DU-21 (*One Hundred Symptoms*).
- Deviation of the mouth and eye: Renzhong DU-26, Jiache ST-6, Dicang ST-4, Chengjiang REN-24, Tinghui GB-2 and Hegu L.I.-4 (*Illustrated Supplement*).
- Lockjaw following windstroke: Renzhong DU-26, Jiache ST-6, Baihui DU-20, Chengjiang REN-24 and Hegu L.I.-4 (*Great Compendium*).
- Pain of the lumbar region and leg: Renzhong DU-26 and Weizhong BL-40 (*Great Compendium*).
- Pain of the lumbar region and lateral costal region due to sprain: Renzhong DU-26, Chize LU-5 and Weizhong BL-40 ... afterwards needle Kunlun BL-60, Shugu BL-65, Zhigou SJ-6 and Yanglingquan GB-34 (*Great Compendium*).

DUIDUAN DU-27

Extremity of the Mouth

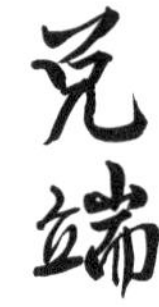

LOCATION

On the midline, at the junction of the margin of the upper lip and the philtrum.

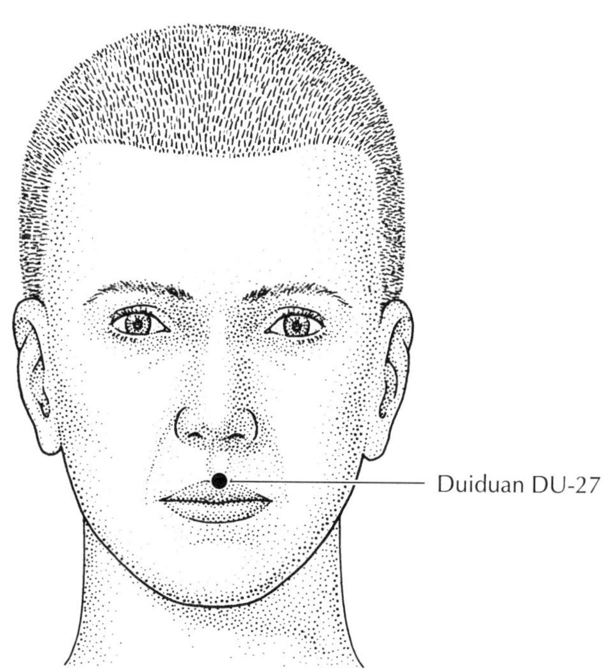

LOCATION NOTE

The philtrum is the marked indentation found on the midline between the root of the nose and the margin of the upper lip.

NEEDLING

Oblique insertion directed superiorly 0.2 to 0.3 cun.

ACTIONS

Clears heat, generates fluid and benefits the mouth
Calms the spirit

INDICATIONS

- Ulceration of the mouth, foul breath, pain of the gums, dry tongue, wasting and thirsting disorder with much drinking, swelling and stiffness of the lips, ceaseless nosebleed, nasal congestion.
- Mania-depression, epilepsy, lockjaw.
- Dark urine, vomiting of foam.

COMBINATIONS

- Stiffness of the lips and pain from tooth decay of the upper jaw: Duiduan DU-27, Muchuang GB-16, Zhengying GB-17 and Ermen SJ-21 (*Thousand Ducat Formulas*).
- Vomiting of foam: Duiduan DU-27, Shaohai HE-3 and Benshen GB-13 (*Supplementing Life*).
- Incessant nosebleed: Duiduan DU-27, Kouheliao L.I.-19 and Laogong P-8 (*Supplementing Life*).

YINJIAO DU-28

Gum Intersection

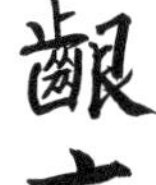

Meeting point of the Governing vessel with the Conception vessel and Stomach channel

LOCATION

Inside the mouth, in the superior frenulum, at the junction of the upper lip and the gum.

LOCATION NOTE

The superior frenulum is the midline band of fibrous tissue connecting the upper lip and gum.

NEEDLING

i. Oblique insertion directed superiorly 0.2 to 0.3 cun; ii. Prick to bleed.

ACTIONS

Clear heat and benefits the gums
Benefits the nose and eyes

INDICATIONS

- Redness, swelling and pain of the gums, erosion of the gums, bleeding from the gums.
- Nasal polyps, nasal sores, nasal congestion, pain of the forehead and glabella.
- Excessive lacrimation, redness, itching and pain of the inner canthus, pain of the eyes and lack of clarity of vision, superficial visual obstruction.
- Red face with agitation, jaundice, stiffness of the neck with inability to turn the head.

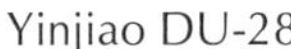

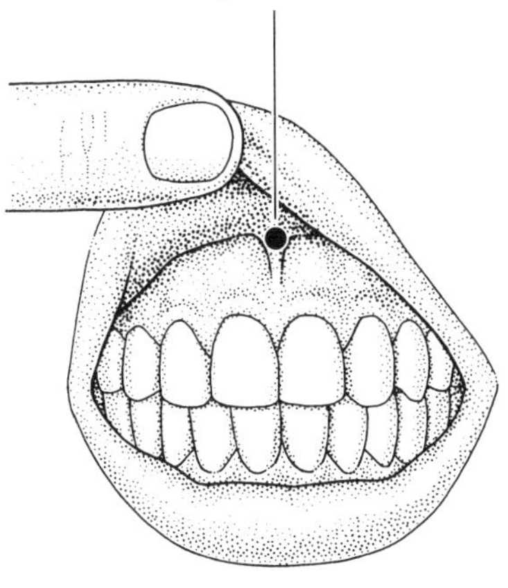

COMBINATIONS

- Stiffness and pain of the neck with inability to turn the head: Yinjiao DU-28 and Fengfu DU-16 (*Supplementing Life*).
- Madness: Yinjiao DU-28 and Renzhong DU-26 (*Systematic Classic*).

NOTES

1 Translated by Giovanni Maciocia.
2 *Essential Questions* Chapter 32.
3 *Spiritual Pivot* Chapter 8.
4 *Spiritual Pivot* Chapter 54.
5 *Spiritual Pivot* Chapter 71.
6 *Essential Questions* Chapter 62.
7 *Essential Questions* Chapter 17.
8 *Ten Works on Practice Toward the Attainment of Truth* (Xiuzhen Shishu), a qigong compendium in 64 volumes from the Qing dynasty; editor and exact date of publication unknown. This text combines important Daoist works on qigong practice from the Sui, Tang and Song dynasties, including the *Classic on the Central Void in the Inner Sphere* (Huangting Neijing Jing). Passage translated by Heiner Fruehauf.
9 *Daoist Internal Mirror* (Neijing). Not the *Yellow Emperor's Inner Classic* but part of the work Che Sheng Ba Bian written by Liu Sijing around 1647. Passage translated by Heiner Fruehauf.

10 *Essentials of Materia Medica* by Wang Ang, 1694.

11 For example *Guanzi*, a 4th century BCE meditation text.

12 *Essential Questions* Chapter 11. Passage translated by Heiner Fruehauf.

13 Some medical historians also hold the opinion that early contact with Jesuit missionaries may have played a part in the revival of the theory of the brain as the centre of consciousness. Wang Qing-ren in the chapter 'On the Brain' (in *Correcting the Errors of Medicine* 1830) cited three people who had previously held the same opinion as himself on the brain: Li Shi-zhen, Jin Sheng and Wang Ang. Jin Sheng was a friend of Jesuit missionaries in the Ming court in the sixteenth century and a convert to Roman Catholicism, whilst Wang Ang was his close colleague. See Andrews, B.J., *Wang Qingren and the History of Chinese Anatomy*, Journal of Chinese Medicine, No. 36, May 1991.

14 B.J.Andrews in *Wang Qingren and the History of Chinese Anatomy*, Journal of Chinese Medicine, No. 36, May 1991, however, believes that Wang Qingren's contact with Western medicine is unproven, and that his refutation of classical Chinese anatomical theories was much influenced by the radical 'evidential research' movement then prevalent amongst Chinese scholars.

15 *Spiritual Pivot* Chapter 33.

16 *Spiritual Pivot* Chapter 8.

17 *Classic of Categories* (Lei Jing) by Zhang Jie-bin, People's Health Publishing House, Beijing, 1982, p. 49. First published in 1624. Passage translated by Giovanni Maciocia.

18 *A Record of Nourishing Xing and Extending Ming* (Yang Xing Yan Ming Lu) written by Tao Hongjing 456-536. This was a compilation of different theories on nourishing life in fashion at that time. Passage translated by Heiner Fruehauf.

19 *Differentiation and Treatment of Disease* (Lei Zheng Zhi Zai) written by Lin Peiqin in 1839. Passage translated by Heiner Fruehauf.

20 *Collected Wisdom by Master Magic Sword* (Ling Jian Zi), attributed to the Daoist Master Xu Sun of the Jin dynasty. One chapter of this book describes how Master Xu slayed a wicked demon hiding in the body of a snake by decapitating the snake with a magic (ling) sword (jian). The actual authors of the book were members of the Zhengming School of Daoism who wrote the book during the Song dynasty at the end of the 10th century. Passage translated by Heiner Fruehauf.

21 Both from the *Classic on the Central Void in the Inner Sphere* (Huangting Neijing Jing). The Huangting Jing is divided into the Neijing Jing and the Waijing Jing. Both books were transmitted by the Jin dynasty (4th century or earlier) Daoist scholar and adept Wei Furen. Its origins, however, go back to Lao Zi. Passages translated by Heiner Fruehauf.

22 *Zheng Li Lun*. Passage translated by Heiner Fruehauf.

23 Translated by Giovanni Maciocia.

24 *Spiritual Pivot* Chapter 10.

25 *Essential Questions* Chapter 17.

26 *Essential Questions* Chapter 61.

27 *Classic of Difficulties* 38th Difficulty.

28 *Classic of Difficulties* 29th Difficulty.

29 *Classic of Difficulties* 36th Difficulty.

30 *Essential Questions* Chapter 32.

31 Ibid.

32 Ibid.

33 Ibid.

34 *Spiritual Pivot* Chapter 33.

35 *Treatment Strategies for Assorted Syndromes* (Lei Zheng Zhi Cai) by Lin Pei-qin, 1839, quoted in *The Practice of Chinese Medicine* by Giovanni Maciocia, Churchill Livingstone, 1994, p. 561.

36 *Spiritual Pivot* Chapter 33.

37 *Essential Questions* Chapter 60.

38 *Spiritual Pivot* Chapter 33.

39 *Spiritual Pivot* Chapter 9 and *Essential Questions* Chapter 70.

40 *Essential Questions* Chapter 17.

41 *Spiritual Pivot* Chapter 33.

42 *The Heart & Essence of Dan-xi's Methods of Treatment*, A Translation of Zhu Dan-xi's Dan Xi Zhi Fa Xin Yao, Blue Poppy Press, p. 99.

43 *Spiritual Pivot* Chapter 9 and *Essential Questions* Chapter 70.

44 *Essential Questions* Chapter 62.

45 *Essential Questions* Chapter 17.

46 *Spiritual Pivot* Chapter 24.

47 0.5 cun posterior to Toulinqi GB-15.

48 Both from the *Classic on the Central Void in the Inner Sphere*. Passages translated by Heiner Fruehauf.

49 *Collected Wisdom by Master Magic Sword*. Passage translated by Heiner Fruehauf.

50 *Spiritual Pivot* Chapter 9 and *Essential Questions* Chapter 70.

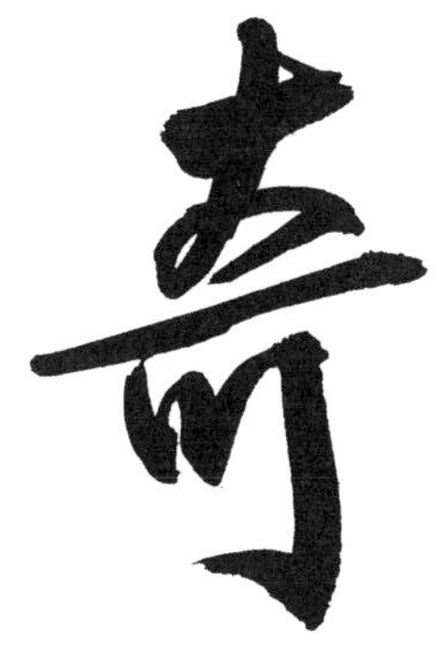

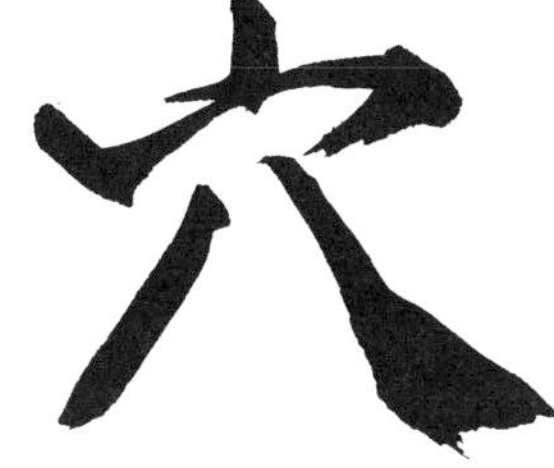

THE EXTRAORDINARY POINTS

EXTRA POINTS OF THE HEAD AND NECK

SISHENCONG (M-HN-1)

Four Alert Spirit

LOCATION

Four points at the vertex of the scalp, grouped around Baihui DU-20 and located 1 cun anterior, posterior and lateral to it.

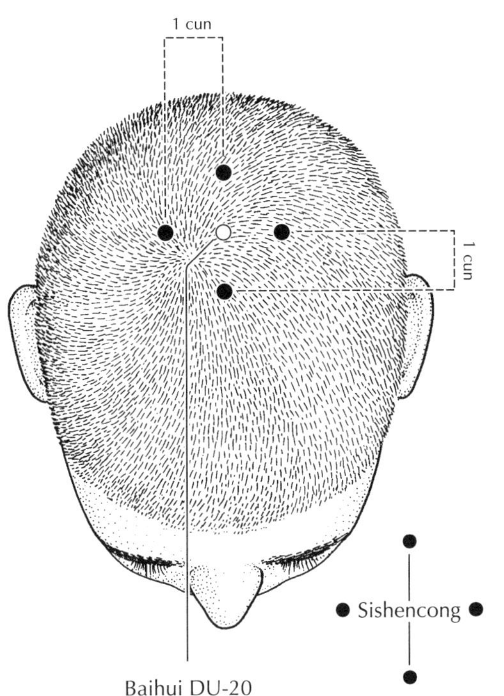

LOCATION NOTE

The distance between Baihui DU-20 and the anterior hairline is 5 cun. If the anterior hairline is indistinct, the distance between Baihui DU-20 and the glabella is measured as 8 cun.

NEEDLING

Transverse insertion 0.5-1.5 cun.

ACTIONS

Calms the spirit
Pacifies wind
Benefits the eyes and ears

INDICATIONS

- Windstroke, epilepsy, mania-depression, insomnia, poor memory.
- One-sided and generalised headache, dizziness, deafness, disorders of the eyes.

COMMENTARY

The four points Sishencong were first discussed in the *Sagelike Prescriptions from the Taiping Era.* (10th century CE). As the name (Four Alert Spirit) implies, these four points are able to pacify interior wind which rises to harass the head and brain (windstroke, epilepsy, dizziness etc.) and to calm the spirit (mania-depression, insomnia etc.). In clinical practice these points are either used as a group, all four being needled together, or through-needled from Baihui DU-20.

YINTANG (M-HN-3)

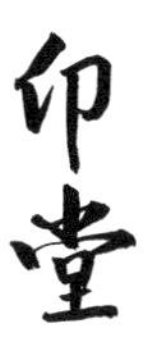

Hall of Impression

LOCATION

At the glabella, at the midpoint between the medial extremities of the eyebrows.

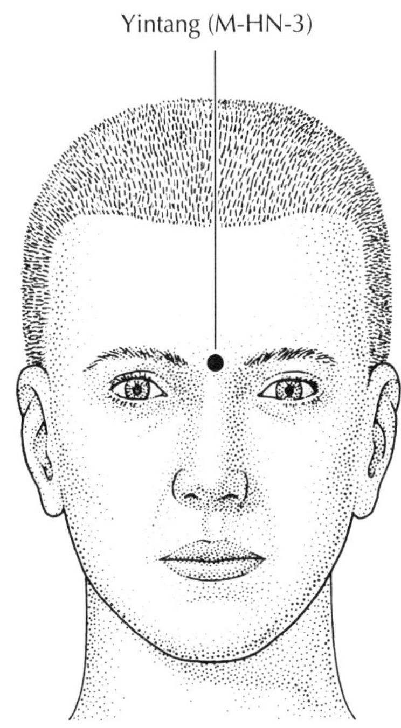

NEEDLING

With the fingers of one hand pinch up the skin over the point, and with the other hand needle transversely in an inferior or lateral direction, 0.3-0.5 cun.

ACTIONS

Pacifies wind and calms the shen
Benefits the nose
Activates the channel and alleviates pain

INDICATIONS

- Chronic and acute childhood fright wind, fright spasm, frontal headache, dizziness, dizziness following childbirth, insomnia, agitation and restlessness.
- Nasal congestion and discharge, rhinitis, nosebleed, disorders of the eyes, hypertension, pain of the face.

COMMENTARY

The extra point Yintang (M-HN-3) was first discussed in the *Essential Questions*. It is curious however, that such an important and commonly used point was not classified as a point of the Governing vessel, on whose pathway it lies. Lying between the eyebrows, in the area ascribed to the 'third eye' by many traditional cultures, Yintang (M-HN-3) has been considered by some qigong authorities to be the location of the upper dantian.

Yintang (M-HN-3) is commonly used in four clinical situations: i. as a powerful and effective point to calm the spirit in the treatment of insomnia, anxiety and agitation; ii. to activate the channel and alleviate pain in the treatment of frontal headache; iii. to benefit the nose in the treatment of nasal congestion and discharge, rhinitis, sinus pain, nosebleed etc. and iv. to pacify wind in the treatment of chronic and acute childhood fright wind (infantile convulsions).

COMBINATIONS

- Head wind following intoxication: Yintang (M-HN-3), Zanzhu BL-2 and Zusanli ST-36 (*Great Compendium*).
- Insomnia: Yintang (M-HN-3), Shenmen HE-7 and Sanyinjiao SP-6.
- Hypertension: Yintang (M-HN-3), Quchi L.I-11 and Zusanli ST-36.
- Headache: Yintang (M-HN-3), Fengchi GB-20, Taiyang (M-HN-9) and Hegu L.I-4.
- Rhinitis: Yintang (M-HN-3), Yingxiang L.I.-20 and Hegu L.I-4.

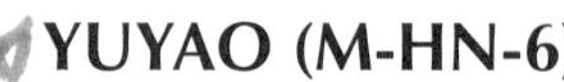

YUYAO (M-HN-6)

Fish Waist

魚腰

LOCATION

In the centre of the eyebrow, in the depression directly above the pupil when the eyes are looking straight forwards.

LOCATION NOTE

Yuyao (M-HN-6) is traditionally located lateral to the supraorbital notch from which the supraorbital nerve emerges.

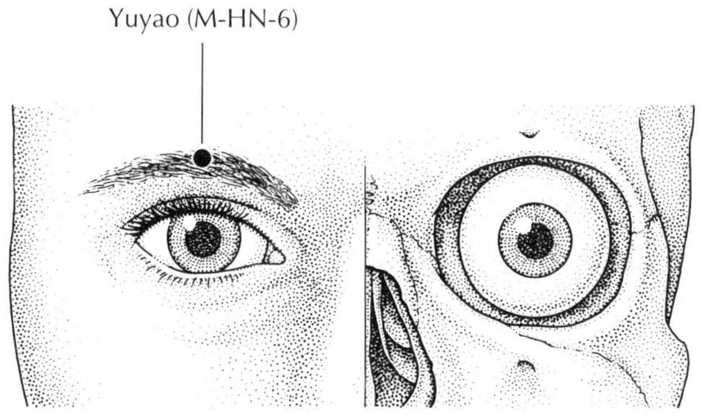

NEEDLING

Transverse insertion medially or laterally, 0.5 to 1 cun.

ACTIONS

Benefits the eyes

Relaxes the sinews and alleviates pain.

INDICATIONS

- Redness, swelling and pain of the eyes, superficial visual obstruction, twitching of the eyelids, drooping of the eyelid, frontal headache.

COMMENTARY

This point first appeared in the *Classic of the Jade Dragon*. In clinical practice it is mostly selected in the treatment of supraorbital pain and diseases of the eyes and eyelids, and is stimulated by through-needling from either Yangbai GB-14 or Zanzhu BL-2.

QIUHOU (M-HN-8)

Behind the Ball

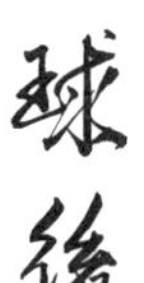

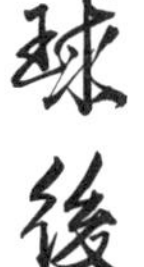

LOCATION

Along the inferior border of the orbit, at the junction of the lateral one quarter and medial three quarters of the infra-orbital margin.

NEEDLING

Ask the patient to close their eyes and look upwards. Use a finger to push the eyeball upwards and insert the needle, first slightly inferiorly, then perpendicularly, between the eyeball and the inferior wall of the orbit, 0.5 to 1 cun.

Caution: i. the needle should be inserted slowly without lifting, thrusting or rotating; ii. immediately on withdrawal of the needle, press firmly with a cotton wool ball for about a minute to prevent haematoma; iii. this needling method should not be attempted by those who have not had appropriate clinical supervision.

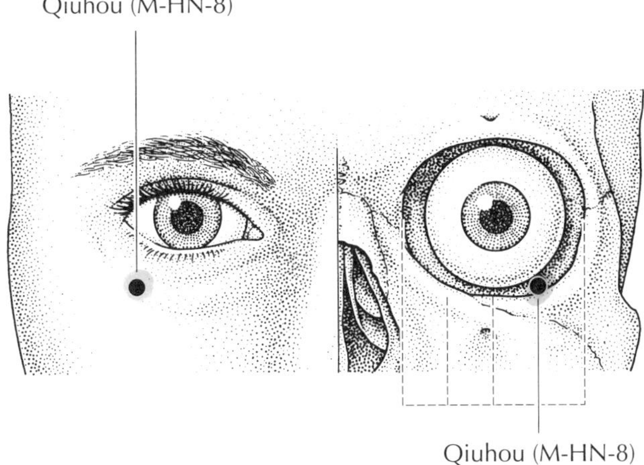

ACTIONS
Benefits the eyes

INDICATIONS
- All eye diseases.

COMMENTARY
Qiuhou (M-HN-8) is a modern addition to the extra points and is used in the treatment of a wide variety of eye diseases including short-sightedness, inflammation or atrophy of the optic nerve, glaucoma, retinitis pigmentosa and convergent strabismus.

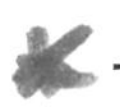

TAIYANG (M-HN-9)
Sun (Supreme Yang)

太陽

LOCATION
At the temple, in the tender depression approximately 1 cun posterior to the midpoint between the lateral extremity of the eyebrow and the outer canthus of the eye.

NEEDLING
i. Perpendicular needling 0.5 to 0.8 cun; ii. Transverse insertion posteriorly towards Shuaigu GB-8, 1 to 1.5 cun; iii. Oblique insertion anteriorly 0.3 to 0.5 cun; iv. Prick to bleed.

ACTIONS
Eliminates wind and clears heat
Reduces swelling and stops pain,
Activates the channel and alleviates pain

INDICATIONS
- One-sided headache, dizziness, toothache, trigeminal neuralgia.
- Disorders of the eyes, dimness of vision, redness and swelling of the eyes, pain of the eyes, deviation of the mouth and eye.

COMMENTARY
Taiyang (M-HN-9) is one of the most important and commonly-used of the extra points. It was first discussed in the *Sagelike Prescriptions from the Taiping Era* (10th century CE), although considering its importance in the martial arts tradition (as a vital spot where a blow may be fatal) it was almost certainly known much earlier than this date.

Taiyang (M-HN-9) is commonly needled or pricked to bleed in two clinical situations: i. in the treatment of one-sided headache and dizziness, in which case it is frequently joined to Shuaigu GB-8; and ii. in the treatment of diseases of the eyes such as redness, swelling and pain. The *Ode of the Jade Dragon* recommends bleeding bilateral Taiyang (M-HN-9) for dimness of vision, and also surprisingly needling it in combination with Shaoze SI-1 for swelling of the breasts.

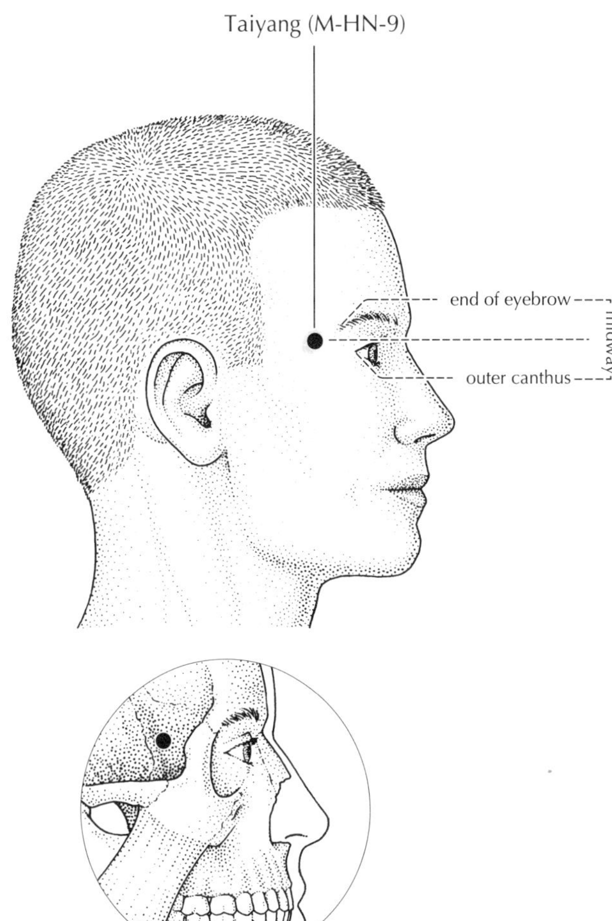

COMBINATIONS

- Disorders of the eyes: Taiyang (M-HN-9), Jingming BL-1 and Yuwei (M-HN-7) (*Ode of the Jade Dragon*).
- Redness, swelling and unbearable pain of both eyes with photophobia: needle Jingming BL-1 and Yuwei (M-HN-7) and bleed Taiyang (M-HN-9) (*Song of the Jade Dragon*).
- Swelling of the breasts: Taiyang (M-HN-9) and Shaoze SI-1 (*Ode of the Jade Dragon*).

ERJIAN (M-HN-10)

耳尖

Tip of the Ear

LOCATION

When the ear is folded forwards, this point lies at the apex of the ear.

LOCATION NOTE

Fold the ear so that the posterior part of the upper helix directly covers the anterior part of the upper helix. Take care not to push the whole of the ear forwards.

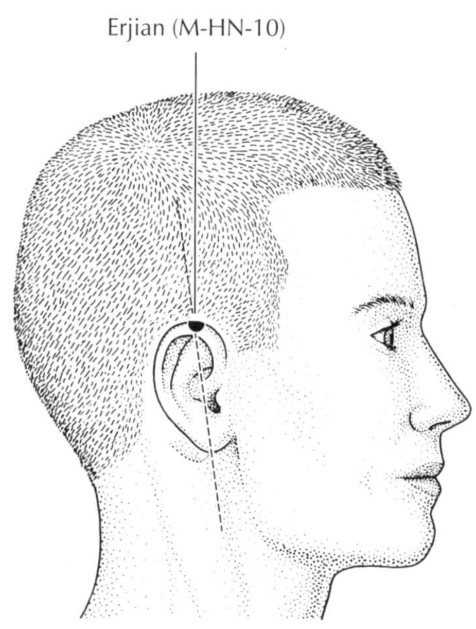

NEEDLING

i. Perpendicular insertion 0.1 cun or prick to bleed; ii. moxibustion 3-5 cones.

ACTIONS

Clears heat and dissipates swelling
Benefits the eyes and throat

INDICATIONS

- Redness, swelling and pain of the eyes, superficial visual obstruction, pain and swelling of the throat, mumps, one-sided headache, high fever.

COMMENTARY

This point was first discussed in the *Great Compendium of Acupuncture and Moxibustion*, which recommended the application of five cones of moxa for the treatment of superficial visual obstruction.

BITONG (M-HN-14)

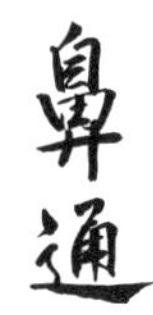

Penetrating the Nose

LOCATION

At the highest point of the naso-labial groove.

LOCATION NOTE

Run the finger along the naso-labial groove into the depression immediately below the nasal bone.

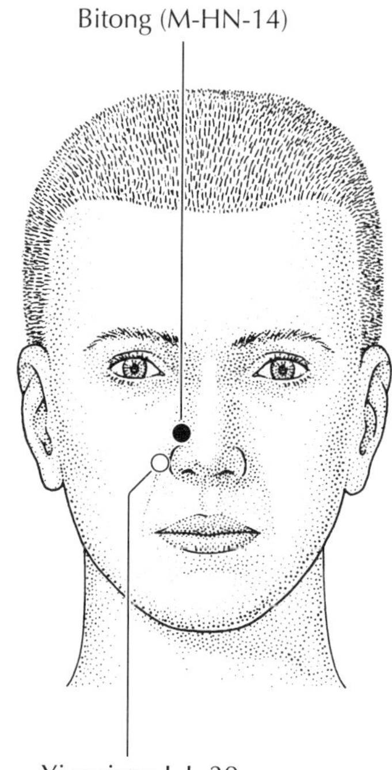

NEEDLING

Transverse insertion towards the bridge of the nose 0.3 to 0.5 cun.

ACTIONS

Benefits the nose

INDICATIONS

- Rhinitis, allergic rhinitis, nasal congestion and discharge, nosebleed, nasal polyps.

COMMENTARY

Bitong (M-HN-14) is a modern addition to the extra points and is commonly used for the treatment of nose disorders, especially by through-needling from Yingxiang L.I.-20.

COMBINATIONS

- Chronic rhinitis: Bitong (M-HN-14), Hegu L.I-4, Shangxing DU-23 and Tongtian BL-7.

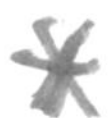

BAILAO (M-HN-30)

Hundred Taxations

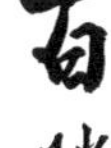

LOCATION

At the back of the neck, 2 cun superior to Dazhui DU-14, 1 cun lateral to the midline.

LOCATION NOTE

The distance between the inferior border of the spinous process of C7 and the posterior hairline is 3 cun.

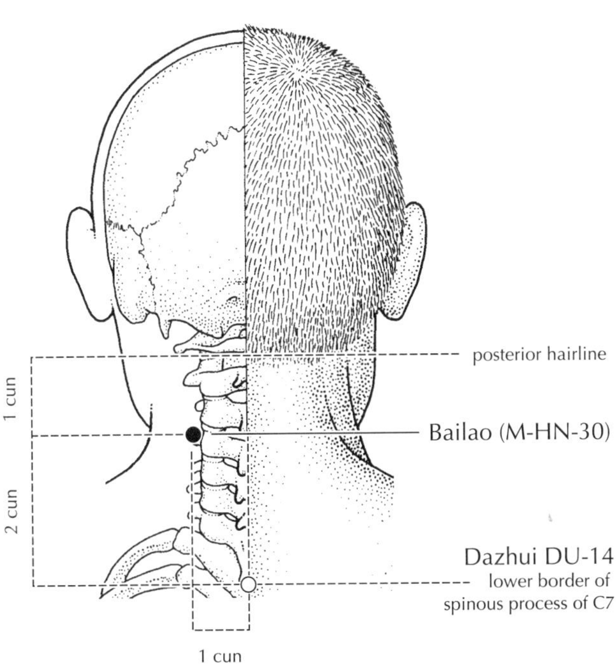

NEEDLING

Perpendicular insertion 0.5 to 0.8 cun.

ACTIONS

Transforms phlegm and dissipates nodules
Stops cough and calms dyspnoea

INDICATIONS

- Scrofula, cough, dyspnoea, Lung consumption, night sweating, spontaneous sweating, steaming bone disorder with tidal fever, stiffness and pain of the neck.

COMMENTARY

This point was first discussed in the *Compilation of Acupuncture and Moxibustion*. Note that the name Bailao (One Hundred Taxations) is also an alternative name for Dazhui DU-14.

COMBINATIONS

- Scrofula: Bailao (M-HN-30) and moxa Zhoujian (M-UE-46) one hundred times (*Compilation*).

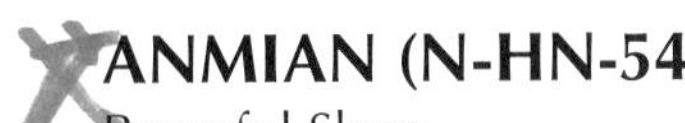

ANMIAN (N-HN-54)

Peaceful Sleep

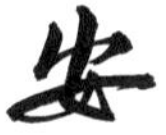

LOCATION

Behind the ear, midway between Fengchi GB-20 and Yifeng SJ-17.

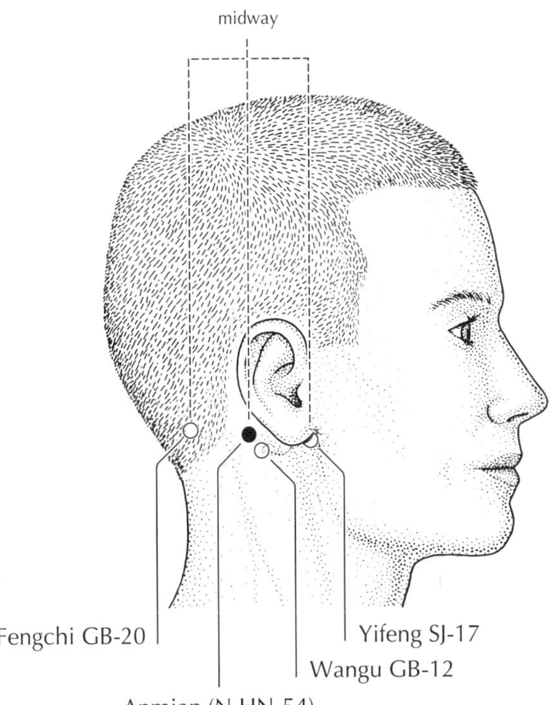

LOCATION NOTE

This point is found close to Wangu GB-12, but posterior and slightly superior to it.

NEEDLING

Perpendicular insertion 0.5 to 1 cun.

ACTIONS
Calms the spirit and pacifies the Liver

INDICATIONS
- Insomnia, agitation and restlessness, palpitations, epilepsy, dizziness, headache, tinnitus, hypertension.

COMMENTARY
Anmian (N-HN-34) is a modern addition to the extra points and is commonly used for the treatment of insomnia. It is located close to Wangu GB-12 which is similarly indicated for insomnia, as well as for mania and agitation of the Heart.

COMBINATIONS
- Insomnia: Anmian (M-HN-34), Neiguan P-6 and Sanyinjiao SP-6.

JIACHENGJIANG (M-HN-18)
Adjacent to Container of Fluids

夾承漿

LOCATION
1 cun lateral to Chengqiang REN-24, over the mental foramen.

NEEDLING
i. Perpendicular-oblique insertion medially and inferiorly into the mental foramen, 0.3 to 0.5 cun; ii. Transverse insertion 0.5 to 1.5 cun.

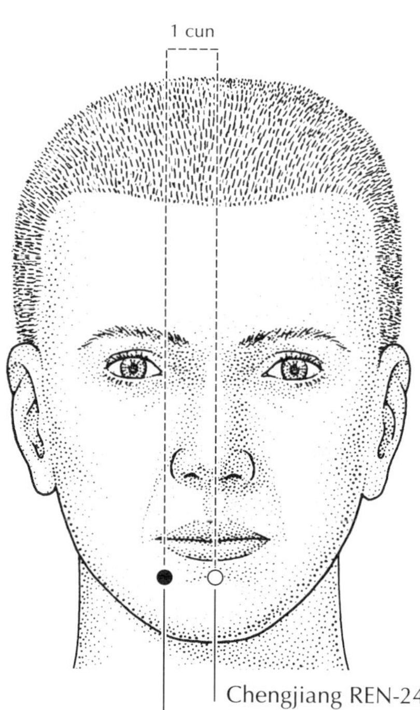

ACTIONS
Eliminates wind, activates the channel and alleviates pain

INDICATIONS
- Deviation of the mouth and eye, pain of the face, toothache, swelling of the gums, jaundice.

COMMENTARY
The point Jiachengqiang (M-HN-18) was first mentioned in the *Thousand Ducat Prescriptions*. Clinically it is most commonly used for facial paralysis and trigeminal neuralgia.

JINJIN YUYE (M-HN-20)
Golden Liquid & Jade Fluid

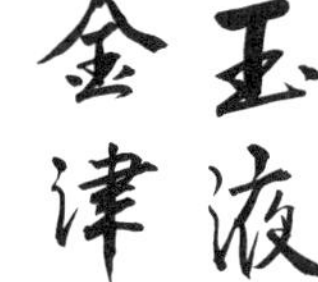

LOCATION
These paired points are located on the veins either side of the frenulum of the tongue, Jinjin to the left and Yuye to the right.

LOCATION NOTE
The tongue should be rolled back to locate and treat these points. If required the practitioner should roll the tongue back using a gauze swab or wooden spatula.

NEEDLING
Prick to bleed.

ACTIONS
Clears heat and reduces swelling
Generates fluids

INDICATIONS
- Lotus flower tongue, pain and swelling of the tongue, mouth ulcers, throat painful obstruction, loss of voice, loss of voice following windstroke.
- Wasting and thirsting disorder, vomiting, nausea and vomiting of pregnancy, diarrhoea.

COMMENTARY
These points were first mentioned in the *Essential Questions*. Several centuries later Sun Si-miao wrote in the *Thousand Ducat Prescriptions* "Sudden swelling of the tongue like an inflated pig's bladder obstructs the respiration and can kill the patient if not treated promptly. Prick the two large vessels on either side of the frenulum". Although not commonly used in clinical practice due to their location beneath the tongue, these points may be used in severe and recalcitrant disorders of the tongue,

including stiffness of the tongue and difficulty in speaking following windstroke. Other disorders that these points may be considered for are parched mouth associated with wasting and thirsting disorder, and severe and unremitting nausea and vomiting of pregnancy.

COMBINATIONS

- Swelling of the tongue with difficulty speaking: Jinjin (M-HN-20), Yuye (M-HN-20) and Lianquan REN-23 (*Great Compendium*).

EXTRA POINTS OF THE BACK AND WAIST

DINGCHUAN (M-BW-1)

定喘

Calm Dyspnoea

LOCATION

0.5 to 1 cun lateral to the depression below the spinous process of the seventh cervical vertebra (Dazhui DU-14).

NEEDLING

Perpendicular-oblique insertion towards the spine, 0.5 to 1 cun.

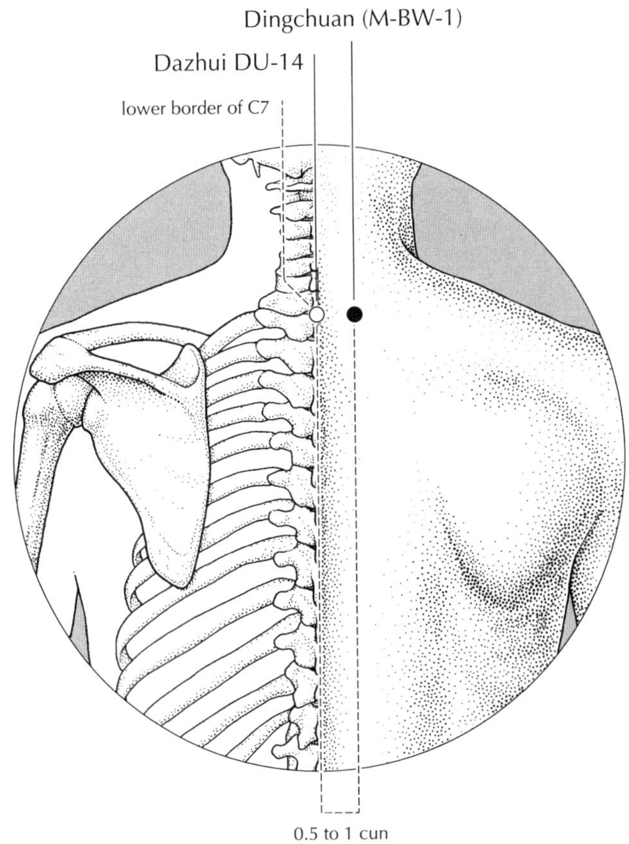

ACTIONS

Calms dyspnoea and wheezing and stops cough

INDICATIONS

- Asthma, wheezing, cough, urticaria, pain of the upper back.

COMMENTARY

Dingchuan (M-BW-1) is a modern addition to the extra points and is one of the primary points for the treatment of acute wheezing, dyspnoea and asthma.

COMBINATIONS

- Acute asthma: Dingchuan (M-BW-1), Tiantu REN-22 and Kongzui LU-6.

WEIGUANXIASHU (M-BW-12)

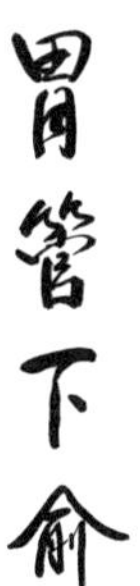

Stomach Controller Lower Shu

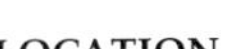

LOCATION

1.5 cun lateral to the lower border of the spinous process of the eighth thoracic vertebra (T8).

LOCATION NOTE

Locate at the visible highest point of the paraspinal muscles.

NEEDLING

Oblique insertion towards the spine, 0.5 to 1 cun, or transverse-oblique insertion 1 to 1.5 cun.

Caution: perpendicular needling or oblique needling away from the spine carries a substantial risk of causing a pneumothorax.

ACTIONS

Clears heat and generates fluid

INDICATIONS

- Wasting and thirsting disorder, dry throat, pain of the chest and lateral costal region, epigastric pain, vomiting.

COMMENTARY

This point, nowadays known as Yishu (Pancreas Shu) was first mentioned in the *Thousand Ducat Formulas*. It was recommended by Sun Si-miao for wasting and thirsting disorder (i.e. diabetes mellitus) and the accompanying symptoms of dryness of the throat.

COMBINATIONS

- Wasting and thirsting disorder and dry throat: Weiguanxiashusanxue (i.e. Weiguanxiashu [M-BW-12] plus the point found inferior to the spinous process of the eighth thoracic vertebra) 100 moxa cones (*Thousand Ducat Formulas*).

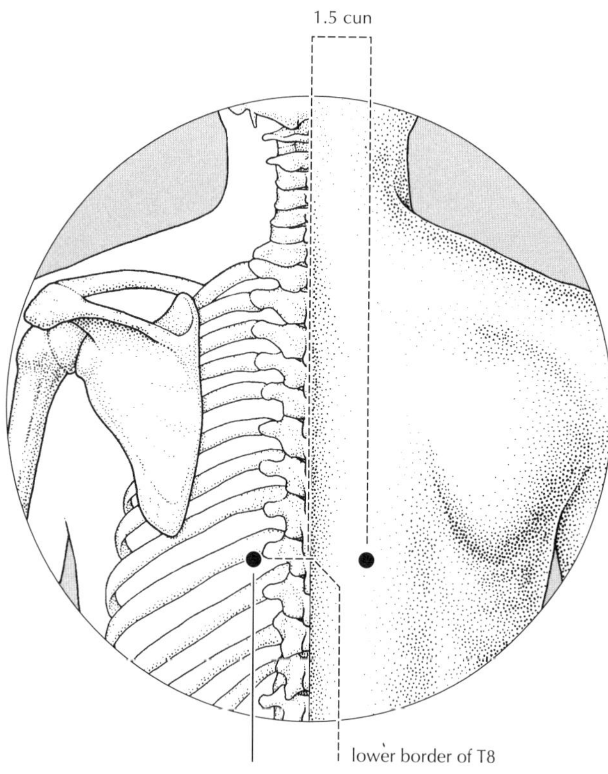

YAOYAN (M-BW-24)

Lumbar Eyes

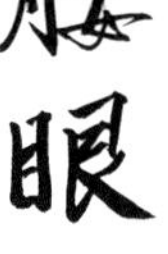

LOCATION

In the depression approximately 3.5 cun lateral to the lower border of L4 (Yaoyangguan DU-3).

LOCATION NOTE

The 'eyes' referred to in the point name are the visible hollows found in many people, just over one handbreadth either side of the lumbar spine, below the level of the iliac crest.

NEEDLING

Perpendicular insertion, 1 to 1.5 cun.

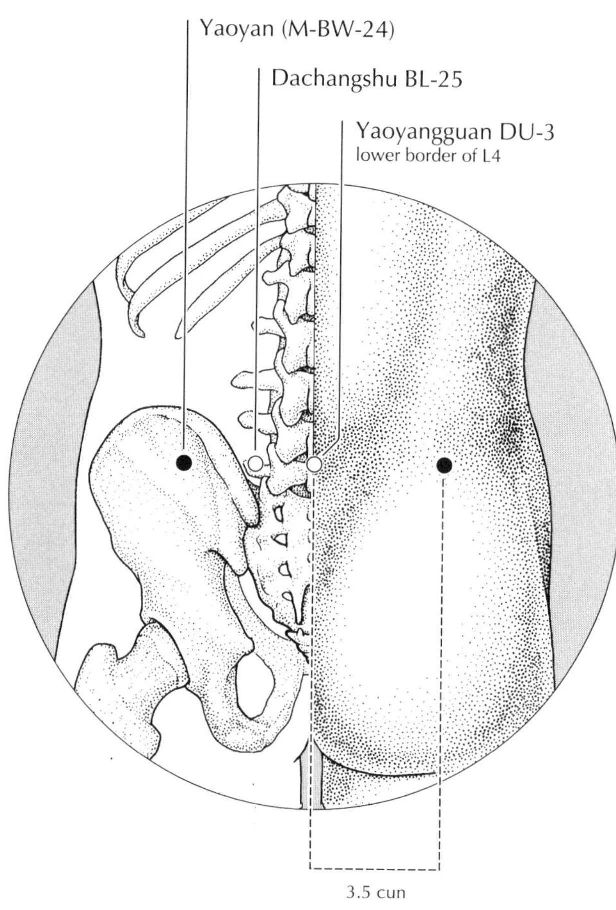

ACTIONS

Strengthens the Kidneys and benefits the lumbar region

INDICATIONS

- Kidney deficiency lumbar pain, lumbar pain, consumption.

COMMENTARY

This point was first mentioned in *Song to Keep Up Your Sleeve*. It is commonly selected as a local point for acute or chronic lumbar pain due to any aetiology.

COMBINATIONS

- Lumbar pain: seven cones of moxa on Yaoyan [M-BW-24] (*Song to Keep Up Your Sleeve*).

SHIQIZHUIXIA (M-BW-25)

Below the Seventeenth Vertebra

十七椎穴

LOCATION

On the midline of the lower back, in the depression below the spinous process of the fifth lumbar vertebra.

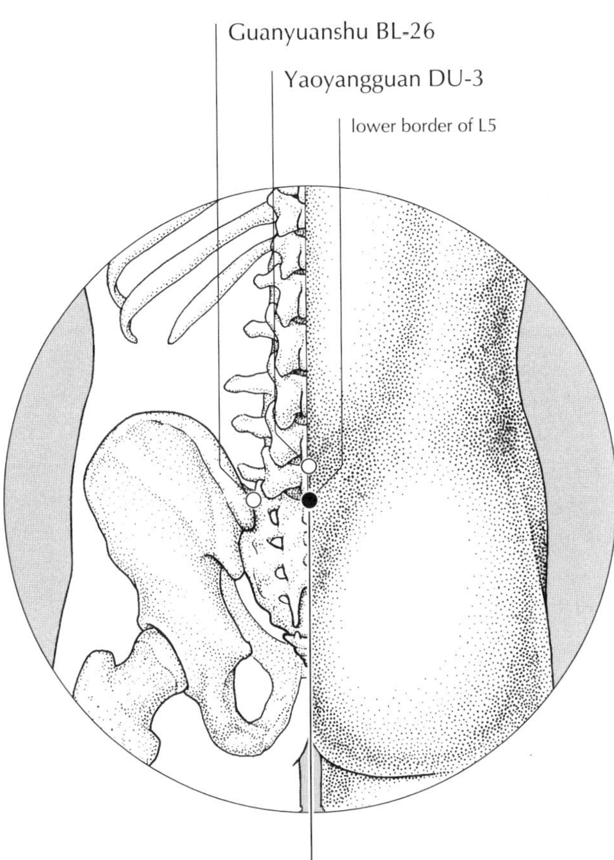

LOCATION NOTE

Slide a finger upwards along the midline of the sacrum until it meets the significant depression inferior to the lumbar spine.

NEEDLING

Perpendicular insertion 0.5 to 1 cun.
Caution: the spinal canal lies between 1.25 and 1.75 cun deep to the skin surface, varying according to body build.

ACTIONS

Tonifies the Kidneys and promotes urination
Activates the channel and alleviates pain

INDICATIONS

- Pain of the lumbar region and legs, difficult urination, foetus pressing on the bladder.

COMMENTARY

Shiqizhuixia (M-BW-25) was first mentioned in the *Supplement to the Thousand Ducat Formulas*. It is among the most commonly used points for chronic back pain and is very often found to be the focus of tenderness. It may be used in both deficiency and excess patterns, and in the frequently encountered clinical situation where the two are found in combination.

COMBINATIONS

- Chronic lumbar pain: Shiqizhuixia (M-BW-25), Guanyuanshu BL-26, Baohuang BL-53 and Weizhong BL-40.

HUATUOJIAJI (M-BW-35)

Hua Tuo's Paravertebral Points

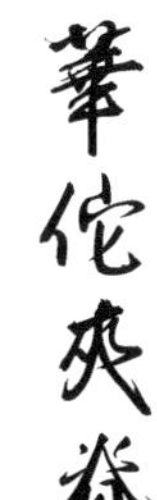

LOCATION

0.5 to 1 cun lateral to the depressions below the spinous processes of the twelve thoracic and five lumbar vertebrae.

LOCATION NOTE

In clinical practice, the points located 0.5 to 1 cun lateral to the depressions below the spinous processes of the seven cervical vertebrae are used as additional Huatuojiaji points.

NEEDLING

Perpendicular-oblique insertion towards the spine, 0.5 to 1 cun. **Note:** the intention of needling these points is to stimulate the appropriate spinal nerve. The superficial location of the point is chosen as 0.5 to 1 cun lateral to the midline according to depth and angle of needle insertion. In some patients a more perpendicular, and in others a more oblique, line of insertion will give easier access to these points.

ACTIONS

Regulates and harmonises the five zang and six fu.

INDICATIONS

- The points from the first to the fourth thoracic vertebrae treat disorders of the Lung and upper limb.
- The points from the fourth to the seventh thoracic vertebrae treat disorders of the Heart.

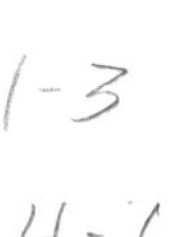

- The points from the seventh to the tenth thoracic vertebrae treat disorders of the Liver and Gallbladder.

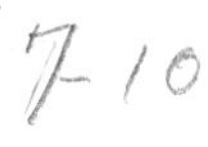

- The points from the tenth to the twelfth thoracic vertebrae treat disorders of the Spleen and Stomach.
- The points from the first to the second lumbar vertebrae treat disorders of the Kidneys.
- The points from the third to the fifth lumbar vertebrae treat disorders of the Bladder, Large and Small Intestines, uterus and lower limbs.
- The points from the first to the seventh cervical vertebrae treat local disorders of the neck.
- All the Huatuojiaji (M-BW-35) points treat herpes zoster at the level of the affected segmental nerve.
- All the Huatuojiaji (M-BW-35) points treat pain and stiffness of the local area.

COMMENTARY

The Huatuojiaji (M-BW-35) points were first mentioned in *Song to Keep Up Your Sleeve*. Their discovery is attributed to the great Han dynasty physician Hua Tuo who was said to use them in preference to the back-shu points.

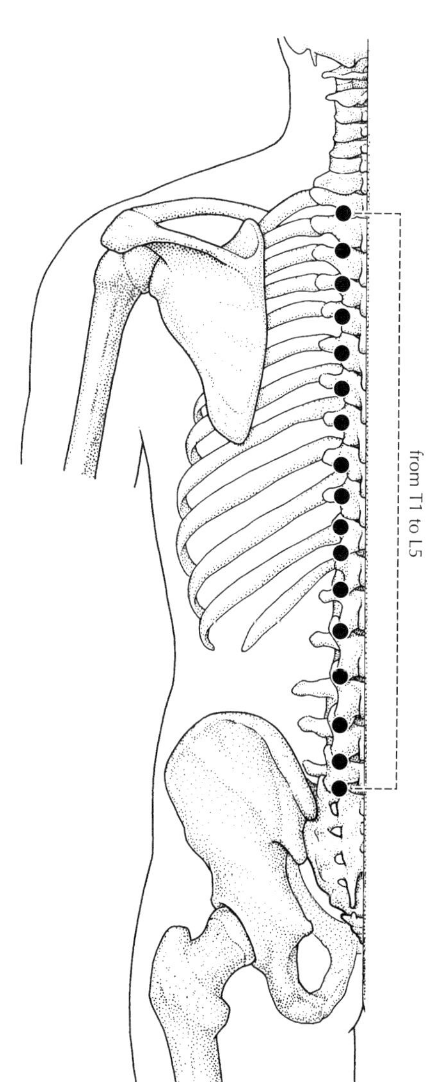

EXTRA POINTS OF THE CHEST AND ABDOMEN

SANJIAOJIU (M-CA-23)

三角灸

Triangle Moxibustion

LOCATION

On the lower abdomen. Construct an equilateral triangle of which the apex is the umbilicus (Shenque REN-8), and the sides are equal to the length of the patient's smile. These points are located at the three points of the triangle.

LOCATION NOTE

It is helpful to describe this location to the patient. This will invariably induce a smile which can then be measured.

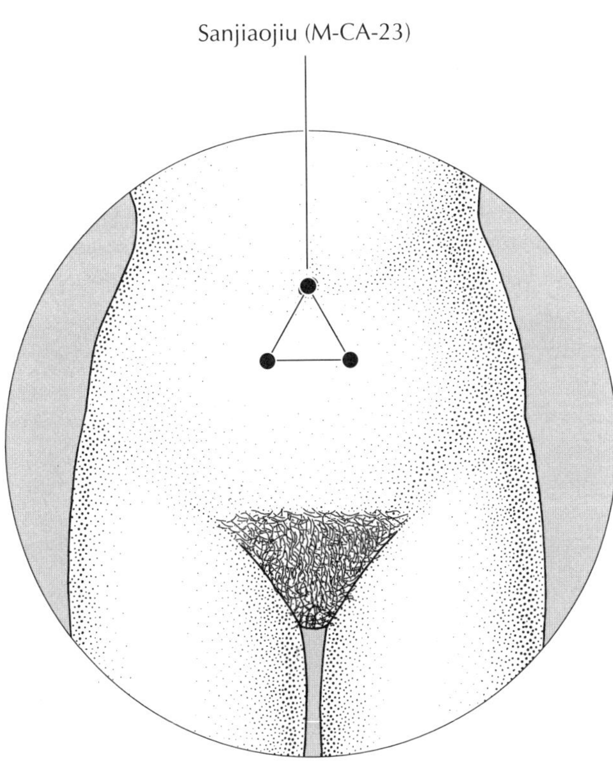

NEEDLING

These points are treated by moxibustion only, whether indirect, mediated by sliced ginger, crushed garlic, aconite cake etc., or by cones placed directly on the skin.

ACTIONS

Regulates qi and alleviates pain

Stops diarrhoea

INDICATIONS

- Chronic diarrhoea, abdominal pain, pain around the umbilicus, shan disorder, running piglet qi arising from the umbilicus.

COMMENTARY

Sanjiaojiu (M-CA-23), also known as Qipang (Beside the Umbilicus) was first described in the *Great Compendium of Acupuncture and Moxibustion* which recommends this point for the treatment of shan disorder, advising that the bottom left point should be treated by moxibustion when the disorder is on the right side, and vice-versa. All three points may be treated for chronic diarrhoea.

ZIGONG (M-CA-18)

子宫

Palace of the Child (Uterus)

LOCATION

On the lower abdomen, 3 cun lateral to the midline, level with Zhongji REN-3.

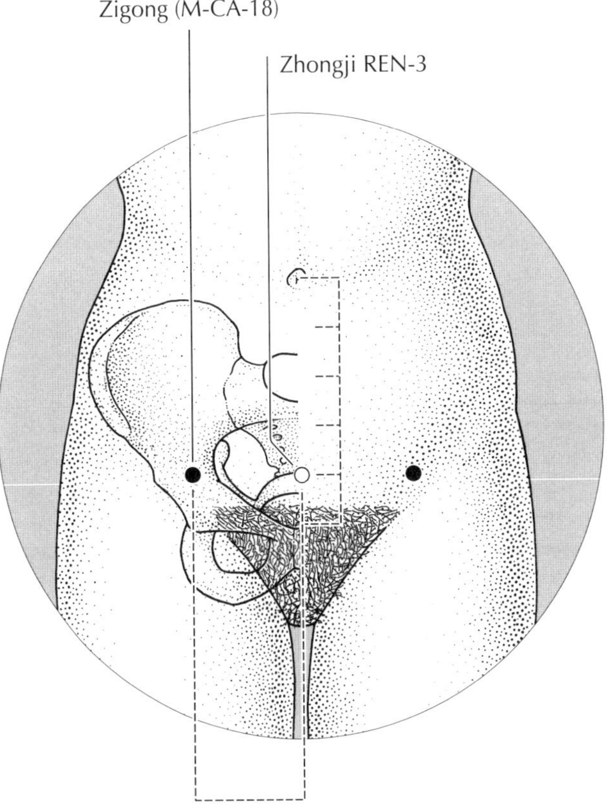

LOCATION NOTE

Zhongji REN-3 lies on the midline of the lower abdomen, 4 cun inferior to the umbilicus and 1 cun superior to the pubic symphysis. Zigong (M-CA-18) is located one handbreadth lateral to this point.

NEEDLING

i. Perpendicular insertion 0.8 to 1.2 cun; ii. For prolapse of the uterus, direct the needle from Zigong (M-CA-18) towards Qugu REN-2 through the muscular layer. Then rotate the needle until it wraps the muscle fibres, firmly pull it upwards and outwards, and tape it to the skin in this raised position for 20-30 minutes.

ACTIONS

Raises and regulates qi
Regulates menstruation and alleviates pain

INDICATIONS

- Prolapse of the uterus, infertility, irregular menstruation, uterine bleeding.

COMMENTARY

Zigong (M-CA-18) was first mentioned in the *Great Compendium of Acupuncture and Moxibustion*.

COMBINATIONS

- Infertility: Zigong (M-CA-18) and Zhongji REN-3 (*Great Compendium*).
- Uterine bleeding: Zigong [Extra] and Zhongji REN-3 (*Great Compendium*).
- Ceaseless uterine bleeding: Zigong (M-CA-18), Zhongji REN-3, Shimen REN-5 and Shenshu BL-23 (*Great Compendium*).

TITUO (N-CA-4)

Lift and Support

提托

LOCATION

On the lower abdomen, 4 cun lateral to the midline, level with Guanyuan REN-4.

LOCATION NOTE

Guanyuan REN-4 lies on the midline of the lower abdomen, 3 cun inferior to the umbilicus and 2 cun superior to the pubic symphysis. Locate Tituo (N-CA-4) 4 cun lateral to this point, medial to the anterior superior iliac spine.

NEEDLING

i. Perpendicular insertion 0.8 to 1.2 cun; ii. For prolapse of the uterus, the following needling method may be employed. Direct the needle from Tituo (N-CA-4) towards Qugu REN-2 through the muscular layer. Then rotate the needle until it wraps the muscle fibres, firmly pull it upwards and outwards, and tape it to the skin in this raised position for 20-30 minutes.

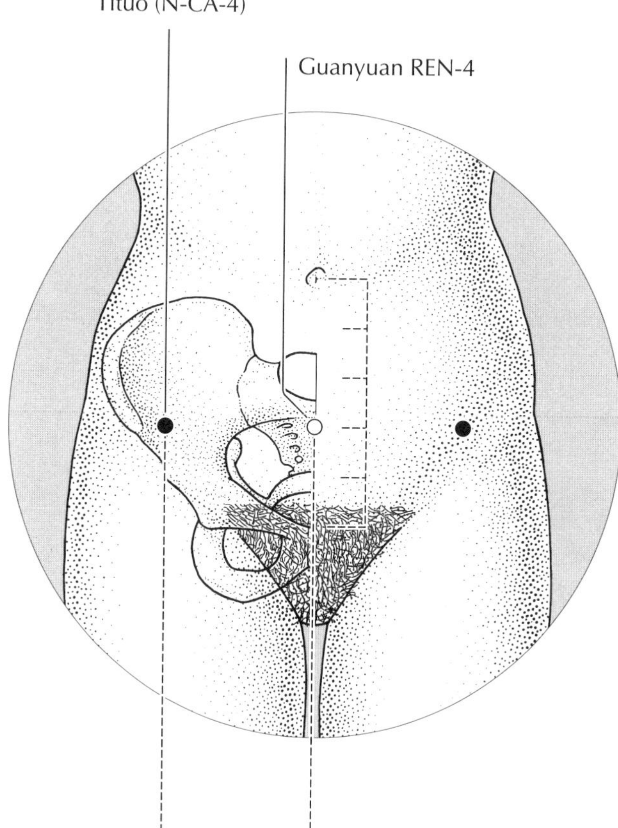

ACTIONS

Raises and regulates qi

INDICATIONS

- Prolapse of the uterus, dysmenorrhoea, abdominal distention and pain.

COMMENTARY

Tituo (N-CA-4) is a modern addition to the extra points and is one of the primary points for the treatment of uterine prolapse.

COMBINATIONS

- Prolapse of the uterus: Tituo (N-CA-4), Baihui DU-20, Zusanli ST-36 and Sanyinjiao SP-6.

EXTRA POINTS OF THE UPPER EXTREMITY

SHIXUAN (M-UE-1)

十宣

Ten Diffusions

LOCATION

On the tips of the ten fingers, approximately 0.1 cun from the fingernail.

NEEDLING

Prick to bleed. This may be followed by moxibustion.

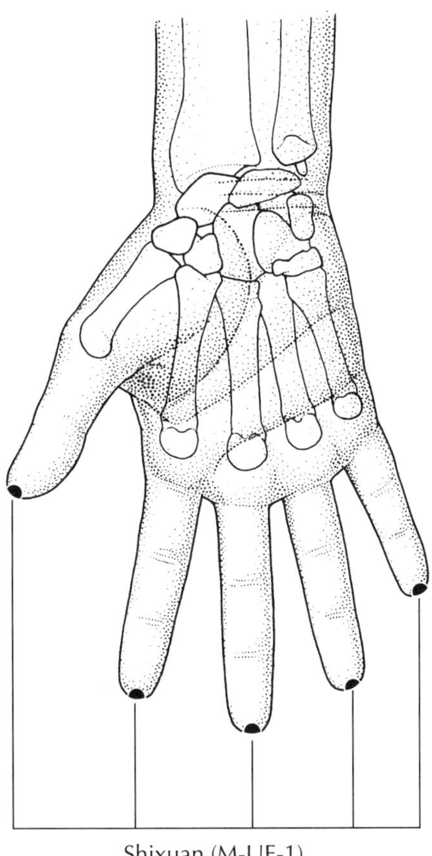

Shixuan (M-UE-1)

ACTIONS

Opens the portals and revives consciousness, drains heat and pacifies wind.

INDICATIONS

- Loss of consciousness, windstroke, summer-heat stroke, febrile disease, swelling and pain of the throat, throat moth, acute childhood fright wind, clonic spasm, epilepsy, mania, vomiting, diarrhoea, numbness or pain of the fingers

COMMENTARY

The points Shixuan (M-UE-1) were first discussed in the *Thousand Ducat Formulas* by the great 7th century physician Sun Si-miao. They are almost exclusively used for acute conditions such as loss of consciousness (including the acute phase of windstroke), epilepsy, heat-stroke, sunstroke etc. They are usually pricked to bleed, a procedure which may occasionally be followed by moxibustion.

SIFENG (M-UE-9)

四缝

Four Seams

LOCATION

On the palmar surface of the hand, at the midpoints of the transverse creases of the proximal interphalangeal joints of the index, middle, ring and little fingers.

LOCATION NOTE

In most subjects two creases will be found at the proximal interphalangeal joints. In this case, Sifeng (M-UE-9) is located on the crease which is more prominent on flexion of these joints.

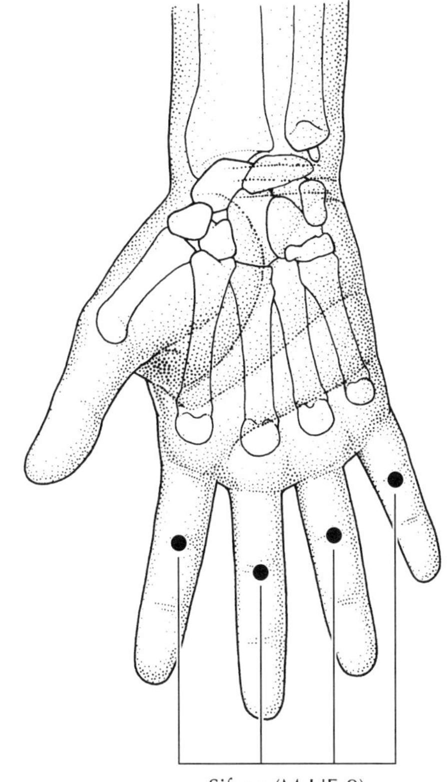

Sifeng (M-UE-9)

NEEDLING
Prick to bleed, or prick and squeeze until a yellow-white liquid appears.

ACTIONS
Fortifies the Spleen and dissipates accumulation

INDICATIONS
- Childhood nutritional impairment, childhood accumulation disorder, childhood diarrhoea, whooping cough.

COMMENTARY
Sifeng (M-UE-9) is an important and commonly used point grouping in the treatment of a wide range of childhood digestive disorders. It is indicated for two important patterns known as childhood nutritional impairment (shao er gan) and childhood accumulation disorder (shao er ji shi). The former refers to childhood malnutrition due to a variety of aetiologies. Its symptoms include emaciation, sallow complexion, impaired digestion, withered hair, exhaustion and enlarged abdomen. The latter, childhood accumulation disorder, more or less corresponds to the pattern of food stagnation in adults and is regarded as a major factor in such varied diseases as constipation, abdominal pain, intestinal parasites, vomiting, diarrhoea, cough and asthma.

The needling method used at these points is very specific, the points being pricked and squeezed to express a few drops of clear yellow fluid.

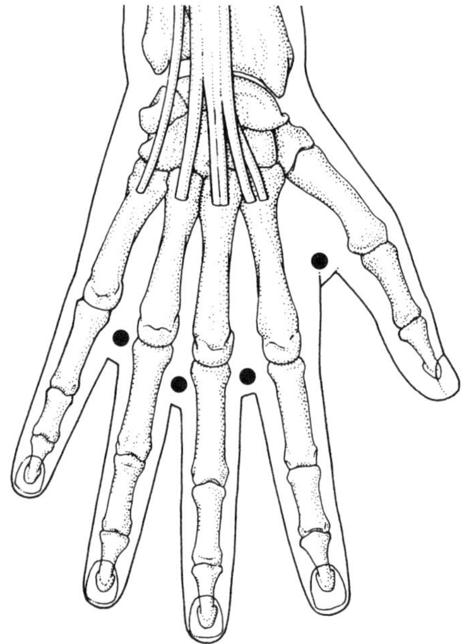

Baxie (M-UE-22)

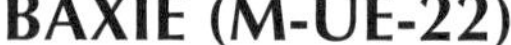

BAXIE (M-UE-22)
Eight Pathogens

八邪

LOCATION
When the hand is made into a fist, six of these points lie in the depressions between the metacarpal heads, proximal to the web margins. The remaining two points lie equidistant between the thumb and index metacarpals, proximal to the web margins.

LOCATION NOTE
To assist location of the first six points described above, with the hand held in a fist draw an equilateral triangle between the prominences of the metacarpal heads and the proximal end of the visible crease formed by the web space. The points lie at the centre of these triangles.

NEEDLING
Perpendicular insertion along the line between the shafts of the metacarpal bones, 0.5 to 1 cun.

ACTIONS
Clears heat and dissipates swelling

INDICATIONS
- Numbness, stiffness, redness, swelling, spasm and pain of the fingers and hand, painful obstruction of the fingers.
- Headache, toothache, pain and swelling of the throat, redness and swelling of the eyes, febrile disease.

COMMENTARY
These points were first discussed as far back as the *Essential Questions* which recommended bleeding them for the treatment of malaria. The name Baxie (Eight Pathogens), however, did not appear until the *Great Compendium of Acupuncture and Moxibustion*. In modern clinical practice they are almost always used for treating pain, swelling, stiffness, numbness or spasm of the fingers and the sur-

rounding area. For disorders of the ring, middle and index fingers, the points either side of the finger are generally needled. For disorders of the little finger the point between the little and ring fingers is needled in combination with points such as Qiangu SI-2 and Houxi SI-3. For disorders of the thumb, the point between the thumb and index finger is needled in combination with points such as Lieque LU-7 and Yuji LU-10.

YAOTONGXUE (N-UE-19) 腰痛穴

Lumbar Pain Point

LOCATION

On the dorsum of the hand, two points located between the second and third and the fourth and fifth metacarpal bones, in the depressions lying immediately distal to the bases of the metacarpals.

LOCATION NOTE

Slide a finger proximally along the back of the hand towards the wrist, in the groove between the metacarpal bones until it reaches the tender depression just proximal to the junction of the metacarpals.

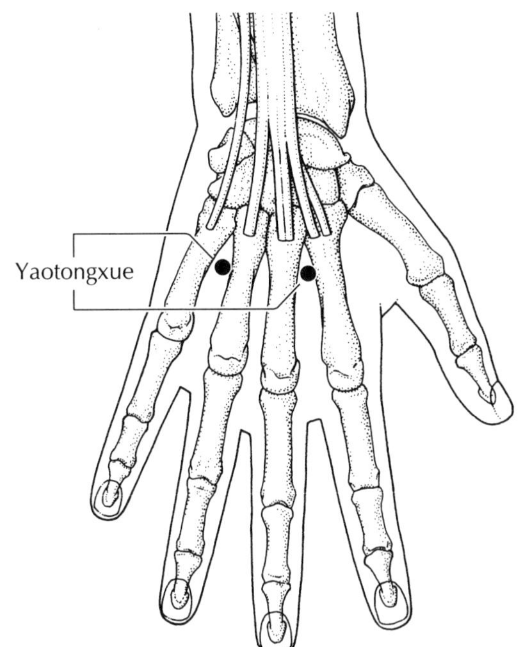

NEEDLING

Perpendicular insertion 0.5 to 1 cun.

ACTIONS

Invigorates qi and blood in the lumbar region

INDICATIONS

- Acute lumbar sprain.

COMMENTARY

Yaotongxue (N-UE-19) is a commonly used point for acute lumbar sprain. It is usually selected when the pain is on either side of the midline and the points on the affected side are manipulated whilst the patient is asked to twist, turn and bend. Note that this point is also known as Yaotongdian (Lumbar Pain Spot).

LUOZHEN (M-UE-24) 落枕

Stiff Neck

LOCATION

On the dorsum of the hand, in the depression just proximal to the second and third metacarpophalangeal joints.

LOCATION NOTE

i. Luozhen (M-UE-24) is usually located and needled with the hand resting in a loose fist; ii. This point may be located at the apex of an equilateral triangle formed by this point and the prominences of the metacarpophalangeal joints of the index and middle fingers; iii. The point is also defined as lying on the dorsum of the hand opposite Laogong P-8.

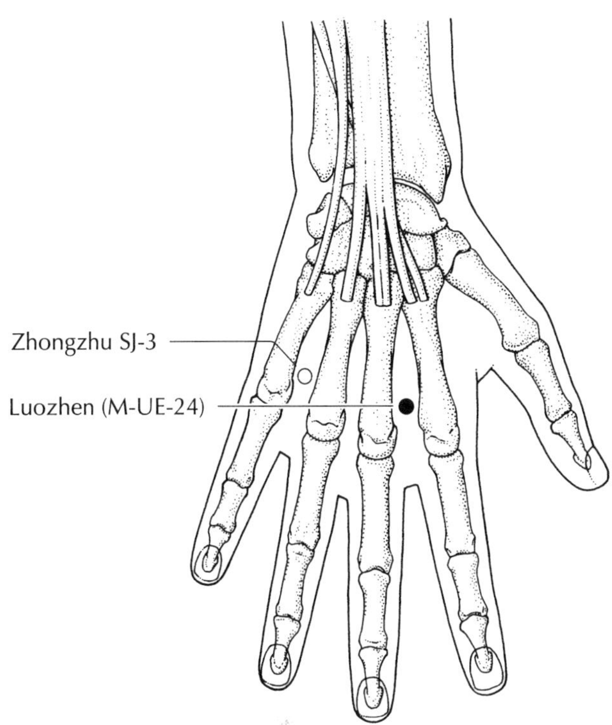

NEEDLING
Perpendicular or oblique insertion directed proximally, 0.5 to 1 cun.

ACTIONS
Invigorates qi and blood in the neck region

INDICATIONS
- Stiffness and pain of the neck, inability to turn the head, headache, pain of the shoulder and arm.
- Pain of the epigastrium, diarrhoea, acute and chronic childhood fright wind

COMMENTARY
Luozhen (M-UE-24) is commonly selected for acute pain and stiffness of the neck. The point on the affected side is manipulated whilst the patient is asked to flex, extend and rotate the neck.

ERBAI (M-UE-29)

二白

Two Whites

LOCATION
On the flexor aspect of the forearm, 4 cun proximal to Daling P-7, either side of the tendon of flexor carpi radialis.

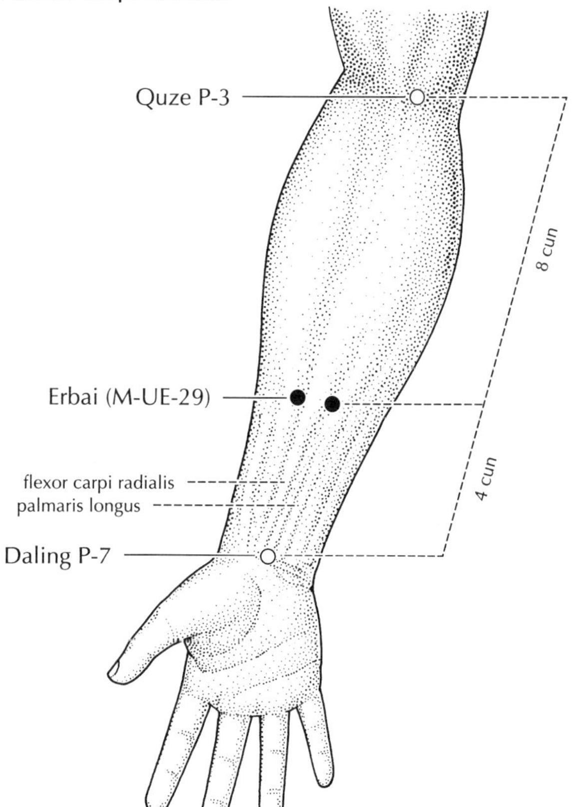

LOCATION NOTE
i. There are two points; one lies on the ulnar side of the tendon of flexor carpi radialis, and between this tendon and the tendon of palmaris longus if this is present, whilst the other lies on the radial side of the tendon of flexor carpi radialis; ii. Divide the distance between the cubital crease and Daling P-7 into thirds and locate this point at the junction of the proximal two thirds and the distal third.

NEEDLING
Perpendicular insertion, 0.5 to 1 cun or oblique proximal insertion 1 to 1.5 cun.

ACTIONS
Treats prolapse of the rectum and haemorrhoids

INDICATIONS
- Haemorrhoids, prolapse of the rectum, itching of the anus, blood in the stool, tenesmus.

COMMENTARY
This point first appeared in the *Classic of the Jade Dragon* and has long been used for the treatment of haemorrhoids and rectal prolapse.

COMBINATIONS
- Chronic haemorrhoids: Erbai (M-UE-29), Chengshan BL-57 and Changqiang DU-1 (*Great Compendium*).
- Prolapse of the rectum and haemorrhoids: Erbai (M-UE-29), Baihui DU-20, Zhishi BL-52 and Changqiang DU-1 (*Great Compendium*).

ZHOUJIAN (M-UE-46)

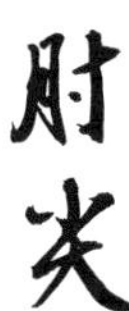

Elbow Tip

LOCATION
On the tip of the olecranon process of the ulna.

NEEDLING
This point is treated by moxibustion only.

ACTIONS
Transforms phlegm and dissipates swelling

INDICATIONS
- Scrofula, carbuncles and furuncles, deep-rooted ulcers, intestinal abscess.

COMMENTARY
This point was first discussed in the *Thousand Ducat Formulas*, particularly in relation to the treatment of intes-

tinal abscess. It has also long been used for scrofula, a term primarily used to describe nodules on the sides of the neck, but also nodules in the axilla and inguinal region. The text *Introduction to Medicine* recommends applying moxibustion to right Zhoujian (M-UE-46) for left-sided scrofula and vice-versa.

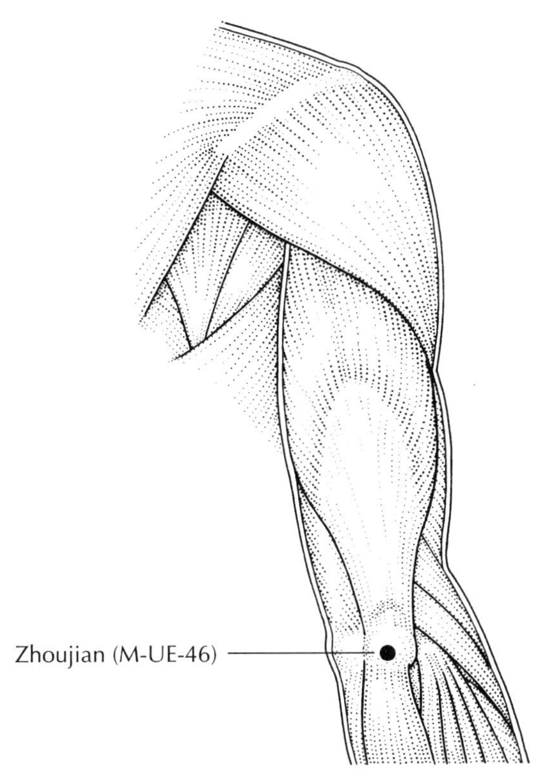

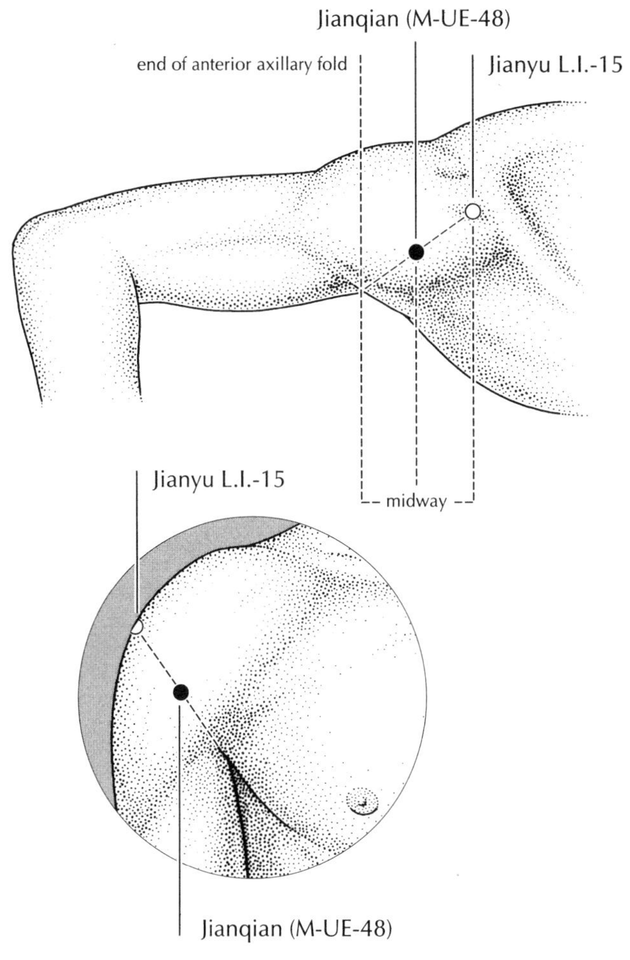

JIANQIAN (M-UE-48)

Front of the Shoulder

肩前

LOCATION

On the anterior aspect of the shoulder joint, midway between the anterior axillary crease and Jianyu L.I.-15.

LOCATION NOTE

This point is usually found to be tender on palpation.

NEEDLING

i. Perpendicular insertion 1 to 1.5 cun; ii. Oblique or oblique-transverse insertion distally towards the elbow, 2 to 3 cun.

ACTIONS

Activates qi and blood and benefits the shoulder joint

INDICATIONS

- Stiffness and pain of the anterior aspect of the shoulder, numbness, paralysis and immobility of the shoulder joint.

COMMENTARY

Jianqian (M-UE-48) also known as Jianneiling (Inner Mound of the Shoulder) is frequently palpated, and needled if tender, for pain in the front portion of the shoulder joint. In clinical practice it is commonly combined with other important points for treating the shoulder such as Jianyu L.I.-15, Juliao L.I.-16, Jianliao SJ-14 and Naoshu SI-10.

EXTRA POINTS OF THE LOWER EXTREMITY

BAICHONGWO (M-LE-34)

Hundred Insect Burrow

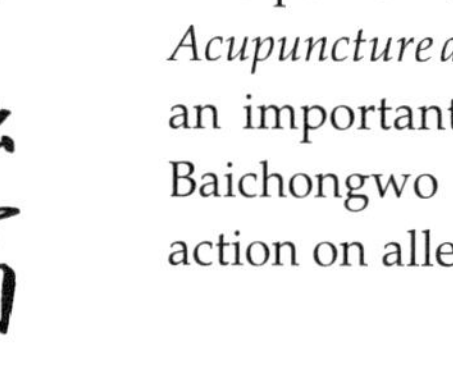

LOCATION

3 cun proximal to the superior border of the patella, in a tender depression on the bulge of the vastus medialis muscle.

LOCATION NOTE

This point lies 1 cun proximal to Xuehai SP-10.

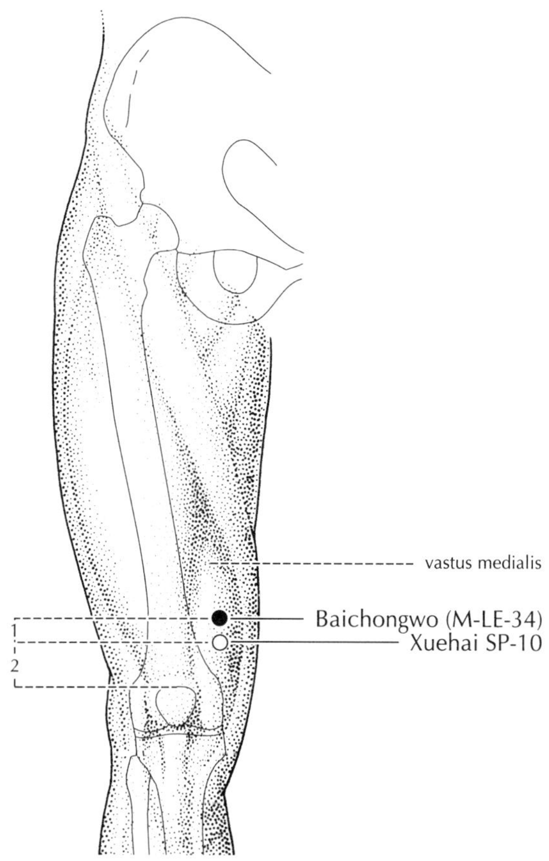

NEEDLING

Perpendicular or oblique insertion 1 to 1.5 cun.

ACTIONS

Clears heat from the blood
Eliminates wind and drains dampness

INDICATIONS

- Sores of the lower region, wind rash, itching of the skin.

COMMENTARY

This point was first discussed in the *Great Compendium of Acupuncture and Moxibustion*. Lying close to Xuehai SP-10, an important point for the treatment of skin diseases, Baichongwo (M-LE-34) is considered to have a special action on alleviating severe itching.

HEDING (M-LE-27)

Crane's Summit

鶴頂

LOCATION

In the depression at the midpoint of the superior border of the patella.

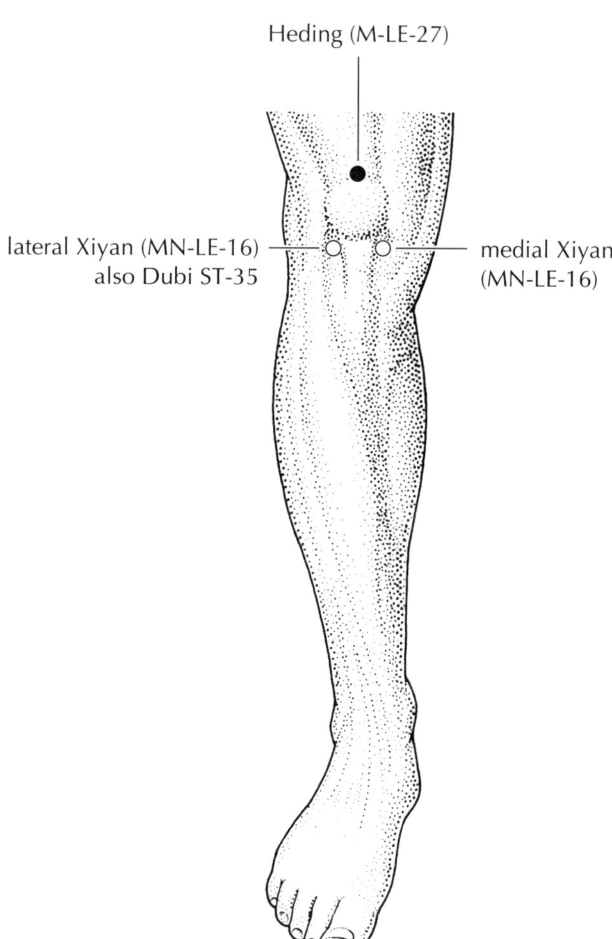

NEEDLING

Perpendicular insertion 0.5 to 1 cun.

ACTIONS

Activates qi and blood and benefits the knee joint.

INDICATIONS
- Crane's knee wind, swelling and pain of the knee, leg qi, weakness of the knee and leg.

COMMENTARY
Heding (M-LE-27) is a valuable secondary point in the treatment of disorders of the knee joint, and is often selected in combination with such points as Xiyan (MN-LE-16), Xuehai SP-10, Liangqiu ST-34, Yanglingquan GB-34 and Yinlingquan SP-9.

XIYAN (MN-LE-16)

膝眼

Eyes of the Knee

LOCATION
On the knee, in the hollows formed when the knee is flexed, immediately below the patella and both medial and lateral to the patellar ligament.

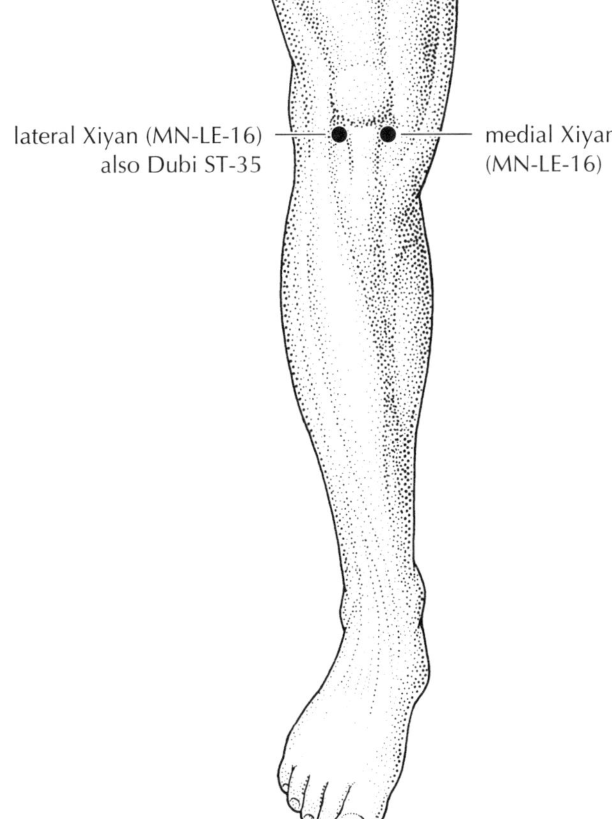

LOCATION NOTE
Lateral Xiyan (MN-LE-16) is identical with Dubi ST-35.

NEEDLING
With the knee flexed and supported by a rolled pillow, i. Perpendicular insertion, directed towards Weizhong BL-40, 1 to 2 cun; ii. Oblique insertion in a medial and superior direction, behind the patella 1 to 2 cun; iii. Through-needling between lateral and medial Xiyan (MN-LE-16), behind the patellar ligament.

ACTIONS
Dispels wind-damp, reduces swelling and alleviates pain

INDICATIONS
- Swelling and pain of the knee joint, difficulty in flexing and extending the knee, weakness of the knee joint, numbness of the knee, numbness of the lower limb, atrophy disorder of the lower limb, leg qi.

COMMENTARY
The Xiyan (MN-LE-16) points were first discussed in the eighth century text *Necessities of a Frontier Official*. Lateral Xiyan (MN-LE-16) corresponds to Dubi ST-35, whilst medial Xiyan (MN-LE-16) is a non-channel point. Used together, these are essential points in the treatment of all knee disorders, whether due to deficiency or excess, heat or cold, and form the basis of any prescription for treating disorders of the knee joint and surrounding tissues.

COMBINATIONS
- Redness, swelling and pain of the knees with inability to walk: Xiyan (MN-LE-16) and Xiguan LIV-7 (*Song of the Jade Dragon*).

LANWEIXUE (M-LE-13)

闌

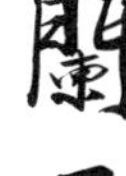

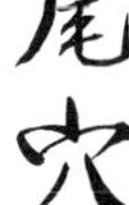

Appendix Point

LOCATION
Approximately 2 cun distal to Zusanli ST-36 on the right leg.

LOCATION NOTE
The exact location of this point is determined by careful palpation to identify the point of maximum tenderness.

NEEDLING
Perpendicular insertion 1 to 1.5 cun.

ACTIONS
Activates qi and blood and clears heat and fire poison from the Large Intestine

INDICATIONS
- Acute and chronic appendicitis, paralysis of the lower limb, drop foot, indigestion.

COMMENTARY
The point Lanweixue (M-LE-13) is famous for its application in the treatment of both acute and chronic appendicitis. In the majority of cases it becomes tender when the appendix is inflamed, and indeed may perform a secondary role in the diagnosis of this condition. Lanweixue (M-LE-13) is one of the few acupuncture points that only exists on one side of the body.

COMBINATIONS
- Acute appendicitis: Lanweixue (M-LE-13), Shangjuxu ST-37 (left), Tianshu ST-25, Quchi L.I.-11.

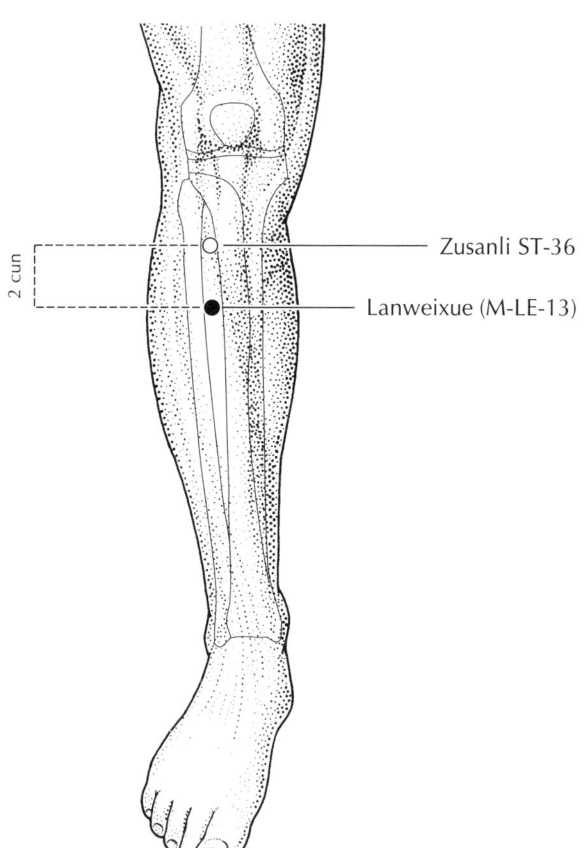

DANNANGXUE (M-LE-23)
Gallbladder Point

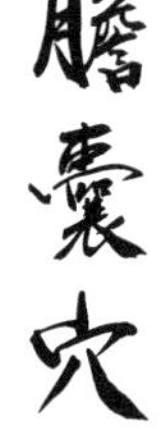

LOCATION
Between 1 and 2 cun distal to Yanglingquan GB-34 on the right leg.

LOCATION NOTE
i. The exact location of this point is determined by careful palpation to identify the point of maximum tenderness; ii. Yanglingquan GB-34 is located below the lateral aspect of the knee, in the tender depression approximately 1 cun anterior and inferior to the head of the fibula.

NEEDLING
Perpendicular insertion 1 to 1.5 cun.

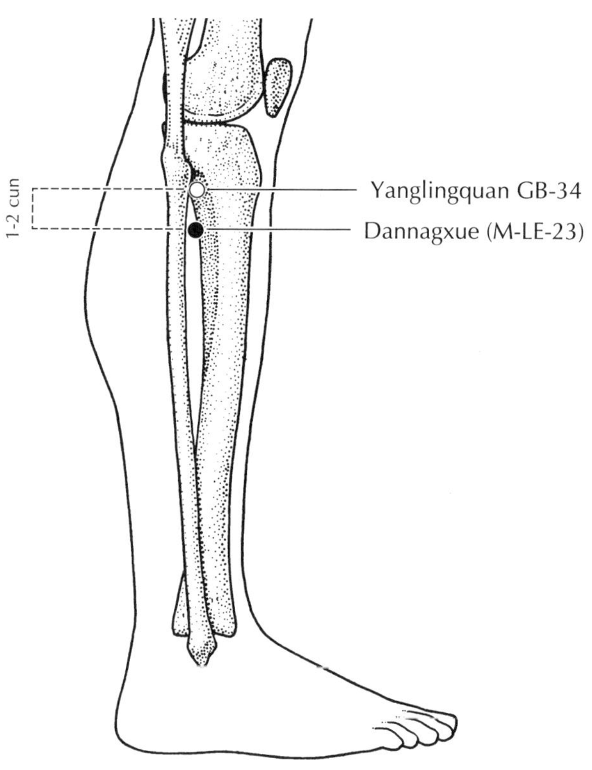

ACTIONS
Clears heat and drains damp

INDICATIONS
- Acute and chronic cholecystitis, acute and chronic cholelithiasis, disease of the bile duct, biliary ascariasis, distention and pain of the lateral costal region, paralysis and numbness of the lower limb.

COMMENTARY

The point Dannangxue (M-LE-23) is famous for its application in the treatment of both acute and chronic cholecystitis and cholelithiasis. In the majority of cases it becomes tender when the gall bladder is inflamed, and indeed may perform a secondary role in the diagnosis of these conditions. Dannangxue (M-LE-23) is one of the few acupuncture points that only exists on one side of the body.

COMBINATIONS

- Acute pain of cholelithiasis: Dannangxue (M-LE-23), Yanglingquan GB-34 (left), Qimen LIV-14 (right), Burong ST-19 (right), Zhongwan REN-12, Hegu L.I.-4 and Taichong LIV-3.

BAFENG (M-LE-8)

Eight Winds

LOCATION

On the dorsum of the foot, between the toes, 0.5 cun proximal to the margin of the web.

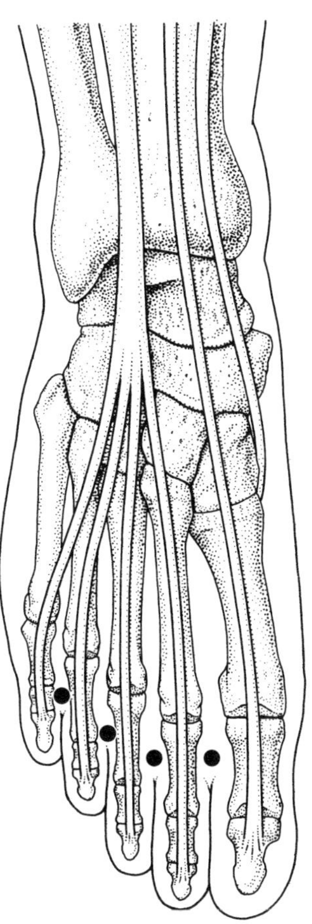

LOCATION NOTE

These eight points include Xingjian LIV-2, Neiting ST-44 and Xiaxi GB-43.

NEEDLING

Oblique insertion directed proximally, 0.5 to 1 cun.

ACTIONS

Clears heat and dissipates swelling

INDICATIONS

- Leg qi, redness, swelling and pain of the dorsum of the foot, malaria, headache, irregular menstruation.

COMMENTARY

The points that comprise Bafeng (M-LE-8) were first mentioned in *Essential Questions*[1], although they were not named Bafeng (Eight Winds) until the Ming dynasty classic *The Great Compendium of Acupuncture and Moxibustion*. The *Thousand Ducat Formulas* of Sun Si-miao named them Bachong (Eight Rushing), reflecting the dynamic qi sensation induced by needling these distal points of the foot. Although indicated for malaria in the *Essential Questions*, and for irregular menstruation in the *Compilation of Acupuncture and Moxibustion*, this group of points is primarily used for disorders of the toes in the same way that the Baxie (M-UE-22) points are used for disorders of the fingers. It should be noted, however, that three of the Bafeng (M-LE-8) points do correspond to channel acupuncture points (Xiaxi GB-43, Neiting ST-44 and Xingjian LIV-2).

NOTES

1 *Essential Questions* Chapter 36.

MAJOR POINTS OF THE EYE REGION

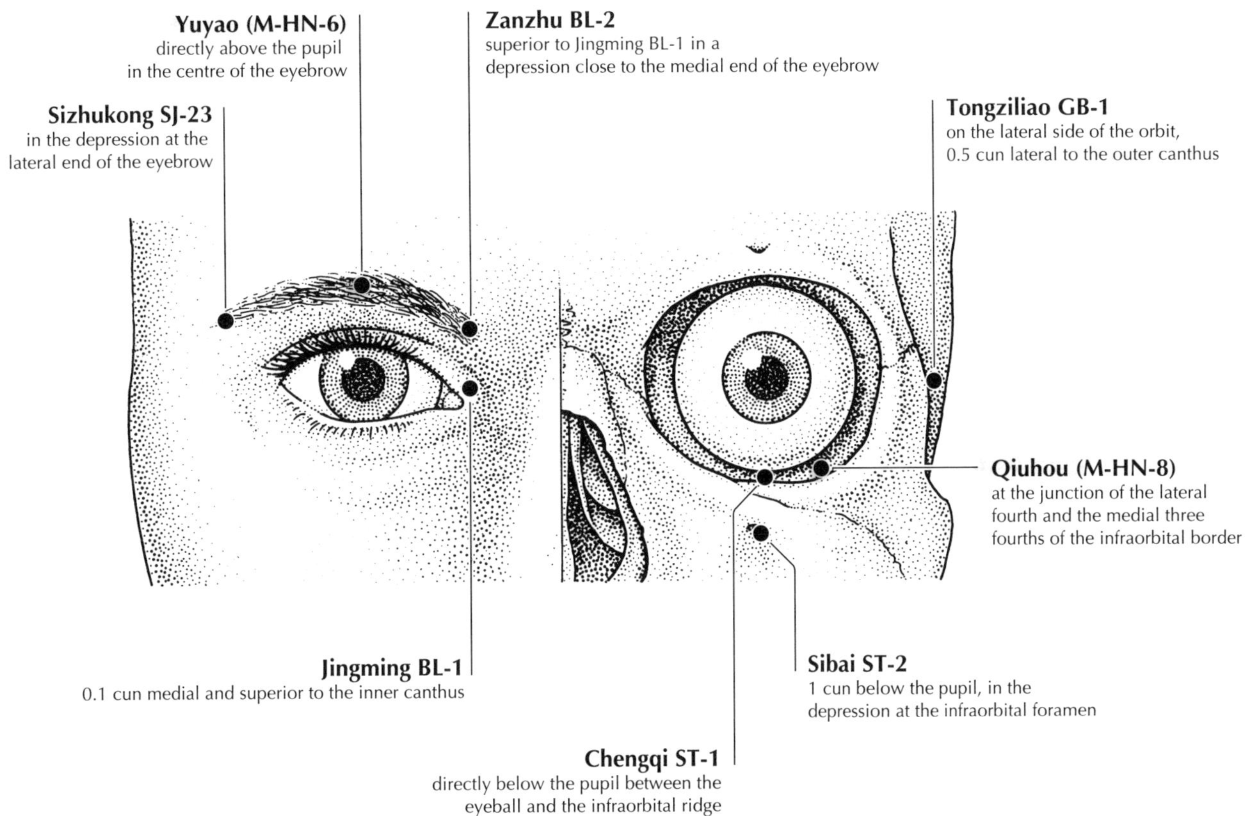
Yuyao (M-HN-6)
directly above the pupil
in the centre of the eyebrow
Zanzhu BL-2
superior to Jingming BL-1 in a
depression close to the medial end of the eyebrow
Sizhukong SJ-23
in the depression at the
lateral end of the eyebrow
Tongziliao GB-1
on the lateral side of the orbit,
0.5 cun lateral to the outer canthus
Qiuhou (M-HN-8)
at the junction of the lateral
fourth and the medial three
fourths of the infraorbital border
Jingming BL-1
0.1 cun medial and superior to the inner canthus
Sibai ST-2
1 cun below the pupil, in the
depression at the infraorbital foramen
Chengqi ST-1
directly below the pupil between the
eyeball and the infraorbital ridge

MAJOR POINTS OF THE FACE

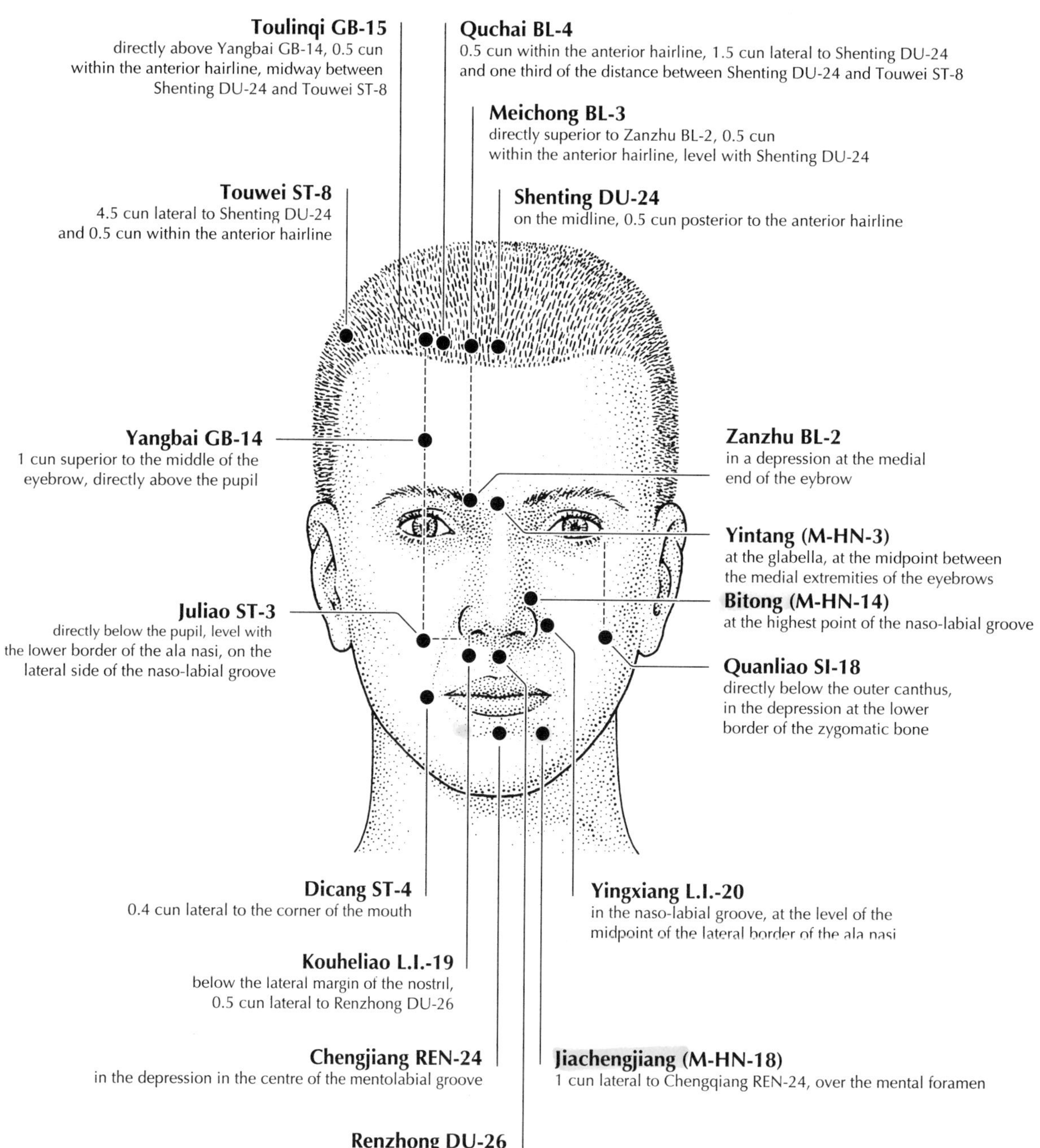
Toulinqi GB-15
directly above Yangbai GB-14, 0.5 cun within the anterior hairline, midway between Shenting DU-24 and Touwei ST-8
Quchai BL-4
0.5 cun within the anterior hairline, 1.5 cun lateral to Shenting DU-24 and one third of the distance between Shenting DU-24 and Touwei ST-8
Meichong BL-3
directly superior to Zanzhu BL-2, 0.5 cun within the anterior hairline, level with Shenting DU-24
Touwei ST-8
4.5 cun lateral to Shenting DU-24 and 0.5 cun within the anterior hairline
Shenting DU-24
on the midline, 0.5 cun posterior to the anterior hairline
Yangbai GB-14
1 cun superior to the middle of the eyebrow, directly above the pupil
Zanzhu BL-2
in a depression at the medial end of the eybrow
Yintang (M-HN-3)
at the glabella, at the midpoint between the medial extremities of the eyebrows
Bitong (M-HN-14)
at the highest point of the naso-labial groove
Juliao ST-3
directly below the pupil, level with the lower border of the ala nasi, on the lateral side of the naso-labial groove
Quanliao SI-18
directly below the outer canthus, in the depression at the lower border of the zygomatic bone
Dicang ST-4
0.4 cun lateral to the corner of the mouth
Yingxiang L.I.-20
in the naso-labial groove, at the level of the midpoint of the lateral border of the ala nasi
Kouheliao L.I.-19
below the lateral margin of the nostril, 0.5 cun lateral to Renzhong DU-26
Chengjiang REN-24
in the depression in the centre of the mentolabial groove
Jiachengjiang (M-HN-18)
1 cun lateral to Chengqiang REN-24, over the mental foramen
Renzhong DU-26
above the upper lip on the midline, at the junction of the upper third and lower two thirds of the philtrum

MAJOR POINTS OF THE SIDE OF THE HEAD

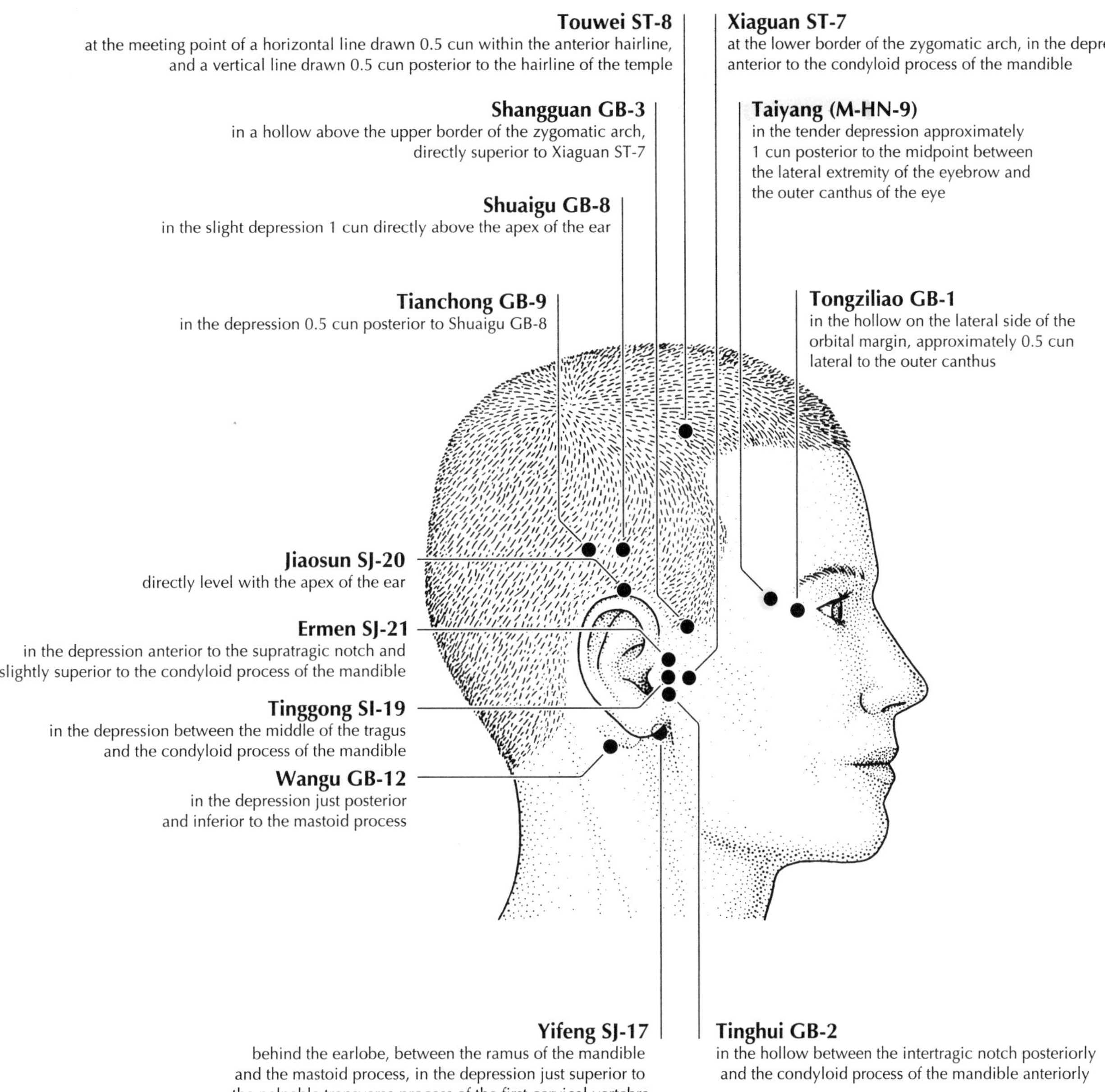
Touwei ST-8
at the meeting point of a horizontal line drawn 0.5 cun within the anterior hairline, and a vertical line drawn 0.5 cun posterior to the hairline of the temple
Xiaguan ST-7
at the lower border of the zygomatic arch, in the depression anterior to the condyloid process of the mandible
Shangguan GB-3
in a hollow above the upper border of the zygomatic arch, directly superior to Xiaguan ST-7
Taiyang (M-HN-9)
in the tender depression approximately 1 cun posterior to the midpoint between the lateral extremity of the eyebrow and the outer canthus of the eye
Shuaigu GB-8
in the slight depression 1 cun directly above the apex of the ear
Tianchong GB-9
in the depression 0.5 cun posterior to Shuaigu GB-8
Tongziliao GB-1
in the hollow on the lateral side of the orbital margin, approximately 0.5 cun lateral to the outer canthus
Jiaosun SJ-20
directly level with the apex of the ear
Ermen SJ-21
in the depression anterior to the supratragic notch and slightly superior to the condyloid process of the mandible
Tinggong SI-19
in the depression between the middle of the tragus and the condyloid process of the mandible
Wangu GB-12
in the depression just posterior and inferior to the mastoid process
Yifeng SJ-17
behind the earlobe, between the ramus of the mandible and the mastoid process, in the depression just superior to the palpable transverse process of the first cervical vertebra
Tinghui GB-2
in the hollow between the intertragic notch posteriorly and the condyloid process of the mandible anteriorly

MAJOR POINTS OF THE TOP OF THE HEAD

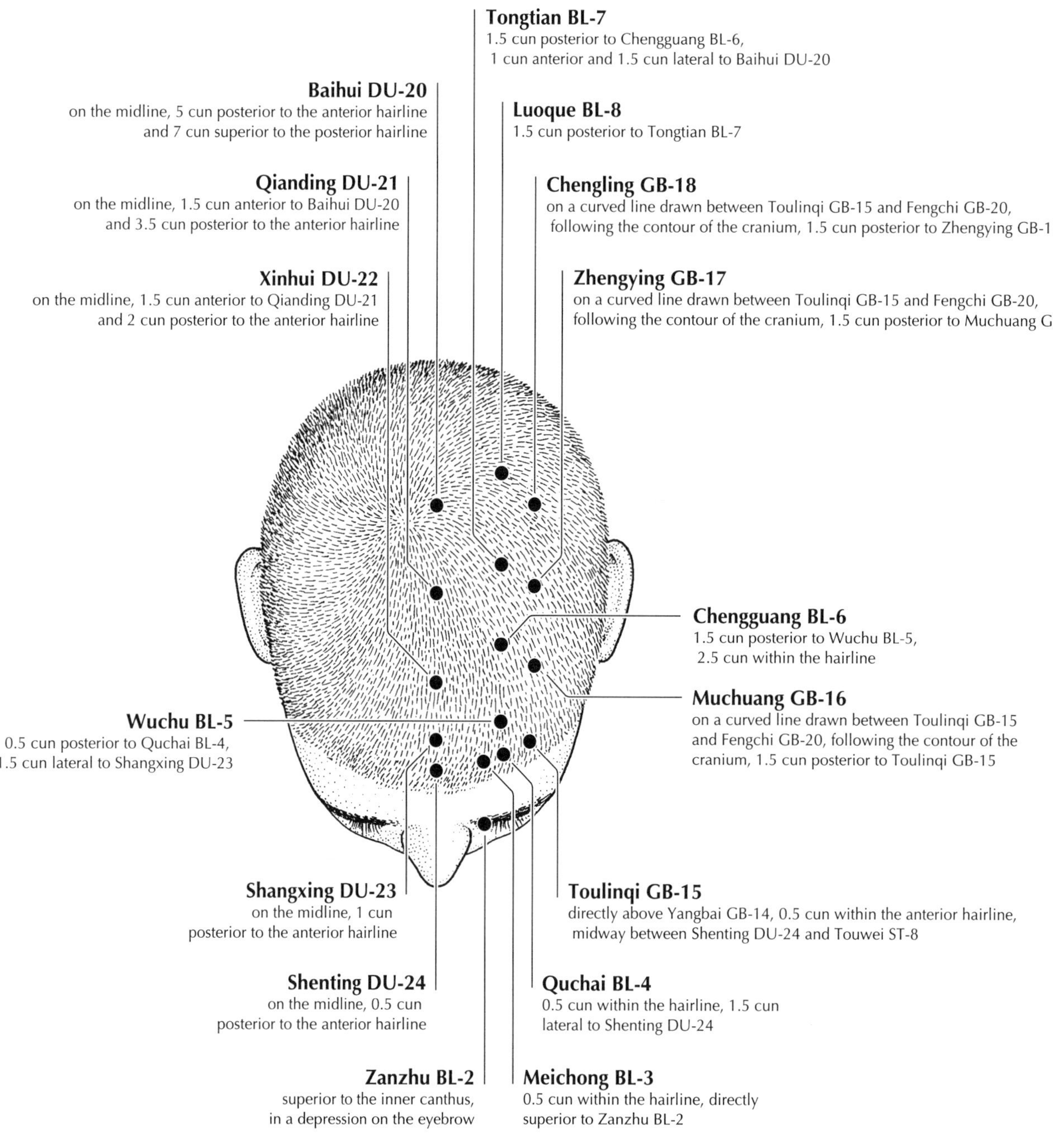

Tongtian BL-7
1.5 cun posterior to Chengguang BL-6,
1 cun anterior and 1.5 cun lateral to Baihui DU-20
Baihui DU-20
on the midline, 5 cun posterior to the anterior hairline
and 7 cun superior to the posterior hairline
Luoque BL-8
1.5 cun posterior to Tongtian BL-7
Qianding DU-21
on the midline, 1.5 cun anterior to Baihui DU-20
and 3.5 cun posterior to the anterior hairline
Chengling GB-18
on a curved line drawn between Toulinqi GB-15 and Fengchi GB-20,
following the contour of the cranium, 1.5 cun posterior to Zhengying GB-17
Xinhui DU-22
on the midline, 1.5 cun anterior to Qianding DU-21
and 2 cun posterior to the anterior hairline
Zhengying GB-17
on a curved line drawn between Toulinqi GB-15 and Fengchi GB-20,
following the contour of the cranium, 1.5 cun posterior to Muchuang GB-16
Chengguang BL-6
1.5 cun posterior to Wuchu BL-5,
2.5 cun within the hairline
Muchuang GB-16
on a curved line drawn between Toulinqi GB-15
and Fengchi GB-20, following the contour of the
cranium, 1.5 cun posterior to Toulinqi GB-15
Wuchu BL-5
0.5 cun posterior to Quchai BL-4,
1.5 cun lateral to Shangxing DU-23
Shangxing DU-23
on the midline, 1 cun
posterior to the anterior hairline
Toulinqi GB-15
directly above Yangbai GB-14, 0.5 cun within the anterior hairline,
midway between Shenting DU-24 and Touwei ST-8
Shenting DU-24
on the midline, 0.5 cun
posterior to the anterior hairline
Quchai BL-4
0.5 cun within the hairline, 1.5 cun
lateral to Shenting DU-24
Zanzhu BL-2
superior to the inner canthus,
in a depression on the eyebrow
Meichong BL-3
0.5 cun within the hairline, directly
superior to Zanzhu BL-2

MAJOR POINTS OF THE BACK OF THE HEAD

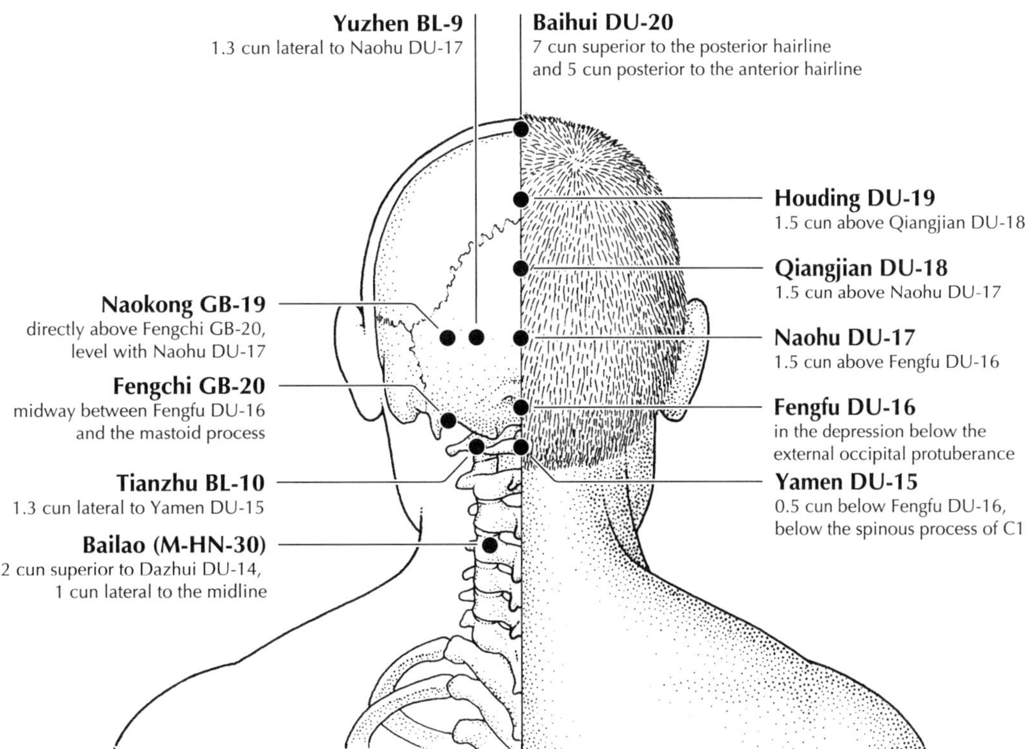
Yuzhen BL-9
1.3 cun lateral to Naohu DU-17
Baihui DU-20
7 cun superior to the posterior hairline
and 5 cun posterior to the anterior hairline
Houding DU-19
1.5 cun above Qiangjian DU-18
Qiangjian DU-18
1.5 cun above Naohu DU-17
Naokong GB-19
directly above Fengchi GB-20,
level with Naohu DU-17
Naohu DU-17
1.5 cun above Fengfu DU-16
Fengchi GB-20
midway between Fengfu DU-16
and the mastoid process
Fengfu DU-16
in the depression below the
external occipital protuberance
Tianzhu BL-10
1.3 cun lateral to Yamen DU-15
Yamen DU-15
0.5 cun below Fengfu DU-16,
below the spinous process of C1
Bailao (M-HN-30)
2 cun superior to Dazhui DU-14,
1 cun lateral to the midline

MAJOR POINTS OF THE NECK REGION

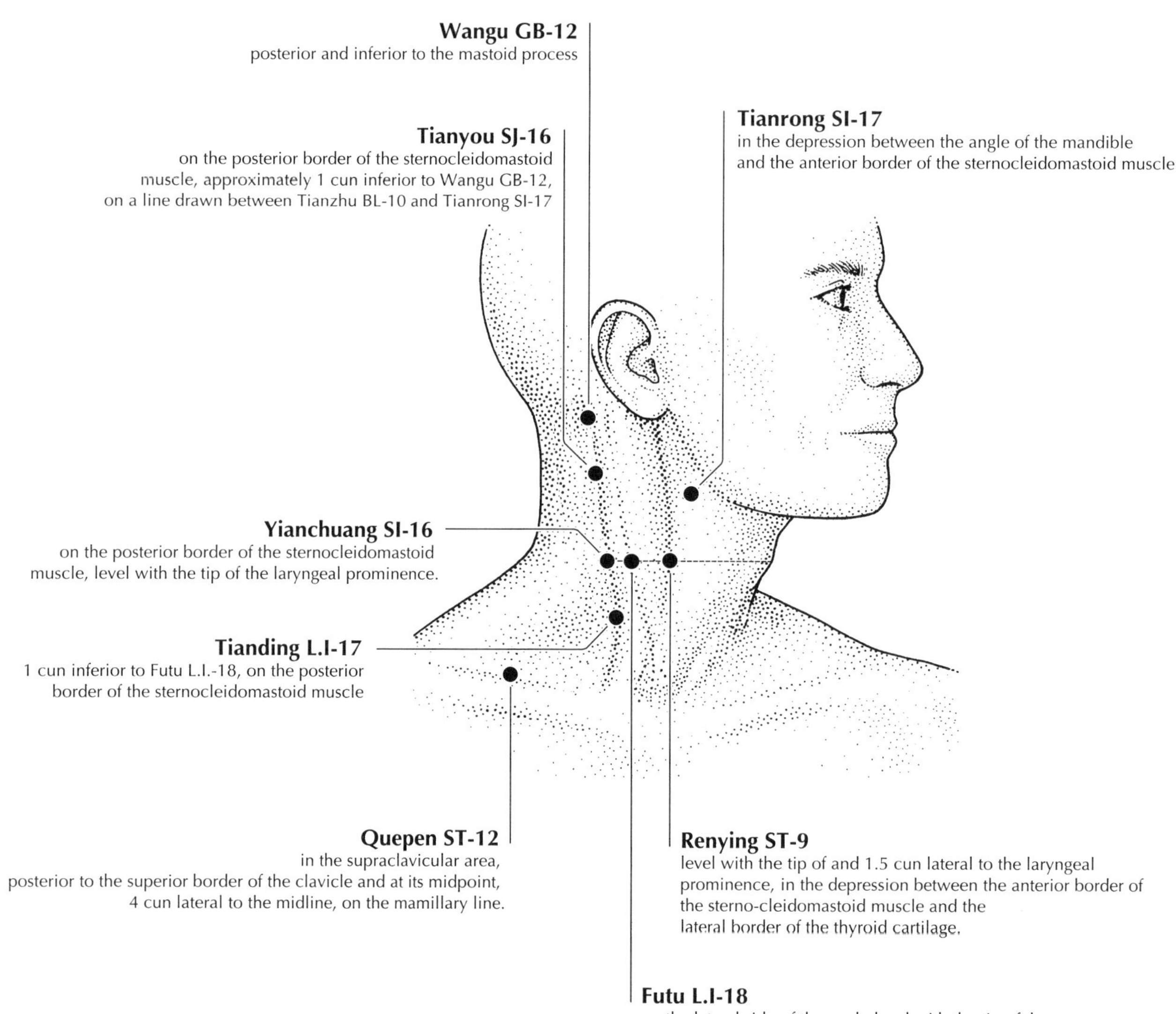
Wangu GB-12
posterior and inferior to the mastoid process
Tianyou SJ-16
on the posterior border of the sternocleidomastoid muscle, approximately 1 cun inferior to Wangu GB-12, on a line drawn between Tianzhu BL-10 and Tianrong SI-17
Tianrong SI-17
in the depression between the angle of the mandible and the anterior border of the sternocleidomastoid muscle.
Yianchuang SI-16
on the posterior border of the sternocleidomastoid muscle, level with the tip of the laryngeal prominence.
Tianding L.I-17
1 cun inferior to Futu L.I.-18, on the posterior border of the sternocleidomastoid muscle
Quepen ST-12
in the supraclavicular area, posterior to the superior border of the clavicle and at its midpoint, 4 cun lateral to the midline, on the mamillary line.
Renying ST-9
level with the tip of and 1.5 cun lateral to the laryngeal prominence, in the depression between the anterior border of the sterno-cleidomastoid muscle and the lateral border of the thyroid cartilage.
Futu L.I-18
on the lateral side of the neck, level with the tip of the laryngeal prominence, between the sternal and clavicular heads of the sternocleidomastoid muscle.

MAJOR POINTS OF THE SHOULDER REGION AND LATERAL UPPER ARM

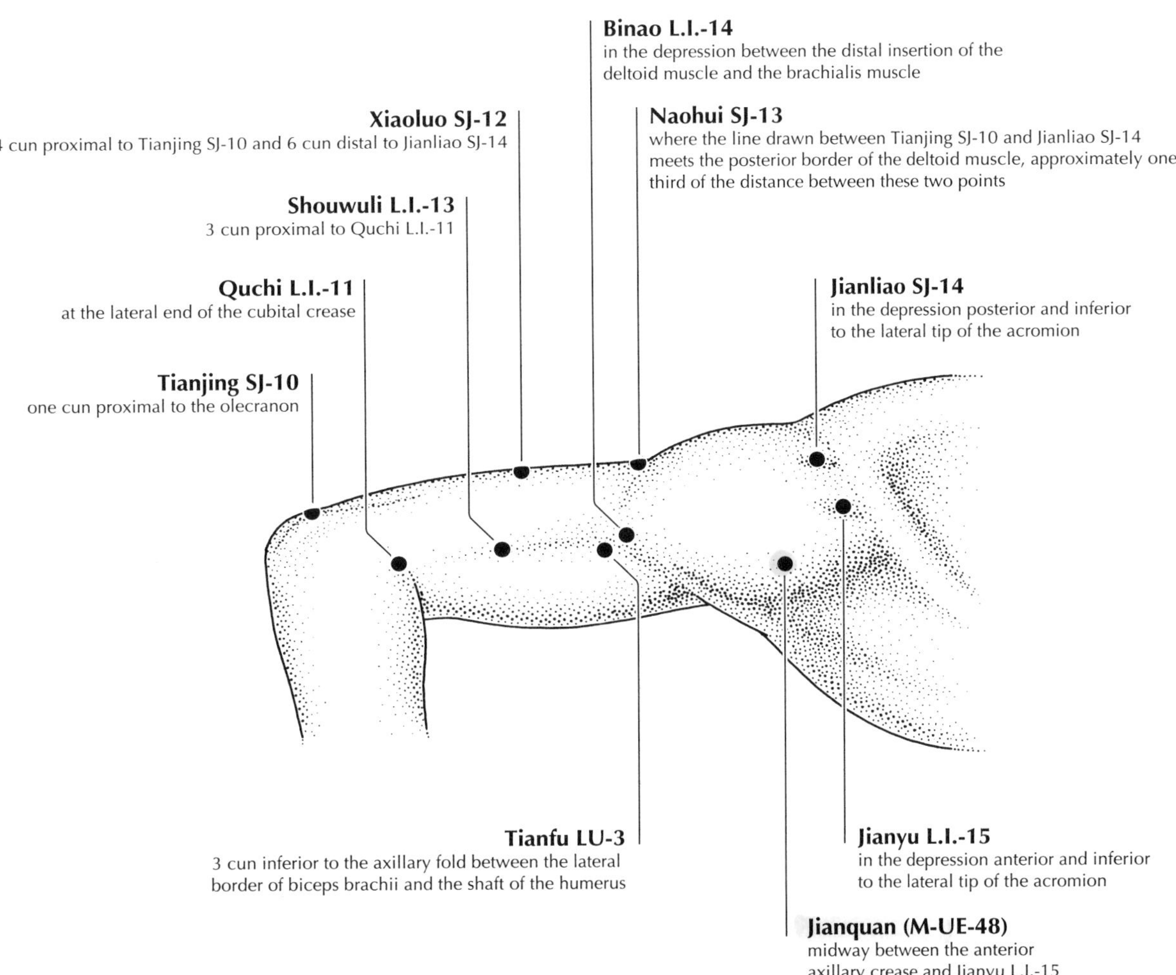
Binao L.I.-14
in the depression between the distal insertion of the deltoid muscle and the brachialis muscle
Xiaoluo SJ-12
4 cun proximal to Tianjing SJ-10 and 6 cun distal to Jianliao SJ-14
Naohui SJ-13
where the line drawn between Tianjing SJ-10 and Jianliao SJ-14 meets the posterior border of the deltoid muscle, approximately one third of the distance between these two points
Shouwuli L.I.-13
3 cun proximal to Quchi L.I.-11
Quchi L.I.-11
at the lateral end of the cubital crease
Jianliao SJ-14
in the depression posterior and inferior to the lateral tip of the acromion
Tianjing SJ-10
one cun proximal to the olecranon
Tianfu LU-3
3 cun inferior to the axillary fold between the lateral border of biceps brachii and the shaft of the humerus
Jianyu L.I.-15
in the depression anterior and inferior to the lateral tip of the acromion
Jianquan (M-UE-48)
midway between the anterior axillary crease and Jianyu L.I.-15

MAJOR POINTS OF THE UPPER ARM

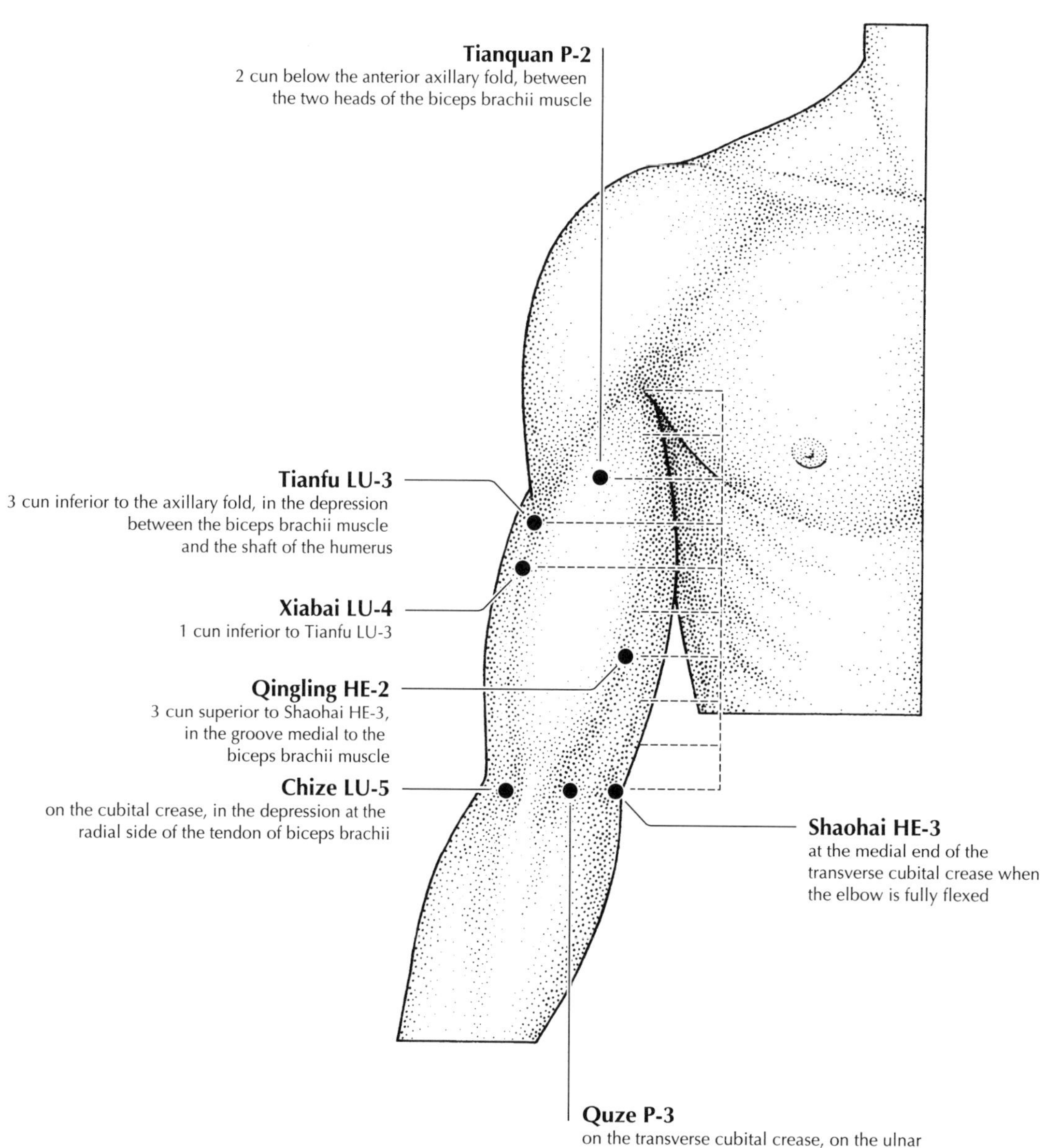
Tianquan P-2
2 cun below the anterior axillary fold, between the two heads of the biceps brachii muscle
Tianfu LU-3
3 cun inferior to the axillary fold, in the depression between the biceps brachii muscle and the shaft of the humerus
Xiabai LU-4
1 cun inferior to Tianfu LU-3
Qingling HE-2
3 cun superior to Shaohai HE-3, in the groove medial to the biceps brachii muscle
Chize LU-5
on the cubital crease, in the depression at the radial side of the tendon of biceps brachii
Shaohai HE-3
at the medial end of the transverse cubital crease when the elbow is fully flexed
Quze P-3
on the transverse cubital crease, on the ulnar side of the aponeurosis of the biceps brachii muscle

MAJOR POINTS OF THE CHEST

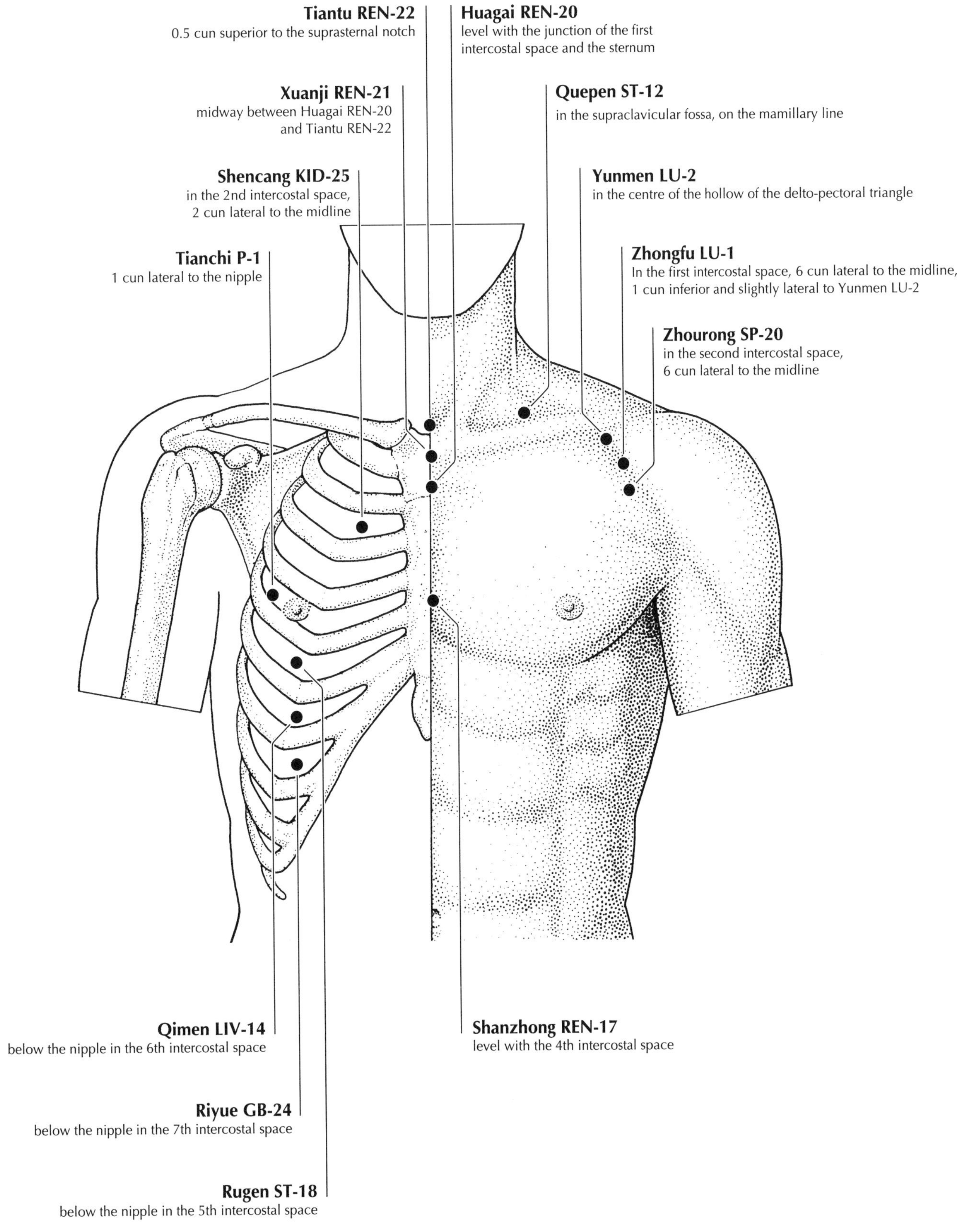
Tiantu REN-22
0.5 cun superior to the suprasternal notch
Huagai REN-20
level with the junction of the first intercostal space and the sternum
Xuanji REN-21
midway between Huagai REN-20 and Tiantu REN-22
Quepen ST-12
in the supraclavicular fossa, on the mamillary line
Shencang KID-25
in the 2nd intercostal space, 2 cun lateral to the midline
Yunmen LU-2
in the centre of the hollow of the delto-pectoral triangle
Tianchi P-1
1 cun lateral to the nipple
Zhongfu LU-1
In the first intercostal space, 6 cun lateral to the midline, 1 cun inferior and slightly lateral to Yunmen LU-2
Zhourong SP-20
in the second intercostal space, 6 cun lateral to the midline
Qimen LIV-14
below the nipple in the 6th intercostal space
Shanzhong REN-17
level with the 4th intercostal space
Riyue GB-24
below the nipple in the 7th intercostal space
Rugen ST-18
below the nipple in the 5th intercostal space

MAJOR POINTS OF THE UPPER ABDOMEN

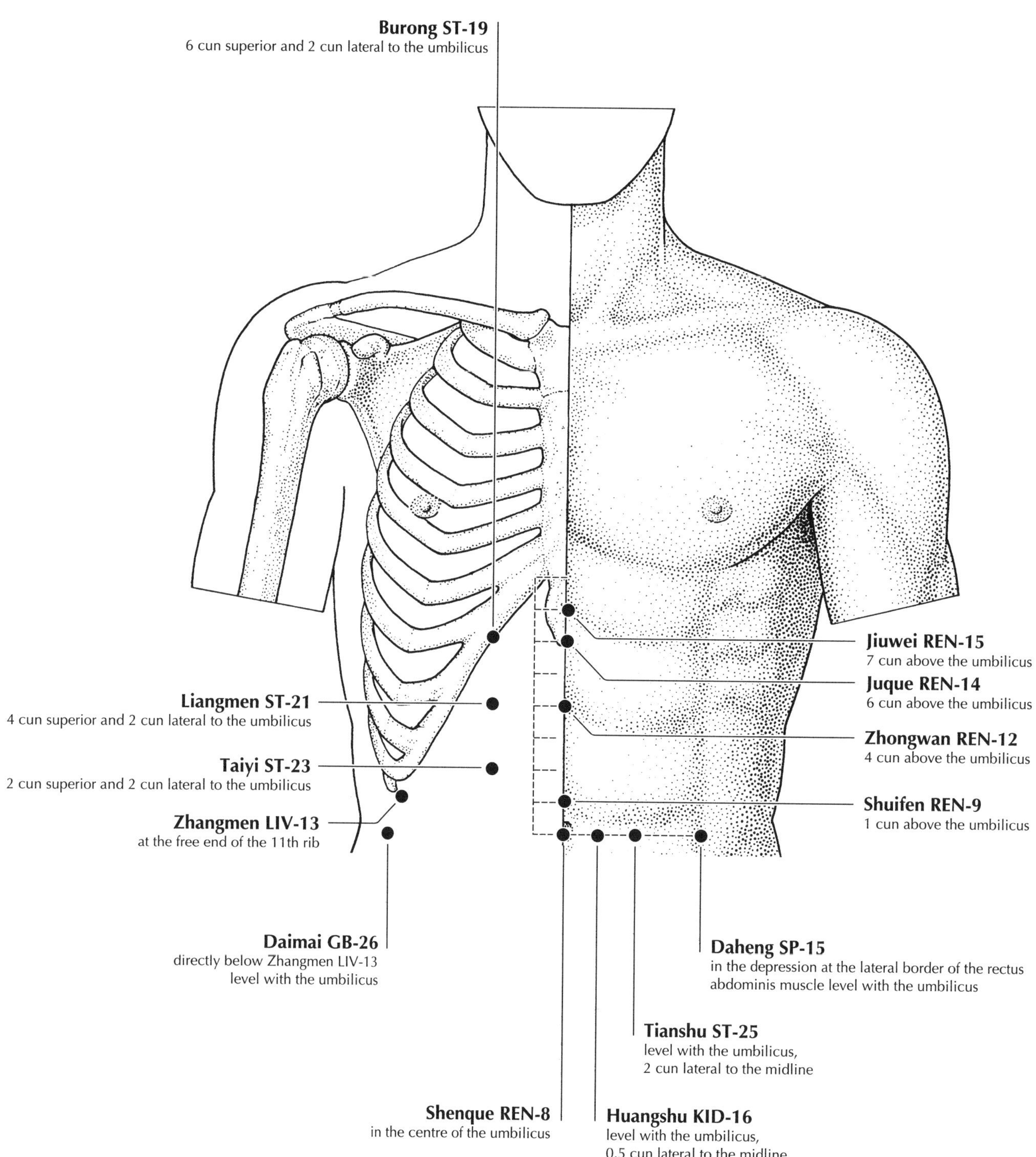
Burong ST-19
6 cun superior and 2 cun lateral to the umbilicus
Jiuwei REN-15
7 cun above the umbilicus
Juque REN-14
6 cun above the umbilicus
Liangmen ST-21
4 cun superior and 2 cun lateral to the umbilicus
Zhongwan REN-12
4 cun above the umbilicus
Taiyi ST-23
2 cun superior and 2 cun lateral to the umbilicus
Shuifen REN-9
1 cun above the umbilicus
Zhangmen LIV-13
at the free end of the 11th rib
Daimai GB-26
directly below Zhangmen LIV-13
level with the umbilicus
Daheng SP-15
in the depression at the lateral border of the rectus
abdominis muscle level with the umbilicus
Tianshu ST-25
level with the umbilicus,
2 cun lateral to the midline
Shenque REN-8
in the centre of the umbilicus
Huangshu KID-16
level with the umbilicus,
0.5 cun lateral to the midline

MAJOR POINTS OF THE LOWER ABDOMEN

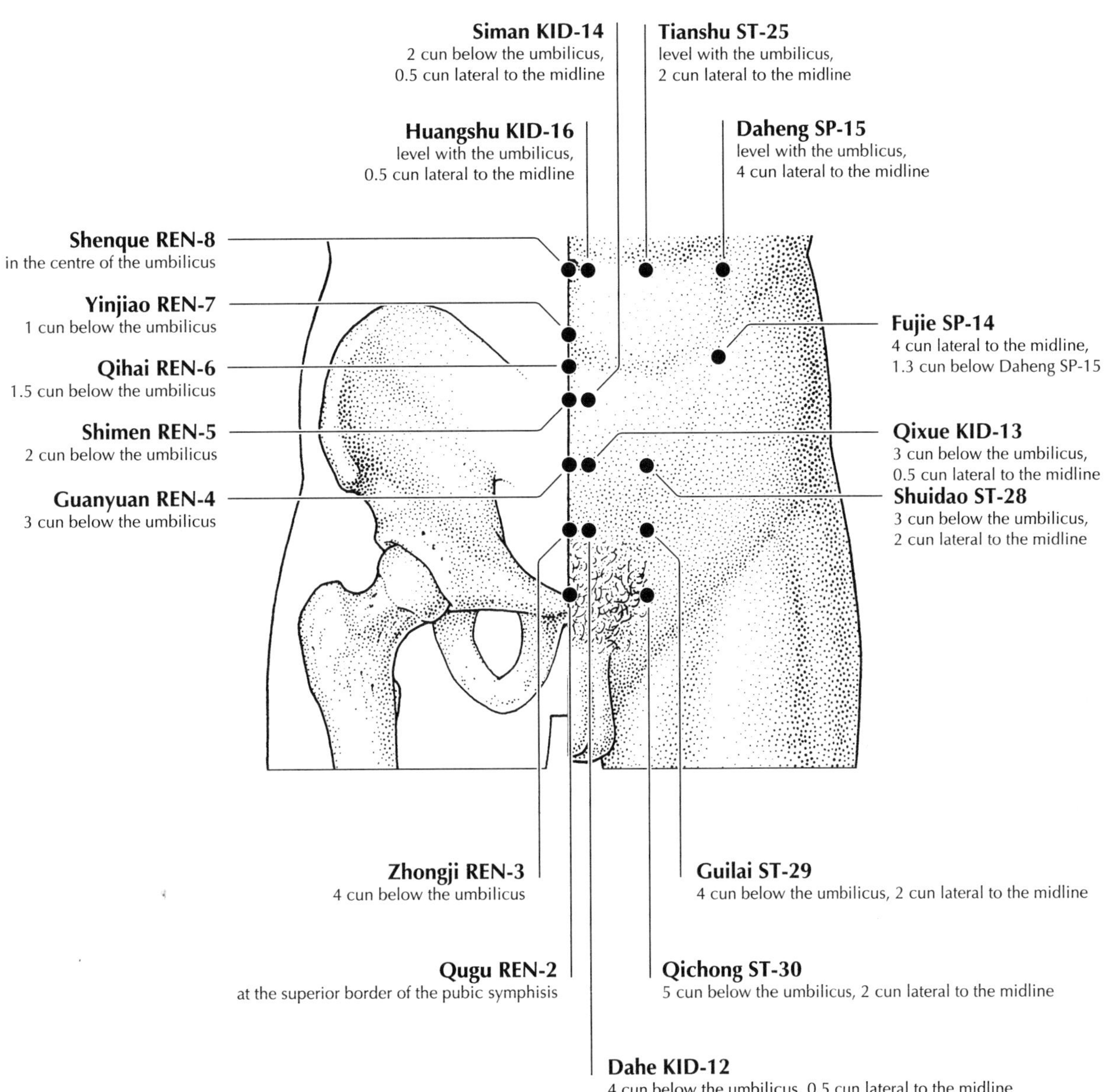
Siman KID-14
2 cun below the umbilicus,
0.5 cun lateral to the midline
Tianshu ST-25
level with the umbilicus,
2 cun lateral to the midline
Huangshu KID-16
level with the umbilicus,
0.5 cun lateral to the midline
Daheng SP-15
level with the umblicus,
4 cun lateral to the midline
Shenque REN-8
in the centre of the umbilicus
Yinjiao REN-7
1 cun below the umbilicus
Fujie SP-14
4 cun lateral to the midline,
1.3 cun below Daheng SP-15
Qihai REN-6
1.5 cun below the umbilicus
Shimen REN-5
2 cun below the umbilicus
Qixue KID-13
3 cun below the umbilicus,
0.5 cun lateral to the midline
Guanyuan REN-4
3 cun below the umbilicus
Shuidao ST-28
3 cun below the umbilicus,
2 cun lateral to the midline
Zhongji REN-3
4 cun below the umbilicus
Guilai ST-29
4 cun below the umbilicus, 2 cun lateral to the midline
Qugu REN-2
at the superior border of the pubic symphisis
Qichong ST-30
5 cun below the umbilicus, 2 cun lateral to the midline
Dahe KID-12
4 cun below the umbilicus, 0.5 cun lateral to the midline

MAJOR POINTS OF THE UPPER BACK

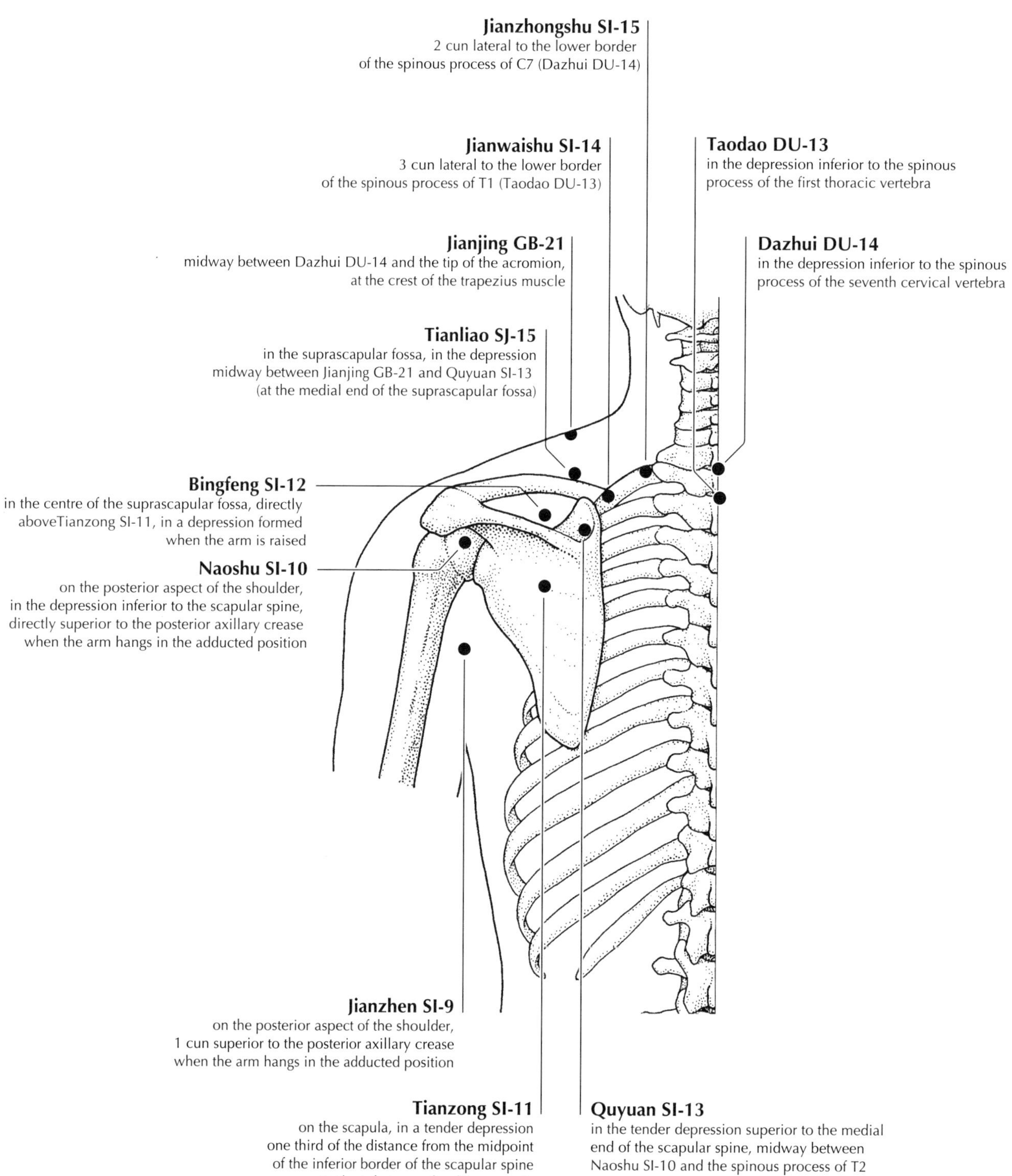
Jianzhongshu SI-15
2 cun lateral to the lower border
of the spinous process of C7 (Dazhui DU-14)
Jianwaishu SI-14
3 cun lateral to the lower border
of the spinous process of T1 (Taodao DU-13)
Taodao DU-13
in the depression inferior to the spinous
process of the first thoracic vertebra
Jianjing GB-21
midway between Dazhui DU-14 and the tip of the acromion,
at the crest of the trapezius muscle
Dazhui DU-14
in the depression inferior to the spinous
process of the seventh cervical vertebra
Tianliao SJ-15
in the suprascapular fossa, in the depression
midway between Jianjing GB-21 and Quyuan SI-13
(at the medial end of the suprascapular fossa)
Bingfeng SI-12
in the centre of the suprascapular fossa, directly
aboveTianzong SI-11, in a depression formed
when the arm is raised
Naoshu SI-10
on the posterior aspect of the shoulder,
in the depression inferior to the scapular spine,
directly superior to the posterior axillary crease
when the arm hangs in the adducted position
Jianzhen SI-9
on the posterior aspect of the shoulder,
1 cun superior to the posterior axillary crease
when the arm hangs in the adducted position
Tianzong SI-11
on the scapula, in a tender depression
one third of the distance from the midpoint
of the inferior border of the scapular spine
to the inferior angle of the scapula
Quyuan SI-13
in the tender depression superior to the medial
end of the scapular spine, midway between
Naoshu SI-10 and the spinous process of T2

MAJOR POINTS OF THE LOWER BACK

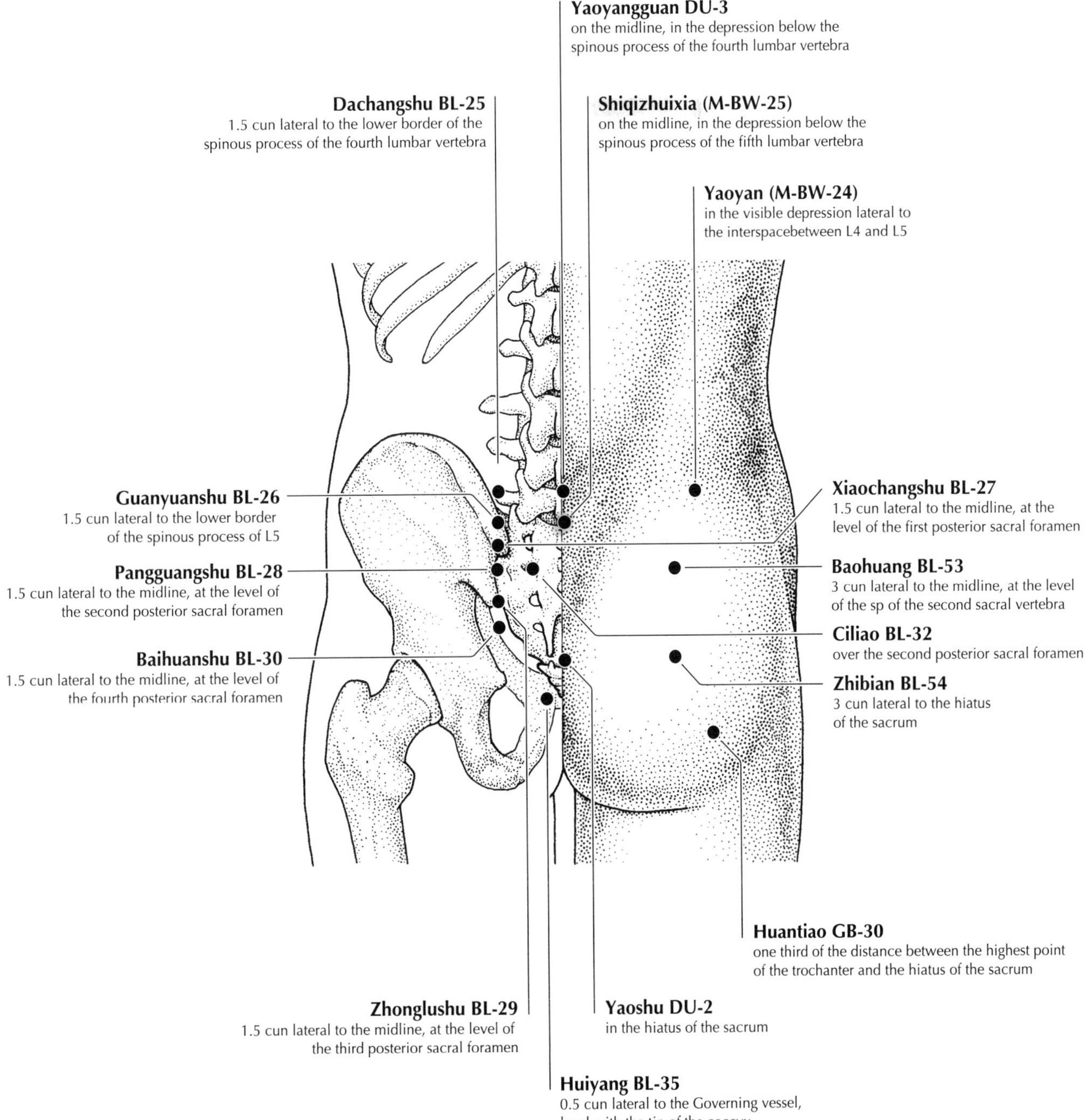
Yaoyangguan DU-3
on the midline, in the depression below the spinous process of the fourth lumbar vertebra
Dachangshu BL-25
1.5 cun lateral to the lower border of the spinous process of the fourth lumbar vertebra
Shiqizhuixia (M-BW-25)
on the midline, in the depression below the spinous process of the fifth lumbar vertebra
Yaoyan (M-BW-24)
in the visible depression lateral to the interspacebetween L4 and L5
Guanyuanshu BL-26
1.5 cun lateral to the lower border of the spinous process of L5
Xiaochangshu BL-27
1.5 cun lateral to the midline, at the level of the first posterior sacral foramen
Pangguangshu BL-28
1.5 cun lateral to the midline, at the level of the second posterior sacral foramen
Baohuang BL-53
3 cun lateral to the midline, at the level of the sp of the second sacral vertebra
Ciliao BL-32
over the second posterior sacral foramen
Baihuanshu BL-30
1.5 cun lateral to the midline, at the level of the fourth posterior sacral foramen
Zhibian BL-54
3 cun lateral to the hiatus of the sacrum
Huantiao GB-30
one third of the distance between the highest point of the trochanter and the hiatus of the sacrum
Zhonglushu BL-29
1.5 cun lateral to the midline, at the level of the third posterior sacral foramen
Yaoshu DU-2
in the hiatus of the sacrum
Huiyang BL-35
0.5 cun lateral to the Governing vessel, level with the tip of the coccyx

POINTS OF THE BACK (GOVERNING VESSEL AND BLADDER CHANNEL)

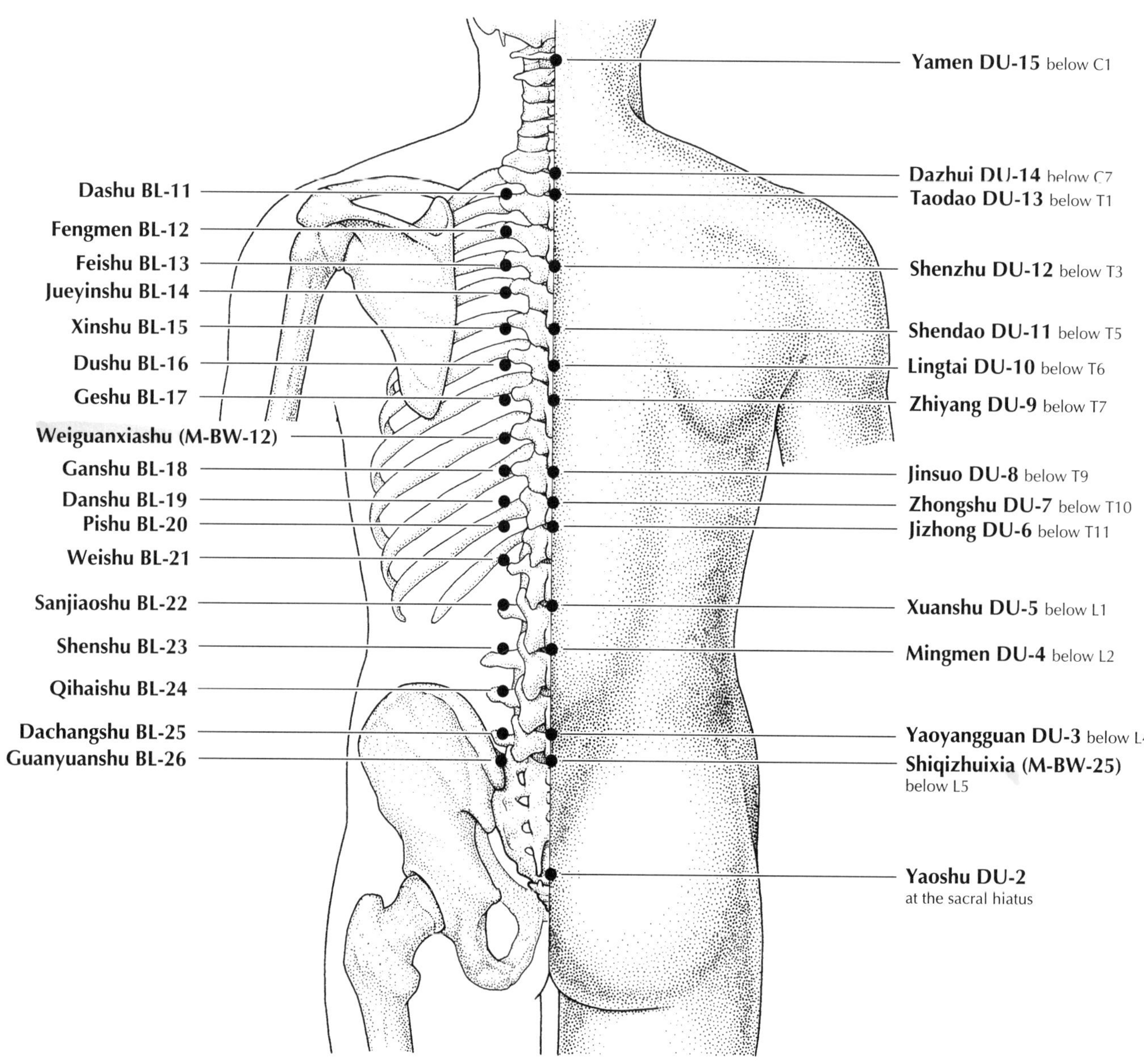
Yamen DU-15 below C1
Dazhui DU-14 below C7
Taodao DU-13 below T1
Shenzhu DU-12 below T3
Shendao DU-11 below T5
Lingtai DU-10 below T6
Zhiyang DU-9 below T7
Jinsuo DU-8 below T9
Zhongshu DU-7 below T10
Jizhong DU-6 below T11
Xuanshu DU-5 below L1
Mingmen DU-4 below L2
Yaoyangguan DU-3 below L4
Shiqizhuixia (M-BW-25) below L5
Yaoshu DU-2 at the sacral hiatus
Dashu BL-11
Fengmen BL-12
Feishu BL-13
Jueyinshu BL-14
Xinshu BL-15
Dushu BL-16
Geshu BL-17
Weiguanxiashu (M-BW-12)
Ganshu BL-18
Danshu BL-19
Pishu BL-20
Weishu BL-21
Sanjiaoshu BL-22
Shenshu BL-23
Qihaishu BL-24
Dachangshu BL-25
Guanyuanshu BL-26

MAJOR POINTS OF THE ANTERIOR THIGH

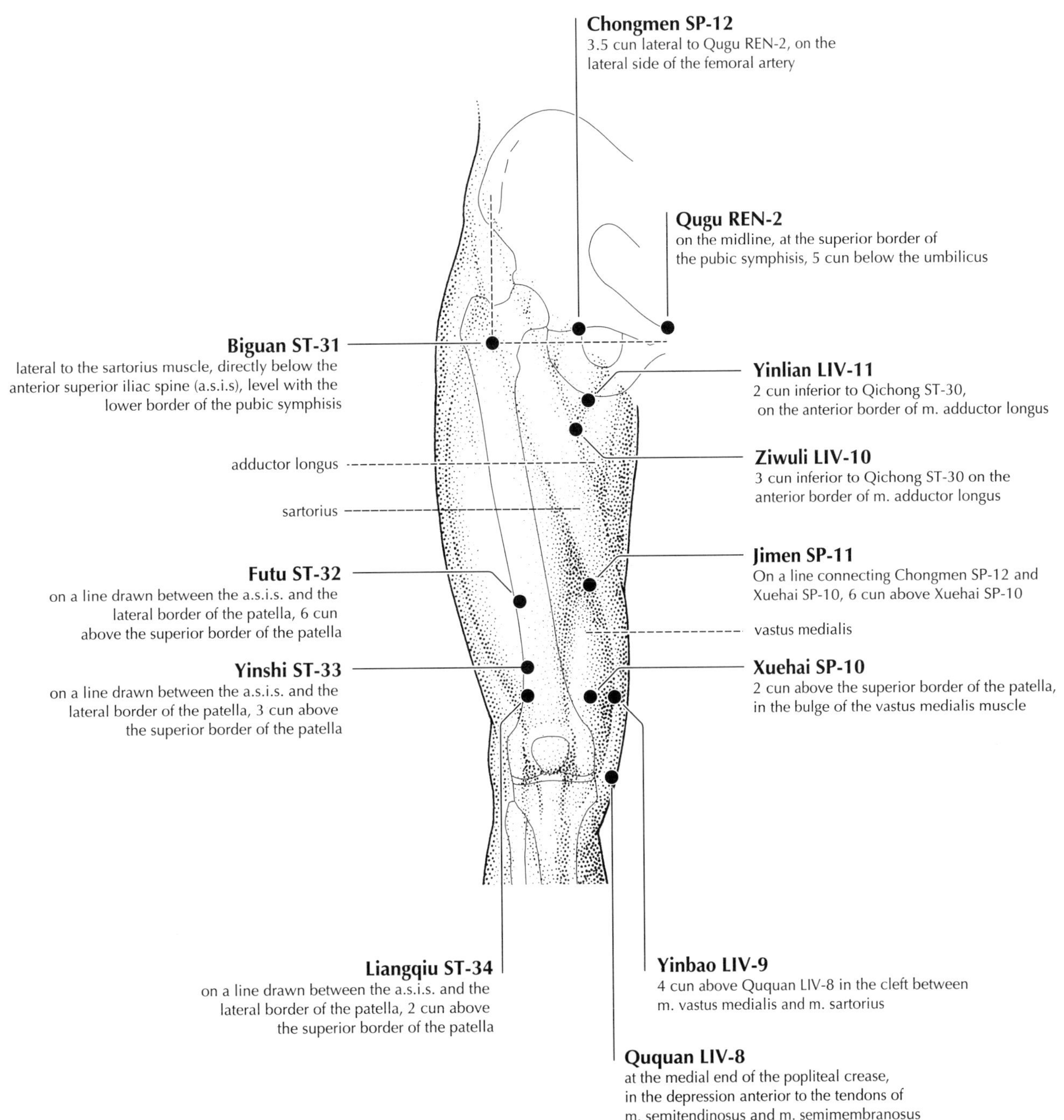
Chongmen SP-12
3.5 cun lateral to Qugu REN-2, on the lateral side of the femoral artery
Qugu REN-2
on the midline, at the superior border of the pubic symphisis, 5 cun below the umbilicus
Biguan ST-31
lateral to the sartorius muscle, directly below the anterior superior iliac spine (a.s.i.s), level with the lower border of the pubic symphisis
Yinlian LIV-11
2 cun inferior to Qichong ST-30, on the anterior border of m. adductor longus
adductor longus
Ziwuli LIV-10
3 cun inferior to Qichong ST-30 on the anterior border of m. adductor longus
sartorius
Futu ST-32
on a line drawn between the a.s.i.s. and the lateral border of the patella, 6 cun above the superior border of the patella
Jimen SP-11
On a line connecting Chongmen SP-12 and Xuehai SP-10, 6 cun above Xuehai SP-10
vastus medialis
Yinshi ST-33
on a line drawn between the a.s.i.s. and the lateral border of the patella, 3 cun above the superior border of the patella
Xuehai SP-10
2 cun above the superior border of the patella, in the bulge of the vastus medialis muscle
Liangqiu ST-34
on a line drawn between the a.s.i.s. and the lateral border of the patella, 2 cun above the superior border of the patella
Yinbao LIV-9
4 cun above Ququan LIV-8 in the cleft between m. vastus medialis and m. sartorius
Ququan LIV-8
at the medial end of the popliteal crease, in the depression anterior to the tendons of m. semitendinosus and m. semimembranosus

MAJOR POINTS OF THE ANTERIOR LOWER LEG

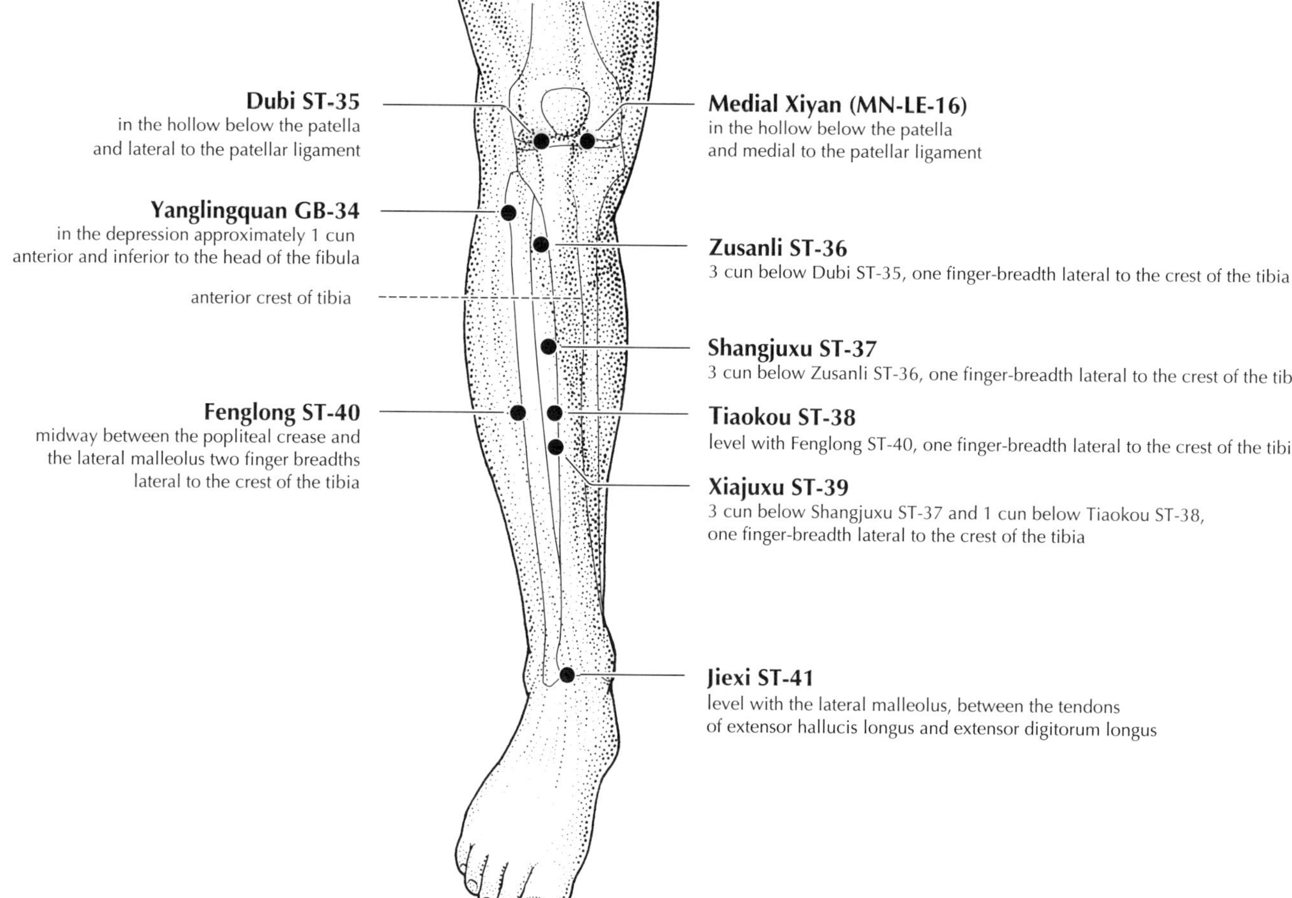
Dubi ST-35
in the hollow below the patella
and lateral to the patellar ligament
Yanglingquan GB-34
in the depression approximately 1 cun
anterior and inferior to the head of the fibula
anterior crest of tibia
Fenglong ST-40
midway between the popliteal crease and
the lateral malleolus two finger breadths
lateral to the crest of the tibia
Medial Xiyan (MN-LE-16)
in the hollow below the patella
and medial to the patellar ligament
Zusanli ST-36
3 cun below Dubi ST-35, one finger-breadth lateral to the crest of the tibia
Shangjuxu ST-37
3 cun below Zusanli ST-36, one finger-breadth lateral to the crest of the tibia
Tiaokou ST-38
level with Fenglong ST-40, one finger-breadth lateral to the crest of the tibia
Xiajuxu ST-39
3 cun below Shangjuxu ST-37 and 1 cun below Tiaokou ST-38,
one finger-breadth lateral to the crest of the tibia
Jiexi ST-41
level with the lateral malleolus, between the tendons
of extensor hallucis longus and extensor digitorum longus

MAJOR POINTS OF THE LATERAL LOWER LEG

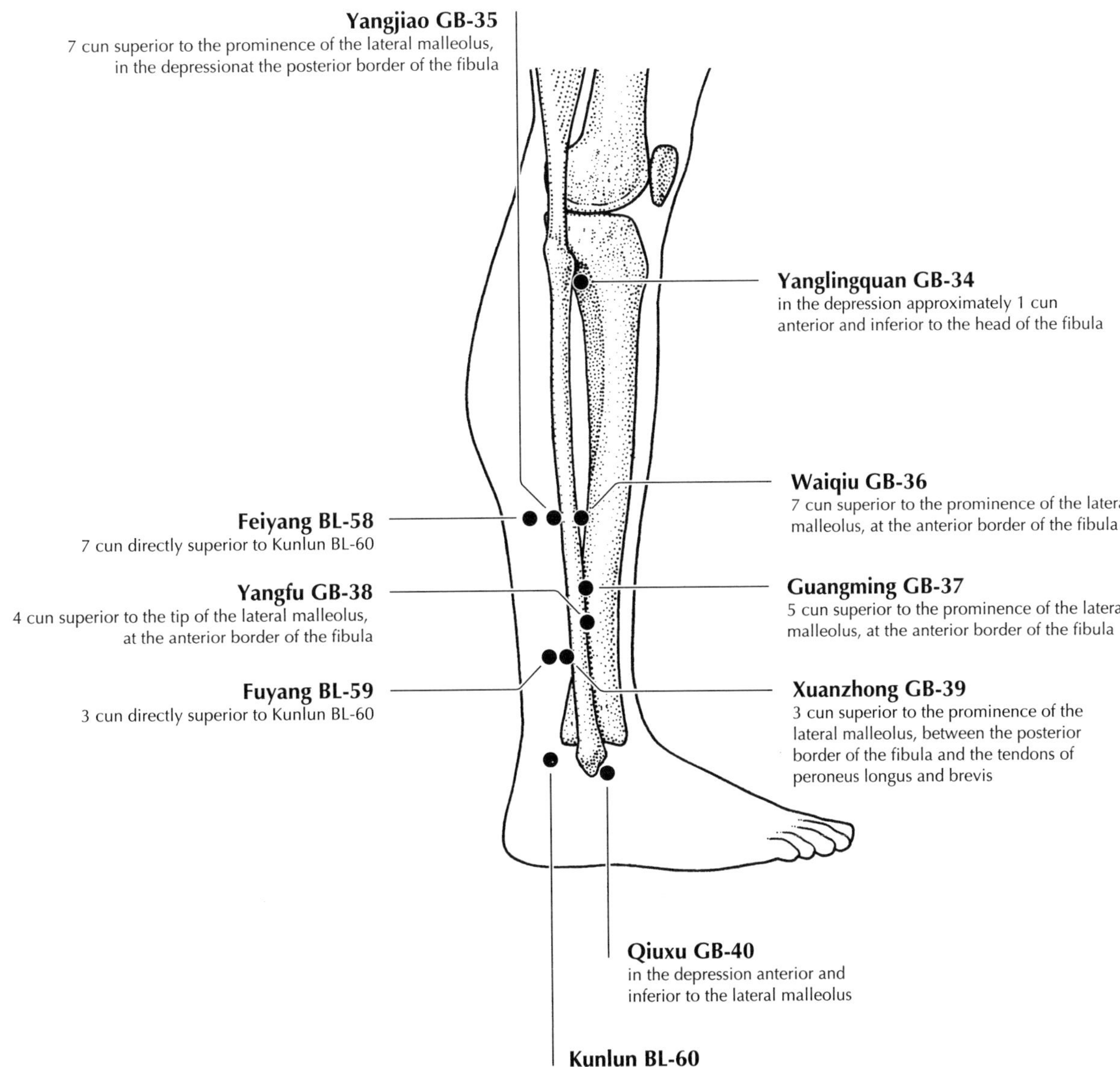
Yangjiao GB-35
7 cun superior to the prominence of the lateral malleolus, in the depressionat the posterior border of the fibula
Yanglingquan GB-34
in the depression approximately 1 cun anterior and inferior to the head of the fibula
Waiqiu GB-36
7 cun superior to the prominence of the lateral malleolus, at the anterior border of the fibula
Feiyang BL-58
7 cun directly superior to Kunlun BL-60
Guangming GB-37
5 cun superior to the prominence of the lateral malleolus, at the anterior border of the fibula
Yangfu GB-38
4 cun superior to the tip of the lateral malleolus, at the anterior border of the fibula
Xuanzhong GB-39
3 cun superior to the prominence of the lateral malleolus, between the posterior border of the fibula and the tendons of peroneus longus and brevis
Fuyang BL-59
3 cun directly superior to Kunlun BL-60
Qiuxu GB-40
in the depression anterior and inferior to the lateral malleolus
Kunlun BL-60
in the depression between the prominence of the lateral malleolus and the Achilles tendon

MAJOR POINTS OF THE MEDIAL LOWER LEG

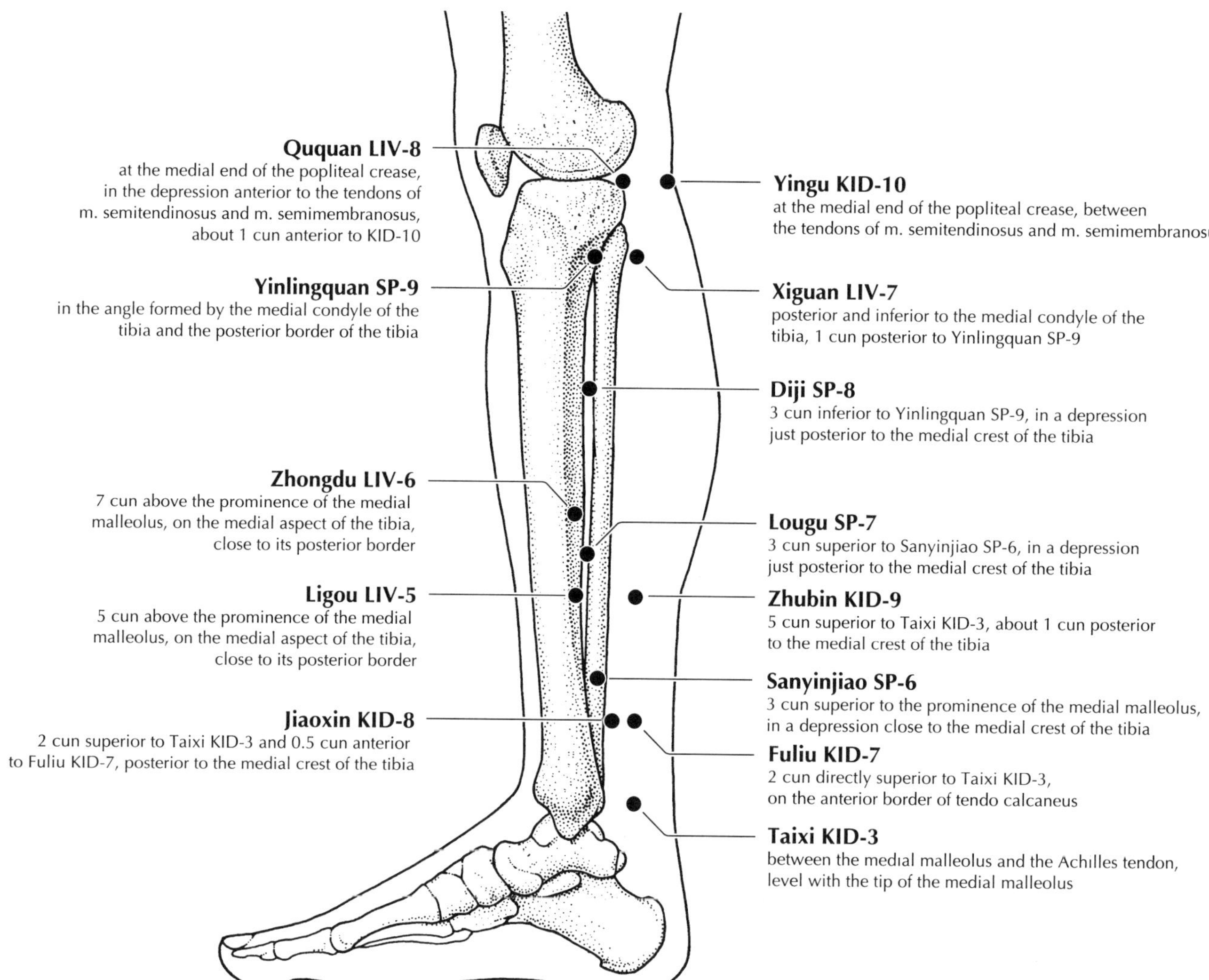
Ququan LIV-8
at the medial end of the popliteal crease, in the depression anterior to the tendons of m. semitendinosus and m. semimembranosus, about 1 cun anterior to KID-10
Yinlingquan SP-9
in the angle formed by the medial condyle of the tibia and the posterior border of the tibia
Zhongdu LIV-6
7 cun above the prominence of the medial malleolus, on the medial aspect of the tibia, close to its posterior border
Ligou LIV-5
5 cun above the prominence of the medial malleolus, on the medial aspect of the tibia, close to its posterior border
Jiaoxin KID-8
2 cun superior to Taixi KID-3 and 0.5 cun anterior to Fuliu KID-7, posterior to the medial crest of the tibia
Yingu KID-10
at the medial end of the popliteal crease, between the tendons of m. semitendinosus and m. semimembranosus
Xiguan LIV-7
posterior and inferior to the medial condyle of the tibia, 1 cun posterior to Yinlingquan SP-9
Diji SP-8
3 cun inferior to Yinlingquan SP-9, in a depression just posterior to the medial crest of the tibia
Lougu SP-7
3 cun superior to Sanyinjiao SP-6, in a depression just posterior to the medial crest of the tibia
Zhubin KID-9
5 cun superior to Taixi KID-3, about 1 cun posterior to the medial crest of the tibia
Sanyinjiao SP-6
3 cun superior to the prominence of the medial malleolus, in a depression close to the medial crest of the tibia
Fuliu KID-7
2 cun directly superior to Taixi KID-3, on the anterior border of tendo calcaneus
Taixi KID-3
between the medial malleolus and the Achilles tendon, level with the tip of the medial malleolus

MAJOR POINTS OF THE LATERAL FOOT

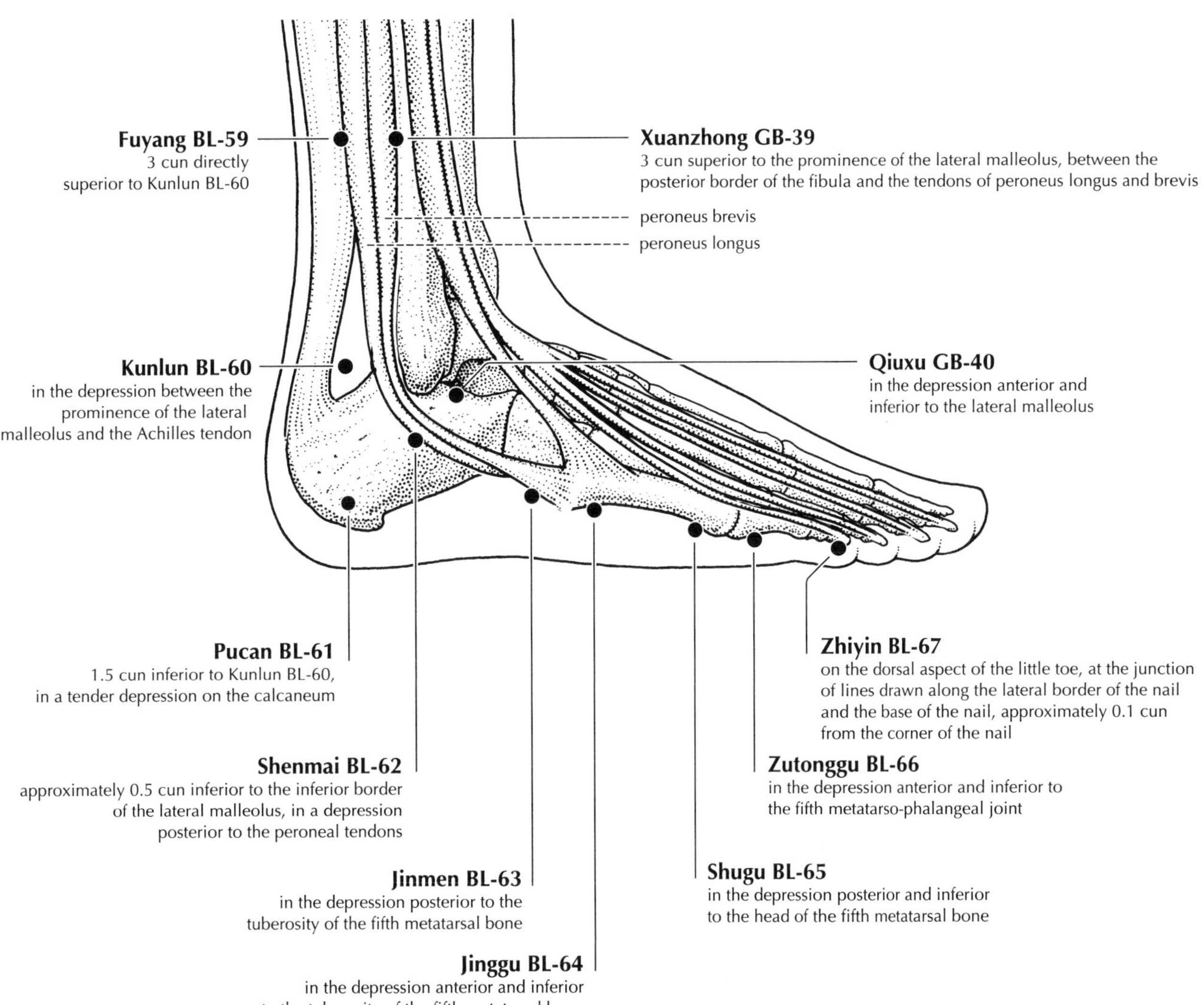
Fuyang BL-59
3 cun directly superior to Kunlun BL-60
Xuanzhong GB-39
3 cun superior to the prominence of the lateral malleolus, between the posterior border of the fibula and the tendons of peroneus longus and brevis
peroneus brevis
peroneus longus
Kunlun BL-60
in the depression between the prominence of the lateral malleolus and the Achilles tendon
Qiuxu GB-40
in the depression anterior and inferior to the lateral malleolus
Pucan BL-61
1.5 cun inferior to Kunlun BL-60, in a tender depression on the calcaneum
Zhiyin BL-67
on the dorsal aspect of the little toe, at the junction of lines drawn along the lateral border of the nail and the base of the nail, approximately 0.1 cun from the corner of the nail
Shenmai BL-62
approximately 0.5 cun inferior to the inferior border of the lateral malleolus, in a depression posterior to the peroneal tendons
Zutonggu BL-66
in the depression anterior and inferior to the fifth metatarso-phalangeal joint
Jinmen BL-63
in the depression posterior to the tuberosity of the fifth metatarsal bone
Shugu BL-65
in the depression posterior and inferior to the head of the fifth metatarsal bone
Jinggu BL-64
in the depression anterior and inferior to the tuberosity of the fifth metatarsal bone

MAJOR POINTS OF THE MEDIAL FOOT

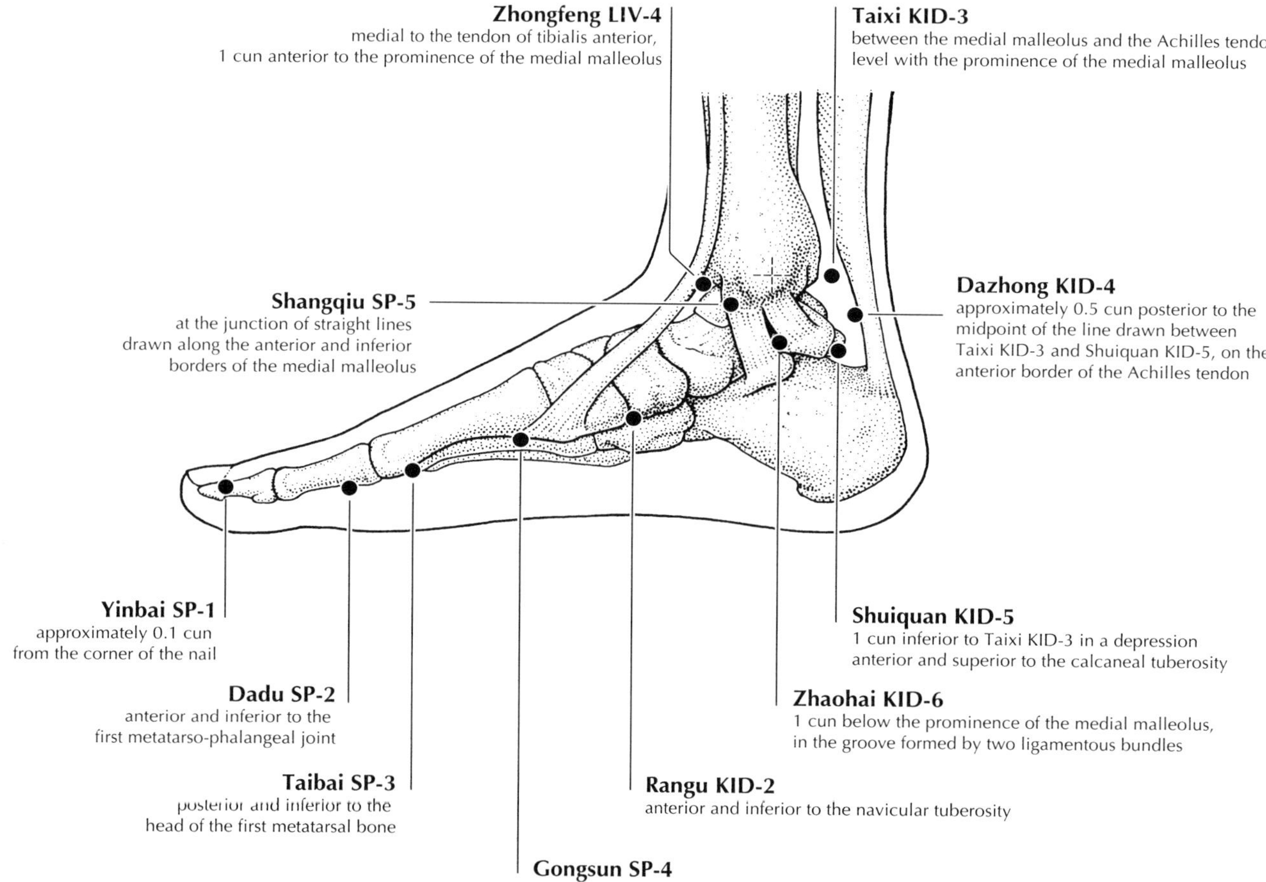
Zhongfeng LIV-4
medial to the tendon of tibialis anterior,
1 cun anterior to the prominence of the medial malleolus
Taixi KID-3
between the medial malleolus and the Achilles tendon,
level with the prominence of the medial malleolus
Shangqiu SP-5
at the junction of straight lines
drawn along the anterior and inferior
borders of the medial malleolus
Dazhong KID-4
approximately 0.5 cun posterior to the
midpoint of the line drawn between
Taixi KID-3 and Shuiquan KID-5, on the
anterior border of the Achilles tendon
Yinbai SP-1
approximately 0.1 cun
from the corner of the nail
Shuiquan KID-5
1 cun inferior to Taixi KID-3 in a depression
anterior and superior to the calcaneal tuberosity
Dadu SP-2
anterior and inferior to the
first metatarso-phalangeal joint
Zhaohai KID-6
1 cun below the prominence of the medial malleolus,
in the groove formed by two ligamentous bundles
Taibai SP-3
posterior and inferior to the
head of the first metatarsal bone
Rangu KID-2
anterior and inferior to the navicular tuberosity
Gongsun SP-4
anterior and inferior to the base of the first metatarsal bone

MAJOR POINTS OF THE TOP OF THE FOOT

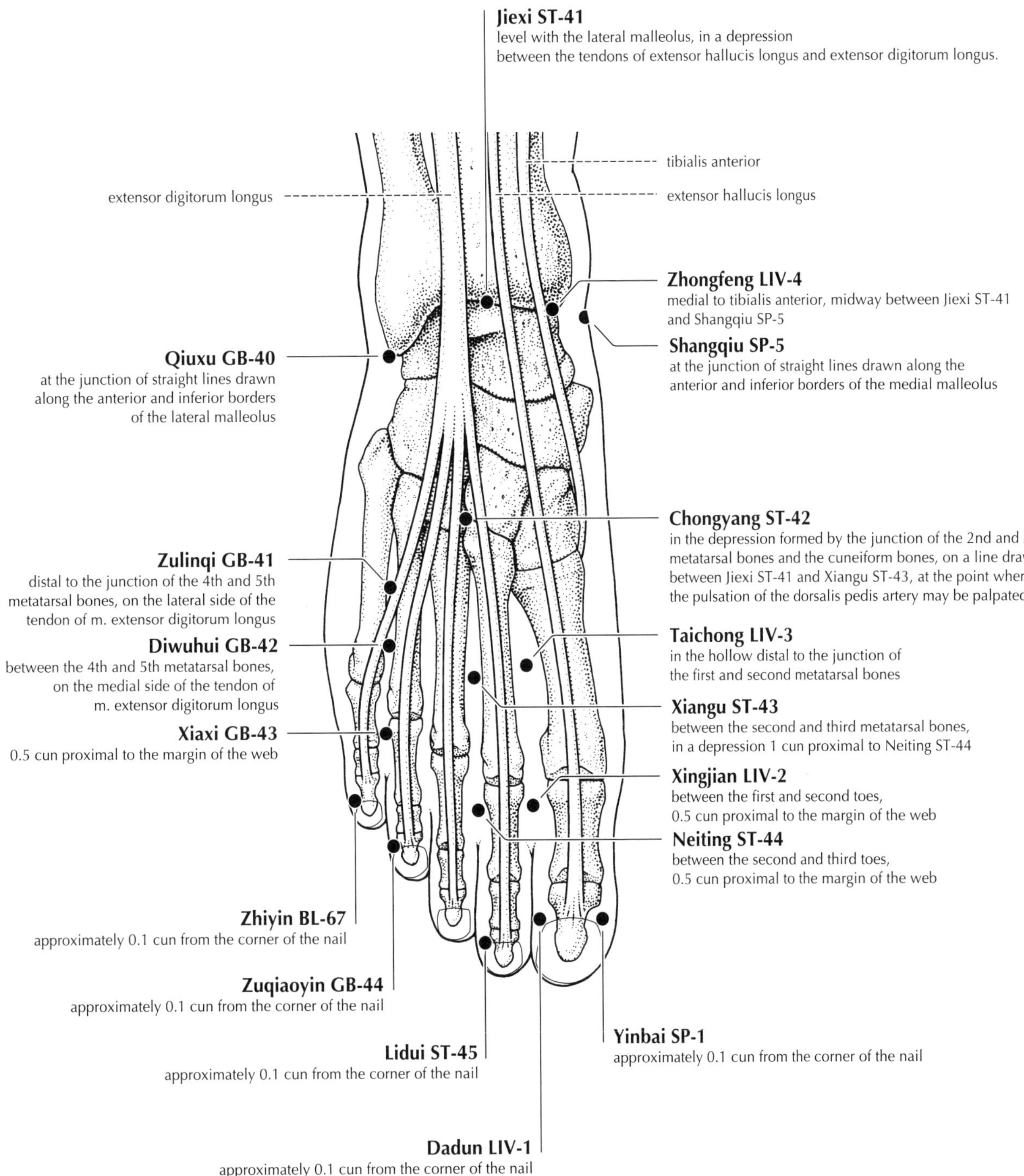
Jiexi ST-41
level with the lateral malleolus, in a depression
between the tendons of extensor hallucis longus and extensor digitorum longus.
tibialis anterior
extensor digitorum longus
extensor hallucis longus
Zhongfeng LIV-4
medial to tibialis anterior, midway between Jiexi ST-41
and Shangqiu SP-5
Shangqiu SP-5
at the junction of straight lines drawn along the
anterior and inferior borders of the medial malleolus
Qiuxu GB-40
at the junction of straight lines drawn
along the anterior and inferior borders
of the lateral malleolus
Chongyang ST-42
in the depression formed by the junction of the 2nd and 3rd
metatarsal bones and the cuneiform bones, on a line drawn
between Jiexi ST-41 and Xiangu ST-43, at the point where
the pulsation of the dorsalis pedis artery may be palpated
Zulinqi GB-41
distal to the junction of the 4th and 5th
metatarsal bones, on the lateral side of the
tendon of m. extensor digitorum longus
Diwuhui GB-42
between the 4th and 5th metatarsal bones,
on the medial side of the tendon of
m. extensor digitorum longus
Taichong LIV-3
in the hollow distal to the junction of
the first and second metatarsal bones
Xiangu ST-43
between the second and third metatarsal bones,
in a depression 1 cun proximal to Neiting ST-44
Xiaxi GB-43
0.5 cun proximal to the margin of the web
Xingjian LIV-2
between the first and second toes,
0.5 cun proximal to the margin of the web
Neiting ST-44
between the second and third toes,
0.5 cun proximal to the margin of the web
Zhiyin BL-67
approximately 0.1 cun from the corner of the nail
Zuqiaoyin GB-44
approximately 0.1 cun from the corner of the nail
Yinbai SP-1
approximately 0.1 cun from the corner of the nail
Lidui ST-45
approximately 0.1 cun from the corner of the nail
Dadun LIV-1
approximately 0.1 cun from the corner of the nail

REGIONS OF THE BODY REACHED BY THE CHANNELS

Anus
- The Bladder divergent channel.
- The Governing vessel.

Axilla
- The Lung divergent channel.
- The Lung sinew channel enters the chest below the axilla.
- The Heart primary channel emerges from the axilla.
- The Heart sinew channel binds at the axilla.
- The Heart divergent channel
- The Small Intestine divergent channel.
- The Small Intestine sinew channel binds at the axilla.
- The Bladder sinew channel crosses beneath the axilla.
- The Pericardium primary channel arches over the axilla.
- The Pericardium sinew channel binds below the axilla.
- The Gall Bladder primary channel descends to the anterior aspect of the axilla.
- The Gall Bladder sinew channel travels anteriorly to the axilla.
- The Yang Motility vessel passes the posterior axillary fold.

Bladder
- The Bladder primary channel.
- The Bladder divergent channel.
- The Kidney primary channel.

Brain
- The Bladder primary channel.
- The Governing vessel.
- The Yin Motility vessel.
- The Yang Motility vessel.

Breast
- The Large Intestine divergent channel.
- The Stomach primary channel descends along the mamillary line.
- The Heart sinew channel travels medially across the breast region.
- The Sanjiao primary channel disperses midway between the breasts at Shanzhong REN-17
- The Gall Bladder sinew channel.

Buttock
- The Bladder primary channel crosses the buttock to join with Huantiao GB-30
- The Bladder sinew channel binds at the buttock.
- The Gall Bladder primary channel emerges on the buttock at Huantiao GB-30

Cheek
- The Large Intestine primary channel.
- The Large Intestine luo-connecting channel.
- The Large Intestine sinew channel.
- The Stomach primary channel.
- The Heart primary channel.
- The Small Intestine primary channel.
- The Bladder sinew channel binds at the cheek bone.
- The Sanjiao primary channel.
- The Gall Bladder divergent channel.
- The Gall Bladder sinew channel.
- The Liver primary channel.
- The Yang Motility vessel.

Chest
- The Lung divergent channel passes anterior to the Heart channel in the chest.
- The Lung sinew channel enters the chest below the axilla, emerges from the supraclavicular fossa and subsequently descends into the chest again.
- The Spleen great luo-connecting channel spreads through the chest and lateral costal region.
- The Spleen sinew channel spreads in the chest, and from inside the chest a branch attaches to the spine.
- The Heart divergent channel enters the chest and connects with the Heart.
- The Heart sinew channel goes to the centre of the chest.
- The Pericardium primary channel originates in the centre of the chest.
- The Sanjiao luo-connecting channel converges with Pericardium channel in the chest.

Disperse in the chest
- The Kidney primary channel.
- The Pericardium sinew channel.
- The Sanjiao divergent channel.
- The Penetrating vessel.

Ascend the chest
- The Stomach sinew channel.
- The Bladder sinew channel.
- The Conception vessel.
- The Yin Motility vessel.

Descend into the chest
- The Large Intestine divergent channel.
- The Gall Bladder primary channel.

Diaphragm
- The Lung sinew channel spreads over the diaphragm.
- The Pericardium sinew channel binds at the diaphragm.

All the following channels traverse the diaphragm
- The Lung primary channel.
- Large Intestine primary channel.
- The Stomach primary channel.
- The Spleen primary channel.
- The Heart primary channel.
- The Heart sinew channel.
- The Small Intestine primary channel.
- The Kidney primary channel.
- The Pericardium primary channel.
- The Sanjiao primary channel.
- The Gall Bladder primary channel.
- The Liver primary channel.

Ear

- The Large Intestine luo-connecting channel enters the ear to join the 'zong mai' (where the channels of the Large Intestine, Stomach, Small Intestine, Gall Bladder and Sanjiao gather).
- The Stomach primary channel ascends anterior to the ear.
- The Stomach sinew channel binds in front of the ear.
- The Small Intestine primary channel enters ear at Tinggong SI-19.
- The Small Intestine sinew channel separates behind the ear, enters the ear, emerges above the ear and passes anterior to the ear.
- The Bladder sinew channel binds behind the ear.
- The Pericardium divergent channel emerges behind the ear.
- The Sanjiao primary channel ascends to the posterior aspect of the ear and circles behind the ear, and a branch separates behind the ear and enters the ear and emerges in front of the ear.
- The Sanjiao sinew channel ascends anterior to the ear.
- The Gall Bladder primary channel passes behind the ear, emerges behind the ear and enters the ear at Yifeng SJ-17 to surface in front of the ear (intersecting the Small Intestine channel at Tinggong SI-19 and the Stomach channel at Xiaguan ST-7).
- The Gall Bladder sinew channel.
- The Yang Linking vessel.

Elbow

- The Lung primary channel goes to the cubital fossa.
- The Lung sinew channel binds at the centre of the elbow.
- The Large Intestine primary channel goes to the lateral aspect of the elbow at Quchi L.I.-11.
- The Large Intestine sinew channel binds at the lateral aspect of the elbow.
- The Heart primary channel goes to the elbow.
- The Heart sinew channel binds at the medial aspect of the elbow.
- The Small Intestine primary channel goes to the medial aspect of the elbow.
- The Small Intestine sinew channel binds at the medial condyle of the humerus.
- The Pericardium primary channel goes to the cubital fossa of the elbow.
- The Pericardium sinew channel binds at the medial side of the elbow.
- The Sanjiao primary channel.
- The sanjiao luo-connecting channel.
- The Sanjiao sinew channel binds at the tip of the elbow.

Eye

- The Stomach primary channel ascends to the medial canthus and descends laterally along the infraorbital ridge.
- The Stomach divergent channel connects with the eye.
- The Stomach sinew channel joins with the Bladder sinew channel to form a muscular net around the eye (the Bladder sinew channel forms the 'upper net' of the eye and the Stomach sinew channel forms the 'lower net' of the eye).
- The Heart primary channel connects with the tissues surrounding the eye.
- The Heart luo-connecting channel goes to the eye.
- The Heart divergent channel connects with the Small Intestine channel at the inner canthus.
- The Small Intestine primary channel goes to the inner and outer canthus.
- The Small Intestine sinew channel connects at the outer canthus.
- The Bladder primary channel originates at the inner canthus.
- The Bladder sinew channel circles the eye.
- The Sanjiao primary channel ascends to the inferior aspect of the eye.
- The Sanjiao primary channel terminates at the outer canthus of the eye at Sizhukong SJ-23.
- The Sanjiao sinew channel goes to the outer canthus.
- The Gall Bladder primary channel originates at the outer canthus of the eye, a branch terminates behind the outer canthus and a branch rises to the infraorbital region.
- The Gall Bladder divergent channel connects with the eye.
- The Gall Bladder sinew channel binds at the outer canthus.
- The Liver primary channel links with the tissues surrounding the eye.
- The Governing vessel ascends to below the middle of the eye and emerges at Jingming BL-1.
- The Conception vessel terminates below the eye at Chengqi ST-1.
- The Yang Motility vessel passes to the inner canthus and communicates with the Yin Motility vessel and the Bladder channel at Jingming BL-1.
- The Yin Motility vessel meets Yang Motility vessel and the Bladder channel at the inner canthus at Jingming BL-1.

Face

- The Heart primary channel.
- The Heart divergent channel emerges on the face.
- The Gall Bladder divergent channel disperses in the face.

Finger

- The Lung primary branch travels to the index finger.
- The Large Intestine primary originates at the index finger.
- The Large Intestine sinew channel originates at the index finger.
- The Heart primary channel originates at the little finger.
- The Heart sinew channel originates at the little finger.
- The Small Intestine primary channel originates at the little finger.
- The Small Intestine sinew channel originates at the dorsum of the little finger.
- The Pericardium primary channel travels from the palm along the middle finger to terminate at its tip at Zhongchong P-9.
- A branch of the Pericardium primary channel arises from the palm at Laogong P-8 and follows the radial aspect of the ring finger to its tip at Guanchong SJ-1.
- The Pericardium sinew channel originates at the tip of the middle finger.
- The Sanjiao primary channel originates at the ulnar aspect of the tip of the fourth finger.
- The Sanjiao sinew channel originates at the ulnar aspect of the tip of the fourth finger.

Foot
- The Stomach primary channel separates on the dorsum of the foot at Chongyang ST-42 and travels to Yinbai SP-1.
- The Stomach sinew channel binds on the dorsum of the foot.
- The Spleen primary channel runs along the medial aspect of the foot.
- The Spleen sinew channel ascends the foot.
- The Kidney primary channel crosses the sole of the foot to Yongquan KID-1.
- The Gall Bladder luo-connecting channel descends and disperses over the dorsum of the foot.
- The Gall Bladder primary channel follows the dorsal surface of the foot.
- The Liver primary channel runs along the foot.
- The Liver divergent channel separates from the primary channel on the dorsum of the foot.
- The Penetrating vessel terminates on the sole of the foot

Forehead
- The Large Intestine sinew channel crosses the temple to the corner of the forehead.
- The Bladder primary channel ascends along the forehead.
- The Small Intestine sinew channel.
- The Sanjiao sinew channel binds at the corner of the forehead.
- The Gall Bladder primary channel ascends to the corner of the forehead.
- The Liver primary channel ascends across the forehead to the vertex where it intersects with the Governing vessel at Baihui DU-20.
- A branch of the Governing vessel follows the Bladder channel bilaterally along the forehead.
- The Yang Motility vessel ascends to the forehead.
- The Yang Linking vessel ascends to the forehead at Benshen GB-13.

Gall bladder
- The Gall Bladder primary channel.
- The Gall Bladder divergent channel.
- The Liver primary channel.

Genitals
- The Stomach sinew channel binds in the pelvic region above the genitals.
- The Spleen sinew channel converges at the external genitalia.
- The Kidney sinew channel binds at the genitals.
- The Gall Bladder primary channel encircles the genitals and runs superficially along the margin of the pubic hair.
- The Liver primary channel encircles the genitals.
- The Liver sinew channel connects with the other sinew channels at the genitals.
- The Liver luo-connecting channel ascends to the genitals.
- The Governing vessel winds around the external genitalia.
- The Yin Motility vessel ascends to the external genitalia.

Gums (see Teeth and Gums)

Heart
- Stomach divergent channel.
- The Spleen primary channel.
- The Heart primary channel originates in the Heart and emerges from the system of blood vessels surrounding the Heart.
- The Heart luo-connecting channel.
- The Heart divergent channel.
- The Small Intestine primary channel.
- The Small Intestine divergent channel.
- The Bladder divergent channel disperses in the cardiac region.
- The Kidney primary channel.
- The Pericardium luo-connecting channel.
- The Gall Bladder divergent channel.
- A branch of the Governing vessel.

Heel
- The Bladder sinew channel binds at the heel.
- The Kidney luo-connecting channel encircles the heel.
- The Kidney primary channel enters the heel.
- The Kidney divergent channel binds at the heel.
- The Kidney sinew channel binds at the heel.
- A branch of the Penetrating vessel branch passes to the heel.
- The Yang Motility vessel originates at the heel at Shenmai BL-62.
- The Yang Linking vessel originates near the heel at Jinmen BL-63.

Hip
- Stomach sinew channel ascends to bind at the hip joint.
- The Spleen sinew channel binds in the anterior region of the hip.
- The Gall Bladder primary channel enters deeply in the hip at Huantiao GB-30.
- The Gall Bladder divergent channel crosses over the hip joint.
- The Yang Motility vessel ascends to the hip at Juliao GB-29.
- The Yang Linking vessel passes through the hip region.

Intestines
- The Spleen luo-connecting channel connects with the intestines.

Large Intestine
- The Lung primary channel.
- The Lung divergent channel.
- The Large Intestine primary channel.
- The Large Intestine divergent channel.

Small Intestine
- The Heart primary channel.
- The Small Intestine primary channel.
- The Small Intestine divergent channel.

Jaw
- The Large Intestine luo-connecting channel.
- The Stomach primary channel.
- The Stomach sinew channel.
- The Small Intestine sinew channel.

Jaw (continued)
- The Sanjiao sinew channel.
- The Gall Bladder primary channel.
- The Gall Bladder divergent channel.
- The Conception vessel.
- The Yang Linking vessel.

Kidneys
- The Bladder primary channel.
- The Bladder divergent channel.
- The Kidney primary channel.
- The Kidney divergent channel.
- The Governing vessel.

Knee
Lateral aspect
- The Stomach sinew channel.
- The Bladder sinew channel.
- The Gall Bladder primary channel.
- The Gall Bladder sinew channel.

Medial aspect
- The Spleen primary channel.
- The Spleen sinew channel.
- The Kidney sinew channel.
- The Liver primary channel.
- The Liver sinew channel.

Anterior aspect
- The Stomach primary channel.

Posterior aspect (popliteal fossa)
- The Bladder primary channel.
- The Bladder divergent channel diverges from the primary channel in the popliteal fossa.
- A branch of the Bladder sinew channel ascends to the lateral aspect of the popliteal fossa.
- A branch of the Bladder sinew channel ascends to the medial aspect of the popliteal fossa.
- The Kidney primary channel passes through the medial side of the popliteal fossa.
- The Kidney divergent channel separates from the Kidney primary channel in the popliteal fossa.
- A branch of the Penetrating vessel.

Lips
- The Large Intestine primary channel curves around the upper lip.
- The Stomach primary channel circles around the lips.
- The Liver primary channel encircles the inner surface of the lips.
- The Governing vessel descends to the philtrum and terminates at the junction of the upper lip and the gum.
- The Penetrating vessel curves around the lips.

Liver
- The Kidney primary channel.
- The Gall Bladder primary channel.
- The Gall Bladder divergent channel.
- The Liver primary channel.

Lung
- The Lung primary channel.
- The Lung divergent channel.
- The Large Intestine primary channel.
- The Large Intestine divergent channel.
- The Heart primary channel.
- The Kidney primary channel.
- The Liver primary channel.

Mastoid
- The Small Intestine sinew channel.
- The Bladder sinew channel.
- The Gall Bladder primary channel.

Mouth
- The Stomach divergent channel emerges at the mouth.
- The Stomach sinew channel ascends to the mouth.

Wind around the mouth
- The Governing vessel.
- The Conception vessel.

Pass the corner of the mouth
- The Large Intestine primary channel.
- The Stomach primary channel.
- The Yin Motility vessel.
- The Yang Motility vessel.

Neck
- The Large Intestine primary channel.
- The Large Intestine sinew channel.
- The Stomach luo-connecting channel.
- The Small Intestine primary channel.
- The Stomach sinew channel.
- The Small Intestine sinew channel.
- The Bladder primary channel splits into two branches at the nape.
- The Bladder divergent channel.
- The Bladder sinew channel.
- The Kidney divergent channel.
- The Kidney sinew channel.
- The Sanjiao primary channel.
- The Sanjiao sinew channel joins the Small Intestine sinew channel at the neck.
- The Gall Bladder primary channel.
- The Liver primary channel.
- The Governing luo-connecting channel ascends bilaterally along the sides of the spine to the nape of the neck.
- The Governing vessel ascends along the interior of the spinal column to Fengfu DU-16 at the nape.
- The Yang Motility vessel.
- The Yang Linking vessel.

Nose
- The Stomach primary channel begins beside the nose at Yingxiang L.I.-20 and ascends to the root of the nose.
- The Stomach sinew channel binds below the nose.
- The Bladder sinew channel binds at the bridge of the nose.
- The Liver primary channel ascends to the nasopharynx.
- The Governing vessel descends along the midline of the head to the bridge of the nose.

Lateral aspect of the nose
- The Large Intestine primary channel.
- The Large Intestine sinew channel.
- The Stomach divergent channel.
- The Small Intestine primary channel.
- The Bladder sinew channel.
- The Gall Bladder sinew channel.
- The Yang Motility vessel.
- The Yin Motility vessel.

Occiput
- The Bladder sinew channel binds at the occipital bone.
- The Kidney sinew channel binds at the occipital bone.
- The Gall Bladder primary channel.
- The Governing luo-connecting channel spreads over the occiput.

Oesophagus
- The Stomach divergent channel.
- The Spleen primary channel.
- The Heart primary channel.
- The Small Intestine primary channel.
- The Gall Bladder divergent channel.

Palm
- The Lung luo-connecting channel follows the Lung channel into the palm and spreads through the thenar eminence.
- The Lung sinew channel binds at the thenar eminence.
- The Heart primary channel travels through the palm.
- The Pericardium primary channel travels through the palm.
- A branch of the Pericardium primary channel arises from the palm at Laogong P-8.

Parietal region
- The Gall Bladder primary channel.
- The Yang Motility vessel.

Pericardium
- The Kidney luo-connecting channel ascends to (a point below) the Pericardium.
- The Pericardium primary channel.
- The Pericardium luo-connecting channel.
- The Sanjiao primary channel.
- The Sanjiao luo-connecting channel.

Perineum
- The Governing vessel.
- The Conception vessel.
- The Penetrating vessel.

Ribs
- The Lung primary channel emerges at Zhongfu LU-1.
- The Lung sinew channel converges in the region of the floating ribs.
- The Stomach sinew channel passes through the lower ribs.
- The Spleen primary channel passes through the lateral ribs.
- The Spleen sinew channel binds at the ribs.
- The Pericardium primary channel emerges in the costal region three cun inferior to the anterior axillary fold.
- The Pericardium sinew channel disperses over the anterior and posterior aspects of the ribs.
- The Gall Bladder primary channel descends along the inside of the ribs.
- The Gall Bladder divergent channel crosses between the lower ribs.
- The Gall Bladder sinew channel ascends across the ribs.
- The Liver primary channel spreads in the costal and hypochondriac region.
- The Girdling vessel originates in the region of Zhangmen LIV-13.
- The Yang Motility vessel passes through the postero-lateral costal region.
- The Yin Linking vessel ascends the ribs to Qimen LIV-14.

Sacrum
- The Bladder primary channel.
- The Kidney primary channel.
- The Gall Bladder primary channel.
- The Gall Bladder sinew channel.
- The Governing vessel.

Shoulder
- The Lung primary channel emerges at Zhongfu LU-1.
- The Lung sinew channel travels laterally to the shoulder, anterior to Jianyu L.I.-15.
- The Large Intestine sinew channel.
- The Small Intestine primary channel ascends to the posterior aspect of the shoulder joint.
- The Small Intestine divergent channel.
- The Sanjiao primary channel ascends to the shoulder at Jianliao SJ-14.
- The Sanjiao luo-connecting channel.
- The Sanjiao sinew channel.
- The Gall Bladder primary channel.
- The Yang Linking vessel.
- The Yang Motility vessel zig-zags across the top of the shoulder.

Meet at Jianyu L.I.-15
- The Large Intestine primary channel.
- The Large Intestine divergent channel.
- The Small Intestine luo-connecting channel.
- The Bladder sinew channel.

Spine
- The six yang channels meet with the Governing vessel at Dazhui DU-14.
- The Large Intestine divergent channel.
- The Large Intestine sinew channel attaches to the upper thoracic spine.
- The Stomach sinew channel.
- The Spleen sinew channel.
- The Bladder primary channel descends alongside the spine.
- The Bladder divergent channel ascends along the spine.
- The Bladder sinew channel ascends laterally along the spine to the nape of the neck.
- The Kidney primary channel threads through the spine.
- The Kidney luo-connecting channel spreads into the lumbar vertebrae.

Spine (continued)

- The Kidney sinew channel travels internally to the spinal vertebrae and ascends the inner aspect of the spine to the nape of the neck.
- The Gall Bladder primary channel.
- The Sanjiao primary channel.
- The Governing vessel ascends the interior of the spinal column.
- A branch of the Governing vessel descends either side of the spine to the Kidneys.
- The Governing luo-connecting channel ascends bilaterally alongside the spine, and subsequently threads through the spine at the level of the scapulae.
- The Conception vessel enters the spine and ascends along the back.
- A branch of the Penetrating vessel ascends inside the spinal column.

Spleen

- The Stomach primary channel.
- The Stomach divergent channel.
- The Spleen primary channel.

Stomach / middle jiao

- The Lung primary channel originates in the middle jiao (Stomach) and ascends past the cardiac orifice of the Stomach.
- The Stomach primary channel enters the Stomach.
- A branch of the Stomach primary channel originates from the pyloric orifice of the Stomach.
- The Stomach divergent channel.
- The Spleen primary channel.
- The Spleen luo-connecting channel.
- The Small Intestine primary channel.
- The Pericardium primary channel descends through the middle jiao.
- The Sanjiao primary channel descends through the middle jiao.
- The Sanjiao divergent channel descends through the middle jiao.
- The Liver primary channel curves round the Stomach.

Supraclavicular fossa

- The Lung divergent channel.
- The Lung sinew channel.
- The Large Intestine primary channel.
- The Large Intestine divergent channel.
- The Stomach primary channel.
- The Stomach sinew channel.
- The Small Intestine primary channel.
- The Bladder sinew channel.
- The Sanjiao primary channel.
- The Sanjiao divergent channel.
- The Gall Bladder primary channel.
- The Gall Bladder sinew channel.
- The Yin Motility vessel.

Teeth and gums

- The Large Intestine primary channel enters the gums of the lower teeth.
- The Large Intestine luo-connecting channel connects with the teeth.
- The Stomach primary channel descends to enter the upper gum.
- The Small Intestine sinew channel ascends across the teeth.
- The Governing vessel terminates at the junction of the upper lip and gum.

Temple

- The Large Intestine sinew channel crosses the temple to the corner of the forehead.
- The Stomach primary channel ascends within the hairline of the temporal region to Touwei ST-8.
- The Bladder primary channel descends to the temples, meeting the Gall Bladder channel at points Qubin GB-7 through to Xuanlu GB-5.
- The Sanjiao primary channel goes to temples, meeting the Gall Bladder channel at Xuanli GB-6 and Hanyan GB-4.
- The Sanjiao sinew channel.
- The Gall Bladder sinew channel descends from the temple.

Throat

- The Lung primary channel.
- The Lung divergent channel.
- The Large Intestine divergent channel.
- The Stomach primary channel.
- The Stomach luo-connecting channel.
- The Spleen divergent channel.
- The Heart divergent channel.
- The Kidney primary channel.
- The Pericardium divergent channel.
- The Liver primary channel ascends along the posterior aspect of the throat.
- The Governing vessel.
- The Conception vessel.
- The Penetrating vessel.
- The Yin Motility vessel.
- The Yin Linking vessel meets the Conception vessel at Tiantu REN-22 and Lianquan REN-23.

Toes

- A branch of the Stomach sinew channel originates at the middle three toes.

Big toe

- A branch of the Stomach primary channel.
- The Spleen primary channel.
- The Spleen sinew channel.
- A branch of the Gall Bladder primary channel.
- The Liver primary channel.
- The Liver sinew channel.
- A branch of the Penetrating vessel.

Second toe

- The Stomach primary channel.

Middle toe

- A branch of the Stomach primary channel.

Fourth toe

- The Gall Bladder primary channel.
- The Gall Bladder sinew channel originates at the fourth toe.

Little toe
- The Bladder primary channel.
- The Bladder sinew channel.
- The Kidney primary channel.
- The Kidney sinew channel.

Tongue
- The Spleen primary channel spreads over the lower surface of the tongue.
- The Spleen divergent channel penetrates the tongue.

Root of the tongue
- The Heart luo-connecting channel.
- The Bladder sinew channel.
- The Kidney primary channel.
- The Kidney divergent channel.
- The Sanjiao sinew channel.

Umbilicus
- The Spleen sinew channel.
- The Heart sinew channel.
- The Governing vessel.
- The Conception vessel.

Uterus
- The Conception vessel.
- The Penetrating vessel.

Vertex
- The Bladder primary channel.
- The Sanjiao divergent channel.
- The Gall Bladder sinew channel.
- The Liver primary channel.
- The Governing vessel.

CHINESE DYNASTIES

Xia Dynasty			21st - 16th c. BCE
Shang Dynasty			16th - 11th c. BCE
Zhou Dynasty	Western Zhou Dynasty		11th c. BCE - 771 BCE
	Eastern Zhou Dynasty		770 - 256 BCE
	Spring & Autumn period		770 - 476 BCE
	Warring States		475 - 221 BCE
Qin Dynasty			221 - 207 BCE
Han Dynasty	Western Han		206 BCE - 24 CE
	Eastern Han		25 - 220 CE
Three Kingdoms	Wei		220 - 265 CE
	Shu Han		221 - 263 CE
	Wu		222 - 280 CE
Western Jin Dynasty			265 - 316 CE
Eastern Jin Dynasty			317 - 420 CE
Northern and Southern Dynasties	Southern Dynasties	Song	420 -479 CE
		Qi	479 - 502 CE
		Liang	502 - 557 CE
		Chen	557 - 589 CE
	Northern Dynasties	Northern Wei	386 - 534 CE
		Eastern Wei	534 - 550 CE

Northern and Southern Dynasties	Northern Qi	550 - 577 CE
	Western Wei	535 - 556 CE
	Northern Zhou	557 - 581 CE
Sui Dynasty		581 - 618 CE
Tang Dynasty		618 - 907 CE
Five Dynasties	Later Liang	907 - 923 CE
	Later Tang	923 - 936 CE
	Later Jin	936 - 946 CE
	Later Han	947 - 950 CE
	Later Zhou	951 - 960 CE
Song Dynasty	Northern Song Dynasty	960 - 1127 CE
	Southern Song Dynasty	1127 - 1279 CE
Liao Dynasty		916 - 1125 CE
Jin Dynasty		1115 - 1234 CE
Yuan Dynasty		1271 - 1368 CE
Ming Dynasty		1368 - 1644 CE
Qing Dynasty		1644 - 1911 CE
Republic of China		1912 - 1949 CE
People's Republic of China		1949 CE

BIBLIOGRAPHY

ABBREVIATIONS

The bracketed abbreviations have been used for the following classical texts in the point combinations.

- Classic of Supplementing Life with Acupuncture and Moxibustion (*Supplementing Life*).
- Compilation of Acupuncture and Moxibustion (*Compilation*).
- Complete Collection of Acupuncture and Moxibustion (*Complete Collection*).
- Illustrated Classic of Acupuncture Points on the Bronze Man (*Bronze Man*).
- Illustrated Supplement to the Classic of Categories (*Illustrated Supplement*).
- Methods of Acupuncture and Moxibustion from the Golden Mirror of Medicine (*Golden Mirror*).
- Ode of One Hundred Symptoms (*One Hundred Symptoms*).
- Precious Mirror of Oriental Medicine (*Precious Mirror*).
- Principles of Divine Moxibustion (Divine Moxibustion).
- Song of Ma Dan Yang's Twelve Heavenly Star Points (*Heavenly Star Points*).
- Song of Points for Miscellaneous Diseases (*Miscellaneous Diseases*).
- Song of the Primary Points of the Fourteen Channels (*Song of Points*).
- The Classic of Categories (*Classic of Categories*).
- The Glorious Anthology of Acupuncture and Moxibustion (*Glorious Anthology*).
- The Great Compendium of Acupuncture and Moxibustion (*Great Compendium*).
- The Secrets of the Celestial Star (Celestial Star).
- The Systematic Classic of Acupuncture and Moxibustion (*Systematic Classic*).
- Thousand Ducat Formulas (*Thousand Ducats*).
- Yellow Emperors Inner Classic, Essential Questions (*Essential Questions*).
- Yellow Emperors Inner Classic, Spiritual Pivot (*Spiritual Pivot*).

SOURCE TEXTS

- *Achieving Longevity by Guarding the Source*
  (Shòu shì bǎo yuán)
  壽世保元
  Gong Ting Xian, 17 Century.
- *Book of Bian Que's Secrets*
  (Biǎn què xīn shū)
  扁鵲心書
  Dou Cai, Song, 1146.
- *Case Histories from the Guide to Clinical Patterns*
  (Lín zhèng zhǐ nán yī àn)
  臨証指南醫案
  Ye Gui, Qing, 1766.
- *Classic of the Jade Dragon (Bian Que`s Spiritual Guide to Acupuncture and Moxibustion, Jade Dragon Classic)*
  (Yù lóng jīng / Biǎn què shēn yīng zhēn jiǔ yù lóng jīng)
  玉龍經 (扁鵲神應針灸玉龍經)
  Wang Guo Rui, Yuan, 1329.
- *Compilation of Acupuncture and Moxibustion*
  (Zhēn jiǔ jí chéng)
  針灸集成
  Liao Run Hong, Qing, 1874.
- *Comprehensive Medicine According to Master Zhang*
  (Zhāng dī yī tōng)
  張氏醫通
  Zhang Lu Zhuan, Qing, 1695.
- *Confucians' Duties to Their Parents*
  (Rú mén shì qīn)
  儒門事親
  Zhang Cong Zheng, Jin-Tartar, 1228.
- *Correcting Errors in Medicine*
  (Yī lín gǎi cuò)
  醫林改錯
  Wang Qing Ren, Qing, 1830.
- *Discourse into the Origin and Development of Medicine*
  (Yī xué yuán liú lūn)
  醫學源流論
  Xu Da Cun, Qing, 1704.
- *Disease Mechanisms According to Master Sha*
  (Bìng jī shā zhuàn)
  病機沙篆
  Anon.
- *Essential Questions*
  (Sù wèn)
  素問
  See the *Yellow Emperor's Inner Classic.*
- *Essential Readings from the Medical Tradition*
  (Yī zōng bì dú)
  醫宗必讀
  Li Zhong Zi, Ming, 1637.
- *Essentials from the Golden Cabinet*
  (Jīn guì yào luè)
  金匱要略
  Zhang Zhong Jing, Eastern Han.
- *General Treatise on the Aetiology and Symptomatology of Disease*
  (Zhū bìng yuán hòu lùn)
  諸病源候論
  Chao Yuan Fang, Sui, 610.
- *Guide to the Classic of Acupuncture*
  (Zhēn jīng zhǐ nán)
  針經指南
  Dou Han Qing, Jin-Yuan, 1241.
- *Helpful Questions in Medical Cases*
  (Wèn zhāi yī àn)
  問齊醫案
  Anon.
- *Illustrated Classic of Acupuncture Points on the Bronze Man*
  (Tóng rén zhēn jiǔ shū xué tú jīng)
  銅人針灸俞穴圖經
  Wang Wei Yi, Song, 1026.

- *Illustrated Supplement to the Classic of Categories*
  (Lèi jīng tú yì)
  類經圖翼
  Zhang Jie Bin, Ming, 1624.
- *Introduction to Medicine*
  (Yī xué rù mén)
  醫學入門
  Li Yan, Ming, 1575.
- *Investigation into Points along the Channels*
  (Xún jīng kǎo xué biān)
  循經考穴編
  probably by Yan Zhen Shi, Ming, c. 1575.
- *Laws for Physicians*
  (Yī mén fǎ lù)
  醫門法律
  Yu Chang, Qing, 1658.
- *Medical Revelations*
  (Yī xué xīn wù)
  醫學心悟
  Cheng Guo Peng, Qing, 1732.
- *Meeting the Source of Acupuncture and Moxibustion*
  (Zhēn jiǔ féng yuán)
  針灸逢源
  Li Xue Chuan, Qing.
- *Method of Moxibustion at Gaohuangshu*
  (Gāo huāng shū jiǔ fǎ)
  膏肓俞灸法
  Zhuang Zhuo, Song, 1128.
- *Methods of Acupuncture and Moxibustion from the Golden Mirror of Medicine*
  (Yī zōng jīn jiàn cì jiǔ xīn fǎ)
  醫宗金鑑刺灸心法
  Wu Qian, Qing, 1742.
- *Ode of One Hundred Symtoms*
  (Bǎi zhèng fù)
  百症賦
  Gao Wu, Ming, 1529.
- *Ode of Spiritual Brightness*
  (Líng guāng fù)
  靈光賦
  First recorded in *The Complete Collection of Acupuncture and Moxibustion*, Xu Feng, Ming, c. 1439.
- *Ode of the Essentials of Understanding*
  (Tōng xuán zhǐ yào fù)
  通玄指要賦
  First recorded in *The Great Compendium of Acupuncture and Moxibustion*, Yang Ji Zhou, Ming, 1601.
- *Ode of the Golden Needle*
  (Jīn zhēn fù)
  金針賦
  First recorded in *The Complete Collection of Acupuncture and Moxibustion*, Xu Feng, Ming, c. 1439.
- *Ode of the Jade Dragon*
  (Yù lóng fù)
  玉龍賦
  First recorded in *The Glorious Anthology of Acupuncture and Moxibustion*, Gao Wu, Ming, 1529.
- *Ode of the Obstructed River*
  (Lán jiāng fù)
  攔江賦
  First recorded in *The Glorious Anthology of Acupuncture and Moxibustion*, Gao Wu, Ming, 1529.
- *Ode of Xi Hong*
  (Xí hóng fù)
  席弘賦
  First recorded in *The Complete Collection of Acupuncture and Moxibustion*, Xu Feng, Ming, c. 1439.
- *Ode to Elucidate Mysteries*
  (Biāo yōu fù)
  標幽賦
  First recorded in *The Guide to Acupuncture and Moxibustion*, Song, 241.
- *Outline of Medicine*
  (Yī xué gāng mù)
  醫學綱目
  Lou Ying, Ming, 1565.
- *Precious Mirror of Oriental Medicine*
  (Dōng yī bǎo jiàn)
  東醫寶鑑
  Xu Sun (Korean), 1611.
- *Principles of Divine Moxibustion*
  (Shén jiǔ jīng lùn)
  神灸經論
  Wu Yang Cheng, Qing.
- *Sagelike Prescriptions from the Taiping Era*
  (Tài píng shèng huì fāng)
  太平聖惠方
  Wang Huai Yin, Song, 987.
- *Secrets of a Frontier Official*
  (Wài tái mì yào)
  外台秘要
  Wang Tao, Tang, 752.
- *Secrets of the Master of Cinnabar Creek*
  (Dān xī xīn fǎ)
  丹溪心法
  Zhu Zhen Xiang, Yuan, 1347.
- *Song More Precious Than Jade*
  (Shèng yù gē)
  胜玉歌
  First recorded in *The Great Compendium of Acupuncture and Moxibustion*, Yang Ji Zhou, Ming, 1601.
- *Song of Ma Dan Yang's Twelve Heavenly Star Points*
  (Mǎ dān yáng tīan xīng shí èr xué gē)
  馬丹陽天星十二穴歌
  First recorded in *Bian Que`s Spiritual Guide to Acupuncture and Moxibustion, Jade Dragon Classic*, Wang Guo Rui, Yuan, 1329.
- *Song of Points for Miscellaneous Diseases*
  (Zá bìng xué fǎ gē)
  雜病穴法歌
  First recorded in *The Glorious Anthology of Acupuncture and Moxibustion*, Gao Wu, Ming, 1529.
- *Song of the Jade Dragon*
  (Yù lóng gē)
  玉龍歌
  First recorded in *Bian Que`s Spiritual Guide to Acupuncture and Moxibustion, Jade Dragon Classic*, Wang Guo Rui, Yuan, 1329.
- *Song of the Nine Needles for Returning the Yang*
  (Húi yáng jiǔ zhēn xué) 回陽九針穴
  First recorded in *The Glorious Anthology of Acupuncture and Moxibustion*, Gao Wu, Ming, 1529.

- *Song of the Primary Points of the Fourteen Channels*
  (Shí sì jīng yào xué zhǔ zhì gē)
  十四經要穴主治歌
- *Song to Keep Up Your Sleeve*
  (Zhǒu hòu gē)
  肘後歌
  First recorded in *The Glorious Anthology of Acupuncture and Moxibustion*, Gao Wu, Ming, 1529.
- *Spiritual Pivot*
  (Líng shū)
  靈樞
  See the *Yellow Emperor's Inner Classic.*
- *Standards of Patterns and Treatments*
  (Zhèng zhì zhǔn shéng)
  証治准繩
  Wang Ken Tang, Ming, 1602.
- *Supplement to the Thousand Ducat Formulas*
  (Qiān jīn yí fāng)
  千金翼方
  Sun Si Miao, Tang, c. 682.
- *Systematic Differentiation of Warm Diseases*
  (Wēn bìng tiáo biàn)
  溫病條辨
  Wu Ju Tong, 1798.
- *The Classic of Categories*
  (Lèi jīng)
  類經
  Zhang Jie Bin, Ming, 1624.
- *The Classic of Difficulties*
  (Nán jīng)
  難經
  Anon., Han.
- *The Classic of Supplementing Life with Acupuncture and Moxibustion*
  (Zhēn jiǔ zī shēng jīng)
  針灸資生經
  Wang Zhi Zhong, Song, 1220.
- *The Classic of the Pulse*
  (Mài jīng)
  脈經
  Wang Shu He, Jin, c. 300.
- *The Complete Collection of Acupuncture and Moxibustion*
  (Zhēn jiǔ dà quán)
  針灸大全
  Xu Feng, Ming, c. 1439.
- *The Complete Works of Jing Yue*
  (Jǐng yuè quán shū)
  景岳全書
  Zhang Jie Bing (Jing Yue), Ming, 1624.
- *The Glorious Anthology of Acupuncture and Moxibustion*
  (Zhēn jiǔ jù yīng)
  針灸聚英
  Gao Wu, Ming, 1529.
- *The Great Compendium of Acupuncture and Moxibustion*
  (Zhēn jiǔ dà chéng)
  針灸大成
  Yang Ji Zhou, Ming, 1601.
- *The Secrets of the Heavenly Star*
  (Tiān xīng mì jué)
  天星秘訣
- *The Systematic Classic of Acupuncture and Moxibustion*
  (Zhēn jiǔ jiá yǐ jīng)
  針灸甲乙經
  Huang Fu Mi, Jin, 282.
- *Thousand Ducat Formulas*
  (Qiān jīn yào fāng)
  千金要方
  Sun Si Miao, Tang, 625.
- *Treatise on Disorders of Blood*
  (Xué zhèng lūn)
  血証論
  Tang Rong Chuan, Qing, 1884.
- *Treatise on Epidemic Warm Febrile Disease*
  (Wēn yì lùn)
  溫疫論
  Wu You Ke, 1642.
- *Treatise on Injury by Cold*
  (Shāng hán lùn)
  傷寒論
  Zhang Zhong Jing, Eastern Han.
- *Treatise on the Spleen and Stomach*
  (Pí wèi lùn)
  脾胃論
  Li Ao, Song, 1249.
- *True Lineage of Medicine*
  (Yī xué zhèng chuán)
  醫學正傳
  Yu Tuan, Ming, 1515.
- *Warp and Woof of Warm Febrile Disease*
  (Wēn rè jīng wěi)
  溫熱經緯
  Wang Meng Ying, Qing, 1852.
- *Yellow Emperor's Inner Classic*
  (Huáng dì neì jīng)
  黃帝內經
  (Consisting of the *Spiritual Pivot* and the *Essential Questions*)

TRANSLATORS' TEXTS

- *A Complete Contemporary Handbook on the Practical Use of Chinese Herbs in External Medicine*
  (Dāng dài zhōng yào wài zhì lín chuáng dà quán)
  當代中葯外治臨床大全
  Jia Yi Jiang, et al
  China Traditional Chinese Medical Press, 1991.
- *A Concise Dictionary of Classical Chinese*
  (Jiǎn míng gǔ hàn yù cí diǎn)
  簡明古漢語詞典
  Shi Dong
  Yunnan People's Press, 1985.
- *Acupuncture and Moxibustion*
  (Zhēn jiǔ xué)
  針灸學
  He Shu Huai
  Traditional Chinese Medical Classics Press, 1986.
- *Acupuncture and Moxibustion*
  (Zhēn jiǔ xué) 針灸學
  Nanjing College of Traditional Chinese Medicine
  People's Medical Press, 1985.

- *Acupuncture Points*
  (Zhēn jiǔ yū xué xué)
  針灸腧穴學
  Yang Jia San, et al
  Shanghai Science and Technology Press, 1989.
- *Collected Explanations on Points*
  (Jīng xué shì yì huì jiě)
  經穴釋义彙解
  Zhang Cheng Xing
  Shanghai Translation Publishing Company, 1984.
- *Comentary on the Systematic Classic of Acupuncture and Moxibustion*
  (Zhēn jiǔ jiā yǐ jīng jiào shì)
  針灸甲乙經校釋
  Shandong College of Traditional Chinese Medicine
  People's Medical Press, 1979.
- *Common Terms of Traditional Chinese Medicine in English*
  (Hàn yīng cháng yòng zhōng yī yào cí huì)
  漢英常用中醫葯詞彙
  Xie Zhu Fan, et al
  Beijing Medical College, 1980.
- *Concise Dictionary of Traditional Chinese Medicine*
  (Jiǎn míng zhōng yī cí diǎn)
  簡明中醫辭典
  College of Traditional Chinese Medical Research, et al
  Joint Publishing Co. Hong Kong, 1979.
- *Dictionary of Acupuncture and Moxibustion*
  (Zhēn jiǔ xué cí diǎn)
  針灸穴辭典
  Wang Xue Tai, et al
  Shanghai Science and Technology Press, 1987.
- *Differentiation and Diagnosis of Symptoms in Traditional Chinese Medicine*
  (Zhōng yī zhèng zhuàng jiàn bié zhěn duàn xué)
  中醫症狀鑑別診斷學
  Zhao Jin Duo, et al
  People's Medical Press, 1985.
- *Essential Compilations from the Treatise on the Spleen and Stomach*
  (pí weì lùn zǔan yaò)
  脾胃論纂要
  Shanxi College of Traditional Chinese Medicine
  Shanxi Science and Technology Press, 1983.
- *Encyclopaedia of Traditional Chinese Medicine*
  (Zhōng yī dà cí diǎn)
  中醫大辭典
  Li Yong Chun, et al
  People's Medical Press, 1986.
- *Great Fundamentals of the Yellow Emperor's Inner Classic*
  (Huáng dì nèi jīng tài sù)
  黃帝內經太素
  Yang Shang Shan
  People's Medical Press, 1965.
- *History of Chinese Acupuncture and Moxibustion*
  (Zhōng guó zhēn jiǔ shǐ)
  中國針灸史
  Dun Shi Yu
  Tianjin Science and Technology Press, 1989.
- *Point Combinations of Chinese Acupuncture and Moxibustion*
  (Zhōng guó zhēn jiǔ chǔ fāng xué)
  中國針灸楚方學
  Xiao Shao Qing
  Ningxia People's Press, 1986.
- *Practice of External Traditional Chinese Medicine*
  (Shí yòng zhōng yī wài kē xué)
  實用中醫外科學
  Gu Bai Hua, et al
  Shanghai Science and Technology Press, 1985.
- *Practice of Internal Traditional Chinese Medicine*
  (Shí yòng zhōng yī nèi kē xué)
  實用中醫內科學
  Huang Wen Dong, et al
  Shanghai Science and Technology Press, 1985.
- *Practical Foundations of Traditional Chinese Medicine*
  (Shí yòng zhōng yī jī chǔ xúe)
  實用中醫其礎學
  Li De Xin
  Liaoning Science and Technology Press, 1985.
- *Questions and Answers in Traditional Chinese Medicine*
  (Zhōng yī xué wèn dá shàng hé xià cè)
  中醫學問答 上和下冊
  Yang Yi Ye
  People's Medical Press, 1985.
- *Quintessential Compilation on Chinese Acupuncture and Moxibustion*
  (Zhōng guó zhēn jiǔ huì cuì)
  中國針灸薈萃
  Wang Xue Tai, et al
  Hunan Science and Technology Press, 1988.
- *Skin Disease in Traditional Chinese Medicine.*
  (Zhōng yī pí fū bìng xué)
  中醫皮膚病學
  Zhu Ren Kang
  People's Medical Press, 1979.
- *Terminology of Traditional Chinese Medicine*
  (Cháng yòng zhōng yī míng cí shù yù)
  常用中醫明詞術語
  Sung J. Liao, et al
  Hunan Science and Technology Press, 1983.
- *The Great Compendium of Acupuncture and Moxibustion Elucidated*
  (Zhēn jiǔ dà chéng jiào shì)
  針灸大成校釋
  Heilongjiang College of Research on Native Medicinal Plants, et al
  People's Medical Press, 1984.
- *The Yellow Emperor's Inner Classic, Spiritual Pivot, corrected and annotated version*
  (Huáng dì neì jīng líng shū jiaò zhù yǔ dì)
  黃帝內經靈樞 校注語諦
  Dun Ai Chun
  Tianjin Science and Technology Press, 1989.
- *Treatment with Traditional Chinese Moxibustion*
  (Zhōng guó jiǔ liáo xué)
  中國灸療學
  Zhang Feng Run, et al
  People's Medical Press, 1989.
- *Wu's Annotations to the Essential Questions of the Inner Classic*
  (Neì jīng sù wèn wú zhù)
  內經素問吳注
  Wu Kun, Ming Dynasty
  Shandong Science and Technology Press, 1984.

ENGLISH TEXTS

- *A Colour Atlas of Surface Anatomy*
  Backhouse, Kenneth., Hutchings, Ralph
  Wolfe Medical Publications Ltd, 1991.
- *Acupuncture A Comprehensive Text*
  O'Connor, John and Bensky, Dan (trans.)
  Shanghai College of Traditional Medicine, Eastland Press, 1981.
- *Acupuncture Cases from China*
  A Digest of Difficult and Complicated Case Histories
  Dengbu, Zhang
  Churchill Livingstone, 1994.
- *Acupuncture in the Treatment of Children*
  Scott, Julian
  Eastland Press, 1991.
- *An Outline of Chinese Acupuncture*
  Academy of Traditional Chinese Medicine
  Foreign Languages Press, Beijing, 1975.
- *Anatomical Atlas of Acupuncture Points*
  Co-Operative Group of Shandong Medical College and Shandong College of Traditional Chinese Medicine
  Shandong Science and Technology Press, Jinan, China 1982.
- *Anatomy of the Human Body*
  Lockhart, L.D, Hamilton, G.F, Fyfe, F.W.
  Faber and Faber Limited, 1959.
- *Anatomy, Regional and Applied*
  Last, R.J.
  Churchill Livingstone, 1978.
- *Celestial Lancets*
  A History and Rationale of Acupuncture and Moxa
  Gwei-Djen, Lu and Needham, Joseph
  Cambridge University Press, 1980.
- *Chinese Acupuncture and Moxibustion*
  Mao-liang, Qiu
  Churchill Livingstone, 1993.
- *Chinese Acupuncture and Moxibustion*
  Xinnong, Cheng (ed.)
  Foreign Languages Press, Beijing, 1987.
- *Churchill's Illustrated Medical Dictionary*
  Churchill Livingstone, 1989.
- *Essentials of Chinese Acupuncture*
  Beijing College of Traditional Chinese Medicine et. al.
  Foreign Languages Press, Beijing, 1980.
- *Extra Treatises Based on Investigation and Enquiry*
  A Translation of Zhu Dan-xi's Ge Zhi Yu Lun
  Shou-zhong, Yang and Wu-jin, Duan
  Blue Poppy Press, 1994.
- *Fluid Physiology and Pathology in Traditional Chinese Medicine,*
  Clavey, Steven
  Churchill Livingstone, 1995.
- *Fundamentals of Chinese Acupuncture*
  Ellis, Andrew., Wiseman, Nigel., Boss, Ken
- *Glossary of Chinese Medical Terms & Acupuncture Points*
  Wiseman, Nigel., Boss, Ken
  Paradigm Publications.
- *Grant's Atlas of Anatomy*
  Boileau Grant, J.C.
  The Williams & Wilkins Co., 1972.
- *Grasping the Wind*
  An Exploration into the Meaning of Chinese Acupuncture Point Names
  Ellis, Andrew., Wiseman, Nigel., Boss, Ken
  Paradigm Publications, 1989.
- *Health Preservation and Rehabilitation*
  Enqin, Zhang (ed.)
  Publishing House of Shanghai College of Traditional Chinese Medicine, 1988.
- *Illustrated Dictionary of Chinese Acupuncture*
  Zhang Rui-fu; Wu Xiu-fen (compiled)
  Sheep's Publications (HK) Ltd. & People's Medical Publishing House, China.
- *Li Dong-yuan's Treatise on the Spleen and Stomach*
  A Translation of the Pi Wei Lun
  Shou-zhong, Yang and Jian-yong, Li
  Blue Poppy Press, 1993.
- *Master Hua's Classic of the Central Viscera*
  A Translation of Hua Tuo's Zhong Zang Jing
  Shou-zhong, Yang
  Blue Poppy Press, 1993.
- *Surface Anatomy*
  The Anatomical Basis of Clinical Examination
  Lumley, John S.
  Churchill Livingstone, 1990.
- *The English-Chinese Encyclopaedia of Practical Traditional Chinese Medicine*
  Medical Qigong
  Xiangcai, Xu (ed.)
  Higher Education Press, Beijing, 1989.
- *The Foundations of Chinese Medicine*
  A Comprehensive Text for Acupuncturists and Herbalists
  Maciocia, Giovanni
  Churchill Livingstone, 1989.
- *The Heart and Essence of Dan-xi's Methods of Treatment*
  A Translation of Zhu Dan-xi's Dan Xi Zhi Fa Xin Yao
  Shou-zhong, Yang
  Blue Poppy Press, 1993.
- *The Location of Acupoints*
  State Standard of the People's Republic of China
  State Administration of Traditional Chinese Medicine
  Foreign Languages Press, Beijing, 1990.
- *The Practice of Chinese Medicine*
  The Treatment of Diseases with Acupuncture and Chinese Herbs
  Maciocia, Giovanni
  Churchill Livingstone, 1994.

GLOSSARY OF TERMINOLOGY

This glossary is designed for two purposes: i. to explain some of the more difficult terminology used in this text, and ii. to refer readers to the original Chinese terms.

Abdominal masses (see Masses).

Abdominal urgency (lí jí 裡急) Abdominal cramping and pain and urgency in the need to defecate that is most commonly seen in dysenteric disorder. The term is usually used in combination in the phrase 'abdominal urgency and tenesmus' (lí jí hòu zhòng 裡急後重).

Agitation and restlessness (fán zào 煩躁) When used together the terms agitation and restlessness denote an uneasy, restive and anxious state of mind. Agitation is usually accompanied by a warm or hot oppressive sensation in the chest, whilst restlessness suggests a fidgety and restless movement of the limbs. The implication is that agitation is usually generated by internal heat, whilst restlessness comes about from external invasion of heat.

Agitation of the Heart (xīn fán 心煩) An uneasy and anxious state of mind that is commonly accompanied by a warm or hot oppressive sensation in the chest.

Atrophy disorder (wěi zhèng 痿證) A disorder characterised primarily by flaccidity and weakness of the limbs. In more severe cases and with the passage of time there is increasing loss of control over the movement of the limbs, progressive loss of muscle tone, wasting and atrophy.

Biting of the tongue (niè shé 嚙舌, 囓舌, 齧舌).

Brain wind (nǎo fēng 腦風) A form of head wind which is characterised by aversion to cold in the neck and back and a cold sensation of the head and brain, accompanied by severe pain that is hard to endure.

Chain and lock point association method (liàn sǔo pèi xué fǎ 鏈鎖配穴法).

Chest painful obstruction (xiōng bì 胸痹) Stuffiness, oppression and pain of the chest (and breast) usually due to weakness of circulation of yang qi in the chest, obstruction by phlegm or blood stasis.

Childhood accumulation disorder (xiǎo ér jī shí 小兒積食).

Childhood fright epilepsy (xiǎo ér jīng xián 小兒驚癇) This term has two meanings : i. One form of epilepsy seen in children that is triggered by sudden fright; ii. Acute childhood fright wind.

Childhood fright wind (xiǎo ér jīng fēng 小兒驚風) A disorder of infants and children characterised by convulsive spasm of the limbs and loss of consciousness. It is generally subdivided into acute and chronic fright wind. Acute childhood fright wind is far more commonly encountered and often develops during the course of an acute illness such as dysentery, meningitis etc. There is usually rapid onset of a very high temperature, great restlessness, redness of the face and lips, coarse breathing, lockjaw, stiffness and pain of the neck and back progressing to convulsive spasms, opisthotonos and finally loss of consciousness. Chronic childhood fright wind is a term reserved for disorders characterised by slow and weak periodic attacks of convulsive spasms. It is often accompanied by a slightly elevated temperature, general lethargy, and a sallow complexion.

Childhood nutritional impairment (xiǎo ér gān jī 小兒疳積) Malnutrition due to a variety of disorders. Manifestations include sallow complexion, emaciation, poor digestion, withered hair, enlarged abdomen with pronounced veins, exhaustion, spiritless demeanour etc.

Childhood umbilical wind (xiǎo ér qí fēng 小兒臍風 ; qí fēng 臍風; fēng chù 風搐; qì rì fēng 七日風; qì rì kǒu jìn 七日口噤) Convulsions, opisthotonos, and lockjaw following infection of the umbilicus in the new born.

Clonic spasm (chì zòng, chè zòng 瘈瘲) A disorder characterised by brief muscular contractions followed immediately by muscular relaxation. It is seen in a range of conditions including: i. Febrile disease due to injury by exterior pathogens, where severe heat injures the yin leading to stirring up of wind and fire and accumulation of phlegm-fire; ii. Epilepsy and tetanus characterised by wind-phlegm and phlegm-fire; iii. Summer heat which injures the qi and body fluids.

Clove sore (dīng chuāng 疔瘡) A small hard deep-rooted clove-shaped purulent lesion. It is primarily due to unregulated diet or external wind and fire poison which invade the superficial portion of the body. The condition tends to develop very rapidly with severe localised pain, redness and swelling, often accompanied by fever.

Cold inversion (hán jué 寒厥) This is one form of inversion pattern (see Inversion counterflow below) that comes about as a result of deficiency of yang and excess of yin.

Cold or damp (dong) diarrhoea (dòng xiè 洞泄) There are two meanings to this term: i. Cold diarrhoea which occurs soon after eating, with undigested food in the stools; ii. Diarrhoea due to invasion of the Spleen by dampness which leads to frequent watery diarrhoea or frequent passing of loose stools, accompanied by a thick greasy tongue coating and a soggy (rú 濡) pulse etc.

Corporeal soul (pò 魄).

Correct qi (zhèng qì 正氣) i. Refers to the totality of a person's qi that is derived from pre- and post- heaven qi (also known as true qi, zhēn qì 真氣); ii. Contrasted to pathogenic qi, it denotes the body's general resistance to disease.

Counterflow qi (nì qì 逆氣) Qi that flows counter to its normal direction. This term is sometimes used to mean the same as rebellious qi (shàng qì 上氣) of the Lung or Stomach, or else as a general term denoting abnormal movement of qi, for example in the limbs where it manifests as coldness due to warming qi not reaching the extremities (see Inversion counterflow).

Crane's knee wind (hè xī fēng 鶴膝風) Also known by a variety of names including 'wandering knee wind', 'crane's joint' and 'eyes of the knee wind'. The disorder is characterised by swelling and enlargement of one or both knees with subsequent atrophy of the area above and below the knee, hence the resemblance to the legs of a crane.

Defensive qi (wèi qì 衛氣) A form of yang qi that circulates outside the channels in the superficial, exterior portion of the body. Its primary functions include defending the body against exterior pathogenic factors, warming the body and controlling the opening and closing of the pores.

Deficiency taxation (xū láo 虛勞) A general term used to describe a variety of disorders associated with injury to and depletion of qi, blood and the zangfu. The aetiology may be deficiency of the pre- or post- heaven qi, prolonged illness, improper diet, excessive sexual activity, improper treatment etc. Symptoms and signs will vary depending on the severity and location of the deficiency.

Dementia (dāi bìng 呆病; dāi 呆; chī dāi 痴呆; bái chī 白痴) A disorder due to phlegm-damp which obscures the portals of the Heart. It is primarily caused by stagnation of Liver qi due to emotional depression that overacts on the Spleen and Stomach, or by injury to the Spleen and Stomach from improper diet or lifestyle. The clinical manifestations are many and varied and include an inability or lack of desire to speak, eat or drink for days on end, neglect of appearance and cleanliness, crying and laughing inappropriately, remaining in the same position for hours on end, indulging in bizarre and obsessional behaviour etc.

Diarrhoea containing undigested food (sūn xiè 飧泄; shŭi gŭ lì 水谷利) Diarrhoea with undigested food in the stools. Most commonly due to Spleen yang deficiency, but may also be due to exterior invasion of wind, damp, cold or heat.

Diarrhoea due to injury by food (shí xiè 食泄).

Diarrhoea with thin stools (táng xiè 溏泄).

Difficult ingestion (shí bú xià 食不下; yǐn shí bú xià 飲食不下; bú xià shí 不下食).

Difficult urination (xiăo biàn bú lì 小便不利) Difficulty in passing diminished amounts of urine.

Diminished qi (shăo qì 少氣) A broad term used to indicate weakness and feebleness of the voice, shortness of breath and general listlessness. Although theoretically weakness of qi of any of the zang may give rise to this condition, it is primarily associated with deficiency of Lung qi.

Disorientation (huăng hū 恍惚) A term that is used to describe a distracted state of mind; the patient is flurried, bewildered, alarmed, and unable to manage basic tasks. It mostly originates from long-term emotional strain, exterior pathogens that injure the interior, or excessive sweating that injures Heart qi and disrupts the mind.

Drum distention (gŭ zhàng 鼓脹; gŭ 臌; gŭ zhàng 臌脹) A disorder characterised by drum-like swelling and distention of the abdomen with a marked and prominent network of veins clearly visible. If present, oedema of the limbs is usually slight, whilst jaundice is usually pronounced. The primary aetiological factors include prolonged emotional strain that leads to stagnation, irregular diet, excessive consumption of alcohol, and chronic parasitic disease. The subsequent damage to the Spleen and Liver caused by the above factors will give rise to stagnation of qi, stasis of blood, accumulation of damp and poor circulation of fluids.

Dysenteric disorder (lí jì 痢疾; xià lí 下痢; lí 痢) This term is used to describe a variety of diseases ranging from acute dysentery to chronic disorders such as ulcerative colitis and Crohn's disease. The principal symptoms are diarrhoea several times a day with relatively little quantity of stools passed, accompanied by abdominal pain and tenesmus. Pus, mucus or blood may frequently be mixed with the stools. If pus or mucus predominate it is known as white dysentery (bái lí 白痢). If blood predominates it is known as red dysentery (chì lí 赤痢). This condition is usually differentiated into excess type, and deficiency complicated with excess type. It is primarily due to damp-heat, heat, epidemic poison or stagnant food. Chronic forms are mainly due to Spleen and Kidney yang deficiency and cold, usually complicated with heat.

Erysipelas [cinnabar toxin] (dān dú 丹毒) A skin disorder that broadly corresponds to erysipelas and cellulitis in western medicine. Initially there is a well-circumscribed fresh-red, burning hot lesion that quickly spreads. It is accompanied by chills and fever, headache and thirst. In severe cases fire poison invades the interior leading to high fever, agitation and restlessness, delirium, incoherent speech, nausea and vomiting. This condition primarily affects the head and face, or alternatively the lower limbs. When in the upper region it is mostly due to wind-heat transforming into fire; when in lower region it is mostly due to damp-heat transforming into fire.

Essence (jīng 精) The vital material basis of the human body which maintains the fundamental activities of life. It includes the essence of the Kidney (pre-heaven essence) and the essence of water and grain (post-heaven essence).

Ethereal soul (hún 魂).

Fifth-watch diarrhoea (wŭ gēng xiè 五更泄).

Five accumulations (wŭ jī 五積) A group of disorders mostly characterised by the formation of masses (subjective or objective) in the chest or abdomen. They are differentiated into five types according to the mode of development, disease mechanism, location and nature: Heart accumulation, Liver accumulation, Lung accumulation, Spleen accumulation and Kidney accumulation.

Five palms agitated and hot (wŭ xīn fā rè 五心煩熱) A hot sensation felt in the palms of the hands and soles of the feet, usually accompanied by heat and agitation of the chest. This symptom is primarily due to deficiency of yin with blazing of fire although it may also be seen in cases of deficiency of blood, stagnant heat or as a sequela of febrile disorders.

Five taxations (wŭ láo 五勞) According to the *Spiritual Pivot* (Chapter 18) the five taxations are: i. Excessive use of the eyes which injures the blood; ii. Excessive lying down which injures the qi; iii. Excessive sitting which injures the flesh; iv. Excessive standing which injures the bones, and v. Excessive walking which injures the sinews. In later texts, the term five taxations was also used to refer to taxation of the five zang, thus: i. Heart taxation, principally involving damage to Heart blood; ii. Spleen taxation due to overeating or excessive worry and pensiveness which injure the Spleen qi; iii. Lung taxation involving depletion of Lung qi or yin; iv. Kidney taxation involving damage to Kidney qi from excessive sexual activity; v. Liver taxation involving injury to Liver qi by mental excitement, with such signs as unclear vision, pain of the chest and hypochondrium, flaccid muscles and sinews and difficulty of movement.

Flaccid tongue (shé huǎn 舌緩) The sudden onset of a slack or limp tongue accompanied by rumbling phlegmy-sounding speech and an inability to speak coherently. It is primarily due to wind-phlegm obstructing the channels.

Focal distention (pǐ qì 痞氣) Focal distension is one of the five accumulations, pertaining to the Spleen. It is characterised by a sensation of a localised lump like an upturned cup in the epigastric or chest region accompanied by a feeling of distention and fullness. It comes about as a consequence of stagnation of the circulation of qi, usually due to deficiency of Spleen qi. As the condition progresses there is wasting of the muscles, lack of strength in the limbs and eventually jaundice.

Four command points (sì zǒng xué 四總穴) A pre-Ming dynasty grouping of points that first appeared in print in *The Glorious Anthology of Acupuncture and Moxibustion* by the Ming dynasty author Gao Wu. The four command points are: Zusanli ST-36 for disorders of the abdomen; Weizhong BL-40 for disorders of lumbar region and back; Lieque LU-7 for disorders of the head and nape, and Hegu L.I.-4 for disorders of the face and mouth. The six command points were derived from Gao Wu's four command points by later commentators who added Neiguan P-6 for disorders of the chest and lateral costal region, and Renzhong DU-26 to rescue urgent situations.

Fright palpitations (jīng jì 驚悸) A form of palpitations that may either be triggered by fright, or in which fright may be an accompanying symptom.

Gathering qi (zōng qì 宗氣) Formed by the combination of the essence of food and drink and the qi of air. By nourishing the Lung and Heart, it has two principle actions: i. To control respiration and the voice, and ii. To circulate the blood.

Grain qi (gǔ qì 谷氣).

Head wind (tóu fēng 頭風) i. Severe, long-standing and repetitive headaches (for example migraine) that are recalcitrant to treatment, in contrast to a single incident of headache. Such headaches are considered to be mostly due to external invasion of wind-cold or wind-heat that lodge in the head, or to stagnation of phlegm and/or blood that obstruct the channels; ii. A condition deriving from attack by exterior wind which invades the channels of the head and gives rise to headache, dizziness and deviation of the mouth and eye.

Heart painful obstruction (xīn bì 心痹) One form of painful obstruction (bi) pattern that affects the zang. It may be due to: I. Exterior pathogens that lodge in the body for a long period of time, eventually entering the Heart; or ii. Excessive deliberation that injures and depletes Heart qi and blood and predisposes to repeated injury by exterior pathogens that may then easily invade the Heart. The result is obstruction of the Heart qi and channels of the chest. Symptoms include an oppressive sensation of the chest, palpitations, heart pain, sudden dyspnoea, a propensity to be easily frightened, dry throat, belching and a deep and thready pulse.

Hot inversion (rè jué 熱厥) One form of inversion pattern. It has two meanings: i. Inversion pattern that comes about as a result of excessive heat which depletes the yin; ii. Inversion pattern due to severe heat that creates stagnation of yang on the interior which is then unable to reach the exterior.

Insufficiency of spirit qi (shén qì bù zú 神氣不足).

Internal eye obstruction (nèi zhàng 內障).

Interstices (còu lǐ 腠理).

Inversion counterflow (jué nì 厥逆) i. Inversion frigidity of the four limbs (severe cold either of part of the limb or of the entire limb); ii. Severe pain of the chest and abdomen with sudden frigidity of the legs and feet, agitation and inability to eat; iii. One form of chronic headache.

Inversion counterflow of the four limbs (sì jué nì 四厥逆) A broad term that is used to describe coldness of the hands and feet that comes about as a result of disruption in the flow of qi. It may be due to deficiency (for example yang deficiency where the cold sensation tends to extend further up the limbs towards the elbows or knees) or excess (for example heat or qi stagnation, in which case only the tips of the extremities are affected).

Inversion qi (jué qì 厥氣) Disordered and contrary flow of qi.

Leg qi (jiǎo qì 腳氣) A disorder characterised by numbness, pain and weakness of the legs and feet. Alternatively there may be spasm and swelling, redness and heat of legs and feet. In severe cases the pathogen attacks more deeply, affecting the abdomen and Heart, in which case there is also discomfort of the abdomen, vomiting, no desire to eat, palpitations, oppression of the chest, dyspnoea, disorientation and deranged speech. Leg qi is primarily due to exterior attack of pathogenic dampness and wind poison, or else due to excessive consumption of rich and greasy foods that generate dampness and heat which will slowly flow downwards to the legs.

Loss of speech, inability to speak (yán yǔ bù néng 言語不能).

Loss of voice (shī yīn 失音; shī yīn bù yǔ 失音不語; yīn bìng 瘖病; yīn yǎ 音啞; wú yīn 無音).

Lotus flower tongue (zhòng shé 重舌; zǐ shé 子舌; zhòng shé fēng 重舌風; lían hūa shé 蓮花舌) A condition characterised by distention and protrusion of dark-red or purple coloured blood vessels below the tongue. Little growths may form resembling little tongues, hence the alternative name of baby tongue (子舌). These may join together to form larger growths resembling lotus flowers. Systemic symptoms may include tidal fever, headache with stiffness of the neck, difficulty in swallowing food, inability to speak and drooling. Over a period of time erosion may develop. This condition is usually attributed to Heart and Spleen damp-heat compounded by attack of exterior wind.

Lung atrophy (fèi wěi 肺痿) A chronic deficiency disorder where the lungs are said to wither and shrivel, in the same way that the limbs are seen to wither in atrophy syndrome. The clinical symptoms and signs include persistent cough and dyspnoea with expectoration of thick glue-like and frothy sputum, emaciation, listlessness, dryness of the mouth, throat and lips, tidal fever, withered dry skin and body hair, and a rapid and deficient pulse. Most cases are due to deficiency of yin with blazing of fire.

Lung consumption (fèi láo 肺痨) A chronic disease characterised by progressive emaciation, cough with blood-streaked sputum, low grade tidal fever, night sweats, lethargy etc. It corresponds to pulmonary tuberculosis.

Malign blood (è xuè 惡血).

Mania-depression (diān kuáng 癲狂) A broad term for insanity and mental derangement bridging the spectrum from depressive behaviour (dian) to manic episodes (kuang). Depressive behaviour includes depression, melancholy, dislike of talking or incoherent speech, mumbling to oneself and slow movements. Manic behaviour includes wild frenzied movement and speech, hallucinations, feelings of boundless strength, violent behaviour, insomnia etc. Most cases are due to accumulation of phlegm or phlegm-heat in the Heart that disrupts the spirit.

Manic ghost talk (kuáng guǐ yǔ 狂鬼語).

Masses (zhēng jiǎ jī jù 癥瘕 積聚) A collective term for abdominal masses. Masses are considered to develop as a result of emotional stagnation, depression and frustration or internal injury by food. These lead in turn to injury of the Liver and Spleen and eventually to insufficiency of correct qi. The terms zhēng and jī (癥積) refer to hard, immovable masses with fixed pain which are generally associated with disorder of the zang and blood. The terms jiǎ and jù (瘕聚) refer to masses of indefinite form which tend to accumulate and dissipate relatively rapidly giving rise to pain of no fixed location. They are generally associated with disorder of the fu and qi. Most commonly in classical texts however, these terms are found in combination, for example zheng jia and ji ju, reflecting the commonly encountered clinical pattern of combined qi stagnation and blood stasis. Zhēng jiǎ (癥瘕) masses mostly occur in the lower jiao and are closely associated with gynaecological disorders, whereas jī jù (積聚) masses tend to occur in the middle jiao and are closely associated with digestive disorders.

Melancholy crying ghost talk (bēi kū gǔi yǔ 悲哭鬼語).

Nasal congestion and discharge (bí yuān 鼻淵).

Nutritive qi (yíng qì 營氣) A form of yin qi that circulates within the vessels of the body. Its primary functions include nourishment of the body and the formation of blood.

Obstructed urination (lóng bì 癃閉; lóng 癃 ; bì lóng 閉癃) Reduced urinary flow, with difficulty in urination. In milder cases (lóng 癃) there is difficulty in passing urine, that comes out in drops. In severe cases (bì 閉) there is total retention of urine.

Oesophageal constriction (yē gé 噎膈; gé 鬲; yē sāi 噎塞; yē zhōng 噎中; gé yān 鬲咽) This condition is characterised by a sensation of blockage of the throat on swallowing, and/or a blockage further down at the level of the diaphragm. In advanced cases food that is ingested gets stuck between the throat and diaphragm or else is vomited up soon after ingestion. Oesophageal constriction comes about as a result of emotional constraint leading to stagnation of qi, excessive anger, excessive consumption of alcohol or rich, sweet foods that generate phlegm. It is usually differentiated into: i. Stagnation of qi and phlegm; ii. Knotting of heat with exhaustion of fluids; iii. Stasis of blood; iv. Consumption of qi and yang.

Original qi (yuán qì 原氣; 元氣) Denotes the original yin and original yang of the body. It originates in the Kidneys and is formed from pre-heaven essence, although it is dependent on nourishment from the post-heaven essence derived from the Stomach and Spleen. Original qi is stored in the 'cinnabar field' (Dāntián 丹田) and flows to all parts of the body via the sanjiao, gathering at the yuan-source points and acting as the source of all transformation and movement in the body and as the promoter of the activity of the zangfu.

Painful obstruction (bì 痹) A disorder characterised by obstruction of the circulation of qi (primarily due to penetration of wind, cold and damp) that leads to pain. The pain most frequently occurs in the muscles, sinews, joints and bones, although any part of the body may be affected, including the internal organs. In terms of modern medicine it corresponds to rheumatic and arthritic disease.

Painful urinary dysfunction (lín zhèng 淋症) A general term referring to urinary difficulty, urgency and frequency. Urination is accompanied by some degree of pain of the urethra and in some cases the hypogastrium. Dribbling of urine often follows urination. Painful urinary dysfunction is usually classified into one of five types depending on presentation: i. Qi painful urinary dysfunction; ii. Blood painful urinary dysfunction; iii. Stone (or sand) painful urinary dysfunction; iv. Turbid painful urinary dysfunction, and v. Taxation painful urinary dysfunction. Note that hot painful urinary dysfunction is not included in this classification, primarily because in practice it is considered to be present in most types of painful urinary dysfunction.

Pathogenic qi (xíe qì 邪氣) i. Disease causing factors that originate outside the body namely wind, cold, damp, dryness, fire, summer heat and epidemic pestilential qi; ii. A general term for all disease causing factors.

Plumstone qi (méi hé qì 梅核氣) A subjective sensation of a lump obstructing the throat. Efforts to cough it up or swallow it are futile. It is frequently exacerbated by emotional upset, and diminished by relaxation and emotional ease. It is often accompanied by an oppressive sensation of the chest, frequent sighing, nausea and depression. It corresponds to globus hystericus in modern medicine.

Pounding of the heart (zhēng chōng 怔忡) A form of severe palpitations. The pulsation and pounding tends to be intense and can often be felt in a broad area ranging from the chest to the umbilicus. It is considered to be a more serious and advanced condition than the other forms of palpitations (palpitations and fright palpitations), from which it often develops.

Protrusion of the tongue (shé zòng 舌縱 ; shēn shé 伸舌) The tongue is extended out of the mouth and the patient finds it difficult or impossible to retract it. It is often accompanied by a scorching hot sensation of the tongue and mental disturbance. This condition is considered to be primarily due to phlegm-heat agitating the Heart.

Purple-white wind blotches [pityriasis versicolor] (zǐ baí diàn fēng 紫白癜風).

Restless zang disorder (zàng zào 臟躁) An episodic mental disorder most commonly occurring in women, characterised by a variety of symptoms such as agitation, restlessness, oppression of the chest, disturbed sleep, irritability, rash and impetuous behaviour, abnormal speech, frequent yawning and stretching, disorientation, worry, grief, weeping, sighing and even convulsions without complete loss of consciousness. It is generally considered to come about as a consequence of emotional frustration which impairs the smooth flow of Liver qi, or worry which injures Heart yin and blood. Historically this condition was also associated specifically with blood deficiency of the uterus, drawing parallels with the original Western concept of hysteria which is how zang zao is sometimes translated.

Rhinitis (bí qiú 鼻鼽) Clear nasal discharge, often accompanied by stuffy nose, itching of the nose and sneezing. It is mostly due to Lung qi deficiency resulting in weakness of the ability of the defensive qi to firm the exterior which in turn will lead to invasion of exterior wind.

Sabre lumps (mǎ dāo 馬刀) Scrofulus tumours that appear on the body in the shape of a sabre.

Scrofula (lǔo lì 瘰癧) This term is primarily used to describe nodules on the sides of the neck, but includes also the axilla and inguinal region. Small nodules are known as lǔo (瘰), large ones as lì (癧). They come about as a consequence of: i. Deficiency of Lung and Kidney yin; ii. Long term stagnation of Liver qi and iii. Deficiency fire that condenses the body fluids to form phlegm. In the early stages of the disorder small bean-sized nodules that are neither hot nor painful emerge. As the disorder develops the nodules often enlarge, form into a linear pattern and become firm and immovable. If the nodules burst, a thin clear liquid is usually discharged. Occasionally a thicker (bean-dreg like) liquid is discharged. In chronic cases an open sinus forms with continual exudation.

Seven injuries (qī shāng 七傷) 1. The seven disease causing factors: i. Injury to the Spleen from excessive eating; ii. Injury to the Liver from excessive anger; iii. Injury to the Kidneys from excessive labour and lifting, as well as extended periods of time spent sitting on damp ground; iv. Injury to the Lung from cold or retention of cold fluid; v. Injury to the Heart from prolonged anxiety and worry as well as excessive deliberation; vi. Injury to the body from wind, rain, cold and summer heat and vii. Injury to the emotions from great fear and dread. 2. A collective term for the seven manifestations of depletion of the Kidneys in men: i. Cold genitals; ii. Impotence; iii. Abdominal urgency; iv. Seminal emission; v. Insufficiency of essence (semen) with dampness of the genitals, vi. Thin semen; vii. Frequency of urination, dribbling of urine or interrupted urination.

Sexual taxation (fáng láo 房勞; nǔ láo 女勞; fáng shì shāng 房室傷) Exhaustion due to depletion of the Kidneys by excessive sexual activity.

Shan disorder (shàn 疝) There are three general definitions for this term: i. The protrusion of an organ or tissue through an abdominal opening; ii. Severe pain of the abdomen accompanied by constipation and retention of urine or difficult urination and iii. A general term denoting disease of the external genitalia, testicles and scrotum.

Six extremes (lìu jí 六极) A collective term for six types of extreme deficiency disorders. According to the *Thousand Ducat Formulas* the six extremes are: i. Qi extreme; ii. Vessel extreme; iii. Sinew extreme; iv. Flesh extreme; v. Bone extreme, and vi. Essence extreme.

Six command points (lìu zǒng xué 六總穴) see Four command points.

Slippery diarrhoea (huá xiè 滑泄) Chronic diarrhoea that gives rise to the downward collapse of qi, which in turn will lead to such symptoms as ceaseless diarrhoea (both at night and during the day), diminished appetite, inversion counterflow of the four limbs or oedema of the limbs, generalised sensation of cold, shortness of breath, emaciation and deficiency fever. It is usually differentiated into hot and cold types.

Spirit (shén 神).

Steaming bone disorder (gǔ zhēng 骨蒸) A feverish sensation that feels to the patient as if it emanates from deep inside the bones and marrow. It is mostly due to deficiency of yin with blazing fire. It is commonly accompanied by tidal fever, night sweats, agitation and restlessness, insomnia, heat sensation of the palms, dyspnoea and dark urine.

Stiffness of the tongue (shé qiáng 舌強) Stiffness of the tongue and loss of ability to control fine movement of the tongue. It is often accompanied by difficulty in speaking, or by total inability to form coherent words. It is most frequently encountered as a sequela of wind-stroke.

Stone oedema (shí shǔi 石水) One form of oedema that is mostly due to yin cold of the Liver and Kidneys, with stagnation and accumulation of fluids in the lower jiao. Symptoms include swelling of the hypogastrium that feels hard like a stone, distention and pain below the lateral costal regions, fullness of the abdomen and a deep pulse.

Sudden fright disorder in children (xiǎo ér kè wǔ 小兒客忤) A disorder of children that is due to weakness or immaturity of the spirit qi. On being startled (for example by seeing a stranger, or suddenly hearing an unexpected or unfamiliar noise) the child suddenly becomes very frightened and begins to weep. Wind-phlegm, generated by the shock, will subsequently disrupt the Spleen and Stomach giving rise to vomiting, diarrhoea and abdominal pain, and ultimately to clonic spasm.

Sudden turmoil disorder (huò luàn 霍亂) A disorder characterised by sudden onset of simultaneous and severe diarrhoea and vomiting, accompanied by abdominal discomfort and pain. It is most commonly associated with unclean food, injury by cold, summer heat and dampness, or epidemic qi.

Superficial visual obstruction (mù yì 目翳; yì zhàng 翳障 ; mù zhōng yì zhāng 目中翳障) A thin membranous growth on the eyeball that impedes vision.

Taxation fever (láo rè 勞熱) A form of fever associated with deficiency taxation patterns. It is frequently accompanied by steaming bone disorder, agitation and heat of the five palms, dryness of the mouth etc. It is primarily due to yin deficiency with blazing fire, although other possibilities include deficiency of yang, blood or qi.

Tetany (jìng 痙) A disorder characterised by stiffness and rigidity of the neck and back, lockjaw, twitching of the limbs, opisthotonos etc. It can usefully be differentiated into excess and deficiency types. The excess type is mostly the result of wind, damp, cold, phlegm, and fire pathogens stagnating and obstructing the channels and collaterals. The deficiency type is mostly the result of excessive sweating, loss of blood, deficiency of qi and blood or depletion of fluids giving rise to malnourishment of the sinews and the generation of internal deficiency wind.

The eight therapeutic methods (bā fǎ 八法) The therapeutic use of the confluent points of the eight extraordinary channels.

Thought (yì 意).

Three corpse possession disorder (sān shī zǒu zhù 三尸走疰).

Throat Moth (rǔ è 乳蛾; hóu è 喉蛾) This is one-sided or bilateral redness, swelling and pain of the tonsils, which is usually accompanied by foul breath, constipation, chills and fever and a thick greasy tongue coating. Yellow-white coloured pus is clearly discernible on the surface of the tonsils. Throat moth is primarily due to: i. Stagnant heat in the Stomach and Lung; ii. Fire poison; iii. Qi and blood stagnation; iv. Old phlegm and Liver fire knotting up and forming blood stasis (malign blood), or v. Depletion of Liver and Kidney yin with blazing fire.

Throat painful obstruction (hóu bì 喉痹, 喉閉) A general term for swelling, congestion and pain of the throat. The term implies that the disorder is relatively mild and will not develop into a critical condition. Accompanying symptoms can include a mild sensation of blockage, hoarseness of the voice, chills and fever etc. Throat painful obstruction can come about as a result of injury by exterior pathogens (mostly wind-heat) or from interior disharmony (mostly deficiency of yin).

Thunder head wind (léi tóu fēng 雷頭風) A type of headache that is primarily due to exterior attack of wind, or internal phlegm-fire that generates wind. The headache tends to be severe with a thundering sound in the head. It may be accompanied by swelling and heat of the face and head.

Tian gui (tiān gǔi 天癸) i. The essential substance responsible for promoting growth, development and reproductive function as well as the maintenance of the menstrual cycle and pregnancy. It is formed from the combined essence of the parents and slowly develops with constant supplementation from the post-heaven qi. ii. In the *Classic of Categories* tian gui is used as an alternative term for original qi; iii. Occasionally used as an alternative name for menstruation.

Tidal fever (cháo rè 潮熱) A feverish sensation (subjective or objective) that occurs at regular intervals, often in the afternoon and evening. Although deficiency cases are most frequently seen in practice, it may also come about as a consequence of excess patterns.

Tongue thrusting (nòng shé 弄舌; tù shé 吐舌; shū shé 舒舌) This is a disorder where the tongue is repeatedly thrust out of the mouth, then immediately drawn back in and moved up and down, left and right, like a snake's tongue. It is most commonly seen in the pattern of Spleen and Heart accumulated heat, though it is also differentiated into Spleen and Kidney deficiency heat. It is frequently seen during the course of a febrile disease or during an epileptic attack, and is often accompanied by a red distended tongue, ulceration of the tongue and thirst with desire for cold fluids.

Uterine masses (see Masses).

Visual dizziness (mù xuàn 目眩) A type of dizziness that initially starts as cloudy vision before developing into dizziness. This is usually contrasted to vertex dizziness (diān xuàn 巔眩) which is used to describe dizziness followed by cloudy vision.

Wasting and thirsting disorder (xiāo kě 消渴) A disorder characterised by excessive thirst, hunger and urination as well as progressive loss of weight and emaciation. It broadly corresponds to diabetes mellitus.

Water binding the chest (shǔi jié xiōng 水結胸) Accumulation of fluid in the chest and costal region leading to pain below the heart, with fullness and hardness on palpation.

Watery diarrhoea (zhù xiè 注泄; shǔi xiè 水瀉, 水泄; xiè zhù 泄注 zhù xià 注下) Diarrhoea that is the consistency of water. It is usually differentiated into damp, cold, and hot types.

White turbidity (bái zhuó 白濁) i. Turbid white urine; ii. White urethral discharge; even though pain on urination and hesitant urinary flow is present, the urine itself is not turbid.

Will (zhì 志).

Wind dizziness (fēng xuàn 風眩 ; fēng tóu xuàn 風頭眩) i. One type of dizziness due to underlying deficiency that predisposes to injury by wind, which then penetrates to the brain giving rise to dizziness, cloudy vision and vomiting. In severe cases there may be continual dizziness, pain of the body and even collapse. ii. In the *Thousand Ducat Formulas* the term wind dizziness is used to denote epilepsy.

Wind rash (fēng zhěn 風疹) A skin disorder that mostly occurs in winter and spring in children aged between one and five. It is due to invasion of exterior wind-heat that becomes blocked at the superficial portion of the Lung (skin). The lesions primarily consist of pink or pale-red macular papules. The condition resolves within one and three days.

Wind taxation (fēng láo 風勞) A disorder where exterior wind-cold enters and lodges in the channels and collaterals, giving rise to painful obstruction. If untreated or severe, the pathogen will enter more deeply reaching the fu and subsequently the zang. The consequent injury to the qi and blood will eventually lead to taxation.

Wind-taxation lumbar pain (fēng láo yāo tòng 風勞腰痛) Lumbar pain due to attack and injury by exterior pathogenic factors which lodge in the back and over time lead to deficiency.

CHINESE POINT NAMES INDEX

Italicised names are alternative names

Qūbìn GB-7 (Crook of the Temple) 曲鬢
Qūchāi BL-4 (Crooked Curve) 曲差
Qūchí L.I.-11 (Pool at the Crook) 曲池
Quēpén ST-12 (Empty Basin) 缺盆
Qūgǔ REN-2 (Curved Bone) 曲骨
Qūquán LIV-8 (Spring at the Crook) 曲泉
Qūyuán SI-13 (Crooked Wall) 曲垣
Qūzé P-3 (Marsh at the Crook) 曲澤

Rángǔ KID-2 (Blazing Valley) 然谷
Rényíng ST-9 (Man's Welcome) 人迎
Rénzhōng DU-26 (Man's Middle) 人中
Rìyuè GB-24 (Sun and Moon) 日月
Rǔgēn ST-18 (Root of the Breast) 乳根
Rǔzhōng ST-17 (Middle of the Breast) 乳中

Sānjiān L.I.-3 (Third Space) 三間
Sānjiǎojiǔ M-CA-23 (Triangle Moxibustion) 三角灸
Sānjiāoshū BL-22 (Sanjiao Shu) 三焦俞
Sānjiéjiāo REN-4 (Triple Intersection) 三結交
Sānyángluò SJ-8 (Three Yang Luo) 三陽絡
Sānyángwǔhuì DU-20 (Three Yang Five Meetings) 三陽五會
Sānyīnjiāo SP-6 (Three Yin Intersection) 三陰交
Shàngguān GB-3 (Above the Joint) 上關
Shàngguǎn REN-13 (Upper Controller) 上管
Shàngjùxū ST-37 (Upper Great Void) 上巨虛
Shànglián L.I.-9 (Upper Angle) 上廉
Shàngliáo BL-31 (Upper Crevice) 上髎
Shàngqìhǎi REN-17 (Upper Sea of Qi) 上氣海
Shāngqiū SP-5 (Shang Mound) 商丘
Shāngqū KID-17 (Shang Bend) 商曲
Shàngtiāntī DU-1 (Stairway to Heaven) 上天梯
Shàngwǎn REN-13 (Upper Cavity) 上脘
Shàngxīng DU-23 (Upper Star) 上星
Shāngyáng L.I.-1 (Shang Yang) 商陽
Shānzhōng REN-17 (Chest Centre) 膻中
Shàochōng HE-9 (Lesser Rushing) 少沖
Shàofǔ HE-8 (Lesser Palace) 少府
Shàohǎi HE-3 (Lesser Sea) 少海
Shàoshāng LU-11 (Lesser Shang) 少商
Shàozé SI-1 (Lesser Marsh) 少澤
Shéncáng KID-25 (Spirit Storehouse) 神藏
Shéndào DU-11 (Spirit Pathway) 神道
Shénfēng KID-23 (Spirit Seal) 神封
Shēnmài BL-62 (Extending Vessel) 申脈
Shénmén HE-7 (Spirit Gate) 神門
Shénquè REN-8 (Spirit Gateway) 神闕
Shènshū BL-23 (Kidney Shu) 腎俞
Shéntáng BL-44 (Hall of the Spirit) 神堂
Shéntáng DU-23 (Hall of the Spirit) 神堂
Shéntíng DU-24 (Courtyard of the Spirit) 神庭
Shēnzhù DU-12 (Body Pillar) 身柱
Shídòu SP-17 (Food Cavity) 食竇
Shíguān KID-18 (Stone Pass) 石關
Shímén REN-5 (Stone Gate) 石門
Shíqīzhuīxià M-BW-25 (Below the Seventeenth Vertebra) 十七椎下
Shíxuān M-UE-1 (Ten Diffusions) 十宣
Shǒusānlǐ L.I.-10 (Arm Three Miles) 手三里
Shǒuwǔlǐ L.I.-13 (Arm Five Miles) 手五里
Shuàigǔ GB-8 (Leading Valley) 率谷
Shūfǔ KID-27 (Shu Mansion) 俞府
Shùgǔ BL-65 (Restraining Bone) 束骨
Shuǐdào ST-28 (Water Passage) 水道
Shuǐfēn REN-9 (Water Separation) 水分
Shuǐquán KID-5 (Water Spring) 水泉
Shuǐtú ST-10 (Water Prominence) 水突
Sìbái ST-2 (Four Whites) 四白
Sìdú SJ-9 (Four Rivers) 四瀆
Sìfèng M-UE-9 (Four Seams) 四縫
Sìmǎn KID-14 (Four Fullnesses) 四滿
Sìshéncōng M-HN-1 (Four Alert Spirit) 四神聰
Sīzhúkōng SJ-23 (Silken Bamboo Hollow) 絲竹空
Sùliáo DU-25 (White Crevice) 素髎

Tàibái SP-3 (Supreme White) 太白
Tàichōng LIV-3 (Great Rushing) 太沖
Tàixī KID-3 (Supreme Stream) 太谿
Tàiyáng M-HN-9 (Sun/Supreme Yang) 太陽
Tàiyǐ ST-23 (Supreme Unity) 太乙
Tàiyuān LU-9 (Supreme Abyss) 太淵
Táodào DU-13 (Way of Happiness) 陶道
Tiānchí P-1 (Heavenly Pool) 天池
Tiānchōng GB-9 (Heavenly Rushing) 天沖
Tiānchuāng SI-16 (Heavenly Window) 天窗
Tiāndǐng L.I.-17 (Heaven's Tripod) 天鼎
Tiānfǔ LU-3 (Palace of Heaven) 天府
Tiānjǐng SJ-10 (Heavenly Well) 天井
Tiānliáo SJ-15 (Heavenly Crevice) 天髎
Tiānquán P-2 (Heavenly Spring) 天泉
Tiānróng SI-17 (Heavenly Appearance) 天容
Tiānshū ST-25 (Heaven's Pivot) 天樞
Tiāntíng DU-24 (Courtyard of Heaven) 天庭
Tiāntú REN-22 (Heavenly Prominence) 天突
Tiānwǔhuì ST-9 (Heaven's Five Meetings) 天五會
Tiānxī SP-18 (Heavenly Stream) 天谿
Tiānyǒu SJ-16 (Window of Heaven) 天牖
Tiānzhù BL-10 (Celestial Pillar) 天柱
Tiānzōng SI-11 (Heavenly Gathering) 天宗
Tiáokǒu ST-38 (Lines Opening) 條口
Tīnggōng SI-19 (Palace of Hearing) 聽宮
Tīnghuì GB-2 (Meeting of Hearing) 聽會
Títūo N-CA-4 (Lift and Support) 提托
Tōnglǐ HE-5 (Penetrating the Interior) 通里
Tōngtiān BL-7 (Heavenly Connection) 通天
Tóngzǐliáo GB-1 (Pupil Crevice) 瞳子髎
Tóulínqì GB-15 (Head Governor of Tears) 頭臨泣
Tóuqiàoyīn GB-11 (Yin Portals of the Head) 頭竅陰
Tóuwéi ST-8 (Head's Binding) 頭維

Wàiguān SJ-5 (Outer Pass) 外關
Wàilíng ST-26 (Outer Mound) 外陵
Wàiqiū GB-36 (Outer Hill) 外丘
Wángǔ GB-12 (Mastoid Process) 完骨
Wàngǔ SI-4 (Wrist Bone) 腕骨
Wèicāng BL-50 (Stomach Granary) 胃藏
Wéidào GB-28 (Linking Path) 維道
Wèiguǎnxiàshū M-BW-12 (Stomach Controller Lower Shu) 胃管下俞
Wèishū BL-21 (Stomach Shu) 胃俞

ENGLISH POINT NAMES INDEX

Italicised names are alternative names

INDICATIONS INDEX

This is an index of the Indications found for each point. See also the General Index.

Diarrhoea with blood (and pus) SP-3, BL-24, LIV-8

Difficult ingestion LU-1, L.I.-17, ST-11, ST-20, ST-25, ST-36, SP-1, SP-20, BL-15, BL-17, BL-19, BL-21, BL-22, BL-46, BL-47, BL-48, BL-49, BL-50, KID-21, P-8, REN-12, REN-13, REN-15, REN-16, REN-17, REN-18, REN-19, REN-20, REN-21

Difficulty in bending BL-28

Discards clothing and runs around ST-40, ST-42, ST-45, DU-24

Diseases of the eight regions in women ST-32

Disorientation HE-7, BL-8, BL-15, KID-20, GB-2, DU-11, DU-20, REN-14
- and forgetfulness LU-3

Dizziness LU-3, L.I.-8, L.I.-11, ST-8, ST-9, ST-36, ST-40, ST-41, ST-45, SP-6, SI-1, SI-7, BL-3, BL-5, BL-8, BL-9, BL-10, BL-11, BL-17, BL-18, BL-43, BL-58, KID-1, KID-6, P-6, SJ-3, SJ-5, SJ-12, SJ-19, SJ-23, GB-8, GB-11, GB-14, GB-18, GB-20, GB-39, GB-41, GB-43, GB-44, LIV-2, LIV-3, DU-4, DU-11, DU-16, DU-20, DU-22, DU-24, REN-4, Anmian (N-HN-54), Sishencong (M-HN-1), Taiyang (M-HN-9), Yintang (M-HN-3)
- accompanied by vomiting DU-24
- and headache BL-56, SJ-1
- due to phlegm-fluid GB-17
- following childbirth, Yintang (M-HN-3)
- with agitation DU-18
- wind dizziness SI-8, BL-2, BL-6, BL-12, BL-62, SJ-5, SJ-16, GB-19, DU-17, DU-19, DU-20, REN-4

Dreams
- confused SJ-16
- excessive ST-45, SP-1, BL-15, KID-3
- nightmares SP-5, KID-6, GB-44

Drooling ST-4, ST-39, SI-1, BL-46, KID-26
- following windstroke P-5

Drum distention ST-25, SP-4, BL-20, LIV-13

Dysenteric disorder (see also Diarrhoea) L.I.-4, L.I.-11, ST-22, ST-25, ST-37, ST-39, ST-44, SP-3, SP-4, SP-8, SP-9, SP-15, SP-16, BL-20, BL-22, BL-25, BL-27, BL-29, BL-35, BL-40, KID-7, KID-8, KID-14, KID-15, KID-21, P-3, REN-4, REN-5, REN-6, REN-12

Dysmenorrhoea ST-25, ST-26, ST-28, SP-6, SP-8, SP-10, BL-24, BL-25, BL-30, BL-31, BL-32, BL-34, KID-5, KID-6, KID-8, P-5, LIV-5, REN-2, REN-6, Tituo N-CA-4
- blood and qi pain in women BL-62

Dyspnoea LU-1, LU-3, LU-4, LU-5, LU-7, LU-8, LU-9, L.I.-9, L.I.-20, ST-10, ST-11, ST-12, ST-13, ST-14, ST-15, ST-18, ST-19, ST-40, SP-1, SP-21, BL-3, BL-4, BL-7, BL-11, BL-12, BL-13, BL-42, BL-44, BL-45, BL-60, KID-1, KID-2, KID-3, KID-22, KID-25, KID-26, KID-27, SJ-19, GB-18, GB-23, LIV-8, LIV-13, LIV-14, DU-9, DU-10, DU-12, DU-24, DU-25, REN-6, REN-12, REN-15, REN-17, REN-20, REN-23, Bailao (M-HN-30)

Dyspnoea (continued)
- and cough L.I.-1, KID-26, P-3
- chronic with cough BL-23
- deficient ST-36
- due to diminished qi KID-4
- sudden REN-22
- with agitation and fullness ST-8
- with difficulty in walking ST-37
- with heat in the body HE-7
- with inability to lie down LU-2, SP-9, REN-4
- with inability to speak REN-20, REN-21
- with inability to stand for long ST-36

Ears
- blocked GB-20
- burning sensation in front of ST-39
- discharge of pus from SJ-17, SJ-19, SJ-20, SJ-21
- earache SJ-1, SJ-2, SJ-3, SJ-17, SJ-21, GB-4
- itching of ST-7, SJ-5, GB-2
- redness, swelling, pain and purulent discharge GB-2
- sores SJ-21
- purulent discharge from ST-7, SI-19, GB-3
- redness and swelling of the back of SJ-20
- redness and swelling of the auricle SJ-20
- swelling of SJ-21
- withered REN-4

Ear pain L.I.-5, ST-7, SI-16, SJ-5, SJ-19, GB-11, GB-12, GB-43
- behind the ear SJ-18
- in the front of the ear LU-11, L.I.-11
- with redness and swelling SJ-5, SJ-17
- with swelling of the root of the ear SJ-5

Eating (see also Difficult Ingestion)
- eats a lot but remains thin BL-20, BL-23, BL-25
- eats little but is easily full REN-12
- excessive SP-5
- desire to eat despite difficult ingestion LIV-14
- difficulty in masticating GB-2
- difficulty in swallowing ST-9
- inability to chew ST-6, SI-18
- inability to eat and drink BL-25, KID-27
- inability to eat ST-4, BL-17, GB-8, DU-9
- inability to taste food or drink ST-13, DU-20
- lack of appetite ST-19, ST-20, ST-21, ST-22, ST-23, ST-25, ST-36, ST-45, SP-6, SP-8, BL-20, BL-21, KID-24
- no desire to eat BL-48, BL-64, KID-22, KID-23, GB-28, GB-39, LIV-4, LIV-8, LIV-13, DU-7 or drink ST-39, SP-1, SP-4, SP-9, SJ-1, REN-9, REN-10

Eczema SP-6, SP-10, BL-40, GB-30
- acute weeping of the face L.I.-2
- and tinea of the hand P-8
- of the hand P-7
- of the scrotum SP-11

Elbow
- difficulty in raising LU-5, L.I.-5, HE-9, GB-44
- emaciation and weakness of L.I.-11
- cold and pain of the elbow and arm HE-1

GENERAL INDEX

This index refers to discussions of the subjects listed, either within the point commentaries or in the introductory discussions to each channel. The bracketed numbers refer to page numbers.

POINT NUMBERS INDEX

This index lists the points by number and gives the page number they appear on

ABOUT THE AUTHORS

Peter Deadman

Peter Deadman spent several years travelling before settling down to hard work, founding Infinity Foods natural foods shop, bakery and warehouse in 1969. He graduated in acupuncture at The International College of Oriental Medicine in East Grinstead, England in 1978 and followed this with post graduate training in Nanjing, China in 1981. He has been in practice in Brighton for 19 years. In 1979 he founded The Journal of Chinese Medicine which he publishes, edits and writes for. In 1991 he qualified at The London School of Chinese Herbal Medicine and followed this with clinical studies in Nanjing. He has taught Chinese medicine and acupuncture since 1979, and has been the principal lecturer at the Skolen for Traditionel Kinesisk Medicine, Denmark, and guest lecturer for the following organisations: The Acupuncture Foundation of Ireland, The Anglo-Dutch College of TCM, The Australian Acupuncture Association, The Deutsche Arztegesellschaft fur Akupunktur, The Israeli School of Acupuncture and Shiatsu, The London School of Acupuncture and TCM, The London School of Chinese Herbal Medicine, The Norskacupunkturskole, Oslo and The Northern College of Acupuncture.

Mazin Al-Khafaji

Mazin Al-Khafaji began his studies in acupuncture as well as modern and classical Chinese in 1979. After graduating in acupuncture at the International College of Oriental Medicine, England in 1983, he attended the post graduate course in acupuncture in Nanjing, China and followed this with intensive studies in modern and medical Chinese at the Taipei Language Institute in Taiwan. His thorough study of the Chinese language earned him the first Sino-British scholarship to study internal medicine at the Shanghai College of Traditional Chinese Medicine alongside Chinese students. He graduated as Doctor of Chinese Medicine in 1987. Since his return to England he has been in private practice in Brighton. In 1991 he returned to China to work in the dermatology department of the Affiliated Hospital in Nanjing, and subsequently established The Skin Clinic for the treatment of dermatological disorders with Chinese herbal medicine. Over the last ten years he has taught Chinese Medicine at graduate and post graduate level in Britain as well as Denmark, Norway, Italy, Germany and Switzerland.

Kevin Baker

Kevin Baker qualified in Medicine from Cambridge University and St George's Hospital Medical School in 1979. He subsequently specialised in Accident and Emergency Medicine and Surgery, obtaining his Membership of the Royal College of Physicians in London in 1983 and his Fellowship of the Royal College of Surgeons in Edinburgh in 1986. He obtained his Diploma in Acupuncture and Traditional Chinese Medicine at the London School of Acupuncture and Traditional Chinese Medicine in 1989 and undertook post graduate training at the Nanjing College of Traditional Chinese Medicine in 1991. Since 1992 he has been Lecturer in Western Medical Pathology at the LSATCM. He currently runs a private Acupuncture practice in Lewes and Brighton and maintains part time Psychotherapy and NHS GP practices.